BING'S LOCAL DIAGNOSIS IN NEUROLOGICAL DISEASES

Bing's Local diagnosis in neurological diseases

Webb Haymaker, M.D.

Senior Scientist, National Aeronautics and Space Administration, Ames Research Center, Moffett Field, California; previously Chief, Neuropathology Section, Armed Forces Institute of Pathology; Associate Professor of Neurology, Georgetown University School of Medicine; Professorial Lecturer in Anatomy, George Washington University School of Medicine, Washington, D. C.

Fifteenth edition

With 395 illustrations, including 8 in color

Saint Louis

The C. V. Mosby Company

1969

Fifteenth edition

Printed in the United States of America

Standard Book Number 8016-2108-9

Library of Congress Catalog Card Number 69-17488

Distributed in Great Britain by Henry Kimpton, London

CB/CB/B 9 8 7

To

Robert Wartenberg

In whose presence no student could be lethargic

Contributors

BERNARD S. EPSTEIN, M.D.

Clinical Professor of Radiology, The Albert Einstein College of Medicine, New York; Department of Radiology, The Long Island Jewish Hospital, New Hyde Park, Long Island, New York

JORGE HUERTAS, M.D.

Research Scientist, National Aeronautics and Space Administration, Ames Research Center, Moffett Field, California

WILLIAM F. MEHLER, Ph.D.

Research Scientist, National Aeronautics and Space Administration, Ames Research Center, Moffett Field, California

HANS R. MÜLLER, M.D.

Head, Department of Electroencephalography and Diagnostic Ultrasound, Neurosurgical Clinic, Bürgerspital, Basel, Switzerland

FRANCIS SCHILLER, M.D.

Associate Clinical Professor of Neurology, University of California Medical School, San Francisco, California

PAUL I. YAKOVLEV, M.D.

Department of Neurology and Warren Anatomical Museum, Harvard Medical School, Boston, Massachusetts

Preface

As this volume appears it marks the sixtieth anniversary of the first edition of Bing's *Kompendium.* This is the fifteenth edition in its long history. Although bearing little resemblance to the original, the present edition nonetheless contains the kernel of Professor Bing's text as well as much of his illustrative material.

Since the appearance of the last edition in English some 12 years ago there has been an explosion of new findings through which localization of lesions can be better understood. The H fields of Forel, once reserved for anatomists, now form part of the vocabulary of neurologists; the gamma (or reticulospinal) system has come into its own alongside the alpha (or pyramidal) system in the performance of motor function; "serotonin cells" are currently considered to be of importance in temperature regulation; time-honored "association areas" of the cerebral cortex are now suspect; the "olivospinal tract" appears now to be a reticulospinal tract. Clinically, "disconnection syndromes" have come into prominence, and "steal syndromes" have supplanted what was once a nebulous area. Korsakoff's syndrome is being created in the course of operating on anterior communicating artery aneurysm; thus this subject is one with which we are coming closer to grips. In many ways, neurophysiology and neuropathology have kept pace with these and other new developments. In the present volume the objective has been to lay out the anatomy and physiology in sufficient detail so that localization of lesions within the nervous system becomes apparent. Illustrations of pathological conditions have been provided in some abundance in order to make localization more realistic.

I cannot forego saying a word about Professor Robert Wartenberg, to whom this edition is dedicated. His art in localization and his contributions as a teacher (he could not have held higher rank in the affection of his students) are well documented in a volume prepared to honor him (J. Nerv. Ment. Dis. **116**:469-480, 1952). He and Professor Bing were close friends, constantly exchanging letters on this or that new finding or new idea in clinical neurology. It was through Professor Wartenberg that our first translation of the "Bing" came about.

I owe much to others in the preparation of this edition. Most of their names are listed on the contributors' page. Major credit goes to Dr. Francis Schiller (San Francisco) for his help in the preparation of some of the chapters and for his suggestions in reorganizing the text. Dr. William F. Hoyt (San Francisco), after going over the chapter concerned with visual disturbances, wrote: "I know from experience how difficult it is to get energetic criticism of even small sections of book manuscripts." Happily, his criticism was indeed energetic! Dr. Hartwig Kuhlenbeck (Philadelphia) wrote passages in the areas in which he is well known. Dr. Kenneth Anderson (Sunnyvale, Calif.) helped in the chapter dealing with disorders involving the trigeminal nerve. Dr. Hans R. Müller (Basel) proved very helpful in his review of the chapter on electroencephalography. I am also thankful to Dr. William F. Mehler (Ames Research Center) for his assistance in the preparation of the chapters on the spinal cord and cerebellum.

For illustrations I am indebted to Dr. Richard Lindenberg (Baltimore), Dr. A. Ornsteen (Philadelphia), Prof. W. Scholz (Munich), Prof. K. J. Zülch (Cologne), Prof. J. François (Ghent), Dr. Sten Graffman (Uppsala), Prof. O. Hassler (Umeå), Prof. I. M. Turnbull (Vancouver), Dr. Wilder Penfield (Montreal), Dr. H. Kuhlenbeck (Philadelphia), Dr. W. F. Hoyt (San Francisco), Dr. R. Raskind (Oakland), Dr. A. Torvik and Dr. L. Jörgensen (Oslo), Dr. L. Roberts (Gainesville, Fla.), Prof. A. Gastaut (Marseilles), Dr. A. Earl Walker (Baltimore), Dr. William F. Mehler (Ames Research Center), Dr. Irving Cooper (New York City), Dr. C. C. Grossman (Pittsburgh), Dr. Herbert H. Jasper (Montreal), and The Director, Armed Forces Institute of Pathology (Washington, D. C.). Here at Ames Research Center, Mrs. Virginia Hughes and Mrs. Betty Sherwood were very helpful in seeing the manuscript through.

Webb Haymaker

Contents

1 Cell groups, tracts, and blood supply of the spinal cord, 1

2 Sensory, motor, trophic, and autonomic function; disturbances in function, 23
With a section by Jorge Huertas

3 Innervation in terms of spinal cord segments, 47

4 Localization of segments involved in spinal cord lesions, 51

5 Localization of lesions of the spinal cord in general, 72

6 Localization of lesions of cervical and upper thoracic segments; autonomic disturbances, 97

7 Localization of lesions involving lower spinal segments and the cauda equina, 105

8 Electromyography, 114
Jorge Huertas

9 Roentgenographic localization of spinal tumors, 123
Bernard S. Epstein

10 Structure of the brainstem, 130

11 Localization of lesions involving the brainstem and emergent nerves, 145

12 Localization of lesions involving cranial nerves IX through XII, 170

13 Localization of lesions involving the statoacoustic nerve, 186
Jorge Huertas and Webb Haymaker

14 Localization of lesions involving the facial nerve, 217

15 Localization of lesions involving the trigeminal nerve, 234
William F. Mehler and Webb Haymaker

16 Localization of lesions involving the extraocular nerves, 251

17 Disorders of cerebellar origin, 277

18 Syndromes of arterial occlusion, circulatory insufficiency, and aneurysms in the region of the brainstem and cerebellum, 294

19 Cerebral landmarks; organization of the cerebral cortex and descending and ascending pathways, 311
Webb Haymaker and Francis Schiller

20 Motor, sensory, reflex, and related disturbances of cerebral cortical and subcortical origin, 329

21 Localization of visual and associated reflex disturbances, 349

22 Disturbances of behavior, memory, awareness, smell, taste, and hearing, 379
Francis Schiller and Webb Haymaker

23 Dysarthria, aphasia, and apraxia, 397
Francis Schiller

24 Extrapyramidal motor disorders, 404
Webb Haymaker, William F. Mehler, and Francis Schiller

25 Localization of lesions of the thalamus, 441
Paul I. Yakovlev

26 Hypothalamus, pituitary gland, midbrain, and related regions, 465

27 Cerebral artery occlusion, aneurysms, and arteriovenous malformations, 497

28 Trauma, brain shifts, intracranial neoplasms, and hematomas, 525

29 Roentgenographic localization of intracranial lesions, 549
Bernard S. Epstein

30 Echoencephalography, 565
Hans R. Müller and Jorge Huertas

31 Electroencephalography, 570
Jorge Huertas

32 Radioactive-nuclide scanning, 584
Jorge Huertas

Color illustrations

Topographic subdivisions of the base of the skull, p. 159

Mechanism by which caloric nystagmus is induced, p. 195

"Onion peel" sensory distribution in the head and neck, p. 247

Bitemporal heteronymous hemianopia, p. 362

Ipsilateral blindness and contralateral temporal hemianopia, p. 364

Nasal heteronymous hemianopia, p. 365

Homonymous hemianopia, p. 366

Connections at various levels, with ultimate innervation of muscle, p. 408

Chapter 1

Cell groups, tracts, and blood supply of the spinal cord

Two aspects of localization should be considered when one is confronted with clinical evidence of damage of the spinal cord. The *first* is the site of the lesion in the transverse plane. Here one has to determine whether the lesion is situated in the central or the peripheral part of the cord, whether it lies dorsally or ventrally, and whether it is on the right or the left side. One needs also to determine the extent to which the gray matter may be damaged and the tracts affected. The *second* aspect to consider is the site of the lesion in the longitudinal plane. The problem is to locate the segment or segments involved. In the text that follows, the principles of localization are considered from these two standpoints.

NERVE CELL GROUPS IN THE SPINAL CORD

Groups of nerve cells form longitudinal columns in the interior of the spinal cord. Some groups are present at all levels of the cord; others are limited to certain segments. As seen in the transverse plane the pattern of the gray differs at different levels. At any level the gray is divisible, however, into three horns: posterior, intermediate, and anterior.

A feature common to all levels is a suggestion of lamination from dorsal to ventral. Such lamination is far more clear cut in the spinal cord of the cat, with laminae I through VI making up the posterior horn, lamina VII the intermediate horn, and laminae VIII and IX different cell groups in the anterior horn (Rexed, 1954, 1964).

Occupying the apex of the posterior horn is the *substantia gelatinosa* (Fig. 1-1), with the tract of Lissauer lateral to it. The substantia gelatinosa is composed of small ovoid and polygonal nerve cells. Along its outer edge, next to the tract of Lissauer, are medium-sized stellate and polygonal cells known collectively as the *posteromarginal nucleus* (or pericornual nucleus). Lying along the inner border of the substantia gelatinosa are small stellate cells and medium-sized polygonal cells known collectively as the *nucleus proprius.* Much of the intermediate part of the posterior horn contains rather diffuse cells, referred to as the *posterior funicular gray.* A prominent and discrete cell group, situated at the base of the posterior horn medially, is the *nucleus dorsalis* (Clarke's nucleus), composed of medium-sized and large, rounded or oval cells. It is located in segments C8 through L2. Situated approximately in the same position as Clarke's nucleus, but at different levels, is an aggregate of rather small cells known as *Stilling's nucleus.* It is present in upper cervical segments (where it enlarges to become continuous with the lateral cuneate nucleus in the medulla oblongata) and also lower in the cord, approximately from segment L3 to S4. Lying ventral and somewhat medial to the nucleus dorsalis

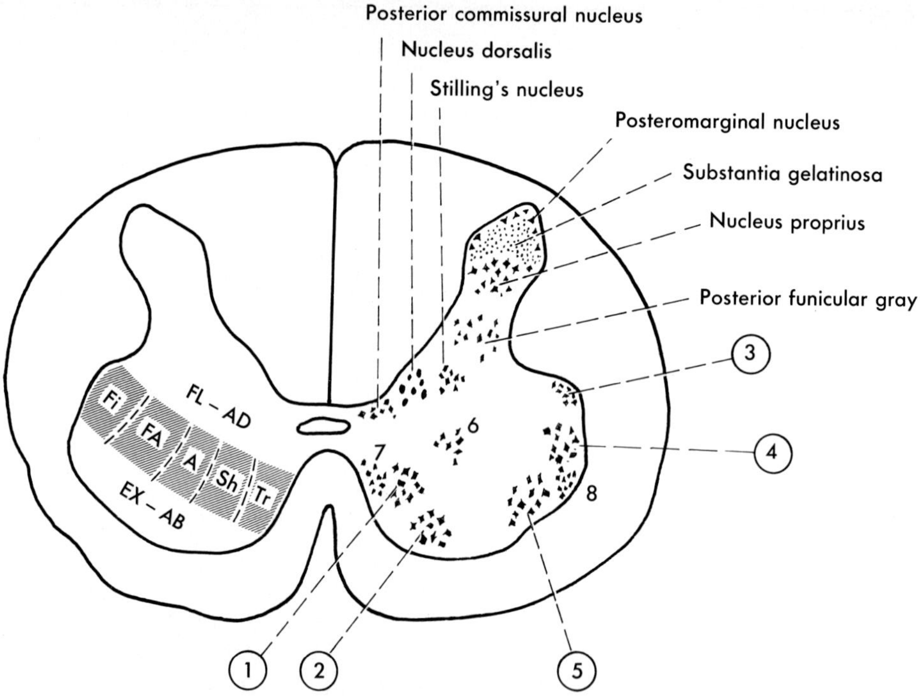

Fig. 1-1. Composite of cell groups of the spinal cord. In the anterior horn the cell groups are as follows: (1) dorsomedial, (2) ventromedial, (3) retrodorsolateral, (4) dorsolateral, (5) ventrolateral, (6) lumbosacral, (7) phrenic, and (8) accessory.

Represented to the left are cell groups innervating the fingers *(Fi)*, forearm *(FA)*, arm *(A)*, shoulder *(Sh)*, and trunk *(Tr)*. Cell groups through which flexor and adductor muscles are innervated *(FL-AD)* are located dorsally, and cell groups innervating extensors and abductors *(EX-AB)*, ventrally. (Redrawn from Austin, G. 1961. The spinal cord. Springfield, Illinois, Charles C Thomas, Publisher.)

is a small group of cells known as the *posterior commissural nucleus.* It is made up of small to medium-sized spindle or polymorphic cells.

The *intermediate horn,* as the name implies, is situated between the posterior and anterior horns. The cell group that concerns us in the subsequent text is situated laterally in the horn, in a region called the *intermediolateral horn.* The cells are small and medium-sized. Distinct intermediolateral horns composed of these cells are present at levels Th1 through L1. Cells of the same type and in the same location in the transverse plane are present in segments C7–C8 and L2–L3. All these cells, from C7 down to L3, are components of the sympathetic nervous system. In a corresponding position, at levels S2–S4, are cells of similar appearance comprising the sacral parasympathetic gray.

The anterior horn contains large multipolar nerve cells disposed in columnar groups, each of which innervates certain functionally related muscles. The cell groups vary in number and composition depending on the segmental level, with the greatest number in the cervical and lumbosacral enlargements. A composite of anterior horn nuclear groups is shown in Fig. 1-1. The grouping used was obtained from various sources, not always in agreement on details (Bok, 1928; Bruce, 1901; Jacobsohn, 1908; Olszewski and Baxter, 1954; Woodburne, 1957).

The major medial cell groups may be subdivided into a dorsomedial and a ventromedial component (Fig. 1-1). *(1)* The dorsomedial component supplies the small deep muscles of the spine. *(2)* The ventromedial component supplies the superficial muscles, such as the latissimus dorsi; it also supplies some of the muscles of the abdominal wall, such as the oblique. The lateral cell groups are also subdivided in accordance with their position: *(3)* the retrodorsolateral, which supplies the muscles of the hand, fingers, foot, and toes; *(4)* the dorsolateral, which supplies the muscles of the forearm, hand, leg, and foot; and *(5)* the ventrolateral, which apparently supplies the muscles of the shoulder girdle, upper arm, hip, and thigh. Thus from medial to lateral these anterior horn cell groups innervate trunk muscles, shoulder and hip muscles, upper arm and thigh muscles, forearm and leg muscles, and hand, finger, foot, and toe muscles. Flexor and adductor muscles are innervated by dorsal cell groups or by dorsal components of individual cell groups or components. A schema bringing this out for the upper limb is illustrated to the left in Fig. 1-1. For a schema with respect to the lower limb, the papers by Romanes (1964) and Sharrard (1955) and the book by Austin (1961) should be consulted.

Another cell group in the anterior horn is *(6)* the lumbosacral nucleus, situated centrally in the horn at levels L2–S2. Its territory of muscular innervation seems unknown. *(7)* The phrenic nucleus is located medially in the horn at levels C3–C5 (Keswani and Hollinshead, 1956), and *(8)* the accessory nucleus in the ventrolateral part of the anterior horn in segments C1–C4 (Pearson, Sauter, and Herrin, 1964).

In addition to large multipolar cells, or alpha motoneurons (Figs. 2-1 and 24-3), the anterior horn contains great numbers of small and medium-sized neurons. Included among them are gamma motoneurons, which innervate muscle spindles. Present also are interneurons, whose axons synapse with alpha and gamma motoneurons. Further, there are Renshaw cells (Renshaw, 1941, 1946), situated in the region of emergence of the motoneuron axons from the gray matter. They receive recurrent collaterals from the outgoing axons of the alpha motoneurons, and also from muscle via posterior root fibers. They have the function of inhibiting the motoneurons through suppression by a negative feedback mechanism. The approximate location of gamma motoneurons and Renshaw cells has been established through electrophysiological studies, but neither of these cells has as yet been clearly identified histologically (Eccles, 1967).

TRACTS OF THE SPINAL CORD

Fiber pathways in the spinal cord are divisible into descending tracts, ascending tracts, and intersegmental tracts.

Descending tracts

Corticospinal, or pyramidal, tract. The fibers comprising the corticospinal tract originate from the cerebral cortex (Fig. 1-2), most of them from the precentral gyrus (p. 315). The fibers course downward through the brain and brainstem; on reaching the lower aspect of the medulla oblongata most of them cross the midline, thus forming the pyramidal decussation. After crossing, these fibers descend in the lateral column of the spinal cord as the lateral corticospinal, or lateral pyramidal, tract. At each spinal segmental level to almost the bottom of the spinal cord, fibers depart from the tract and synapse with interneurons at the base of the posterior horn, and monosynaptically with alpha motoneurons of the anterior horn (Eccles, 1967).

The remainder (about 20 percent) of the corticospinal fibers do not cross in the pyramidal decussation. Instead, they proceed directly down the cord, ipsilateral to their site of origin. Some of these fibers course downward in the anterior column of the cord, near the anterior median fissure; they comprise the anterior corticospinal, or anterior pyramidal, tract. In some cords the tract has been found to course downward only to the upper thoracic segments (Weil and Lassek, 1929), while in others they descend to sacral levels. At various levels fibers depart from the tract, some terminating in the ipsilateral anterior horn, while most cross the midline via the anterior white commissure and terminate in the medial part of the contralateral anterior horn (Kuypers, 1964; Nathan and Smith, 1955; Schoen, 1964; Stewart, 1901). Other fibers proceed downward in the lateral column of the cord as the uncrossed lateral corticospinal tract (Barnes, 1901; Dejerine, 1901). Such fibers are relatively few (Weil and Lassek, 1929).

Frequently the pyramidal crossing is asymmetric; in such cords more fibers cross from one side than from the other. Consequently the anterior column of the cord on one side is much larger than the other, and half of the cord contains a much greater number of pyramidal fibers than the other. Now and then the fibers in a pyramid, without crossing, proceed into the ipsilateral half of the cord downward in the anterior column. Some pyramidal fibers in such cases may cross at midbrain or pontile levels. Fur-

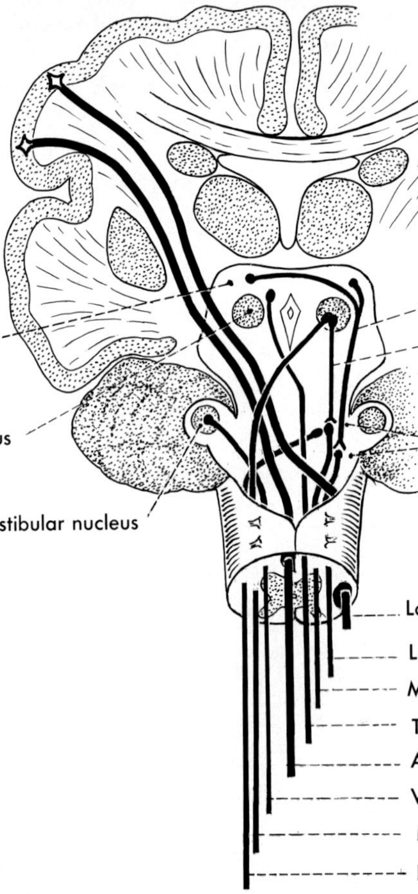

Fig. 1-2. Major descending tracts of the spinal cord.

ther, in a small proportion of cords the anterior corticospinal tract is absent (Verhaart and Kramer, 1952; Weil and Lassek, 1929). (For these and other variations and abnormalities, see Nathan and Smith, 1955.) In a case of hemiplegia in which both the lesion and the paresis were on the same side, no pyramidal decussation was found (Zenner, 1898).

In short, most of the corticospinal fibers originating from the hemisphere of one side influence the activity of anterior horn cells of the opposite side.

Tracts descending from subcortical structures. The chief fiber systems descending into the spinal cord from cell aggregates in the brainstem are illustrated in Fig. 1-2. All of these cell aggregates receive fibers from higher levels.

Tectospinal tract. The tectospinal tract arises in the tectum of the midbrain at the level of the superior colliculus. It curves ventrally around the periaqueductal gray matter to reach the median plane, which it crosses in the dorsal tegmental decussation (Fig. 10-15). Maintaining a median position just ventral to and intermixed with the medial longitudinal fasciculus, it descends through the pons and the medulla oblongata to reach the medial part of the anterior column of the spinal cord (Collier and Buzzard, 1901). Its fibers terminate at cervical levels near intercalated cells whose axons proceed to anterior horn motor cells (Szentágothai, 1948). Another connection between the tectum and the spinal cord is by way of the tectotegmentospinal pathway. Fibers originate in the superior colliculus of both the ipsilateral and the contralateral side, pursue a course downward to the pons, and end in synaptic relation with tegmental cells. The axons of these tegmental cells course down the spinal cord in the region ventral to the rubrospinal tract. The depth to which the tract descends in the spinal cord remains to be ascertained; some fibers may proceed to anterior horns, others to the intermediolateral (sympathetic) horns (Crosby, Humphrey, and Lauer, 1962).

Rubrospinal tract. The rubrospinal tract is poorly developed in man. It takes its origin in the red nucleus, which is situated in the tegmentum of the midbrain. Its fibers arise from the magnocellular part of the nucleus. Shortly after leaving the red nucleus, the fibers cross to the opposite side in the ventral tegmental decussation (Fig. 10-15). They pass downward in the more lateral part of the pons and medulla oblongata and the lateral column of the spinal cord. Stern (1938) traced them caudally into the upper thoracic region. According to Kuypers (1964) they extend all the way down the cord, decreasing in number as they descend, and terminate mainly in the intermediate part of the gray matter, with some spilling over into dorsomedial parts of the anterior horn. According to Eccles (1967), all fibers of the rubrospinal tract terminate on interneurons, the latter being inhibitory to extensor motoneurons and excitatory to flexor motoneurons.

Vestibulospinal tract. The vestibulospinal tract, of very small size in man, takes origin in the lateral vestibular nucleus (of Deiters), situated in the pons–medulla oblongata junctional area (Fig. 10-10). Without decussating, the vestibulospinal tract descends in the anterior column of the spinal cord to sacral levels, giving off fibers to anterior horns en route (Collier and Buzzard, 1901; Foerster and Gagel, 1932; Langworthy, 1930; Pompeiano, 1967). The principal terminations are directly on extensor motoneurons and on interneurons having connections with flexor motoneurons (Eccles, 1967).

Reticulospinal tracts. There are two reticulospinal tracts, lateral and medial. The *lateral reticulospinal tract* arises in the tegmentum of the pons, immediately decussates, and extends downward in the medulla oblongata and the lateral column of the cord ventral to the rubrospinal tract. At upper spinal levels the fibers of the lateral reticulospinal and rubrospinal tracts are somewhat intermingled. The *medial reticulospinal tract* arises chiefly in the medial, large-celled portion of the medullary reticular formation and, without decussating, passes dorsal to the inferior olivary nucleus and descends in the anterior column of the cord adjacent to the anterior fasciculus proprius. (Brodal, 1958; Collier and Buzzard, 1901; Kuypers, 1964.) Some of these fibers probably originate in the medullary "respiratory center." In Fig. 1-1, this tract is shown as a component of the rubroreticulospinal tract (the rubroreticular component originates in the parvocellular portion of the red nucleus). Reticulospinal fibers in general reach all levels of the cord, terminating in dorsal parts of the anterior horn but not in regions in which motoneurons are located (Jansen and Brodal, 1954; Nyberg-Hansen, 1965).

Olivospinal tract. Since the turn of the century there has been an argument about the polarity of the so-called triangular tract of Helweg, situated in the anterior column of the spinal cord. Some have contended that it is an olivospinal tract, others that it is spino-olivary. Experimental evidence in animals has not supported the view that it originates in the inferior olivary nucleus and descends (Mehler, Feferman, and Nauta, 1960). Reevaluation in human material indicates that the fibers in question probably originate from cell aggregates in the reticular formation (Mehler, 1969; Okamoto and others, 1965).

Ascending exogenous tracts

A number of tracts are referred to as "exogenous" because they originate in the "periphery," that is, both in the somatic periphery and in the viscera. Their cell stations are in the posterior root ganglia. Their central processes extend into the spinal cord by way of the posterior spinal roots. The incoming posterior root fibers may be subdivided into short, intermediate, and long systems, according to the distance they travel prior to synapse. The short system is carried by the *lateral* division of the root, the intermediate and long systems by the *medial* division (Fig. 1-3).

Short posterior root fibers; lateral spinothalamic tract. The short posterior root fibers course centrally in the lateral division of the root. They extend into the tract of Lissauer (posterolateral fasciculus) (Fig. 1-3), which they may directly traverse to end in the substantia gelatinosa (Wall, 1964). Or, while in the tract, the fibers give off collaterals that reach the substantia gelatinosa (and neighboring cells) either directly or after ascending or descending in the tract of Lissauer for a segment or two (Pearson, 1952). Only about 25 percent of the fibers in the tract

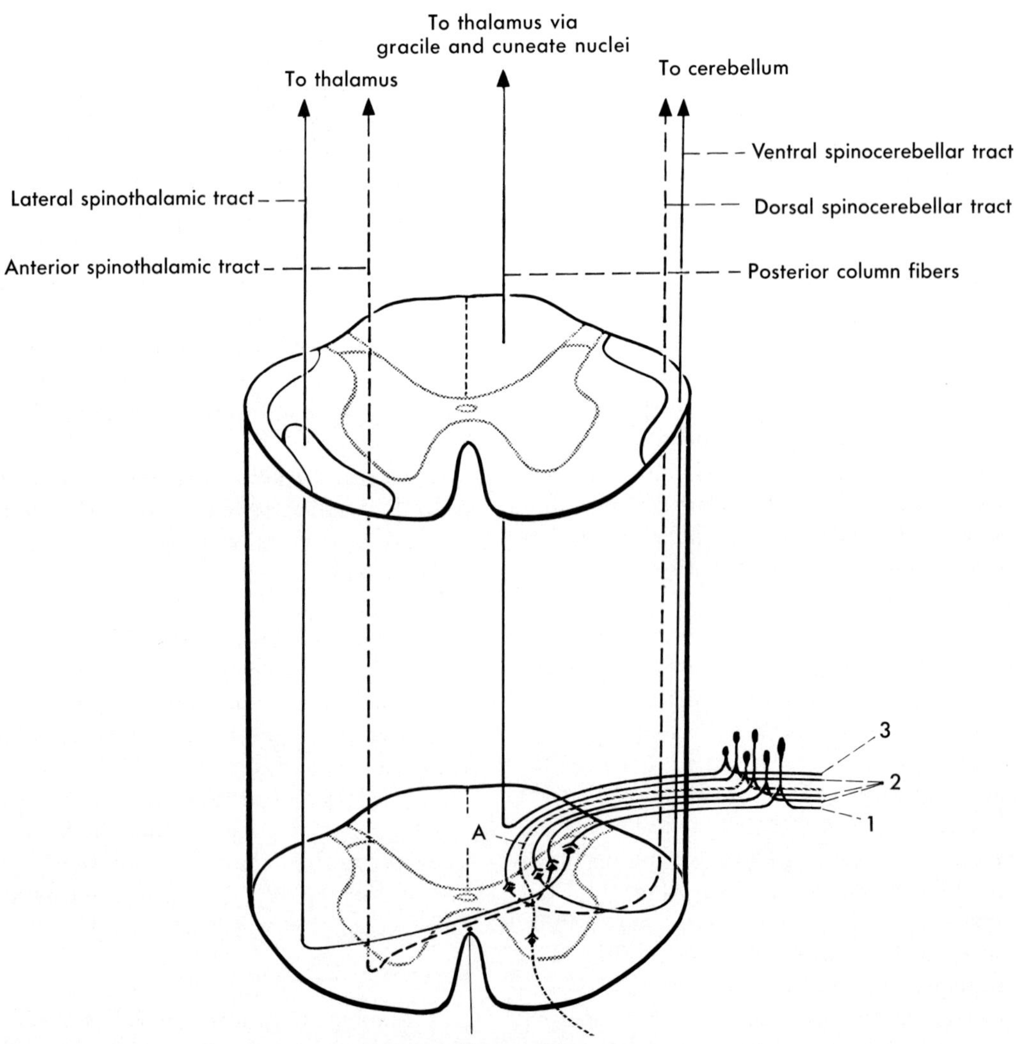

Fig. 1-3. Short (*1*), intermediate (*2*), and long (*3*) posterior root fiber systems and their respective courses in the spinal cord. *A* refers to monosynaptic reflex fibers.

of Lissauer are of posterior root origin; the others (fibrae spinospinales) link the substantia gelatinosa of various spinal levels (Earle, 1952).

The short posterior root fibers carry impulses aroused by noxious stimuli—impulses from somatic sources interpreted at higher levels as painful or thermal in nature, also impulses from visceral sources interpreted as painful or otherwise. Posterior root fibers conveying "pain impulses" outnumber the cells that give rise to the lateral spinothalamic tract. These cells thus constitute a "pool" for the reception of incoming pain impulses. Fibers reach this pool not only from the posterior roots but also from higher sources, the latter probably acting in an inhibitory capacity (Mehler, 1962).

Some posterior root fibers reaching this pool are known, others are postulated.

According to Pearson (1952), incoming fine fibers (conveying pain impulses) traverse Lissauer's tract and synapse with cells of the posteromarginal nucleus, while collaterals of larger fibers (also conveying pain impulses) course to cells of the nucleus proprius. Both the posteromarginal nucleus and the nucleus proprius, according to Pearson, contain second-order neurons whose axons ascend in the contralateral lateral spinothalamic tract. By contrast, Wall (1964) and Melzack and Wall (1965), in fostering the view that no pain fibers as such exist, proposed the following: (1) Both finer and coarser incoming fibers terminate in the substantia gelatinosa, the coarser giving rise, en route, to collaterals that proceed up the posterior columns to the gracile and cuneate nuclei. (2) Cells of the nucleus proprius—"central transmission cells"—have dendrites in the substantia gelatinosa and axons that extend across the cord to make up the contralateral lateral spinothalamic tract. (3) The cells of the substantia gelatinosa mediate control over entering sensory information; in other words, the substantia gelatinosa functions as a *gate control system* that modulates the afferent patterns before they influence the central transmission cells. (4) The afferent patterns in the posterior column act, at least in part, as a central control trigger that activates selective brain processes that influence the modulating properties of the gate control system. The central transmission cells activate neural mechanisms that comprise the action system responsible for response and perception. (5) Pain phenomena are determined by interactions among these three systems—the substantia gelatinosa, the posterior column system, and the central transmission system.

Although considerable doubt exists that there are "pain fibers" as such in the peripheral and the central nervous system, or that "pain impulses" occur, nonetheless these and similar expressions will be used in the following text for purposes of ease in description.

Sites of termination of somatic pain fibers and visceral pain fibers are assumed to differ in some degree. According to the Sherrington neuron pool concept, while somatic pain afferents come into synaptic relation with one group of cells in the posterior horn, and visceral pain afferents with another group, a field of overlap exists in which *both* the somatic afferents and the visceral afferents enter into synaptic relation with the same cells of the pool. This proposed system comes into consideration later in the text in connection with the problem of referred pain (pp. 63-66).

Fibers of the second order issuing from the posteromarginal nucleus and from the nucleus proprius cross the midline of the cord via the anterior white commissure and reach the lateral spinothalamic tract (Pearson, 1952). The fibers enter the tract in its ventral part (in the anterior column). Then, gradually shifting dorsolaterally, the tract ascends mainly into the ventral half of the lateral column. Lamination of these fibers occurs, with the cervical fibers situated medially and the thoracic, lumbar, and sacral segments more and more laterally, in that order (Fig. 1-4). Within the region of the lateral spinothalamic tract the fibers conveying temperature sensibility are located more dorsally than those conveying pain sensibility. (Foerster, 1936; Foerster and Gagel, 1932; Sjöqvist, 1949; Walker, 1940.)

At lower levels of the medulla oblongata pain and temperature fibers proceed upward just dorsal to the inferior olivary nucleus. In this area the lateral spinothalamic tract possesses much the same somatotopic pattern that it has in the spinal cord. At the level of the medulla oblongata the tract is joined by fibers coming from the spinal nucleus of the trigeminal nerve; they convey pain im-

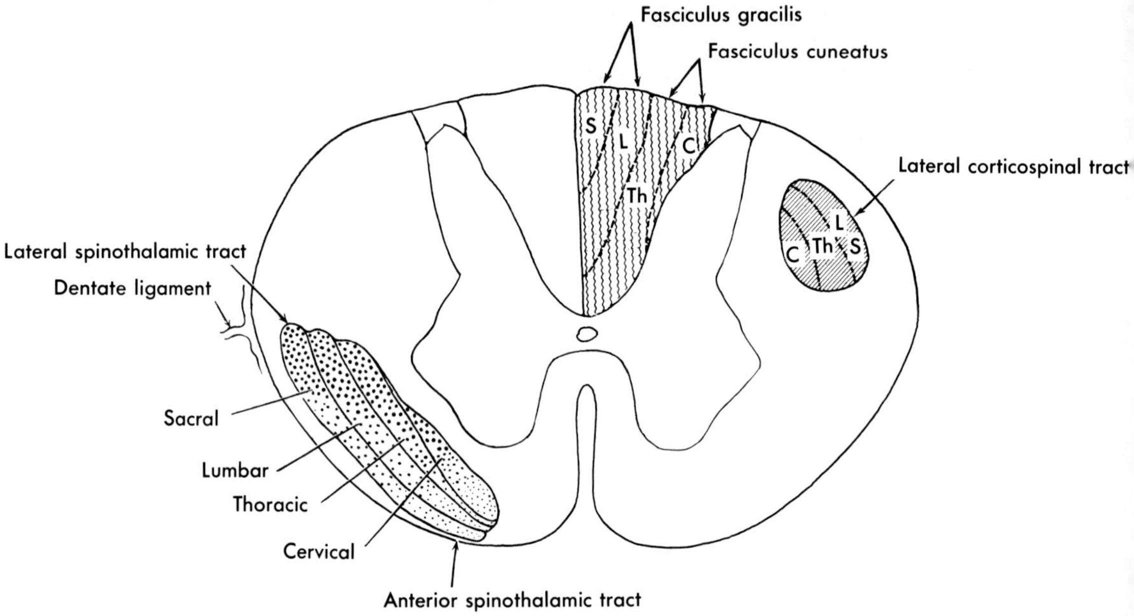

Fig. 1-4. Lamination of the posterior column, lateral corticospinal tract, and spinothalamic tracts. In the lateral spinothalamic tracts the *coarse dots* indicate the fibers conveying heat and cold impulses; the *medium-sized dots,* those carrying pain impulses, and the *fine dots,* those carrying tactile impulses. The lateral thalamic tract reaches dorsally to the level of the dentate ligament. *C,* Cervical, *Th,* thoracic, *L,* lumbar, and *S,* sacral segments. (From Foerster and Gagel, 1932, and Walker, 1940.)

pulses from the face. The tract extends upward in the midbrain, where it is situated laterally, ventral to the quadrigeminal plate; here the tract is somatotopically organized, the fibers transmitting impulses from the lower limb being situated most dorsally (Walker, 1942). The tract terminates in the thalamus; the fibers from the spinal cord end in the ventral posterolateral nucleus (VPL), those from the face in the ventral posteromedial nucleus (VPM). Pain fibers are conventionally included in this tract, but at levels approaching the thalamus their number dwindles (Bowsher, 1957). Fibers of the medial lemniscus supplant them, to end also in VPL. What proportion of the fibers terminating in VPL are pain fibers is not evident; VPL projects to the somesthetic cortical area, where pain is not known to be represented.

In addition to this "lateral" pain system, there is another, the "medial" pain system. Its components and its precise location are largely inferential, as the information available on this pathway has been obtained through studies of the spinal cord and brainstem of persons subjected to anterolateral cordotomy, in which fibers additional to pain fibers were severed. Nonetheless, there is ample electrophysiological evidence from animal studies that great numbers of the severed spinal cord fibers in point are, in fact, pain fibers. Some of these fibers may constitute a diffuse spinoreticulothalamic system (Bowsher, 1957; Spiegel and Wycis, 1962). At the level of the medulla oblongata, some "pain" fibers apparently leave the lateral spinothalamic tract to reach the reticular formation. Fibers terminate in the lateral reticular nucleus of the medulla oblongata, and great numbers of collaterals extend dorsomedially into the reticular formation and terminate in various other medullary reticular nuclei (Mehler, 1962). It has been postulated that the pain pathway from this general region upward consists of diffuse, multisynaptic systems of neurons collectively referred to as the reticulothalamic tract (Bishop, 1959; Noordenbos, 1959). In the upper midbrain this system is situated largely in the dorsal part of the tegmentum (just ventral to the quadrigeminal plate), medial to the lateral spinothalamic tract, and in the lateral part of the periaqueductal gray as well (Nashold, Wilson, and Slaughter, 1969). In this region, they are joined by trigeminal fibers (quintothalamic tract) issuing chiefly from the principal sensory trigeminal nucleus, decussating, and ascending dorsally in the tegmentum. From both areas—dorsomedial tegmentum and lateral periaqueductal gray—the fibers ascend into medial, basal regions of the thalamus. Joined by spinal and trigeminal fiber systems of the lateral spinothalamic tract, they terminate in medial intralaminar thalamic nuclei as well as in lateral thalamic relay nuclei. Neurophysiological studies (Collins, Nulsen, and Shealy, 1966) provide support for the presence of loci of pain fibers in these regions. Nonetheless, the site(s) of termination of many of the pain fibers needs yet to be established. Also remaining to be settled is the nature of the interrelationship that may exist between the "two" pain pathways. Bishop (1962) has suggested that the lateral spinothalamic tract exerts an inhibitory influence on the medial pain conducting system, and Spiegel and Wycis (1967) have suggested the reverse.

Studies carried out in the course of mesencephalic tractotomy or thalamotomy in man provide support for the location of the pain pathways as just described. Nashold, Wilson, and Slaughter (1969), in electrically stimulating the midbrain (prior to tractotomy), noted differing responses from the lateral and medial areas (defined in the foregoing). On stimulation of the lateral area (mainly the lateral spinothalamic tract) the patients complained of sharp pain, burning sensation, and numbness on the contralateral side (mainly face, arm, or chest), while on stimulation of the medial area, the patients complained of sensations in central portions of the head and body (face, nasal and oral cavities, neck, center of the chest [near the heart], or the abdomen), namely, diffuse pain, burning sensation, vibration, and cold.

That the thalamic loci indicated in the foregoing are, actually, sites in which pain fibers run is suggested by the relief from intractable pain experienced by patients following stereotactically placed lesions in the posterior or basal thalamus (Spiegel and Wycis, 1966) or in the internal medullary lamina (Mark, Ervin, and Hackett, 1960).

Intermediate posterior root fibers and ascending pathways

Anterior spinothalamic tract. As viewed in cross sections of the cord, intermediate posterior root fibers skirt the dorsal surface of the posterior horn, then synapse with small cells of the nucleus proprius (Pearson, 1952). These are collaterals of fibers proceeding up the (ipsilateral) posterior column for a considerable but varying distance from the level of root entry, then turning ventrally and terminating in the nucleus proprius. Fibers of the second order pursue the same course across the cord as that described for the pain and temperature fibers; they reach the dorsal part of the anterior column. Here they form the anterior spinothalamic tract. The fibers of this tract intermix with fibers of the lateral spinothalamic tract, and they undergo lamination in the same manner as for the lateral spinothalamic tract (Fig. 1-4). Tactile fibers are carried by this tract. At the level of the lower pons these fibers join the medial lemniscus and terminate in the ventral posterolateral nucleus (VPL) of the thalamus. In their spinal course the anterior spinothalamic tract and the lateral spinothalamic tract are known jointly as the spinal lemniscus.

Dorsal spinocerebellar tract (of Flechsig). Incoming posterior root fibers also take a course along the ventral edge of the posterior column, and reach the nucleus dorsalis (Clarke's nucleus), situated at the base of the posterior horn. This nucleus, which is somatotopically organized (Szentágothai and Albert, 1955), is present in segments Th2 to L2 inclusive (Bruce, 1910; Pass, 1933). From the nucleus dorsalis the fibers pass laterally to the periphery of the cord where they form the dorsal spinocerebellar tract. They continue upward in this tract to the medulla oblongata, where they enter and traverse the

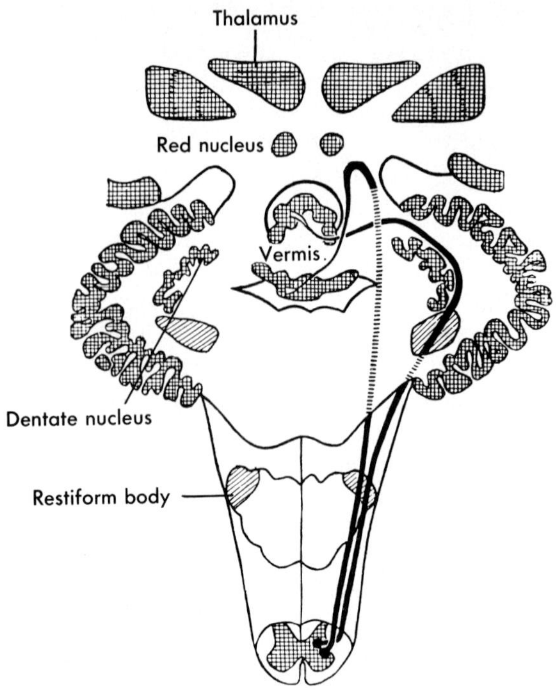

Fig. 1-5. Course and termination of the dorsal and ventral spinocerebellar tracts. The ventral spinocerebellar tract goes the highest.

inferior cerebellar peduncle to end in rostral and caudal parts of the vermis. Termination in the vermis is both contralateral (Fig. 1-5) and ipsilateral. (Ferraro and Barrera, 1935; Smith, 1957).

Accompanying these fibers in their course through the inferior cerebellar peduncle are fibers from the lateral cuneate nucleus (for the position of this nucleus, see Figs. 10-8 and 10-9). These fibers reach the ipsilateral peduncle after taking a course dorsally and laterally (as dorsal superficial arcuate fibers), then proceed to the cerebellar cortex. The lateral cuneate nucleus receives fibers from the cervical and upper thoracic roots by way of the fasciculus cuneatus. The fibers of this system convey proprioceptive and tactile impulses to the cerebellum from the region of the neck, upper limb, and upper trunk.

Ventral spinocerebellar tract (of Gowers). Posterior root fibers, after proceeding through the posterior column, terminate rather diffusely in the posterior funicular gray at all spinal levels, chiefly in Stilling's nucleus and the posterior commissural nucleus. Some of the fibers originating in these nuclei pass directly laterally to form the ventral spinocerebellar tract, but most of them course in the anterior white commissure to the contralateral ventral spinocerebellar tract. (For clinical reasons such as lack of cerebellar disturbance contralateral to a spinal lesion, the decussating fibers, which form the majority, are not illustrated in Fig. 1-3.) At successively higher levels the tract as a whole shifts dorsalward, a displacement brought about by the entrance of fibers from successively higher levels into the ventral part of the tract (Yoss, 1953). These fibers pass near the lateral edge of the medulla oblongata, dorsal to the inferior olivary nucleus. In the lower pons they maintain much the same position. Reaching the midpons, they curve around the ventral aspect of the incoming fibers of the root of the fifth nerve. On reaching the uppermost portion of the pons, the fibers enter the superior cerebellar peduncle and terminate in the cerebellum, mainly in the vermis and paravermian regions; here the fibers overlap with terminal fibers of the dorsal spinocerebellar tract (Yoss, 1953). The tract carries proprioceptive impulses.

Spino-olivary tract. The existence of spinal projections to the inferior olive has been confirmed in a large number of experimental animals, including several species of monkeys (Brodal, Walberg, and Blakstad, 1950; Mehler, Feferman, and Nauta, 1960). The evidence indicates that in all of these species spino-olivary fibers originate mainly in lumbar levels, ascend in the anterior column, and terminate consistently in the older, accessory portions of the inferior olive (the dorsal and parts of the medial accessory nuclei). In man, Bowsher (1962) described connections with the caudal part of the principal olive. However, in another study carried out on a large number of human cordotomy and medullotomy cases, no spino-olivary connections of any kind were found (Mehler, 1962; Mehler, Feferman, and Nauta, 1960). Similarly, failure to demonstrate spino-olivary connections in control cordotomy studies in the chimpanzee has led Mehler (1969) to conclude that no spino-olivary tract exists in man or any other truly biped primate species. Its appearance only in quadruped species suggests that it might function as a coordinator of hind- and forelegs (Mehler, 1969).

Spinotectal tract. Spinal fiber connections with cells in the deeper layers of the superior colliculus and cells in adjacent parts of the periaqueductal gray have long been recognized, and their presence in animal and man has recently been reaffirmed (Mehler, 1962). The fibers arise at various levels of cord down to lower thoracic segments. Their site of origin in the posterior horn remains unknown, nor is it known whether they arise ipsilaterally or contralaterally. In the spinal cord they ascend in the anterior and lateral columns and in their ascent through the medulla oblongata and pons they accompany the spinothalamic systems. Because of this association, the spinotectal tract has been implicated as a possible component of the central pain pathway.

Spinoreticular systems. Ascending in the anterior and lateral columns from all levels of the spinal cord, fibers proceed to the reticular formation of the medulla oblongata. They are numerous in man as well as in lower mammals (Batten and Holmes, 1913; Brodal, 1958; Mehler, 1962; Mehler, Feferman, and Nauta, 1960). A major portion of these fibers are of fine caliber. They have been considered to be collaterals of longer coursing fiber tracts such as the ventral spinocerebellar and the spinotectal and spinothalamic tracts. However, the strong decrement of spinal fibers in their ascent through the medulla oblongata suggests that separate spinoreticular systems or tracts exist. Some spinoreticular fibers have been shown to extend upward for considerable distances; for example, ascending fibers of single neurons, giving off a wealth of arborizations en route, have been traced from the spinal cord to the diencephalon (Scheibel and Scheibel, 1958). Functionally, the longer spinoreticular fibers are thought to convey proprioceptive impulses to the reticular formation. They have also been viewed as visceral sensory tracts and, possibly, as components of the central pain pathway.

Posterolateral tract. The posterolateral tract (of Morin, 1955) originates in spinal gray matter, ascends in the lateral column, and terminates in the lateral cervical nucleus; in man this nucleus consists of a small group of cells lying lateral to the posterior horn (Kircher and Ha, 1968; Truex, Taylor, and Smythe, 1968). Second-order fibers decussate and join the medial lemniscus in the latter's ascent to the thalamus. Fibers of the tract may originate as collaterals of fibers of the dorsal spinocerebellar tract. They may carry tactile and pressure impulses, also proprioceptive impulses originating from joint movement (Morin, 1955; Oswaldo-Cruz and Kid, 1964).

Long posterior root fibers; pathways in the posterior column. Fibers of this posterior root system enter the lateral aspect of the posterior column as part of the medial division of the posterior root system (Fig. 1-3). They pass upward to the superior end of the column where they terminate in the nucleus gracilis and the nucleus cuneatus. As the fibers from lower spinal levels ascend in the posterior column, they are displaced medially by fibers entering the column from successively higher posterior roots (Fig. 1-6). Thus lamination of posterior column fibers occurs.

In the cervical cord, a division of the posterior column into two parts demarcated by the posterior intermediate sulcus can be seen macroscopically. The medial division is the fasciculus gracilis, which contains posterior root fibers which have arisen in the lower half of the body, from segment Th4 and below. The lateral division is the fasciculus cuneatus, composed

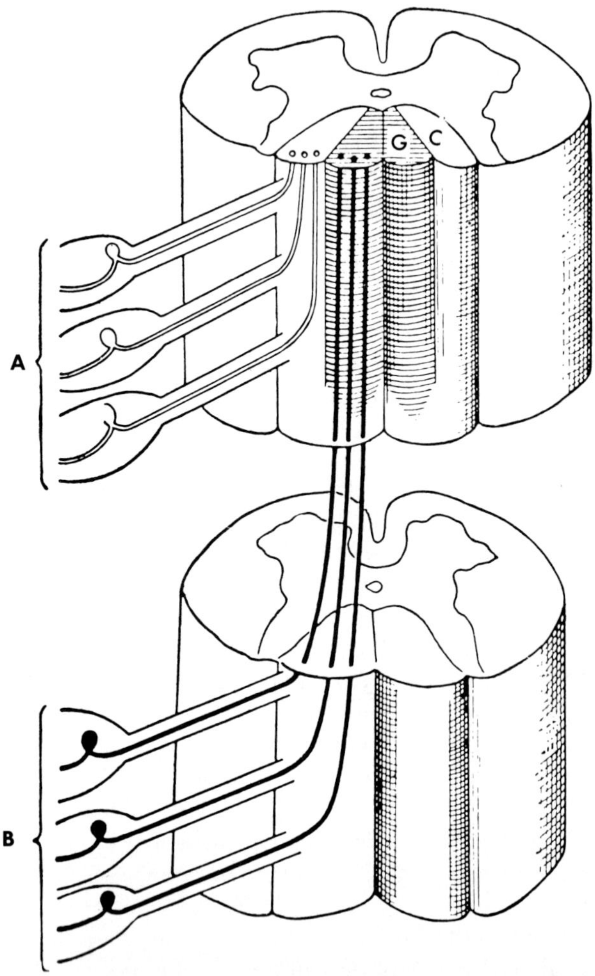

Fig. 1-6. Arrangement of fibers in the posterior column. *C,* Fasciculus cuneatus; *G,* fasciculus gracilis; **A** and **B,** long posterior root fibers arising in the upper half and lower half of the body, respectively.

of fibers which have originated in the upper half of the body from segment Th3 and above.

In addition to the fiber systems mentioned, the posterior column carries fibers that originate at cervical and upper thoracic levels and terminate in the lateral cuneate nucleus, with relay to the cerebellum (p. 10).

Traditionally, the posterior column and its upward continuation, the medial lemniscus, serve touch and pressure sense, position sense, kinesthesis, pallesthesia (appreciation of vibration), and discriminative forms of sensation (Poggio and Mountcastle, 1960; White and others, 1950). However, since posterior cordotomy leads to little or no sensory disturbance in man (Cook and Browder, 1965) or monkey (Schwartzman and Bogdonoff, 1969), there must be *alternate routes* by which the various forms of sensation under discussion are also mediated. Morin's tract (p. 11) is assumed to have the same functional capacity as the posterior column–medial lemniscal system. The anterolateral column may convey, from the ipsilateral side, impulses concerned in discriminative functions, such as two point discrimination, as concluded from a study of anterolateral cordotomy cases (Schiller, 1956). The medial part of the lateral column may carry vibratory stimuli from the ipsilateral side of the body, as concluded from findings in syringomyelia (Netsky, 1953).

The posterior columns have also been accorded motor function. Through fibers descending in the posterior column and making synaptic connections in the posterior horn (such as were mentioned on p. 7), the posterior columns constitute an essential part of the mechanism for projected movement into space, in particular the fine contactual orienting reactions of the upper limbs (Gilman and Denny-Brown, 1966).

Intersegmental tracts

Cell bodies situated along the border of the spinal gray give off axons (fibrae propriae, or fibrae spinospinales) which, collected in bundles (proprius bundles), pass upward, and others downward, in the adjoining white matter for varying distances, bringing the various segments of gray matter into communication with one another. The bundles are found in the lateral and anterior columns immediately adjacent to the corresponding columns of gray matter, in the posterolateral fasciculus of Lissauer ventrally, and in the posterior column. Dorsal to the spinal gray commissure these fibers form the cornucommissural tract, made up chiefly of ascending intersegmental fibers (Fig. 1-7). Cell bodies in the cord having both efferent and afferent affiliations run in the proprius bundles. Possibly some fibrae propriae decussate.

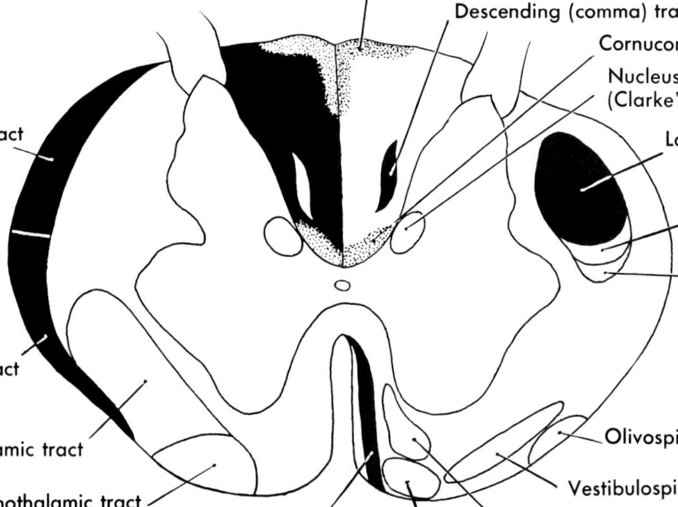

Fig. 1-7. The long spinal cord tracts and some intersegmental tracts. The long spinal tracts indicated in black are compact and well defined, while those in white are loosely arranged and poorly demarcated. On the right side of the figure the descending tracts are indicated, and on the left, the ascending tracts. The dotted areas represent intersegmental tracts. The tectospinal tract illustrated is the medial one.

The spinal white matter contains certain other endogenous groups of fibers. One is the septomarginal tract (Fig. 1-7), composed of descending branches of the fibers of the fasciculus gracilis. At sacral levels it is located in the dorsomedial angle of the posterior column (triangular field of Gombault and Phillippe), at lumbar levels it takes a position along the septum (oval field of Flechsig), while at thoracic levels it is situated along the dorsal border of the cord and the adjacent part of the median septum. Individual fibers coursing in the septomarginal tract descend two or three segments, then turn ventralward, and end in relation to anterior horn cells, ipsilaterally and perhaps also contralaterally. Some of the fibers possibly terminate in the posterior funicular gray.

Another group of fibers in the posterior column is the fasciculus interfascicularis (or comma field of Schultze), situated between the fasciculus gracilis and fasciculus cuneatus (Fig. 1-7). It is made up of descending branches of fibers entering the posterior column and is best developed at thoracic levels. Its fibers terminate in the same manner as those of the septomarginal tract. (Nathan and Smith, 1959.)

TOPOGRAPHY OF THE LONG SPINAL TRACTS

The cross-sectional topography of most of the long spinal tracts is shown in Fig. 1-7: the left half of the diagram illustrates the ascending tracts, and the right half the descending. The fiber groups indicated by black are compact, well-defined tracts, while the others are diffuse and their borders ill-defined. The levels of termination of these tracts have been indicated in the previous text.

The lateral corticospinal tract (lateral pyramidal tract) is largest at cervical levels and decreases steadily in size as it descends the cord; it expends itself as groups of its fibers terminate in each succeeding spinal segment. At upper levels of the cord the tract has the form and position indicated in Fig. 1-7; it is oval and is situated in the more dorsal part of the lateral column. Below segment L3 the pyramidal tract shifts laterally to the periphery of the cord, and thus it assumes the position occupied at higher levels by the dorsal spinocerebellar tract. In lower spinal segments there is no dorsal spinocerebellar tract.

The anterior corticospinal tract (anterior pyramidal tract) is situated adjacent to the anterior median fissure. The lower limit of the tract is at a lower cervical or an upper thoracic level.

The tectospinal and tectotegmentospinal tracts are situated peripherally in the anterior column.

The rubrospinal tract is to be found immediately ventral to the lateral corticospinal tract.

The vestibulospinal tract occupies a narrow zone near the periphery of the anterior column.

The reticulospinal tracts have a predominantly central location in the lateral and anterior columns of the cord, respectively.

The fasciculi of the posterior column (gracilis and cuneatus) contain the ascending long posterior root fibers. They are present at all levels of the spinal cord. Descending collaterals from the fasciculus gracilis form the septomarginal tract and the fasciculus interfascicularis, and at certain levels the collaterals are intermixed with intersegmental fibers.

The lateral and anterior spinothalamic tracts are contiguous; the lateral lies in the more ventral part of the lateral column, the anterior in the more dorsal part of the anterior column. As the spinothalamic tracts ascend they are displaced more and more dorsalward in the lateral column.

The dorsal spinocerebellar tract is present only in the segments above L3, while the ventral spinocerebellar tract is present at all spinal levels. The two tracts lie adjacent to each other in the peripheral zone of the lateral column, and at higher cervical levels they are intermixed.

The spinotectal tract is detectable from

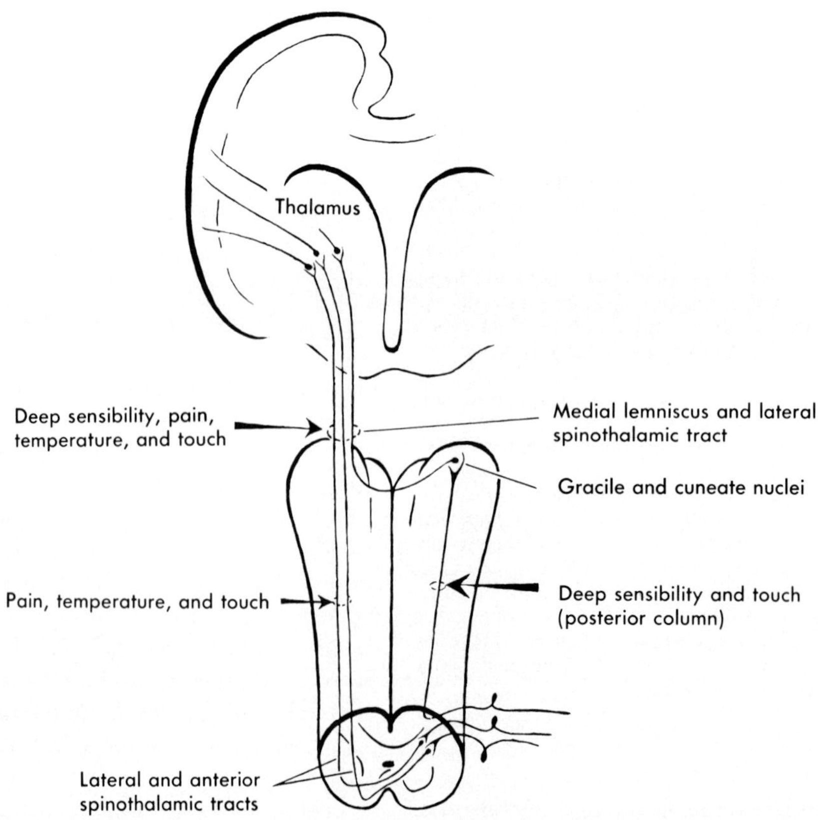

Fig. 1-8. Conventional spinal pathways conveying sensory impulses to the thalamus, thence to the cerebral cortex.

lower thoracic levels upward. It occupies the anterolateral part of the cord.

Spinoreticular systems also run upward in the anterolateral part of the cord, and they are found at all cord levels.

SUMMARY OF SPINAL PATHWAYS CONVEYING AFFERENT IMPULSES

Pathways conveying impulses concerned in the various forms of sensibility may be summarized as follows (conventional pathways are illustrated in Fig. 1-8).

Fibers transmitting pain and thermal impulses from the periphery reach the substantia gelatinosa. Collaterals ascend and descend a segment or two in Lissauer's tract before terminating in the posterior horn. Fibers of neurons of the second order cross to the opposite side and ascend in the lateral spinothalamic tract. "Medial" and "lateral" pain pathways reach the thalamus via divergent routes.

Fibers conveying tactile impressions pass up the ipsilateral posterior column. Some terminate in the nucleus gracilis and nucleus cuneatus, but most of them end in the nucleus proprius of the posterior horn at the level of root entry and at successively higher segments, after having ascended in the posterior column. Fibers of the second order cross the midline of the cord and ascend in the anterior spinothalamic tract.

Position sense and kinesthesis are transmitted centralward via the ipsilateral posterior column. An alternate pathway is Morin's tract, which runs in the ipsilateral lateral column, lateral to the posterior horn.

Fibers concerned in discriminative sensibility ascend in the ipsilateral posterior column. Evidence exists that Morin's tract and the ipsilateral lateral column (its medial aspect) are utilized as alternate routes for the passage of these fibers.

Vibratory stimuli may be transmitted in the ipsilateral posterior column. They may also travel in the medial aspect of the ipsilateral lateral column.

Proprioceptive fibers reaching the cerebellum take three routes, all ipsilateral: (1) from the nucleus dorsalis via the dorsal spinocerebellar tract and, in turn, the inferior cerebellar peduncle; (2) from the nucleus of Stilling and the postcommissural nucleus, via the ventral spinocerebellar tract and, in turn, the superior cerebellar peduncle; (3) from the lateral cuneate nucleus via the dorsal superficial arcuate fibers, then the inferior cerebellar peduncle.

ANTERIOR ROOT FIBERS

Most fibers of the anterior root arise from cells of the anterior horn; they extend into the peripheral nerves and supply somatic muscles. Others originate in cells of the intermediolateral horns (from C7 to L3, inclusive), pass through the anterior roots, and then take various courses to innervate smooth muscle, arterioles, and sweat glands. Still another group, which enters the cord by way of the posterior root (with cell bodies in the dorsal root ganglion), synapses with anterior horn cells. These two neurons make up the monosynaptic reflex arc (Fig. 1-3). Many other reflex pathways ultimately connect posterior root systems with anterior horn cells. Some that have been mentioned come from fibers ascending in the posterior column.

BLOOD SUPPLY OF THE SPINAL CORD

Arterial supply

The major arteries contributing to the blood supply of the spinal cord are indicated in Table 1-1 and Fig. 1-9. Most of the cervical cord is supplied from the vertebral arteries, either from the region where they merge to form the basilar artery or through their radicular branches (Fig. 1-9, *A*). Segments C7–Th2 receive their supply from radicular vessels coming off the cervical branches of the inferior thyroid artery or the costocervical trunk. Tributaries for all segments below Th2 are provided by vessels arising from the aorta or the internal iliac arteries.

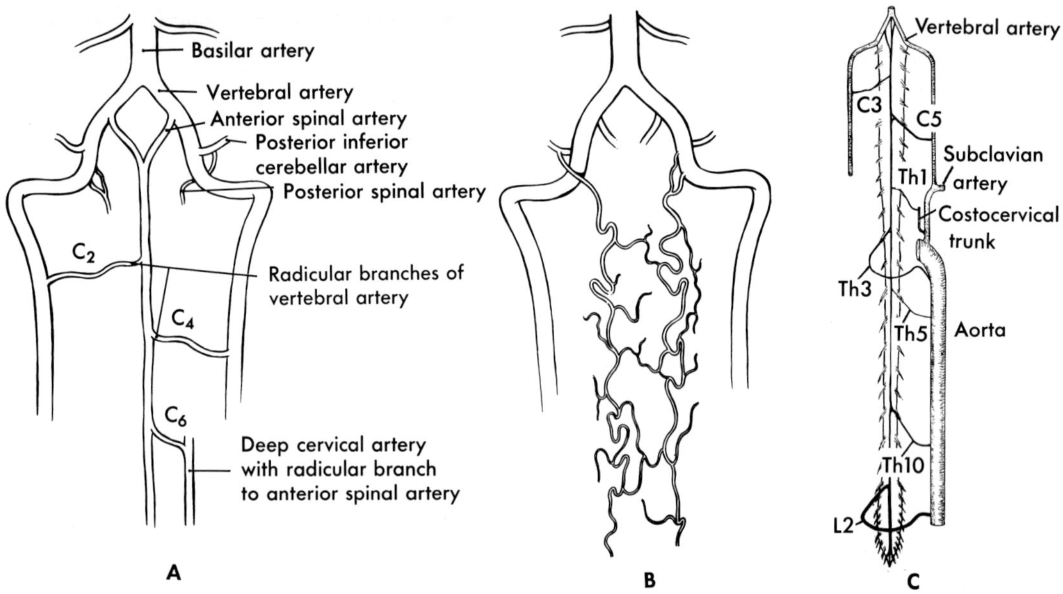

Fig. 1-9. Arterial supply of the spinal cord. **A,** Sources of cervical arteries which join the anterior spinal artery. **B,** Plexus formed by the posterior spinal arteries. (**A** and **B** from Schechter and Zingesser, 1966.) **C,** Sources of radicular arteries extending to the anterior spinal artery. (From Lindenberg, 1957.)

Table 1-1. Sources of arterial supply of the spinal cord

Main arteries	*Branches*
Subclavian artery	Vertebral artery Ascending cervical branches of the inferior thyroid artery Deep cervical branch of the costocervical (or costovertebral) trunk Superior intercostal branches of the costocervical trunk
Aorta	Intercostal arteries Lumbar arteries
Internal iliac arteries	Iliolumbar arteries Lateral sacral arteries

The anterior spinal artery originates from the intracranial part of both vertebral arteries or, occasionally, from only one of these arteries or directly from the basilar artery. It is situated at the mouth of the anterior median fissure and extends all the way down the cord (Adams and van Geertruyden, 1956; Bolton, 1939). The anterior spinal artery may be doubled down to the C5 segmental level or further caudalward (Turnbull, Brieg, and Hassler, 1966).

According to Gillilan (1958), from seven to ten arteries extend inward along anterior roots to merge with the anterior spinal artery (according to Corbin [1961] the maximum is fourteen arteries). These are the anterior radicular branches of radicular arteries. At least one major radicular artery sends branches to the cervical cord (usually along root C6 or C7); two major arteries send them to the thoracic cord, and one major artery to a lower level. Individual variations in radicular arterial pattern exist particularly for the cervical and upper thoracic spinal regions, as will be noted for the cervical cord in Figs. 1-9, *A* and 1-9, *C*, depicted by two different observers. In 10 percent of cases (Turnbull, Brieg, and Hassler, 1966), anterior roots C7, C8, and Th1 carry no radicular arteries. As few as three anterior radicular arteries have been noted in the cervical region (Lazorthes and others, 1957).

The artery extending to the lower part

of the cord—the great anterior radicular artery of Adamkiewicz—is the most constant and the largest. Fig. 1-9, *C* shows it coursing inward along anterior root L2. It usually runs along root L1 or L2, but it may be found on any anterior root at levels between Th8 and L3 (Craigie, 1961). It is never paired, and in two-thirds of observed cases it runs along an anterior root of the left side. When coursing along a root on the right side, it originates from the left side (from the aorta) and passes over the ventral surface of the body of the vertebra, as shown in Fig. 1-9, *C*. Thus, in about a third of cases it is subject to compression by any mass that happens to be situated in the vicinity. The lower the artery of Adamkiewicz, the more numerous and the smaller the other radicular arteries (Adams and van Geertruyden, 1956). This artery is an important vessel, since it provides a copious blood supply for a fourth of the cord in 50 percent of cases, and half the cord in the other 50 percent. In its course, the anterior spinal artery is of widest caliber at levels at which it receives radicular tributaries; its caliber is smallest at cord levels Th7 and Th8. The artery extends down to the conus where, according to Bolton (1939) and Craigie (1961), it divides into two branches, one on either side merging with the corresponding posterior spinal artery.

As a rule, the relatively small posterior spinal arteries originate directly from the intracranial part of the vertebral artery, though in some instances they come from the posterior inferior cerebellar artery (Figs. 1-9, *A* and 1-9, *B*). At upper cervical levels they are situated along the medial edge of the posterior roots, one on each side of the cord. In the midcervical region, these arteries meander and give off plexiform vessels (Fig. 1-9, *B*) that are fed by arteries coming in along cervical posterior roots. At upper thoracic levels the plexiform arrangement dissipates and the posterior spinal arteries straighten out. All told, according to Lindenberg (1957), the posterior spinal artery of each side receives branches from thirty to forty radicular arteries; according to Corbin (1961), they receive twenty-three at most, and according to Hassler (1966), no more than fifteen. Variability in the number of radicular arteries is greatest at the cervical level (Turnbull, Brieg, and Hassler, 1966).

Each segment of the spinal cord is supplied by sulcocommissural arteries, the posterior spinal arteries, and arteries running along the lateral and anterior sides of the cord.

The sulcocommissural arteries, of which there are some two hundred altogether (Craigie, 1961; Herren and Alexander, 1939; Lindenberg, 1957), are derived from the anterior spinal artery. According to most descriptions, these arteries are given off alternately, one artery to the right and the next to the left, in supplying successively higher levels. The sulcocommissural arteries are fewest in the thoracic region (sometimes one per segment) and most numerous in the lumbar region. Each sulcocommissural artery arborizes in the anterior and intermediolateral gray horns. Moreover, each provides branches for the supply of much of the lateral column of the cord, and, according to Mair and Druckman (1953), each arborizes in the ventral part of the posterior white columns.

The two posterior spinal arteries anastomose in the pia in the region of the midline. The artery of one side sends branches into the posterior white column, the largest branch being in the posterior median septum. Some of these vessels arborize in the posterior column; others continue on and arborize in the central gray (Craigie, 1961). Another branch, entering the cord just lateral to the posterior root, arborizes in the posterior horn, down to (and perhaps including) the nucleus dorsalis.

Arteries running alongside the lateral aspect of the cord are, in part, branches of the radicular arteries (Fig. 1-10) (Schechter and Zingesser, 1966; Suh and Alexander, 1939; Tureen, 1938). Others (few, according to Gillilan, 1958) originate from the arteriae corona, formed by the anastomosis of branches from the anterior and posterior spinal arteries (Fig. 1-10). The system often contains a longitudinally running lateral spinal artery and also a longitudinally running ventrolateral spinal artery (Craigie, 1961). This anastomotic system is present at cervical, thoracic, lumbar, and sacral levels; however, in the longitudial plane little or no communication appears to exist between them (Lazorthes and others, 1958). This anterolateral system of arteries, whether fed by the arteriae corona or not, sends branches into the adjoining white matter including the lateral pyramidal tract, which also receives a supply from the sulcocommissural artery. Some of the penetrating vessels also extend into gray matter (Craigie, 1961).

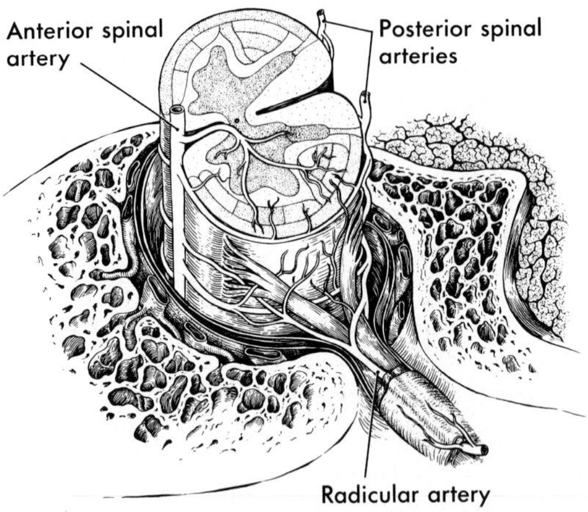

Fig. 1-10. Arterial supply of spinal cord segment. (From Schechter and Zingesser, 1966.)

As already indicated, much of the border of the gray matter and the adjoining part of the white receive a blood supply jointly from central and peripheral arterial branches. Hassler (1966) and Turnbull, Brieg, and Hassler (1966) have emphasized this point. They observed that the central and peripheral arterial beds within the cord are discrete, but that they overlap ("like the branches of two trees growing side by side"). This occurs in the areas indicated in Fig. 1-11.

By way of summary, the spinal gray re-

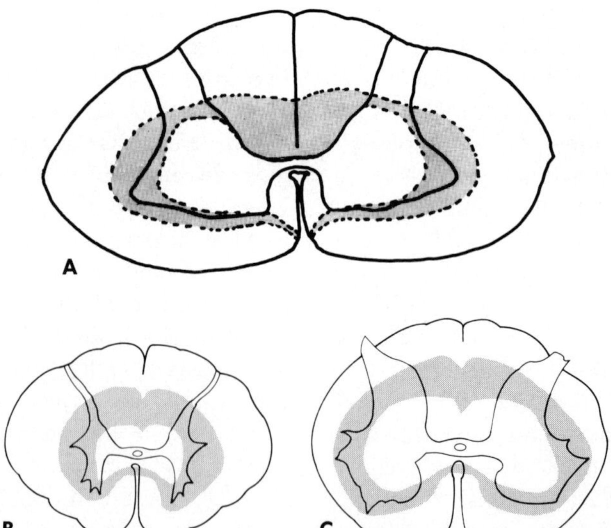

Fig. 1-11. A, Cervical cord; **B,** thoracic cord; **C,** lumbar cord. Distribution of central and peripheral arterial systems. The areas indicated in white are supplied by one system, the shaded areas by both. Capillary distribution in the upper sacral cord resembles that in the lumbar cord, the latter having a larger central area and a proportionately smaller peripheral area than the thoracic cord. Overlap in the posterior columns in the cervical cord is more ventrally situated than at the other levels. (From Hassler, 1966, and Turnbull, Brieg, and Hassler, 1966.)

ceives its arterial supply from three sources: the sulcocommissural artery, the posterior spinal artery, and the anterolateral (coronal) arterial system.

In general, the anterior spinal artery feeds the anterior two-thirds of a cord segment, and the posterior spinal artery the remainder. In the gray matter, all arteries constitute end-arteries in the sense that no anastomosis occurs except at the capillary level. In the transverse plane, certain regions of apposition of capillary beds are particularly susceptible to ischemia (Fig. 5-11). The susceptibility may be attributable to the slenderness of the coronal arterial connections between the posterior and anterior spinal arteries, with the result that effective shunting cannot occur. In other words, the coronal arteries do not comprise an efficient safeguard against reduced blood flow in either system, at least not at some spinal levels. Longitudinally considered, certain levels are particularly susceptible to general reduction in blood flow (p. 84), owing apparently to sparsity of collateral circulation between segments. Moreover, these and other levels may be directly affected by occlusion of larger radicular arteries (pp. 87 and 98).

Venous return from the spinal cord

Veins of the spinal cord run alongside the arteries and pass outward by way of the anterior and posterior roots (Craigie, 1961; Turnbull, Brieg, and Hassler, 1966). They drain into the voluminous spinovertebral venous plexus, which is continuous upward into the intracranial cavity (Fig. 1-12). At thoracic and upper lumbar levels this venous plexus drains into the azygos vein. Moreover, it has a free and rich anastomosis with veins of the thoracic, abdominal, and pelvic cavities, and a direct venous connection exists between the lungs and the spinovertebralazygos system. The blood pressure in the spinovertebral venous plexus is relatively low; since blood flow in the plexus is altered with every compression of the trunk such as in lifting, coughing, or holding the breath, the plexus offers a potential means for the transport of tumor cells and other embolic material (or gas bubbles) upward from the pelvic or femoral venous system (Batson, 1940). It has been contended that puerperal dural sinus thrombosis may be due to the lodgement, in dural sinuses, of material originating in the pelvic region and carried upward via this venous system (Martin, 1941; Stewart, 1942). However, in one case no thrombus was found in the pelvic veins in association with puerperal sinus thrombosis (Kendall, 1948), and it has been argued that thrombosis of intracranial veins and sinuses in the puerperium takes place in situ for the same reason that thrombosis of the pelvic and femoral

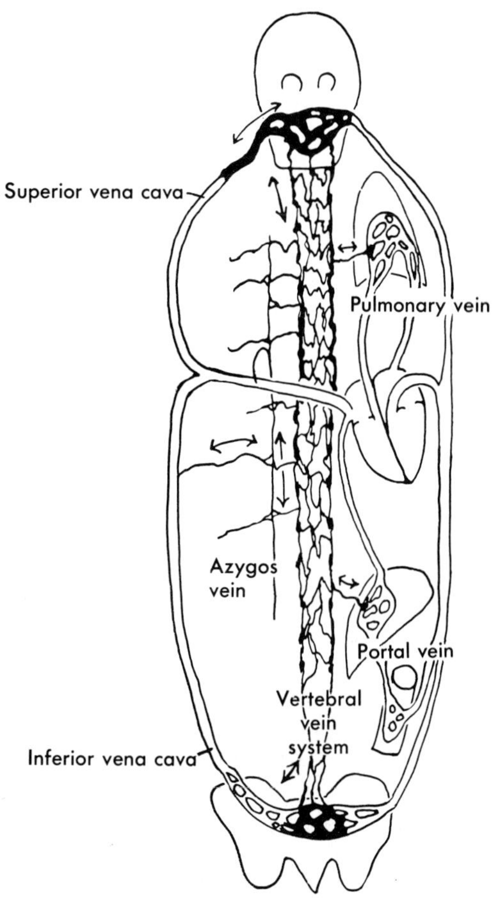

Fig. 1-12. The spinovertebral system of veins and its connections. Directions of blood flow are indicated. (From Batson, 1940.)

veins occurs (Barnett and Hyland, 1953; Kalbag and Woolf, 1967).

REFERENCES

Adams, H. D., and van Geertruyden, H. H. 1956. Neurologic complications of aortic surgery. Ann. Surg. **144**:574-609.

Austin, G. 1961. The spinal cord: basic aspects and surgical considerations. Springfield, Illinois, Charles C Thomas, Publisher.

Barnes, S. 1901. Degeneration in hemiplegia, with special reference to a ventrolateral pyramidal tract. Brain **24**:463-501.

Barnett, H. J. M., and Hyland, H. H. 1953. Non-infective intracranial venous thrombosis. Brain **76**:36-49.

Batson, O. V. 1940. The function of the vertebral veins and their role in the spread of metastases. Ann. Surg. **112**:138-149.

Batten, F. E., and Holmes, G. 1913. The endogenous fibers of the human spinal cord. Brain **35**: 259-275.

Bishop, G. H. 1959. The relation between nerve fiber size and sensory modality: phylogenetic implications of the afferent innervation of cortex. J. Nerv. Ment. Dis. **128**:89-114.

Bishop, G. H. 1962. Pain. In Grenell, R. G., editor: Neural physiopathology: some relationships of normal to altered nervous system activity. New York, Harper & Row, Publishers, pp. 95-133.

Bok, S. T. 1928. Das Rückenmark. In von Möllendorff, W., editor: Handbuch der mikroskopischen Anatomie des Menschen, vol. 4, part 1. Berlin, Springer-Verlag, pp. 478-578.

Bolton, B. 1939. The blood supply of the human spinal cord. J. Neurol. Neurosurg. Psychiat. **2**:137-148.

Bowsher, D. 1957. Termination of the central pain pathway in man: the conscious appreciation of pain. Brain **80**:606-622.

Bowsher, D. 1962. The topographical projection of fibers from the anterolateral quadrant of the spinal cord to the sub-diencephalic brain stem in man. Psychiat. Neurol. (Basel) **143**:75-99.

Brodal, A. 1958. The reticular formation of the brain stem: anatomical aspects and functional correlations. Springfield, Illinois, Charles C Thomas, Publisher.

Brodal, A., Walberg, F., and Blackstad, T. 1950. Termination of spinal afferents to inferior olive in cat. J. Neurophysiol. **13**:431-454.

Bruce, A. N. 1901. A topographical atlas of the spinal cord. London, Williams & Norgate.

Bruce, A. N. 1910. The tract of Gowers. Quart. J. Exp. Physiol. **3**:391-407.

Collier, J., and Buzzard, F. 1901. Descending mesencephalic tracts in cat, monkey and man; Monakow's bundle; the dorsal longitudinal bundle; the ventral longitudinal bundle; the pontospinal tracts, lateral and ventral; the vestibulospinal tract; the central tegmental tract (centrale Haubenbahn); descending fibers of the fillet. Brain **24**:177-221.

Collins, W. F., Nulsen, F. E., and Shealy, C. N. 1966. Electrophysiological studies of peripheral and central pathways conducting pain. In Knighton, R. S., and Dumke, P. R., editors: Pain. Boston, Little, Brown and Company, pp. 33-45.

Cook, A. W., and Browder, E. J. 1965. Functions of the posterior columns in man. Arch. Neurol. **12**:72-79.

Corbin, J. L. 1961. Anatomie et pathologie artérielles de la moelle. Paris, Masson & Cie.

Craigie, E. H. 1961. Vascular supply of the spinal cord. In Austin, G., editor: The spinal cord: basic aspects and surgical considerations. Springfield, Illinois, Charles C Thomas, Publisher, pp. 217-243.

Crosby, E. C., Humphrey, T., and Lauer, E. W. 1962. Correlative anatomy of the nervous system. New York, The Macmillan Company.

Dejerine, J. 1901. Anatomie des centres nerveux. Paris, Reuff.

Earle, K. M. 1952. The tract of Lissauer and its possible relation to the pain pathway. J. Comp. Neurol. **96**:93-109.

Eccles, J. C. 1967. Functional organization of the spinal cord. Anesthesiology **28**:31-45.

Ferraro, A., and Barrera, S. E. 1935. Posterior column fibers and their terminations in Macacus rhesus. J. Comp. Neurol. **62**:507-530.

Foerster, O. 1936. Symptomatologie der Erkrankungen des Rückenmarks und seiner Wurzeln. In Bumke, O., and Foerster, O., editors: Handbuch der Neurologie, vol. 5. Berlin, Springer-Verlag, pp. 1-400.

Foerster, O., and Gagel, O. 1932. Die Vorderseitenstrangdurchschneidung beim Menschen. Zbl. Ges. Neurol. Psychiat. **138**:1-92.

Gillilan, L. A. 1958. The arterial blood supply of the human spinal cord. J. Comp. Neurol. **110**: 75-103.

Gilman, S., and Denny-Brown, D. 1966. Disorders of movement and behavior following dorsal column lesions. Brain **89**:397-418.

Hassler, O. 1966. Blood supply of the human spinal cord: a microangiographic study. Arch. Neurol. Psychiat. **15**:302-307.

Herren, R. Y., and Alexander, L. 1939. Sulcal and intrinsic blood vessels of the human spinal cord. Arch. Neurol. Psychiat. **41**:678-687.

Jacobsohn, L. 1908. Über die Kerne des menschlichen Rückenmarks. Königlich-preussische Akademie der Wissenschaften zu Berlin. Physikalisch-mathematische Klasse. Abhandlungen, pp. 1-73.

Jansen, J., and Brodal, A. 1954. Aspects of cerebellar anatomy. Oslo, Johan Grundt Tanum.

Kalbag, R. M., and Woolf, A. L. 1967. Cerebral venous thrombosis, with special reference to primary aseptic thrombosis. London, Oxford University Press.

Kendall, D. 1948. Thrombosis of intracranial veins. Brain **71**:386-402.

Keswani, N. H., and Hollinshead, W. H. 1956. Localization of the phrenic nucleus in the spinal cord of man. Anat. Rec. **125**:683-700.

Kircher, C., and Ha, H. 1968. The nucleus cervicalis lateralis in primates, including the human. Anat. Rec. **106**:376.

Kuypers, H. G. J. M. 1964. The descending pathways to the spinal cord, their anatomy and function. Progr. Brain Res. **11**:178-202.

Langworthy, O. R. 1930. Medullated tracts in the brain stem of a seventh month human fetus. Contributions to Embryology (Publications of the Carnegie Institution) **21**:37-52.

Lazorthes, G., Poulhes, J., Bastide, G., Roulleau, J., and Chancholle, A. R. 1957. Recherches sur la vascularisation artérielle de la moelle; applications à la pathologie médullaire. Bull. Acad. Nat. Med. **141**:464-477.

Lazorthes, G., Poulhes, J., Bastide, G., Roulleau, J., and Chancholle, A. R. 1958. La vascularisation artérielle de la moelle; recherche anatomiques et applications à la pathologie médullaire et à la pathologie aortique. Neurochirurgie **4**:3-19.

Lindenberg, R. 1957. Die Gefässversorgung und ihre Bedeutung für Art und Ort von kreislaufbedingten Gewebsschäden und Gefässprozessen. In Lubarsch, O., Henke, F., and Rössle, R., editors: Handbuch der speziellen pathologischen Anatomie, vol. 13, edited by Scholz, W., pt. 1A. Berlin, Springer-Verlag, pp. 1071-1164.

Mair, W. G. P., and Druckman, R. 1953. The pathology of spinal cord lesions and their relation to the clinical features in protrusion of cervical intervertebral discs (a report of four cases). Brain **76**:70-91.

Mark, V. H., Ervin, F. R., and Hackett, T. 1960. Clinical aspects of stereotactic thalamotomy in the human: the treatment of chronic severe pain. Arch. Neurol. **3**:351-367.

Martin, J. P. 1941. Thrombosis in the superior longitudinal sinus during childbirth. Brit. Med. J. **2**:537-540.

Mehler, W. R. 1962. The anatomy of the so-called "pain tract" in man: an analysis of the course and distribution of the ascending fibers of the fasciculus anterolateralis. In French, J. D., and Porter, R. W., editors: Basic research in paraplegia. Springfield, Illinois, Charles C Thomas, Publisher, pp. 26-55.

Mehler, W. R. 1969 (in press). Some neurological species differences—a posteriori. In Petras, J. M., and Noback, C. R., editors: Comparative and evolutionary aspects of the vertebrate central nervous system. New York, New York Academy of Sciences.

Mehler, W. R., Feferman, M. E., and Nauta, W. J. H. 1960. Ascending axon degeneration following anterolateral cordotomy: an experimental study in the monkey. Brain **83**:718-750.

Melzack, R., and Wall, P. D. 1965. Pain mechanisms: a new theory. Science **150**:971-979.

Morin, F. 1955. A new spinal pathway for cutaneous impulses. Amer. J. Physiol. **183**:245-252.

Nashold, B. S., Jr., Wilson, W. P., and Slaughter, D. C. 1969. Sensations evoked by stimulation in the midbrain in man. J. Neurosurg. **30**:14-24.

Nathan, P. W., and Smith, M. C. 1955. Long descending tracts in man: review of present knowledge. Brain **78**:248-303.

Nathan, P. W., and Smith, M. C. 1959. Fasciculi proprii of the spinal cord in man: review of present knowledge. Brain **82**:610-668.

Netsky, M. G. 1953. Syringomyelia: a clinicopathologic study. A.M.A. Arch. Neurol. Psychiat. **70**:741-777.

Noordenbos, W. 1959. Pain: problems pertaining to the transmission of nerve impulses which give rise to pain. Amsterdam, Elsevier Publishing Company.

Nyberg-Hansen, R. 1965. Sites and modes of termination of reticulospinal fibers in the cat; an experimental study with silver impregnation methods. J. Comp. Neurol. **124**:71-100.

Okamoto, M., Kanaseki, T., Hamase, T., and Mizuno, N. 1965. Studies of the human triangular tract of Helweg. Okajimas Folia Anat. Jap. **40**:861-887.

Olszewski, J., and Baxter, D. 1954. Cytoarchitecture of the human spinal cord. Basel, S. Karger AG.

Oswaldo-Cruz, E., and Kid, C. 1964. Functional properties of neurons in the lateral cervical nucleus of the cat. J. Neurophysiol. **27**:1-14.

Pass, I. J. 1933. Anatomic and functional relationships of the nucleus dorsalis (Clarke's column) and of the dorsal spinocerebellar tract (Flechsig's). Arch. Neurol. Psychiat. **30**:1025-1045.

Pearson, A. A. 1952. Role of gelatinous substance of spinal cord in conduction of pain. Arch. Neurol. Psychiat. **68**:515-529.

Pearson, A. A., Sauter, R. W., and Herrin, G. R. 1964. The accessory nerve and its relation to the upper spinal nerves. Amer. J. Anat. **114**:371-392.

Poggio, G. F., and Mountcastle, V. B. 1960. A study of the functional contributions of the lemniscal and spinothalamic systems to somatic sensibility: central nervous mechanisms in pain. Bull. Johns Hopkins Hosp. **106**:266-316.

Pompeiano, O. 1967. Functional organization of the cerebellar projections to the spinal cord. Progr. Brain Res. **25**:282-321.

Renshaw, B. 1941. Influence of discharge of motoneurons upon excitation of neighboring motoneurons. J. Neurophysiol. **4**:167-173.

Renshaw, B. 1946. Observations on the interactions of nerve impulses in the gray matter and the nature of central inhibition. Amer. J. Physiol. **146**:443-448.

Rexed, B. 1954. Cytoarchitectonic atlas of the spinal cord of the cat. J. Comp. Neurol. **100**:297-379.

Rexed, B. 1964. Some aspects of the cytoarchitectonics and synaptology of the spinal cord. Progr. Brain Res. **11**:58-92.

Romanes, G. J. 1964. The motor pools of the spinal cord. Progr. Brain Res. **11**:93-119.

Schechter, M. M., and Zingesser, L. H. 1966. The spinal arteries. Acta Radiol. **5**:1124-1131.

Scheibel, M. E., and Scheibel, A. B. 1958. Structural substrates for integrative patterns in the brain stem reticular core. In Jasper, H. H., and others, editors: Reticular formation of the brain. Boston, Little, Brown and Company, pp. 31-55.

Schiller, F. 1956. The cutaneous sensory modalities: a critique of their "specificity." A.M.A. Arch. Neurol. Psychiat. **75**:203-219.

Schoen, J. H. R. 1964. Comparative aspects of

the descending fibre systems in the spinal cord. Progr. Brain Res. **11**:203-222.
Schwartzman, R. J., and Bogdonoff, M. D. 1969. Proprioception and vibration sensibility discrimination in the absence of the posterior columns. Arch. Neurol. **20**:349-353.
Sharrard, W. J. W. 1955. The distribution of the permanent paralysis in the lower limb in poliomyelitis. J. Bone Joint Surg. **37B**:540-558.
Sjöqvist, O. 1949. Surgical section of pain tracts and pathways in the spinal cord and brain stem. IVe Congrès neurologique international, Paris, 5-10 Septembre, 1944, **1**:119-132.
Smith, M. C. 1957. Observations of the topography of the lateral column of the human cervical spinal cord. Brain **80**:263-272.
Spiegel, E. A., and Wycis, H. T. 1962. Stereoencephalotomy: clinical and physiological applications. New York, Grune & Stratton.
Spiegel, E. A., and Wycis, H. T. 1966. Present status of stereoencephalotomies for pain relief. Confin. Neurol. **27**:527-717.
Spiegel, E. A., and Wycis, H. T. 1967. Multiple representation of various functions in the human subcortex. Confin. Neurol. **29**:163-167.
Stern, K. 1938. Note on nucleus ruber magnocellularis and its efferent pathway in man. Brain **61**:284-289.
Stewart, P. 1901. Degenerations following a traumatic lesion of the spinal cord, with an account of a tract in the cervical region. Brain **24**: 222-237.
Stewart, R. H. M. 1942. Primary cerebral sinus thrombosis. Brit. Med. J. **2**:455.
Suh, T. H., and Alexander, L. 1939. Vascular system of the human spinal cord. Arch. Neurol. Psychiat. **41**:659-677.
Szentágothai, J. 1948. Anatomical considerations of monosynaptic reflex arcs. J. Neurophysiol. **11**: 445-454.
Szentágothai, J., and Albert, A. 1955. The synaptology of Clarke's column. Acta Morph. Acad. Sci. Hung. **5**:43-51.
Truex, R., Taylor, M., and Smythe, M. 1968. The lateral cervical nucleus of the human spinal cord. Anat. Rec. **160**:443.
Tureen, L. L. 1938. Circulation of the spinal cord and the effect of vascular occlusion. Res. Publ. Ass. Res. Nerv. Ment. Dis., Proc. **18**:394-437.
Turnbull, I. M., Brieg, A., and Hassler, O. 1966. Blood supply of cervical spinal cord in man. A microangiographic cadaver study. J. Neurosurg. **24**:951-965.
Verhaart, W. J. C., and Kramer, W. 1952. The uncrossed pyramidal tract. Acta Psychiat. Scand. **27**:181-200.
Walker, A. E. 1940. The spinothalamic tract in man. Arch. Neurol. Psychiat. **43**:284-298.
Walker, A. E. 1942. Somatotopic localization of spinothalamic and secondary trigeminal tracts in mesencephalon. Arch. Neurol. Psychiat. **48**:884-889.
Wall, P. D. 1964. Presynaptic control of impulses at the first central synapse in the cutaneous pathway. Progr. Brain Res. **12**:92-118.
Weil, A., and Lassek, A. 1929. Quantitative distribution of pyramidal tract in man. Arch. Neurol. Psychiat. **22**:495-510
White, J. C., Sweet, W. H., Hawkins, R., and Nilges, R. G. 1950. Anterolateral cordotomy: results, complications and causes of failure. Brain **73**:345-367.
Woodburne, R. T. 1957. Essentials of human anatomy. New York, Oxford University Press.
Yoss, R. E. 1953. Studies of the spinal cord: topographic localization within the ventral spino-cerebeller tract in the macaque. J. Comp. Neurol. **99**:613-638.
Zenner, P. 1898. Ein Fall von Hirngeschwulst in der linken motorischen Sphäre; linkseitige Lähmung, Abwesenheit der Pyramidenkreuzung. Neurol. Zentralbl. **17**:202-203.

Chapter 2

Sensory, motor, trophic, and autonomic function; disturbances in function

SENSORY FUNCTION

Various classifications of body sensation have been proposed. Source of stimulus and site of receptor are the basis of a classification proposed by Sherrington (1906): *exteroceptors,* present in the skin, provide information on changes in the ambient environment; *proprioceptors,* present in muscles, tendons, and the region of joints, give information as to position in space and movement of the body or its voluntarily movable parts; and *interoceptors* convey impulses from the viscera. Other terms refer to mediation through some agent, for example, mechanoreceptor, pressoreceptor (Merkel's disks, pacinian corpuscles, and others), and chemoreceptor.

Somatic sensibility includes cutaneous (or superficial) sensations; deep sensations, that is, those originating from joints, muscles, and tendons *(bathesthesia);* and sensations classed as deep pain and pressure-touch. With respect to deep sensations, the appreciation of passive and active movement is served by different receptors: capsular receptors in the first instance, and muscle and tendon receptors in the second (Browne, Lee, and Ring, 1954). This difference accounts for the fact that active movement can still be perceived after the appreciation of passive movement is lost. The term *kinesthesis* usually refers to the appreciation of movement alone. *Proprioception* signifies perception of position, sometimes of movement as well. *Somesthesis* includes both superficial and deep sensibility and excludes visceral sensation.

Protopathic sensibility and *epicritic sensibility* are terms introduced by Henry Head in 1905, based on studies following complete nerve section (his own posterior cutaneous nerve of the forearm). Head's summation of his findings appeared in 1920.

After section, deep sensibility remained, and with it the capacity to feel and localize deep pain. Superficial sensibility was absent. After several months, pain and temperature sensations returned to a zone lying between the central area of complete anesthesia and the surrounding area of normal sensation. In this intermediate zone, however, pain from pinprick was far more unpleasant than before nerve section (Head's *hyperesthesia*), and it was difficult to localize the pain. "Pain spots" and "cold spots" responded only to intense stimulation, and in an explosive fashion. These characteristics he called "protopathic." Also, in the intermediate zone, touch by cotton was not perceived, nor was discrimination of two points or smaller changes in temperature. About 1 year after the section, fine grades of sensitivity returned to the intermediate zone and with them the capacity to distinguish between moderate temperatures and to localize tactile stimuli. A state of "epicritic" sensibility—as he called it—was reestablished. Head postulated that sensory impressions are carried by three sets of nerves or nerve fibers: (1) deep pain, by motor nerves; (2)

cutaneous pain and extremes of temperature (below 68° and above 113° F.), by superficial nerves originating from a relatively wide cutaneous field *(the protopathic system)*; and (3) localization and discrimination of tactile stimuli and appreciation of finer grades of temperature, by superficial nerves originating from a relatively small cutaneous field *(the epicritic system)*.

Trotter and Davies, taking up the problem, reported (in 1909) that the thresholds for all kinds of cutaneous sensation in the intermediate zone rose gradually as the central area of complete sensory loss was approached. The gradation, they asserted, was indicative of the presence of fewer and fewer nerve fibers centralward. Hence, the loss in endings and fibers was quantitative, not qualitative, and the facts at variance with Head's concept of separate systems of fibers. Weddell (1962) concluded: "The terms 'protopathic' and 'epicritic' should no longer be used to imply a belief in Head's original hypothesis which Trotter and Davies demolished many years ago. The term 'protopathic' . . . should be used . . . merely to imply that incomplete sensory information is reaching the brain, if it is to remain meaningful."

However, according to Denny-Brown (1965), Trotter and Davies underestimated the importance of the hyperesthesia in the intermediate zone. In reinnervation studies following complete nerve section, Denny-Brown observed not only the hyperesthesia of Head, but also, of a more troublesome nature and more widespread in the denervated area, an intense deep throbbing pain (much like "cold" pain) induced by deep contact, which he called *posttraumatic neuralgia.* Moreover, he found that the size of the area stimulated, hence the element of spatial summation, was important to sensory perception. Acuity of thermal appreciation was very poor for the fingertip alone as compared with the immersed whole terminal phalanx, and was maximal when the entire hand was immersed. The same applied to tactile sensation. On the basis of these findings and the observation that tactile sensation from small cutaneous fields and from very large ones could be recorded from different areas of the cerebral cortex (see Chapter 20), Denny-Brown concluded that two types of cutaneous neural arrangements exist by which the more highly differentiated (more localized, more specific) receptors of each sensory mode have, in the course of phylogenesis, acquired an additional pathway in the neuraxis and an additional representation in the cortex. According to this theory, specialized function (epicritic) evolved from the more general (protopathic), a view originally put forward by Head (1905). The distinction, according to Schiller (1956), is comparable to that made between the pyramidal and extrapyramidal systems.

In current clinical usage, "protopathic" denotes the appreciation of pain and of extremes in heat and cold; "epicritic," the appreciation of minor temperature differences, light touch, nature of the object touched, and distance between two points.

A *receptor unit* may be defined as being made up of a nerve fiber and its specialized terminals. Each nerve fiber bears only one kind of nerve ending (the endings on a fiber "are as alike as the flowers on the same stalk"). The number of receptors belonging to a nerve fiber varies from one or two for the pacinian corpuscle, to thirty or more for fibers bearing other receptors. Touch and pressure, pain, warm, and cold are generally considered the elementary sensations. For each of these forms of sensation, varied peripheral receptors have been identified or postulated as having functional specialization (Iggo, 1968). Whether such specialization actually exists or whether information transmitted to the spinal cord by the receptor is of the crudest kind, it is agreed that as the information ascends in the central nervous system it is coded in the form of impulse patterns until it assumes a form increasingly specific (as contended, for example, by Melzack and Wall, 1965). Through the mediation of central mechanisms, "touch" comes to include other sensations, such as tickle (when touch is lightly applied and brief), warm, cold, wet, rough, and so on. Similarly, "touch" and "pain" will vary in quality with the objects producing them and with the areas stimulated. "Warm," too, has its associated sensations. (Schiller, 1956.)

The following deals with the peripheral mechanisms considered to be concerned in the different classes of sensibility.

Superficial, or exteroceptive, sensibility

Tactile sensibility. The appreciation of touch is tested by touching or stroking the skin lightly with cotton wool, a piece of soft paper, or the like. Tested areas are compared with corresponding or adjacent areas. Diminution in the appreciation of touch is known as *tactile hypesthesia;* its complete loss, *tactile anesthesia.* Exaggerated perception of touch, usually of an unpleasant nature, is loosely spoken of as *tactile hyperesthesia* (discrimination is usually reduced and paresthesia present).

Some of the impulses initiated by touch originate from contact with hairs. Through leverage brought about by a touch stimulus to a hair, the hair transmits oscillations to the nerve plexus surrounding the hair root. Hairy parts of the skin also contain Merkel's disks (or corpuscles), which are a form of touch receptor. Here, deformation of the epidermis is transmitted to the epidermal peg, which acts as the arm of a lever in stimulating the disk. Merkel's disks are also present in hairless areas such as the hands and feet. Instead of hairs, the skin in such areas contains a number of subepidermal receptor organs. Included among them is Meissner's corpuscle. This corpuscle is activated by compression brought about by deformation of the papillary ridges coinciding with the long axis of the corpuscle. The Meissner corpuscle is particularly altered as a consequence of the aging process and under conditions of inactivity. In all likelihood these various end-organs serve only a very localized tactile function—for example, those in the fingertips—while touch elsewhere is mediated mostly by a diffuse plexus, separate from the plexuses receptive to cold, warmth, and painful stimuli. (Cauna, 1956, 1965; Cauna and Ross, 1960; Denny-Brown, 1965.)

Appreciation of vibration. The appreciation of vibration *(pallesthesia)* implicates both superficial sensibility and deep sensibility, that is, somesthesis generally. A vibrating tuning fork is applied to fingertip, ankle, tibia, knee, malleolus, crest of ilium, or spinous process of the vertebral column. Normal subjects are most sensitive to vibrations of 200 to 400 c.p.s./sec. Where only continuous contact is felt, the subject is said to have *pallanesthesia.*

Pallesthesia appears to depend on the rapid adaptation of mechanoreceptors; pacinian corpuscles are the end-organs most likely involved. These corpuscles are situated in the subcutaneous connective tissue, particularly that in the fingertips, palms, toes, and soles; they are also found in the periosteum, in fascial planes, and around joints. Whether the effective stimulus is "tactile" or "vibratory" is, according to Calne and Pallis (1966), "irrelevant." Whereas most receptors code the intensity of a stimulus in an appropriate frequency of impulses, in the case of vibration two distinct parameters must be coded: the amplitude and the frequency of mechanical displacement. The temporal discrimination of amplitude means vibration. Further, the signalling of amplitude probably depends on spatial coding, that is, the number of fibers activated. Recruitment of receptors and a suitable range of thresholds exist in any population of pacinian corpuscles. (Calne and Pallis, 1966; Gray, 1966; Winkelmann, 1960.)

As shown by a vibrogram technique, men have lower thresholds for the appreciation of vibration than women. Men older than forty-five exhibit a general rise in the threshold curve at all frequencies, while in women the effect of age is to increase the thresholds at higher frequencies after age twenty, with little change in the perception of lower frequencies. (Goff and others, 1965.)

Superficial pain sensibility. Superficial pain sensibility is tested by pricking the skin with a pin or by using a pinwheel. Diminution of pain sensibility is known as *hypalgesia;* its absence, *analgesia;* and its exaggeration, *hyperalgesia.*

Free nerve endings emanate from the superficial corial plexus situated in epithelium and are present also in deeper connective tissue, periosteum, joint surfaces, the adventitia of blood vessels, and the viscera. There is no consensus regarding the function(s) of these endings. However, evidence is strong that free nerve endings in the epidermis are activated by pain-provoking stimuli. Sherrington (1906) promulgated this view and, in accordance with his concept of *nociception,* concluded that any stimulus of a noxious character—whether mechanical, chemical, or extremes of heat or cold—constituted an adequate stimulus for pain, and that "the responsive range is supplied by the naked nerve itself." Lim (1966), noting the regularity with which a peptide such as bradykinin (when injected intra-arterially into the skin) will provoke the same manifestations of pain as physical nociception and pointing to the ability of some analgesics to block pain peripherally, suggested that the primary neurons mediating pain possess nerve endings that can transduce chemical stimuli in physiological concentrations. It would seem to follow, according to Lim, that cutaneous (and visceral) receptors for pain (free nerve endings) are primarily chemosensitive.

Pain impulses are carried by small myelinated fibers and by smaller nonmyelinated fibers. Both a "fast" and a "slow" system of pain fibers exist. Brief exposure of the dorsum of the hand to a hot object, such as an electric light bulb, brings out this difference; a first peak of pain is followed shortly by a second ("first and second pain," "double pain," "echo pain"). The pricking of normal skin with a pin to 0.25 mm. depth induces a brief, slightly painful sensation; when the depth pierced is increased to 1.0 mm., a stinging or burning pain of increasing intensity occurs and reaches a maximum in a second or two. In different cutaneous areas these two qualities of pain may be recognized separately or blended (Weddell, Guttmann, and Gutman, 1941). In all likelihood these two qualities of pain can be accounted for by the passage of the impulses over the different sized fibers at differing velocities.

Causalgia may occur within a few weeks after median nerve, brachial plexus, or sciatic nerve injury when the interruption is partial. The pain occurs spontaneously; it is intense, usually of a burning quality (as though the part were on fire), constant, and persistent. The pain is subject to violent exacerbation (for example, by sudden movement) and may be relieved or aggravated either by warming or cooling the part. In some cases the pain is described as crushing, tearing, or "like a toothache." The hand or foot is glossy and moist, and usually pink and warm at first, and moist and cold and blue later on. Causalgia is not entirely a clear-cut entity, for it has many gradations in quality and intensity. Abnormal activity of the internuncial neuronal pool in the posterior horn of the spinal cord may be a significant factor in the occurrence of the pain. (Sunderland, 1968.)

The *hyperesthesia of Head* and its special subtype, *posttraumatic neuralgia* (both already mentioned), are, by contrast, observed under conditions in which nerve interruption is complete. When occurring in the upper limb, the fingers become cold and blue in the third week after denervation, at a time when increased sensitivity to the action of circulating epinephrine appears. The skin becomes dry and undergoes scaling, and anhidrosis may occur. The hyperesthesia (to pinprick, heat, and cold) and the neuralgia are not due to a change in conduction, but, instead, appear to represent a summated mass effect resulting from the absence of a damping, or inhibiting, effect which, under normal conditions, is exercised by specific localized touch receptors on all other neighboring receptors. (Denny-Brown, 1965.)

Anesthesia dolorosa refers to the condition in which hypesthesia and pain coexist in the same area. *Dysesthesia* is a term signifying sensations of tingling, a feeling of warmness or wetness, prickling ("pins and needles" sensation), and formication (as if ants were running over the skin); it is noted in varied disorders involving peripheral nerves. *Paresthesia,* almost a synonym of dysesthesia, is the term sometimes used in referring to sensations of discomfort induced by contact with an object, for instance, garments or bedclothes.

By *acroparesthesia* is meant a state characterized by intense pain in the tips of the fingers, also by burning when the hand is warm. It is a mild kind of causalgia. The pain commonly awakens the patient, and relief is obtained by vigorously exercising the limb. The fingers may be shiny, hot, or red. Motor loss and muscle wasting rarely occur. The condition may be a feature of the *carpal tunnel syndrome,* brought about by constriction of the median nerve through thickening of the transverse carpal ligament secondary to wrist injury or by a space-occupying lesion in the carpal tunnel. Under other conditions involving the upper limb, acroparesthesia may not be limited to the field of the median nerve. Reference is made to stretching, compression, and/or friction of neurovascular structures passing from the neck to the arm. Abnormal ribs, scalenus anterior deformation, and costoclavicular compression are among the numerous conditions that may be responsible. In the lower limb, acroparesthesia may occur in connection with the *tarsal tunnel syndrome.* (Sunderland, 1968.)

Temperature sensibility. Temperature sensibility is tested by having the patient distinguish cold and warm objects. For this purpose two tubes, one containing pieces of ice (40° F.) and the other, heated water (110° F.) may be used. Diminution of this form of sensibility is called *thermohypesthesia,* and its complete absence, *thermoanesthesia.* An increase in thermal appreciation is called *thermohyperesthesia.* Different temperatures are normally recognizable when 5° to 10° or more apart.

Krause's corpuscles, superficially located, have been thought to respond selectively to cold stimuli, and the Ruffini type of ending, more deeply situated, selectively to warmth, but supportive evidence is lacking. The areal nature of cold and warm spots suggests that branching fibers serve as temperature receptors. The earlier view that mechanoreceptors (pacinian corpuscle, hair follicle receptors) may have some temperature receptive capability (Zotterman, 1959) no longer holds, as it has been shown that they are only weakly excited (if at all) by temperature change, thus representing, apparently, a confusing experimental artifact (Iggo, 1969). Both "warm" and "cold" cutaneous spot-like receptive fields have been identified, and the view put forward that each has a very high degree of selective sensitivity to natural stimuli delivered to the surface of the skin. Both temperature and rate of change of temperature of the skin are detected by receptors in the skin, supplanting the older view that the threshold stimulus of cold reception is rapid fall in temperature alone. Myelinated fibers convey temperature-induced impulses from the skin, except for a small proportion from glabrous skin, which is nonmyelinated. (Iggo, 1969.)

Deep, or proprioceptive, sensibility

Deep sensibility refers to the sum of the consciously perceived centripetal impulses streaming into the central nervous system from the proprioceptor end-organs of the muscles, tendons, periosteum, and joints. These impulses provide information regarding the position that a limb has assumed and the degree to which a finger or other member is flexed, extended, abducted, or in some other position *(sense of position)*, also the extent to which a movement is carried out *(sense of movement, kinesthesis)*.

Sense of position is tested by passively moving a member such as a finger or a toe, then halting the movement and asking the subject (with eyes closed from the start of the test) to state its new position. In carrying out the test the examiner lightly grasps the sides of the fingers or toes to minimize cues from pressure. Another maneuver is the finger-to-finger test. The arm to be tested is passively moved and brought to rest with the forefinger extended. The subject is then asked to touch the extended forefinger with the forefinger of the other hand. A quantitative estimate of the error can be obtained by interposing a notebook between the two fingers and marking their positions of contact (for the purpose of obtaining a record); or the integrity of the sense of position may be determined (in the subject with eyes closed) by placing a limb in an unusual position and asking him to duplicate the posture with his other limb. *Sense of movement* may be tested by moving the subject's finger or toe (with the examiner's fingers placed as indicated) and asking him to state the direction in which it was moved. A normal person is aware of quite small angular displacements.

End-organs concerned include muscle spindles (see p. 30). Also responsive are corpuscles of lamellar structure (pacinian, or Vater-pacinian, corpuscles, and Golgi, or Golgi-Mazzoni, corpuscles) situated in the vicinity of joints and in muscle tendons and periosteum (Hromada, 1960; Ralston, Miller, and Kasahara, 1960; Stilwell, 1956b, 1957a, b).

Deep pain, or *pressure pain*, is elicited by applying pressure over nerve trunks, by firmly grasping superficial muscles such as the gastrocnemius, or by pinching tendons. Like superficial pain, it is characterized by two peaks of pain (Weddell and Harpman, 1940).

Pressure-touch, or *light pressure*, is also in the realm of deep sensibility. Between pressure sense and light touch there is no sharp line of demarcation: pressure sensibility gradually replaces tactile sensibility as the deforming force increases in intensity. Deep nerves conduct the impulses, for it has been found that pressure-touch can still be appreciated after sectioning all the superficial nerves to the area in question (Head, 1905). "The touch of a finger [on the skin] is a test of deep sensibility" (Head, 1920). Corpuscles of lamellar structure in many locations are responsive to the pressure. Laterality differences in the perception of pressure-touch (for example, greater sensitivity in the right hand in the left-handed) has been described by some (Semmes and others, 1960; Weinstein and Sersen, 1961) but has not been noted by others (Fennell, Satz, and Wise, 1967).

Combined sensibility (cortical sensory function)

In this category are included various kinds of sensibility of a discriminative nature.

Stereognosis. "Stereognosis" refers to the ability to identify familiar objects by feeling or handling them. A key, pen, or coin can serve as a test object. The perception is in the realms of form, size, and texture. In astereognosis, although objects cannot be identified by handling, the patient is fully able to recognize them by sight. If motor deficit is such that the patient has great difficulty in manipulating objects, the status of stereognosis can, of course, not be judged. Impulses originating from various nerve terminals, including Meissner's corpuscle, contribute to the patterning through which form, size, and texture are perceived.

Disturbances in stereognostic recognition are most commonly encountered in parietal lobe lesions; they have, however, also been noted in interruption of the medial lemniscus, the posterior columns of the cervical spinal cord, the posterior spinal roots, and the brachial plexus (Halpern, 1968). For semantic reasons, use of the term *stereoanesthesia* has been suggested when the responsible lesion is situated peripherally. Here, the inability of the patient to recognize an object by feeling it is due, in part at least, to reduction in tactile sensibility.

Three different gradations of disturbed stereognostic recognition, from high to low levels, have been distinguished: (1) tactile agnosia, in which, in spite of the capacity to recognize form, the ability to identify the handled object is lost (usually due to a cortical lesion); (2) astereognosis with or without associated impairment in the sense of position and with the inability to recognize form (observed in cortical lesions or in interruption of sensory pathways); and (3) disturbed stereognostic recognition as a result of impairment of superficial sensibility. (Halpern, 1968.)

Localization of tactile stimuli. A way to test the capacity to localize tactile stimuli *(topagnosis)* is to place the part to be tested, for example the hand, out of sight of the subject, touch a point on the skin, and have the subject indicate the point on a drawing beside him. After each response the examiner indicates the correct spot on the drawing and thus obtains a record. Duration and intensity of the stimuli influence the result. Another way to test is to touch various areas of skin and ask the subject to indicate where he was touched. In the hand, error in point localization is maximal in the distal direction (Semmes and others, 1960).

Somatic sense of space. Two point discrimination, like passive joint movement, is a function of the somatic sense of space. Appreciation of differing distances between two applied points involves space sense in the plane parallel to the skin. In "depth-sense aesthesiometry," by contrast, space perception in the right-angle plane to the skin is involved.

To test tactile discrimination, two blunt ends of a compass are applied simultaneously to the skin at varied distances apart (2.5 mm. to 100 mm. at 2.5 mm. intervals). The patient is asked whether he feels one or two points. Both duality and spatial cutaneous perception are thus tested. The *two point threshold* (the shortest distance between the two points at which they are still perceived as two contacts) is smaller for tactile than for warm or cold stimuli. Regional differences in responsiveness are pronounced. For the hand, the threshold for two point discrimination is less along the transverse than along the longitudinal axis (Semmes and others, 1960).

The difficulties encountered in testing two point discrimination in the fingertip with the two point compass are obviated with the use of the "depth-sense aesthesiometer." The instrument is, moreover, a more sensitive indicator of neurological lesions than the two point discrimination aesthesiometer, for with the "depth-sense" instrument, abnormalities may be detected where two point discrimination appears normal. (Renfrew, 1969.)

Meissner's corpuscle, together with the papillary ridge (which coincides with the long axis of the corpuscle), constitutes a specialized receptor for tactile discrimination of two separated points. The corpuscles are so assembled in groups in sites such as the fingertip as to constitute an organ remarkably adapted to this role. Both two point discrimination and tactile localization are probably dependent on the geometrical pattern of the Meissner corpuscles. (Cauna, 1958; Cauna and Ross, 1960; Critchley, 1953.)

Discrimination of weights. Objects of equal weight are placed in the two hands to see if the weight appears lighter or heavier in one hand than in the other. Another way of testing is to place objects of different weight such as coins, one after another, in the hand. Both touch and pressure are involved. A cold object feels heavier than a warm object of the same weight (Weber's illusion), perhaps because of the presence of certain mechanoreceptors that possess cold receptive capacity (Ruch and others, 1965).

Figure writing. For the assessment of the spatial aspect of cutaneous sensibility, figure writing on the skin constitutes a simple test. With the subject's eyes closed, the examiner slowly traces numerals from 0 to 9 on larger surfaces of skin, either with his finger or with a blunt object. A record of the responses can easily be made. *Graphesthesia* is thus tested.

Ataxia as a sensory disturbance

Ataxia of peripheral origin ("sensory ataxia") is caused partly by the interruption of fibers concerned in postural sensibility (by way of posterior columns to thalamus) and partly by the interruption of afferent fibers concerned in the (subconscious) regulation of posture and movement that proceed to the cerebellum (by way of posterior columns and spinocerebellar pathways). The importance of the latter route is particularly evident in patients with ataxia in whom no impairment in postural sensibility or in the appreciation of passive movement is detectable. In posterior root–posterior column disease, ataxia usually begins in the lower limbs and is manifested by slight unsteadiness on walking and turning. To lessen the unsteadiness, the patient stands or walks on a wide base. Since the patient can to some extent compensate for the deficit by means of vision, his ataxia becomes more pronounced when he closes his eyes or when he is in the dark. For example, he may fall into the sink when washing his face with his eyes closed.

The ataxia can be brought out in various ways (described elsewhere): by having the subject slide his heel down his opposite tibia from knee to ankle, and noting whether the movement is smooth or wavering; by having the prone subject flex his leg so that it is vertical, and observing whether the leg sways or not; or by having him walk along a line by placing one heel in front of the opposite toe and seeing how much he swerves. Another means of detecting ataxia is *Romberg's test.* In tabes dorsalis, the patient begins to sway when he closes his eyes, the swaying being most pronounced when the test is carried out with the patient's feet close together. In cerebellar ataxia, by contrast, the patient sways whether his eyes are open or shut; in a lesion involving a cerebellar hemisphere, he sways toward that side, and if the vermis is the site of the lesion he will sway backward and forward. If swaying occurs from the hips rather than from the ankles, hysteria is to be suspected.

SOMATIC MOTOR FUNCTION

Jorge Huertas

The term *motility,* which is commonly used in connection with somatic motor function, includes muscle strength, muscle tonus, reflex activity, and the execution of movements. In addition to voluntary movements, the term embraces irritative, autochthonous, and automatic movements.

As an example of *irritation-induced movements,* jacksonian attacks may be cited. These are usually brought about through irritative lesions involving motor neurons of cortex but may also result from irritation of descending motor tracts.

Inspiration is an example of *autochthonous movement.* During the pause following expiration, CO_2 collects in the blood and is carried to the pons, where it directly induces inspiration by heightening the irritability of the respiratory center (Gellhorn, 1953). Acceleration of respiration brought about under pathological conditions may be explained on the basis of a continuous CO_2-induced hyperirritability of the center. Such phenomena are called "autochthonous" because, in contrast to reflexes, the stimulus is applied locally within the central nervous system rather than being transmitted from peripheral parts of the body via nerve pathways. Lowered oxygen tension in the blood has a similar effect on the initiation of inspiration, but here the action is directly on the sino-auricular receptors (Hugelin, Bonvallet, and Dell, 1959), through which impulses reach the respiratory center by way of the ninth and tenth nerves.

Under the term *automatic movements* are included tremor, fibrillary twitchings, myoclonus, chorea, athetosis, muscle spasms, and tics.

Muscle tonus, muscle contraction, reflexes

By *muscle tonus* is meant the elastic tensions and forces inherent in muscle. These qualities make muscle resistant to stretch. This resistance of muscle is generated and graded by the action of the central nervous system through anterior horn cells. These cells do not, however, discharge impulses to muscles in a resting state. During "easy standing," for example, involving gravity alone, no electrical activity can be recorded from muscles, not even from such postural muscles as the erector spinae; however, if the person sways, short bursts occur in the muscles and position is restored (Inman and others, 1952).

The genesis of muscle tonus, which is a function of muscle contraction, has been clarified through identification of the *gamma efferent system* and its effect on the *muscle spindle* (Granit, 1959; Granit, Holmgren, and Merton, 1955).

Tonus is maintained through the activity of reflex arcs and is modulated by supraspinal mechanisms through the mediation of anterior horn cells. Two kinds of muscle fiber come into consideration: the fusiform muscle fiber with its spindle and annulospiral and flower-spray endings, and the striated muscle fiber. Each of the fusiform fibers is continuous at both ends with a striated muscle fiber. Numerous variations exist (Cooper and Daniel, 1963). The sensory components or feedback mechanisms are the annulospiral and

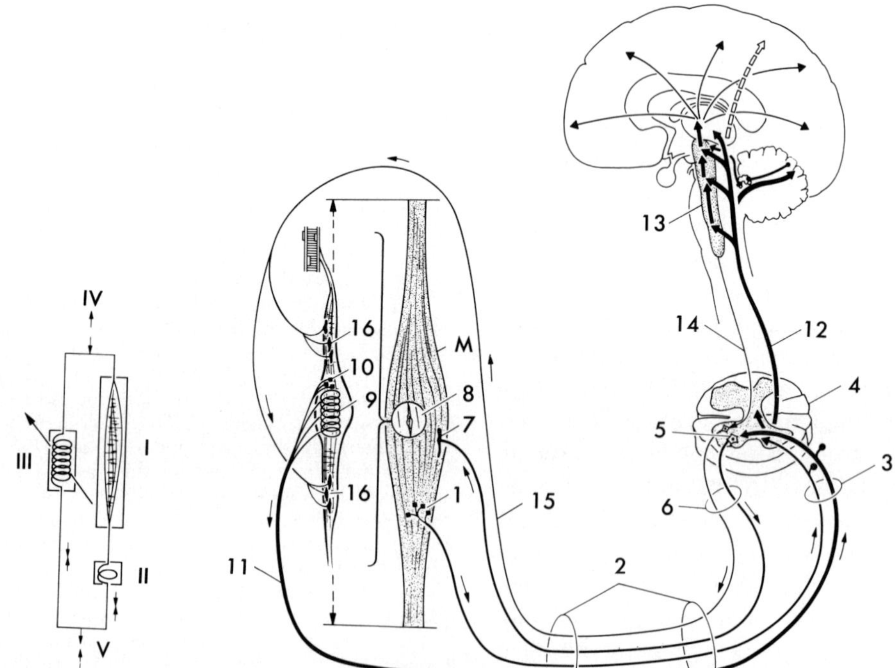

I. Striated muscle
II. Force gauge Golgi tension in series
III. Length gauge connected in parallel to the muscle (muscle spindle)
IV and V. Fixation points (bone)

1. Golgi tendon organ
2. Mixed nerve
3. Dorsal root
4. Spinal cord
5. Anterior horn cell (motor)
6. Ventral root
7. Motor end plate
8. Muscle spindle
9. γ primary ending
10. γ secondary ending
11. γ afferent (AI fiber)
12. Spinal cord (ascending tracts)
13. Reticular formation
14. Reticulospinal tract
15. γ efferent nerve
16. Spindle motor endplates (large or small)

M. Striated muscle

Fig. 2-1. Diagrammatic representation of neuromuscular control system.

flower-spray endings and their centrally coursing fibers (Figs. 2-1 and 24-3). The spindle is attached to and lies parallel with the striated muscle fibers. Through this arrangement, the annulospiral ending measures the length of the striated muscle fibers in the muscle bundle. Thus if the muscle is lengthened, the annulospiral organ will be discharging accordingly; if the muscle is stretched further the number of electrical discharges will become more frequent, yielding information to the central nervous system about the degree of muscle stretching. The spindle thus functions as a sensing element of a proprioceptive servo system. It can be shortened or elongated by neural activity. The length of the spindle in relation to the length of the striated muscle fiber sets the resolution of the sensory endings in the spindle. The spindle together with its annulospiral ending functions in the *dynamic* sphere, and the flower-spray ending serves a *static* function, responding to the force of gravity (Bessou and Laporte, 1966).

Making up another set of receptors are the *Golgi tendon organs* (Figs 2-1 and 24-3). These organs are located at the ends of the striated muscle fibers. Physically they act as though they were connected in series, and they will therefore generate electrical potentials whenever the force of tension at the tendon, either isometric or isotonic, is increased. The Golgi tendon organ is responsive to *load* on a muscle, the spindle to *length* of the muscle. All these endings and their fibers—annulospiral, flower-spray, and Golgi tendon organ—are components of the *gamma* system.

The central nervous system responds to the load borne by the muscle expressed as force, as sensed by the Golgi organ, and it also responds to the relative length of the muscle fibers, sensed by the spindles.

Taking into consideration the principles just mentioned, tonus may be explained as follows. The interaction occurring between the load on the muscle and the muscle spindle generates a response from the spindle as it is being stretched. To obviate a tendency of the central nervous system to keep contracting the muscle further, the cycle is broken by an automatic reset of the muscle spindle carried by the gamma efferent system. The response from the muscle spindle generates in turn a new contraction of the striated muscle (stretch reflex) (9, 11, 5, 7 in Fig. 2-1). A braking mechanism is necessary to interrupt this potentially vicious cycle. This mechanism is situated in suprasegmental structures of the central nervous system. The reticular substance (13), through the gamma efferent system (14, 15), grades the length of the muscle spindle. If the spindle is rather long it will respond to long stretch. If the spindle is shortened or contracted it will respond to less stretch. The main role of the gamma efferent system is to set the length of the spindle in such a way that the contraction generated at the muscle is exactly the amount necessary to cope with the work that is being performed. For instance, the pull of gravity without motion will generate the basic tonus of the muscular system.

Responses by the central nervous system affect muscle activity in two ways: (1) automatic, *static* (equilibratory) and (2) voluntary or semiautomatic, *dynamic* (translatory or expressive).

Static activity is mostly reflex activity and depends upon the gamma feedback mechanisms already described. The expression of this system is the stretch reflex, which controls posture by contracting or relaxing antagonistic groups of muscles concerned in responding to gravitational forces. Static motions are further influenced by vestibular and visual inputs into the central nervous system.

Dynamic (semiautomatic and voluntary) *responses* operate upon the physiological "anlage" laid out by the static system. Purely voluntary movement appears to be carried out largely through the mediation of the pyramidal system; in the performance of semiautomatic movements such as walking, the extrapyramidal system appears to play a role in the modulation of the motions. The two systems involved are the following.

(a) Fibers of the pyramidal tract (or alpha route) terminate on the large motoneurons *(alpha motoneurons)* in the anterior horn. Axons of the motoneurons pass through the anterior spinal root and end on striated muscle fibers as end-plates. (b) Fibers of *COEPS* (p. 318) descend, through multisynaptic pathways, to the upper brainstem, from which the (medial) reticulospinal and related tracts (the gamma route) descend to reach small motoneurons *(gamma motoneurons)* in the anterior horn. Axons of these motoneurons also pass through the anterior root but they end on the fusiform muscle fiber at both poles of the spindle.

Pyramidal tract activation appears to facilitate the excitability of alpha motoneurons (Jinnai and others, 1964a, b). On interruption of the pyramidal tract anywhere along its course or on interruption of the afferent limb of the stretch reflex arc, the muscle becomes flaccid or atonic and offers little resistance to stretch. The muscle thus exhibits *paresis.* Not only is there a reduction in motor power but also a slowing in the tempo of muscle contraction. Muscle paralysis does not occur under these conditions, since a continuity between spinal cord and muscle remains. With the passage of time following pyramidal tract interruption, the activity of gamma motor neurons comes to predominate and *muscle spasticity* develops. Concurrently, activity of the stretch reflex becomes increased. For example, when the patellar tendon is tapped, the quadriceps femoris contracts more vigorously than normal; the quadriceps femoris reflex ("patellar reflex," "knee jerk") is thus said to be increased. Clinically, the term "increased *deep* reflex" is commonly used.

On the other hand, the final neuron in the chain for the innervation of the muscles is situated in the anterior horn of the spinal cord. Each individual muscle receives its nerve supply from a circumscribed group of alpha neurons. Near its termination, the axon of each of these neurons undergoes repeated division, so that any given cell innervates from three to one hundred and fifty individual muscle fibers. The end-organ is the motor end-plate (Fig. 24-3). The alpha motoneuron and the muscle fibers it innervates are called the *motor unit.* Such units overlap to some extent in the sense that muscle fibers supplied by one unit may also be supplied by another (Feindel, 1954). Total destruction of anterior horn cells of sufficient scope causes *paralysis* of the muscles they supply. Associated deep reflexes are lost.

The localizing value of tonus and reflexes may be summarized as follows:

1. *Lesions of the posterior root system*—hypotonia and hyporeflexia, or atonia and areflexia, together with sensory deficits.
2. *Lesions of the anterior root system*—hypotonia and hyporeflexia, or atonia and areflexia, together with motor deficits (sensory alterations are lacking).
3. *Lesions of suprasegmental systems*—the responses vary in accordance with the function of the system, the extent to which it is involved, and the nature of the system (inhibitory or facilitatory). Interruption of the pyramidal tract system, which, when activated, has a facilitating action on alpha motoneurons, leads initially to muscle paresis. Subsequently, owing to the action of gamma motoneurons, muscle spasticity occurs. Lesions of the extrapyramidal system produce muscle rigidity, also involuntary movements while the patient is at rest and awake: parkinsonism, athetosis, chorea, and so on. Lesions of the cerebellar system produce alterations in the range of movements when the patient moves: adiadochokinesis, ataxia, past-pointing.

Muscle fibrillation, fasciculation, and atrophy

In diseases involving certain motor units, muscles exhibit "spontaneous" contractions. These are known as *fibrillation* and *fasciculation.*

Fibrillation, occurring during degeneration of the motoneuron in the region of its cell body, cannot be observed through the skin. Electrophysiological studies reveal, however, that the disturbances are irregular and asynchronous and produce no shortening of the muscle. Only single muscle cells or muscle fibers are involved. The activity reaches a peak in about 2 to 3 weeks and ceases either when innervation is reestablished or when sufficient muscle fiber degeneration has occurred. The fibrillation is enhanced by neostigmine (Prostigmin). The fact that the fibers fire in the absence of nerve stimulation suggests that the fibrillation is an expression of denervation sensitivity to acetylcholine, which presumably is the stimulus.

Fasciculation, by contrast, is visible through the skin or mucosa. It represents a "spontaneous" discharge of motor units. The discharge time is longer than for fibrillation, owing to the somewhat asynchronous firing of the individual muscle fibers, and amplitude is much greater. Triggering of fasciculation probably originates in cell bodies in the anterior horn. However, there are cases in which procaine block fails to halt fasciculation, indicating peripheral origin. Possibly the end-plate of a fiber is involved, with antidromic conduction to the branching point of the motor axon and from there to all fibers of a motor unit ("axon reflex") (Woodbury and Ruch, 1961).

A decrease in muscle volume is referred to as *muscle atrophy.* Following section of a motor nerve, subsarcolemmal nuclei of extrafusal muscle fibers increase in size and number, starting from the ninth to sixteenth day, and this activation persists for some weeks or months. However, the earliest and most characteristic change is a loss of sarcoplasm and a reduction in muscle fiber caliber. By 60 days, the average cross-sectional area of the fiber has decreased 70 percent, and by 120 days, another 10 percent (Sunderland, 1968). Cross-striations persist until the muscle cells become quite small, that is, well after a year following denervation. Degenerative changes in muscle fibers apparently do not succeed the atrophy, at least not in 1 to 3 years after nerve severance. Motor end-plates undergo little if any recognizable change. Not long after nerve section, connective tissue in muscle bundles undergoes an increase. Similar though far less severe atrophic changes occur in intrafusal muscle fibers. All this constitutes a progressive reaction known as *denervation atrophy.* In the muscle atrophy following limb immobilization or occurring as a feature of the spastic syndrome *(disuse atrophy),* the muscle changes seldom advance to so extreme a degree. In spinal cord transection much the same muscle changes are noted as after nerve section, however, with these differences: the initial nuclear proliferation does not occur, and there is a smaller decrease in total nitrogen content in the muscle. (Adams, Denny-Brown, and Pearson, 1962; Bowden and Gutmann, 1944; Gutmann, 1962; Pellegrino and Franzini, 1963; Sunderland, 1968.)

Myokymia. The term *myokymia* was first used to describe a rare syndrome characterized by continuous, slow, undulating, rippling muscular contractions. In this form of the disorder, strips of muscles contract independently of the others, each contraction lasting 2 to 15 seconds, giving an overall undulating effect that can be likened to the "movement of an army of parallel earthworms." The contractions are slower than the fasciculations observed in anterior horn disease. Calf, thigh, and arm muscles may thus be affected. There may also be associated muscle cramps and painful muscle spasms. No weakness or wasting of muscles occurs. Other forms based on differences in electromyographic findings have been described. Site(s) of the basic disturbance appears unknown. However, facial myokymia has been found associated with pontile tumor and other central pathological processes (p. 227). (Gardner-Medwin and Walton, 1969.)

VISCERAL MOTOR FUNCTION

Autonomic nervous system

An overall view of the autonomic system—its sympathetic and parasympathetic components—is provided in Fig. 2-2. The cell bodies of *sympathetic* preganglionic neurons (in man) are situated in the intermediolateral horns of spinal segments C7 through L2 or L3 (Gagel, 1928). Classically, the preganglionic fibers arising from these sources traverse the anterior roots, the mixed spinal nerves, the white rami communicantes, and synapse in the chain of sympathetic ganglia (Fig. 2-3), from

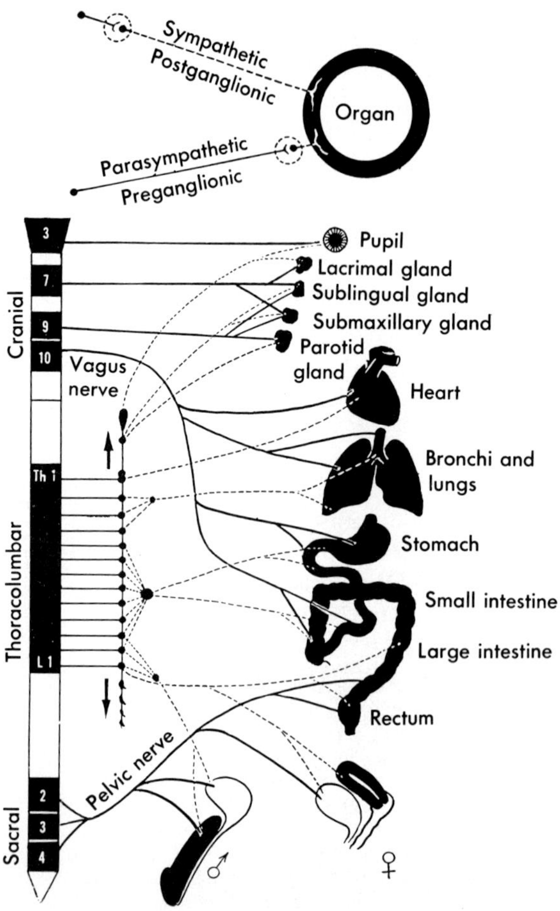

Fig. 2-2. Diagram of the autonomic nervous system. The parasympathetic system has cranial and sacral subdivisions. The sympathetic system arises largely from segments Th1 through L1. The respective lengths of the preganglionic and postganglionic fibers are indicated in the upper diagram. Some of the preganglionic sympathetic fibers synapse in the ganglionated chain, others in the prevertebral ganglia. (Modified from Abbie, 1950.)

which postganglionic fibers proceed via the gray rami communicantes to the peripheral nerve trunks, in which they course distally. However, some preganglionic fibers—from spinal segments C8, Th1, and Th2 (for the upper limb) and from Th12 through L3 (for the lower limb)—terminate in "intermediate" ganglia situated in the corresponding spinal roots, and, without traversing the ganglionic chain, the postganglionic fibers proceed directly via the segmental nerves to the periphery (Alexander and others, 1949; Kuntz and Alexander, 1950; Leivy, Tovi, and Krueger, 1968). Yet another system of sympathetic preganglionic fibers extends directly to prevertebral ganglia, whence postganglionic fibers extend to viscera. They probably are accompanied by postganglionic fibers that have originated from accessory ganglia situated in the sympathetic roots (Kuntz and Alexander, 1950).

Postganglionic sympathetic fibers, on coursing distally in somatic nerve trunks, take one of two routes. Those fibers extending to sweat glands and to the arrectores pilorum muscles run their course as components of the peripheral nerves. By contrast, vasomotor fibers leave the nerve trunks or nerves at intervals and extend to the larger arteries, along which they run and eventually reach the vessels of the skin and subcutaneous tissue over an area similar to that assigned to the nerve as its territory of sensory distribution (Woollard and Phillips, 1932).

The *parasympathetic* division of the autonomic system supplies certain structures of the head and pelvis. The *cranial* part arises from nuclei in the brainstem and has its synaptic stations in the ciliary, sphenopalatine, submaxillary, and otic ganglia. The *sacral* part takes origin from segments S2, S3, and S4 and has its synaptic stations in or near the organ or structure supplied. The pelvic nerve joins sympathetic fibers in the inferior hypogastric plexus to reach the pelvic organs. Vasodilator fibers arise from the sacral segments (White, Smithwick, and Simeone, 1952).

Through its numerous central nervous mechanisms the autonomic system is concerned in integrated reactions in response to changes in the internal and the external milieu. However, in some regions the neural pathways serving these functions run in more or less separate contingents, allowing localization of lesions when one contingent, or a combination of contingents, is interrupted. This subject is dis-

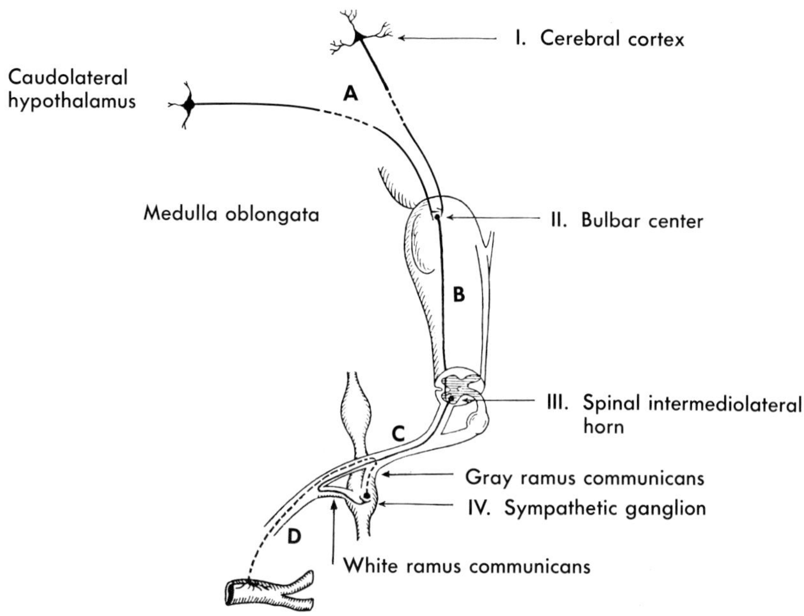

Fig. 2-3. Some of the descending fiber systems concerned in vasomotility. **A,** Cerebrobulbar and hypothalamobulbar pathways; **B,** bulbospinal pathways; **C,** spinosympathetic (preganglionic) pathway; **D,** sympathicovascular (postganglionic) pathway.

cussed in Chapter 4, and to some extent in the following paragraphs.

Vasomotor function

Vasomotor control systems are distributed throughout much of the central nervous system.

In the cerebrum, autonomic pathways originate largely from the cortex and the hypothalamus (Fig. 2-3). Vasomotor neural mechanisms have been detected in the motor (area 4) and premotor cortex (areas 6, 8, and 44), prefrontal cortex, insula, orbitofrontal cortex, and temporal cortex, on the basis of electrical stimulation studies (Peiss, 1962). Vasomotor fibers, particularly from areas 4 and 6, course downward in close relation to the pyramidal and extrapyramidal pathways (Spiegel and Hunsicker, 1936; Wall and Davis, 1951). Fibers from other areas, particularly the more rostral parts of the convexity of the frontal cortex, extend to the hypothalamus (Nauta, 1964; Ward and McCulloch, 1947), where both vasodepressor (Folkow, Johansson, and Öberg, 1959) and vasoactivator areas (Magoun, 1940) are located. Another input into the hypothalamus, reaching the lateral preoptic and lateral hypothalamic areas, is from the orbitofrontal cortex, with a third coming from the septal area. Fibers originating in the caudolateral part of the hypothalamus extend into the tegmentum of the midbrain, some by way of the prerubral field (field H of Forel). The descending vasomotor system contains a *vasodilator pathway* that originates in the lateral part of the hypothalamus; it is functionally discrete with respect to the vasomotor area in the medulla oblongata, and extends downward in the lateral column of the spinal cord, in the region of the corticospinal tract. On electrical stimulation of this pathway vasodilatation occurs in skeletal muscle, and vasoconstriction in the skin; capillary blood flow in muscle is, however, not altered (Lindgren and others, 1956; Uvnäs, 1960a).

Pressor activity and depressor activity have also been recorded from different areas in the midbrain. Moreover, vasoconstrictor and vasodepressor areas have been located in the reticular formation of the medulla oblongata at the level of the olive (McQueen, Browne, and Walker, 1954; Wang and Ranson, 1939). Vasodilation mediated through bulbar mechanisms is brought about by inhibition of sympathetic vasoconstrictor outflow, not by the action of a medullary "vasodilator center" (Uvnäs, 1960b).

The influence of higher levels of the central nervous system on vasomotility is generally considered to be brought about through a modification of the activity of the medullary vasomotor center. However, it is likely that descending pathways, originating from all brainstem levels, bypass the medullary integrative cells through the mediation of collaterals. Bypass systems as well as systems for the medullary center would proceed downward, spread diffusely in the spinal cord, and terminate about preganglionic sympathetic cells in the intermediolateral horns. Situated here are two sets of cells, which through their postganglionic fibers are both vasoconstrictors (norepinephrine-responsive) and vasodilators (acetylcholine-responsive). The fibers proceeding to the skin of the hands and feet are vasoconstrictors, those reaching the skin of the forearm have both vasoconstrictor and vasodilator function (Blair, Glover, and Roddie, 1960; Doupe, Cullen, and Macaulay, 1943).

As a working model for the integration of vasomotor outflow, it has been proposed that all vasomotor levels in the central nervous system are reached by ascending fiber systems from the spinal preganglionic cell bodies upward to the cerebral cortex. A central internuncial system in the reticular core (excitatory and inhibitory) would be activated by the inflow. The efferent vasomotor outflow from each area within the central internuncial system would be the result of the interaction of afferent input, specific excitability, cell population, and the excitatory and inhibitory interconnections between each level. (Peiss, 1962.)

Clinically, vasomotor skin disturbances have been noted in the presence of lesions at various levels of the central nervous system. In cortical lesions such disturbances are uncommon, but they have been detected particularly in premotor and parietal lesions. In hemiplegia of internal capsular origin, pallor from vasoconstrictor spasm may occur in the contralateral side of the body as well as in the face and ear during the first few hours after the ictus and may persist for the next few days. Later on, the temperature of these parts may be increased by 0.5° to 3.5° F. Circulatory disturbances observed in hemiplegic limbs long after the ictus are almost certainly caused by a vasomotor disorder, not by muscular inactivity (Kennard, 1935). Reflex vasodilatation occurring in parkinsonism appears to be mediated by an arc reaching to a level well above the brainstem (Appenzeller and Schneiden, 1963).

In lesions involving the tegmentum of the pons or the reticular formation of the medulla oblongata the vasomotor disturbances vary; in some cases pallor and coldness are noted on the side contralateral to the lesion, with the skin temperature falling 2° to 5° F., and in other cases vasoconstrictor phenomena, without alteration in skin temperature, occur on the ipsilateral side.

Lesions at the spinal level give rise more frequently to a disturbance in vasomotor function than lesions situated elsewhere in the central nervous system. Somatotopic representation exists. The spinal vasomotor center for the face and ear is situated in the intermediolateral cell column in segments Th3 and Th4, the center for the upper limb in segments Th2-Th6, with fibers issuing in part from anterior root C8 (Coldwater and others, 1957), and the center for the lower limb in segments Th10 through L1 (Fulton, 1938; Smithwick, 1937; Telford, 1938). Because of this representation, an injury of the midthoracic cord, for example, may give rise to cyanosis of the upper limbs without altering sensibility or motor function in those limbs. In general, lesions involving gray matter of the spinal cord in which vasomotor cells are situated (the intermediolateral horns) give rise to vasomotor paralysis. This occurs, however, only when the pathological process is acute. Cutaneous cyanosis and coldness usually prevail from the outset, but they may be preceded by redness and increased warmth. The skin temperature may fall to as low as 50° F. The most dramatic vasomotor disturbances occur in traumatic spinal cord transection. With transection in the region of C7–Th1, vasoconstriction at the periphery of the upper limb may be so powerful that blood flow in the fingers almost stops; under these conditions, circulation through the forearm muscles is greatly increased, and the neck and face become intensely flushed. In transection at levels above Th5 or Th6 much the same change occurs in the fingers and, in addition, both systolic and diastolic pressure undergo great increase. In transection at any spinal level vasoconstriction occurs in the toes. All these disturbances are reflexly enhanced by distension of the abdominal viscera, particularly the urinary bladder. (Peiss, 1962.)

Vasomotor reflexes are a counterpart of motor reflexes. Of these, *reflex erythema* (also called *dermographia dolorosa*) is of considerable clinical importance, as is the more rarely occurring *reflex ischemia*, caused by vasoconstriction. Reflex erythema occurs as three successive reactions when the skin of any region of the body, but especially the thorax, is scratched or pricked with a pin. These three reactions are: (1) a tongue-like or flame-like reddening of the area irritated, (2) a spreading of the flush to the adjacent skin *(flare)*, and (3) the development of a white or pale pink elevation of the skin (wheal). This triple response is caused by histamine or a histamine-like substance liberated by the tissues as a result of the stimulus (Lewis, 1927). In a lesion involving sympathetic fibers, whether in the spinal cord or peripheral nervous system, the flare is more pronounced and of longer duration the more recent the lesion. Following interruption of a peripheral nerve, an exaggerated flare may be induced in the innervated area of skin up to about the sixth day after the injury. The flare component gradually fades and then disappears in about 14 to 21 days (Doupe, 1943). If there is cutaneous anesthesia, and if after the twenty-first day a flare can still be produced, the lesion must lie in the spinal cord or brain (Tolnick and Beck, 1945).

Reflex erythema is to be distinguished from *dermographia peripherica*, a cutaneous phenomenon consisting in the development of a narrow white, rose-red, or red stripe when the skin is stroked with a blunt object. Soon the stripe widens. If the reaction is more intense and involves a wider area than in the average individual, and if it lasts more than 2 or 3 minutes, the reaction is to be regarded as abnormal, particularly if a urticaria-like elevation develops. This form of dermographia, aroused through an axon reflex having limbs situated entirely at the periphery, is evidence of "autonomic imbalance," and frequently is observed in association with clammy, moist hands, increased mechanical nerve irritability, tremor of the outstretched fingers, and hyperirritable reflexes. In short, abnormal dermographia provides a clue as to the autonomic constitution of the subject.

Vasomotility also suffers in *peripheral nerve injury*. When a nerve is completely divided, vasodilatation occurs immediately in the denervated region owing to elimination of vasoconstrictor tone, and the skin is pink and warm. After about 3 weeks, vasoconstriction tends to develop in the anesthetic area; the skin becomes pale, and the part affected is abnormally susceptible to cold. In partial nerve division, vasomotor disturbances are more prolonged, especially when causalgia exists (Richards, 1954).

Sudomotor function

Sudomotor postganglionic sympathetic fibers, in contrast to vasomotor and pilomotor fibers, are cholinergic. Sweating is inhibited by atropine and other anticholinergic drugs and is stimulated by acetylcholine. Epinephrine has no effect on the sweat glands. From these observations it can be concluded that although sweating may accompany peripheral vasodilation, the two occur independently of each other.

Sudomotor fibers have their cell bodies in the intermediolateral horns of the spinal cord at levels indicated in the previous text.

Sudomotor function appears to be represented in area 6: ablation of this part of the cortex (in monkeys and chimpanzees) results in hypohidrosis on the opposite side of the body (Kennard, 1935); moreover, if the lesion produces paresis of the arm or the leg, hypohidrosis may be limited to the paretic limb (Kennard, 1949). In persons affected with unilateral frontal lobe lesions, hyperhidrosis rather than hypohidrosis occasionally occurs on the contralateral side of the body (Darrow, 1936). Where lesions are widespread the pattern of disturbed sweating is of course highly variable. Multiple sclerosis is an apt example; loss or reduction of sweating may be noted over the lower limbs, the lower half of the body, or even the entire body (Noronha, Vas, and Aziz, 1968).

In lesions involving the prerubral field, anhidrosis of the ipsilateral part of the body over a rather wide area has been noted (p. 102). Where lesions involve the lateral tegmentum of the pons or the ventrolateral part of the reticular formation of the medulla oblongata, hypohidrosis or anhidrosis is also commonly observed.

This was evident in a series of cases reported by List and Peet (1939). Unilateral or predominantly unilateral tumor involving the tegmentum and pars basilaris at upper and middle pontile levels was manifested by bilateral symmetrical hypohidrosis or anhidrosis with sparing of the face and neck. Lesions of vascular origin occupying the lateral tegmentum resulted either in minimal hypohidrosis in the contralateral leg and side of the trunk or in ipsilateral hypohidrosis, most striking in the face. Where the dorsolateral part of tegmentum of the lower pons and the corresponding part of the reticular formation of the upper medulla oblongata were damaged, ipsilateral hemihypohidrosis was noted; the disturbance was most pronounced in the face and neck, and least in the lower limbs. When the dorsolateral, retro-olivary area of the medulla oblongata was the site of vascular occlusion, ipsilateral hemihypohidrosis was noted; face, neck, and upper limb were most affected. Hyperhidrosis occurring contralaterally in some of these cases was considered a compensatory phenomenon. In one case, *hemihypohidrosis cruciata* was observed (hypohidrosis of the leg ipsilaterally and arm and trunk contralaterally).

From these data, List and Peet (1939) suggest that sudomotor fibers for the body and limbs decussate in the upper half of the pons, and that bilateral hypohidrosis occurring with lesions at this level may be attributable to a unilateral lesion that interrupts the decussating fibers of both sides. As to the lower pons and the medulla oblongata, the findings suggested that sudomotor fibers course chiefly ipsilaterally. The patterning of the hypohidrosis also suggested that fibers for the innervation of the facial sweat glands run in a separate path in the upper pons, and that at the medullary level they are situated ipsilaterally in the lateral part of the reticular formation, with the fibers for the ipsilateral lower limb situated more medially. Sudomotor fibers were assumed to be carried largely in reticulospinal pathways.

In regard to the *spinal cord,* Guttmann (1954) is of the opinion that two major sudomotor centers exist, one cervicothoracic, the other lumbosacral. Destruction of a sufficient proportion of the intermediolateral column or, more commonly, interruption of the respective fibers extending downward in the cord to reach it, results either in *hypohidrosis* or *anhidrosis* in the area of skin concerned. Sudomotor fibers descending in the cervical cord appear to have a somatotopic arrangement; the fibers for the upper limb lie in the most medial part of the lateral and adjacent anterior columns, while those for the lower limb are more laterally situated, along the ventral border of the lateral pyramidal tract (Foerster, 1936a).

Traumatic transection of the cervical cord gives rise to varying alterations in sweating capacity. With body temperature in the normal range, complete transection results in anhidrosis of much of the body surface and of the neck and face and, in hemisection of the cord, either in hypohidrosis or anhidrosis on the corresponding side, even for months after the injury (Guttmann, Silver, and Wyndham, 1958; List and Peet, 1939). When, however, in acute cervical cord injury the body temperature reaches a high peak, the patient may suddenly break into a sweat, including the region beneath the level of transection, with the result that the temperature falls to a normal or subnormal level. Furthermore, in long-standing cases in which chills and fever occur as the result of a complicating infection, the skin in the region below the level of the transection remains dry and pallid during a chill, but when the fever reaches a high level, sweating and vasodilation occur over the entire body (Foerster, 1935). While these responses have been taken as evidence that the spinal cord has thermoregulatory function (Seckendorf and Randall, 1958), it has also been contended that the sweating is a nonthermoregulatory manifestation of the spinal mass reflex (Head and Riddoch, 1917). These views have been brought into harmony by List and Pimenta (1944), who showed that thermoregulatory sweating and spinal sweating are separate phenomena that may occur simultaneously.

In occasional cases, spinal cord injury may result in *hyperhidrosis.* For example, injury at spinal level Th10 may, in early stages, result in distressing perspiration over the lower abdomen, groin, and legs, and it persists indefinitely. The cause is not apparent. (Leivy, Tovi, and Krueger, 1968.)

In *peripheral nerve injury,* anhidrosis is a sign of loss of nerve function. Areas of anhidrosis are slightly larger than areas of sensory deficit. Sweating occurring in the presence of total paralysis and anesthesia may be taken as dependable evidence of partial integrity of the nerve and/or as a sign of impending restoration of motor and sensory functions.

For testing sudomotor function, sweating may be induced by external heat, drinking of hot fluids, taking acetylsalicylic acid, or injecting pilocarpine subcutaneously. Sweating under such conditions can be demonstrated by painting the area of skin to be investigated with a 1.5% alcoholic solution of iodine, allowing it to dry, then sprinkling the area with starch. The area in which sweating occurs becomes deep blue. Another substance frequently used is chinizarin 2-6 disulfonate, a powder sprinkled on the skin after the affected part has been warmed. Areas of sweating take on a deep red–purple hue. (Guttmann, 1940.) Use may also be made of a sodium electrode for the measurement of electrical changes induced by varying electrolyte content of the skin surface (Goldbloom and Sekelj, 1963).

Pilomotor function

The arrectores pilorum are solely under the control of the sympathetic nervous system. The postganglionic fibers are adrenergic. Contraction of the arrectores brings the papillae into prominence ("goose flesh").

Neural mechanisms concerned in pilomotor function are situated in the cerebrum, brainstem, spinal cord, and ganglia of the sympathetic chain. Following ablation of area 6 of the cortex of one side (in the monkey), persistent piloerection has been found to occur bilaterally (Kennard, 1949). In man, piloerection can sometimes be observed in lesions involving the intermediolateral horns of spinal segments C8–L1. For example, piloerection may be evident in the upper limb in lesions of the upper thoracic cord. If not occurring spontaneously, piloerection may be induced reflexly (by cooling, scratching, or pinching the skin of the neck) or through direct stimulation (by stroking the cutaneous area involved with a blunt object). However, the response is so variable in its occurrence, intensity, and manner of development that it has little localizing value. Loss of the pilomotor reflex may be detectable in restricted areas. For example, in upper thoracic cord lesions the pilomotor reflex may be lost only in a limited cutaneous area of the upper limbs.

In severance of a peripheral nerve a pilomotor reaction can still be produced by electrical stimulation of the affected area, but only during the first few days after the severance, while the nerve endings are still intact. Thereafter the pilomotor reflex is lost.

Trophic function

Profound alterations of a trophic (nutritional) nature occur in skin, fingernails, digits, muscles, and bones in association with lesions of the central or the peripheral nervous system, and also, in some instances, under conditions in which no lesions of the nervous system are demonstrable.

In *multiple sclerosis,* trophic changes may, in some cases, take the form of abnormal brittleness of the fingernails, loss of hair, epidermolysis, effusion within joint capsules, and, occasionally, in final stages, decubital ulceration.

Poliomyelitis may, in the acute stage, be characterized by mottling or flushing of the skin in the affected parts, while in later stages the skin tends to be cool, either livid or mottled, strikingly thin and smooth, and often unusually hairy. Muscle atrophy occurs, and the bones of the affected parts become demonstrably rarefied. In children, bone growth lags, and in some cases the bones of the affected limbs become smaller and so rarefied that the slightest accident may cause a fracture.

Syringomyelia has far more serious consequences. When occurring at the cervicothoracic level, as usually it does, the back of the hand may be cold, glossy, livid, and edematous. The skin generally in the affected parts is abnormally dry, scaly, fissured ("toad skin"); layers of the epidermis separate. Fingernails fall out, cutaneous hair disappears, and the palmar aponeurosis may undergo contraction such that Dupuytren's contracture ensues. The soft tissues of the hand may proliferate (chiromegaly). Whether the syrinx is in the cervicothoracic or the lumbosacral region, the trophic sores that develop may progress to leprosy-like mutilations, for example, partial or complete loss of fingers or toes. Osteoarthropathies are common. Osteosclerotic changes occur in some cases, osteoporosis in others.

Another disease characterized by the occurrence of trophic changes is *tabes dorsalis.* The compact layer of bone is thinned, and the haversian canals become enlarged. Brittleness of bones may be such that spontaneous (painless) fractures occur; fracture of the neck of the femur can result from stepping off the curb into the street and fracture of the radius from striking an arm against the back of a chair. In the repair process, callus formation may be deficient or excessive. Further, there may be complete destruction of the head of the femur or humerus. Arthropathies develop; secretory disturbances occur in synovia (giving rise to a globular joint "comparable to the swollen abdomen of a dropsical child") and articular cartilagenous tissue proliferates. Perforating ulcer, most commonly involving the sole of the foot, is also characteristic of tabes dorsalis.

Lesions of the *peripheral nervous system* may result in profound trophic disturbances. Advanced lysis of bones and joints of the feet may occur, for example, in radiculitis involving the cauda equina (Fig. 7-1). In peripheral nerve injury, a "warm phase" lasts about 3 weeks (the skin is dry, warm, and flushed) and, during this time, the disturbances are not responsive to cooling. This phase is succeeded by a "cold phase," at which time trophic disturbances become evident. Most affected are the digits. In some incomplete lesions of the median and sciatic nerves with causalgia, the warm phase may persist and be accompanied by sweating. In causalgia, the alterations observed in skin and bone are more striking than in nonpainful nerve injury of equivalent degree (Richards, 1946; Sunderland, 1968), but they may occasionally be minimal (Haymaker and Woodhall, 1953).

Trophic alterations may even occur in "functional" conditions: digital atrophy, nail changes, and indolent ulceration can develop in *hysterical palsy,* with complete cure achieved by psychotherapy alone (Hurst, 1920).

Interruption of the motoneuron, interruption of sympathetic fibers resulting in circulatory disturbances, and interruption of sensory fibers have been invoked as responsible for trophic changes. Experimental studies in animals have allowed only inferences as to trophic function in man to be drawn, as the studies were necessarily carried out under conditions not duplicating disease states in man.

Muscle. Following cord section (in dogs), a profound metabolic change occurs in the muscles situated distal to the level of the transection. Normally, muscle does not give up creatine (instead, it gives up creatinine), but in the spinal cord-transected dog, creatine "bleeds" from the muscle; this occurs either immediately or after a day or two, and may last 2 or 3 weeks. A disturbance in vascular permeability associated with the metabolic disturbance was assumed, but the mechanism(s) through which this was brought about was not investigated (Anderson and others, 1962). There has been the question as to whether the axon supplies muscle with substances in addition to the acetylcholine (ACh) released at synaptic endings. Axoplasmic migration distalward has been established with the use of ^{3}H-labeled amino acids (Droz and LeBlond, 1963; Singer and Salpeter, 1966). In an experiment carried out by Wheeler, Boyarsky, and Brooks (1966), glutamic acid (but none of the other amino acids tested) was found to be released at a greater rate during electrical stimulation than during the resting state, from which it was considered probable that an active system for specifically transmitting this amino acid across the membrane exists. Whether the glutamic acid crossed the myoneural junction was not studied in this experiment. That such transport can occur was, however, ascertained in another experiment. ^{32}P-inorganic phosphate or ^{14}C-amino acids applied to the hypoglossal nucleus (in rabbits) proceeded down the hypoglossal nerve at a rate of 5.5 mm. per day, and by the eighth day reached the tongue musculature, in which it was localized radioautographically. No radioactivity could be found in the tongue if the nerve had been sectioned. (Korr, Wilkinson, and Chornock, 1967.) Thus, as Guth (1968) comments, evidence is beginning to accumulate that substances other than ACh are transported across the myoneural junction.

Bones, joints, periarticular surfaces, and other tissues. Both myelinated (somatic sensory) and nonmyelinated (postganglionic autonomic and somatic sensory) fibers, running partly along with vessels, extend to the vertebrae, supplying periosteum and endosteum; among the terminations found are endings on vessel walls, free endings in the periosteum and endosteum, encapsulated end-organs in periosteum, and Ruffini endings in diarthrodial joints. (Stilwell, 1956a.) Nonmyelinated fibers have also been observed in the periosteum, endosteum, and haversian and Volkmann canal systems of long bones, and terminals resembling pacinian corpuscles, in the lining of the medullary canal (Budy, 1968; Urist, 1967). In classic studies, de Castro (1925, 1930) traced "emigrant fibers" which, after becoming detached from the vascular adventitia, crossed the bone marrow spaces without establishing new connections with vessels, and ending near osteoblasts. His conclusion was that nerves exert a trophic influence on bone formation—an opinion not tenable on morphological evidence alone. Thus far there has been no evidence that nerves have any influence in inducing stem cells (osteoprogenitor cells) to differentiate into osteoclasts instead of osteoblasts. A crucial experiment similar to that carried out with respect to muscle has, however, not been carried out.

Bone resorption occurring in nonneurological states (for example, following prolonged bed rest) is generally thought to represent a "disuse" form of atrophy, in which deficit in mechanical stress is the initiating factor and circulatory disturbances a subsequent pathogenic factor. Altered circulation in relation to muscle inactivity brought about by severing the Achilles tendon has been found instrumental in inducing trophic changes, as shown in an experiment in rabbits by Geiser and Trueta (1958), in which a micro-opaque material was injected to show up the vascular tree. Bone structure deteriorated very rapidly, and within 6 weeks there was grossly visible reduction in bone mass. Bone resorption was accompanied by great enlargement of blood vessels in the vicinity. (Urist, 1967.) Presumably, reduction in rate of blood flow through the bone tipped the scales toward initiation of the mechanism of bone resorption. Bone cell mechanisms are presumed to be influenced by way of diffusion pathways. Oxygen tension is of importance: in bone cultures, osteoprogenitor cells differentiate into osteoclasts (with clastic function) instead of osteoblasts if the oxygen concentration in the culture is increased from 35 percent to 95 percent (Urist, 1967).

Naturally the question raised by these results is whether interruption of sympathetic nerve supply may so alter blood flow that trophic disturbances result. Tower (1935) could find no significant changes in muscle in sympathectomized limbs. However, according to the evidence accumulated by Sunderland (1968), the matter is not settled. Poor peripheral circulation brought about mostly by disuse of the limb was thought by Richards (1954) to be the chief basis of tissue changes, though in some cases alterations in vasa nervorum, he believed, may be an additional and perhaps a decisive factor. Atlas (1938, 1941) sought to explain late tissue and associated vascular changes on the basis that sensitivity of the vessels to epinephrine is increased (a sensitivity not abolished by preganglionic sympathectomy), and concluded that "such sensitization to vasoconstrictive influences could be the etiology of the vasomotor and nutritional changes in denervated tissues."

In regard to the possibility that afferent impulses sustain trophic function, Tower (1937a, b) observed that no trophic disturbances in muscle or other tissue followed interruption of posterior roots.

Considering the evidence derived experimentally, the real basis of trophic changes in such conditions as multiple sclerosis, poliomyelitis, syringomyelia, tabes dorsalis, and peripheral nerve injuries remains something of an enigma. Trauma has clearly been shown to be a significant factor. In animals with a limb completely denervated, Corbin and Hinsey (1939) found that those allowed the freedom of a large area soon showed bone and joint changes, while those confined to small cages remained free from such changes. Under such conditions trauma can, however, be considered only an *inciting* factor, not a causative factor. Under disease conditions, it is likely that all three factors cited at the beginning of this discussion—motoneuronal, circulatory, and sensory—combine to produce trophic changes, the relative importance of each factor depending on the site of the lesion(s) in the nervous system. On the question of neural influence on tissue, whether direct or through vascular nerves, Sherrington (1900) reached the conclusion that "Every nerve and nerve cell that can influence the proper and specific activity of a tissue—and that is the sole function of nerves—possesses, in so far, a trophic influence on that tissue."

Respiratory function

Respiration as it relates to thermoregulatory and other integrated viscerosomatic responses is under the influence particularly of the orbitofrontal cortex, hypothalamus, and midbrain tegmentum (Bailey and Sweet, 1940; Delgado and Livingston, 1948; Kennard, 1949). A respiratory inhibiting (pneumotaxic) center is situated in the tegmentum of the lateral part of the pons, and an apneustic center (which exerts a tonic effect on the bulbar inspiratory center) is present in the middle and caudal pontile tegmentum. A current hypothesis on respiratory neurogenesis states that both respiratory rhythmicity and respiratory responses to stimuli originate in reciprocally related populations of inspiratory and expiratory neurons occupying these parts of the brainstem. (Plum and Alvord, 1964.) Lesions at different levels are manifested by varied disturbances in respiration. Sequences of respiratory waxing and waning with intermittent apnea *(Cheyne-Stokes respiration)*, with over-all *hyperventilation*, result from mass lesions situated at levels above the medulla oblongata. By contrast, lack of a consistent pattern between breaths and lack of a consistent pattern between deep and shallow tidal volume *(atactic respiration)*, with over-all *hypoventilation*, signifies dysfunction of medullary respiratory centers (Brown and Plum, 1961). Respiration arrested in tonic inspiration *(apneustic respiration)* appears to be an extreme form of respiratory ataxia and to be the outcome of unequal forces acting on either pole of the pontile inspiratory-expiratory center. Apneustic respiration has been noted in patients in whom infarction (resulting from basilar artery thrombosis) almost completely transected the brainstem at a level just rostral to the motor nucleus of the fifth nerve. (Plum and Alvord, 1964.) With interruption of pathways at upper cervical levels pulmonary tidal volume is temporarily reduced (p. 100).

Pupillary dilatation

Pupillary dilatation is brought about through corticohypothalamic and corticomesencephalic mechanisms that discharge through descending pathways into the sympathetic system. Another mechanism, which is responsive to pain and which extends from upper thoracic segments of the spinal cord upward to the mesencephalon (ciliospinal reflex pathway), serves to inhibit pupilloconstriction (dealt with in Chapter 16).

Pupillary responses in the monkey have been obtained by electrically stimulating the cerebral cortex in the region from which eye and lid movements can be elicited (*caudal part of the middle frontal gyrus,* in area 6). Pupillary dilatation occurred upon stimulation of some foci in this area, and pupillary constriction upon stimulation of others. Dilatation was most easily elicited by stimulating the part of area 6 situated adjacent to the medial border of the hemisphere (Kennard, 1949; Smith, 1949). In cats, dilatation of the pupils occurs on stimulation of the caudolateral part of the hypothalamus. Unilateral stimulation causes pupillary dilatation bilaterally, with the reaction most pronounced ipsilaterally. Pupillary constriction could be induced by stimulating rostral hypothalamic areas. Inasmuch as the pupillary changes were accompanied by other autonomic responses during stimulation, it was concluded that no isolated pupillary centers exist in the hypothalamus (Hess, 1948). In monkeys, continuous stimulation of the hypothalamus through implanted electrodes could maintain mydriasis up to 30 to 40 minutes, and miosis for as long as 24 hours (Delgado, 1959).

In man, according to Foerster (1931, 1936b), no change in pupillary size occurs upon electrical stimulation of the cerebral cortex. However, pupillary responses have been obtained in man by electrically stimulating certain foci in the *diencephalon* and *mesencephalon* through chronically implanted electrodes (prior to thalamotomy), also when lesions were made. Pupillary dilatation resulted from diencephalic stimulation (in thalamus and subthalamus), and constriction from mesencephalic stimulation. Dilatation was most readily brought about by stimulation in regions of the subthalamus adjacent to the ventral lateral thalamus and in a region that included the fields of Forel and mesencephalic tegmentum. On stimulation in these regions, the ipsilateral pupil would dilate, then, in a second or two, the contralateral pupil would dilate. The pupils would remain dilated many seconds after cessation of the stimulus but would constrict quickly to direct light. Bilateral pupillary constriction could also be elicited by unilateral stimulation, most commonly from the tegmental region adjacent to the aqueduct at the level of the posterior commissure. Focal destruction of tissue in the region of the mesencephalon extending from the level of the posterior commissure cephalad to the level of the pineal recess (a distance of 2 mm.) led to transient dilatation of the ipsilateral pupil, the latter reacting slowly to direct light but briskly in accommodation. Bilateral miosis lasting two weeks resulted from lesions in the cephalic portion of the mesencephalic tegmentum. Focal destruction in field H of Forel was usually without effect on the pupil, except for the rare occurrence of miosis or paralysis of accommodation. (Nashold and Gills, 1967.)

From the mesencephalic tegmental region, fibers concerned in pupillodilatation proceed downward through the brainstem to the intermediolateral horns at spinal cord levels C8 and Th1. From here, impulses are projected to dilator mechanisms of the pupil through the cervical sympathetic chain in the manner already described.

The pupils may respond reflexly to painful stimuli applied locally to the region of the eyeball or coming from more distant parts. They may also respond to anxiety or pain through epinephrine secretion.

The *oculosensory reflex* consists either in constriction of the pupil or in dilatation followed by constriction in response to painful stimuli of the eye or its adnexa.

The *ciliospinal reflex* consists in dilatation of the ipsilateral pupil when the skin of the neck is pinched or otherwise stimulated. The reflex is inconstant. The afferent impulses appear to be transmitted by somatic sensory nerves. The pupillodilatation is brought about through inhibition of the pupillary constrictor tonus maintained by parasympathetic fibers coursing in the third nerve; the inhibitory pathway in point reaches the Edinger-Westphal nucleus by ascending in the lateral column of the spinal cord, the reticular formation of the medulla oblongata, and the dorsal part of the tegmentum of the pons and midbrain (Harris, Hodes, and Magoun, 1944). The reflex is not mediated through the sympathetic system, since it remains unaltered following interruption of sympathetic fibers descending in the lateral part of the medulla oblongata and is not affected by sympathetic blocking agents (McNealy and Plum, 1962). The ciliospinal reflex is thus a means of testing the integrity of the brain stem up to and including mesencephalic levels.

Pain-induced reflex pupillary dilatation may be mediated through the intermediolateral horns, but it probably represents an epinephrine effect (Langworthy, 1943).

REFERENCES

Abbie, A. A. 1950. The principles of anatomy: an introduction to human biology, ed. 3. Sydney, Angus & Robertson, Ltd., p. 187.

Adams, R. D., Denny-Brown, D., and Pearson, C. 1962. Diseases of muscle: a study in pathology, ed. 2. New York, Harper & Row, Publishers.

Alexander, W. F., Kuntz, A., Henderson, W. P., and Ehrlich, E. 1949. Sympathetic conductor pathways independent of sympathetic trunks—their surgical implications. J. Int. Coll. Surg. **12**:111-119.

Anderson, E., Kedda, L. H., and Knowlton, K. 1962. A preliminary investigation of the source of the creatinuria following transection of the spinal cord. Proc. Soc. Exp. Biol. Med. **110**:690-694.

Appenzeller, O., and Schneiden, H. 1963. Neurogenic pathways concerned in reflex vasodilation in the hand with especial reference to stimuli affecting the afferent pathway. Clin. Sci. **25**:413-421.

Atlas, L. N. 1938. Etiology of vasomotor and nutritional changes following peripheral nerve section. Surgery **4**:718-721.

Atlas, L. N. 1941. Further observations on etiology of vasomotor disturbances following peripheral nerve section. Surgery **10**:318-322.

Bailey, P., and Sweet, W. R. 1940. Effects of respiration, blood pressure and gastric motility of stimulation of orbital surface of frontal lobe. J. Neurophysiol. **3**:276-281.

Bessou, P., and Laporte, Y. 1966. Observations on static fusiform fibres. In Granit, R., editor: Muscular afferents and motor control. New York, John Wiley & Sons, Inc., pp. 81-89.

Blair, D. A., Glover, W. E., and Roddie, I. C. 1960. Vasomotor fibres to skin in the upper arm, calf and thigh. J. Physiol. **153**:232-238.

Bowden, R. E. M., and Gutmann, E. 1944. Denervation and re-innervation of human voluntary muscle. Brain **67**:273-313.

Brown, H. W., and Plum, F., 1961. The neurologic basis of Cheyne-Stokes respiration. Amer. J. Med. **30**:849-860.

Browne, K., Lee, K., and Ring, P. A. 1954. Sensation of passive movement at metatarso-phalangeal joint of great toe in man. J. Physiol. **126**:448-458.

Budy, A. M., editor. 1968. Biology of hard tissue. Washington, D. C., National Aeronautics and Space Administration, pp. 285-289.

Calne, D. B., and Pallis, C. A. 1966. Vibratory sense: a critical review. Brain **89**:723-746.

Cauna, N. 1956. Nerve supply and nerve endings in Meissner's corpuscles. Amer. J. Anat. **99**:315-350.

Cauna, N. 1958. Structure of digital touch corpuscles. Acta Anat. (Basel) **32**:1-23.

Cauna, N. 1965. The effects of aging on the receptor organs of the human dermis. In Montagna, W., editor: Advances in biology of skin, vol. 6. New York, Pergamon Press, Inc., pp. 63-96.

Cauna, N., and Ross, L. L. 1960. The fine structure of Meissner's touch corpuscles of human fingers. J. Biophys. Biochem. Cytol. **8**:467-482.

Coldwater, K. B., Alexander, W. F., Cox, J. W., and Randall, W. C. 1957. The functional significance of the first thoracic ganglion in sympathectomy of the upper extremity in man. Ann. Surg. **145**:530-539.

Cooper, S., and Daniel, P. M. 1963. Muscle spindles in man; their morphology in the lumbricals and the deep muscles of the neck. Brain **86**:563-586.

Corbin, K. B., and Hinsey, J. C. 1939. Influence of the nervous system on bone and joints. Anat. Rec. **75**:307-317.

Critchley, M. 1953. Tactile thought, with special reference to the blind. Proc. Roy. Soc. Med. **46**:27-30.

Darrow, C. W. 1936. The galvanic skin reflex (sweating) and blood pressure as preparatory and facilitative functions. Psychol. Bull. **33**:73-94.

de Castro, F. 1925. Technique pour la coloration du système nerveux quand il est pourvu de ses étuis osseux. Trab. Lab. Invest. Biol. Univ. Madrid **23**:427-446.

de Castro, F. 1930. Quelques observations sur l'intervention du système nerveux autonome dans l'ossification: innervation du tissu osseux et de la moelle osseuse. Trab. Lab. Invest. Biol. Univ. Madrid **26**:215-244.

Delgado, J. M. R., 1959. Prolonged stimulation of brain in awake monkeys. J. Neurophysiol. **22**:458-475.

Delgado, J. M. R., and Livingston, R. B. 1948. Some respiratory, vascular and thermal responses to stimulation of orbital surface of frontal lobe. J. Neurophysiol. **11**:39-55.

Denny-Brown, D. 1965. The release of deep pain by nerve injury. Brain **88**:725-738.

Doupe, J. 1943. Studies in denervation: mechanism of axonal vasodilatation. J. Neurol. Psychiat. **6**:115-120.

Doupe, J., Cullen, C. H., and Macaulay, L. J. 1943. Studies in denervation: the circulation in the skin of the proximal parts of the limbs. J. Neurol. Psychiat. **6**:129-132.

Droz, B., and LeBlond, C. P. 1962. Migration of proteins along the axons of the sciatic nerve. Science **137**:1047-1048.

Feindel, W. 1954. Anatomical overlap of motor-units. J. Comp. Neurol. **101**:1-17.

Fennell, E., Satz, P., and Wise, R. 1967. Laterality differences in the perception of pressure. J. Neurol. Neurosurg. Psychiat. **30**:337-340.

Foerster, O. 1931. The cerebral cortex in man. Lancet **2**:309-311.

Foerster, O. 1935. Ueber Störung der Thermoregulation bei Erkrankungen des Gehirns und Rückenmarks und bei Eingriffen am Zentralnervensystem. Jahrb. Psychiat. Neurol. **52**:1-14.

Foerster, O. 1936a. Symptomatologie der Erkrankungen des Rückenmarks und seiner Wurzeln. In Bumke, O., and Foerster, O., editors: Handbuch der Neurologie, vol. 5. Berlin, Springer-Verlag, pp. 1-403.

Foerster, O. 1936b. Motorische Felder und Bahnen; Sensible corticale Felder. In Bumke, O., and Foerster, O., editors: Handbuch der Neurologie, vol. 6. Berlin, Springer-Verlag, pp. 1-448.

Folkow, B., Johansson, B., and Öberg, B. 1959. A hypothalamic structure with a marked inhibitory effect on tonic sympathetic activity. Acta Physiol. Scand. **47**:262-270.

Fulton, J. F. 1938. Physiology of the nervous system. London, Oxford University Press.

Gagel, O. 1928. Zur Histologie und Topographie der vegetativen Zentren im Rückenmark. Z. Ges. Anat. (Abt. 1) **85**:213-250.

Gardner-Medwin, D., and Walton, J. N. 1969. Myokymia with impaired muscular relaxation. Lancet **1**:127-130.

Geiser, M., and Trueta, J. 1958. Muscle action, bone rarefaction, and bone formation. J. Bone Joint Surg. **40B**:282-311.

Gellhorn, E. 1953. On the physiological action of carbon dioxide on cortex and hypothalamus. EEG Clin. Neurophysiol. **5**:401-413.

Goff, G. D., Rosner, B. S., Detre, T., and Kennard, D. 1965. Vibration perception in normal man and medical patients. J. Neurol. Neurosurg. Psychiat. **28**:503-509.

Goldblum, R. B., and Sekelj, P. 1963. Cystic fibrosis of the pancreas: diagnosis by application of a sodium electrode to the skin. New Eng. J. Med. **269**:1349-1352.

Granit, R. 1959. Circuit analysis of postural reflexes and the relative significance of alpha and gamma motoneurones. Proc. Internat. Congr. Physiol. Sci., Buenos Aires, pp. 93-100.

Granit, R., Holmgren, R., and Merton, P. A. 1955. Two routes for excitation of muscle and their subservience to the cerebellum. J. Physiol. **130**: 213-224.

Gray, J. A. B. 1966. The representation of information about rapid changes in a population of receptor units signalling mechanical events. In de Reuck, A. V. S., and Knight, J., editors: Ciba Foundation Symposium on Touch, Heat and Pain. London, Churchill, pp. 219-315.

Guth, L. 1968. "Trophic" influences of nerve on muscle. Physiol. Rev. **48**:645-687.

Gutmann, E. 1962. Denervation and disuse atrophy in cross-striated muscle. Rev. Canad. Biol. **21**:353-365.

Guttmann, L. 1940. Topographic studies of disturbances of sweat secretion after complete lesions of peripheral nerves. J. Neurol. Psychiat. **3**:197-210.

Guttmann, L. 1954. Visceral activity and peripheral circulation in spinal man. In Wolstenholm, G. E. W., and Freeman, J. S., editors: Peripheral circulation in man, Ciba Found. Sympos. Boston, Little, Brown and Company, pp. 192-203.

Guttmann, L., Silver, J., and Wyndham, C. H. 1958. Thermoregulation in spinal man. J. Physiol. **142**:406-419.

Halpern, L. 1968. Astereognosis not of cortical origin. J. Neurol. Sci. **7**:245-250.

Harris, A. J., Hodes, R., and Magoun, H. W. 1944. The afferent path of the pupillodilator reflex in the cat. J. Neurophysiol. **7**:321-343.

Haymaker, W., and Woodhall, B. 1953. Peripheral nerve injuries: principles of diagnosis, ed. 2. Philadelphia, W. B. Saunders Co.

Head, H. 1905. The afferent nervous system from a new aspect. Brain **28**:99-115.

Head, H. 1920. Studies in neurology, vol. 2. London, Oxford University Press.

Head, H., and Riddoch, G. 1917. The automatic bladder, excessive sweating and some other reflex conditions, in gross injuries of the spinal cord. Brain **40**:188-263.

Hess, W. R. 1948. Die funktionelle Organisation de vegetativen Nervensystems. Basel, Benno Schwabe and Co.

Hromada, J. 1960. Beitrag zur Kenntnis der Entwicklung und der Variabilität der Lamellenkörperchen in der Gelenkkapsel und im periartikulären Gewebe beim menschlichen Fetus. Acta Anat. (Basel) **40**:27-40.

Hugelin, A., Bonvallet, M., and Dell, P. 1959. Activation réticulaire et corticale d'origine chémoreceptive au cours de l'hypoxie. EEG Clin. Neurophysiol. **11**:325-340.

Hurst, A. 1920. War neuroses and neuroses of civil life. Guy's Hosp. Rep. **70**: (pt. 3): 125-155.

Iggo, A. 1968. Electrophysiological and histological studies of cutaneous mechanoreceptors. In Ken-

shalo, D. R., editor: The skin senses. Springfield, Illinois, Charles C Thomas, Publisher, pp. 84-105.
Iggo, A. 1969. Cutaneous thermoreceptors in primates and sub-primates. J. Physiol. **200**:403-430.
Inman, V. T., Ralston, H. J., Saunders, J. B. de C. M., Feinstein, B., and Wright, E. W., Jr. 1952. Relation of human electromyogram to muscular tension. EEG Clin. Neurophysiol. **4**: 187-194.
Jinnai, D., Nishimoto, A., Numoto, M., and Adachi, I. 1964a. Electrophysiological studies in stereotaxic surgery for extrapyramidal disorders: electrophysiological study of globus pallidus, thalamus and their vicinity. Confin. Neurol. **24**: 281-284.
Jinnai, D., Nishimoto, A., Numoto, M., and Adachi, I. 1964b. Electrophysiological studies in stereotaxic surgery for extrapyramidal disorders: mechanism of parkinsonism tremor. Confin. Neurol. **24**:289-300.
Kennard, M. 1935. Vasomotor disturbances resulting from cortical lesions. Arch. Neurol. Psychiat. **33**:537-545.
Kennard, M. 1949. Autonomic function. In Bucy, P. C., editor: The precentral motor cortex, ed. 2. Urbana, University of Illinois Press.
Korr, I. M., Wilkinson, P. N., and Chornock, F. W. 1967. Axonal delivery of neuroplasmic components to muscle cells. Science **155**:342-345.
Kuntz, A., and Alexander, W. F. 1950. Surgical implications of lower thoracic and lumbar independent sympathetic pathways. Arch. Surg. **61**:1007-1018.
Langworthy, O. R. 1943. General principles of autonomic innervation. Arch. Neurol. Psychiat. **50**:590-602.
Leivy, D. M., Tovi, D., and Krueger, E. G. 1968. Failure of lumbar sympathectomy in the relief of hyperhidrosis. J. Neurosurg. **29**:65-69.
Lewis, T. 1927. The blood vessels of the human skin and their responses. London, Shaw & Son, Ltd., pp. 23-80.
Lim, R. K. S. 1966. A revised concept of the mechanism of analgesia and pain. In Knighton, R. S., and Dumke, P. R., editors: Pain. Boston, Little, Brown and Company, pp. 117-154.
Lindgren, P., Rosen, A., Strandberg, P., and Uvnäs, B. 1956. The sympathetic vasodilator outflow—a new cortico-spinal autonomic pathway. J. Comp. Neurol. **105**:95-109.
List, C. F., and Peet, M. M. 1939. Sweat secretion in man: disturbances of sweat secretion with lesions of the pons, medulla and cervical portion of cord. Arch. Neurol. Psychiat. **42**: 1098-1127.
List, C. F., and Pimenta, A. DeM. 1944. Sweat secretion in man: spinal reflex sweating. Arch. Neurol. Psychiat. **51**:501-507.
Magoun, H. W. 1940. Descending connections from the hypothalamus. Res. Publ. Ass. Res. Nerv. Ment. Dis., Proc. **20**:270-285.
McNealy, D. E., and Plum, F. 1962. Brainstem dysfunction with supratentorial mass lesions. Arch. Neurol. Psychiat. **7**:10-32.
McQueen, J. D., Browne, K. M., and Walker, A. E. 1954. Role of the brainstem in blood pressure regulation in the dog. Neurology **4**:1-13.
Melzack, R., and Wall, P. D. 1965. Pain mechanisms: a new theory. Science **150**:971-979.
Nashold, B. S., Jr., and Gills, J. P. 1967. Ocular signs from brain stem stimulation and lesions. Arch. Ophthal. **77**:609-618.
Nauta, W. J. H. 1964. Some afferent connections of the prefrontal cortex in the monkey. In Warren, J. M., and Akert, K., editors: The frontal granular cortex and behavior. New York, McGraw-Hill Book Company, pp. 397-409.
Noronha, M. J., Vas, C. J., and Aziz, H. 1968. Autonomic dysfunction (sweating responses) in multiple sclerosis. J. Neurol. Neurosurg. Psychiat. **31**:19-22.
Peiss, C. N. 1962. Sympathetic innervation of the arterial tree. In Abramson, D. I., editor: Blood vessels and lymphatics. New York, Academic Press, Inc., pp. 96-104.
Pellegrino, C., and Franzini, C. 1963. An electron microscope study of denervation atrophy in red and white skeletal muscle fibers. J. Cell. Biol. **17**:327-349.
Plum, F., and Alvord, E. C., Jr. 1964. Apneustic breathing in man. Arch. Neurol. **10**:101-112.
Ralston, H. J., III, Miller, M. R., and Kasahara, M. 1960. Nerve endings in human fasciae, tendons, ligaments, periosteum and joint synovial membrane. Anat. Rec. **136**:137-148.
Renfrew, S. 1969. Fingertip sensation: a routine neurological test. Lancet **1**:396-397.
Richards, R. L. 1946. The peripheral circulation in health and disease. Edinburgh, E. & S. Livingstone Ltd.
Richards, R. L. 1954. Vasomotor and nutritional disturbances after injuries to peripheral nerves. In Seddon, H. J., editor: Peripheral nerve injuries. London, Her Majesty's Stationery Office, pp. 25-56.
Ruch, T. C., Patton, H. D., Woodbury, J. W., and Towe, A. L. 1965. Neurophysiology, ed. 2. Philadelphia, W. B. Saunders Company.
Schiller, F. 1956. The cutaneous sensory modalities: a critique of their "specificity." Arch. Neurol. Psychiat. **75**:203-219.
Seckendorf, R., and Randall, W. C. 1958. Thermal reflex sweating in paraplegic man. Fed. Proc. **17**:144.
Semmes, J., Weinstein, S., Ghent, L., and Teuber, H.-L. 1960. Somatosensory changes after penetrating brain wounds in man. Cambridge, Mass., Harvard University Press.
Sherrington, C. S. 1900. Trophic functions of the spinal cord. In Schäfer, E. A.: Text-book of physiology, vol. 2. Edinburgh, Pentland, p. 878.
Sherrington, C. S. 1906. The integrative action of the nervous system. New Haven, Conn., Yale University Press, p. 411.
Singer, M., and Salpeter, M. M. 1966. The transport of ^{3}H-l-histidine through the Schwann and myelin sheath into the axon, including a reevaluation of myelin function. J. Morph. **120**: 281-316.
Smith, W. K. 1949. The frontal eye fields. In

Bucy, P. C., editor: The precentral motor cortex, ed. 2. Urbana, University of Illinois Press, pp. 307-342.

Smithwick, R. H. 1937. The value of sympathectomy in the treatment of vascular disease. New Eng. J. Med. **216**:141-150.

Spiegel, E. A., and Hunsicker, W. C., Jr. 1936. Conduction of cortical impulses to autonomic system. J. Nerv. Ment. Dis. **83**:252-274.

Stilwell, D. L., Jr. 1956a. The nerve supply of the vertebral column and its associated structures in the monkey. Anat. Rec. **125**:139-169.

Stilwell, D. L. 1956b. The innervation of deep structures of the hand. Amer. J. Anat. **101**: 75-99.

Stilwell, D. L. 1957a. The innervation of deep structures of the foot. Amer. J. Anat. **101**:59-73.

Stilwell, D. L. 1957b. Regional variations in the innervation of deep fasciae and aponeuroses. Anat. Rec. **127**:635-653.

Sunderland, S. 1968. Nerves and nerve injuries. Edinburgh, E. & S. Livingstone Ltd.

Telford, E. D. 1938. Sympathetic denervation of the upper extremity. Lancet **1**:70-72.

Tolnick, B., and Beck, W. C. 1945. Histamine flare in evaluation of peripheral nerve lesions. War Med. **8**:386-388.

Tower, S. S. 1935. Atrophy and degeneration in skeletal muscle. Amer. J. Anat. **56**:1-43.

Tower, S. S. 1937a. Function and structure in chronically isolated lumbosacral spinal cord of dog. J. Comp. Neurol. **67**:109-131.

Tower, S. S. 1937b. Trophic control of nonnervous tissues by the nervous system: a study of muscle and bone innervated from an isolated and quiescent region of spinal cord. J. Comp. Neurol. **67**:241-268.

Trotter, W., and Davies, H. M. 1909. Experimental studies in the innervation of the skin. J. Physiol. **38**:134-246.

Urist, M. R. 1967. Bone-body fluid continuum as influenced by prolonged inactivity. In Calloway, D. H., editor: Human ecology in space flight II. New York, New York Academy of Sciences, pp. 109-223.

Uvnäs, B. 1960a. Sympathetic vasodilator system and blood flow. Physiol. Rev. **40** (suppl. 4): 69-80.

Uvnäs, B. 1960b. Central cardiovascular control. In Field, J., Magoun, H. W. and Hall, V. E., editors: Handbook of physiology, sect. 1, vol. 2. Washington, D. C., Amer. Physiol. Soc., pp. 1131-1162.

Wall, P. D., and Davis, G. D. 1951. Three cerebral cortical systems affecting autonomic function. J. Neurophysiol. **14**:507-517.

Wang, S. C., and Ranson, S. W. 1939. Autonomic responses to electrical stimulation of the lower brain stem. J. Comp. Neurol. **71**:437-455.

Ward, A. A., and McCulloch, W. S. 1947. The projection of the frontal lobe to the hypothalamus. J. Neurophysiol. **10**:309-314.

Weddell, A. G. M. 1962. Normal and abnormal sensory patterns: pain: "activity pattern" hypothesis for sensation of pain. In Grenell, R. G., editor: Neural physiopathology: some relationships of normal to altered nervous system activity. New York, Paul B. Hoeber, Inc., pp. 134-177.

Weddell, A., Guttmann, L., and Gutman, E. 1941. Local extension of nerve fibers into denervated areas of the skin. J. Neurol. Psychiat. **4**:206-225.

Weddell, G., and Harpman, J. A. 1940. The neurohistological basis for the sensation of pain provoked from deep fascia, tendon, and periosteum. J. Neurol. Psychiat. **3**:319-328.

Weinstein, S., and Sersen, E. A. 1961. Tactile sensitivity as a function of handedness and laterality. J. Comp. Physiol. Psychol. **54**:665-669.

Wheeler, D. D., Boyarsky, L. L., and Brooks, W. H. 1966. The release of amino acids from nerve during stimulation. J. Cell. Physiol. **67**: 141-148.

White, J. C., Smithwick, R. H., and Simeone, F. A. 1952. The autonomic nervous system; anatomy, physiology and surgical application, ed. 3. New York, The Macmillan Company, pp. 51-52, 384-390.

Winkelmann, R. K. 1960. Nerve endings in normal and pathologic skin: contributions to the anatomy of sensation. Springfield, Illinois, Charles C Thomas, Publisher.

Woodbury, J. W., and Ruch, T. C. 1961. Muscle. In Ruch, T. C., and others: Neurophysiology. Philadelphia, W. B. Saunders Company, pp. 96-127.

Woollard, H. H., and Phillips, R. 1932. The distribution of sympathetic fibers in the extremities. J. Anat. **67**:18-27.

Zotterman, Y. 1959. Thermal sensations. In Field, J., Magoun, H. W., and Hall, V. E., editors: Handbook of physiology, sect. 1, vol. 1. Washington, D. C., American Physiological Society, pp. 431-458.

Chapter 3

Innervation in terms of spinal cord segments

It is well known that an embryo is composed of individual more or less transversely situated units known as somites or metameres. In the spinal region, each somite contains a unit of nervous tissue (a neurotome or neuromere), a unit of integument (a dermatome or dermatomere), and a unit of muscle tissue (a myotome or myomere), all three of which become more and more intricately interrelated. Each embryonic spinal cord segment gives rise to motor fibers that pass through the respective anterior roots to the corresponding muscle segment of the two sides. In an analogous manner, each spinal cord segment receives centripetal fibers by way of its posterior roots from the corresponding cutaneous segment of the two sides. The fact that the cutaneous radicular zones in the limbs are longitudinal in arrangement, in contrast to the trunk, in which they are circular, is explicable on an ontogenetic basis. During embryonic development the radicular zones of the limb buds lie at a right angle to the trunk (Fig. 3-1), but as the limbs grow, these zones become displaced peripherally in varied degree. In principle, however, the radicular zones still possess their original circular distribution (Figs. 4-15 and 4-16).

In the fully developed body, most of the components have lost their strict segmental arrangement. This holds for most of the musculature. Thus the arrangement may be such that four adjacent myotomes (which we shall designate A, B, C, and D) give rise to three muscles (I, II, and III), as follows: *muscle I,* from myotomes A, B, C, and D; *muscle II,* from myotomes A, B, and C; *muscle III,* from myotomes A and B. To cite a concrete example of such an arrangement: the biceps femoris and the gluteus maximus (each an example of muscle I) are derived from myotomes L4 through S2; the semitendinosus and semimembranosus (each an example of muscle II) from myotomes L4, L5, and S1; and the tibialis anterior (an example of muscle III) from myotomes L4 and L5. These various *myotomes* receive their nerve supply from corresponding *neurotomes.* In the fully developed body the biceps femoris and gluteus maximus are innervated by way of the anterior roots of spinal segments L4 through S2, the semitendinosus and semimembranosus from L4, L5, and S1, and the tibialis anterior from L4 and L5. What has just been described is the *radicular innervation* of muscles.

Regarding the *peripheral innervation* of the muscles in question, the biceps femoris, semitendinosus, semimembranosus, and tibialis anterior are supplied by the deep peroneal branch of the common peroneal nerve, while the gluteus maximus is innervated by the inferior gluteal. Thus, both

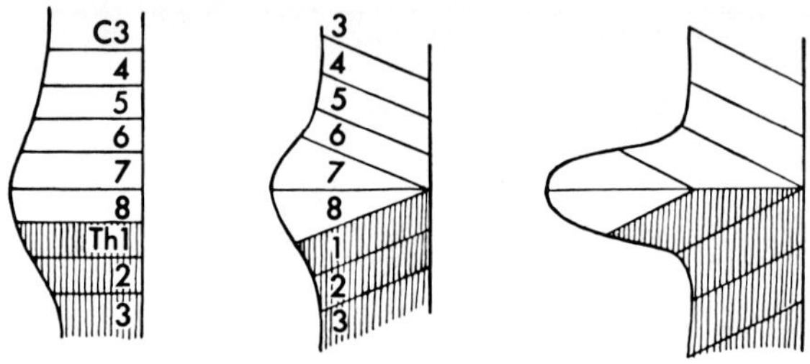

Fig. 3-1. Displacement of dermatomes in the formation of the upper limb. (From study by Bolk, 1968.)

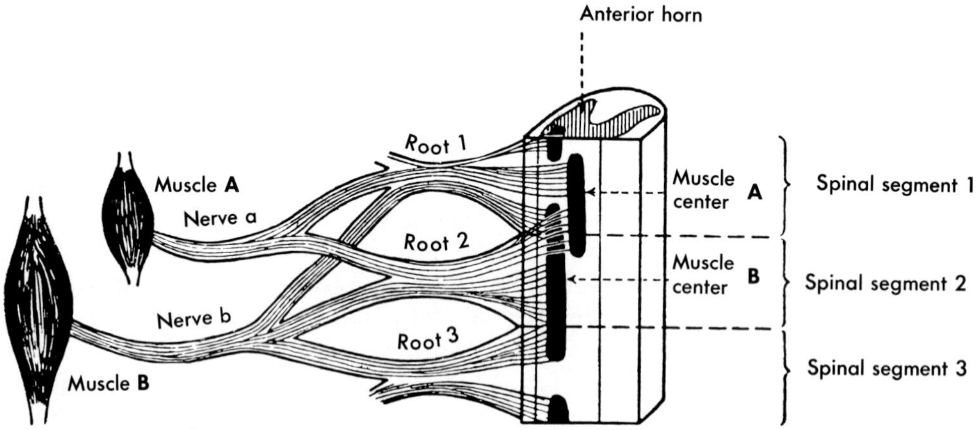

Fig. 3-2. Radicular and peripheral nerve supply of muscles. Muscle **A** is supplied from spinal segments 1 and 2; muscle **B**, from spinal segments 1, 2, and 3.

these nerves carry motor fibers that have emerged from spinal roots L4 through S2. This arrangement of innervation, mediated through nerve plexuses, applies to all peripheral motor nerves. The branching of a motor nerve permits it to supply numerous muscle fibers, with the smaller muscles and the muscles employed in delicate movements receiving relatively the greater number.

The ultimate distribution of nerve fibers to muscles (and to the skin as well) is dependent upon their regrouping not only in the brachial and lumbosacral plexuses but also in the peripheral nerves. Through the mediation of *intraneural plexuses,* the several funiculi that comprise a nerve trunk constantly divide and anastomose with one another, so much so that the funicular pattern differs greatly at levels only a few millimeters apart. (Foerster, 1929; Sunderland, 1952, 1968; Sunderland and Ray, 1948.)

The principles of radicular and peripheral motor innervation are illustrated in Fig. 3-2. In this diagram it will be noted that individual muscles receive their innervation from nerve cell columns lying either side by side or above or below one another. These various columns are composites of the cell groups illustrated in Fig. 1-1.

Immediately outside the spinal canal but within the intervertebral foramina, the anterior and posterior roots unite to form mixed nerves (mixed spinal nerves). Passing peripherally, the mixed spinal nerves are continuous with plexuses, and the plexuses, in turn, with peripheral nerves. Thus, both the plexuses and the peripheral nerves contain motor fibers having their cell bodies in anterior horns, and sensory fibers having their cell bodies in the various posterior root ganglia. Moreover, just as an individual anterior horn sends its fibers into several peripheral nerves, so

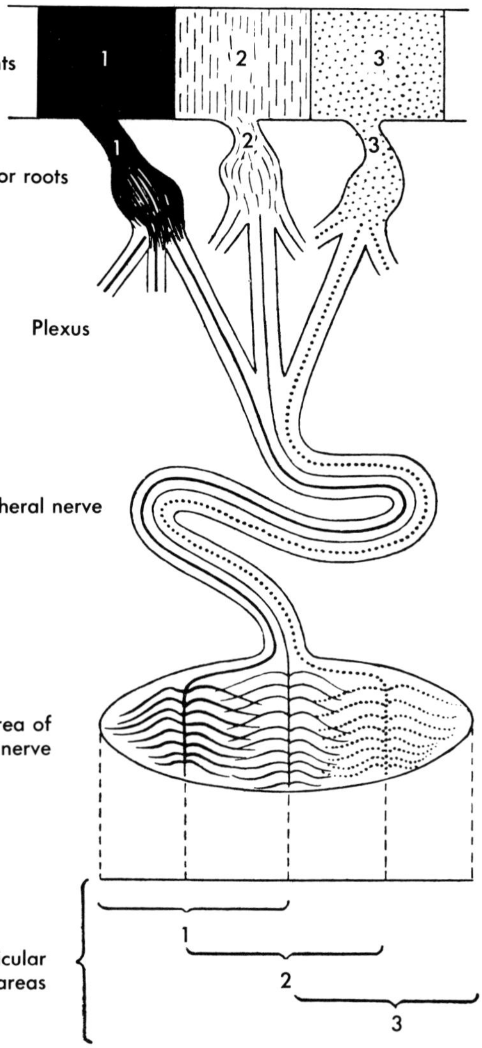

Fig. 3-3. Radicular nerve supply of skin. The adjoining radicular fields overlap.

also does an individual posterior root ganglion receive fibers from several peripheral nerves.

Taking into consideration these anatomical features, it becomes apparent that complete flaccid paralysis of a muscle may be brought about not only by a lesion of the spinal cord that completely destroys the muscle's nuclear center but also by one that interrupts the muscle's nerve supply either at the root, plexus, or peripheral nerve level. Interruption of a single anterior root, however, results in only partial loss of motor power in the muscles it supplies because each muscle (of the limbs at least) is innervated from two or more spinal segments. For complete radicular paralysis of a muscle to occur it is necessary that two or more anterior roots be interrupted.

Turning to the sensory side of the peripheral nervous system, though the pathways of radicular sensory fibers through peripheral nerves and plexus are rather intricate, the pattern of their termination at the periphery is simple; fibers of any given posterior spinal root almost invariably supply the same cutaneous region. To reach the periphery the sensory fibers of a root become scattered in various plexus components and peripheral nerve trunks and then reunite peripherally to form a dermatome (Fig. 3-3). From these considerations it might be assumed that destruction of a single posterior root would result in a sharply circumscribed zone of cutaneous anesthesia. In reality, however, this is not the case, for the individual radicular zones overlap one another like tiles on a roof, each area of the skin being innervated by two posterior roots. However, overlap is not complete, for at the level of the limb plexus interruption of a single posterior root leads to a reduction of sensibility, as is evident in compression of a posterior root by a herniated nucleus pulposus. Only by interruption of two or more adjacent roots does *radicular anesthesia* occur. If, however, a peripheral nerve is interrupted, cutaneous anesthesia will occur, and the zone of anesthesia will occupy much of the region of distribution of the peripheral nerve interrupted. Such an area of anesthesia covers two or more contiguous radicular zones.

REFERENCES

Bolk, L. 1898. Die Segmentaldifferenzirung des menschlichen Rumpfes und seiner Extremitäten. Beiträge zur Anatomie und Morphogenese des menschlichen Körpers. Die Segmente der oberen Extremität. Morph. Jb. **26**:91-211.

Foerster, O. 1929. Die Symptomatologie der Schussverletzungen der peripheren Nerven. In Bumke, O., and Foerster, O., editors: Handbuch der Neurologie, vol. 2, pt. 2, Ergänzungsband. Berlin, Springer-Verlag, pp. 975-1508.

Sunderland, S. 1952. A classification of peripheral nerve injuries producing loss of function. Brain **74**:491-516.

Sunderland, S. 1968. Nerves and nerve injuries. Edinburgh, E. & S. Livingstone Ltd.

Sunderland, S., and Ray, L. J. 1948. The intraneural topography of the sciatic nerve and its popliteal divisions in man. Brain **71**:242-273.

Chapter 4

Localization of segments involved in spinal cord lesions

LOCALIZATION OF MOTOR DISTURBANCES

The muscles affected by a lesion of the anterior horn or anterior root of any given spinal cord segment are indicated in Tables 4-1 and 4-2. In order to be able to distinguish between radicular paralysis and peripheral nerve paralysis, it is necessary to keep in mind the pattern of peripheral nerve innervation, such as presented in Table 4-3. In the first column of Table 4-3 will be found the names of the individual peripheral nerves, in the second the muscles they supply, and in the third the movements performed.

A study of the tables makes it clear that if there is paralysis of a group of muscles, each of which is supplied by the same peripheral nerve, the site of the lesion must be peripheral. On the other hand, if there is paralysis of a group of muscles, each of which has the same radicular innervation, the lesion must then be located in the anterior roots or spinal cord.

In Figs. 4-1 through 4-8 the most important muscles of the arm, forearm, thigh, and lower leg are illustrated in cross section. Various shadings are used for muscle groups in order to distinguish radicular and peripheral nerve supplies.

Following are some examples of peripheral nerve paralysis as contrasted with radicular paralysis. In *radial nerve paralysis* resulting from injury of the nerve in its course in the upper forearm, the extensors of the forearm and fingers and the brachioradialis are affected. In the *forearm type of spinal paralysis,* the extensors and flexors of the forearm and fingers are also involved, but the brachioradialis usually escapes because it derives its nerve supply partly from segment C5. Isolated *paralysis of both the deltoid and the teres minor* is frequent in injury of the axillary nerve, though the teres minor may be spared because it is supplied in part by the suprascapular nerve. Circumscribed paralysis of one or both of these muscles never results from a spinal or a radicular lesion. Actually, a spinal lesion that causes deltoid and teres minor paralysis also affects the scapular muscles, the biceps, and the brachioradialis (the *arm type of spinal paralysis*). This pattern of involvement is observed in lesions of spinal segments or roots C5 and C6; it is also characteristic of lesions of the upper trunk of the brachial plexus, which is formed by the union of the anterior primary rami of segments C5 and C6. Since this plexus trunk is superficially located it is prone to traumatic injury; interruption of the trunk gives rise to so-called *Duchenne-Erb upper plexus paralysis.*

The various constituents of the brachial plexus are shown in Fig. 4-9, and those of the lumbosacral plexus in Fig. 4-10.

Paralysis of spinal or radicular origin may involve any part of a limb. Fig. 4-11 illustrates *radicular finger paralysis* caused by trauma of the anterior roots of segments C7 and C8; some of the affected muscles are supplied by the radial nerve and others by the ulnar. Shown in Fig. 4-12 is an example of *ulnar paralysis.*

If the lesion not only destroys anterior horns but also interrupts the adjoining lateral pyramidal tract, there will be paralysis of the muscles at the level or levels

Text continued on p. 56.

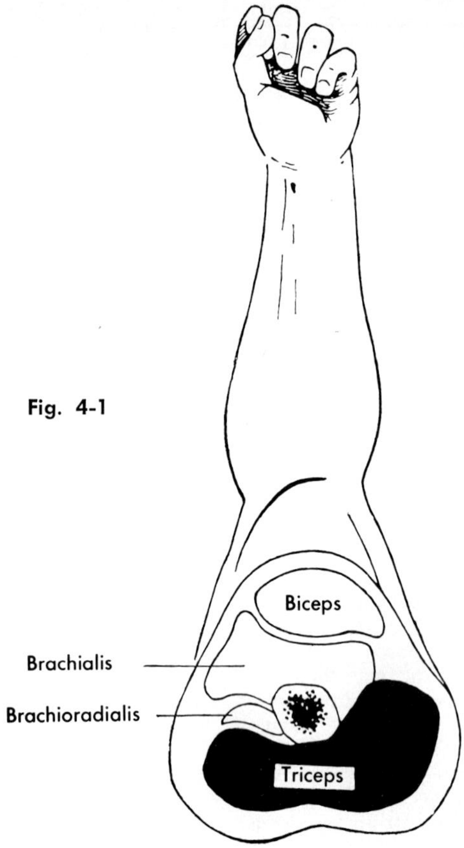

Fig. 4-1

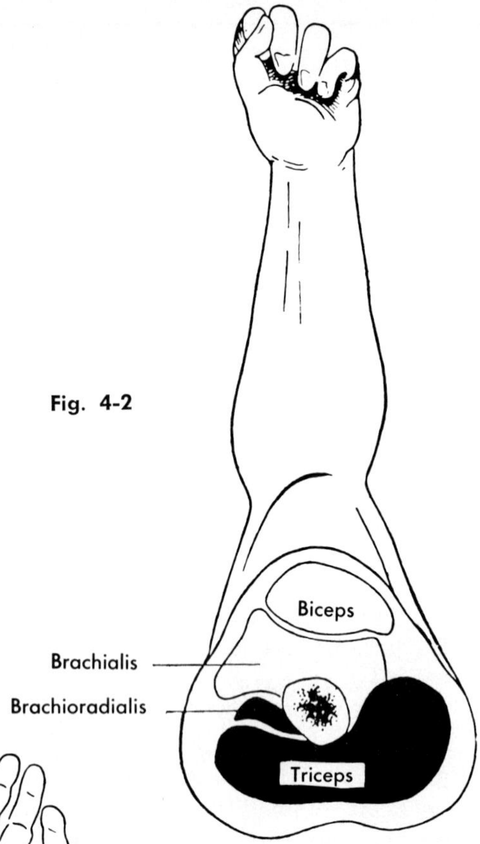

Fig. 4-2

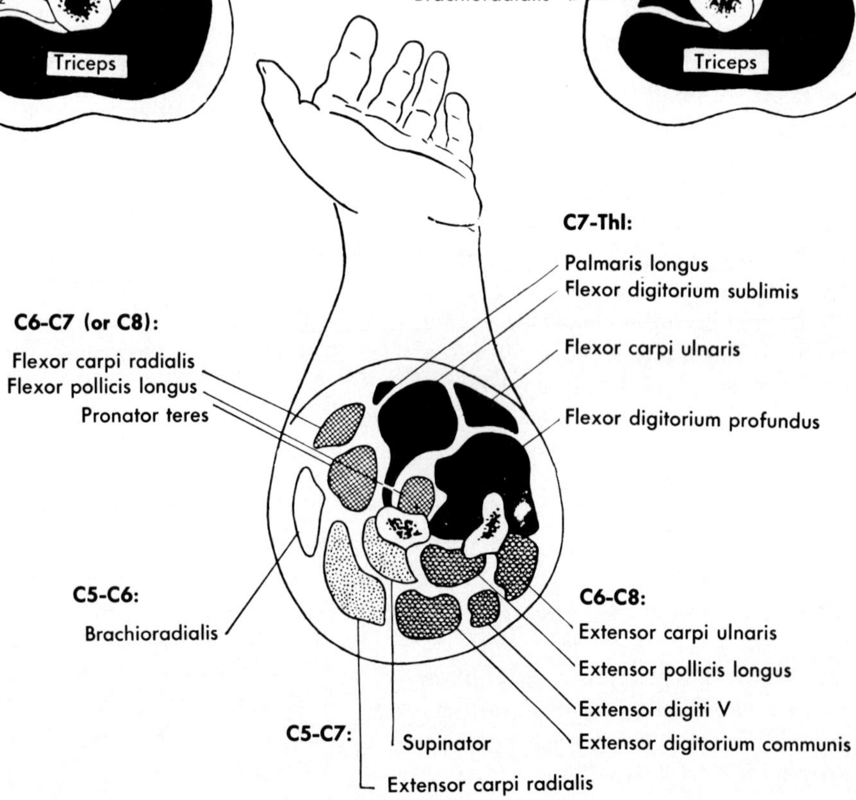

Fig. 4-3

Fig. 4-1. Radicular innervation of the arm muscles. *White,* C5 and C6; *black,* C6, C7, and C8.
Fig. 4-2. Peripheral nerve supply of the arm muscles. *White,* musculocutaneous nerve; *black,* radial nerve.
Fig. 4-3. Radicular innervation of the forearm muscles.

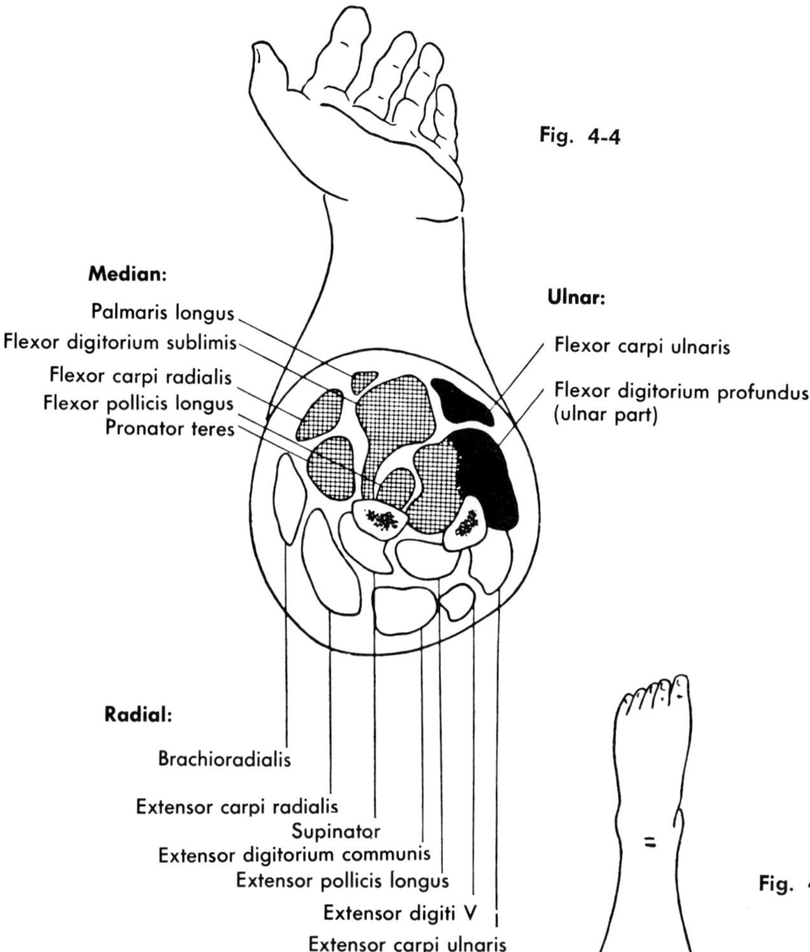

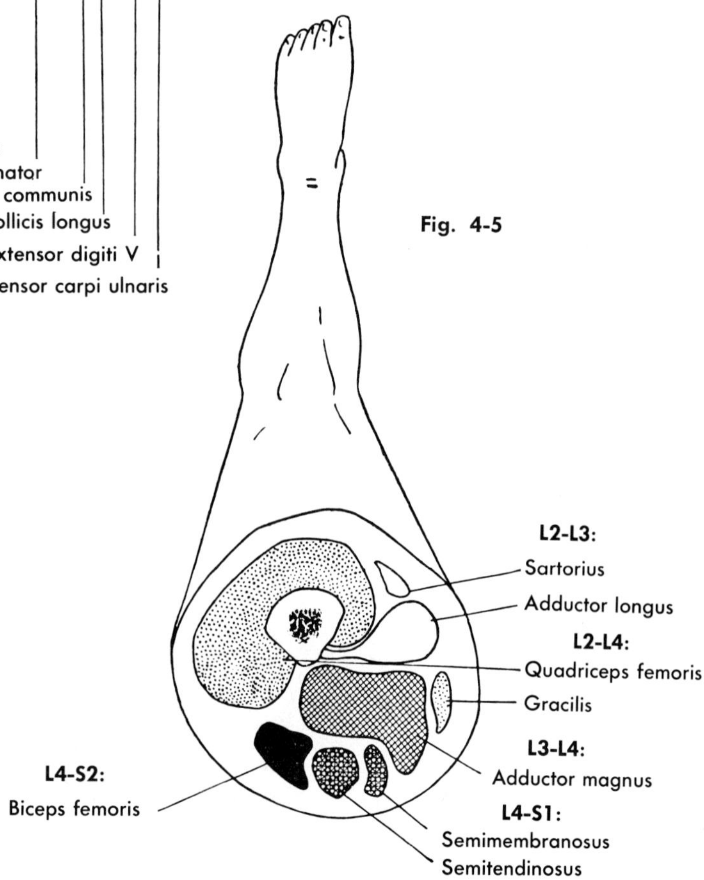

Fig. 4-4. Peripheral nerve supply of the forearm muscles.
Fig. 4-5. Radicular innervation of the thigh muscles.

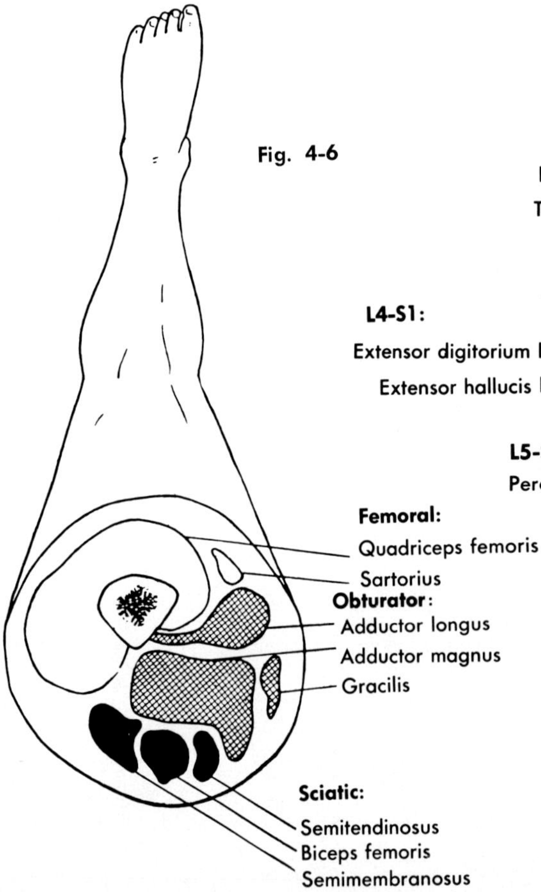

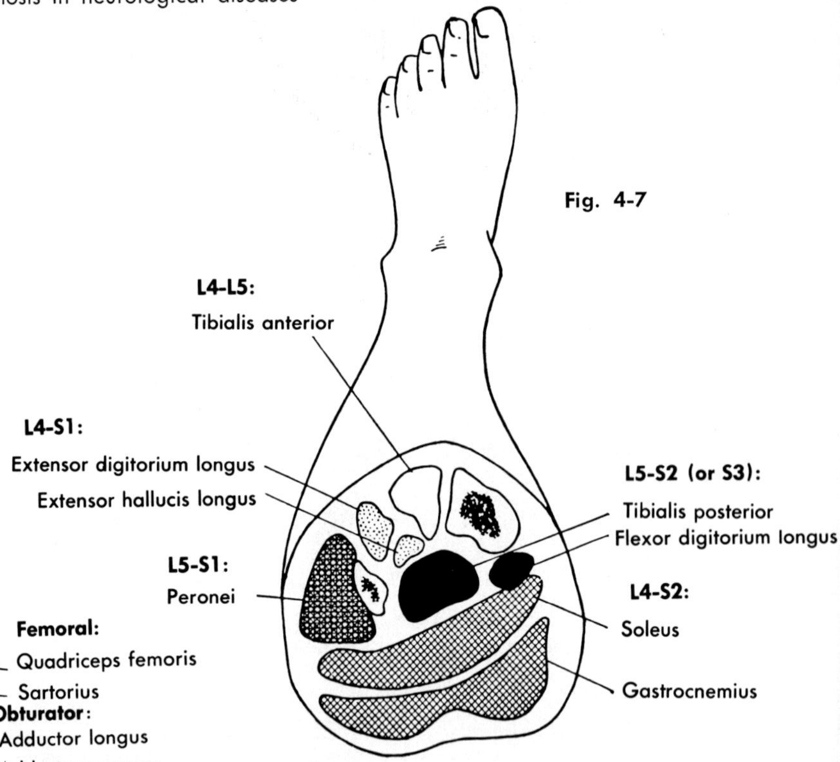

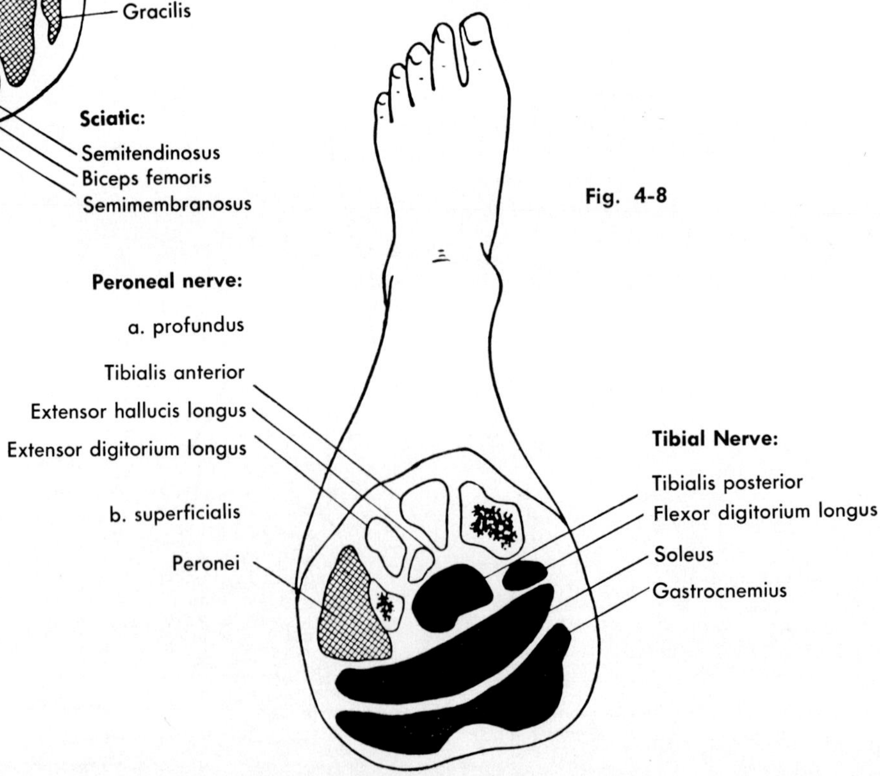

Fig. 4-6. Peripheral nerve supply of the thigh muscles.
Fig. 4-7. Radicular innervation of the calf muscles.
Fig. 4-8. Peripheral nerve supply of the calf muscles.

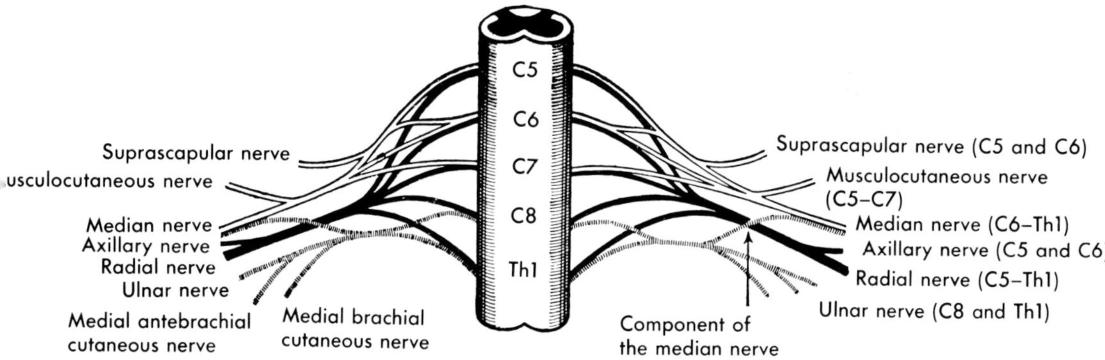

Fig. 4-9. The constituents of the brachial plexus. *White,* lateral cord; *black,* posterior cord; *hatched,* medial cord.

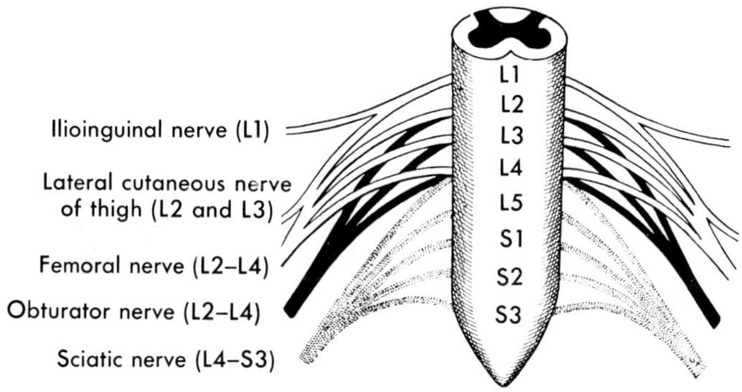

Fig. 4-10. The components of the lumbosacral plexus.

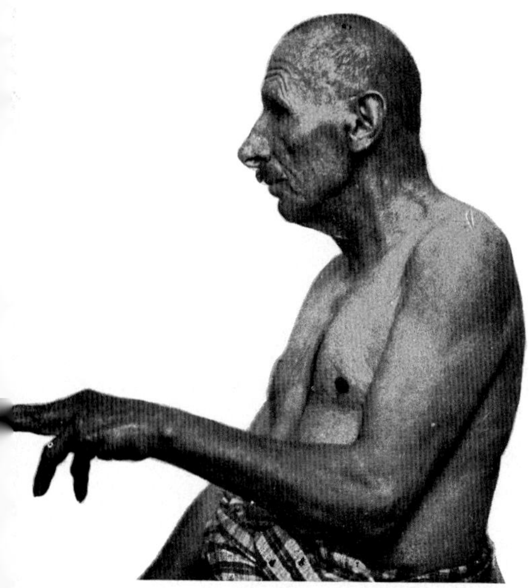

Fig. 4-11

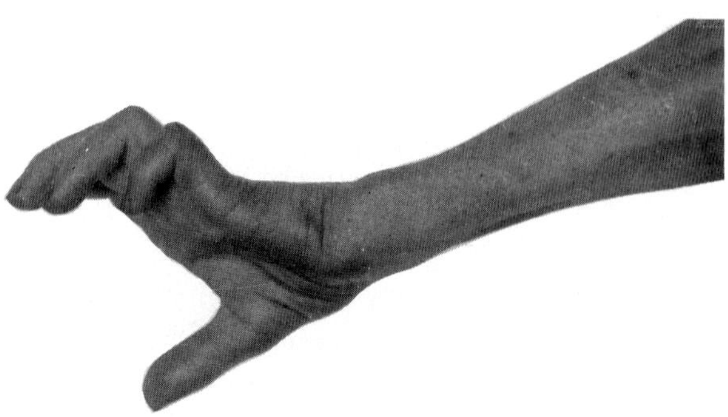

Fig. 4-12

Fig. 4-11. Traumatic radicular paralysis of the ring and little fingers.
Fig. 4-12. Traumatic ulnar nerve palsy.

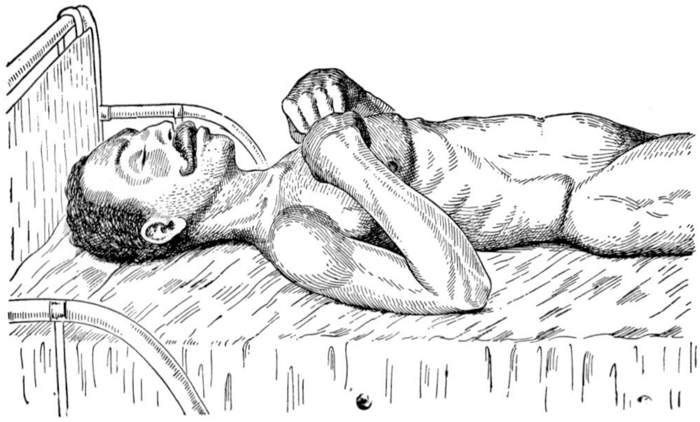

Fig. 4-13. Contracture-in-flexion of the arms due to a lesion of spinal segment C7.

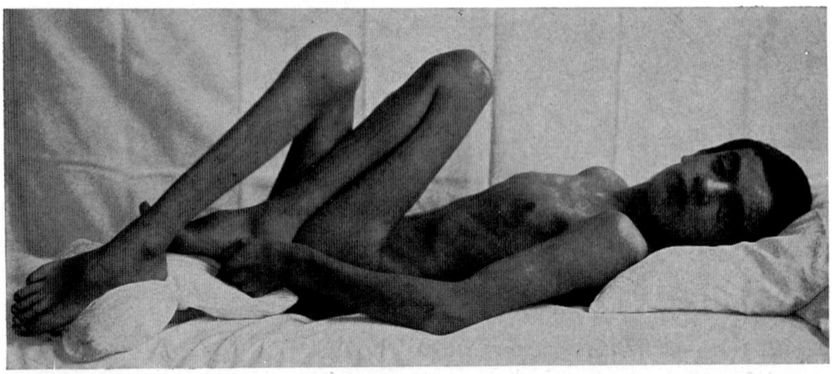

Fig. 4-14. Contracture-in-flexion at the hip in a lesion of lower thoracic segments.

of the destroyed anterior horn cells (radicular paralysis) together with paresis of the muscles deriving their nerve supply from anterior horns below the level of the lesion. The extent of the paralysis and paresis resulting from a lesion at any given spinal level is indicated in Tables 4-1 and 4-2. The muscles that will undergo complete or partial paralysis are those boxed off, while the muscles that will be rendered paretic (as a result of the pyramidal tract lesion) are all those to the right of the boxes. Table 4-4 will serve as a means of quick orientation of the part of the cord affected in paralysis in any location.

Spinal cord injury resulting from fracture or dislocation of a vertebra or from pressure exerted by a tumor in the spinal canal causes paralysis of muscles of the damaged segments, paralytic contracture, and spasticity of muscles below the level of the lesion. The contracture, if developed in opposing muscle groups, is most pronounced in the more powerful group. A few examples will serve to illustrate the point.

A transverse lesion of spinal segment *C8* gives rise to contracture of muscles of the hand such that the hand assumes the attitude of a claw *(claw hand)*; however, the other parts of the upper limb are normal in all respects. The contracture is the outcome of persistent contraction of the flexors of the fingers (from C7) resulting from paralysis of the finger extensors (C8). In destruction of segment *C7*, the upper limb is flexed at the elbow as if by force (Figs. 4-13 and 5-10); in such instances the biceps brachii and brachialis are persistently contracted because their antagonist, the triceps brachii, is paralyzed. In destruction of segment C6, extension, abduction, and external rotation of the arm are frequently encountered. This results from contracture of the supraspinatus, teres minor, deltoid, and infra-

Table 4-1

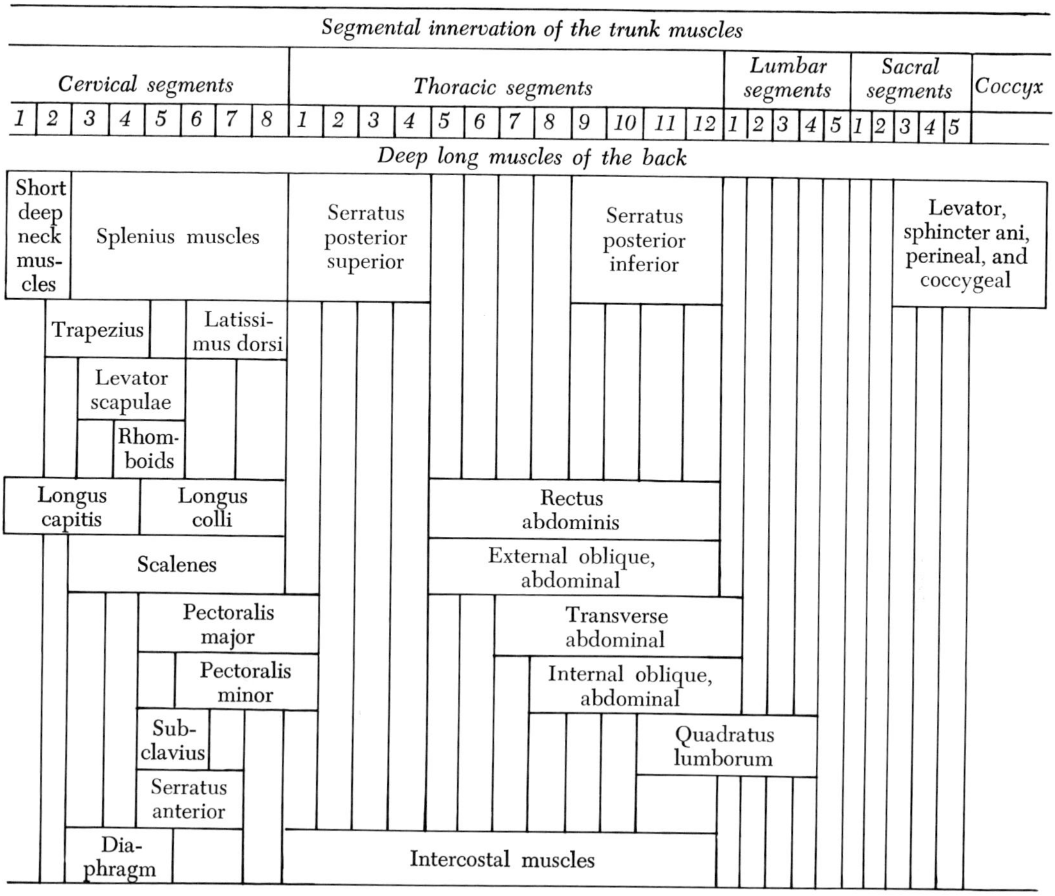

spinatus muscles, and flaccidity of the biceps brachii and brachialis. In interruption of the *lower thoracic* spinal cord, flexion-contracture at the hip is common (Fig. 4-14). This is the result of unopposed action of the iliopsoas muscle, supplied chiefly through segments L1 and L2. The question of whether flexion-contracture or extension-contracture will occur following transverse lesions of the spinal cord is discussed on pages 85 and 86.

LOCALIZATION OF SENSORY DISTURBANCES

In the preceding section attention was drawn to the fact that the distribution of paralysis of radicular origin is different from the paralysis of peripheral nerve origin. This difference is still more striking in the realm of sensibility. The cutaneous radicular and peripheral nerve fields are indicated in Figs. 4-15 through 4-18. These illustrations reveal the great difference that exists in radicular and peripheral nerve distribution. In regard to the extent of the radicular fields, Figs. 4-15 and 4-16 show that each field is located on either side of a line bearing the respective segment number. Each of these fields overlaps with the adjoining two radicular fields. The overlap is such that anesthesia can occur only when two or more posterior roots have been interrupted; hypesthesia but not anesthesia may occur when one root is interrupted.

The factor of overlap of adjacent radicular fields may lead to inaccuracy in the assessment of the exact upper level of the responsible lesion. Thus it is mandatory that in carrying out exploratory operation

Text continued on page 63.

Table 4-2

Segmental innervation of muscles of extremities

		Cervical segments					*Thoracic segments*
		4	*5*	*6*	*7*	*8*	*1*
Shoulder	Supraspinatus	+	+				
Shoulder	Teres minor	+	+				
Shoulder	Deltoid	(+)	+	+			
Shoulder	Infraspinatus	(+)	+	+			
Shoulder	Subscapular		+	+			
Shoulder	Teres major		(+)	+	+		
Arm	Biceps brachii		+	+			
Arm	Brachialis		+	+			
Arm	Coracobrachialis		+	+	+		
Arm	Triceps brachii			+	+	+	
Arm	Anconaeus				+	+	
Forearm	Brachioradialis		+	+			
Forearm	Supinator		+	+	+		
Forearm	Extensor carpi radialis		+	+	+		
Forearm	Pronator teres			+	+		
Forearm	Flexor carpi radialis			+	+		
Forearm	Flexor pollicis longus			+	+	+	
Forearm	Abductor pollicis longus			+	+	+	
Forearm	Extensor pollicis brevis				(+)	+	+
Forearm	Extensor pollicis longus			+	+	+	
Forearm	Extensor digitorum communis			+	+	+	
Forearm	Extensor indicis proprius			+	+	+	
Forearm	Extensor carpi ulnaris			+	+	+	
Forearm	Extensor digiti V proprius			+	+	+	
Forearm	Flexor digitorum sublimis				+	+	+
Forearm	Flexor digitorum profundus				+	+	+
Forearm	Pronator quadratus				+	+	+
Forearm	Flexor carpi ulnaris				+	+	+
Forearm	Palmaris longus				(+) +	+	+ (+)
Hand	Abductor pollicis brevis				+	+	+
Hand	Flexor pollicis brevis				+	+	+
Hand	Opponens pollicis			+	+	(+)	(+)
Hand	Flexor digiti V				+	+	+
Hand	Opponens digiti V				+	+	+
Hand	Adductor pollicis					+	+
Hand	Palmaris brevis					+	+
Hand	Abductor digiti V					+	+
Hand	Lumbricals					+	+
Hand	Interossei					+	+

Table 4-2—cont'd

Region	Muscle	Thoracic 12	Lumbar 1	Lumbar 2	Lumbar 3	Lumbar 4	Lumbar 5	Sacral 1	Sacral 2	Sacral 3
Hip	Iliopsoas	X	X	X	X					
Hip	Tensor fasciae latae					X	X			
Hip	Gluteus medius					X	X	X		
Hip	Gluteus minimus					X	X	X		
Hip	Quadratus femoris					X	X	X		
Hip	Gemellus inferior					X	X	X		
Hip	Gemellus superior					(X)	X	X		
Hip	Gluteus maximus					(X)	X	X	(X)	
Hip	Obturator internus						X	X		
Hip	Piriformis						X	X		
Thigh	Sartorius			X	X					
Thigh	Pectineus			X	X					
Thigh	Adductor longus			X	X					
Thigh	Quadriceps femoris			(X)	X	X				
Thigh	Gracilis			X	X	X				
Thigh	Adductor brevis			X	X	X				
Thigh	Obturator externus				X	X				
Thigh	Adductor magnus				X	X				
Thigh	Adductor minimus				X	X				
Thigh	Articularis genu				X	X				
Thigh	Semitendinosus					X	X	X		
Thigh	Semimembranosus					X	X	X		
Thigh	Biceps femoris					(X)	X	X	X	
Leg	Tibialis anterior					X	X			
Leg	Extensor hallucis longus					X	X	(X)		
Leg	Popliteus					X	X	X		
Leg	Plantaris					X	X	X		
Leg	Extensor digitorum longus					X	X	X		
Leg	Soleus					(X)	X	X	(X)	
Leg	Gastrocnemius					(X)	X	X	X	
Leg	Peroneus longus						X	X		
Leg	Peroneus brevis						X	X		
Leg	Tibialis posterior						X	X	(X)	
Leg	Flexor digitorum longus						X	X	X	X
Leg	Flexor hallucis longus						X	X	X	X
Foot	Extensor hallucis brevis					X	X	X		
Foot	Extensor digiti brevis					X	X	X		
Foot	Flexor digiti brevis						X	X		
Foot	Abductor hallucis						X	X		
Foot	Flexor hallucis brevis						X	X	X	X
Foot	Lumbricals						X	X	X	
Foot	Adductor hallucis							X	X	
Foot	Abductor digiti V							X	X	
Foot	Flexor digiti V brevis							X	X	
Foot	Opponens digiti V							X	X	
Foot	Quadratus plantae							X	X	
Foot	Interossei							X	X	

Table 4-3. Motor functions of the spinal nerves*

Nerves	*Muscles*	*Function*
A. *Cervical plexus* (C1–C4)	Deep cervical	Flexion, extension, and rotation of the neck
Cervical	Scalene	Elevation of the ribs (inspiration)
Phrenic	Diaphragm	Inspiration
B. *Brachial plexus* (C5–Th1)		
Anterior thoracic	Pectorales major and minor	Adduction and depression of the arm downward and medially
Long thoracic	Serratus anterior	Fixation of scapula on raising the arm
Dorsal scapular	Levator scapulae	Elevation of scapula
	Rhomboid	Drawing the scapula upward and inward
Suprascapular	Supraspinatus	Elevation and outward rotation of the arm
	Infraspinatus	Outward rotation of the arm
Subscapular	Latissimus dorsi } Teres major }	Inward rotation and adduction of the arm toward the back
	Subscapularis	Inward rotation of the arm
Axillary	Deltoid	Raising of arm to the horizontal
	Teres minor	Outward rotation of the arm
Musculocutaneous	Biceps brachii	Flexion and supination of the forearm
	Coracobrachialis	Elevation and adduction of the arm
	Brachialis	Flexion of the forearm
Median	Flexor carpi radialis	Flexion and radial deviation of the hand
	Palmaris longus	Flexion of the hand
	Flexor digitorum sublimis	Flexion of the middle phalanges of IId through Vth fingers
	Flexor pollicis longus	Flexion of the distal phalanx of the thumb
	Flexor digitorum profundus (radial half)	Flexion of the distal phalanges of IId and IIId fingers
	Pronator quadratus	Pronation
	Pronator teres	Pronation
	Abductor pollicis brevis	Abduction of metacarpus I at right angles to palm
	Flexor pollicis brevis	Flexion of proximal phalanx of thumb
	Lumbricals I, II, III	Flexion of the proximal phalanges and extension of the other phalanges of Ist, IId and IIId fingers
	Opponens pollicis brevis	Opposition of metacarpus I
Ulnar	Flexor carpi ulnaris	Flexion and ulnar deviation of the hand
	Flexor digitorum profundus (ulnar half)	Flexion of distal phalanges of IVth and Vth fingers
	Adductor pollicis	Adduction of metacarpus I
	Hypothenar	Abduction, opposition, flexion of the little finger
	Lumbricals III, IV	Flexion of the first phalanx and extension of the other phalanges of IVth and Vth fingers
	Interossei	Same action as preceding. Also spreading apart of fingers and bringing them together

*Various muscles may receive still other nerve supplies than those mentioned. The following are the principal accessory nerve supplies: the *brachial muscle* receives fibers from the radial nerve; the *flexor digitorum sublimis,* from the ulnar; the *adductor pollicis,* from the median; the *pectineus,* from the femoral; the *adductor magnus,* from the tibial.

Table 4-3. Motor functions of the spinal nerves—cont'd

Nerves	*Muscles*	*Function*
Radial	Triceps brachii	Extension of the forearm
	Brachioradialis	Flexion of the forearm
	Extensor carpi radialis	Extension and radial flexion of the hand
	Extensor digitorum communis	Extension of proximal phalanges of IId through Vth fingers
	Extensor digiti quinti proprius	Extension of the proximal phalanx of the little finger
	Extensor carpi ulnaris	Extension and ulnar deviation of the hand
	Supinator	Supination of the forearm
	Abductor pollicis longus	Abduction of metacarpus I
	Extensor pollicis brevis	Extension of the proximal phalanx of the thumb
	Extensor pollicis longus	Abduction of Ist metacarpus and extension of the distal phalanges of the thumb
	Extensor indicis proprius	Extension of the proximal phalanx of the index finger
C. Thoracic nerves		
Thoracic	Thoracic and abdominal	Elevation of the ribs, expiration, abdominal compression, etc.
D. Lumbar plexus (Th12–L4)		
Femoral	Iliopsoas	Flexion of the leg at the hip
	Sartorius	Inward rotation of the leg together with flexion of the upper and lower leg
	Quadriceps femoris	Extension of the lower leg
Obturator	Pectineus Adductor longus Adductor brevis Adductor magnus Gracilis	Adduction of the leg
	Obturator externus	Adduction and outward rotation of the leg
E. Sacral plexus (L5–S5)		
Superior gluteal	Gluteus medius Gluteus minimus	Abduction and inward rotation of the leg, also under certain circumstances, an outward rotation
	Tensor fasciae latae	Flexion of the leg at the hip
	Piriformis	Outward rotation of the leg
	Gluteus maximus	Extension of leg at the hip
Inferior gluteal		
Sciatic	Obturator internus Gemelli Quadratus femoris	Outward rotation of the leg
	Biceps femoris Semitendinosus Semimembranosus	Flexion of the leg at the hip
(1) Peroneal (a) deep	Tibialis anterior	Dorsiflexion and supination of the foot
	Extensor digitorum longus	Extension of the toes
	Extensor hallucis brevis	Extension of the great toe
(b) superficial	Peroneus	Pronation of the foot

Continued.

Table 4-3. Motor functions of the spinal nerves—cont'd

Nerves	*Muscles*	*Function*
(2) Tibialis	Gastrocnemius } Soleus }	Plantar flexion of the foot
	Tibialis posterior	Adduction of the foot
	Flexor digitorum longus	Flexion of the distal phalanges II through V
	Flexor hallucis longus	Flexion of distal phalanx I
	Flexor digitorum brevis	Flexion of middle phalanges II through V
	Flexor hallucis brevis	Flexion of middle phalanx I
	Plantar	Spreading and bringing together and flexion of the proximal phalanges of the toes
Pudendal	Perineal and sphincters	Closure of sphincters of the pelvic organs. Also participation in the sexual act. Contraction of pelvic floor

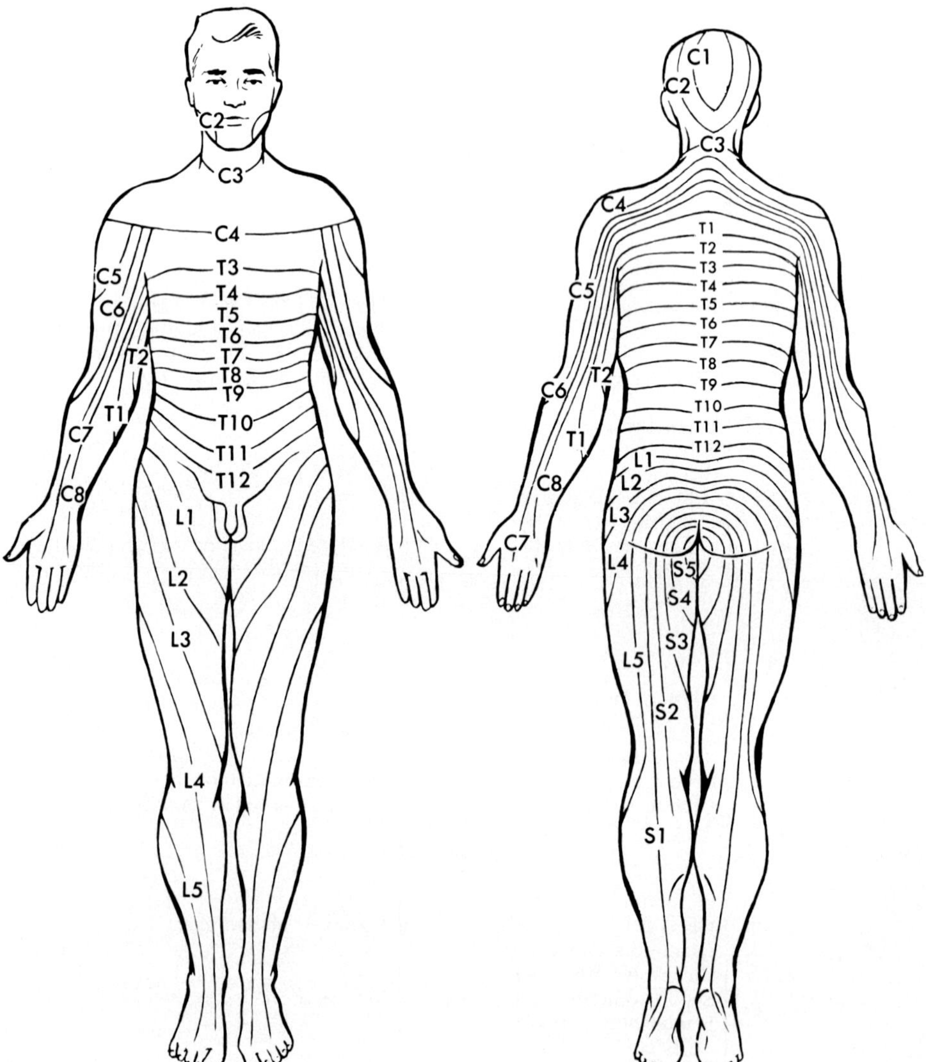

Fig. 4-15 **Fig. 4-16**

Figs. 4-15 and **4-16.** Radicular cutaneous fields. (After Edinger, 1904.)

Table 4-4. Movements and muscles affected in damage of the spinal cord at various levels

Cervical cord			*Thoracic cord*	*Lumbar cord*		*Sacral cord*
Upper	*Middle*	*Lower*		*Upper*	*Lower*	
Neck and head movements; elevation of the shoulders	Diaphragmatic breathing; movements of the upper arm; movements of the forearm	Hand and finger movements	Intercostal muscles in respiratory movements; contraction of abdominal muscles	Flexion of leg at hip; adduction of thigh	Other movements of thigh; movements of lower leg	Movements of foot and toes; contraction of sphincters and perineal muscles

Table 4-5. Sites to which pains of radicular origin are projected

Spinal root involved by lesion	*Region to which pains are projected*	*Spinal root involved by lesion*	*Region to which pains are projected*
C2	Occiput	L1	Inguinal region
C3	Ear	L2	Anterior aspect of upper thigh
C4	Neck, upper shoulder	L3	Middle anterior aspect of thigh, inner knee
C5	Lower shoulder, lateral side of upper arm	L4	Lateral aspect of thigh, front and medial side of leg, great toe
C6	Lateral side of forearm, thumb, and index finger	L5	Lateral side of leg, dorsum and lateral sole of foot
C7	Index and middle fingers	S1	Back of thigh, lateral side of leg and foot
C8	Ring and little fingers	S2	Back of medial side of thigh and leg, medial side of heel
Th1	Uppermost thorax, inner side of arm	S3	Medial side of thigh
Th2	Medial side of upper arm, upper thorax	S4	Saddle region, external genitalia
Th4	Nipple zone	S5	Perianal region
Th6	Submammary girdle zone		
Th10	Umbilical girdle zone		

on the spinal cord, one or two segments (or sometimes three or four) higher than the upper level of the anesthesia be exposed.

The rule that anesthesia does not result from interruption of one root does not apply to *irritative phenomena* (spontaneous pains, dysesthesias), since they often occur when one root is involved, for example, by a herniated intervertebral disk, neoplasm, or spondylitic process. The location of pains originating from damaged individual spinal roots is given in Table 4-5. Some of the data used in this table were derived from the map of Keegan and Garrett (1948).

The pains and dysesthesias just mentioned, when originating from an "irritable" focus in a posterior spinal root, are projected to the periphery through the corresponding peripheral nerves. The brain misinterprets the source of the incoming pain impulses and, as a result, the pain is projected to the dermatome supplied by the affected spinal root, not to the region of the irritable focus in the root. Since the pain is projected along a natural course, that is, through the root-nerve system, it does not fall into the category of referred pain.

Referred pain is also projected to the periphery, but is designated as "referred" because it originates from structures outside the territory of the root-nerve system, that is, from viscera or muscles. Like any other projected pain, referred pain is projected to dermatomes. However, referred pain does not have a fixed anatomi-

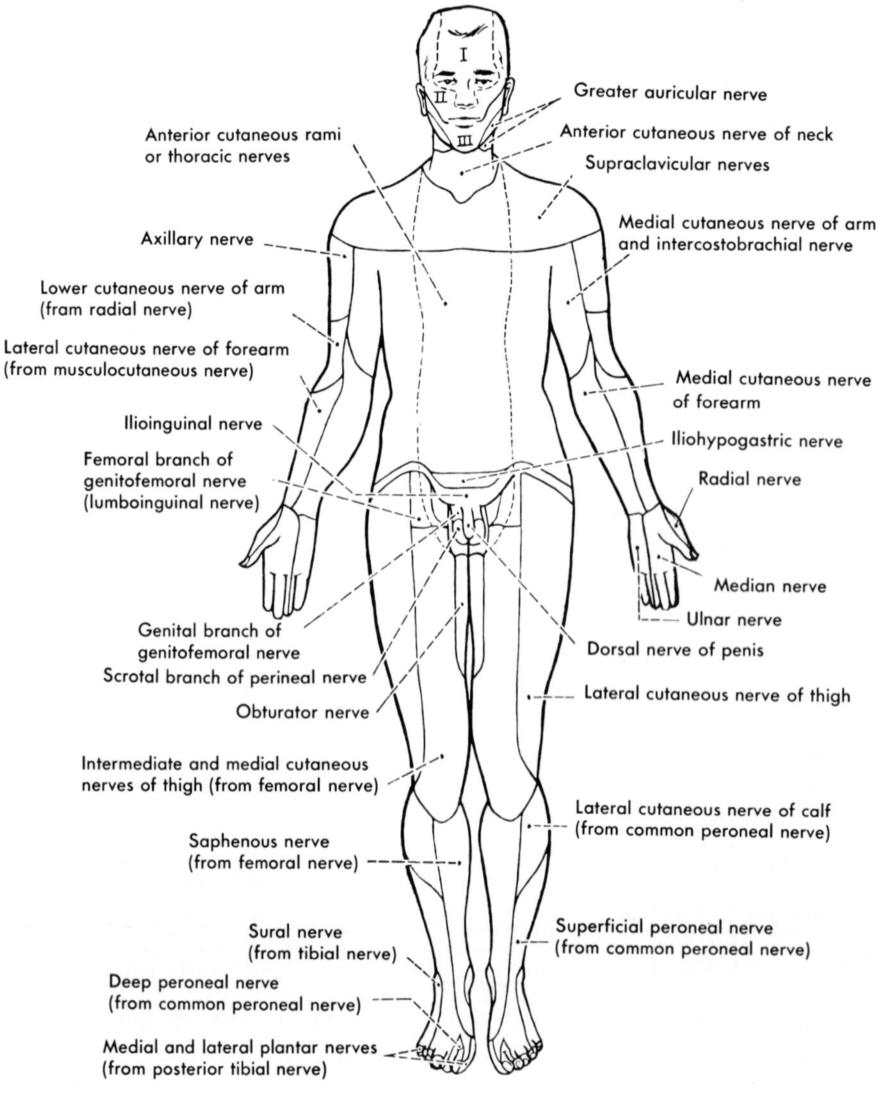

Fig. 4-17. Peripheral nerve supply of the skin.

cal substrate, nor is the referral of pain necessarily confined to the segment(s) of innervation. This is brought out in a study of pain reference in normal subjects receiving injections of hypertonic saline into interspinous ligaments (Hockaday and Whitty, 1967).

Three mechanisms proposed for the referral of pain are:

1. *Convergence-facilitation.* Impulses from the viscera create an "irritable focus" in the segment at which they enter the cord, magnifying afferent impulses from the skin, such that the patient feels pain in the corresponding radicular cutaneous area. In other words, the impulses from the viscera "facilitate" somatic pain (the view of Mackenzie, 1918). This view could account for the cutaneous hyperesthesia that occurs under these conditions, not necessarily the pain reference.

2. *Convergence-projection.* Some visceral afferents converge on the same neurons upon which cutaneous afferents converge, either at the spinal (p. 7), thalamic, or cortical level. The brain interprets the impulses as coming from the skin, since the brain has "learned" to do so through previous experience (view based on Sherrington's neuron-pool concept; see Ruch and others, 1965).

3. *Set-point view.* A presynaptic filter that can be "set" by the activity of supraspinal structures or in response to the afferent barrage preceding sensation is postulated to exist at the spinal cord

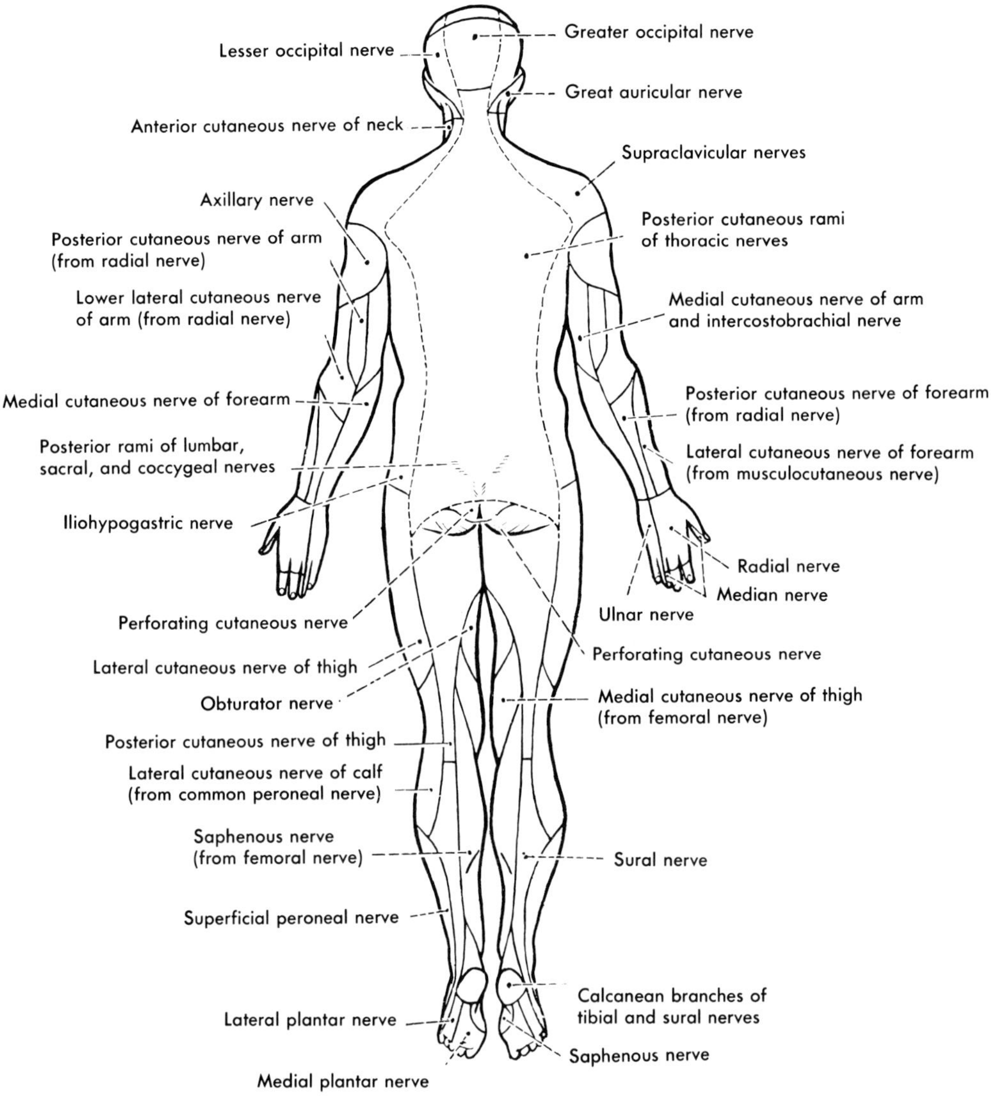

Fig. 4-18. Peripheral nerve supply of the skin.

level. Pain is assumed to result when the total of afferent barrage in all fibers exceeds a preset level (Melzack and Wall, 1966).

Both somatic afferent and visceral afferent fibers carry impulses centrally from viscera. Under pathological conditions involving visceral structures both nonprojected and referred pain occur. Only referred pain concerns us here. *Somatic* afferent fibers originating in the lining of visceral cavities and from certain visceral structures, and the sites to which the pain is referred, are indicated in Table 4-6. Corresponding data on the referral of pain via *visceral* afferents are given in Table 4-7. The visceral afferents conveying these impulses course into the central nervous system via certain components of the cranial parasympathetic system, the sympathetic system, or the sacral parasympathetic system.

Before leaving the subject, mention should be made of the converse of what has been said. Pain originating superficially may be referred to deep structures. For example, in herpes zoster involving upper

Table 4-6. Somatic afferents from visceral structures and sites of pain projection (partly from Ruch and associates, 1965)

Structure	*Nerves carrying pain impulses to central nervous system*	*Radicular segments involved in pain projection*	*Site(s) of referred pain*
Central zone of diaphragm (pleural and peritoneal sides) Portions of pericardium Biliary tract	Phrenic nerve	C3–C4	Region of junction of neck and shoulder
Borders of diaphragm	Intercostal nerves	Th6–Th12	Anterior abdominal wall laterally; occasionally to back
Parietal pleura Parietal peritoneum Roots of mesentery	Thoracic and upper lumbar nerves	Th1–L2	Anterior thorax and abdomen; occasionally to posterior thorax

thoracic segments, pain may be felt in the region of the heart, and the diagnosis of angina made and then changed when the vesicles begin to appear (see Keele, 1957, for discussion).

Fig. 4-19 is provided for quick orientation as to the levels of the spinal cord (or the posterior roots) involved when one is confronted by disturbances of sensibility of radicular distribution. The four straight lines correspond to the upper limit of the following spinal segments:

Verticoauricular line, segment C2
Scapulodigital line, segment Th1
Ilio-inguinal line, segment L1
Perianal line, segment S3

Other landmarks that serve in segmental orientation are the nipples (in the male), which are situated in the field of segment Th4, and the umbilicus, located in the field of segment Th10. Occasionally there are individual variations in the position of these landmarks; what has been stated applies to the average.

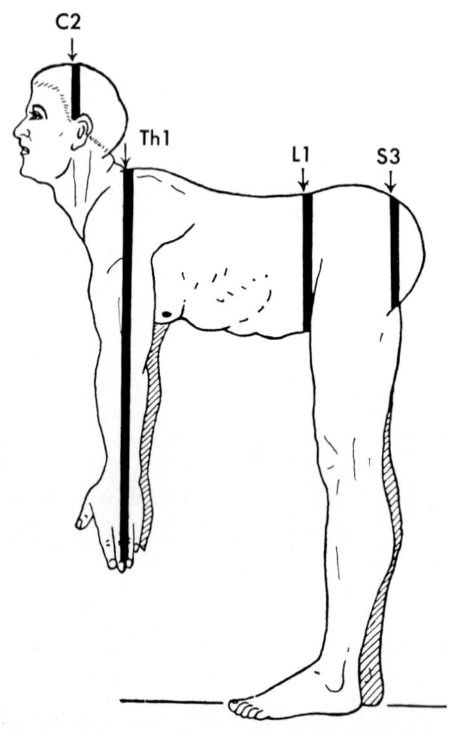

Fig. 4-19. Plan for remembering the cutaneous distribution of spinal cord segments.

LOCALIZATION OF REFLEX CHANGES

Next in importance to paralyses and disturbed sensibility in the localization of spinal lesions are changes in the reflexes. Reflexes are abolished at the levels at which the reflex arcs are broken. The pathways of the various reflex arcs through the spinal cord, based as they are on clinical and pathological observations, are well known; a compilation is given in Table 4-8.

Normally, the *quadriceps femoris reflex* is always present. The *triceps humerus re-*

Table 4-7. Sources of visceral afferents; sites of referred pain*

Structure	Nerves carrying afferent pain impulses	Radicular Segments involved in pain projection	Site(s) to which pain is referred
Cranial parasympathetic system			
Larynx	Tenth	—	No referred pain; pain felt in superior or inferior laryngeal area
Upper esophagus, trachea, bronchi	Tenth	—	Midline, lowermost neck, and xiphoid
Sympathetic system			
Apical pleura	Brachial plexus	—	—
Heart	Cardiac	Th1–Th5	Thorax and inner upper arm
Asc. aortic arch (aneurysm)	Cardiac	Th1, Th2	Right shoulder and neck
Gallbladder	Right splanchnic	Th7–Th9	Above umbilicus on right side
Pancreas	Splanchnic	Th7–Th9	Anterior upper abdomen, occasionally through to back
Lower esophagus, gastric cardia, duodenal cap	Splanchnic	Th7	Region of xiphoid
Duodenum	Splanchnic	Th7–Th10	Midline and deep, from xiphoid to umbilicus
Jejunum, ileum	Splanchnic	Th10	Region of umbilicus
Appendix	Splanchnic	Th11, Th12	Right lower quadrant of abdomen (2nd stage pain)
Upper colon	Splanchnic	Th11–L1	Side of abdomen below umbilicus
Kidney pelvis	Lower splanchnic	Th10–L1	Region of costovertebral angle, occasionally to glans penis
Ureter	Renal, spermatic, and hypogastric plexus	Th11–L1	Lateral border of rectus muscle, suprapubic region up to umbilicus, groin, down the leg, occasionally to glans penis
Bladder fundus	Hypogastric	Th11–L1	Suprapubic region
Testis	Spermatic plexus	Th10	Groin
Uterine fundus	Superior hypogastric plexus	Th11–L1	Lower lateral quadrants of abdomen
Ovary, fallopian tube	Along ovarian arteries	Th10	Small of back, also lateral to and below umbilicus
Sacral parasympathetic system			
Lower colon, rectum	Pelvic	S2–S4	Lower midabdomen
Prostate	Pelvic	S2–S4	Glans penis, lumbar region
Bladder neck	Pelvic	S2–S4	Hard to define zone; maximal pain in region of buttock; may radiate from sacral region, around ilium, to lower abdomen
Seminal vesicles	Pelvic	S2–S4	Lumbar region
Uterine cervix, upper vagina	Pelvic	S2–S4	Lumbar region

*From Behan (1914), Capps and Coleman (1932), Jones (1938, 1943), McLellan and Goodell (1943), Ray and Neill (1947), White (1943), and White and Sweet (1955).

Table 4-8. Spinal reflexes

Deep muscle reflexes	*Superficial reflexes*	*Methods of elicitation*	*Results*	*Segments traversed*
Biceps reflex	—	Tapping the biceps tendon	Flexion of forearm at elbow	C5–C6
Forearm pronator reflex	—	Tapping the palmar aspect of the forearm just medial to the styloid process of the radius	Pronation	C6
Triceps reflex	—	Tapping the triceps tendon	Extension of forearm at elbow	C6–C7
Brachioradialis reflex	—	Tapping the styloid process of the radius, with forearm held in semipronation	Flexion of forearm at elbow	C7–C8
Finger-flexion reflex	—	Tapping the palmar surface of the tip of the fingers	Flexion of the fingers	C7–Th1
Abdominal reflex	—	Tapping the lowermost portion of thorax, the abdominal wall, or the symphysis pubis	Contraction of the abdominal wall and when the symphysis pubis is tapped, adduction of the leg	Th8–Th12
—	Abdominal reflex	Stroking skin of the upper, middle or lower portion of the abdomen	Contraction of abdominal muscles with retraction of the umbilicus to the stimulated side	Th8–Th12
—	Cremasteric reflex	Stroking the adductor region in the upper aspect of the leg	Upward movement of the testicle	L1–L2
Adductor reflex	—	Tapping the medial condyle of the tibia	Adduction of the leg	L2–L4
Quadriceps reflex	—	Tapping the tendon of the quadriceps femoris	Extension of the lower leg	L2–L4
Triceps sural reflex	—	Tapping the tendo Achillis	Plantar flexion of the foot	L5–S2
—	Plantar reflex	Stroking the sole of the foot	Plantar flexion of the toes	S1–S2

flex and the *triceps sural reflex* ("ankle jerk") are usually present, though the latter may be unelicitable in older persons or where myxedema exists (Appenzeller, Imarisio, and Gilbert, 1966). The *abdominal reflex* can almost always be elicited in normal persons 5 months to 50 years of age. The *cremaster and plantar reflexes* are also usually elicitable. The localizing value of superficial reflexes is limited because the level at which they are unelicitable may be far below the level of the causative lesion. Superficial reflexes may be abolished, for example, by cerebral lesions. The neural mechanisms instrumental in the maintenance of the superficial reflexes are much more complicated than those mediating deep reflexes. In regard to the abdominal reflex, its centripetal impulses enter the lower thoracic spinal segments by way of the corresponding posterior roots, and its centrifugal impulses leave the lower thoracic segments by way of the corresponding anterior roots. The impulses subserving these reflexes utilize direct reflex arcs as well as arcs made up of connector neurons. Axons of these connector neurons pass up the cord, presumably to the region of the motor cortex, where synapse occurs. Descending axons course into the spinal cord in a region in or near the pyramidal tracts. The existence of this pathway would serve to explain why the abdominal reflexes (the principle applies also to the other superficial reflexes) are abolished not only by a lesion of lower thoracic segments but also by lesions at much higher levels. Under normal conditions, superficial reflexes can at times be obtained by stimulating areas more distant from the usual reflexogenous zone. For instance, the cremaster reflex may be elicited by stimulating the sole of the foot.

The *flexor withdrawal reflex* is an important aid in localizing an involved segment. The *upper border of the reflexogenous zone* is never above the level of the lower end of the lesion; actually it may be detected up to the very level of the radicular field corresponding to the lower end of the lesion.

The *vasomotor reflex*, or reflex erythema, may in some cases be utilized to determine the level of a spinal lesion. It is of localizing value only when absent in the region of the radicular field corresponding to a spinal cord lesion, and present above and below this radicular field. The absence of a *pilomotor reflex* in a radicular field has the same significance.

ALIGNMENT OF SPINAL CORD SEGMENTS AND VERTEBRAL SPINOUS PROCESSES

Alignment of the individual spinal cord segments and root pairs with the spinous processes of the vertebral column is illustrated in Fig. 4-20. In the uppermost part of the spinal canal the roots tend to pass horizontally to gain their respective intervertebral foramina. Thus, the upper cervical segments of the cord are covered more or less by the corresponding spinous processes; for instance, cord segments C1 and C2 lie beneath spinous process C I, and cord segment C3 beneath spinous process C II. From the midcervical region downward, the successive spinal roots pursue longer and longer courses caudalward through the spinal canal before they pass through intervertebral foramina. Generally speaking, cord segment Th1 is in alignment with spinous process C VI, cord segment L1 with spinous process Th X, and cord segment S1 with spinous process Th XII. All five sacral spinal segments and the coccygeal segment lie beneath spinous processes Th XII and L I. From the level of the second lumbar vertebra downward there is no spinal cord; the spinal canal contains only the roots comprising the cauda equina.

These data illustrate that in the operative approach to spinal cord tumors, laminectomy must be performed at a level above that of the upper border of the anesthetic zone, with the distance above the anesthetic zone varying with the vertebral level. One may, however, perform laminectomy for an extramedullary tumor at too high a level. This is under conditions in which, for example, circumscribed adhesive arachnoiditis develops above the level of the tumor and interferes with cord function through circulatory deficit. Occasionally the damming of spinal fluid by high cervical tumors leads to symptoms and signs referable to the brain stem or its nerves—a syndrome of involvement, for instance, of the twelfth, eleventh, tenth, and ninth cranial nerves, or even paresis of the seventh and sixth nerves with facial anesthesia, nystagmus, and vertigo.

Two other conditions under which symptoms and signs above the level of the lesion may develop are the following:

1. Extramedullary tumor, especially tumor in the lumbosacral region, may compress adjacent roots that have originated at higher levels and thus give rise to clinical disturbances referable to segments higher than that of the tumor.
2. Above the level of an intramedullary

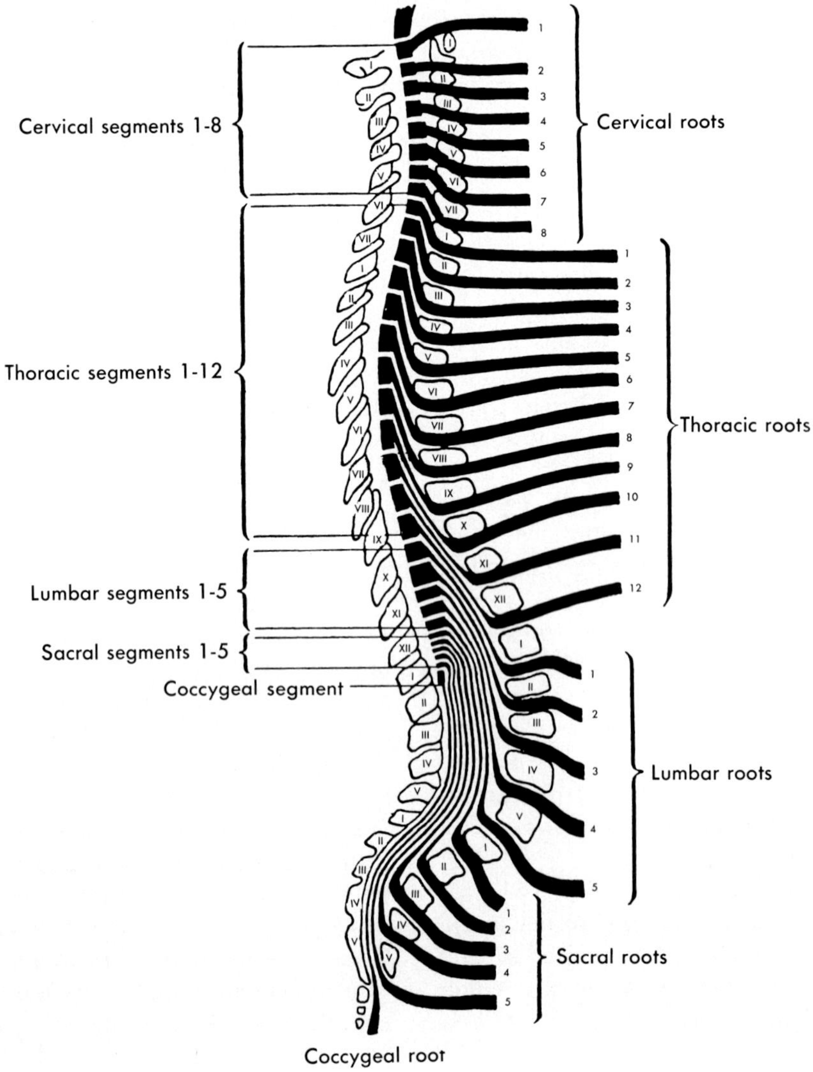

Fig. 4-20. Topographical correlation between spinal cord segments and vertebral bodies, spinous processes, and intervertebral foramina.

tumor the gray matter may be destroyed by a syringomyelia-like excavation that implicates the anterior white commissure, giving rise to sensory disturbances (analgesia and thermoanesthesia) at a level higher than the sensory disturbances produced by the tumor itself.

REFERENCES

Appenzeller, O., Imarisio, J. J., and Gilbert, J. J. 1966. The effect of age and neurological disease on the ankle jerk. Arch. Neurol. **15**:147-150.

Behan, R. J. 1914. Pain: its origin, conduction, perception and diagnostic significance. New York, Appleton & Co.

Capps, J. A., and Coleman, G. H. 1932. An experimental and clinical study of pain in the pleura pericardium and peritoneum. New York, The Macmillan Company.

Edinger, L. 1904. Vorlesungen über den Bau der nervösen Zentralorgane des Menschen und der Tiere, vol. 1. Leipzig, F. C. W. Vogel, p. 91.

Hockaday, J. M., and Whitty, C. W. M. 1967. Patterns of referred pain in the normal subject. Brain **90**:481-496.

Jones, C. M. 1938. Digestive tract pain: diagnosis and treatment; experimental observations. New York, The Macmillan Company.

Jones, C. M. 1943. Pain from the digestive tract. Res. Publ. Ass. Res. Nerv. Ment. Dis., Proc. **23**: 274-288.

Keegan, J. J., and Garrett, F. D. 1948. The segmental distribution of the cutaneous nerves in the limbs of man. Anat. Rec. **102**:409-437.

Keele, K. D. 1957. Anatomies of pain. Oxford, Blackwell Scientific Publications Ltd.

Mackenzie, J. 1918. Symptoms and their interpretation, ed. 3. London, Oxford University Press.

McLellan, A. M., and Goodell, H. 1943. Pain from the bladder, ureter and kidney pelvis. Res. Publ. Ass. Res. Nerv. Ment. Dis., Proc. **23**:252-262.

Melzack, R., and Wall, P. D. 1965. Pain mechanisms: a new theory. Science **150**:971-979.

Ray, B. S., and Neill, C. L. 1947. Abdominal visceral sensation in man. Ann. Surg. **126**:709-724.

Ruch, T. C., Patton, H. D., Woodbury, J. W., and Towe, A. L. 1965. Neurophysiology, ed. 2. Philadelphia, W. B. Saunders Company.

White, J. A. 1943. Sensory innervation of the viscera: studies on visceral afferent neurones in man based on neurosurgical procedures for the relief of intractable pain. Res. Publ. Ass. Res. Nerv. Ment. Dis., Proc. **23**:373-390.

White, J. A., and Sweet, W. H. 1955. Pain: its mechanism and neurosurgical control. Springfield, Illinois, Charles C Thomas, Publisher.

Chapter 5

Localization of lesions of the spinal cord in general

Spinal cord diseases and injuries manifest themselves in localizable disturbances of motility (including alterations of the reflexes) or sensibility or both. The trophic and vasomotor changes that occur are, by contrast, of relatively little help in localizing a lesion.

DISTURBANCES IN MOTILITY

Motor disability—paresis or paralysis—results when either corticospinal fibers (upper motor neurons) or spinomuscular fibers (lower motor neurons) are interrupted. Corticospinal fibers are affected when lesions interrupt the central part of the lateral column, and spinomuscular fibers when anterior horns or anterior roots are damaged. Hence, when confronted with motor impairment of spinal origin, it is necessary to determine whether the causative lesion is in the lateral column or the anterior horns (or roots) or in both.

Disturbances due to lesions of the pyramidal tract

The clinical disturbances resulting from a lesion involving the pyramidal tract are known collectively as the *spastic syndrome*. Its characteristics are as follows.

Spasticity. A feature of the spastic syndrome is that the tension, or tonus, of paretic muscles is greatly increased; the muscles are hypertonic, or spastic, and on palpation they are found to be hard and unyielding. On passive movement their resistance is increased, especially when the movement is rapid. This applies particularly to the flexors of the arm and the extensors of the leg. The resistance is greatest at the beginning of the movement, after which it rapidly gives way, as in opening a jackknife. Spastic muscles also exhibit increased irritability to direct mechanical stimuli, such as tapping them with a reflex hammer.

Deep muscle reflexes. Due to the increase in muscle tension, the deep reflexes ("tendon" reflexes) in the domain of paretic muscles are exaggerated. The more common reflexes and their localizing significance are listed in Table 4-8.

Muscle clonus. Muscle clonus can usually be elicited when hyperreflexia exists. When the examiner suddenly dorsiflexes the patient's foot and keeps it dorsiflexed under elastic pressure, a rhythmic oscillation of the foot occurs and persists as long as the gastrocnemius muscle is maintained in a state of tension. This is known as *ankle clonus. Patellar clonus* may occasionally be elicited by suddenly displacing the patella downward and holding it in that position. In exceptional cases, wrist, finger, or elbow clonus can be elicited.

Crossed reflexes. In the presence of pyramidal tract lesions, crossed reflexes can sometimes be elicited. For instance, the adductor femoris of the left side contracts when the medial condyle of the right tibia is tapped. Some crossed reflexes occurring in the lower limbs are attributable to transmission of the concussion by way of the pelvis. In limbs with normal muscle tonus the response to tapping a tendon is ipsilateral; any crossed reflexes that may occur are scarcely perceptible.

Superficial muscle reflexes. In pyramidal tract lesions, superficial muscle reflexes ("cutaneous" reflexes) are not as consistently altered as are the deep reflexes. The former are usually either diminished or lost, but there are cases of spasticity of pyramidal tract origin in which they are unaltered.

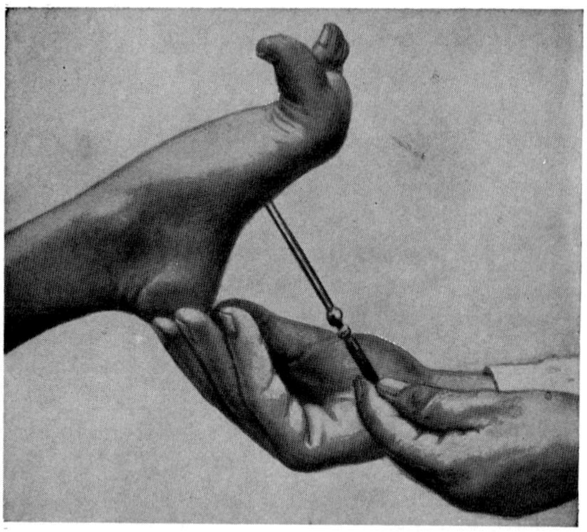

Fig. 5-1. The Babinski reflex: dorsiflexion of the great toe on stroking the lateral side of the plantar surface of the foot.

Toe responses. The reflexogenous zone for tonic dorsal flexion of the great toe extends a considerable distance beyond the sole of the foot. The reflex can be induced by stroking the dorsum of the foot with a pin, by kneading the gastrocnemius muscle, by squeezing the Achilles tendon, by repeatedly tapping the region of the metatarsophalangeal joints just medial to the tendon of the extensor hallucis longus muscle, and by widely abducting the little toe. All these reflexes may be grouped together as *extensor responses.*

The most important sign of a pyramidal tract lesion is the *Babinski reflex* or *sign.* It is characterized by rather slow, tonic hyperextension (dorsal flexion) of the great toe when the lateral part of the sole of the foot is stroked (Fig. 5-1). This constant and obligatory feature of the Babinski reflex may be accompanied by various other movements such as plantar flexion or hyperextension of the other four toes, or by a sluggish spreading apart of the toes (the *fanning phenomenon*) (Fig. 5-2). There may be simultaneous reflex contractions of flexor muscles at the hip,

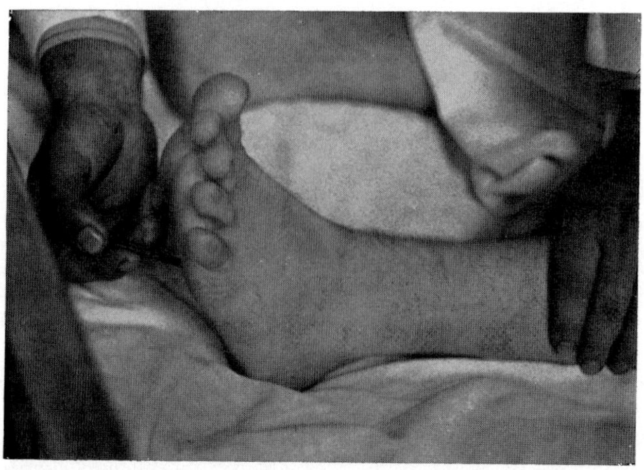

Fig. 5-2. Fanning of the toes as a component of the Babinski reflex. (Courtesy Dr. A. Ornsteen, Philadelphia.)

knee, and ankle. All are part of the *flexor withdrawal reflex*—an ipsilateral mass flexion movement—except the Babinski reflex, which is foreign to the flexor withdrawal reflex.

Latent reflexes. Interruption of the pyramidal tract not only results in an increase in deep muscle reflexes but also brings to the fore some latent reflexes that normally are not easily elicitable. When obtained, they are indicative of a pyramidal tract lesion only if they are very pronounced or if unilateral.

To elicit the *finger flexor reflex,* the examiner places his middle and index fingers across the tips of the patient's slightly bent four fingers and taps his own fingers lightly with a percussion hammer (Fig. 5-3). The ensuing flexion of the patient's four fingers as well as the end-phalanx of the thumb can be seen and felt (*Wartenberg's sign*). Another way of eliciting the finger flexor reflex is for the examiner to hold the middle phalanx of the patient's middle finger between his own second and third fingers and with a rapid flick of his thumb nip the nail of the patient's finger, thus suddenly flexing the finger; then the examiner releases it. The reflex consists in flexion of the other fingers, including the thumb (*Hoffmann's sign*). The response may also be obtained by tapping the distal end of the radius.

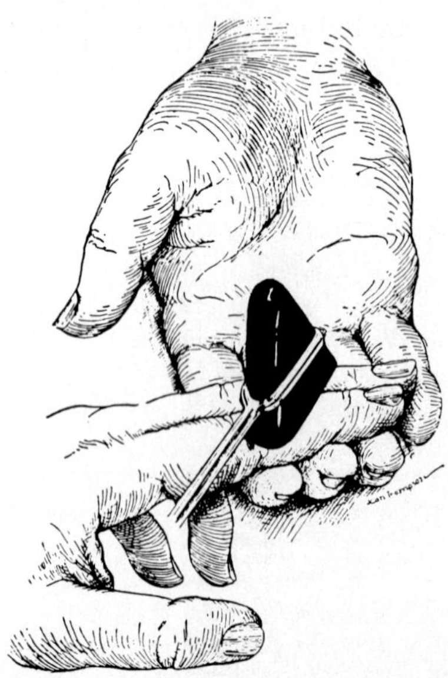

Fig. 5-3. Method of elicitation of the finger-flexion reflex. (From Wartenberg, 1945.)

To elicit the *toe flexor reflex* (latent deep plantar muscle reflex), the examiner taps the lateral aspect of the dorsum of the patient's foot *(Mendel-Bechterew's sign)* or taps the pulps of the patient's toes, displacing them upward *(Rossolimo's sign).* Stretching of the toe flexors is thus brought about; the response consists in flexion of the toes.

Associated movements. Associated movements are involuntary accompaniments of all normal voluntary motor acts. For instance, on making a fist, dorsal flexion of the hand occurs. Pathological associated movements occur as components of the spastic syndrome. Impulses from (intact) subcorticospinal tracts appear to bring the movements about. Examples of pathological associated movements of lateralizing or localizing importance are given in the following.

The patient, lying supine with his legs outstretched, is asked to lift the affected leg against resistance. The examiner opposes the movement by placing his hand on the patient's knee. In spastic paresis the foot assumes a position of dorsiflexion and supination during this maneuver; the tendon of the tibialis anterior muscle stands out sharply *(tibialis sign of Strümpell).* In a normal person thus tested the foot undergoes plantar flexion.

The patient, lying supine with his legs abducted and his arms across his chest, attempts to rise to a sitting position. In the unilateral spastic syndrome the thigh of the paretic side flexes in association with flexion of the trunk, and as a result the limb rises involuntarily and the heel is raised from the bed. Normally during this maneuver the legs remain motionless and the heels are kept pressed down. In the bilateral spastic syndrome both legs rise (*trunk-thigh sign of Babinski*).

When the patient bends his four fingers firmly against resistance offered by the examiner (or flexes his fingers around an object), the thumb undergoes adduction, flexion, and opposition (*Wartenberg's sign*). Normally the thumb remains in abduction and extension.

When the patient elevates and extends his paretic arm, involuntary hyperextension and spreading of the fingers occur (*interosseous phenomenon of Souques*). This does not normally occur.

Muscle atrophy. See p. 33.

Chronic circulatory disturbance. See p. 36.

Pathological processes giving rise to the spastic syndrome. Spinal cord compression by anteriorly situated tumor may affect the pyramidal tract selectively and thus give rise to the spastic syndrome. The same is true for prolapsed intervertebral disk; an explanation offered is that the lateral pyramidal tract is affected because of traction exerted on the lateral part of the cord through stretching of dentate ligaments incident to disk prolapse (Kahn, 1947). Multiple sclerosis may also be responsible for selective pyramidal tract involvement; occasionally, stiffness of the limbs is complained of as an initial symptom (Carter, Sciarra, and Merritt, 1950). In lathyrism the pyramidal tracts are characteristically affected. Paraplegia usually develops suddenly. Sensory loss is said not to occur, although lesions have been noted in the anterior and posterior columns postmortem (Pentschew, 1958). Intrinsic degeneration of the pyramidal tract bilaterally (primary lateral sclerosis) can also be a basis of the spastic syndrome in cases in which amyotrophic lateral sclerosis does not subsequently develop (Stark and Moersch, 1945). Strümpell-Lorrain's familial spastic paraplegia also falls under the category of selective involvement of the corticospinal tracts (Fontaine and others, 1969; Ozsváth, 1968; Schwarz and Liu, 1956).

Manifestations of anterior horn lesions

The muscles affected by anterior horn lesions are at first completely paralyzed. In time, however, a certain degree of restitution of function occurs in those muscle fibers innervated by anterior horn cells which were not directly damaged.

Seldom do anterior horn lesions implicate all the muscles of an extremity. The reasons are the following: (1) at any given transverse level the anterior horns contain segregated cell groups scattered over a considerable area, each supplying its separate groups of muscles—no lesion is likely to destroy all the cell groups; (2) the cell groups supplying the muscle of a limb may be separated in the longitudinal plane by as much as a few centimeters—lesions of the spinal cord are seldom that widespread.

A lesion situated in an anterior horn frequently spares the neighboring pyramidal tracts and thus gives rise to an uncomplicated paralysis of the peripheral type. This is true for certain virus infections such as poliomyelitis and Japanese B encephalomyelitis and for certain degenerative diseases such as hereditary spinal muscular atrophy (*Werdnig-Hoffmann disease*) (Byers and Banker, 1961).

Motoneuron damage from anterior horn lesions is characterized as follows.

Flaccid paralysis. There is weakness of voluntary movement owing to a reduction in the number of available functioning motor units. The paralyzed muscles are atonic due to interruption of nerve impulses necessary for the maintenance of the inherent elastic tension of muscle. Atonia manifests itself by decreased resistance to passive movements, by looseness of movements at joints owing to deprivation of muscular support, by the ease with which passive hyperextension at various joints can be performed, and by an increased range of movement that allows the examiner to place the patient's limbs in contortionist positions. Muscles that are completely atonic no longer manifest irritability in response to direct mechanical stimuli.

Abolition of reflexes. Abolition of reflexes is due to interruption of the centrifugal limb of the spinal reflex arc.

Lack of pathological reflexes. The Babinski reflex, for example, is not elicitable.

Lack of pathological associated movements. Such movements are dependent on integrity of the lower motor neuron.

Vasomotor disturbances. Vasomotor disturbances occur much more frequently and are far more pronounced in anterior horn lesions than in pyramidal tract lesions. One reason is that the (sympathetic) vaso-

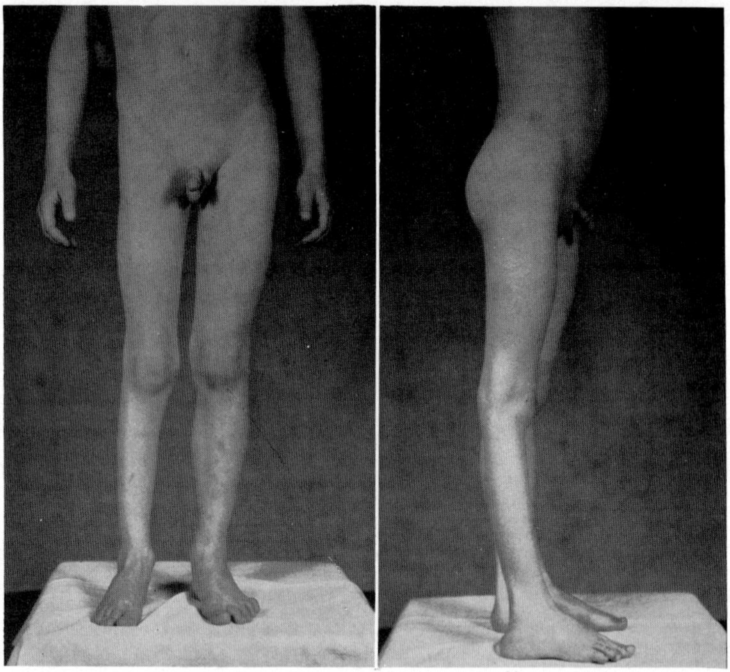

Fig. 5-4. Muscular atrophy of the right hip, thigh, and lower leg due to destruction of anterior horn cells in acute poliomyelitis. Pelvic tilt is also visible. (From 98th Gen. Hosp.; Negs. 777—1 and 2.)

motor cell groups in the gray matter of the cord are more compact than the vasomotor fibers in the lateral column and thus are more vulnerable.

Muscle atrophy, fasciculation, and reaction of degeneration. Degenerative atrophy, fasciculation, and reaction of degeneration develop fairly rapidly in the muscles supplied by the damaged anterior horn cells but are preceded by weakness in voluntary movement. Atrophy of the muscles of the lower limb in poliomyelitis is illustrated in Fig. 5-4.

Disturbances due to combined pyramidal tract and anterior horn lesions

Combined pyramidal tract and anterior horn involvement is exemplified in *amyotrophic lateral sclerosis* (Fig. 5-5). In this disorder the clinical picture is dominated by muscle paralysis. Most of the affected muscles are completely paralyzed and show atrophy and reaction of degeneration (R.D.). Before the R.D. has given way to a complete lack of reaction, certain phenomena indicate that the pyramidal tracts and, in about a third of cases, cells in areas 4 and 6 of the cerebral cortex (Davison, 1949) are undergoing degeneration. Thus, in relatively early stages the reflexes are exaggerated and irritability to direct mechanical stimuli is increased. When the lower limb is involved, various pathological reflexes such as the Babinski reflex may be elicitable for a time. As to the anterior horns in earlier stages, degenerative changes in their cells are associated with successive, isolated contractions of fiber bundles (fasciculations). The contractions have the rapidity of lightning and are plainly perceptible both by inspection and palpation.

Degeneration of bulbar nuclei and of the corticobulbar system is part of this disorder, the structures most affected being the tongue, orbicularis oris, palate, and extrinsic muscles of the pharynx and larynx (p. 164). The disease may be hereditary and appear as an entity (Kurland and Mulder, 1955; Thomson and Alvarez, 1969)

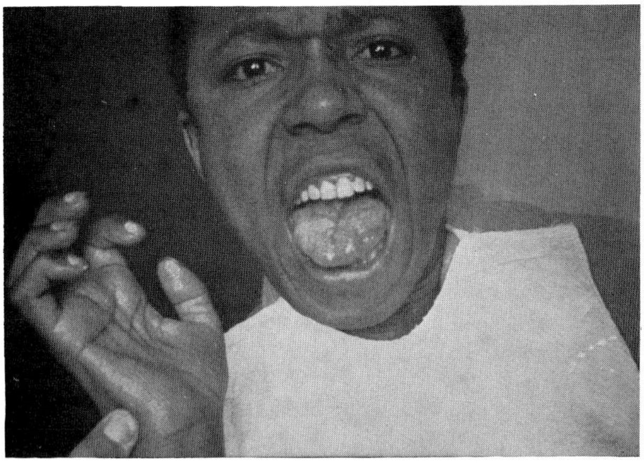

Fig. 5-5. Amyotrophic lateral sclerosis. Predominant atrophy of the extensor muscles has resulted in "claw hand." The tongue is also atrophic. (Courtesy Dr. A. Ornsteen, Philadelphia.)

Table 5-1. Clinical features of lesions of the lateral column, anterior horn, both lateral column and anterior horn

Lateral column	*Anterior horn*	*Combined*
Paresis	Paralysis	Paralysis predominates
Diffuse distribution	Distribution confined to individual muscles	Diffuse distribution
Hypertonia	Atonia	Suggestive hypertonia initially, then atonia
Hyperreflexia	Areflexia	Hyperreflexia giving way to areflexia
No muscle fasciculation	Muscle fasciculation	Muscle fasciculation
Associated movements frequent	No associated movements	Occasional associated movements
Pathological reflexes usually elicitable (Babinski, etc.)	No pathological reflexes	Pathological reflexes; subsequently not elicitable
No muscle atrophy	Muscle atrophy	Muscle atrophy
No reaction of degeneration	Reaction of degeneration	Reaction of degeneration

or in combination with parkinsonism (p. 429) or other disorders.

Differential diagnosis between lateral column lesions, anterior horn lesions, and a combination of the two is listed in Table 5-1.

DISTURBANCES IN SENSIBILITY

Some spinal pathways conveying sensory impulses are illustrated in Figs. 1-3 and 1-8. The essential points are the following:

1. Tactile fibers pass up the ipsilateral posterior column and the contralateral anterolateral column.
2. Pain and temperature fibers ascend in the contralateral lateral spinothalamic tract.
3. Fibers conveying deep sensibility extend up the ipsilateral posterior column.
4. Proprioceptive impulses not reaching the level of consciousness pass up the ipsilateral lateral and posterior columns to reach the cerebellum.

From these data the sites of lesions can be deduced as follows.

Posterior root lesions. In complete interruption of posterior roots all forms of sensibility in the innervated region are lost. If interruption is incomplete, sensibility will merely be diminished. The disturbances are in the realm of cutaneous sensibility (faulty appreciation of touch, pain, and temperature) and deep sensibility (ataxia, stereoanesthesia, faulty appreciation of passive movement, defective two-point discrimination, inability to appreciate vibration, and impairment of the ability to recognize numerals written on the skin). Appreciation of vibration of a tuning fork may be diminished or lost when all other forms of sensibility are intact, and thus pallanesthesia is a particularly sensitive index of posterior root and posterior (or lateral) column lesions.

Spinal cord lesions involving tracts carrying pain and thermal impulses. Interruption of these tracts in their course through the gray matter or in the lateral column is manifested by analgesia and thermoanesthesia. Since fibers carrying tactile impulses accompany the pain and temperature fibers through the gray matter and lie adjacent to them in the white matter, it might be expected that a lesion in either location would interfere with tactile as well as with pain and temperature sensibility. Because of the double route taken by tactile fibers up the cord (Fig. 1-8), this is, however, usually not the case. Loss of pain and temperature sensibilities and preservation of all other forms of sensibility are pathognomonic of a lesion situated centrally in the spinal cord or in the posterior horn. Conditions under which this form of dissociated sensibility is observed include syringomyelia (Fig. 5-6), hematomyelia, and certain intramedullary tumors.

So far as *syringomyelia* is concerned, the syrinx usually develops in the gray matter in the region dorsolateral to the central canal and spreads into the ventral part of posterior horn and/or the dorsal part of the anterior horn, and across the midline dorsal to the central canal. The lower cervical region is the site usually affected initially. With enlargement of the syrinx, other structures become affected such as the posterior column and the anterior horn. In early stages, pains, which may be severe, commonly occur in various af-

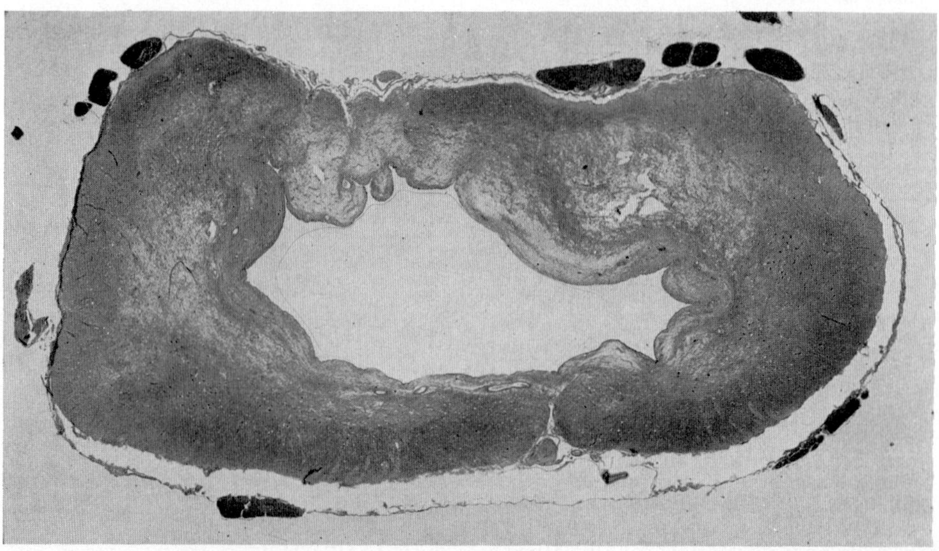

Fig. 5-6. Far advanced syringomyelia. Lower cervical region. In earlier stages the patient had dissociated anesthesia and atrophy of muscles of the hand. At the stage illustrated, signs of pyramidal tract and posterior column damage were also evident. (From the Scholz Collection, AFIP Acc. 312166-V14.)

fected regions such as the fingers or arm. Soon thereafter pain and thermal sensibility are lost, while tactile and deep sensibility are little if at all altered. Not uncommonly, all fingers and the hands are affected up to the wrist. The basis of this peculiar distribution is obscure but can perhaps be attributed to interruption of pain and temperature fibers (from the three or four segments implicated) both in the posterior horn and in the region ventral to the central canal.

Occasionally only the perception of deep pain is lost, the distribution being the same as already mentioned—not limited to the distribution of specific dermatomes. In such a case, in which the hands were involved, it was suggested that fibers conveying deep pain sensibility up the cord, might, like other sensory fibers, be laminated, with the lamina conveying deep sensibility situated nearer the anterior horn than the lamina conveying superficial pain, thus more vulnerable (Magee and Schneider, 1967). In this connection it is proposed that some fibers conveying deep sensibility are situated ventromedially in the lateral spinothalamic tract at the cervical level (Yoss, 1953). Moreover, in cases of syringomyelia in which the lateral column of the cord was compressed by the syrinx, pallanesthesia was noted in association with intact position sense, from which it was concluded that vibratory stimuli are conveyed upward in the more medial part of the lateral column (Netsky, 1953).

Insensitivity to pain and defective appreciation of warm or cold may occur congenitally.

In such a case, in which the loss was universal, Lissauer's tract was found absent, and the spinal tract of the fifth nerve much depleted. On the other hand, the substantia gelatinosa and the nucleus of the spinal tract of the fifth nerve appeared normal. Large myelinated fibers were found in the posterior roots but hardly any smaller fibers, an observation consistent with the clinical findings. (Swanson, 1963; Swanson, Buchan, and Alvord, 1963.)

Lateral spinothalamic tract lesions. The position of the spinothalamic tracts shifts dorsally as the tracts ascend. Lamination of the lateral spinothalamic tract is such that at a high cervical level the fibers from the sacral region are most lateral in the tract; medial to them, in turn, are the fibers from the lumbar and the thoracic regions, and most medial the fibers from the lower cervical region (Fig. 1-4). Thus the lateral fibers of the tract convey impulses from the lower extremity, the intermediate fibers from the trunk, and the medial fibers from the upper extremity and neck. This anatomical arrangement accounts for the fact that in progressively enlarging extraspinal intradural masses that compress the lateral aspect of the cervical cord, reduction in pain and temperature sensibility occurs initially in the lower limb, then upward in the order indicated. Moreover, fibers conveying thermal impulses occupy the dorsal half of the lateral spinothalamic tract and pain-conveying fibers occupy the ventral half, so that either one or the other or both groups of fibers may be chiefly affected by an extraspinal compressive mass.

Disturbances in tactile sensibility. In a destructive lesion limited to the posterior column, the appreciation of touch may be reduced. If in high cord lesions the damage is limited to the fasciculus gracilis, the reduction in tactile sensibility will be noted only over the lower half of the body, and if limited to the fasciculus cuneatus, then only over the upper half of the body (Fig. 1-4). Tactile anesthesia is most often due to interruption of peripheral nerves or spinal posterior roots. For tactile anesthesia over one side of the body to occur as a result of intramedullary injury, the posterior column ipsilaterally and the anterior spinothalamic tract contralaterally would have to be interrupted.

Ataxia together with loss of deep sensibility. This combination occurs in degenerative states involving the posterior column—ataxia from interruption of fibers passing to the cerebellum via the lateral cuneate nucleus, and loss of deep sensibility from interruption of fibers passing up to the thalamus.

Friedreich's ataxia is an apt example, both ataxia and loss of deep sensibility being characteristic of the disorder. Although Friedreich (1863) emphasized posterior column degeneration as the basis of the disorder, reports by subsequent workers have indicated that the spinocerebellar tracts and sometimes the pyramidal tracts are also affected. A variant is illustrated in Fig. 5-7. In Friedreich's ataxia, a degenerative process in large cell bodies in posterior root ganglia occurs initially. In time, these cell bodies undergo atrophy and disappear. Proximally and distally, thin myelinated fibers are no longer seen, large myelinated fibers become strikingly depleted, then vanish, whereas nonmyelinated fibers persist and appear normal.

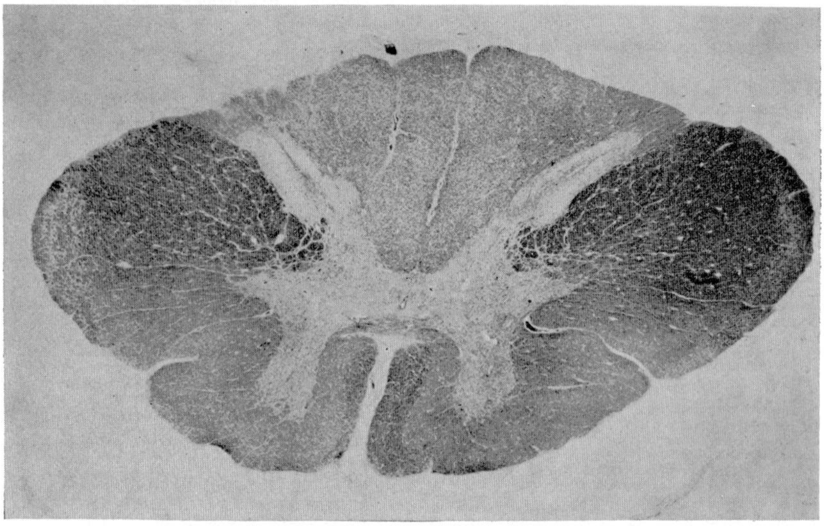

Fig. 5-7. Hereditary ataxia, with manifestations of Friedreich's ataxia. Lower cervical level. Myelin has disappeared from the posterior columns, anterior columns (especially in the anterior corticospinal tracts), ventral part of the dorsal spinocerebellar tract, and ventral spinocerebellar tract. (From Schut and Haymaker, 1951.)

Posterior roots become fibrosed. Appreciation of joint position, two-point distances, and pallesthesia all suffer heavily in this disease; recognition of shape and form and appreciation of size and weight are less affected; while appreciation of touch, pain, and temperature is little if at all altered. (Hughes, Brownell, and Hewer, 1968.)

Ataxia of spinal cord origin is distinguishable from ataxia of cerebellar origin. In cerebellar ataxia, individual movements are performed with much more accuracy than in the posterior column ataxia; however, in cerebellar ataxia the ability to coordinate individual movements (to produce synergic movement), is more severely compromised. Such coordination (or mutual participation of muscles in a movement) is requisite to the performance of locomotion, as it is also to the maintenance of static relationships. Thus, the patient with cerebellar ataxia walks on a broad base in zigzag fashion, and his trunk sways when he sits upright.

In interruption of posterior column fibers both postural sensibility and pallesthesia (appreciation of vibration) suffer. One may, however, be more affected than the other. Thus, in lesions involving thoracic and lumbar segments, pallesthesia may be impaired earlier and more strikingly than position sense, while in lesions involving the upper cervical cord or the dorsal part of the lower medulla oblongata, the reverse may be true (Weinstein and Bender, 1940). In destructive lesions limited to the nuclei gracilis and cuneatus and immediate environs there may be ataxia together with disturbances of deep sensibility, including stereoanesthesia. Tumors in the lower part of the fourth ventricle may give rise to the same syndrome (David and Askenasy, 1937).

Sensory irritative phenomena. Disease processes involving posterior root fibers up to their zone of entry into the spinal cord or in their course up the cord tend to induce spontaneous severe pains that are often cutting or tearing in nature. Such pains, present in early stages when interruption is minimal, are projected not to the overlying spine but to the periphery, that is, to the area of skin (later also to the regional musculature and periosteum) in which the sensory end-organs of the irritated fibers are situated. A patient having such pains is best able to indicate their location when an individual spinal root, or a pair of roots,

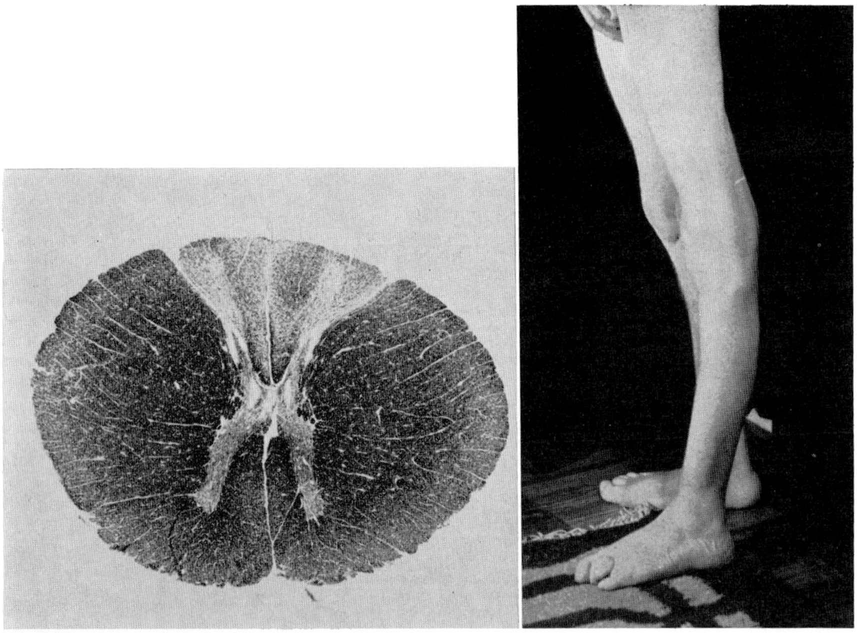

Fig. 5-8. Tabes dorsalis. **A,** Degeneration of the posterior columns as seen at a thoracic level. The site of origin of the degeneration in this disease is in the posterior roots. (From the Scholz Collection, AFIP Acc. 312166-V14.) **B,** Genu recurvatum in tabes dorsalis. (Courtesy Dr. A. Ornsteen, Philadelphia.)

is involved, as in circumscribed neoplasms in the vicinity or in such conditions as cervical hypertrophic pachymeningitis or tuberculous spondylitis.

Posterior root involvement is frequently bilateral, as may be expected from the closeness of the roots to the median plane. When roots at lower thoracic levels are implicated, girdle pains frequently occur. The root pains of herpes zoster are of posterior root ganglion origin. In hemorrhagic or traumatic lesions within the spinal cord, the site of pain at the periphery is ill defined; a rather wide cutaneous area is painful because of involvement of fibers at several root levels.

Root pains are projected to totally anesthetic cutaneous regions only rarely, and then only briefly, coincident with acute root damage. Under such circumstances, even though conduction from the periphery is interrupted, the central stumps of the interrupted posterior roots are sensitive to irritative influences and hence are capable of transmitting pain impulses. Such a state, known as *anesthesia dolorosa,* may persist for a day or two until wallerian degeneration sets in. Anesthesia dolorosa may also be due to acute lesions of sensory tracts of the spinal cord.

Dysesthesias and paresthesias are also included among sensory irritative disturbances.

Combined ataxia, sensory loss, and sensory irritative phenomena. Tabes dorsalis is a classic example of this combination of disorders. Lower thoracic and lumbar roots are chiefly affected. Large myelinated (fast conducting) fibers suffer, as manifested by degenerative changes in the posterior column (Fig. 5-8, *A*), and reflected in pallanesthesia and disturbances in the appreciation of the position of a toe or other part. Fibers concerned in reflex activity passing from the posterior roots to the anterior horn cells are also interrupted, resulting in loss of the ankle-jerk, then the knee-jerk and other deep reflexes. The hypotonia that occurs may also be due to interruption of these fibers. Hypotonia predominating in the muscles of the anterior part of the thigh leads to *genu recurvatum* (Fig. 5-8, *B*). Deep pain sensibility suffers early. The Achilles tendon is no longer painful to pinching (*Abadie's sign*), and the same applies to the ulnar nerve (*Biernacki's sign*) and the testes. Superficial pain sensibility is also impaired, the loss occurring initially in such areas as the side of the nose, the ulnar border of the upper limb, the outer border of the leg, and the dorsum and sole of the foot. Even when pain can be appreciated in such areas, it is felt only after a delay of several seconds following application of a painful stimulus. The inference is that the "fast" pain fibers are selectively interrupted, and that the "slow" pain fibers convey the pain impulses. Reduction in tactile sensibility in the feet and legs is noted ultimately in about a third of cases (Leimbach, 1895). Lancinating pains, usually in the lower limbs and less commonly in the trunk (girdle pains) and upper limbs, and "crises," especially gastric, are common in tabes dorsalis. Progressive destruction of pain fibers, causing bursts of impulses to be generated in fibers that remain viable, may be the basis.

COMBINED MOTOR AND SENSORY DISTURBANCES

Lesions involving both the posterior and the lateral column

A familiar example of selective involvement of the posterior and lateral columns is subacute combined degeneration of the cord, occurring as a complication of pernicious anemia (Fig. 5-9). Much the same change may be encountered in alimentary vitamin B_{12} deficiency (Verjaal and Timmermans-van den Bos, 1967), as it may in total or partial gastrectomy (Olivarius and Roos, 1968). Several years usually

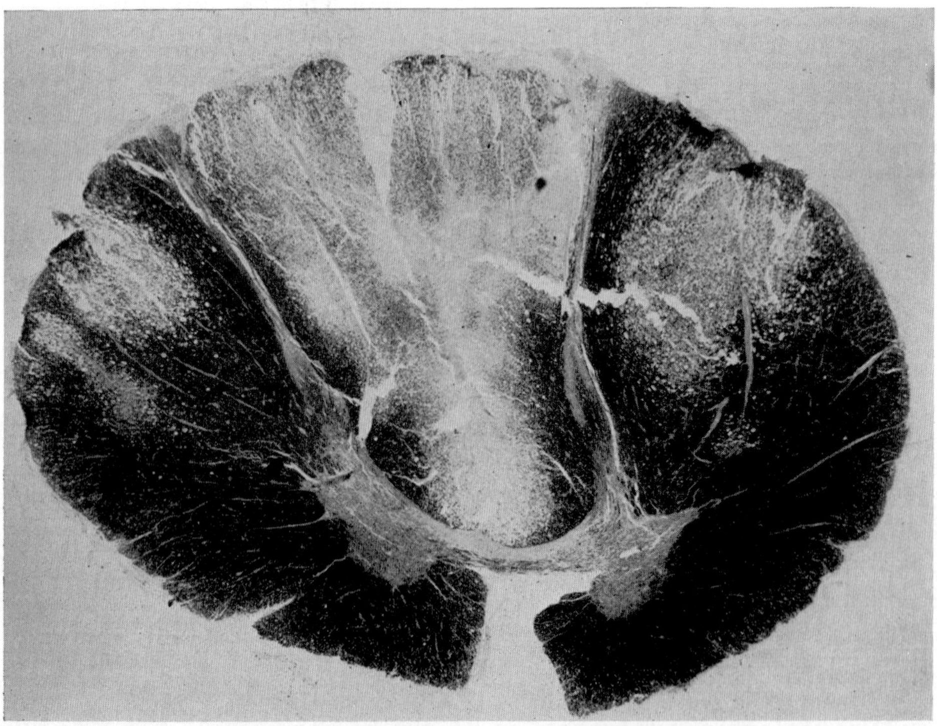

Fig. 5-9. Subacute combined degeneration of the cord in association with pernicious anemia. Lower cervical level. There is severe degeneration of the posterior columns and the lateral pyramidal tracts. (From the Scholz Collection, AFIP Acc. 312166-T 13.)

pass before the myelopathy sets in. Similarly, in chronic meningitis the posterior and lateral columns may be the most vulnerable. Clinically, the dominant manifestations under any of these conditions are ataxia, reduction in deep sensibility, and muscle paresis. If the pyramidal tracts are predominantly affected, there will be spastic-ataxic paraplegia with relatively less pronounced disturbances of sensibility, and if the posterior columns are most affected there will be ataxia, motor weakness, areflexia, and disturbances in deep sensibility. Under either condition, reflexes pathognomonic of a pyramidal tract lesion may be elicited. Their elicitation in a patient with signs of advanced posterior column damage provides the evidence that the lateral column is also damaged.

Transverse lesions of the spinal cord

"Distant" effects. Damage of the cord in the transverse plane may present difficulties in localization of the level primarily affected when occurring in missile wounds, spinal concussion, fracture-dislocation of a vertebra, and in other forms of acute injury. This is because of "distant" effects.

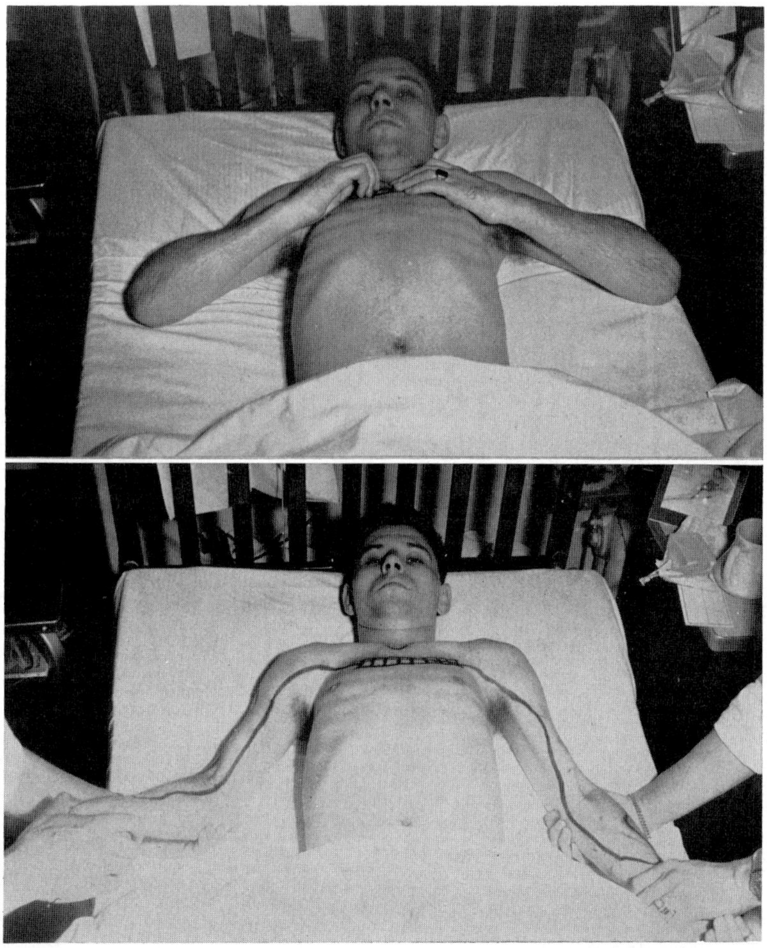

Fig. 5-10. Upper level of sensory loss at cord segment C6, in fracture-dislocation of vertebra C2. There is flexion-contraction of the upper limbs owing to contraction of the unaffected biceps brachii and brachialis (innervated mainly by cord segment C5) in the presence of paralysis of their antagonist, the triceps brachii (innervated mainly by cord segment C7). (From Walter Reed Army Hospital.)

Sensory and motor functions above the level of spinal transection are commonly suppressed—for example, in the region of supply of segments Th4 to C7 when the transverse lesion is at Th5. Such suppression, the cause of which is obscure (perhaps damage of spinal roots in the region of their ascent), usually last no longer than 2 weeks. By contrast, the site of greatest cord damage may lie a considerable distance below the injured level—for example, an upper level of sensory loss at C6 following fracture-dislocation of vertebra CII (Fig. 5-10). Such "distant" effects appear to be contingent on circulatory deficit in regions of apposition of arterial beds in the cord. Segment Th4 has been found to be the site of predilection of ischemic necrosis under a number of conditions: in vertebral subluxation at cord levels C5 and C6, in spinal concussion, and in tumor of upper cervical segments. L1 is another vulnerable segment. A transverse lesion has been noted at this level following penetration of a bullet into segment Th8. (Garcin and others, 1962; Zülch, 1962, 1967.)

In both the transverse and the longitudinal plane of the spinal cord the base of the posterior column and adjoining gray matter are sites vulnerable to the development of ischemic necrosis; the ventral part of the posterior horn is also vulnerable (Fig. 5-11). Involved are the region of apposition of the beds of the sulcocommissural artery (derived from the anterior spinal artery) and the dorsal penetrating branches of the posterior spinal artery. The closer the involved segments to a major segmental artery, the smaller the infarct (Zülch, 1967). Fairly often in occlusion of superficial spinal arteries consequent to spinal cord compression or to local trauma, hemorrhagic infarction of the central part of the cord extends for a considerable distance, usually a greater distance downward than upward. This condition may be misdiagnosed as hematomyelia. In cases of this kind the white matter of the periphery of the cord, particularly that of the lateral columns, may also suffer (Bartsch, 1954; Zülch, 1967).

"Distant" effects may also complicate traumatic paraplegia. A year or more (even 14 years) may pass, following injury of the thoracic or lumbar cord, before manifestations of a lesion involving contiguous lower or higher levels appear. This was noted in paraplegics in World War I by Holmes (1915). In transection at L1-L2, for instance, pain may first appear in the hand, and be followed by hypalgesia at levels below C5. Thermoanesthesia and hypalgesia at the new levels may accompany the pain. In some cases the spinal nucleus of the fifth nerve becomes affected, and Horner's syndrome may be noted, as in syringomyelia. All the changes may be unilateral or bilateral. Delayed distant effects such as these occur in 1 to 2 percent of patients with traumatic paraplegia. The

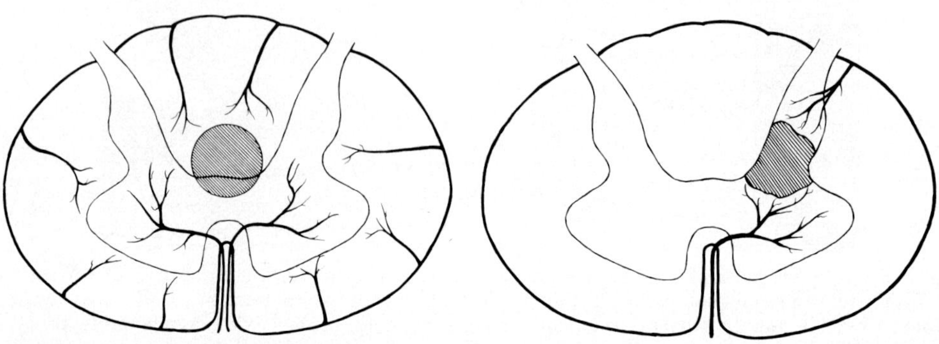

Fig. 5-11. Sites of predilection of infarction in the cord in ischemic states. (From Zülch, 1967.)

disorder is not known to occur in persons with nontraumatic paraplegia. The base of the posterior horn and adjoining posterior column and corticospinal tract appear most affected; a syrinx may be found in this region. Pathogenesis is obscure. Apparently, transuded fluid accumulates in the traumatized part of the cord and, under pressure, extends upward (or downward) along planes of least resistance, causing perceptible damage only with the passage of time. (Barnett and others, 1966; Holmes, 1915; Klawans, 1968; Rossier and others, 1968.)

Traumatic paraplegia. Immediately following complete transection of the spinal cord, and also following partial transection if the cord is blocked, all voluntary movement is abolished. Sensibility up to the level of the transection and reflex activity as well are also lost. This is during the period of *spinal shock,* which appears to be due to loss of facilitation from descending tracts, persisting inhibition exercised by spinal segments beneath the level of transection acting upon extensor reflexes, and degeneration of the axons of interneurons. Spinal shock usually lasts 2 to 3 weeks, may vanish in 3 to 4 days, or may persist for as long as 6 weeks. Reflex activity is restored earliest (usually in 1 to 3 weeks): flexor earlier than extensor reflexes, superficial earlier than deep reflexes, distal earlier than the proximal reflexes. Crossed reflexes usually require about 3 months to appear. If the transection is partial, muscle function first returns proximally in the limbs. (Austin, 1961.)

Paraplegia-in-flexion or paraplegia-in-extension ultimately develops. Neither is an index of completeness or incompleteness of transection. Cervical transection tends to be succeeded by paraplegia-in-extension, upper thoracic transection by either type, and midthoracic transection by paraplegia-in-flexion (Austin, 1961). However, previous position assumed by the paralyzed limbs may determine the pattern of the reflex synergy. Prolonged fixation of the paralyzed limbs in adduction and semiflexion (by placing pillows under the knees) promotes flexor spasms and thus favors the development of paraplegia-in-flexion. Conversely, factors effectual in facilitating extensor activity are: maintaining the paralyzed limbs in a position of abduction and extension, with the patient lying supine; keeping the patient in a prone position; instituting passive movements early; and restoring the upright position, in particular having the patient stand between parallel bars. (Guttmann, 1946, 1952.)

Among the reflex synergies that become established soon after spinal transection are movements of the great toe in response to plantar stimulation. Contraction of the extensor hallucis longus following plantar stimulation is one of the regular components both of extensor and flexor synergies (Marshall, 1954; Pollock and others, 1951; Riddoch, 1917), although a flexor response of the great toe may prevail for the first week or two or even longer (Grimby, 1965). Increase in the reflexogenous zone occurs in the paralyzed part after some weeks have passed, such that (in complete transection) plantar stimulation on either side leads to flexion synergy of the entire lower limb (withdrawal movement) and, if the transection is in the lower cervical region, to contraction of the ipsilateral trunk muscles and of the paralyzed finger and thumb extensors of the same or even of the opposite side (Foerster, 1936; Guttmann, 1952; Riddoch, 1917).

Transition from muscle flaccidity to the spasticity of paraplegia appears to be due to the growth of new axons in the affected part of the cord. Boutons terminaux are normally arranged along the surface of the perikaryon of interneurons. Following loss of boutons owing to degeneration of descending tracts, remaining terminals, chiefly those of afferent fibers, appear to sprout new boutons that may fill the gaps. Electrophysiological studies following cord hemisection in animals have indicated that the potential attributed to afferent terminals is significantly increased on the side of the hemisection. (Austin and McCouch, 1955; Liu and Chambers, 1958; McCouch and others, 1958.)

In some cases of paraplegia the paralysis

remains of the flaccid type (the muscles fail to show reflex synergies) and areflexia persists. This adynamia may occur in the region of distribution of a few segments below the level of the transection or in the entire paralyzed region. Under such condition the muscles are severely atrophic and show R.D. to electrical testing, indicating profound damage of the gray matter in the longitudinal plane. Ischemic necrosis of the cord or hematomyelia may be responsible. (Guttmann, 1946, 1952.)

Partial versus complete transection of the spinal cord

Points helpful in distinguishing between partial and total transection of the spinal cord are the following.

In partial transection the paralysis is not as symmetrical as in total transection, and the sensory defects are not as complete. Voluntary movement tends to return during the first week only if the transection is partial. In partial transection, the paralysis and anesthesia are incongruous, the area of paralysis being larger than the area of anesthesia. In complete transection, by contrast, the areas of paralysis and anesthesia tend to be congruous, or identical.

The reflexogenous zone for the elicitation of flexor responses is smaller in partial than in complete transections.

Flexor spasms are infrequent in partial transection but are common in complete transection.

Vasomotor and sphincter disturbances are less pronounced in partial than in complete transection.

In partial transection of higher cord segments the quadriceps femoris reflexes are usually exaggerated. If absent they are soon restored. In partial transection the reflexes on the two sides usually differ in degree.

If the patient exhibits a flexor-withdrawal reflex, the examiner should ascertain whether or not after the withdrawal the limb again extends. Flexor withdrawal only (the one-phase reaction) suggests that the transection is complete. If after the withdrawal the limb returns to its original position (the two-phase reaction) the transection is likely to be incomplete.

If pressure applied to the bottom of the foot of a limb passively flexed at all joints precipitates alternate (marching) movements in the two legs, the transection is, without question, incomplete.

In regions distal to the level of the lesion, irritative phenomena are more pronounced in partial than in complete transection. These are mostly sensory in nature and include pains, paresthesias, anesthesia dolorosa, hyperesthesia, and hyperkinesias. In general, all these disturbances are infrequent.

Complete flaccid paraplegia with areflexia together with complete sensory loss lasting longer than 5 days after injury signifies total transection.

Spinal cord involvement of miscellaneous cause

Neurosyphilis takes on protean forms—tabes dorsalis (already discussed), meningomyelitis, pachymeningitis, spastic paraplegia, and amyotrophy. In the *meningomyelitic form,* occurring in the secondary stage of syphilitic infection, the pathological process is indiscriminate as to spinal level(s) affected. The lumbosacral enlargement tends, however, to be most affected. The infective process extends via vascular sheaths into white matter, also into gray matter. Infarction occurs and may be manifested by the Brown-Séquard syndrome or by disturbances indicating a transverse lesion or lower motoneuron destruction (Sträussler, 1958). *Syphilitic pachymeningitis* is characterized by a hypertrophic gummatous process. Vessels may be occluded, resulting in infarction of the spinal cord, which leads to degeneration of the anterior and posterior roots of the affected segments. Root pains and paresthesias are presenting symptoms and are followed by sensory loss and muscle atrophy. When occurring at the cervical level (*pachymeningitis cervicalis hypertrophica*) the medulla oblongata is also involved, and Horner's syndrome may be evident. In syphilitic pachymeningitis paraplegia usually results (Gellerstedt, 1956). In *syphilitic spastic paraplegia* the posterolateral columns of white matter bear the brunt of the damage. Paraparesis precedes the paraplegia. Bladder function suffers early and may overshadow all other disturbances in severity (Hughes, 1966). *Syphilitic amyotrophy* is usually a complication of meningovasculitis in which anterior spinal roots suffer heavily. The upper limbs are chiefly affected. Here, severe pains often precede the development of muscle atrophy. Sensory loss and sphincter disturbances also occur. The muscle atrophy is unilateral or bilateral and begins in the small muscles of the hand, in the shoulder girdle, or, less commonly, in the legs. The deep reflexes are abolished. In some cases, amyotrophic lateral sclerosis is simulated. In contrast to the muscular state in that disease, in syphilitic amyotrophy the muscles are atonic. (Mackay and Hall, 1933; Martin, 1925.) Syphilitic amyotrophy may occur after apparently successful treatment in primary syphilis (Hewitt, 1967).

Diabetic amyotrophy is manifested by weakness and wasting of proximal muscle groups of rapid onset in patients with poorly controlled diabetes mellitus. The involvement may be either bilaterally equal or asymmetrical on the two sides. Muscles of the pelvic girdle or the shoulder are usually first affected. Distal hypesthesia, paresthesias, and altered pallesthesia (acroneuropathy) may be accompaniments. Extensor plantar responses are elicited in some cases. Protein in the cerebrospinal fluid is usually increased. Muscle fasciculation does not occur, but fibrillation has been noted electromyographically, substantiating the view that the disorder may, in fact, be an amyotrophy, not purely a peripheral nerve degenerative state. (Hamilton, Dobson and Marshall, 1968; Jones and Walsh, 1965.)

Generalized arteriosclerotic disease is a more common cause of myelopathy than previously suspected, especially in the aged. It is not so much the sclerosis involving spinal arteries that leads to myelopathy as it is the atherosclerosis of vessels feeding the spinal cord, such that blood flow to the cord is reduced. Reduction in blood flow in any of the feeding arteries listed in Table 1-1 may be responsible for cord damage. The myelopathy, when it occurs, is characterized by diverse syndromes—distal amyotrophy, atypical paraparesis or quadriparesis without sensory disturbances, and incomplete transverse cord damage. Neuralgic pains in association with monoparesis are occasionally noted. Local atheroma of the anterior spinal artery is infrequent and usually slight (incidence in the aged, 2.6 percent) (Mannen, 1966) but may be a factor in infarction of the cord. In such cases the infarction usually occurs at spinal level C5 or C6 (Garland, Greenberg, and Harriman, 1966; Jellinger, 1967; Zeitlin and Lichtenstein, 1936).

Progressive myelopathy involving white matter or both white and gray matter can occur at various levels of the cord. In lumbosacral segments (Gruner and Lapresle, 1962) the disorder occurs in association with a severely atheromatous abdominal aorta under conditions in which the tributaries are neither thrombosed nor otherwise occluded, although the mouths of the relevant arteries (lumbar arteries) are usually buried in the plaques of ulcerating atheroma (Hughes and Brownell, 1964; Jellinger and Neumayer, 1962). Dissecting aneurysm of the aorta is also a cause of progressive myelopathy involving the lumbosacral region. Surgically induced aortic occlusion may also lead to cord damage if the occlusion is above the renal level (Adams and van Geertruyden, 1956). Lower cervical and upper thoracic segments (C5-Th3) may suffer as a consequence of stenosis of the vertebral arteries (Jellinger, 1967; Mannen, 1966), the result of inadequate blood supply from the vertebrals and subclavian arteries above, and the aorta below. Cord damage may also follow occlusion of intercostal and lumbar arteries during thoracoplasty, pneumonectomy, or thoracolumbar sympathectomy, or may result from obstruction of radicular tributaries by malignant tumor infiltrating intervertebral foramina (Hughes, 1966). A mass in the upper thorax that compresses the artery running along root Th3 (Fig. 1-9) can also be the basis of cord damage, as can trauma of the posterior mediastinum that interferes with blood flow in this artery (Lindenberg, 1957). Furthermore, cord damage can occur in the presence of a mass in the region of the upper thorax that compresses the artery associated with root Th3 (Fig. 1-9), or following trauma involving the posterior mediastinum that interferes with blood flow in this artery (Lindenberg, 1957).

Anterior spinal artery occlusion occurs under a broader set of circumstances than already dealt with. In a case described by Spiller (1909), due to syphilitic disease, in which the proximal part of the artery was most seriously affected, cord damage extended from levels C4 to Th3. In another, described by Zeitlin and Lichtenstein (1936), the occlusion was related to severe sclerosis involving the artery; softening of the cord occurred chiefly in the thoracic region, where three-fourths of the anterior portion of the cord was destroyed. Other conditions in which infarction from decreased blood flow occurs are coarctation of the aorta, aortic collapse, major chest surgery, sympathectomy, traumatic injury, cervical spondylosis, infective processes, and spinal cord hemangioma (Gillilan, 1958; Hughes and Brownell, 1964). Onset of the anterior spinal artery occlusion under any of these conditions is sudden and dramatic. With arterial occlusion at higher levels of the cord, pain occurs in the trunk and dysesthesia and weakness in the upper limbs. Flaccid areflexic paresis involving the upper limbs then develops. There may be dissociated anesthesia, which is of the syringomyelia type. The lower limbs become spastic, and the bladder and bowel paralytic. Later on, improvement sets in but muscle atrophy persists. Or there may be paraplegia with anesthesia from the start, with little recovery. (Hughes, 1966; Zeitlin and Lichtenstein, 1936.)

Posterior spinal artery occlusion is rare and includes pyramidal tract involvement (Chung, 1926).

Spinal thrombophlebitis (Blackwood, 1963), originally called *subacute necrotic myelitis* (Foix and Alajouanine, 1926), is a disorder characterized by great distension and tortuosity of spinal veins commonly associated with systemic vascular disease such as thrombophlebitis or thrombosis involving the inferior vena cava or the pelvic veins. The pathological process is relentless. White matter of the cord becomes progressively necrotic. The initial clinical manifestations often appear in regions innervated from lower thoracic or lumbosacral levels of the cord, and the disturbances then spread.

Myelopathy is associated with *visceral carcinoma* (lung, stomach, prostate, breast, thyroid, and so on) in occasional instances. A patchy and nonsystematized but fairly symmetrical necrotizing process gradually develops both in white and gray matter. Any level, or even the entire cord, may be affected. (Mancall and Rosales, 1964.) The cerebellum is more commonly affected under these conditions (pp. 286-288).

Pott's paraplegia, of tuberculous origin, is due to compression of the cord, the latter brought about directly through vertebral subluxation resulting from caries or through an accumulation of purulent material extending from infected vertebral bodies into the extradural space. The lower thoracic spine is the most vulnerable. Neurologically the disturbances simulate those observed in anteriorly situated intraspinal-extramedullary neoplasm. (Griffiths, Seddon, and Roaf, 1956.)

Herpes zoster, believed to be due to

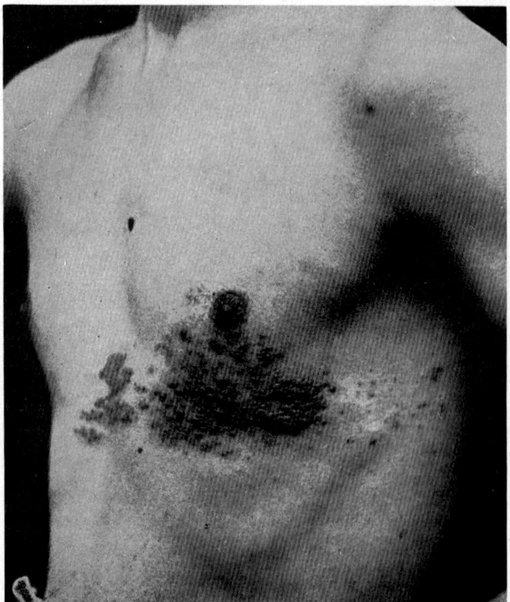

Fig. 5-12. Herpes zoster in dermatomes Th5 and Th6.

activation of varicella zoster virus acquired during a previous attack of chicken pox, primarily affects one or more posterior root ganglia, most commonly thoracic ganglia below Th2. Inflammation and hemorrhagic infarction occur in these ganglia. Cutaneous vesicles appear in the corresponding dermatomes (Fig. 5-12). Intense and persistent pain occurs in the involved dermatomes. The infection may spread to the cord, producing focal myelitis of varied distribution or, rarely, transverse myelitis. Muscle atrophy from anterior horn involvement sometimes occurs, as does also a syringomyelia-like disturbance or a Brown-Séquard syndrome. In some instances, viremia is associated with thrombotic infarction in heart, brain, or spinal cord. Herpes zoster may also be engrafted on preexistent disease, such as syringomyelia, tabes dorsalis, tuberculous caries, and diabetic neuritis. (Denny-Brown, Adams, and Fitzgerald, 1944; Döring, 1955; Kendall, 1957.) Zoster occurring in children is similar to that in adults, but is milder. The cutaneous eruptions appear in crops. Thoracic dermatomes are most frequently involved, lumbar dermatomes next most frequent. Pain occurs but it is seldom severe. When the zoster occurs in the course of leukemia or Hodgkin's disease it may be more widespread than ordinarily. That zoster is contagious is well documented. (Brunell, Miller, and Lovejoy, 1968.)

In *decompression sickness,* whether in caisson disease or in decompression to altitude, the anterior horns are usually damaged, leading to muscle atrophy, which, however, is rather minor. White matter is perhaps more vulnerable; either the lateral or the posterior column is predominantly affected, the anterior rarely. Thoracic segments of the cord tend to suffer the most. (Behnke, 1955; Haymaker, 1955; Haymaker and Johnston, 1955.)

MANIFESTATIONS OF UNILATERAL LESIONS OF THE SPINAL CORD

A purely unilateral transverse lesion of the spinal cord above midlumbar levels gives rise to the *Brown-Séquard syndrome.* Probably the most common cause is trauma, such as a fall on the back from considerable height (Austin, 1961). Stab wound may also be responsible. Spinal laminae prevent entrance of a knife or other sharp-pointed object directly from behind, but when the object is directed into the region slightly lateral to the midline, one side of the cord will be damaged if the spinal canal is penetrated (St. John and Rand, 1953). Laterally situated extramedullary tumor may also give rise to the syndrome, but masses in this location often produce signs and symptoms extraneous to the syndrome (McAlhany and Netsky, 1955). Occlusion of the anterior spinal artery may also be responsible, although paraplegia is the rule (Tureen, 1938). Delayed radionecrosis of the cord is another cause (Dynes and Smedal, 1960; Smithers, Clarkson, and Strong, 1943).

In hemisection of the cord the part of the body lying caudal to the site of the lesion shows the following changes (Fig. 5-13):

Ipsilateral to the lesion: (1) motor paresis, (2) vasomotor paralysis, (3) reduction of deep sensibility, and (4) hyperesthesia to tactile stimuli (transitory).

Contralateral to the lesion: (5) reduction in cutaneous sensibility, particularly for painful and thermal stimuli.

(1) Ipsilateral motor paresis, spastic in character, occurs in the region caudal to the site of the lesion. The deep reflexes are exaggerated, although initially they may be absent. Pathological reflexes such as the Babinski reflex can usually be elicited.

(2) Ipsilateral vasomotor paralysis, reflected in reddening and increased warmth of the skin, occurs in early stages. Later on these changes may revert to normal, or they may be succeeded by cyanosis and coldness, which persist. The disturbance is due to interruption of vasomotor fibers passing down the lateral column of the cord.

(3) Position sense and appreciation of passive movement and of vibration are diminished or lost in the ipsilateral parts of the body caudal to the lesion. Upon recovery of motor power, ataxia may occur owing to interruption of fibers in the posterior column and spinocerebellar tracts.

(4) In early stages there may be cutaneous hyperesthesia of the entire ipsilateral side caudal to the level of the lesion. This is a transient symptom,

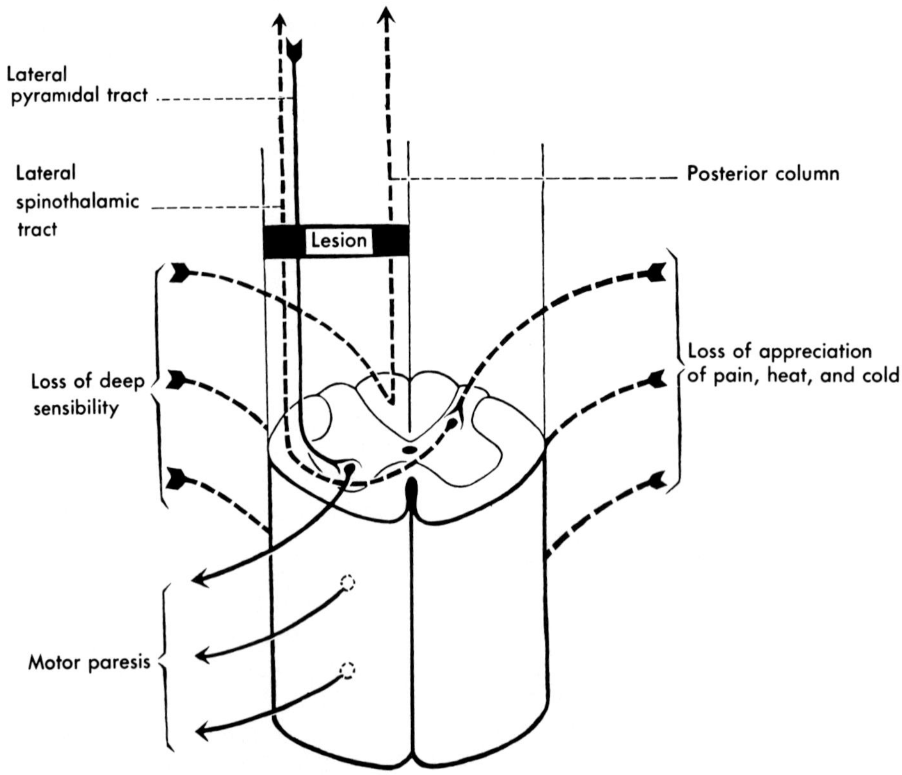

Fig. 5-13. The anatomical basis of the Brown-Séquard syndrome.

the basis of which is obscure. In other instances hyperesthesia is noted in the segmental zone situated just above the level involved in the hemisection—usually only on the side damaged but sometimes on the contralateral side as well. This may be due to the sprouting of new axons from posterior roots at these levels, which find their way to the nucleus proprius of the posterior horn (Liu and Chambers, 1958). In still other instances ipsilateral cutaneous hyperesthesia is lacking.

(5) Pain sensibility and thermal sensibility of the side of the body *contralateral* to the lesion are diminished or lost. The loss is contralateral because the fibers are involved before they have decussated. By contrast, tactile sensibility is little affected despite interruption at the level of hemitransection of all touch fibers passing upward in that half of the cord. This is because touch fibers from one side of the body pass up both sides of the cord.

Unilateral lesions are most common in the thoracic region. They give rise to *spinal hemiplegia.* Fig. 5-14 indicates the nature of the symptoms and signs in such a case. The anesthesia in the narrow zone lying just above "Motor paresis" is the result of interruption of fibers from the posterior roots that enter the spinal cord at the level of the lesion.

Unilateral lesions of lower lumbar or sacral segments do not give rise to the Brown-Séquard syndrome, for in these regions the individual segments lie so close together that few if any sensory fibers pass caudal to the lesion in reaching the opposite side of the cord. The cutaneous anesthesia is found therefore mostly on the side of the cord injury and on the same side as the paralysis (Fig. 5-15).

In some pathological processes, unilateral irritation rather than unilateral destruction of the cord occurs. In such instances, muscle spasms occur ipsilaterally and spontaneous pains contralaterally.

The classical Brown-Séquard syndrome, as just described, is much less common than incomplete forms of the syndrome. As a rule, the lesion either falls short of hemisecting the cord or it encroaches somewhat on the opposite side. When, however,

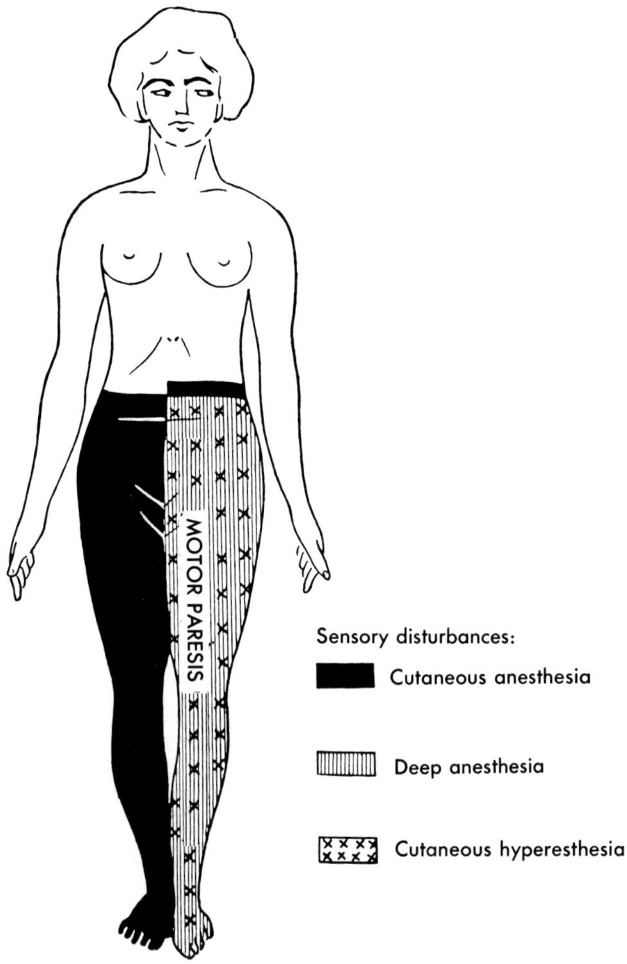

Fig. 5-14. The Brown-Séquard syndrome resulting from a lesion of the left half of the spinal cord in region of segment Th10.

in transverse lesions, muscular paresis dominates the clinical picture on one side of the body, and disturbances of superficial sensibility, especially pain and thermal sensibility, are predominant on the other side, one can without hesitation localize the lesion to the paretic side.

NEOPLASMS INVOLVING THE SPINAL CORD

The most common extramedullary-intradural tumors are neurofibromas and neurinomas. They develop along the course of spinal roots, mainly at cervical and thoracic levels. Meningioma is also

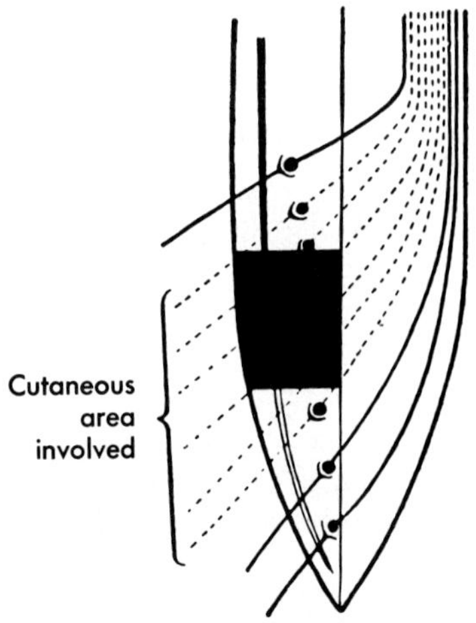

Fig. 5-15. The basis of the widespread ipsilateral sensory loss in the presence of unilateral lesions of lower segments of the spinal cord. A representative lesion is indicated by the black area.

comparatively frequent; it is usually attached to the inner surface of the dura and also predominates at cervical and thoracic levels. Ependymoma is the most frequent intramedullary tumor. It originates mainly in the caudal part of the cord and the filum terminale. Astrocytoma is next in incidence; it is found mainly in upper segments of the cord. Vascular tumors rank third; they tend to involve multiple segments. Most epidural tumors are metastatic in origin and malignant. (Elsberg, 1929, 1941; McAlhany and Netsky, 1955; Russell and Rubinstein, 1963; Schloof, Kernohan and MacCarty, 1964; Tilney and Elsberg, 1926.)

The following points may be taken as criteria for distinguishing extramedullary (*intraspinal*) from intramedullary tumors:

1. In extramedullary tumors prodromal pains of radicular distribution are common because these tumors spring mostly from the region of the posterior roots; the pain may also radiate to adjacent segments. Radicular pain in intramedullary tumor is rare, nonradicular pain common, although less so than in *extradural* tumor. (Pain may also constitute a very early symptom in *extradural* tumor; it is of wider scope than in intradural tumor.) (Austin, 1961.)
2. Dysesthesias and paresthesias are common at all stages of intramedullary tumor growth, while in extramedullary tumors they seldom occur until considerable time has elapsed.
3. Motor irritative phenomena (for example, muscle fasciculations) are fairly common in extramedullary tumors and infrequent in intramedullary tumors. Fasciculations occurring in cervical myotomes jointly with muscle atrophy and long-tract signs may be due to tumor involving anterior roots; amyotrophic lateral sclerosis may be simulated.
4. In rather numerous extramedullary tumors there is a slow but continuous loss of pain, thermal, and deep sensibility. Intramedullary tumors are often characterized by a striking dissociated loss of sensibility, with pain and thermal sensibility suffering the most. However, dissociation equally conspicuous may also occur in extramedullary tumors, especially those situated in the cervical region, and thus this criterion has limited usefulness. In extramedullary compression of the cervical cord, fibers carrying pain and thermal impulses are more often unequally involved than in compression from an intramedullary tumor.
5. Disturbed function of the bladder and rectal sphincters usually occurs late in extramedullary tumors, although the disturbance will be manifested fairly early if the tumor is in the sacral region, and occasionally if the tumor is at the thoracic level. In intramedullary tumors these disturbances tend to occur relatively early.
6. A subjective sensation of intense coldness in one or more limbs in high cervical tumors is characteristic of extramedullary, not intramedullary, tumors.
7. In compression by extramedullary tumor the more caudal dermatomes are preponderantly affected, while in intramedullary growths there is a more even dermatomal involvement. In extramedullary growths a strong tendency exists for the disturbances of motility and sensibility to remain stationary with respect to position even though they are increasing in intensity. The upper limit of these changes usually does not advance cephalad because extramedullary tumors tend to increase in size in the transverse rather than in the longitudinal plane. In intramedullary tumors the upper level of the sensory changes is often indistinct and occasionally may gradually shift cephalad. Symptoms and signs may be precipitated or increased immediately after lumbar puncture, thus making the level of an extramedullary tumor more readily discernible.
8. In extramedullary growths the spastic syndrome is very common and persists even after paraplegia is established. Also, there is an early and pronounced flexor-withdrawal reflex of the lower limbs. In intramedullary growths, spasticity occurs in about 50 percent of cases and is usually less pronounced than in extramedullary growths.
9. In extramedullary tumors there is little or no muscle atrophy. In exceptional instances in which muscles have undergone slight to moderate atrophy, electrical irritability is less altered than might be expected from the degree of atrophy. By contrast, intramedullary tumors are often characterized by muscle atrophy.
10. In extramedullary tumors trophic disturbances of the skin are usually absent, while in intramedullary tumors they are fairly common.
11. Increased sensitiveness of the vertebral column to local pressure is common in extramedullary tumors but not in intramedullary tumors.
12. Alterations of the cerebrospinal fluid are much more frequent in extramedullary than in intramedullary tumor. In extramedullary growths, especially when at lower thoracic or lumbar levels, albumin in the lumbar fluid is often markedly increased, whereas "lymphocytes" are in normal number or only slightly increased (albuminocytological dissociation). In some cases the fluid is xanthochromic because of stagnancy of the spinal fluid brought about by blockage of its circulation at the level of the tumor. Xanthochromic fluid may or may not contain hemoglobin. The xanthochromia is by no means pathognomonic, for it may occur under other conditions such as intracranial chronic subdural hematoma.

In complete blockage of spinal fluid by an extramedullary tumor, the total protein of the fluid is greatly augmented. Both globulin and albumin undergo an increase, the latter by far the most; also, the spinal fluid may coagulate spontaneously upon removal. These abnormalities are all the more pronounced the lower the level of the obliteration of the spinal canal, and they are not observed in fluid taken above the level of the lesion (by suboccipital puncture).

Myelography, also important in differential diagnosis of intramedullary and extramedullary tumors, is discussed in Chapter 9.

The *Queckenstedt test* is helpful in differential diagnosis in that it allows a distinction to be made between high and low extramedullary tumors that block the flow of spinal fluid. Under normal conditions, with the patient lying on his side, the lumbar spinal fluid pressure is 60 to 175 mm. H_2O (children, 45 to 95 mm.), as measured by a manometer. When the patient is in a sitting position the pressure is 190 to 250 mm. H_2O. The Queckenstedt test consists in determining the effect of compression of the jugular veins on the manometric pressure. When the spinal canal is normally patent, compression of the jugular veins (for 10 seconds) causes the lumbar pressure to rise rapidly to 300 to 400 mm. H_2O or more, and on release of pressure from the jugular vein the lumbar pressure falls with equal rapidity. The elevation of pressure occurs as the result of backing up of blood in intracranial veins, the increased intracranial volume thus induced causing a rise in the intracranial pressure and, consequently, in the intraspinal pressure as well.

If an obstruction exists above the site where the lumbar puncture needle is inserted, the rise of pressure in the lumbar fluid following compression of the jugular veins is delayed or pressure increase is absent. Additional evidence of block may be obtained by removing 8 ml. or more of lumbar fluid. Normally the pressure does not fall more than 50 percent, whereas in the presence of block it falls much more. If the obstruction is below the site of entrance of the needle, there will, of course, be a normal increase in spinal pressure on performing the Queckenstedt test.

It is probable that both hydrostatic and vascular factors contribute greatly to the normal pressure of the cerebrospinal fluid. When the CSF pressure is measured with the patient in a horizontal position the lumbar, cisternal, and lateral ventricular pressures are equal. If the patient's feet are raised the lumbar pressure will fall, the ventricular pressure will rise, and the cisternal pressure will be intermediate between the two. Upon elevating the patient's head the pressures will be reversed, with the ventricular and cisternal pressures becoming subatmospheric and the lumbar pressure rising to 200 mm. H_2O or more. Such lability in pressure indicates that the CSF is not in a closed rigid container, but, instead, in a vented (subarachnoid) space. The venous system is the most important factor in the venting. As the head is elevated, the increased volume of blood in the intracranial veins induces CSF to pass into the spinal canal, thus reducing the ventricular pressure and increasing the lumbar pressure. On compression of the jugular veins, the ventricular pressure rises relatively slowly because of the displacement of fluid to the spinal subarachnoid space, and on continued jugular compression the ventricular pressure fails to rise beyond a certain level, probably because of the establishment of a collateral venous circulation between the intracranial and spinal veins by way of the foramen magnum (O'Connell, 1953).

During forced expiration (cough), both the intracranial and the intraspinal pressure rise rapidly and equally. This is due to back pressure in thoracic and abdominal veins that retards the flow of blood from intracranial and spinal veins (Batson, 1940) (Fig. 1-12). With forced expiration or with straining, in which abdominal compression occurs, the lumbar pressure increases even in the presence of spinal block. *A Queckenstedt test signifying an abnormal situation should always be confirmed by testing the response of the lumbar pressure to abdominal compression.* Confirmatory evidence consists in a greater rise of lumbar pressure following abdominal compression than following jugular compression.

REFERENCES

Adams, H. D., and van Geertruyden, H. H. 1956. Neurologic complications of aortic surgery. Ann. Surg. **144**:574-610.

Austin, G. M. 1961. The spinal cord: basic aspects and surgical considerations. Springfield, Illinois, Charles C Thomas, Publisher.

Austin, G. M., and McCouch, G. P. 1955. Presynaptic component of intermediary cord potential. J. Neurophysiol. 18:441-451.

Barnett, H. J. M., Botterell, E. H., Jousse, A. T.,

and Wynn-Jones, M. 1966. Progressive myelopathy as a sequel to traumatic paraplegia. Brain **89**:159-174.

Bartsch, W. 1954. Frühstadien der spinalen Mangeldurchblutung. Nervenarzt **25**:481-486.

Batson, O. V., 1940. The function of the vertebral veins and their role in the spread of metastases. Ann. Surg. **112**:138-149.

Behnke, A. R. 1955. Decompression sickness. Mil. Med. **117**:257-271.

Blackwood, W. 1963. Vascular diseases of the central nervous system. In Greenfield's Neuropathology, ed. 2. London, Edward Arnold (Publishers) Ltd., pp. 71-137.

Brunell, P. A., Miller, L. H., and Lovejoy, F. 1968. Zoster in children. Amer. J. Dis. Child. **115**:432-437.

Byers, R. K., and Banker, B. Q. 1961. Infantile muscular atrophy. Arch. Neurol. **5**:140-164.

Carter, S., Sciarra, D., and Merritt, H. H. 1950. The course of multiple sclerosis as determined by autopsy proven cases. Res. Publ. Ass. Nerv. Ment. Dis., Proc. **28**:471-532.

Chung, M. F. 1926. Thrombosis of spinal vessels in sudden syphilitic paraplegia. Arch. Neurol. Psychiat. **16**:761-771.

David, M., and Askenasy, H. 1937. Ataxia and astereognosis of bulbar origin. Brain **60**:354-360.

Davison, C. 1949. Pathology. In Bucy, P. C., editor: The precentral motor cortex, ed. 2. Urbana, University of Illinois Press, pp. 425-427.

Denny-Brown, D., Adams, R. D., and Fitzgerald, P. J. 1944. Pathologic features of herpes zoster. Arch. Neurol. Psychiat. **51**:216-231.

Döring, G. 1955. Zoster. In Henke, F., Lubarsch, O., and Rössle, R., editors: Handbuch der speziellen pathologischen Anatomie und Histologie, vol. 13 (edited by Scholz, W.), pt. 5. Berlin, Springer-Verlag, pp. 291-312.

Dynes, J. B., and Smedal, M. I. 1960. Radiation myelitis. Amer. J. Roentgen. **83**:78-87.

Elsberg, C. A. 1929. Tumors of the spinal cord. Problems in their diagnosis and localization; procedures for their exposure and removal. Arch. Neurol. Psychiat. **22**:949-965.

Elsberg, C. A. 1941. Surgical diseases of the spinal cord, membranes, and nerve roots. New York, Hoeber.

Foerster, O. 1936. Symptomatologie der Erkrankungen des Rückenmarks und seiner Wurzeln. In Bumke, O., and Foerster, O., editors: Handbuch der Neurologie, Berlin, Springer-Verlag **5**: 1-400.

Foix, C., and Alajouanine, T. 1926. La myélite necrotique subaigüe. Rev. Neurol. **2**:1-42.

Fontaine, G., DuBois, B., Farriaux, J. P., and Maillard, E. 1969. Une observation familiale de maladie de Strümpell-Lorrain. J. Med. Sci. **8**: 183-187.

Friedreich, N. 1863. Ueber degenerative Atrophie der spinalen Hinterstränge. Virchows Arch. Path. Anat. **26**:391-419, 433-459; **27**:1-26.

Garcin, R., Zülch, K.-J., Lazorthes, G., and Gruner, J. 1962. Pathologie vasculaire de la moelle. Paris, Masson et Cie.

Garland, H., Greenberg, J., and Harriman, D. G. F. 1966. Infarction of the spinal cord. Brain **89**:645-662.

Gellerstedt, N. 1956. Erkrankungen der Dura mater (Pachymeningitis haemorrhagica, Pachymeningitis cervicales hypertrophica). In Henke, F., Lubarsch, O., and Rössle, R., editors: Handbuch der speziellen pathologischen Anatomie und Histologie, vol. 13 (edited by Scholz, W.), pt. 4. Berlin, Springer-Verlag, pp. 775-825.

Gillilan, L. A. 1958. The arterial blood supply of the human spinal cord. J. Comp. Neurol. **110**:75-103.

Griffiths, D. L., Seddon, H. J., and Roaf, R. 1956. Pott's paraplegia. London, Oxford University Press.

Grimby, L. 1965. Pathological plantar response. Part I. Flexor and extensor components in early and late reflex parts: loss of significance of stimulus site. J. Neurol. Neurosurg. Psychiat. **28**:469-474.

Gruner, J., and Lapresle, J. 1962. Etude anatomopathologique des medullopathies d'origine vasculaire. Rev. Neurol. **106**:592-631.

Guttmann, L. 1946. Rehabilitation after injuries to spinal cord and cauda equina. Brit. J. Phys. Med. **9**:162-171.

Guttmann, L. 1952. Studies on reflex activity of the isolated cord in the spinal man. J. Nerv. Ment. Dis. **116**:957-972.

Hamilton, C. R., Jr., Dobson, H. L., and Marshall, J. 1968. Diabetic amyotrophy: clinical and electronmicroscopic studies in six patients. Amer. J. Med. Sci. **256**:81-90.

Haymaker, W. 1955. Decompression sickness. In Henke, F., Lubarsch, O., and Rössle, R., editors: Handbuch der speziellen pathologischen Anatomie und Histologie, vol. 13 (edited by Scholz, W.), pt. 1B. Berlin, Springer-Verlag, pp. 1600-1672.

Haymaker, W., and Johnston, A. D. 1955. Pathology of decompression sickness: a comparison of the lesions in airmen with those in caisson workers and divers. Mil. Med. **117**:285-306.

Hewitt, A. B. 1967. Syphilitic amyotrophy: a case occurring after apparently successful treatment in primary syphilis. Brit. J. Vener. Dis. **43**:272-274.

Holmes, G. 1915. The Goulstonian Lectures on spinal injuries of warfare. Brit. Med. J. **2**:769-774.

Hughes, J. T. 1966. Pathology of the spinal cord. London, Lloyd-Luke.

Hughes, J. T., and Brownell, B. 1964. Cervical spondylosis complicated by anterior spinal artery thrombosis. Neurology **14**:1073-1077.

Hughes, J. T., and Brownell, B. 1966. Spinal cord ischemia due to arteriosclerosis. Arch. Neurol. **15**:189-202.

Hughes, J. T., Brownell, B., and Hewer, R. L. 1968. The peripheral sensory pathway in Friedreich's ataxia: an examination by light and electron microscopy of the posterior nerve roots, posterior root ganglia, and peripheral sensory nerves in cases of Friedreich's ataxia. Brain **91**: 803-818.

Jellinger, K. 1967. Spinal cord arteriosclerosis and progressive vascular myelopathy. J. Neurol. Neurosurg. Psychiat. **30**:195-206.

Jellinger, K., and Neumayer, E. 1962. Myélopathie progressive d'origine vasculaire: contribution anatomoclinique aux syndromes d'une hypovascularisation chronique de la moelle. Acta Neurol. Belg. **62**:944-956.

Jones, K. K., and Walsh, J. R. 1965. Diabetic amyotrophy. Postgrad. Med. **37**:342-347.

Kahn, E. A. 1947. The role of the dentate ligaments in spinal cord compression and the syndrome of lateral sclerosis. J. Neurosurg. **4**:191-199.

Kendall, D. 1957. Motor complications of herpes zoster. Brit. Med. J. **2**:616-618.

Klawans, H. L., Jr. 1968. Delayed traumatic syringomyelia. Dis. Nerv. System **29**:525-528.

Kurland, L. T., and Mulder, D. W. 1955. Epidemiologic investigations of amyotrophic lateral sclerosis: familial aggregations indicative of dominant inheritance. Neurology **5**:249-268.

Leimbach, R. 1895. Statistisches zur Symptomatologie der Tabes dorsalis. Dtsch. Z. Nervenheilk. **7**:493-503.

Lindenberg, R. 1957. Die Gefässversorgung und ihre Bedeutung fur Art und Ort von Kreislaufbedingten Gewebsschäden und Gefässprozessen. In Henke, F. Lubarsch, O., and Rössle, R., editors: Handbuch der speciellen pathologischen Anatomie, vol. 13 (edited by Scholz, W.), pt. 1A. München, Springer-Verlag, pp. 1071-1164.

Liu, C. N., and Chambers, W. W. 1958. Intraspinal sprouting of dorsal root axons. A.M.A. Arch. Neurol. Psychiat. **79**:46-61.

Mackay, R. P., and Hall, G. W. 1933. Syphilitic amyotrophy. Arch. Neurol. Psychiat. **29**:241-254.

Magee, K. R., and Schneider, R. C. 1967. Syringomyelia: loss of deep-pain sensation with otherwise normal sensory perception. J.A.M.A. **200**:795-797.

Mancall, E. L., and Rosales, R. K. 1964. Necrotizing myelopathy associated with visceral carcinoma. Brain **87**:639-656.

Mannen, T. 1966. Vascular lesions in the spinal cord in the aged: a clinicopathological study. Geriatrics **21**:151-160.

Marshall, J. 1954. Observations on reflex changes in the lower limbs in spastic paraplegia in man. Brain **77**:290-304.

Martin, J. P. 1925. Amyotrophic meningo-myelitis. Brain **48**:153-183.

McAlhany, H. J., and Netsky, M. G. 1955. Compression of the spinal cord by extramedullary neoplasms: a clinical and pathologic study. J. Neuropath. Exper. Neurol. **14**:276-287.

McCouch, G. P., Austin, G. M., Liu, C. N., and Liu, C. Y. 1958. Sprouting as a cause of spasticity. J. Neurophysiol. **21**:205-216.

Netsky, M. C. 1953. Syringomyelia: a clinicopathologic study. A.M.A. Arch. Neurol. Psychiat. **70**:741-777.

O'Connell, J. E. A. 1953. The cerebrospinal fluid pressure as an aetological factor in the development of lesions affecting the central nervous system. Brain **76**:279-298.

Olivarius, B. de F., and Roos, D. 1968. Myelopathy following partial gastrectomy. Acta Neurol. Scand. **44**:347-362.

Ozsváth, K. 1968. Paralysis spinalis spastica familiaris. Deut. Ztschr. Nervenheilk. **193**:287-323.

Pentschew, A. 1958. Intoxikationen. In Henke, F., Lubarsch, O., and Rössle, R., editors: Handbuch der speziellen pathologischen Anatomie und Histologie, vol. 13 (edited by Scholz, W.), pt. 2. Berlin, Springer-Verlag, pp. 1907-2502.

Pollock, L. J., Boshes, B., Finkelman, I., Chor, H., and Brown, M. 1951. Spasticity, pseudospontaneous spasms, and other reflex activities late after injury to the spinal cord. A.M.A. Arch. Neurol. Psychiat. **66**:537-560.

Riddoch, G. 1917. The reflex functions of the completely divided spinal cord in man, compared with those associated with less severe lesions. Brain **40**:264-402.

Rossier, A. B., Werner, A., Wildi, E., and Berney, J. 1968. Contribution to the study of later cervical syringomyelic syndromes after dorsal or lumbar traumatic paraplegia. J. Neurol. Neurosurg. Psychiat. **31**:99-105.

Russell, D. S., and Rubinstein, L. J. 1963. Pathology of tumours of the nervous system, ed. 2. London, Edward Arnold (Publishers) Ltd.

Schloof, J. L., Kernohan, J. W., and MacCarty, C. S. 1964. Primary intramedullary tumors of the spinal cord and filum terminale. Philadelphia, W. B. Saunders Co.

Schut, J. W., and Haymaker, W. 1951. Hereditary ataxia: a pathologic study of five cases of common ancestry. J. Neuropath. Clin. Neurol. **1**:183-213.

Schwarz, G. A., and Liu, C.-N. 1956. Hereditary (familial) spastic paraplegia. Arch. Neurol. Psychiat. **75**:144-162.

Smithers, D. W., Clarkson, J. R., and Strong, J. A. 1943. The roentgen treatment of cancer of the esophagus. Amer. J. Roentgen. **49**:606-634.

Spiller, W. G. 1909. Thrombosis of the cervical anterior median spinal artery: syphilitic acute anterior poliomyelitis. J. Nerv. Ment. Dis. **36**: 601-613.

St. John, J. R., and Rand, C. W. 1953. Stab wounds of the spinal cord. Bull. Los Angeles Neurol. Soc. **18**:1-24.

Stark, F. M., and Moersch, F. P. 1945. Primary lateral sclerosis; a distinct clinical entity. J. Nerv. Ment. Dis. **102**:332-337.

Sträussler, E. 1958. Die Syphilis des Zentralnervensystem und die progressive Paralyse (quartäre Syphilis). In Henke, F., Lubarsch, O., and Rössle, R., editors: Handbuch der speziellen pathologischen Anatomie und Histologie, vol. 13 (edited by Scholz, W.), pt. 2A. Berlin, Springer-Verlag, pp. 847-994.

Swanson, A. G. 1963. Congenital insensitivity to pain with anhydrosis: a unique syndrome in two male siblings. Arch. Neurol. **8**:299-306.

Swanson, A. G., Buchan, G. C., and Alvord, E. C., Jr. 1963. Absence of Lissauer's tract and small dorsal root axons in familial, congenital, universal insensitivity to pain. Trans. Amer. Neurol. Ass. **88**:99-103.

Thomson, A. F., and Alvarez, F. A. 1969. Hereditary amyotrophic lateral sclerosis. J. Neurol. Sci. **8**:101-110.

Tilney, F., and Elsberg, C. A. 1926. Sensory disturbances in tumors of the cervical spinal cord: arrangement of the fibers in the sensory pathways. Arch. Neurol. Psychiat. **15**:444-454.

Tureen, L. L. 1938. Circulation of the spinal cord and the effect of vascular occlusion. Res. Publ. Ass. Nerv. Dis., Proc. **18**:394-437.

Verjaal, A., and Timmermans-van den Bos, A. H. C. C. 1967. Combined degeneration of the spinal cord due to deficiency of alimentary vitamin B_{12}. J. Neurol. Neurosurg. Psychiat. **30**: 464-467.

Wartenberg, R. 1945. The examination of reflexes: a simplification. Chicago, Year Book Medical Publishers, Inc., p. 38.

Weinstein, E. A., and Bender, M. B. 1940. Dissociation of deep sensibility at different levels of the central nervous system. Arch. Neurol. Psychiat. **43**:488-497.

Yoss, R. E. 1953. Studies of the spinal cord: pathways for deep pain within the spinal cord and brain. Neurology **3**:163-175.

Zeitlin, H., and Lichtenstein, B. W. 1936. Occlusion of the anterior spinal artery: clinicopathologic report of a case and a review of the literature. Arch. Neurol. Psychiat. **36**:96-111.

Zülch, K. J. 1962. Réflexions sur la pathophysiologie des troubles vasculaires médullaires. Rev. Neurol. **106**:632-645.

Zülch, K. J. 1967. Die spinale Mangeldurchblutung und ihre Folgen. Verhandl. deutsch. Gesellsch. inn. Med., 72. Kongr., München, Bergmann.

Chapter 6

Localization of lesions of cervical and upper thoracic segments; autonomic disturbances

TRAUMA, SPONDYLOSIS, PROLAPSED INTERVERTEBRAL DISK, TUMOR

Trauma. Sudden arrest of the body (fixed or not) of a seated person in forward motion causes the head to bend forward rapidly in extreme flexion, then snap back. By contrast, with sudden propulsion of the body forward from a position of rest, motion of the head occurs in the reverse order. The sudden (forward) flexion or (backward) extension of the neck under both conditions may be a sufficient degree to injure the cervical spine. In this "whiplash" type of injury, head impact may be an accompaniment, but is excluded as a factor in the discussion that follows.

In severe whiplash injury pain in the neck and numbness and tingling in the arms and fingers (of dermatomal distribution) are common complaints. Stretching or concussion of posterior spinal roots has been considered the chief basis. When the injury is limited to the region of the axis and atlas, numbness and tingling may occur in the back of the neck and over the occiput, and may be referred to the ear as well. In some cases these sensory disturbances last for months. Slight motor deficit of anterior root origin may also occur but tends to be transitory. Moreover (in the absence of head impact), symptoms of brain concussion originating at the time of the injury have been noted in as many as 62 percent of cases. (Austin, 1961; Cailliet, 1962; Gay and Abbott, 1953.) Dizziness, commonly preceded by positional vertigo, is one of the most distressing symptoms of whiplash injury, and in 50 percent of patients having this complaint, injury of the vestibular system can be substantiated by nystagmography. Ischemia of the vestibular apparatus from vertebral-basilar arterial insufficiency can be a basis, particularly in persons having poor collateral circulation in this region. Thrombosis of the inferior cerebellar artery has been known to result from whiplash injury. (Compere, 1968.)

In monkeys subjected to severe whiplash injury (without head impact), gross hemorrhages and contusions were noted over the surface of the upper cervical cord and the brain. Subdural hematoma was especially common. (Ommaya, Faas, and Yarnell, 1968.) Small hemorrhages have also been found in the brainstem in violent whiplash.

Cervical spondylosis. The formation of osseofibrous ridges or excrescences (osteophytes) at the junction of the disk and the vertebral body (spondylosis) is most frequent at levels C IV–C V, C V–C VI, and C VI–C VII (Taylor, 1964). The critical factor so far as spinal cord compression is concerned is not the height of the ridge, but the distance from the apex of the spondylotic ridge to the roof of the spinal canal (Nugent, 1959). Roentgenographic findings in cervical spondylosis include loss of cervical lordosis and narrowing of the intervertebral disks. (Epstein, Epstein, and Lavine, 1963; Holmes, 1966; Langfitt and Elliott, 1967.) Roentgenographic findings in plain cervical films bear no relation to neurological deficit.

Elderly males are chiefly affected, though in one series the age range was from 25 to 74 years, with an average age of 45 years (Matthews, 1968). Brachialgia, signifying posterior root compression, is a common manifestation (Holmes, 1966). Pain is commonly experienced in the lower back and lower limbs in the absence of signs or symptoms of spinal cord damage and may be the initial complaint. It is of a burning or aching quality and deep, diffuse, and boring. This "spinal cord pain" may be in one leg only, but is usually bilateral and often symmetrical. No complaint is made of limitation of back mobility, nor aggravation of the signs and symptoms by exercise or by coughing or sneezing. Night pain, relieved by getting out of bed, is another characteristic. Intermittent numbness and paresthesias of the lower limbs also occur and may precede the pain. There may be early motor disturbances, such as dragging of one leg or finding it difficult to climb stairs. All these disturbances have been attributed to compression of the cervical spinal cord in the region of the spondylosis. (Langfitt and Elliott, 1967.)

In contrast are overt signs of cervical cord damage in some patients. These may be referable to posterior column, lateral column, or, occasionally, gray matter involvement. Paraplegia may occur (Matthews, 1968). The myelopathy may, in some cases, be shown at operation to be related to spinal cord compression (Nugent, 1959); proof of such has, however, been difficult to establish in numerous other cases. In Taylor's view (1964), the myelopathy is usually due to interference with blood flow in a sizable artery (a main radicular artery) running along a spinal root, an interference brought about either directly through pressure exerted on the root(s) by excrescences or through constriction of the root(s) by thickened, hyalinized fibrous tissue. Cervical osteophytosis may occasionally be manifested by disturbances other than those mentioned—for example, by dysphagia and hoarseness (Facer, 1967). In differential diagnosis, involvement of the cervical cord by prolapsed intervertebral disk, atherosclerotic disease, multiple sclerosis, and (occasionally) meningioma come into consideration, as any of them can masquerade as "cervical spondylosis."

Evidence has been provided that ankylosing spondylitis is in some instances, at least, a part of the *rheumatoid disease complex*. In such a case involving the cervical region, rheumatoid connective tissue changes found in the dura (rheumatoid pachymeningitis) were associated with rheumatoid spondylitis. Compression myelopathy occurred in this patient. (Gutmann and Hable, 1963.)

Besides the cervical region, other levels of the spine and dura may be involved in ankylosing spondylosis and rheumatoid disease. In the former, for example, a cauda equina syndrome may occur (Matthews, 1968).

Prolapsed intervertebral disk. Prolapse of an intervertebral disk may be the outcome of spondylosis, with trauma sometimes the precipitating factor, or the prolapse may be due solely to trauma.

In the cervical region the disks at lower levels are most subject to prolapse. In *chronic midline prolapse* the "distant" symptoms (pains) may be no different from those already described for cervical spondylosis. There may also be dysesthesias or weakness in one or more limbs, most often in all four, and, in 50 percent of cases, ataxia and incoordination of the limbs as well. The paresis of the limbs, when it occurs, is usually of the spastic type. With *acute midline prolapse*, the signs and symptoms are similar to those of any other extramedullary mass impinging on the anterior aspect of the cord. Pain in the neck is experienced on turning the head. With prolapse of the disk between vertebrae C V and C VI, for example, there may be numbness and tingling of the fingers and legs, flaccidity or spasticity of the lower limbs, exaggerated reflexes, and no objective sensory change. In *lateral prolapse* the onset may be characterized by severe lateralized pain on turning the head. Compression of one or more roots results in radicular pain and weakness of the muscles of one or both upper limbs. Signs and symptoms referable to the lower limbs may also occur. The question of whether cord compression or occlusion of a main radicular artery is responsible for these disturbances is the same as for cervical spondylosis. In cases of this kind, Greenfield (1953) thought that the areas of demyelination in the cord he observed were too scattered and circumscribed to be caused by direct pressure. The ataxia without other posterior column signs observed in such cases could be attributed to cerebellar dysfunction (circulatory insufficiency from vertebral artery occlusion brought about by pressure exerted by the disk). (Mair and Druckman, 1953; Mixter and Barr, 1934; Odom, Finney, and Woodhall, 1958; Yuhl and others, 1955.)

Disk prolapse at the *lumbar level* (L IV–L V; L V–S I) is far more common than prolapse elsewhere. Low back tenderness and pain are characteristic initial symptoms. Shortly thereafter pain occurs in one lower limb, usually in the region of distribution of the sciatic nerve; the pain is sharp and shooting, and it radiates. Weakness in dorsal flexion and plantar flexion of the foot also occurs. The ankle jerk is not elicitable if root S1 is compressed. With compression of root L4 the knee jerk is absent and pain is referred to the anterior part of the thigh. Stretching of the affected nerve root(s) aggravates the pain.

Tumor in the region of the foramen magnum. The spinal cord may be compressed at the level of the foramen magnum, most frequently by neoplasm (meningioma, neurofibroma, ependymoma, hemangioblastoma) and basilar artery aneurysm. Neoplasms arising at the level of the lower medulla oblongata may extênd down through the foramen magnum, and those originating from the uppermost cervical levels (usually meningioma and neurofibroma) may extend up into the posterior cranial fossa. Constriction within the foramen magnum gives these tumors an hourglass shape.

Depending on their position and size, tumors situated just above the foramen magnum may give rise to signs and symptoms referable to the lower medulla oblongata and the lower cranial nerves. Thus there may be, singly or in various combinations, nystagmus, trigeminal hypesthesia, facial paresis, protrusion of the tongue to one side together with fibrillary twitching of the other side of the tongue, and weakness of the trapezius and sternocleidomastoid muscles. Increased intracranial pressure together with papilledema may also occur. By contrast, in tumor limited to the region of the foramen magnum or just below the foramen, signs of damage of the medulla oblongata and cranial nerves are rare. Such manifestations, if they occur, are overshadowed by disturbances referable to spinal cord compression.

Suboccipital headache is a consistent complaint in these tumors. Its development long before signs of cord compression become evident suggests that the tumor is originating in the region of the foramen magnum and is growing downward. Frequently the cord compression is manifested first by spastic paresis of the upper limb of the ipsilateral side, then the lower limb of the ipsilateral side, then the contralateral lower limb, and finally the contralateral upper limb. The small muscles of the hand and the muscles of the forearm frequently undergo atrophy, and thus the disorder may simulate amyotrophic lateral sclerosis. Presumably the atrophy is due to compression of one or both vertebral arteries, branches of which form the anterior spinal artery as far down as segment C5 (Fig. 1-9). In some cases, dissociated anesthesia develops, with tactile sensibility preserved and pain and thermal sensibility reduced ipsilaterally over a variable region. There may also be signs referable to the posterior columns of the cord, but they tend to occur late in the clinical course.

Another common manifestation of tumor in the foramen magnum is pain in the region of distribution of segment C2, usually ipsilateral but sometimes bilateral. This may be the first complaint, and it is particularly significant if numbness and dysesthesias develop in the painful region. Numbness and tingling may also occur in the region of the ipsilateral hand and forearm. A common complaint is that of a sensation of intense cold in one or more limbs. Moreover, there may be spasms of the neck muscles, later complicated by contracture. (Bennett and Fortes, 1945; Naffziger and Brown, 1933; Symonds and Meadows, 1937.)

RESPIRATORY, PULSE, VASOMOTOR, AND SUDOMOTOR DISTURBANCES

Serious disturbances in respiration result from lesions of segments C3–C5 that involve the phrenic nucleus (Fig. 1-1). Destruction of this nucleus or its outgoing fibers leads to paralysis of the diaphragm, while irritation (induced by a lesion near the nucleus) results in hiccup, dyspnea, and coughing.

Anterolateral cordotomy at levels C1–C2 for the relief of intractable pain has resulted in immediate reduction in pulmonary tidal volume by more than 50%, with recovery in a few minutes. Loss in diaphragmatic function also occurred in these patients but was less tangible. Most of the descending respiratory pathway believed to be concerned in diaphragmatic function is situated deep in the anterior (white) column in the vicinity of the anterior horn. The remaining fibers are more dorsally situated and possibly merge in some degree with fibers of the lateral spinothalamic tract; they are assumed to innervate the intercostal muscles and the abdominal and lumbar musculature used in respiration. The lateral border of this tract appears to lie about 2 mm. deep in cord surface, and the medial border about 4 mm. (at levels C1-C2). Reticulospinal fibers emerging from the respiratory center, situated mainly in the pons (p. 41), constitute the major component of the respiratory pathway; these fibers are concerned in automatic respiration. Voluntary respiration, on the other hand, is mediated by the lateral pyramidal tract. Death during sleep is known to occur following anterolateral cordotomy at high cervical levels and can be attributed to a combination of reticulospinal tract interruption and abeyance of voluntary respiration. (Hitchcock and Leece, 1967.)

Transitory slowing of the pulse is characteristic of lesions of upper cervical segments. This is apparently due to interruption or irritation of fibers ascending to the cardiovascular center in the medulla oblongata. In occasional instances of upper cervical cord injury, bradycardia is permanent and associated with periodic attacks of generalized muscle spasms.

Vasomotor and sudomotor paralysis involving the face and related areas sometimes occurs in lesions of the brainstem or spinal cord down to about Th2 but much more commonly in interruption of sympathetic nerves peripherally. The pathway concerned is much the same as indicated in Fig. 5-14. The preganglionic neurons have their cell stations in the intermediolateral horns; the axons leave the spinal cord by way of anterior roots Th7–Th2 and synapse in the superior cervical sympathetic ganglion. From here, postganglionic fibers proceed peripheralward by two routes: (1) via the internal carotid artery, ophthalmic artery, and supraorbital and supratrochlear arteries for the innervation of vessels in the orbit and conjunctiva and for the innervation of vessels and sweat glands of the eyelids and forehead, and (2) via the external carotid artery for the innervation of vessels and sweat glands of the face. A lesion interrupting the sympathetic chain or damaging the superior sympathetic ganglion will involve all the cutaneous areas mentioned. At first the skin is hyperemic and warm, and later on cyanotic and cold. Anhidrosis is evident in the areas implicated. In lesions interrupting only the postganglionic fibers coursing along the internal carotid artery, disturbances in vasomotility and sweating occur in the eyelids and forehead but not in the face (see pp. 103 and 104).

In lesions of the upper spinal cord there may occasionally be hyperhidrosis rather than anhidrosis of the face. This suggests that the spinal center of facial sweating lies somewhat apart from the ciliospinal

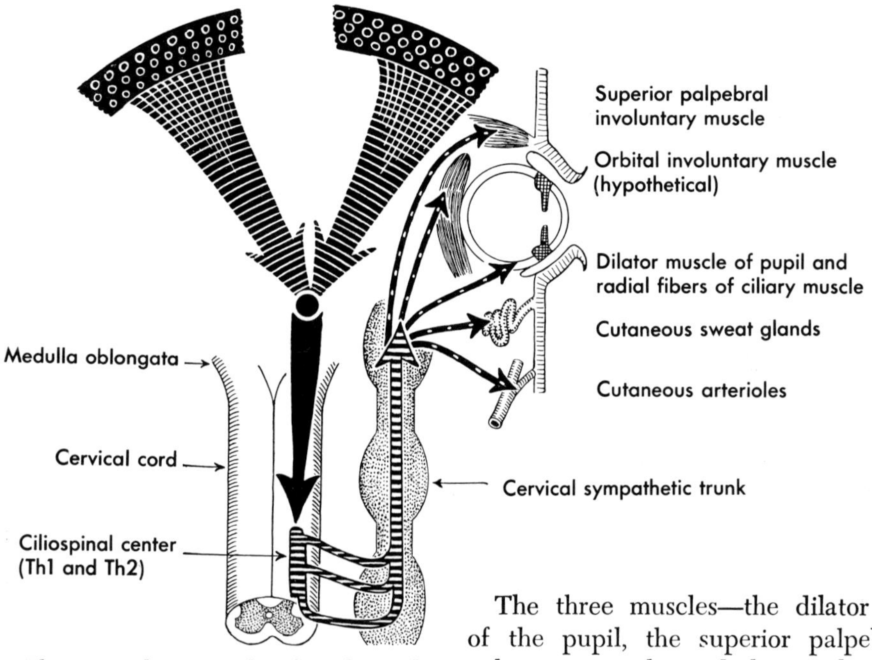

Fig. 6-1. The sympathetic supply of ocular and cutaneous structures.

center, yet sufficiently near so that a lesion may damage the latter and irritate the former.

HORNER'S SYNDROME AND ASSOCIATED DISTURBANCES

Issuing from the superior cervical sympathetic ganglion are fibers that pass craniad along the internal carotid, then the ophthalmic artery, to supply (1) the pupillodilator muscle, (2) the superior palpebral involuntary muscle (Müller's muscle), (3) hypothetically, the orbital involuntary muscle (Landstrom's muscle) (Fig. 6-1), and (4) vasoconstrictor fibers for the orbit, eyelids, and forehead, as already mentioned. The superior palpebral involuntary muscle lies on the undersurface of the levator palpebrae superioris, with which its fibers are interdigitated. In mammals in which the orbits communicate freely with the temporal fossae, the orbital muscle is a well-developed layer that prevents the orbital contents from being displaced backward. Whether it exists in man is questionable.

The three muscles—the dilator muscle of the pupil, the superior palpebral involuntary muscle, and the involuntary orbital muscle—and the vasoconstrictor fibers are under the influence of a group of cells, the ciliospinal center, situated in the intermediolateral horns of segments C7–Th2. As indicated, the preganglionic fibers proceed to the superior cervical sympathetic ganglion, and the postganglionic fibers course from this ganglion to the structures mentioned.

Interruption of the sympathetic fibers to the eye and adjacent region gives rise to disturbances known as *Horner's syndrome.*

Miosis. The affected pupil is smaller than that of the opposite side and does not dilate when the eye is shaded. The inequality of the two pupils (*anisocoria*) is much more evident in dim than in bright light; in bright light the antagonistic sphincter pupillae, innervated by the third nerve, comes into action on both sides. When the responsible lesion involves the sympathetic chain or sympathetic fibers more peripherally the mydriatic, cocaine,* introduced into the conjunctival sac of the miotic eye, does not cause pupillary dilatation; however, when the interruption is in

*Cocaine (4 percent) probably exerts its action by inhibiting the enzyme that normally decomposes epinephrine. Cocaine therefore allows epinephrine to accumulate at the motor end-plate and produces dilatation of the pupil. In the presence of ocular sympathetic paralysis the production of epinephrine is impaired, and consequently cocaine fails to dilate the affected pupil.

the central nervous system, the pupil dilates to cocaine almost as well as the pupil on the normal side (Jaffe, 1950). Epinephrine (1:1000), which does not normally alter pupillary size, may cause pupillary dilatation if pupillary paralysis has lasted for a time, especially when the interruption is peripherally situated (Boniuk and Schlezinger, 1962). Miosis is most pronounced when due to interruption of anterior roots C7–Th1. Miosis resulting from a lesion in the brainstem tends gradually to decrease in severity over a period of months, while miosis of peripheral origin may or may not decrease, depending on the cause of the miosis.

Ptosis. The upper eyelid droops somewhat because of paralysis of the superior palpebral involuntary muscle; the ptosis is less marked than that observed in interruption of the third nerve. The eyelid can be raised voluntarily, but not as well as that on the normal side. In time the ptosis may or may not be reduced, depending on the site of the lesion (Mahoney and Sheehan, 1936).

Enophthalmos. Backward displacement of the eyeball into the orbit is said to be a feature of Horner's syndrome, but measurements of the position of the eye have shown that enophthalmos is only apparent, not real (Boniuk and Schlezinger, 1962; Jaffe, 1950). Approximation of the eyelids brought about by the ptosis accounts for the impression that the eyeball has sunk into the orbit. Frequently there is not even an apparent enophthalmos.

Vasodilation in conjunctiva, forehead, and face, together with anhidrosis. As indicated, these conditions occur depending on the level of interruption of the sympathetic fibers. Hyperhidrosis occurs but is rare (Bodenheimer, 1924; Jung, 1947).

Heterochromia iridis. In the present context this term refers to pigment alteration occurring in the iris as a result of sympathetic denervation. The pigment change is perhaps most pronounced following interruption of sympathetic fibers in the lower brachial plexus in connection with plexus injury occurring during birth. (Walsh and Sloan, 1935.) Heterochromia iridis seems never to occur following sympathetic denervation in older persons.

Horner's syndrome may result from interruption of sympathetic pathways at numerous levels.

The prerubral field. The syndrome has commonly been observed as a complication of thalamotomy for the relief of dyskinesias, and has been considered to be due to interruption of sympathetic fibers emanating from the dorsocaudal part of the lateral hypothalamic area and coursing in the prerubral field, then lateral and ventral to the red nucleus. Ptosis and miosis were frequent in these patients and sometimes occurred in the absence of anhidrosis and, conversely, anhidrosis sometimes occurred when no ptosis or miosis was evident. The anhidrosis involved the side ipsilateral to the lesion—chest, axillary region, and palm of the hand and plantar aspect of the foot. (Carmel, 1968.) Horner's syndrome has also been known to occur in hemiballism; here, too, the sympathetic disturbance was ipsilateral to the lesion (Garcin and others, 1949).

The sympathetic fibers passing down the brainstem and cervical cord to the ciliospinal center. Horner's syndrome of brainstem origin most commonly occurs in lesions situated in the reticular formation in the region dorsolateral to the inferior olivary nucleus. Vascular occlusion and tumor are most frequently responsible (Giles and Henderson, 1958; List and Peet, 1939). Syringomyelia and syringobulbia are also among the causative lesions. The syndrome is frequently dissociated, ptosis being present and miosis absent, or the reverse.

The ciliospinal center. This center is situated in the uppermost thoracic segments.

The anterior roots of segments Th1 and Th2 or the respective white rami communicantes. Interruption of anterior roots C8 and Th1, most often due to trauma or neoplasm, produces not only Horner's syndrome but also lower brachial plexus paralysis (*Dejerine-Klumpke's paralysis*). The small muscles of the hand and the flexors of the forearm are paralyzed. Horner's syndrome together with Dejerine-Klumpke's paralysis (Fig. 6-2) can be produced only by lesions that interrupt anterior root fibers proximal to the point where the white rami communicantes are given off. A lesion distal to this point gives rise to De-

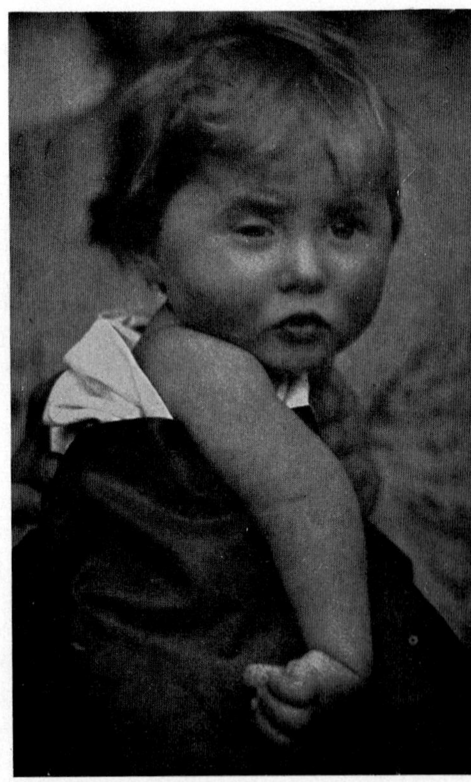

Fig. 6-2. Horner's syndrome in association with lower brachial plexus palsy (Dejerine-Klumpke's paralysis).

jerine-Klumpke's paralysis alone. Encroachment of a cervical rib on the lower cords of the brachial plexus is another cause of Horner's syndrome.

The cervical sympathetic chain. Carcinoma of the apex of the lung ("Pancoast" tumor), compressing the chain, is often first suspected when Horner's syndrome develops (Jaffe, 1950). Trauma may also be responsible (Fig. 6-3). The sympathetic chain or the pericarotid sympathetic plexus may also be interrupted as a consequence of intraoral trauma. For example, this occurred in a child with a dowel stick in his mouth who fell and impaled his left tonsillar fossa; the ptosis and miosis cleared in about 4 months (Pruett, 1967). Horner's syndrome occurring under these conditions is occasionally succeeded by internal carotid artery thrombosis (Acquaviva and others, 1961). Almost any condition in the area, such as cervical adenopathy, may compromise sympathetic fibers and thus give rise to Horner's syndrome.

Postganglionic neurons. The course of postganglionic sympathetic fibers running in the sheath of the internal carotid artery is illustrated in Fig. 14-1. Horner's syndrome may occur as a result of interruption of these fibers anywhere in their postganglionic course. Some of the fibers traverse the ciliary ganglion en route to the superior palpebral involuntary muscle and the dilator pupillae, and others traverse the sphenopalatine ganglion en route to the orbital muscle. Hence a destructive lesion confined to the ciliary ganglion leads to miosis and ptosis.

Overaction of the ciliospinal center is manifested by *spasmodic pupillodilatation and exophthalmos.* This is a rare disturbance that may be due to a lesion in the thoracic segments situated just below the ciliospinal center (at about Th3).

Interruption of postganglionic sympathetic fibers results in *denervation hypersensitivity,* whereby the miotic pupil enlarges when the patient is frightened or is subjected to other emotional excitement. This is due to hypersensitivity of the terminal area to circulating epinephrine.

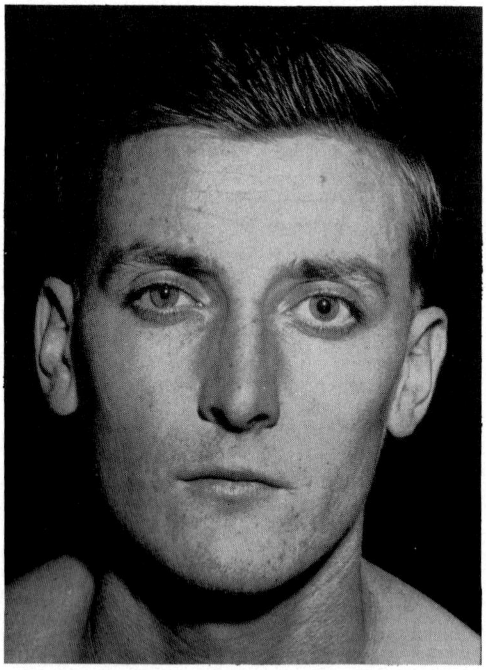

Fig. 6-3. Horner's syndrome due to grenade wound of right side of neck. On that side there is slight ptosis and obvious miosis. (From Walter Reed Army Hosp.; Negs. 4060—1 and 2.)

Raeder's paratrigeminal syndrome is a disorder characterized by ocular sympathetic pathway paralysis with or without alteration in sweating of the face, and associated with involvement of one or more cranial nerves (II, III, IV, V, VI). Causative pathological conditions include metastatic tumor, ophthalmic herpes zoster, trauma, and orbital syphilitic osteitis. Prolonged maxillary sinusitis and chronic otitis media have been noted in some cases. The ptosis and miosis that occur are often less noticeable than in Horner's syndrome due to lesions at more proximal levels. Two groups within the syndrome may be distinguished—those associated with cranial nerve involvement (usually due to a lesion in the middle cranial fossa), and those not. Only the latter will be considered in the following.

Disturbances are variable. Engorgement of conjunctival vessels and excess tear secretion mark some cases, such that the patient may be treated for "acute conjunctivitis." Further, there may be anhidrosis of the forehead and eyelid. Pain in the forehead and/or headache are of common occurrence. The pain is distinguishable from trigeminal neuralgia in that it is most severe within and around the orbit; it is deep and boring and on occasion mounts steadily in severity until it is excruciating; attacks of this kind, which are self-limited, sometimes occur on one side, then the other. Objective changes in the affected area, such as hypesthesia, are lacking. Raeder's syndrome may be misdiagnosed as "atypical facial neuralgia." Damage of the oculosympathetic fibers in the sheath of the internal carotid artery due to dilation of the artery and edema of the sheath have been suggested as causes. (Boniuk and Schlezinger, 1962; Ford and Walsh, 1958.) Occasionally, the syndrome is associated with aneurysm of the extracranial part of the carotid artery, and, rarely, aneurysm of the supracavernous portion of the artery (Davis, Daroff, and Hoyt, 1968).

REFERENCES

Acquaviva, R., Thevenot, C., LeBascle, J., and Tamic, P. M. 1961. Thrombose de la carotide interne après contusion de la loge amygdalienne par appareil de prosthèses dentaire. Maroc Méd. **40**:781-782.

Austin, G. M. 1961. The spinal cord: basic aspects and surgical considerations. Springfield, Illinois, Charles C Thomas, Publisher.

Bennett, A. E., and Fortes, A. 1945. Meningioma obstructing the foramen magnum. Arch. Neurol. Psychiat. **53**:131-134.

Bodenheimer, L. 1924. Zur Symptomatologie der Lähmung der sympathischen Grenzstranges. Z. Ges. Neurol. Psychiat. **92**:597-608.

Boniuk, M., and Schlezinger, N. S. 1962. Raeder's paratrigeminal syndrome. Amer. J. Ophthal. **54**: 1074-1084.

Cailliet, R. 1962. Neck and arm pain. Philadelphia, F. A. Davis Co.

Carmel, P. W. 1968. Sympathetic deficits following thalamotomy. Arch. Neurol. **18**:378-387.

Compere, W. E., Jr. 1968. Electronystagmographic findings in patients with "whiplash" injuries. Laryngoscope **78**:1226-1233.

Davis, R. H., Daroff, R. B., and Hoyt, W. F. 1968. Hemicrania, oculosympathetic paresis, and subcranial aneurysm: Raeder's paratrigeminal syndrome (group 2): case report. J. Neurosurg. **29**:94-96.

Epstein, J. A., Epstein, B. S., and Lavine, L. S. 1963. Cervical spondylotic myelopathy: the syndrome of the narrow canal treated by laminectomy, foramenotomy, and the removal of osteophytes. Arch. Neurol. **8**:307-317.

Facer, J. C. 1967. Osteophytes of the cervical spine causing dysphagia. Arch. Otolaryng. **86**: 117-121.

Ford, F. R., and Walsh, F. B. 1958. Raeder's paratrigeminal syndrome. Bull. Johns Hopk. Hosp. **103**:296-298.

Garcin, R., Bertrand, I., Kipfer, M., Gruner, J., and Pestel, M. 1949. Hemiballismus, étude anatomo-clinique. Rev. Neurol. **81**:964-968.

Gay, J. R., and Abbott, K. H. 1953. Common whiplash injuries of the neck. J.A.M.A. **152**: 1698-1704.

Giles, C. L., and Henderson, J. W. 1958. Horner's syndrome: an analysis of 216 cases. Amer. J. Ophthal. **46**:289-296.

Greenfield, J. G. 1953. Malformations et degenerescences des disques intervertebraux de la region cérvicale. Rév. Méd., Suisse Rom. **73**: 227-250.

Gutmann, L., and Hable, K. 1963. Rheumatoid pachymeningitis. Neurology **13**:901-905.

Hitchcock, E., and Leece, B. 1967. Somatotopic representation of the respiratory pathways in the cervical cord of man. J. Neurosurg. **27**: 320-329.

Holmes, J. T. 1966. Pathology of the spinal cord. London, Lloyd-Luke.

Jaffe, N. S. 1950. Localization of lesions causing Horner's syndrome. Arch. Ophthal. **44**:710-728.

Jung. 1947. Wieso kommt es beim Hornerschen Syndrom zu einer lokalen Hyperhidrosis der Stirnpartie über dem erkrankten Auge? Dtsch. Med. Wschr. **72**:131.

Langfitt, T. W., and Elliott, F. A. 1967. Pain in the back and legs caused by cervical spinal cord compression. J.A.M.A. **200**:382-385.

List, C. F., and Peet, M. M. 1939. Sweat secretion in man: disturbances of sweat secretion with lesions of the pons, medulla and cervical portion of the cord. Arch. Neurol. Psychiat. **42**:1098-1127.

Mahoney, W., and Sheehan, D. 1936. Experimental ptosis in primates. Arch. Neurol. Psychiat. **35**:99-108.

Mair, W. G. P., and Druckman, R. 1953. The pathology of spinal cord lesions and their relation to the clinical features in protrusion of cervical intervertebral discs. (A report of four cases.) Brain **76**:70-91.

Matthews, W. B. 1968. The neurological complications of ankylosing spondylitis. J. Neurol. Sci. **6**:561-573.

Mixter, W. J., and Barr, J. S. 1934. Rupture of the intervertebral disc with involvement of the spinal canal. New Eng. J. Med. **211**:210-214.

Naffziger, H. C., and Brown, H. A. 1933. Hourglass tumors of the spine. Arch. Neurol. Psychiat. **29**:561-584.

Nugent, G. R. 1959. Clinicopathologic correlations in cervical spondylosis. Neurology **9**:273-281.

Odom, G. L., Finney, W., and Woodhall, B. 1958. Cervical disk lesions. J.A.M.A. **166**:23-28.

Ommaya, A. K., Faas, F., and Yarnell, P. 1968. Whiplash injury and brain damage: an experimental study. J.A.M.A. **204**:285-289.

Pruett, R. C. 1967. Horner's syndrome following intra-oral trauma. Arch. Ophthal. **78**:420-421.

Symonds, C. P., and Meadows, S. P. 1937. Compression of the spinal cord in the neighbourhood of the foramen magnum. Brain **60**:52-84.

Taylor, A. R. 1964. Vascular factors in the myelopathy associated with cervical spondylosis. Neurology **14**:62-68.

Walsh, F. B., and Sloan, L. L. 1935. Results of cervical sympathectomy in pigmentary degeneration of the retina. Arch. Ophthal. **14**:699-714.

Yuhl, E. T., Hanna, D., Rasmussen, T., and Richter, R. B. 1955. Diagnosis and surgical therapy of chronic midline disk protrusions. Neurology **5**:494-509.

Chapter 7

Localization of lesions involving lower spinal segments and the cauda equina

INNERVATION AND FUNCTION OF THE URINARY BLADDER

The bladder musculature is a single entity, consisting of bundles of smooth muscle fibers running in many directions, changing planes and orientation in their course, decussating, and, in essence, forming a syncytium. The bladder trigone is the product of blending the ureteric muscle continuing across the midline to form the interureteric fold. The bladder proper has no separate sphincter muscle. Instead, the entire urethra in the female and the prostatic and membranous parts of the urethra in the male constitute the sphincter of the bladder. Sphincteric action by this system is credited (1) to the contraction of two opposing arcades of longitudinal detrusor vesicle muscle bundles that are continuous with the submucosal muscular layer of the urethra, and (2) to the contractile action of elastic tissue, of circular orientation, in the region of the bladder neck and along the length of the urethra. Holding of the vesicle orifice closed as the bladder expands and as the muscular wall is stretched appears to be a function largely of the elastic tissue in these regions. On the other hand, opening of the urethra is initiated at the vesicle neck by the concurrent contraction of the detrusor muscle bundles of the bladder and the longitudinal muscle bundles extending from bladder to urethra. The contraction results in funneling (or opening) of the bladder neck and the proximal urethra and shortening of the urethra. The older concept of opposing actions of the detrusor and internal vesicle sphincter controlled by alternating action of the sympathetic and parasympathetic systems is no longer valid. (Woodburne, 1961, 1968.)

The urinary bladder derives its nerve supply from two chief sources: the parasympathetic nervous system, which transmits impulses of an involuntary nature, and the cerebrospinopudendal pathway, which carries fibers concerned in volitional control. Bladder function is subject to control from several suprasegmental levels. This includes sympathetic mechanisms, the action(s) of which finds, however, little if any clinical expression.

Sympathetic fibers originate from the intermediolateral horns of the lower thoracic and upper lumbar segments (approximately Th11 through L1). They gain exit from the cord via the corresponding anterior roots and traverse the sympathetic chain, which they leave at ganglionic levels L1–L4. (There is no consensus as to their sites of synapse; Mitchell, 1953.) The postganglionic fibers descend along the abdominal aorta to form, at its bifurcation, the superior hypogastric plexus (or the "presacral nerve") This plexus divides to form two groups of nerves, the hypogastric nerves, which course along the anterior surface of the sacrum to reach the bladder wall. The fibers are said to terminate solely in the extension of the ureteral musculature situated in the trigone of the bladder. There is also evidence that central sympathetic mechanisms exert a facilitatory action on bladder contraction (see subsequent text), but considered clinically (as already mentioned), the sympathetic system appears not to be significantly concerned in micturition. (Denny-Brown and Robertson, 1933; Langworthy, Kolb, and Lewis, 1940.)

Parasympathetic preganglionic fibers arise in intermediolateral cell groups of the spinal cord, mainly in segment S3 and less so in S2 and S4, and proceed through the corresponding anterior roots (Heimburger, Freeman, and Wilde, 1948). They pass peripherally by way of the pudendal plexus, the pelvic nerve (Fig. 2-2), and the inferior hypogastric plexus, mingling with the sympathetic fibers, and terminate in ganglia in the outer wall of the bladder, whence arise postganglionic fibers that supply muscle bundles having detrusor action and others, in the urethra, having sphincteric action. The parasympathetic, when stimulated, causes contraction of detrusor muscle bundles and, secondarily, a stretching of the elastic tissue, which results in bladder emptying.

The *cerebrospinopudendal pathway* pursues the following course: The upper motor neurons, which carry voluntary impulses, arise in the paracentral lobule and follow approximately the same route as the parasympathetic fibers in reaching the lower part of the spinal cord. They synapse with anterior horn cells of segments S3 and S4. The fibers of these cells pass peripherally as the pudendal nerve to supply the urethral sphincter mechanism and the accessory urethral and perineal muscles. These fibers carry impulses concerned in voluntary cessation of urination.

Afferent pathways from the bladder can be subdivided into certain functional groups: fibers conveying the feeling of bladder fullness traverse the pelvic nerve; pain impulses from the dome of the bladder pass via the hypogastric nerves, those from the trigone via the pelvic nerve. It can be assumed that afferent fibers enter numerous cord levels, as all sensation of increased bladder tension is abolished only in lesions that completely transect the spinal cord at levels above Th7 (Bors, 1952). Desire to void is mediated by fibers running in the pelvic nerve. This is shown by the fact that patients with sacral cord lesions do not indicate a need to void, and by the observation that neither presacral neurectomy nor pudendal nerve procaine block interferes with the desire to void (Sarnoff and Arrowood, 1947). Fibers conveying sensibility from the bladder pass partly up the posterior column and partly up the spinothalamic tracts of the spinal cord.

In addition to the afferent fibers just mentioned, there are others, passing by way of the pelvic nerve, which are concerned in reflex functioning of the bladder. The basic arc is at the sacral level. The incoming fibers represent the afferent limb of the stretch reflex, initiated in the bladder, upon which micturition mainly depends.

Suprasegmental autonomic fibers originate from several levels. An area situated in the reticular formation of the caudal midbrain and rostral pons is concerned exclusively in the organization of the micturition reflex in all its phases: initiation, continuation, termination (Bradley and Conway, 1966). A center exerting a facilitatory influence on the bladder has been described as situated at the pontile level and another at the intercollicular level. An inhibitory center is located at a slightly higher level. Other neurons, of an autonomic nature, originate in the cerebral cortex and probably pass directly to the hypothalamus; others arising in the orbitofrontal cortex also reach the hypothalamus. Postsynaptic fibers gain the lateral hypothalamic area, where they are joined by fibers from the septal region. Situated in the caudolateral part of the hypothalamus are sympathetic neurons that have a strong facilitatory influence on the bladder. Fibers leaving the hypothalamus and coursing downward synapse at various brainstem levels, possibly in some of the centers already mentioned. Some postsynaptic neurons pass down the spinal cord in close association with the pyramidal tracts. (Hess, 1948; Langworthy, Kolb, and Lewis, 1940; Ruch, 1955.)

Emptying of the bladder is brought about in a manner approximately as follows: When 50 to 150 cc. of urine collects in the bladder, tension receptors in the mucosa and submucosa providing this information initiate impulses that pass via the pelvic nerve to the cord, then to the cerebrum, where, in response to the stimulus, the desire to urinate arises. The voiding begins with an increase in intra-abdominal pressure and a reciprocal relaxation of the perineal and pelvic muscles (including the external sphincter), which induces a "tug" on the vesicle neck. In turn, this tug initiates a contraction of the detrusor muscle bundles situated in the base of the bladder and on into the urethra, and the contraction then spreads upward in the muscle syncytium of the bladder wall to the dome. Emptying of the bladder is brought to a halt through contraction of muscles of the pelvic floor, an action that elevates the entire bladder base in such a manner that the vesicle "snaps shut." (Bradley, 1967; Muellner, 1951.)

In the normal younger person the bladder capacity is 400 to 600 cc. and after micturition the bladder contains no residual urine. Neither does the bladder contract reflexly to small amounts of urine or in response to perineal, rectal, or abdominal stimulation.

DISTURBANCES IN BLADDER FUNCTION

Interruption of higher suprasegmental systems (uninhibited neurogenic bladder). Sites involved include the paracentral lobules (by parasagittal meningioma, thrombosed superior sagittal sinus) and the corticospinal tracts of the two sides (in vascular "accidents," multiple sclerosis). Bladder sensation in such cases is intact. Increased frequency as well as urgency of urination occurs. As the bladder is filled the detrusor contracts, increasing intravesical pressure. Automatic micturition may ultimately develop. At this stage the bladder may become so contracted that a small quantity of urine is capable of inducing micturition.

Uninhibited neurogenic bladder may also be noted in lesions involving the hypothalamus or midbrain. In glioma of the tuber cinereum, involuntary micturition is occasionally an initial manifestation. Involvement of the midbrain in parkinsonism or chronic encephalitis leads in some cases to elevated intravesical pressure combined with increased frequency of micturition, indicating vesicomotor overactivity (Brouwer, 1950).

Uninhibited bladder is common in older people not incontinent. The capacity of the bladder is reduced and the amount of residual urine increased. Thus the bladder neither fills properly nor does it empty properly. Uninhibited bladder contractions may occur during filling, and may be of sufficient strength to empty the bladder suddenly when there is little urine. Precipitancy and nocturia are also common in the elderly. Trabeculation and diverticula are found on examination of the bladder. In some 50 percent of aged women, pelvic floor incompetence and funneling of the bladder outlet are also to be found. These disturbances can occur whether or not the elderly have hemiplegia, multiple strokes, signs of cerebral arteriosclerosis, and so on. (Brocklehurst, 1967.)

Cord lesions above the sacral level (reflex bladder, automatic bladder). With complete spinal transection above segment S1, bladder function is dependent solely on the spinal reflex arc (hence the term "reflex bladder"). Retention occurs first, then overflow incontinence, and finally pronounced automaticity. The automaticity is such that there is no dribbling. The bladder never completely empties itself. Frequently it can be made to empty reflexly by applying a stimulus to the perineum, rectum, or abdomen, or even the lower limb, such as tickling the sole of the foot. Under such conditions, the automatic micturition is part of a mass reflex, which includes priapism and flexion contraction (withdrawal) of the entire lower limb.

Automatic bladder developing in the course of paraplegia due to complete or incomplete traumatic transection of the cervical or upper thoracic cord may be associated with a variety of autonomic manifestations. Occurring at the time of bladder distention, they include marked elevation of blood pressure, bradycardia, varied cardiac arrhythmias with rates as low as 36 per minute, pronounced constriction of the cutaneous blood vessels, decrease in skin temperature (as much as 8° F. in the fingers and toes), and dilatation of the pupils; and above the level of the cord damage, "goose flesh," blotchy redness of the skin, and profuse perspiration. These disorders vanish when the increased elastic tension of the bladder is relieved by section of the anterior and posterior roots of segments S1 through S5. (Guttmann and Whitteridge, 1947; Scheibert, 1955.)

In tumors situated at spinal cord level Th12 or higher, urinary symptoms usually precede the onset of other neurological disturbances. In benign tumor, the time involved before these other neurological disturbances are recognized may be an average of 2 years. The main bladder symptoms in tumors in this location are urgency, incontinence, increased frequency, and nocturia (Campbell, 1967). In extramedullary-intradural tumor involving the cervical cord, sphincter disturbances are often encountered but are highly variable in degree (Craig and Sheldon, 1940).

Lesions involving sacral segments (autonomous neurogenic bladder). Most if not all the afferent and efferent connections are interrupted, decentralizing the bladder. Vesicle disturbances often develop concurrently with symptoms denoting damage of sacral cord systems that supply somatic structures (Campbell, 1967). The stages of retention and overflow incontinence are of the same nature and duration as described earlier. Spontaneous detrusor contractions are lacking, but owing to autorhythmicity of the detrusor musculature, low-level rhythmic contractions can be demonstrated (by cystometry). Because of the lack of spontaneous detrusor action, *(paralytic) incontinence* occurs. The bladder wall becomes greatly hypertrophied. Stimulation of the perineum, rectum, abdomen, or sole of the foot does not induce automatic micturition. Presacral (sympathetic) neurectomy under these conditions does not appreciably improve bladder emptying (Jacobson, Braasch, and Love, 1944). In some cases this procedure does, however, ameliorate intractable bladder pain (Learmonth, 1931; Scott and Schroeder, 1938).

Lesions of the cauda equina. In tumors involving the cauda equina, of which ependymoma is the most common, incontinence may be the only bladder disturbance. This disorder occurs, however, only in about a third of cases, and even then, only after the development of pain (usually sciatica) and weakness and numbness in the gluteal region and lower limbs (Kernohan, Woltman, and Adson, 1933). Surgical section of anterior and posterior roots S1 through S5 for "hypertonic" bladder complicating cervical or upper thoracic traumatic myelopathy has restored bladder function (Scheibert, 1955). When motor outflow is preferentially interrupted (*motor paralytic bladder*), bladder sensation is preserved, while detrusor contraction is lacking. Such findings indicate damage either of the cauda equina or of sacral segments (Austin, 1961).

Lesions of posterior lumbar roots. Tabes dorsalis is a familiar example of a disorder in which the posterior lumbar roots are affected. The functional deficit is thus on the afferent side of the arc. The micturition reflex is lost. The bladder wall becomes markedly stretched, and dribbling incontinence occurs. The patient is not aware that his bladder is filled. Voluntary micturition is possible, but only with great effort.

Diabetes mellitus is another condition in which overfilling of the bladder occurs, and this disturbance may be the initial manifestation of the diabetes. Possibly the responsible lesion is situated in the posterior lumbar roots. In some 50 percent of patients having this condition, and not suspected as having diabetes, the glucose tolerance test reveals a decrease in tolerance. Evidence that bladder sensation is deficient is evident from the fact that as much as 700 cc. (instead of the usual 50 to 150 cc.) of urine may collect before the first desire to void arises. Urinary retention, stress incontinence, the presence of calculi, and recurring infection may be manifestations of the deficit in bladder sensation. (Motzkin, 1968.)

Involvement of lower spinal levels in myelomeningocele. Some 60 percent of children with myelomeningocele have disturbances in voiding. The posterior roots are commonly damaged and sometimes the spinal cord as well. Cystometry in these children has revealed two main types of disturbance (in addition to cutaneous sensory loss): upper motor neuron (or reflex) type of bladder disorder, and lower motor neuron (denervated, or decentralized) type. Although overlap between these two types is common, one or the other usually predominates. A third type is found in children with myelomeningocele who have relatively normal detrusor action; here sensory loss resulting either from posterior root or ascending tract damage is encountered, as is also motor weakness due to partial motor denervation. In all three types significant differences exist from child to child in the rate of continence and in the incidence of upper urinary tract dilatation. (Cooper, 1968 a, b.)

INNERVATION AND FUNCTION OF THE SIGMOID AND RECTUM

The neural connections of the rectum are similar to those of the bladder. Here, too, parasympathetic cells are present in sacral segments 3, 4, and 5. In defecation the parasympathetic system brings about contraction of the sigmoidal and rectal muscles and relaxation of the internal sphincter. The sympathetic nervous system has the reverse function: it is concerned in rectal filling (Learmonth and Markowitz, 1929). Afferent impulses course chiefly in parasympathetic trunks (Goligher and Hughes, 1951). Impulses pass to the cerebrum, supplying it with information as to the degree of rectal filling. On the efferent (voluntary) side, fibers arising in the cerebrum pass down the cord in the lateral columns, transmitting impulses for defecation. These impulses reach mainly the anterior horn cells of Th6 to Th12, which are concerned in contraction of the abdominal muscles. These muscles have a powerful detrusor action on the rectum.

DISTURBANCES IN RECTAL FUNCTION

Spinal lesions above the sacral level. Voluntary control of the sphincter ani and the sensation of rectal urgency are lost. As a result, fecal retention occurs. The constrictor ani continues to contract reflexly and is usually spastic (as can be noted by insertion of a finger into the rectum), a finding which indicates that the site of the lesion is supranuclear. In exceptional cases, and then in total cord transection, reflex sphincter contraction is absent.

In some patients defecation occurs at rather long intervals, involuntarily. This condition is called *reflex intermittent defecation.* In non-neoplastic hypothalamic lesions intrarectal pressure may need to be extraordinarily high before the evacuation reflex is initiated; by contrast, in tumor involving the tuber cinereum there may be highly exaggerated defecation reflex activity (Brouwer, 1950).

Lesions of the sacral cord. In lesions involving segments S3–S5, permanent paralysis of the sphincter ani occurs, with fecal incontinence resulting, though hard fecal masses may be retained. The paralysis may be either partial or complete, depending upon the degree of elasticity of the anal sphincter.

INNERVATION AND FUNCTION OF THE MALE GENITAL ORGANS

In erection two factors play a role: (1) engorgement of the corpora cavernosa with blood due to relaxation of tonus of the arteries of the penis, and (2) inability of the blood in the corpora cavernosa to escape into the venous system because of tonic contraction of the transverse perineal, bulbocavernosus, and ischiocavernosus muscles. Another explanation of the blood retention is that the emergent veins are compressed by the enlarged corpora cavernosa as they pass under the tunica albuginea.

The decrease of the vascular tonus that results in erection is effected partly by inhibition of the vasoconstrictor (sympathetic) center, situated in intermediolateral horns of segments L1 and L2, and partly by excitation of vasodilator (parasympathetic) centers, situated in segments S1, S2, and S3. The vasoconstrictor fibers pass to the external genitalia through the superior hypogastric plexus and are joined by the vasodilator fibers coursing in the inferior hypogastric plexus. The spinal centers receive fibers from the cerebrum and from vasomotor centers of the medulla oblongata via the lateral columns of the cord.

In the ejaculatory act the sperm are brought to the membranous part of the urethra through reflex peristalsis of the ampulla of the ductus deferens, the seminal vesicles, and the ejaculatory duct, then are propelled through the urethral canal by means of clonic spasms of the bulbocavernosus and ischiocavernosus muscles. The reflex arc subserving ejaculation is as follows: The afferent limb, activated by impulses arising in the genital epithelium, extends centrally by way of the dorsal nerve of the penis and the pudendal nerve, thence to the spinal cord predominantly in posterior roots S3 and S4. The impulses reach two spinal centers, from which fibers of the efferent limb of the reflex arc arise: (1) sympathetic centers in segments Th6–L3 (Austin, 1961), which induces peristalsis of the ampulla of the ductus deferens, the seminal vesicles, and the ejaculatory ducts, and (2) a parasympathetic center in segments S3 and S4, which induces clonic spasms of the bulbocavernosus and ischiocavernosus muscles. The peripheral pathway concerned is the perineal branch of the pudendal nerve. Sympathetic ganglion L II is especially important in the ejaculatory act (Retief, 1950).

DISTURBANCES IN SEXUAL FUNCTION

Spinal lesions above the sacral level. Vasoconstrictor fibers that innervate the vessels of the corpora cavernosa are no longer functional. The vessels fill with blood, and thus the penis becomes enlarged. *Priapism* lasting varying periods of time, sometimes over long periods, is commonly met with in lesions of the cord situated above the lower thoracic segments (infectious myelitis, Pott's disease of the spine, and multiple sclerosis) (Wechsler, 1952). In one series of cases of traumatic complete cord section, priapism was common; it was also noted following partial cord transection (Hartwell, 1917). Priapism occurring in lesions partially interrupting the cord is thought to be due to parasympathetic-induced vasodilatation, although an additional factor consists in tonic contraction of the transverse perineal, bulbocavernosus, and ischiocavernosus muscles, preventing the escape of blood into the venous system; mass reflex action has also been postulated as a basis. Under the conditions cited, ejaculatory reflex activity may at times be so increased that the slightest stimulus causes either an ejaculation or the occurrence of clonic contractions of the muscles in question. Normal erection can occur in transection at levels above the sacral segments (Horne, Paull, and Munro, 1948), which can be taken to mean that erection need not be under suprasegmental control.

Lesions of the sacral cord. In lesions involving segments S3–S5, erection of the penis and ejaculation do not occur; in other words, complete impotence prevails. Occasionally, however, there is a dissociated disturbance of potency—normal erection and an inability to ejaculate or to have an orgasm. This is usually due to a very circumscribed sacral cord lesion such as infarct. Histological findings in such cases would lead to the conclusion that the center for erection lies somewhat higher than that for ejaculation, the former at S1 to S3, and the latter at S3 and S4.

OTHER CLINICAL FEATURES OF CONUS MEDULLARIS AND EPICONUS LESIONS

For the sake of clinical convenience, segments S3–Cocl may be regarded as comprising the conus medullaris, and segments L4–S2 the epiconus. The cauda equina classically includes roots L3–Cocl.

Lesions limited to the *conus medullaris,* so defined, give rise to highly characteristic signs:

1. Paralytic incontinence and, usually, bladder distention
2. Fecal incontinence
3. Impotence and, later, a dissociated disturbance of potency
4. Perianogenital, or saddle, anesthesia (sensibility is lost in cutaneous radicular fields S3, S4, and S5)
5. Absence of motor disturbances in the lower limbs and absence of the Babinski and other pathological pyramidal tract signs (The lower limbs derive their innervation from segments of the spinal cord above the conus medullaris. Most of the muscles of the feet are innervated from spinal segments not lower than S2. Only the flexor digitorum longus and the flexor hallucis longus and brevis receive a nerve supply from segments S3, but it is minor. The arc of the "ankle jerk" traverses segments L5, S1, and S2.)

The *conus syndrome* in its pure form offers no diagnostic difficulties. It is not often encountered, and then only in certain lesions such as small intramedullary tumor metastases, hemorrhagic infarct, gliotic foci, and cysts (Nassar, Carrell, and Houspian, 1968; Poser, 1956). When the conus medullaris is heavily damaged by extramedullary processes or by trauma, the conus syndrome is almost never encountered in its pure form, the reason being that surrounding cauda equina is also damaged. Occasionally in fracture or dislocation the cauda equina escapes injury, whereas the conus medullaris, despite being surrounded by the cauda equina, is alone injured. Moreover, fractures of the lower lumbar vertebrae or the sacrum have been known to cause the conus syndrome by selectively injuring the medially located roots of the cauda equina (those that have emerged from the lower sacral segments).

The *epiconus syndrome* is also uncommon. In contrast to the conus syndrome, it is characterized by considerable motor disability. External rotation and extension (dorsal flexion) of the thigh are most affected, and more or less involved are abduction at the hip, flexion at the knee, and flexion and extension at the ankle. The "Achilles jerk" is lost. Disturbances in sensibility occur in radicular fields L4–S2, inclusive. The bladder and rectum function reflexly but not voluntarily.

Owing to differential growth of the vertebral column and the spinal cord during embryonic and fetal life, the lowermost part of the spinal cord comes to lie at the level of vertebra L I or L II. From this level downward the spinal canal is filled with the roots of segments L3 to Coc1, which are coursing to their respective intervertebral foramina (Fig. 4-20).

The close spatial relationship that exists between cauda equina and conus makes it difficult to distinguish cauda equina lesions from conus lesions. Compression of the cauda equina at the level between vertebrae L III and L IV gives rise to much the same signs as compression of the conus, brought about by fracture of vertebra L I. Fracture as the basis is revealed by sensitivity of the vertebral column to digital pressure, by the presence of visible and palpable deformities, and by roentgenography. Sometimes precise localization may be evident only with the passage of time, when complicating edema and hemorrhage involving the cauda and conus have subsided. Differential features are given in Table 7-1. (The characteristics of unilateral lesions of the lower segments of the cord are indicated on p. 90.)

Decubital ulcers are more prone to occur in spinal cord than in cauda equina lesions. In occasional instances severe trophic disorders of the feet develop as the result of polyradiculopathy involving the cauda equina. Edema appears early

Table 7-1. Differential diagnosis of lower spinal cord and cauda equina lesions

Lesions of lower spinal cord	*Lesions of the cauda equina*
In lesions situated in the central part of the cord dissociated anesthesia tends to occur (decrease in pain and temperature sensibility and no change in tactile sensibility).	All forms of sensibility are affected.
Spontaneous pains are uncommon and are usually not marked.	Spontaneous pains occur, especially in the perineum, over the sacrum, and in the region of the bladder; they are usually severe and consist in radicular pains, or there may be anesthesia dolorosa followed by complete sensory loss. These disturbances occur, as a rule, in compressive lesions.
Fibrillary twitchings in the paralyzed muscles are rare. Tonic-clonic contractions occasionally occur.	Fibrillary twitchings in the paralyzed muscles (especially in the peroneus group) are common.
Signs of damage are practically always symmetrical on the two sides.	The signs frequently predominate on one side.

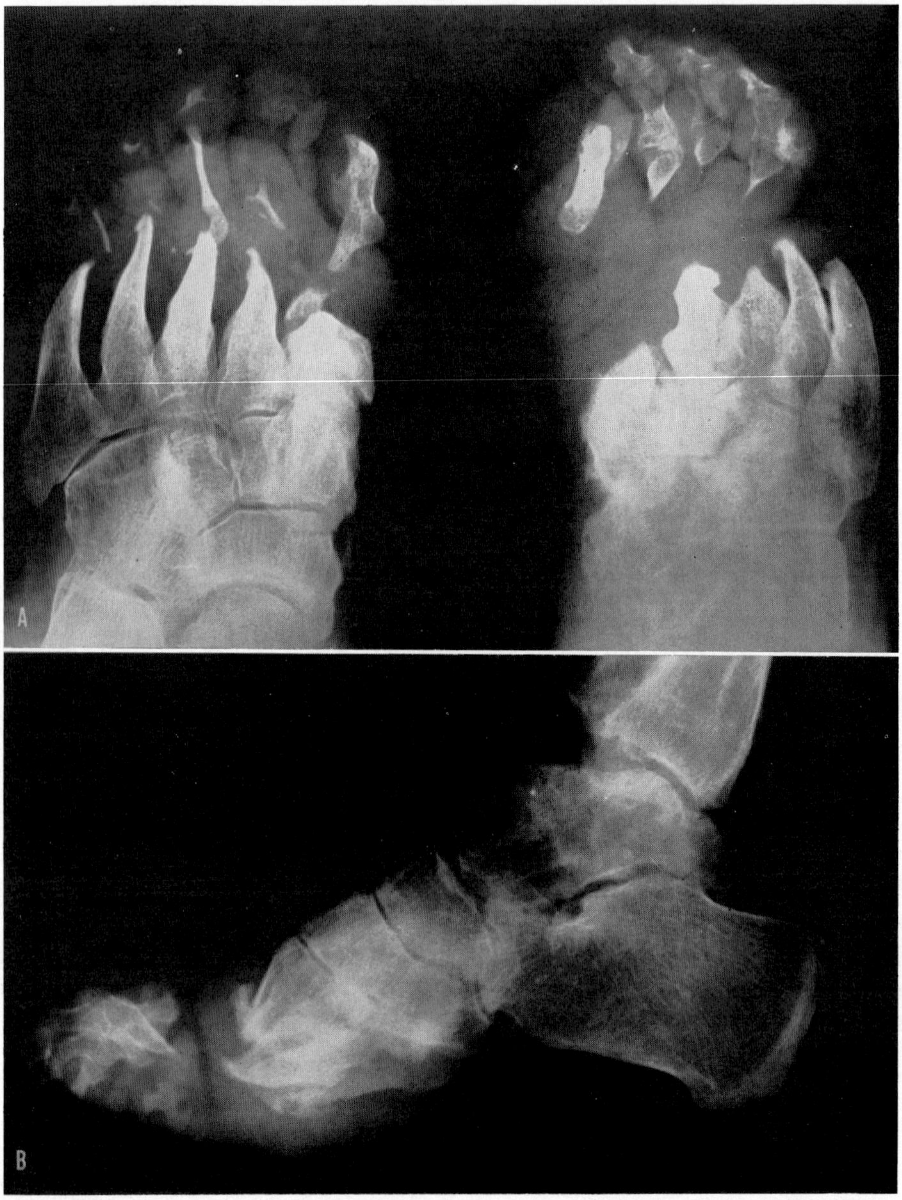

Fig. 7-1. X-ray view of the feet in radiculopathy involving the cauda equina. Osteolysis is intense in the metatarsus and the phalanges. The foot shown on the right side in **A** is illustrated in **B.** (From Barraquer-Ferré and Barraquer-Bordas, 1952.)

and in time the skin ulcerates and the bones of the feet, principally those of the metatarsus, undergo intense lysis resulting in sequestration (Fig. 7-1). As a consequence, the feet and toes become badly deformed (Barraquer-Ferré and Barraquer-Bordas, 1952).

REFERENCES

Austin, G. M. 1961. The spinal cord: basic aspects and surgical considerations. Springfield, Illinois, Charles C Thomas, Publisher.

Barraquer-Ferré, L., and Barraquer-Bordas, L. 1952. Trophic disorders of the feet in acquired lesions of the cauda equina. J. Nerv. Ment. Dis. **116**:902-911.

Bors, E. 1952. Segmental and peripheral innervation of the urinary bladder. J. Nerv. Ment. Dis. **116**:572-578.

Bradley, W. E. 1967. Neurologic aspects of smooth muscle disease: dysfunction of the urinary bladder. Postgrad. Med. **41**:260-262.

Bradley, W. E., and Conway, C. J. 1966. Bladder representation in the pontine-mesencephalic reticular formation. Exper. Neurol. **16**:237-249.

Brocklehurst, J. C. 1967. The management of incontinence. Postgrad. Med. J. **43**:527-533.

Brouwer, B. 1950. Positive and negative aspects of hypothalamic disorders. J. Neurol. Neurosurg. Psychiat. **13**:16-23.

Campbell, E. W., Jr. 1967. Bladder dysfunction related to lesions of the spinal cord. South. Med. J. **60**:364-366.

Cooper, D. G. W. 1968a. Detrusor action in children with myelomeningocele. Arch. Dis. Child. **43**:427-432.

Cooper, D. G. W. 1968b. Bladder studies in children with neurogenic incontinence: with comments on the place of pelvic floor stimulation. Brit. J. Urol. **40**:157-174.

Craig, W. McK., and Shelden, C. H. 1940. Tumors of the cervical portion of the spinal cord. Arch. Neurol. Psychiat. **44**:1-16.

Denny-Brown, D., and Robertson, E. G. 1933. On the physiology of micturition. Brain **56**:149-190.

Goligher, J. C., and Hughes, E. S. R. 1951. Sensibility of the rectum and colon: its role in the mechanism of anal continence. Lancet **1**:543-548.

Guttmann, L., and Whitteridge, D. 1947. Effects of bladder distention on autonomic mechanisms after spinal cord injuries. Brain **70**:361-404.

Hartwell, J. B. 1917. An analysis of 133 fractures of the spine treated at the Massachusetts General Hospital. Boston Med. Surg. J. **177**:31-41.

Heimburger, R. F., Freeman, L. W., and Wilde, N. J. 1948. Sacral nerve innervation of human bladder. J. Neurosurg. **5**:154-164.

Hess, W. R. 1948. Die functionelle Organisation des vegetativen Nervensystems. Basel, Benno Schwabe and Company.

Horne, H. W., Paull, D. P., and Munro, D. 1948. Fertility studies in the human male with traumatic injuries of the cord and cauda equina. New Eng. J. Med. **239**:959-961.

Jacobson, C. F., Braasch, W. F., and Love, J. G. 1944. Presacral neurectomy for intractable vesical pain and neurogenic vesical dysfunction. Surg. Gynec. Obstet. **79**:21-26.

Kernohan, J. W., Woltman, H. W., and Adson, A. W. 1933. Gliomas arising from the region of the cauda equina: clinical, surgical and histologic considerations. Arch. Neurol. Psychiat. **29**:287-307.

Langworthy, O. R., Kolb, L. C., and Lewis, L. G. 1940. Physiology of micturition: experimental and clinical studies with suggestions as to diagnosis and treatment. Baltimore, The Williams & Wilkins Co.

Learmonth, J. R. 1931. Neurosurgery in the treatment of diseases of the urinary bladder: treatment of vesical pain. J. Urol. **25**:531-549.

Learmonth, J. R., and Markowitz, J. 1929. Studies on the function of the lumbar sympathetic outflow: the relation of the lumbar sympathetic outflow to the sphincter ani internus. Amer. J. Physiol. **89**:686-691.

Mitchell, A. G. 1953. Anatomy of the autonomic nervous system. Edinburgh, E. & S. Livingstone, Ltd.

Motzkin, D. 1968. The significance of deficient bladder function. J. Urol. **100**:445-450.

Muellner, S. R., 1951. The physiology of micturition. J. Urol. **65**:805-810.

Nassar, S. I., Correll, J. W., and Housepian, E. M. 1968. Intramedullary cystic lesions of the conus medullaris. J. Neurol. Neurosurg. Psychiat. **31**:106-109.

Poser, C. M. 1956. Relationship between syringomyelia and neoplasm. Springfield, Illinois, Charles C Thomas, Publisher.

Retief, P. J. M. 1950. Physiology of micturition and ejaculation. South African Med. J. **24**:509-512.

Ruch, T. C. 1955. The urinary bladder. In Fulton, J. F., editor: A textbook of physiology, ed. 17. Philadelphia, W. B. Saunders Co., pp. 943-949.

Sarnoff, S. J., and Arrowood, J. J. 1947. Differential spinal block: block of cutaneous and stretch reflexes in the presence of unimpaired position sense. J. Neurophysiol. **10**:205-210.

Scheibert, C. D. 1955. Studies on the sacral reflex arc in paraplegia: surgical therapy of autonomic hyperreflexia in cervical and upper thoracic myelopathy. J. Neurosurg. **12**:468-474.

Scott, W. J. M., and Schroeder, C. F. 1938. Denervation of the bladder for relief of intractable pain. Ann. Surg. **108**:730-740.

Wechsler, I. S. 1952. A textbook of clinical neurology, with an introduction to the history of neurology, ed. 7. Philadelphia, W. B. Saunders Co.

Woodburne, R. T. 1961. The sphincter mechanism of the urinary bladder and the urethra. Anat. Rec. **141**:11-20.

Woodburne, R. T. 1968. Anatomy of the bladder and bladder outlet. J. Urol. **100**:474-487.

Chapter 8

Electromyography

Jorge Huertas

Electromyography is concerned with the recording and interpretation of the electrical potentials produced by muscles during the processes involved in muscular function.

The striated (voluntary) muscles considered altogether constitute the largest organ in mammals. They are concerned in functions that range from the production of heat to locomotion. Histologically speaking, the muscle is a very stereotyped organ. It consists of a series of parallel strands—the muscle cells. CNS action on the muscle produces histochemical changes within the internal structure of the fibers, causing them to contract. Electromyography considers both the muscle and the neural motor system as a unit because both tissues are intimately related and because during activity both produce electrical currents.

Electromyography serves to locate the failing link in the series of electrical events that lead to muscular contraction and to reveal its nature. The muscle contains both sensory and motor end-organs. The neuromuscular system can therefore be considered as a closed loop servo mechanism. However, the afferent and efferent portions of the loop are clear cut only at the peripheral nerve and muscle. The anterior horn cell, which is the functional unit for muscular contraction, is modulated by influences from various sources: vestibular apparatus, pyramidal system, extrapyramidal system, reticular substance, cerebellum, and intersegmental connections (Fig. 8-1).

ELECTROMYOGRAPHIC EXAMINATION AND RESULTS

Methods, general background

In an electromyographic examination at least four sets of observations need to be made: (1) while the exploring electrode is being inserted into muscle, (2) with the electrode in place in a quiescent muscle (both voluntary and passive movement must be excluded), (3) during volitional movement (isotonic and/or isometric), and (4) during electrical stimulation.

Individual muscles vary greatly in dimensions in the same organism. They range in size from the tiny stapedius muscle to giants such as the gastrocnemius. There are over 400 individual muscles in man. An electromyogram can be altered by pathological processes peculiar to the muscle tissue itself, by anomalies in the chemical processes involved in synaptic transmission, as a consequence of pathological changes in the peripheral nerves, and by involvement of the brain and spinal cord. Because of this wide range in possible sites of abnormality, it can be difficult to pinpoint its exact location. No one set of rules can be set down as a guide in the performance of an electromyographic examination. The examiner must take into consideration the clinical history and

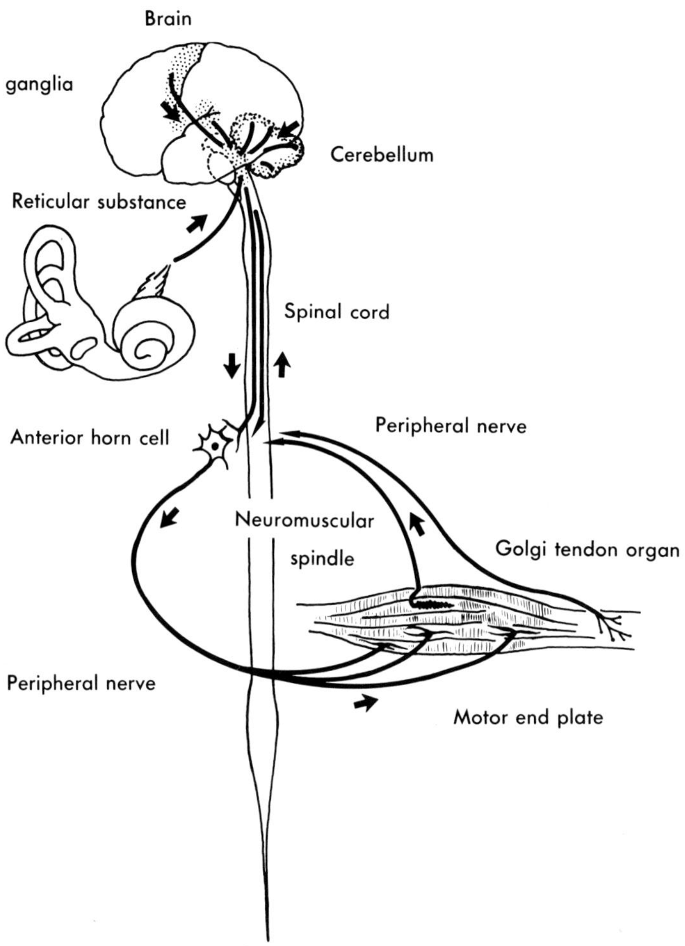

Fig. 8-1. Schematic representation of the neuromuscular system. The dotted areas represent parts of the brain concerned in afferent and efferent aspects of motor function. The anterior horn cell has been placed outside the spinal cord to emphasize the "final common path." The arrows indicate the direction of conduction.

physical findings and then proceed as he sees fit for the particular case. His observations will always be in accordance with the precise location of the recording electrodes. The following points are important to bear in mind during the examination.

Site of the presumed pathological process. The electromyogram is an expression both of muscle and CNS function. As such, the complete motor apparatus of the brain and spinal cord are represented at the muscle terminal. Therefore, during an electromyographic analysis the examiner should be able to manipulate muscle conditions at the recording site in such a way that the suspected link becomes predominantly activated—for example, by placing the extremities in antigravitational positions when parkinsonism is in question or by exercising a muscle in myasthenia gravis. It is also of great importance to choose the appropriate muscles for examination in a given clinical question. In the case of peripheral palsy of a limb it may be possible to localize the site of the lesion within a single nerve root, a plexus, or a peripheral nerve, according to the muscles showing electromyographic signs of denervation.

Physiological status of the muscle. Normally a muscle at rest is electrically quiescent. However, many myoneurological diseases are expressed by electrical activity in the muscle during rest. Special attention and patience should therefore be exercised while examining an individual at rest. Sometimes the searching electrode has to be moved about in the same muscle in order to locate the affected fiber.

Work performed by the muscle. Muscular mechanical activity and muscular electrical activity are related; however, they cannot be correlated. One is a metabolic process involving the muscle tissue in toto and the other a membrane metabolic process only. Profuse electrical activity is not necessarily an expression of a strong mechanical contraction (Kugelberg, 1950).

Recording

Many types of electrodes are available, and interpretation of the record must take into consideration the type of electrode used. Most commonly used is a "monopolar" needle electrode (20-gauge), insulated except at the very tip and long enough to penetrate into the muscle under investigation. The reference electrode is placed at some distance in an electrically silent area (see Chapter 31). A coaxial bipolar needle electrode can also be used. The EMG wave frequencies are much faster (20-5,000 Hz.) than those in EEG. Therefore, if a loudspeaker is connected to the amplifier, the examiner can hear the events as they happen. It is customary to display the record on an oscilloscope and photograph selected parts of it. Some machines have a magnetic tape recorder. EMG amplifiers should have the same general characteristics as the EEG amplifiers, except for minor special adjustments such as a shorter input time constant and a linear frequency response up to 5,000 Hz. (Fisher, 1961.)

Observations

During insertion of the electrode into the muscle. During this maneuver a re-

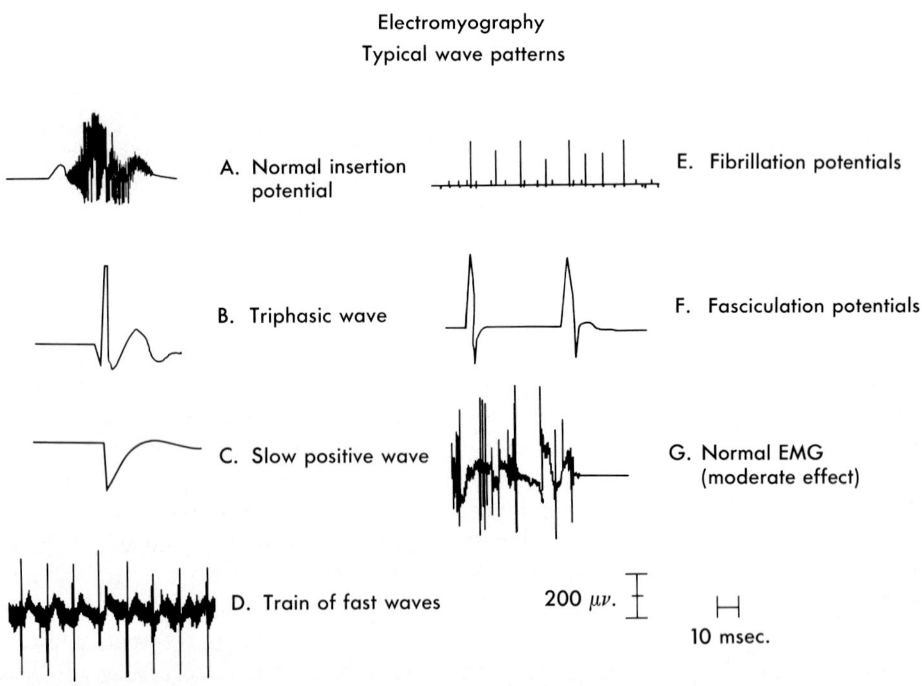

Fig. 8-2. Highly schematic representation of the main wave forms having significance in the electromyogram.

sponse occurs in muscle fibers as the exploring electrode reaches them. It consists of a short "splash" potential that lasts a few milliseconds (Fig. 8-2, *A*). If the electrode is left quiet at that particular location and if the muscle is normal, a steady D.C. potential will dominate the picture thereafter, providing that no motion occurs. If the nerve fiber or the intramuscular nervous tissue is defective, the muscle fiber performance will be altered. A large potential of short duration will be observed that crosses the zero line two or three times. This is called a diphasic or a triphasic wave (Fig. 8-2, *B*). Another characteristic of a lesion of either nerve or muscle is the appearance of a slow, positive wave (Fig. 8-2, *C*). Thus, after insertion of the examining electrode, a repetitive appearance of polyphasic (biphasic or triphasic) waves accompanied by slow positive waves means that the muscle is being affected by malfunction of its innervating nerve (reaction to degeneration; R.D.).

If, however, the pathological process is strictly limited to the muscle (beyond nerve fiber and neuromuscular junction) the insertion of an electrode may produce a train of fast waves that last several seconds (Fig. 8-2, *D*). If the needle is moved again—even slightly—this process will be triggered once more. Over the loudspeaker the sound is characteristic because the process increases and decreases in intensity while the frequency of the spikes, which may wax and wane also, is about 120 Hz. This noise has been compared to the noise made by a fast low-flying airplane passing overhead. The insertion activity thus can differentiate clearly between a muscular disease (myotonia) and peripheral nerve fiber alterations (denervation activity). Many attempts have been made to correlate the most common combinations of high frequency activity subsequent to the insertion of an electrode with a muscle and a specific muscular disease. However, this is currently no more than of academic interest.

Not all intrinsic muscular diseases, however, produce insertion potentials. When muscular atrophy is advanced, or when the muscle tissue has been replaced by another tissue—for example, fat—in spite of the presence of a muscular disease there is no electromyographic expression.

During muscle rest. As already stated, during rest normal muscles are not electrically active. However, some diseases of the CNS and of the lower motor neuron produce random characteristic discharges.

Muscle cramps. Muscle cramps are the least common finding during rest. The cramps are characterized by a sudden involuntary contraction of a muscle or a muscle group that lasts for about a minute and relaxes spontaneously and independently of the subject's wishes. The waves are large because many fibers are contracting synchronously (summation) and the frequency of the waves reaches 150 or more per second. They are well organized and repetitive. The organized synchronous repetition of the waves is in contrast to the disorganized, random, asynchronous activity of normal muscular contractions. Cramps are observed in normal subjects, in electrolyte imbalance particularly of sodium chloride or calcium, or in diseases such as amyotrophic lateral sclerosis.

Fasciculations and fibrillations. These phenomena have received a great deal of semantic attention. For our purpose it suffices to remember that a fascicle consists of a group of fibrils. Fasciculations are spontaneous contractions of whole fascicles or larger parts of them, while fibrillations represent spontaneous contractions of individual muscle fibers. Because the fasciculation is larger than the fibrillation, it is commonly stated that fasciculation can be seen during neurological examination, while fibrillation cannot be seen. This statement is quantitatively accurate; however, the volume of a muscle itself can preclude from the observer's eye a fasciculation when it occurs well beneath the skin. An electromyogram in such cases always proves useful. Since a muscle is innervated by many motor units, selective pathological change in one or a few motor units will result in selective contraction of the muscle fibrils supplied by that unit. The electromyogram will present such a finding only if the electrode is in the affected motor unit.

Fibrillation potentials are most readily obtained by using electrodes with a small tip. Physiologically, the potentials are the discharges of single muscle fibers (Fig. 8-2, *E*). As such, they last from 0.5 to 1.5 milliseconds. They all have approximately the same amplitude (25 to 100 microvolts) and they fire at characteristic rates (2 to 10 per second). If the frequency reaches apparently faster values, it is due to the interposition of several muscular units firing irregularly. Fibrillation potentials occur spontaneously in denervated muscles and can be found in any disease causing degeneration of lower motor neurons. However, purely muscular diseases may sometimes be characterized by fibrillations also, such as in the case in polymyositis and dermatomyositis.

The *fasciculation potential,* which represents the spontaneous discharge of a whole motor unit or a group of muscle fibers, lasts approximately 3 to 5 milliseconds (Fig. 8-2, *F*). It measures from 300 to 1,000 microvolts and characteristically it is a triphasic or multiphasic wave. The waves can appear either in singles or in groups. They are sometimes found in normal people, but they are a characteristic finding in amyotrophic lateral sclerosis. They are also found in progressive muscular dystrophy and in some of the cerebellospinal degenerations.

Repetitive fasciculations are seldom seen in electromyography. They are associated with cramps of nervous origin such as nerve root (disk), plexus, or trunk compression (pregnancy), and in certain metabolic disorders such as tetany.

Examination during voluntary contraction of varied strength. If a muscle has been at rest for some time and is then stimulated by short tetanic stimuli, it will show increased strength of contraction with each consecutive contraction. Yet the action currents at the muscle level are exactly the same. This is the so-called *staircase effect,* in which the mechanical property of the muscle to contract with a certain amount of strength improves with repetition of that function, while the electrical membrane potential remains unaltered throughout the process. This is important to bear in mind during an electromyographic examination of voluntary contraction because electrical activity alone is not indicative of the mechanical properties of the muscle in question. For examination during voluntary contraction, it is customary to ask the patient to contract the muscle being examined. Strictly speaking, it does not matter whether the patient executes an isometric or an isotonic contraction. The important factor is that the muscle be contracted. The examiner can ask the patient to contract slightly, summoning a few motor units, or to contract vigorously, summoning many motor units (recruitment). If voluntary contractions are suspect, it is very important to know when the measured contraction occurred—for example, if in a disease of the myasthenia gravis type the muscles are fatigued, the characteristics of the muscular action potentials change and only a correlation of these potentials with previous potentials obtained in the same locality in the same time sequence can allow a diagnosis to be made.

On slight voluntary muscular contraction only a few motor units are active. If the force of the contraction is increased, more and more units will be summoned until a maximal electromyographical effect will appear. From then on, the force of the muscular contraction can be increased without changing the maximal electrical effect already reached. During muscular contraction, the size and form of the motor unit action potentials vary because the examiner is dealing with a sum of action potentials rather than with isolated muscle fibers. Briefly, the motor unit action potential consists of a larger negative phase preceded sometimes and followed always by a positive phase (Fig. 8-2, *G*). They can be biphasic or polyphasic and they occur continuously as long as the contraction is maintained.

Polyphasic potentials (potentials with more than three phases), when excessive in number, indicate either a muscular abnormality, such as progressive muscular dystrophy, or reinnervation. The amplitude and duration of the action potentials are diminished in some types of muscular pathology, as in progressive muscular dystrophy, polymyositis, and so on. However, to make a diagnosis, this type of change has to be correlated with other clinical symptoms and compared with recordings of analogous muscle groups in the same subject. On the other hand, an increase in the mean duration and amplitude is the characteristic finding in diseases of anterior horn cells, such as in poliomyelitis.

In peripheral palsies of any type the number of motor units firing during maximal effort is decreased, while the rate of discharge of each individual motor unit is compensatively increased. In the case of subtotal denervation, very rapid firings of single motor units can be seen during strong volition.

In primary muscular disease the individual motor units are less efficient than normal, owing to loss of active muscle fibers. To achieve the same muscular strength, more units have to be activated than in normal muscles. It can be seen in these cases that even on minimal contractions, so many motor units are utilized that the EMG shows a pattern of "interference" similar to that produced by a normal muscle on maximal effort.

A special case of abnormality during voluntary contraction consists in alterations in conduction at the level of the neuromuscular junction.

Myasthenia gravis is typical of this group of diseases. Electromyographically, the disorder can be detected in two ways. One method is to ask the patient to exercise vigorously and then observe how the muscle action potentials wane as the patient is exercising. However, this method is not clear cut. A more precise method consists in asking him to perform exercise until the muscle groups in question become tired and weak. At this point a neostigmine-like substance is injected. The response is dramatic because both the patient's strength and muscle action potentials improve almost instantaneously.

ELECTRICAL STIMULATION

Electrical stimulation serves to differentiate nervous disease from muscle disease or to measure certain parameters within the nervous system. Electrical stimulation is best achieved when square waves are used to perform the stimulation. The square waves must be monophasic (deflected only in one direction from the zero line); their frequency, duration, and intensity must be arranged for each particular situation. Some wave generators can produce other types of waves —sine waves, ramps—but these are to be used only for special purposes and not routinely. The use of A.C. for stimulation is becoming obsolete because of the more reliable results obtained by using square waves. A muscle can be stimulated to contract by an electrical current directly, by placing the electrodes over the muscular tissue proper, or indirectly by stimulating parts of the CNS—for example, motor cortex—or by stimulating the peripheral nerves that innervate the muscle under examination.

Stimulation of the CNS

With the advent of stereotaxic techniques in human neurosurgery, stimulation of the pyramidal or the extrapyramidal systems has been carried out in some laboratories for the purpose of determining somatotopographical correlations between muscle groups and brain area stimulated (Hassler and others, 1960). A given muscle group will be activated if the proper anatomical structure is stimulated. This technique is for use in the operating room under expert supervision and therefore is not a routine examination. For physiological reasons, the stimulating electrode is always the anode.

Stimulation of the peripheral nervous system

Conduction time. Stimulation of the peripheral nervous system was first performed to determine the anatomical or physiological integrity of a peripheral nerve. It is possible to stimulate some superficial nerve trunks through the skin. Stimulation of a nerve fiber always occurs at the anode. In applying single shock (single square wave) techniques a few seconds apart, it is possible to determine conduction time (Lambert, 1962). The shock must be delivered at the mixed nerve proximally and recording must be performed distally either at the nerve or, better, at the terminal muscle. Thus, in such conditions as the carpal tunnel syndrome or in interstitial neuritis, conduction time of nerve activity provoked by this technique will be delayed. Sometimes the delay is so small that comparison with the opposite side is necessary. The distance between stimulating and recording electrode must be kept constant. It is advisable that the distance be more than 10 cm. The farther away the stimulating electrode is placed from the recording electrodes, the easier it will be to perform the measurements. Peripheral neuropathies, both interstitial and parenchymatous, will have the effect of delaying conduction time. A change in conduction time alone is not diagnostic; comparative examinations with other nerve groups and with the symmetrical counterpart, together with a good history, are essential for the interpretation of the data.

Conduction velocity. By determining the conduction time from different points on a nerve (for example, by stimulating the median nerve at the elbow and at the wrist), and by measuring the distance between these two points, it is possible to calculate the conduction velocity. This procedure can be repeated at different levels of a nerve (for instance, ulnar nerve at upper arm, elbow, forearm, wrist); in this way the site of a lesion in a given mononeuropathy can be determined. Conduction velocity is slowest at the level of the lesion. (Kaeser and Richter, 1963.)

H-reflex. Each time a nerve trunk (mixed nerve) is stimulated electrically, a response is elicited from the stimulated fibers that will travel in both directions (distal and proximal), starting at the stimulus point

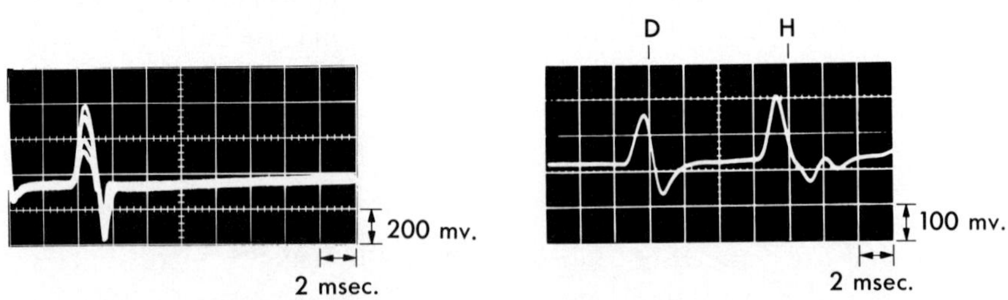

A. Direct muscular response—four different intensities were used.

B. H-reflex

Fig. 8-3. A, Direct response of the adductor pollicis brevis to stimulation of the ulnar nerve in a monkey; 4 msec. elapsed from stimulus discharge until muscular activity started. **B,** Response of the same muscle after stimulating with a higher voltage. A second wave (H wave) appears after a latency of 12 msec. During this time the nervous impulse traveled via the posterior roots to the spinal cord, anterior horn cells, motor nerve, and muscle. Conduction across the anterior horn cell synapse takes about 1 msec.

(anode). Stimulation of a motor fiber will result in contraction of the terminal muscle, as already described, with no effect on the CNS (antidromic volley). The sensory fibers of nerve trunks that are relatively superficially located (ulnar and peroneal) also respond to stimulation. The sensory fibers originating in the muscle spindles are the largest nerve fibers in such nerve trunks. A stimulus applied to these fibers (also called A-1 fibers) will travel through the posterior roots to the anterior horn cells, then on to the muscle and produce a twitch. This is the so-called H-reflex (Fig. 8-3). The physiological characteristics of the H-reflex are those of a monosynaptic reflex. This technique has been used clinically for the accurate measurement of the stretch reflex (Fig. 8-3). Since the H-reflex constitutes a complete reflex arc, a single twitch produced by this mechanism can yield valuable data. The location of the stimulating and recording electrodes can be measured exactly. The time spent by the volley during afferent travel, synaptic delay, efferent travel, neuromuscular delay, and intramuscular travel times can be calculated, and specific failure of one of the systems can be established at least theoretically. This method has gained popularity only recently. The results are not yet clear because of many variants, such as state of consciousness. (Huertas, 1965; Landau and Clare, 1964; Magladery and others, 1952; Magladery and Teasdall, 1958; Paillard, 1960; Takamori, 1967.)

Muscle stimulation

Inasmuch as the nerve fibers in muscle are intimately intermingled with muscle fibers, and since the threshold for electrical stimulation of intramuscular nerve fibers is lower than the threshold for electrical stimulation of the muscle fibers, direct electrical stimulation of the muscle fiber per se cannot normally be achieved. However, in electromyography an advantage has been taken of this discrepancy in threshold for stimulation between intramuscular nerve fiber and muscle proper. If the nerve fibers are degenerating, fewer nerve fibers will be available for stimulation (Fisher, 1939). The result is a release of the denervated muscle fiber to its own stimulation threshold. If the muscle is stimulated and the observed response is plotted, a strength-duration curve can be obtained (Kugelberg, 1950). The strength-duration curve migrates from the typical neuromuscular response to an exclusive muscular response. The chronaxy of the denervated muscle apparently increases as the denervation atrophy increases. At extreme stages it reaches values of 40 times or more those initially found for the muscle fibers. The stages in between the two extremes can show broken strength duration curves. Theoretically, the length of the chronaxy indicates that the denervated muscle fiber is susceptible to stimulation by currents with slow rise times like sinusoidal curves. The classical concept, which states that normal muscle responds to direct current stimulation and that denervated muscle responds to sinusoidal waves, is merely an expression of the tremendous change of chronaxy in the denervated muscle.

If the muscle becomes reinnervated the process described in the foregoing is reversed until the stimulus strength duration curve migrates downward and to the left, until it becomes the response of a nerve.

REFERENCES

Fisher, E. 1939. The effect of faradic and galvanic stimulation upon the course of atrophy in denervated muscles. Amer. J. Physiol. **127**: 605-619.

Fisher, E. 1961. Physiology of skeletal muscle. In Licht, S., editor: Electrodiagnosis and electromyography. New Haven, Licht, pp. 66-112.

Hassler, R., Riechert, T., Mundinger, F., Umbach, W., and Ganglberger, J. A. 1960. Physiological observations in stereotaxic operations in extrapyramidal motor disturbances. Brain **83**: 337-350.

Huertas, J. 1965. The relationship between evoked myography and different states of consciousness. In Proctor, L., and Adey, W. R., editors: Symposium on analysis of CNS and cardiovascular data using computer methods. NASA SP-92, Washington, D. C., National Aeronautics and Space Administration.

Kaeser, H. E., and Richter, H. R. 1963. Technique de la mensuration de la vitesse de conduction par courts segments. Rev. Neurol. **108:** 190-192.

Kugelberg, E. 1950. Electromyography in muscular dystrophies, differentiation between dystrophies and chronic lower motor neuron lesions. J. Neurol. Neurosurg. Psychiat. **12:**129-132.

Lambert, E. H. 1962. Diagnostic value of electrical stimulation of motor nerves. In Pinelli, P., editor: Progress in electromyography. EEG Clin. Neurophysiol., suppl. 22, pp. 9-16.

Landau, W. M., and Clare, M. H. 1964. Fusimotor function: H-reflex, tendon jerk, and reinforcement in hemiplegia. Arch. Neurol. **10:**128-134.

Magladery, J. W., Park, A. M., Porter, W. E., and Teasdall, R. D. 1952. Spinal reflex patterns in man. Res. Publ. Ass. Nerv. Ment. Dis., Proc. **30:**118-151.

Magladery, J. W., and Teasdall, R. D. 1958. Stretch reflexes in patients with spinal cord lesions. Bull. Johns Hopk. Hosp. **103:**236-241.

Paillard, J. 1960. Functional organization of afferent innervation of muscle studied by monosynaptic testing. In Bouman, H. D., and Woolf, A. L., editors: Utrecht symposium on the innervation of muscle. Baltimore, The Williams & Wilkins Co., pp. 31-39.

Takamori, M. 1967. H-reflex study in upper motorneuron disease. Neurology **17:**32-44.

Chapter 9

Roentgenographic localization of spinal tumors

Bernard S. Epstein

The diagnosis of tumors of the vertebral column and the spinal cord requires adequate radiographical investigation, which usually begins with plain film roentgenograms of the suspected area. At least anteroposterior and lateral roentgenograms are made, and oblique views as well are often required. Stereoscopic pairs offer considerable help in demonstrating finer anatomical details and small masses. Additional information is obtainable from body section roentgenograms, cineradiography, myelography, and strontium-85 scans (Charkes and Sklaroff, 1965; Epstein, 1962; Roth, 1963). These are utilized when plain film examinations and the clinical picture indicate the need for additional study. Every effort should be made to obtain adequate and reliable data with a minimum of radiological exposure. However, equal caution should be used to make sure that the study will not mislead the radiologist and his clinical colleagues.

The decision regarding the special procedures to be undertaken requires critical appraisal, because a program requiring myelography, multiple exposures, or the use of radioactive material should not be entered into lightly.

Intraspinal tumors produce changes visible on plain film roentgenograms only when they reach sufficient size to impinge on the bony confines of the spinal canal. This occurs in relatively few patients with spinal cord or nerve root tumor, so that normal radiological findings do not exclude intraspinal tumor. In diffuse swelling of the spinal cord, such as occurs in intramedullary gliomas, gross bony changes in the adjacent vertebrae are infrequent. This is particularly true if the tumor has grown rapidly. In such patients, pain and sudden alteration in posture may, however, be clues to the presence of the tumor. This is noted particularly in children.

If increased bulk of the cord or the cauda equina is slowly attained, bony changes may be visible on scout films. Among the changes encountered are loss of bone of the pedicles with widening of the interpedicular spaces, increase in the sagittal diameter of the spinal canal, erosive changes in the dorsal aspects of the involved vertebral bodies, and thinning of the laminae. Such changes are observed classically in ependymoma involving the cauda equina; occasionally the changes are far advanced (Fig. 9-1). In syringomyelia there may be minimal changes in the cervical or thoracic spinal architecture, but they are difficult to evaluate on plain film examinations alone (McIlroy and Richardson, 1965). Every now and then a suggestive increase in the anteroposterior

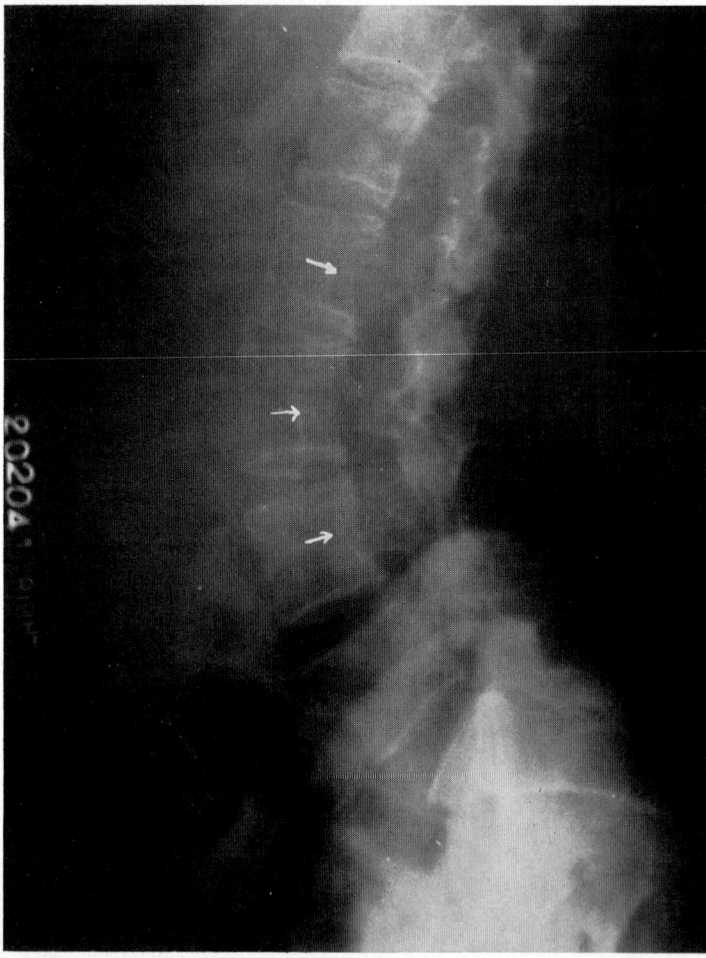

Fig. 9-1. Ependymoma of the cauda equina. The spinal canal is widened and there is atrophy of the pedicles. The posterior aspect of vertebrae L2, L3, and L4 display concavities due to the impression of the tumor (arrows).

diameter of the spinal canal is visible but, by and large, myelography is required for the demonstration of the enlarged cord. The concomitance of bony abnormalities in the vicinity of the foramen magnum or upper cervical vertebrae is regarded as a helpful hint in diagnosis. Diagnosis of an intramedullary tumor is usually based on myelographic demonstration of widening of the spinal cord and thinning of the lateral margins of the iophendylate (Pantopaque) column in that region. The axillary pouches are compressed, so that the combination of thin, flat, lateral streaks and a bulging cord is quite diagnostic. This appearance may be simulated by compressive changes produced by midline spurs, so transcervical studies are necessary, especially in adults.

Atrophy of the spinal cord, a relatively infrequent condition, cannot be identified in positive contrast myelograms. However, syringomyelia associated with a dilated, fluid-filled central canal can be identified in air myelograms as a shrunken cord following withdrawal of the fluid from both the spinal canal and the central canal of the cord (McIlroy and Richardson, 1965).

Localized tumors of nerve roots are usually intradural and extramedullary in position. Some are entirely extradural, while others are occasionally situated both

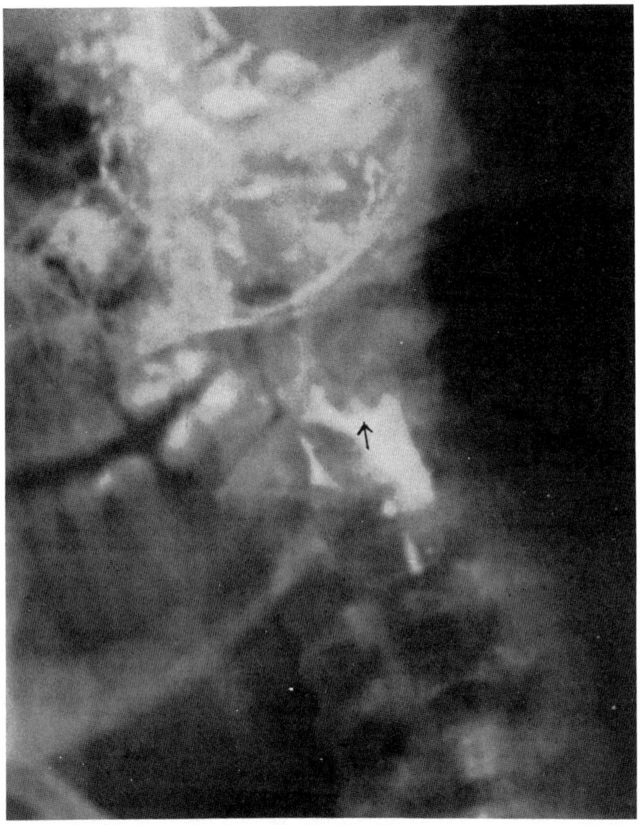

Fig. 9-2. Pantopaque myelogram revealing a semicircular defect at the level of the vertebra C2 due to meningioma (arrow). There was no obstruction to the flow of cerebrospinal fluid.

intradurally and extradurally. If located within the canal, and if quite large, the tumor may impinge on the adjacent pedicle and the dorsal aspect of adjacent vertebral bodies, resulting in partial loss of bone. When the tumor is situated in the intervertebral foramen, the dimensions of the foramen may be increased without visible bone destruction. Tumors on either side of the foramen are referred to as *dumbbell tumors* and, as a rule, are neurofibromas. While usually single, this kind of tumor is so frequently multiple that a careful investigation of the entire spinal canal is warranted.

Neurofibromas are the most common intraspinal tumors, but meningiomas are also quite frequent. These too are usually subdural and extramedullary in position. As a rule they produce no significant changes in the adjacent bone. Occasionally, however, a meningioma can be identified from the psammomatous calcifications it contains. Myelographic investigation discloses neurofibromas and meningiomas far more frequently than do plain films. If there is other evidence of such tumors, myelography usually settles the issue by revealing an intradural, extramedullary type of deformity of the iophendylate (Pantopaque) column. Deformity resulting from meningioma is shown in Fig. 9-2, and from neurofibroma in Fig. 9-3. Care should be taken not to overlook such a tumor at the craniovertebral junction. Myelographic examination of the foramen magnum may be required to investigate this possibility.

Other intraspinal tumors include epidermoids, lipomas, vascular malformations, melanomas, arachnoid cysts, and tumor

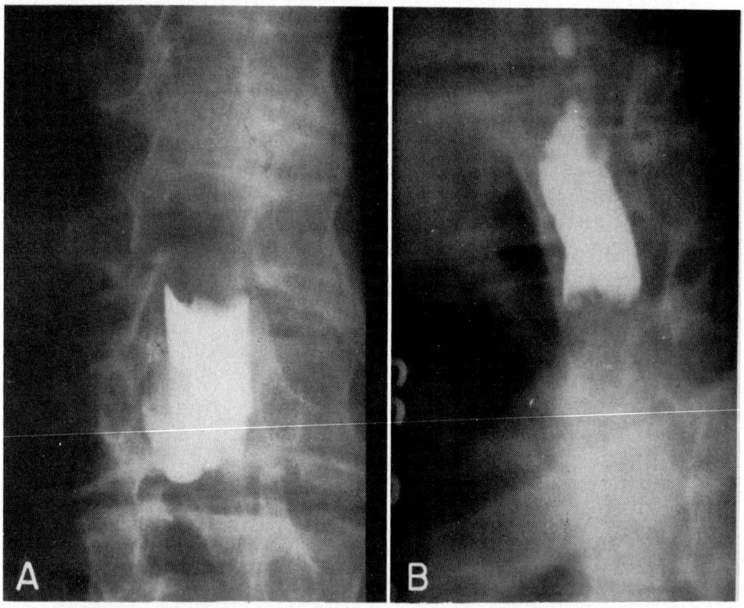

Fig. 9-3. A, The patient had symptoms referable to the lower thoracic spine. Myelography (2 ml. of Pantopaque) discloses a complete block at the level of the inferior aspect of thoracic vertebra X. Note the tent-like configuration of the head of the Pantopaque column. **B,** Same patient in inverted position, lateral projection. The defect is again visible. The finding fits in with an intradural extramedullary mass, which proved to be a large neurofibroma.

Fig. 9-4

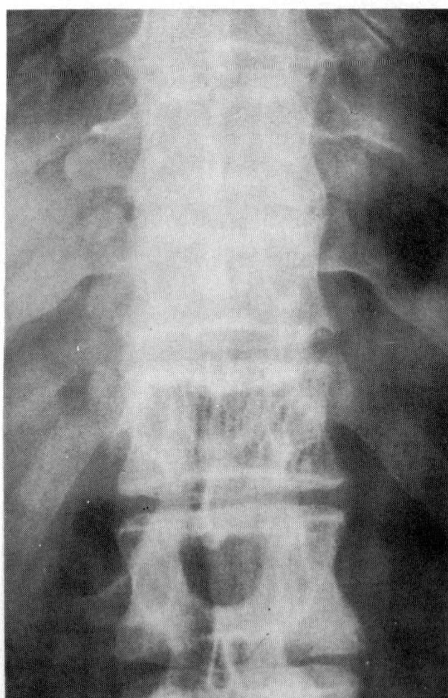

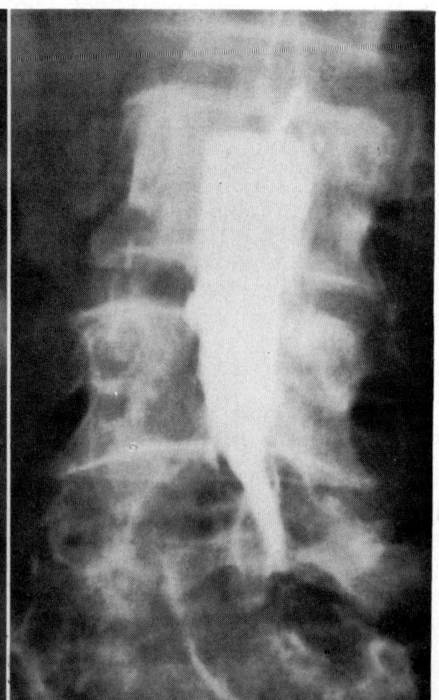

Fig. 9-5

Figs. 9-4 and **9-5. Fig. 9-4.** Hemangioma of the body of thoracic vertebra XII in a 26-year-old woman. This was disclosed incidentally during gastrointestinal examination. The patient did not complain of symptoms referable to this lesion. **Fig. 9-5.** Marked narrowing and shifting of the caudal aspect of the Pantopaque column in a patient with epidural metastases from a bronchogenic carcinoma.

deposits brought to the region by the cerebrospinal fluid (Epstein, 1962). These are not usually demonstrable on plain film roentgenograms; once in a while, however, an arachnoid cyst becomes large enough to cause a widening of the interpedicular spaces with loss of the inner bony margin. These tumors likewise require myelographic examination for diagnosis. Vascular malformations are ideally demonstrated directly by means of aortography, the contrast material entering the spinal circulation and opacifying the abnormal vessels. Viewed in myelograms, the convoluted pattern produced by arteriovenous intraspinal malformations can be equally diagnostic (Epstein, Beller, and Cohen, 1949).

Vertebral tumors appear as primary neoplasms. These include sarcoma, chordoma, osteochondroma, chondrosarcoma, Ewing's sarcoma, hemangioma, osteoblastoma, osteoid osteoma, and aneurysmal bone cyst (Cohen, Dahlin, and MacCarty, 1964). Some, such as hemangioma (Fig. 9-4), aneurysmal bone cyst, and osteoid osteoma, present a change recognizable on plain film roentgenograms. The others, however, cannot be distinguished without histological confirmation.

Metastatic tumors of the vertebral column are relatively frequent. They come mostly from tumors of the breast, lung, and thyroid, and also from myelomas and lymphomas. They are usually visible in plain film roentgenograms. Their intraspinal extension is usually epidural. They may be of sufficient size to obstruct the spinal canal completely or to impinge on nerve roots and give rise to radicular symptoms. Such involvement is best demonstrated by myelography (Fig. 9-5). A fairly large area of bone destruction must be present before vertebral metastases can be demonstrated on plain film roentgenograms. If cortical bone is destroyed, an area of at least 1 to 2 ccm. in size must be lost before the damage is visible. A greater quantity of cancellous bone must be involved before a metastatic tumor limited to that part of the bone can be identified. Body section radiography is often helpful in doubtful cases. Altered configuration of

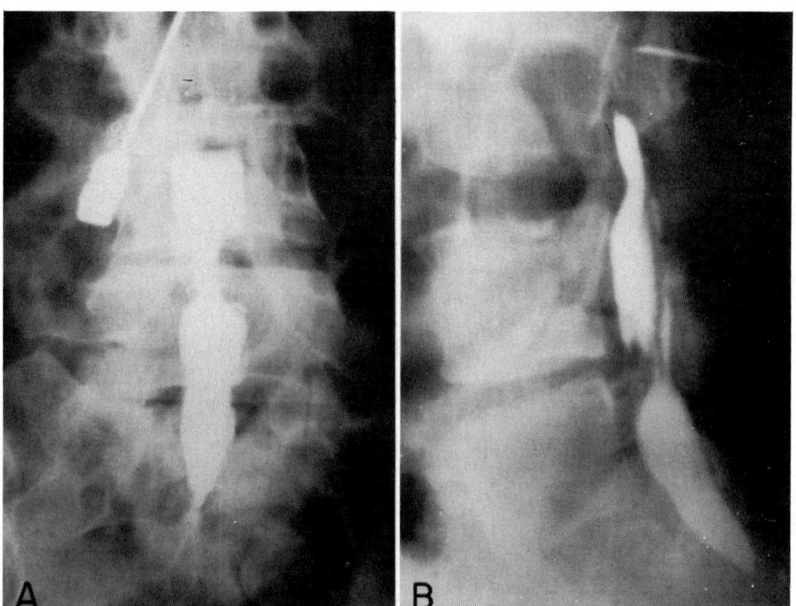

Fig. 9-6. A, A large defect at the fourth lumbar interspace on the left side. **B,** On the lateral projection the defect extends into the anterior aspect of the Pantopaque column. A large extruded intervertebral disk was removed at operation.

vertebrae incident to partial collapse sometimes provides one with a clue in his search for spinal metastases. Extensive metastatic involvement may be present when the plain films appear to be within normal limits (Epstein, 1952). Under such conditions, as well as in other doubtful situations, scanning with strontium-85 can offer useful information (Charkes and Sklaroff, 1965).

The diagnosis of disk herniations and spondylotic spur formations intruding into the spinal canal and the intervertebral foramina requires plain film and myelographic investigations (Holt, 1964). The plain films are, however, often deceptive; patients with extensive spondylosis may present no evidence of radicular or cord involvement, while others with a perfectly normal vertebral column give every clinical indication of such a process. It is particularly in these persons that myelography is required. However, this should not be carried out unless all concerned are prepared to follow through with operation. Myelographic characteristics of an extruded disk are illustrated in Fig. 9-6.

Plain film examinations are often helpful in providing information regarding the sagittal diameter of the spinal canal and especially in the evaluation of spondylosis with "ridge" defects (Fig. 9-7). The anteroposterior measurement in the cervical region at the levels of the lowermost four segments should be more than 1.3 cm., while in the lumbar region the sagittal diameter should be 1.5 cm. or more. The sagittal diameter of the canal is an important factor in determining whether or not an intraspinal protrusion will produce symptoms. It has been found that sagittal narrowing predisposes to cord and nerve root compression (Epstein, Epstein, and Lavine, 1962, 1964).

Myelography is best performed under image intensification control. As a rule, 8 to 10 ml. of iophendylate (Pantopaque) is used. However, if a block is suspected the examination is started with only about 1.5 ml. By and large, no fixed quantity can be

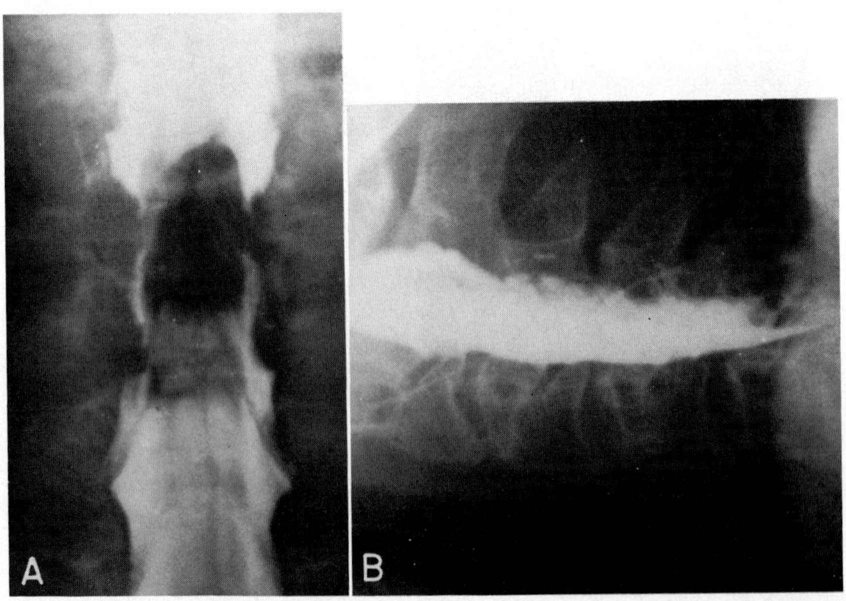

Fig. 9-7. **A,** Marked deformity of the Pantopaque column in the lower cervical area in a 48-year-old patient with an extensive "ridge syndrome." A partial block to the passage of Pantopaque was observed both cephalad and caudad to the involved site. **B,** Transcervical study, showing deep indentation into the dorsal aspect of the Pantopaque column.

recommended. The amount used for lumbar myelography should fill the lumbar canal up to the level of the third lumbar vertebra with the patient erect. Larger quantities are often required for thoracic and cervical examinations (Epstein, 1962). Cineradiographic recording has been found to be most helpful. Removal by siphonage is advantageous in that it is possible to recover most or all of the iophendylate (Pantopaque) with little or no pain (Epstein, 1964; Epstein and Epstein, 1966). I have used this technique in over two hundred fifty patients with great satisfaction.

Air myelography has certain advantages in demonstrating the spinal cord itself, and it may be used for the evaluation of certain congenital malformations such as myelomeningoceles (Roth, 1965). While the technique is one which, in my opinion, should be reserved for such investigations, others have found it quite helpful in the demonstration of intraspinal tumors and atrophy of the spinal cord.

Water soluble substances have also been used for myelography, particularly in the Scandinavian countries. This technique requires spinal anesthesia, so the examination is necessarily limited to the lumbar canal because of the toxic qualities of the contrast agent. Its advantages are that the contrast material is absorbed and that details of the cauda equina are brought out sharply (Harvey and Freiberger, 1965; Turner, Fisher, and Bernstein, 1966). However, the procedure is lengthy and has not found much use in this country. The dangers inherent in the use of intraspinal water soluble contrast agents should not be overlooked, even though reports state that the procedure is safe.

Diskography has its advocates in the diagnosis of disk herniations, but in my opinion this procedure is not as reliable as positive contrast myelography, nor does it permit adequate examination of the entire spinal canal (Holt, 1964). I do not use this method of examination.

REFERENCES

Charkes, N. D., and Sklaroff, D. M. 1965. The radioactive strontium photoscan as a diagnostic aid in primary and metastatic cancer in bone. Radiol. Clin. N. Amer. 3:499-509.

Cohen, D. M., Dahlin, D. C., and MacCarty, C. S. 1964. Apparently solitary tumors of the vertebral column. Mayo Clin. Proc. **39**:509-528.

Epstein, B. S. 1952. Myelographic diagnosis of epidural metastases in the lumbosacral spinal canal. Amer. J. Roentgen. **68**:730-735.

Epstein, B. S. 1962. The spine: a radiological test and atlas, ed. 2. Philadelphia, Lea & Febiger.

Epstein, B. S. 1964. The evacuation of Pantopaque from the lumbar spinal canal by siphon action. Radiology **83**:472-475.

Epstein, B. S., and Epstein, J. A. 1966. Syphonage technique for removal of Pantopaque. Acta Radiol. **5**:1007-1012.

Epstein, B. S., Epstein, J. A., and Lavine, L. 1964. The effect of anatomic variations in the lumbar vertebrae and spinal canal on cauda equina and nerve root syndromes. Amer. J. Roentgen. **91**:1055-1063.

Epstein, J. A., Beller, A. J., and Cohen, L. 1949. Arterial anomalies of the spinal cord. J. Neurosurg. **6**:45-56.

Epstein, J. A., Epstein, B. S., and Lavine, L. 1962. Nerve root compression associated with narrowing of the lumbar spinal canal. J. Neurol. Neurosurg. Psychiat. **25**:165-176.

Harvey, J. P., Jr., and Freiberger, R. H. 1965. Myelography with an absorbable agent. J. Bone Joint Surg. **47A**:397-416.

Holt, E. P. 1964. Fallacy of cervical discography. J.A.M.A. **188**:799-801.

McIlroy, W. J., and Richardson, J. C. 1965. Syringomyelia: a clinical review of 75 cases. Canad. Med. Ass. J. **93**:731-734.

Roth, M. 1963. Gas myelography by the lumbar route. Acta Radiol. **1**:53-65.

Roth, M. 1965. The caudal end of the spinal cord: abnormal pneumographic features: lumbar intumescence artery syndrome and spinal dysraphism. Acta Radiol. **3**:297-304.

Turner, O., Fisher, C. J., and Bernstein, L. L. 1966. Intrathecal sodium diatrizoate. Neurology **16**:230-235.

Chapter 10

Structure of the brainstem

In the present text the term *brainstem* refers to the medulla oblongata, pons, and midbrain. In other texts the diencephalon is included as a part of the brainstem. As defined here, the brainstem gives rise to all the cranial nerves except the olfactory and the optic. Embryologically and anatomically these two nerves are not peripheral nerves like the other ten but are parts of the brain that have been projected peripherally during early embryonic development.

The sites of emergence of the cranial nerves from the brainstem are indicated in Figs. 10-1, 10-2, and 10-6, and the positions of cranial nerve nuclei in the brainstem in Figs. 10-3, 10-4, and 10-5.

Various levels of the brainstem are illustrated in Figs. 10-7 through 10-16. A key figure (Fig. 10-6) showing the plane of the various levels is provided for purposes of orientation.

LOWER MEDULLA OBLONGATA AT LEVEL OF THE PYRAMIDAL DECUSSATION (FIG. 10-7)

The essential features at this level are much the same as in the spinal cord. Minor changes, however, especially in the disposition of the gray matter, have occurred. The posterior horns have lost their connection with the periphery, for no posterior roots are present at this level. The nucleus of the spinal tract of the fifth nerve extends downward, and at a more caudal level (C2) is continuous with the substantia gelatinosa of the posterior horn of the spinal cord. In Fig. 10-7 it can be noted that the spinal tract of the fifth nerve is applied to the lateral aspect of its nucleus like a cap.

Anterior roots are absent at this level; however, one of their homologues, the eleventh nerve, is represented. This nerve arises from a group of cells in the ventrolateral part of the anterior horn, and courses dorsally, then laterally, in gaining exit from the medulla oblongata. The nerve supplies the sternocleidomastoid and trapezius muscles.

The posterior columns of white matter have the same relative position and the same topography as in the spinal cord. Two cell aggregates have appeared: the nucleus gracilis medially and the nucleus cuneatus laterally. These nuclei are synaptic stations for the long fibers of the posterior root system that have passed up the posterior columns. At higher levels of the brainstem, the fibers arising in the gracile and cuneate nuclei course ventrally as internal arcuate fibers to enter and ascend in the contralateral medial lemniscus, through which they reach the thalamus.

Situated along the lateral aspect of the medulla oblongata, in much the same position as in the cord, are the dorsal and ventral spinocerebellar tracts (right side of Fig. 10-7). Just ventral to the nucleus and spinal tract of the fifth nerve and separated from it by fibers of the eleventh nerve is the spinothalamic tract (left side of figure), which contains the fibers of the

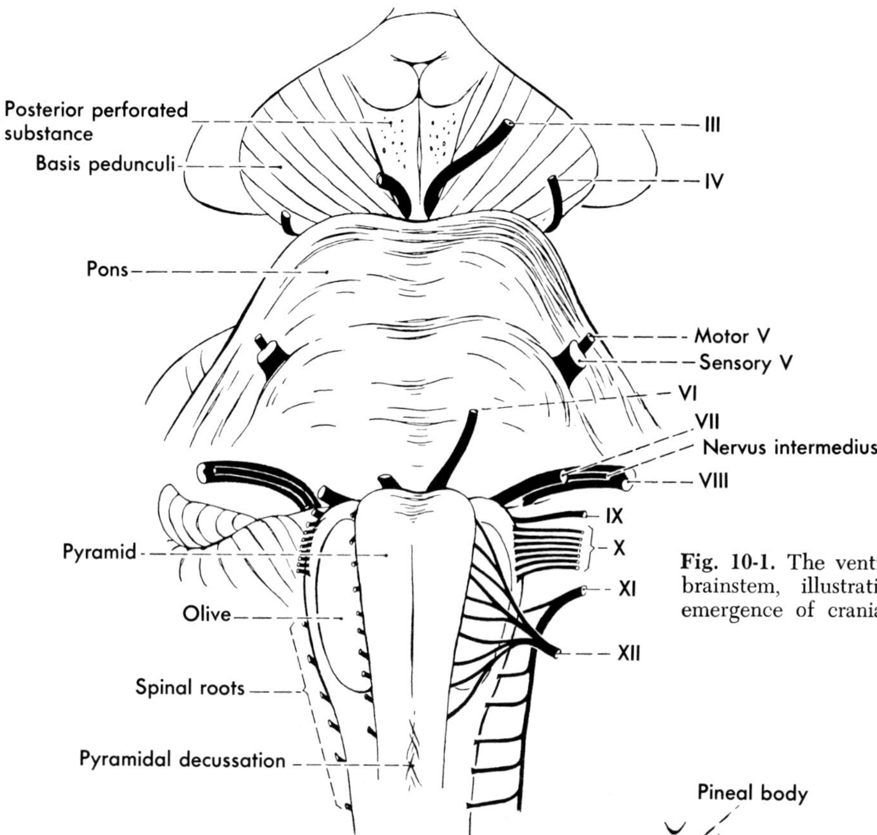

Fig. 10-1. The ventral surface of the brainstem, illustrating the sites of emergence of cranial nerves.

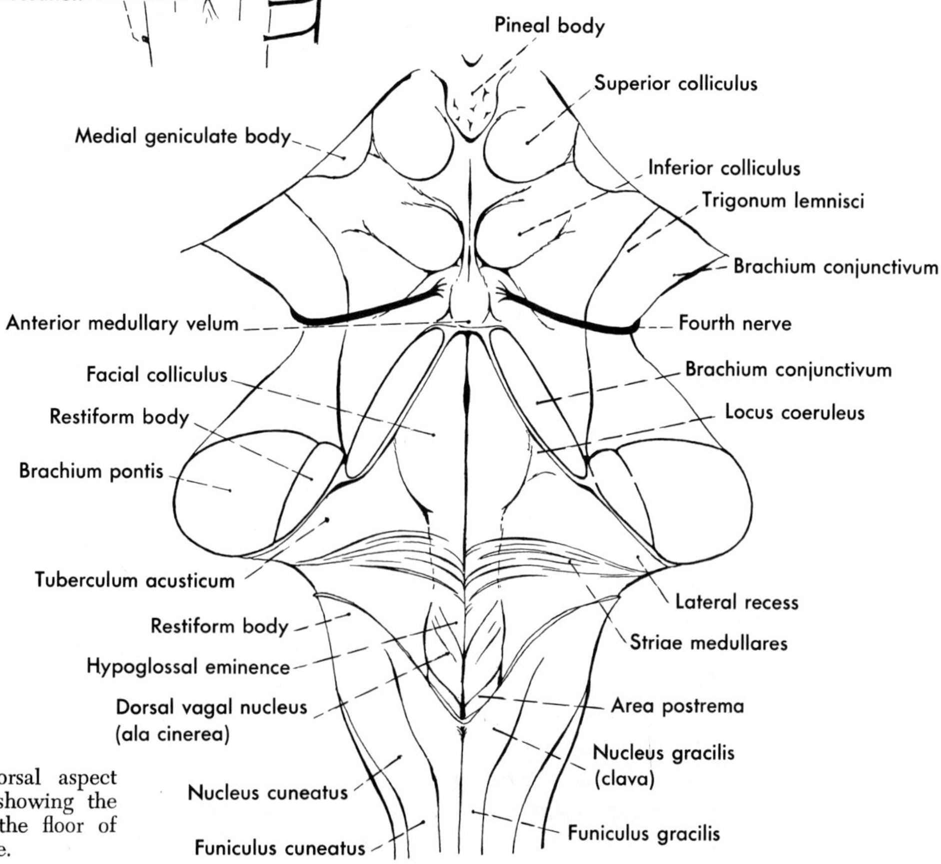

Fig. 10-2. The dorsal aspect of the brainstem, showing the fourth nerve and the floor of the fourth ventricle.

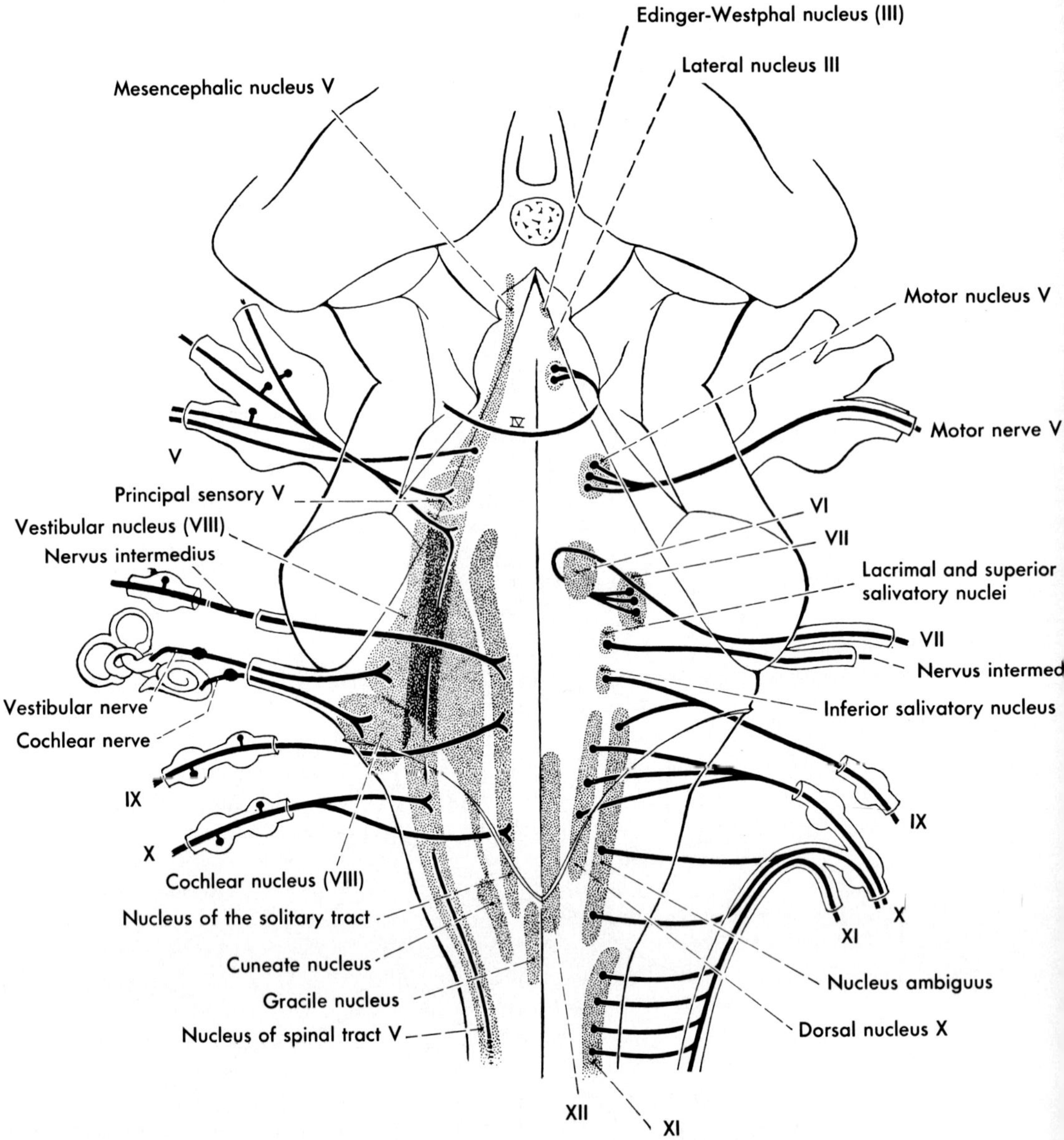

Fig. 10-3. The brainstem nuclei and nerves (dorsal view). *Left,* sensory; *right,* motor.

lateral spinothalamic tract and some fibers of the anterior spinothalamic tract. These fibers convey pain, temperature, and tactile impulses to the thalamus.

An imposing structure at this level is the pyramidal decussation. Here the majority of the corticospinal fibers cross the midline preparatory to passing downward in the spinal cord as the lateral pyramidal tract. The remaining fibers maintain their position with respect to the anterior median fissure, passing down the anterior column of the spinal cord as the anterior pyramidal tract, and decussating at successive levels to make synaptic connections with cells in the anterior horns.

MEDULLA OBLONGATA AT LEVEL OF THE SENSORY DECUSSATION (FIG. 10-8)

At this level the gray matter has undergone still more change. The nucleus and

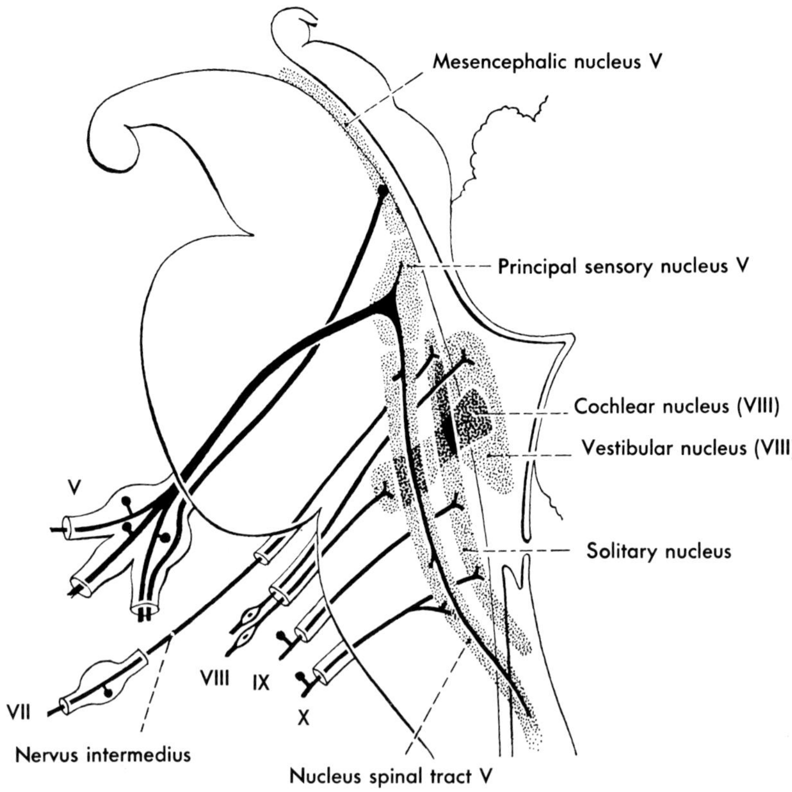

Fig. 10-4. The sensory brainstem nerves and nuclei (lateral view).

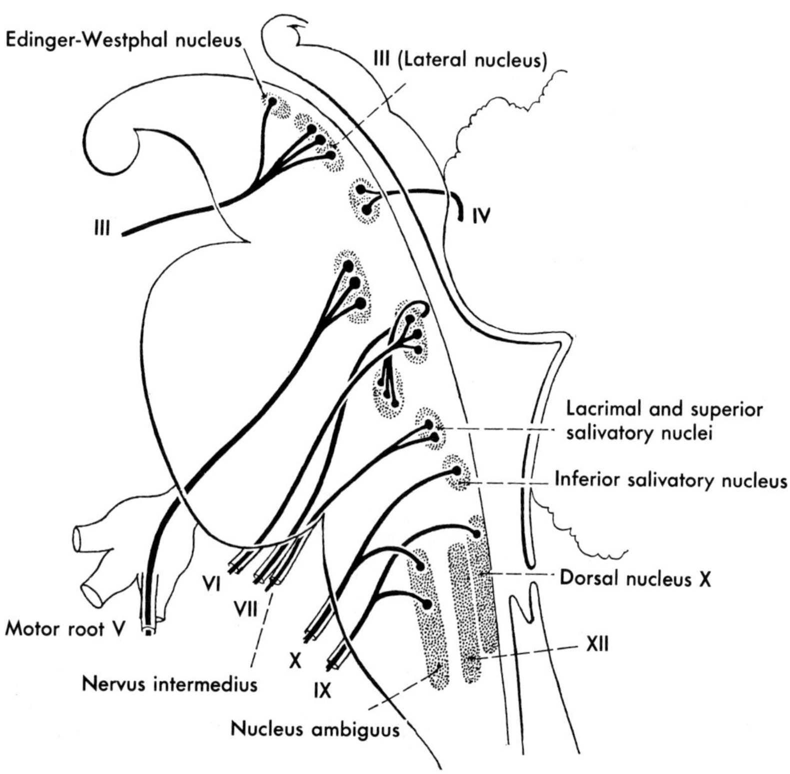

Fig. 10-5. The motor brainstem nerves and nuclei (lateral view).

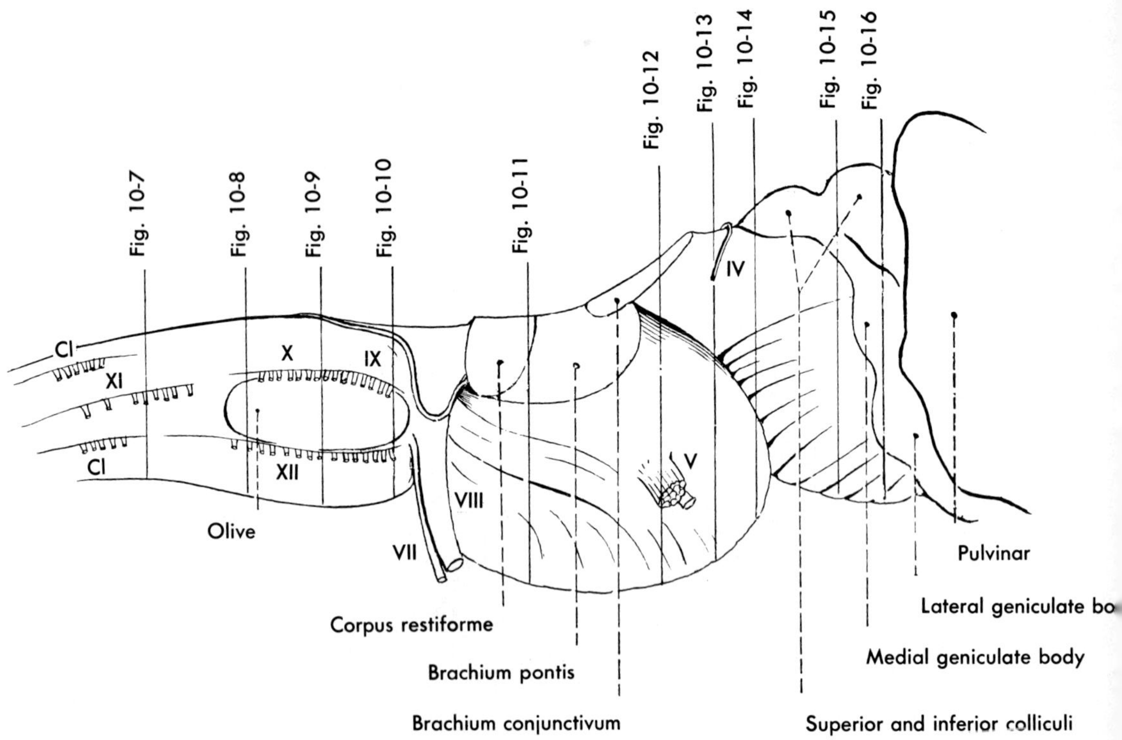

Fig. 10-6. Key to the level of the transverse sections illustrated in Figs. 10-7 through 10-16.

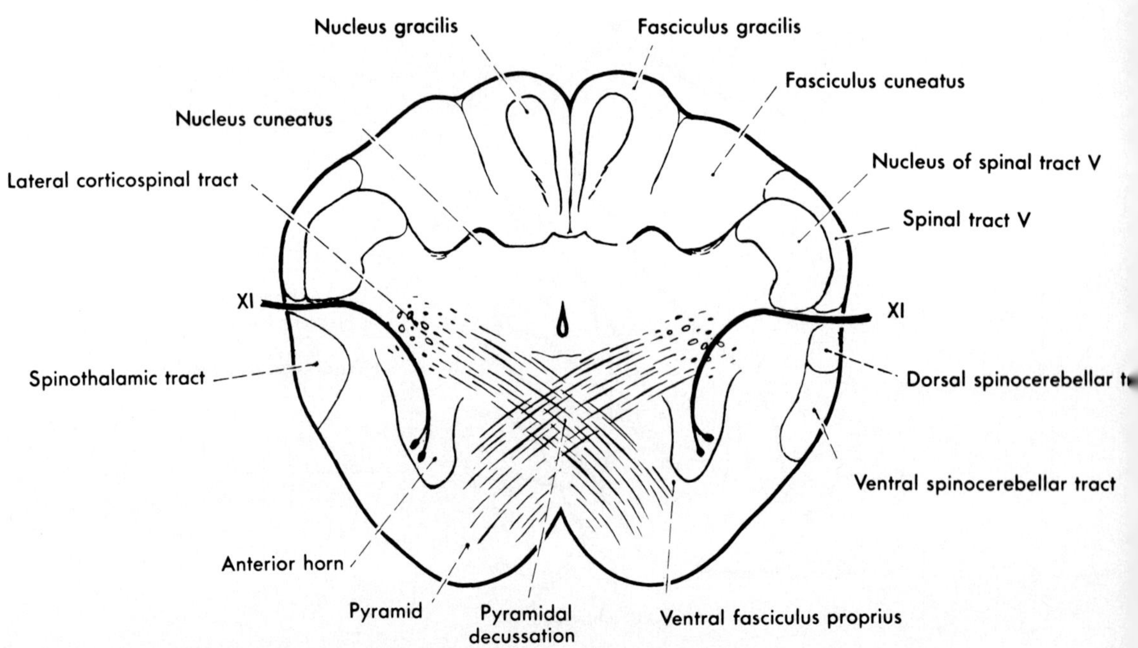

Fig. 10-7. Lowermost medulla oblongata at the level of the pyramidal decussation.

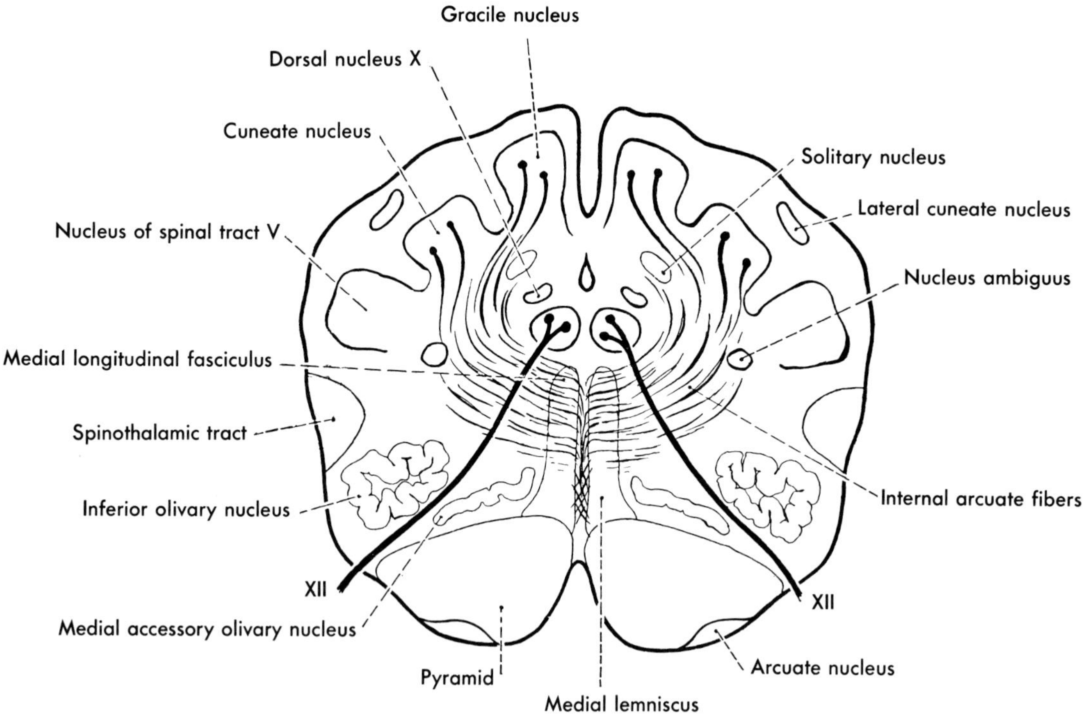

Fig. 10-8. Transverse section through the medulla oblongata at the level of the sensory decussation.

spinal tract of the fifth nerve have been displaced somewhat ventrally by the greatly enlarged gracile and cuneate nuclei, but the relationship of nucleus to tract remains the same as at the level just described. From the gracile and cuneate nuclei, internal arcuate fibers sweep ventrally in a wide arc and cross to the opposite side. After crossing the median plane they turn upward in the medial lemniscus.

Other internal arcuate fibers emanate from the nucleus of the spinal tract of the fifth nerve. Some extend over to the medial edge of the opposite spinothalamic tract, while others course to the region just ventrolateral to the twelfth nucleus and ascend in the bulbothalamic tract (Figs. 10-12 and 11-3). This tract carries fibers of the second order from the nucleus of the spinal tract of the fifth nerve and transmits pain impulses that have reached the nucleus through the fifth nerve, nervus intermedius, and the ninth and tenth nerves. Although on the basis of clinicopathological findings the bulbothalamic tract can be assumed to be present, its existence has not been verified experimentally.

Dorsolateral to the cuneate nucleus is the lateral cuneate nucleus. This nucleus, apparently a homologue of the nucleus dorsalis (Clarke's nucleus) of the spinal cord, receives fibers from cervical and upper thoracic roots by way of the posterior column and sends them through the restiform body of the cerebellum. The lateral cuneate nucleus is also the recipient of fibers from cranial nerves IX and X (via the spinal tract of nerve V) (Rhoton, O'Leary, and Ferguson, 1966); presumably a route (via the restiform body) thus exists through which the cerebellum may exercise an influence over visceromotor activity.

The spinothalamic tract is still situated at the lateral edge of the medulla oblongata, but has moved somewhat ventralward as compared with its position in the previous section. The dorsal and ventral spinocerebellar tracts occupy much the same positions as in the previous section (Fig. 10-8).

No anterior horns as such are to be seen. There are, however, scattered motor nuclei. One is the nucleus ambiguus, the fibers of which pass lateralward as a component of the tenth nerve. At this level the nucleus ambiguus provides the nerve supply for the adductor muscles of the larynx. Fibers for the supply of the abductors are situated at a higher level, and fibers passing to the cricothyroid muscle are still higher. The muscles of the pharynx appear to be innervated from the middle third of the nucleus, and those of the soft palate from the more caudal part of the nucleus.

The solitary nucleus occupies a position ventral to the gracile nucleus. At this level it receives fibers that convey the sensation of taste via nerve IX (from the posterior third of the tongue) and via nerve X (from the epiglottis). Taste sensation transmitted by the nervus intermedius (from the anterior two-thirds of the tongue) is carried by fibers reaching the superior part of the solitary nucleus. Fibers of nerves IX and X carrying impulses concerned in cardiorespiratory and other visceromotor reflex activity reach the inferior part of the solitary nucleus.

Another nucleus found at the level under discussion is the twelfth. Its nerve fibers leave the medulla oblongata as a series of rootlets in the region between the olive and pyramid, then join rootlets from higher levels to form the twelfth nerve. The nerve then pursues its peripheral course and supplies the muscles of the tongue.

Still another of the motor nuclei is the dorsal nucleus of the tenth nerve, whose fibers supply thoracic and abdominal viscera. The inferior olivary nucleus and the medial accessory olivary nuclei are also to be seen at this level.

Instead of the posterior median septum, there is now a posterior median fissure. It extends ventrally toward the central canal. The point at which the posterior median fissure and the central canal merge—namely, at the inferior end of the calamus scriptorius—constitutes the caudal limit of the fourth ventricle.

The pyramids, which are relatively large, lie on both sides of the anterior median fissure. Ventral to the pyramids is the arcuate nucleus, which receives collateral fibers from the corticospinal tract and fibers from the reticular formation of the opposite side. Fibers arising in the arcuate nucleus pass (as ventral external arcuate fibers) along the surface of the medulla oblongata to reach the cerebellum by way of the restiform body. Other fibers originating in the arcuate nucleus (joined by some fibers from the arcuate nucleus of the other side) constitute the so-called arcuatocerebellar pathway: the fibers pass dorsalward along the raphe, and on reaching the floor of the fourth ventricle, course lateralward along its surface (as the striae medullares) to reach the cerebellum by way of the restiform body.

Dorsal to the pyramids is the medial lemniscus. Still further dorsally is the tectospinal tract (not illustrated) and the medial longitudinal fasciculus. At this level the medial longitudinal fasciculus is ill defined owing to admixture with fibers of the tectospinal tract and medial lemniscus. Below this level, the fibers of the fasciculus course in the anterior column of the cord, midway between the anterior horn and median fissure, and terminate in the anterior horns of the cervical segments (Fig. 13-6). These are association fibers that connect the vestibular nuclei with anterior horns; they are concerned in orientation of the head in space.

MEDULLA OBLONGATA AT LEVEL OF LOWER THIRD OF THE FOURTH VENTRICLE (FIG. 10-9)

The fourth ventricle has now appeared. The cranial nerve nuclei occupy a dorsal location; lying immediately beneath the floor of the ventricle is the nucleus of the twelfth nerve. Occupying an intermediate position in the dorsal half of the medulla

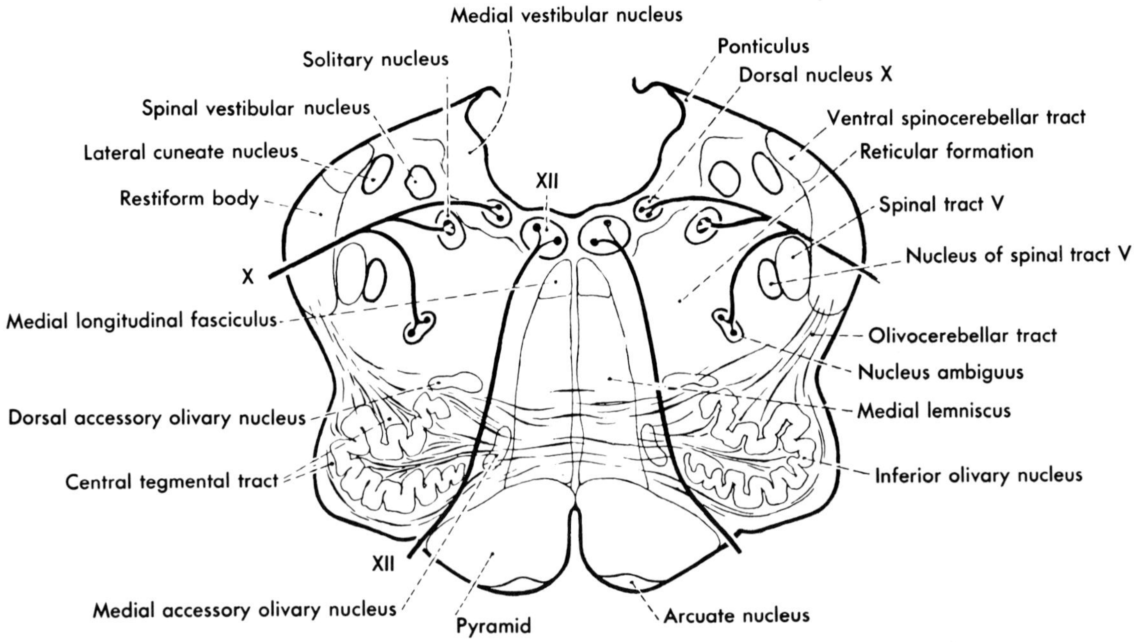

Fig. 10-9. Section through the medulla oblongata at the level of the lower third of the fourth ventricle.

oblongata are the nuclei related to the tenth nerve: the dorsal nucleus, the nucleus (and tractus) solitarius, and the nucleus ambiguus. The dorsal nucleus of the tenth nerve, situated near the floor of the fourth ventricle, imparts a grayness to the region (hence, *ala cinerea*). The fibers from all three nuclei unite to form the vagal rootlets, which leave the lateral aspect of the medulla oblongata by traversing the restiform body. Afferents carrying pain impulses from the viscera leave the vagus nerve in its intramedullary course and pass to the spinal nucleus of the fifth nerve. The solitary nucleus is also to be seen at this level.

Of the two spinocerebellar tracts, the *dorsal* has now become a part of the restiform body, while the *ventral* has shifted dorsally, coming to lie lateral to the lateral cuneate nucleus. The position of the spinal tract and nucleus of the fifth nerve has not changed.

Two vestibular nuclei have appeared at this level, the medial vestibular and the spinal vestibular. The lateral spinothalamic tract (not illustrated) has moved to a position just dorsal to the more lateral part of the inferior olivary nucleus, in a position indicated in Fig. 11-3. As compared with Fig. 10-8, there is no essential change in the position of the medial longitudinal fasciculus, medial lemniscus, pyramid, twelfth nucleus, inferior olivary nucleus, or medial accessory olivary nucleus. Another olivary nucleus, the posterior accessory nucleus, has, however, made its appearance.

MEDULLA OBLONGATA AT LEVEL OF THE NINTH NERVE (FIG. 10-10)

Here the dorsal part of the medulla oblongata is considerably wider than at lower levels because of greater flare of the walls of the fourth ventricle. The section is somewhat tangential. To the right are the dorsal and ventral cochlear nuclei, concerned in hearing. The ventral cochlear nucleus is in the wall of the cerebellopontile angle and forms a prominence on the surface of the brainstem known as the *tuberculum acusticum*. On the left, next to the cochlear nerve, is the vestibular

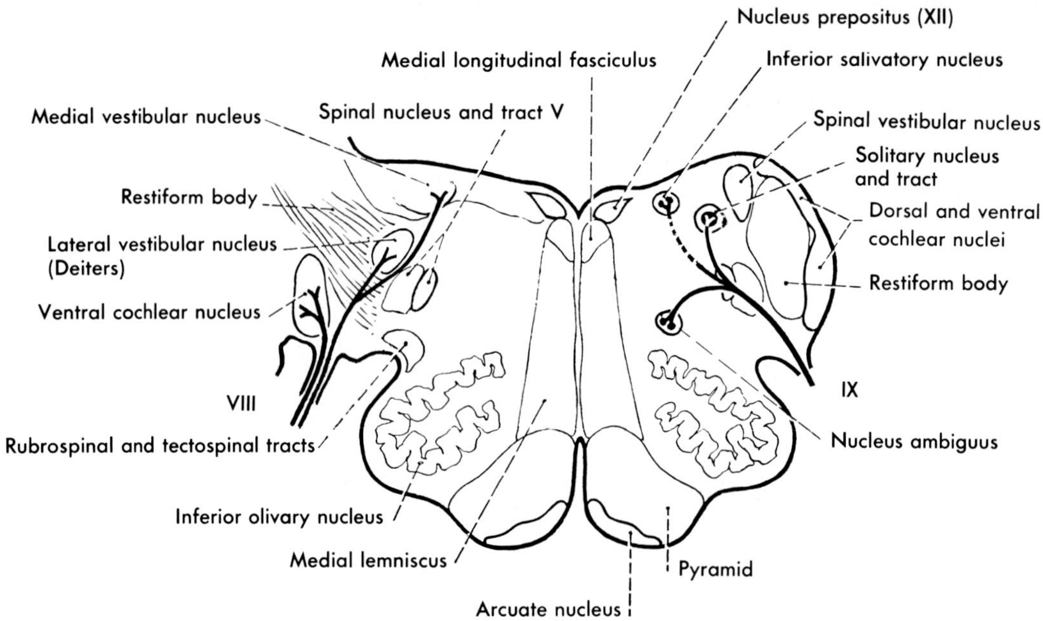

Fig. 10-10. Section through the medulla oblongata at the level of the ninth nerve. The section is somewhat tangential; the level is slightly higher on the left than on the right. The lateral tectospinal tract is illustrated; the medial tectospinal tract lies just ventral to the medial longitudinal fasciculus.

nerve, which serves the function of orientation of the head and body in space. It can be seen ending in the lateral vestibular (Deiters') nucleus and the medial vestibular nucleus; to the right, in the floor of the fourth ventricle, is the spinal vestibular nucleus. Another cell aggregate is the nucleus prepositus, one of a series of nuclei propriae in the floor of the fourth ventricle.

On the right, a rootlet of the ninth nerve is to be seen. Its fibers arise from the nucleus ambiguus and, at a somewhat higher level, from the inferior salivatory nucleus. Its afferent fibers terminate partly in the caudal part of the solitary nucleus (taste), partly in the spinal nucleus of the fifth nerve (pain), and partly in the principal nucleus of the fifth nerve and the (medial) cuneate nucleus (touch).

The restiform body contains all its component fiber systems and on the left side is turning toward the cerebellum. The ventral spinocerebellar tract (not illustrated) occupies a position just dorsal to the restiform body. To the left, in the angle dorsal to the inferior olivary nucleus, is the rubrospinal tract.

Other structures have the same spatial relationships as in the previous section (Fig. 10-9).

PONS AT LEVEL OF THE SIXTH AND SEVENTH NUCLEI (FIG. 10-11)

The pattern at this level is altogether different from that of the medulla oblongata. The dorsal part of the pons, the region beneath the floor of the fourth ventricle, is referred to as the *tegmentum pontis*. It is easily distinguishable from the ventral part, called the *pars basilaris pontis*. The dividing line between tegmentum and the pars basilaris lies just ventral to the medial lemniscus.

Situated in the floor of the fourth ventricle somewhat medial to the superior vestibular nucleus is the superior salivatory nucleus; slightly ventrolateral to it is the lacrimal nucleus.

The tegmentum pontis is occupied by

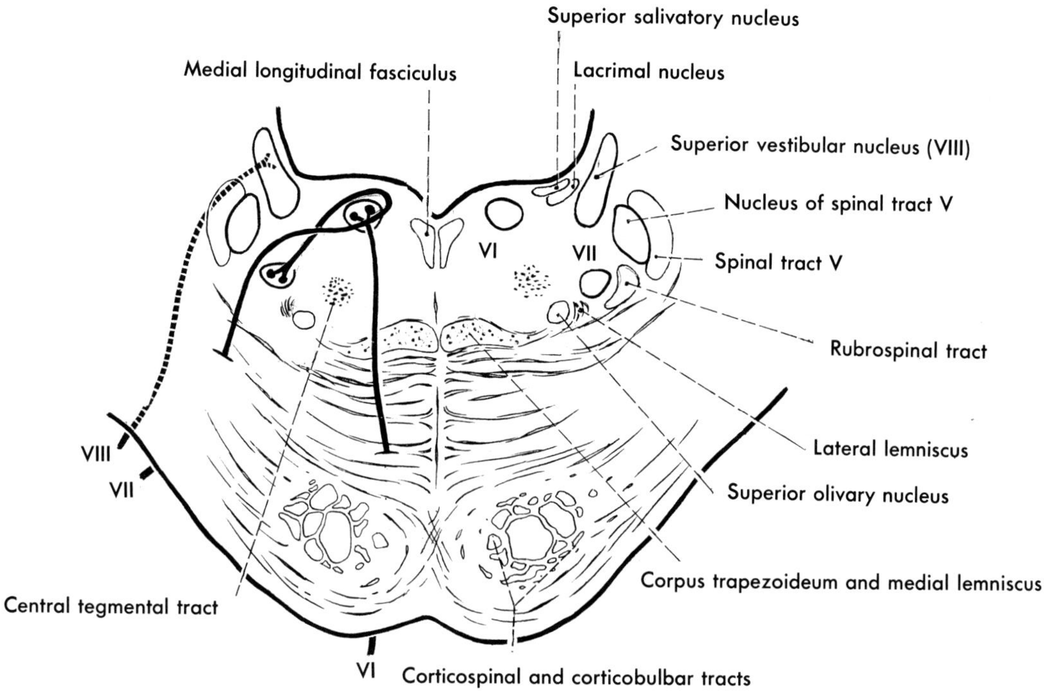

Fig. 10-11. Lower pons at the level of the nuclei of the sixth and seventh nerves. The sites indicated for the superior salivatory and lacrimal nuclei are after Crosby and DeJonge (1963).

a number of nuclei and fiber tracts. Conspicuous is the sixth nucleus. Its fibers emerge at the lower border of the pons, a few millimeters from the midline. The sixth nerve supplies the lateral rectus muscle. In the depth of the tegmentum lies the nucleus of the seventh nerve. Neurons for the supply of the upper facial muscles, including those for the eyelids, appear to be situated ventrally in the nucleus, those for the lower face dorsally (Crosby and DeJonge, 1963). An intermediate group of neurons probably supplies the frontal and orbital muscles (Pearson, 1946). The fibers issuing from the seventh nucleus run a devious course. First they pass dorsalward to a point near the floor of the fourth ventricle, where they partly encircle the sixth nucleus; they then pass ventrolaterally to emerge from the lowermost pontile level in the region of the cerebellopontile angle. Here the seventh nerve is situated just medial to the eighth. In their dorsalmost course the fibers from the seventh nucleus pass dorsal to the sixth nucleus, forming a prominence on the floor of the fourth ventricle known as the *facial colliculus* or *eminentia teres.*

The superior vestibular nucleus is represented at this level. Lateral to it is the restiform body (not illustrated) and just ventrolateral to it are the nucleus and spinal tract of the fifth nerve. The medial longitudinal fasciculus retains its position with respect to the raphe. The rubrospinal tract occupies the same position as in the previous section. The medial lemniscus has shifted its position and now lies ventral in the tegmentum near the midline (represented by dots). It is intermixed with transversely coursing fibers of the corpus trapezoideum. Lateral to the superior olivary nucleus are the fibers of the corpus trapezoideum; they are concerned in the transmission of impulses from the ventral cochlear nucleus; the fibers turn upward in the lateral lemniscus. At higher levels these fibers reach the nucleus of the lateral lemniscus and, in turn, the nucleus of the inferior colliculus and the medial geniculate body; fibers terminate in each of these nuclei (Fig. 13-10).

Also conspicuous at this level is the central tegmental tract, which is composed of fibers from various tegmental sources; it runs downward dorsal and lateral to the inferior olivary nucleus, in which many of its fibers terminate.

In the pars basilaris pontis there are a number of vertically coursing pyramidal fiber bundles, the corticospinal and corticobulbar tracts. The transversely coursing bundles are the pontocerebellar fibers, which form the brachium pontis.

PONS AT LEVEL OF THE FIFTH NERVE (FIG. 10-12)

The brachium conjunctivum (in the superior cerebellar peduncle) is situated lateral to the fourth ventricle and is prominent. It is composed partly of fibers passing from cerebellar nuclei to the red nucleus. Lateral to it is the ventral spinocerebellar tract, passing in the opposite direction to end in the cerebellar cortex. The anterior (or superior) medullary velum forms part of the roof of the fourth ventricle. Lying on the roof is the lingula of the cerebellum. Just ventral to the brachium conjunctivum is a group of fibers comprising the lateral spinothalamic tract; farther medial is the mesencephalic root of the fifth nerve. Another group of fibers in this general region, but lying in the dorsal part of the tegmentum pontis, is the bulbothalamic tract.

The medial longitudinal fasciculus retains the position that it occupied at lower levels. The medial lemniscus has shifted somewhat laterally in the confines of the corpus trapezoideum. The motor and principal sensory nucleus of the fifth nerve are evident, and just ventral to them is the rubrospinal tract.

The pars basilaris pontis has much the same features as in the previous section (Fig. 10-11).

UPPER PONS AT LEVEL OF DECUSSATION OF THE FOURTH NERVE (FIG. 10-13)

This section is through a level of the isthmus, the region of transition of mid-

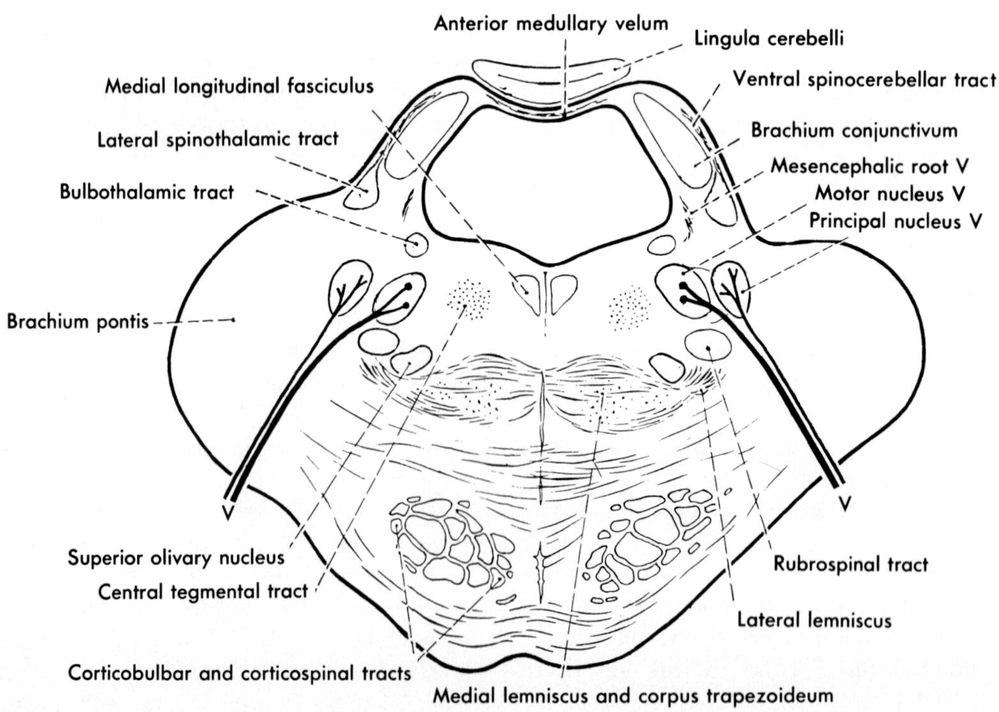

Fig. 10-12. Section through the midpons at the level of the fifth nerve.

brain to pons. The fourth ventricle is about to merge with the aqueduct. Dorsal to the ventricle are the fourth nerves, which have arisen at a somewhat higher level (Fig. 10-14). Each is seen crossing the midline. Ventral to the isthmic cavity is the nucleus of the locus coeruleus. The pigment in cells of this nucleus is brown, as seen microscopically, but in the gross specimen the ependyma filters the color so that it appears a cerulean blue. This nucleus receives collaterals from the dorsal longitudinal fasciculus (not illustrated) and gives off fibers that reach the more ventral part of the reticular formation of the medulla oblongata.

The fibers of the brachium conjunctivum are decussating preparatory to entering the undersurface and medial aspect of the red nucleus. The medial longitudinal fasciculus continues to lie dorsally, near the raphe. The medial lemniscus has moved laterally and is contiguous with the lateral lemniscus, containing fibers of the auditory system. The nucleus of the lateral lemniscus is a synaptic station of auditory fibers. Interposed between medial lemniscus and brachium conjunctivum is the rubrospinal tract.

The pars basilaris pontis retains its characteristic features.

MIDBRAIN AT LEVEL OF THE INFERIOR COLLICULUS (FIG. 10-14)

This is a section through a lower level of the midbrain, to which a part of the pars basilaris pontis is attached. The midbrain is subdivided into: tectum, with its nucleus of the inferior colliculus; tegmentum, which extends ventrally to the substantia nigra; and the basis pedunculi. The substantia nigra is interposed between tegmentum and basis pedunculi. The term *cerebral peduncle* includes tegmentum, substantia nigra, and basis pedunculi, and excludes the lamina quadrigemina.

The nucleus of the fourth nerve has now appeared and ventral to it is the medial longitudinal fasciculus. The fibers of the brachium conjunctivum of each side are

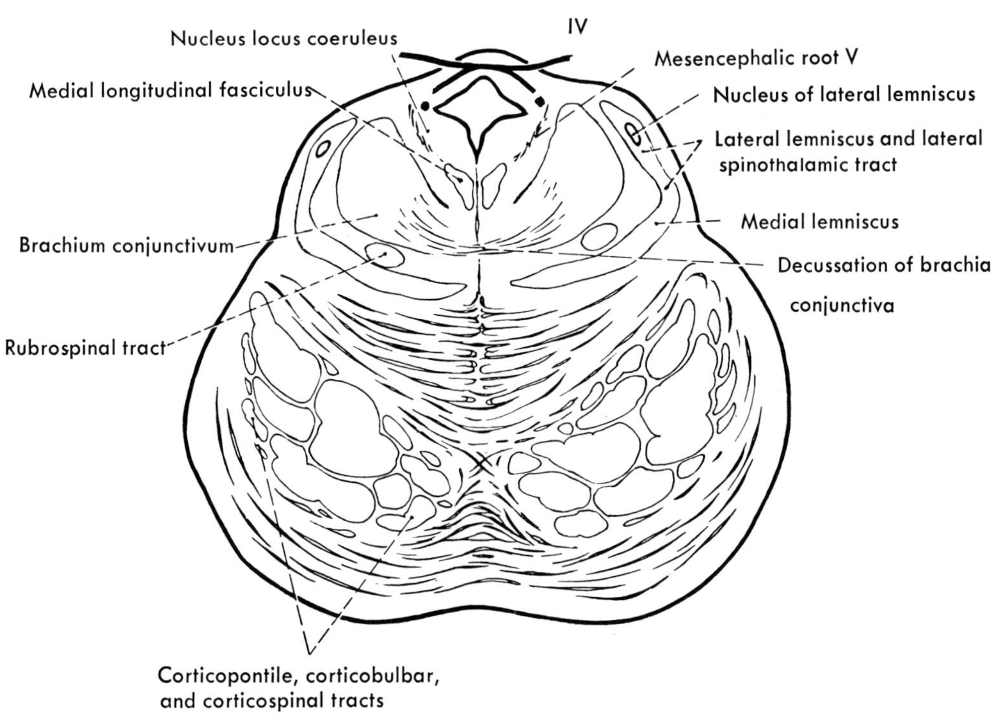

Fig. 10-13. Section through the upper pons at the level of the decussation of the fourth nerve.

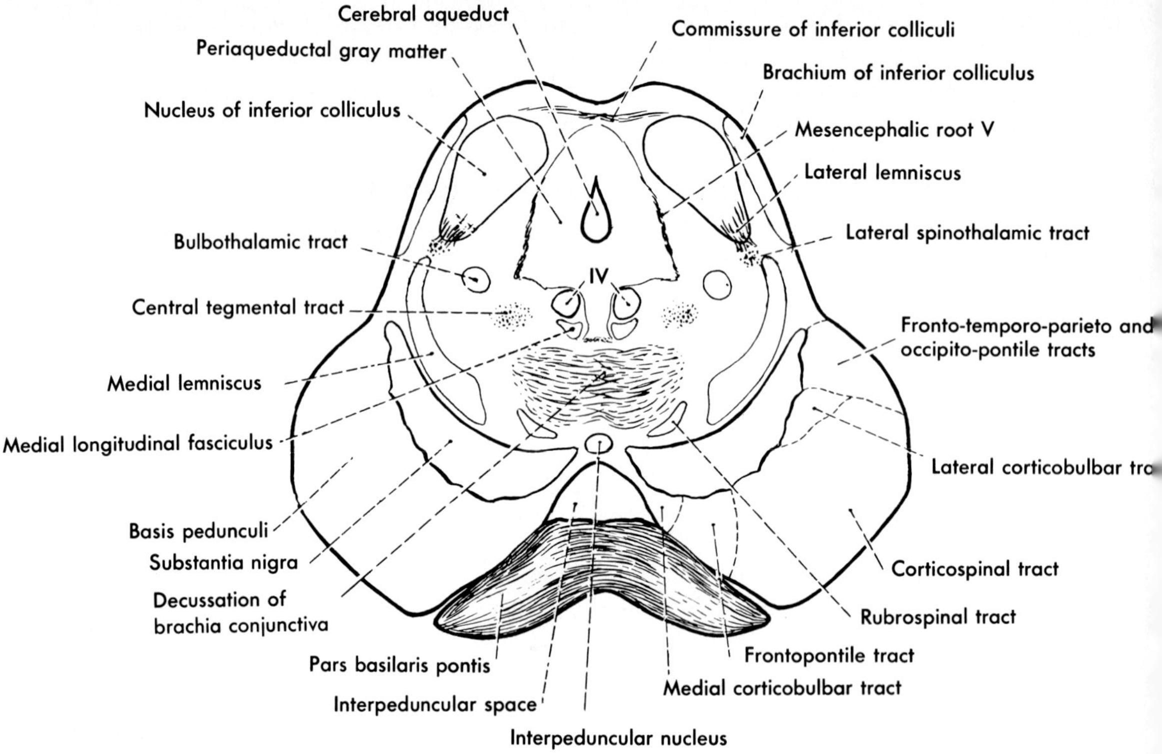

Fig. 10-14. Section through the midbrain at the level of the inferior colliculus.

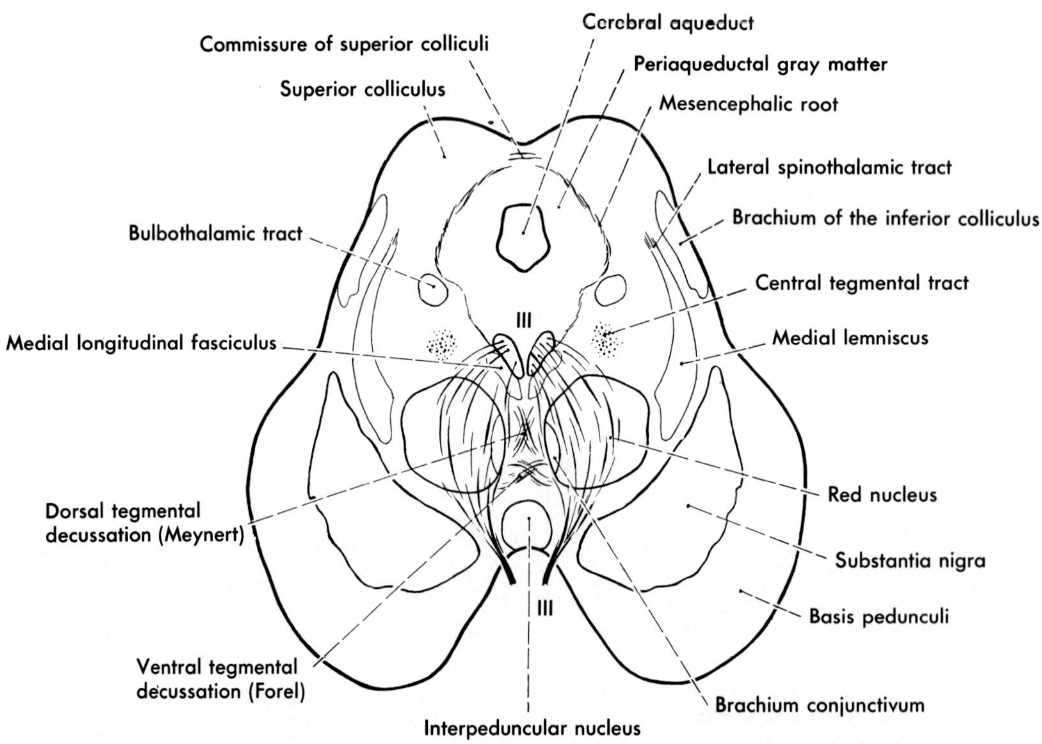

Fig. 10-15. Section through the midbrain at a lower level of the superior colliculus.

decussating prior to ending in the red nucleus, which is to be seen at the next higher level (Fig. 10-15). A few fibers of the lateral lemniscus are extending into the nucleus of the inferior colliculus; others, components of the lateral spinothalamic tract (represented by dots), are ascending to the thalamus. Still others will be turning laterally to traverse the brachium of the inferior colliculus in reaching (in Fig. 10-16) the medial geniculate body. The bulbothalamic tract retains its position, and the rubrospinal tract is to be seen just ventral to the decussation of the brachia conjunctiva. Lying ventrally in the midsagittal plane is the interpeduncular nucleus, which receives fibers from the habenular nucleus; these fibers form a robust bundle known as the habenulo-interpeduncular fasciculus (fasciculus retroflexus of Meynert).

To the right, the subdivisions of the basis pedunculi are indicated; the medial third contains a corticobulbar tract and the frontopontile tract, the middle third the corticospinal tract, and the lateral third another corticobulbar tract and a group of corticopontile tracts arising in the cortex of the frontal, temporal, parietal, and occipital lobes. This subdivision of the fiber pathways is based on degeneration studies. Electrical stimulation in the basis pedunculi (in the human brain) has revealed a somatotopic distribution of its fibers, the face, arm, and leg being represented in that order ventrodorsally, with a wide representation for the arm (Martinez, Bertrand, and Botana-Lopez, 1967).

LEVEL OF THE LOWER MIDBRAIN (FIG. 10-15)

The red nucleus has now appeared. Along its medial border are fibers of the contralateral brachium conjunctivum. Visible in the ventral part of the periaqueductal region is the lateral component of the third nucleus. Fibers of the third nerve pass through the medial longitudinal fasciculus, the red nucleus, skirt the substantia nigra, and leave the midbrain along the medial border of the basis pedunculi. Between the red nuclei is the dorsal teg-

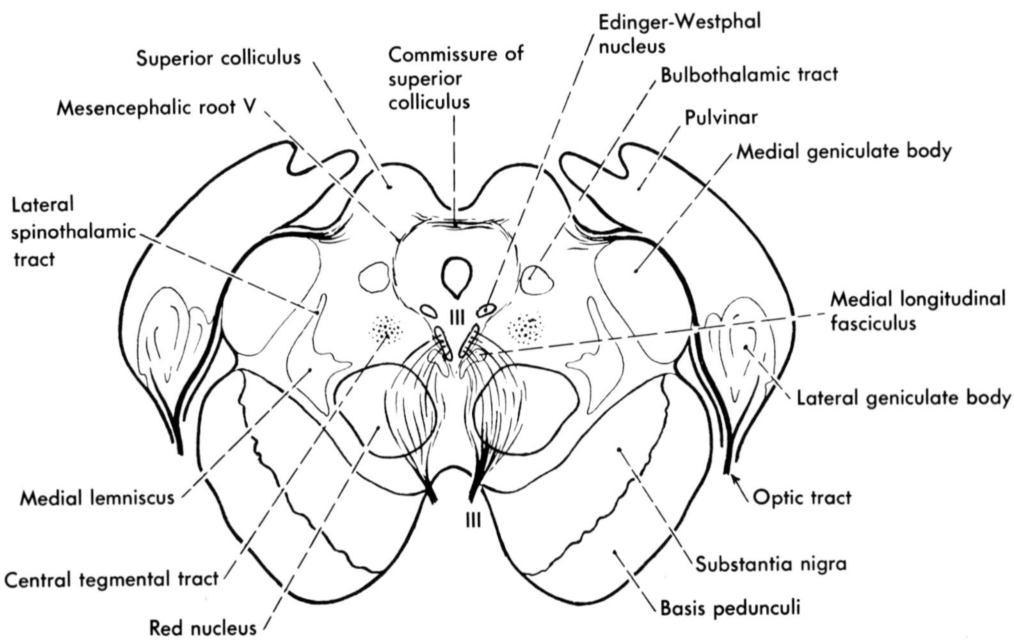

Fig. 10-16. Section through an upper level of the midbrain, which includes the pulvinar of the thalamus.

mental decussation, which carries tectobulbar fibers and the tectospinal tract. Beneath this decussation, carrying the fibers of the rubrospinal tract, is the ventral tegmental decussation. Ventral to these is the interpeduncular nucleus.

LEVEL OF THE UPPER MIDBRAIN (FIG. 10-16)

The pulvinar of the thalamus is included in this section. Ventral to it is the lateral geniculate body, which is receiving fibers from the optic tract. Some fibers from the optic tract run lateral to the medial geniculate body and gain the superior colliculus and the pretectal region. Medial to the medial geniculate body lies the lateral spinothalamic tract; lateral to the periaqueductal gray matter is the bulbothalamic tract. The central tegmental tract is still visible. It draws its fibers mainly from the tegmentum.

REFERENCES

Crosby, E. C., and DeJonge, B. R. 1963. Experimental and clinical studies of the central connections and central relations of the facial nerve. Ann. Otol. **72**:735-755.

Martinez, S. N., Bertrand, C., and Botana-Lopez, C. 1967. Motor fiber distribution within the cerebral peduncle: results of unipolar stimulation. Confin. Neurol. **29**:117-122.

Pearson, A. A. 1946. The development of the motor nuclei of the facial nerve in man. J. Comp. Neurol. **85**:461-476.

Rhoton, A. L., Jr., O'Leary, J. L., and Ferguson, J. P. 1966. The trigeminal, facial, vagal, and glossopharyngeal nerves in the monkey: afferent connections. Arch. Neurol. **14**:530-540.

Chapter 11

Localization of lesions involving the brainstem and emergent nerves

From the anatomical features of the brainstem just outlined, certain structural principles may be derived that serve as a guide in the localization of lesions. Cranial nerve nuclei and their emergent nerves have a close spatial relationship with long, vertically directed fiber tracts at various levels of the brainstem, so that numerous basic anatomical patterns exist. The differing patterns are the key to localization of lesions in terms of syndromes.

STRUCTURAL FEATURES OF THE BRAINSTEM

Brainstem nuclear pattern

The morphogenesis of the vertebrate head region is closely interrelated with the formation of the branchial (visceral) arches and gill clefts (Fig. 11-1).

Within the mesoderm of the branchial arches arises the branchial musculature, the origin of which is not traceable from somites. As the branchial arches and branchial musculature develop, the segmentation of the ancestral head somites, variously estimated to have numbered nine to thirteen, is disturbed: only the three most rostral preotic somites persist to form the eye muscles; the intermediate head somites in the otic region disappear; the most caudal postotic somites remain, and together with the rostral trunk somites provide myotomes from which the hypobranchial, or tongue, musculature develops (Fig. 11-1, *A*).

Corresponding to this subdivision into eye musculature, branchial arches, and hypobranchial musculature, three different groups of greatly modified nerves originate from the deuterencephalon (mesencephalon and rhombencephalon), namely, the eye muscle nerves (III, IV, VI), the branchial nerves (V, VII through XI), and the tongue muscle nerve (XII) (Figs. 11-1, *B* and 11-1, *C*). Although serially homologous with spinal nerves, the cranial nerves of the deuterencephalon differ from them as a result of adaptation to the specific head structures during the course of evolutionary development. Despite this progressive differentiation, certain features of the spinal roots of primitive vertebrates are preserved. Thus, dorsal roots (namely, the branchial nerves, or nerves V, VII, IX, X, XI) and ventral roots (III, IV, VI, XII) remain unconnected and independent of each other as they emerge from the brainstem, and dorsal roots include abundant efferent components—for example, the motor portion of the fifth nerve and the motor and parasympathetic fibers of the tenth. In their peripheral course, branchial and other nerves may, however, anastomose. This is true, for instance, for the third nerve and the ophthalmic division of the fifth. The basic similarity of the cranial nerves in the selachian and the human brain is illustrated in Figs. 11-1, *B* and *C*.

The nuclear pattern of the brainstem may be simplified through a consideration of the formation of nuclear columns from the longitudinal zones of the embryonic brainstem.

Consistent with their specialization, the cranial nerves contain components additional to those found in spinal nerves. Analysis of the cranial nerves in the entire vertebrate series has led to the formulation of the doctrine of functional nerve components, based on concepts as to which structures are somatic and which visceral. Somatic functions are defined as those concerned in the adjustment of the body to its environment, and visceral functions as those concerned in the internal adjustments of the body. It so happens that the somatic musculature is derived mostly from embryonic structures known as somites, and that branchial arches including their musculature (concerned with respiration in fishes) are designated

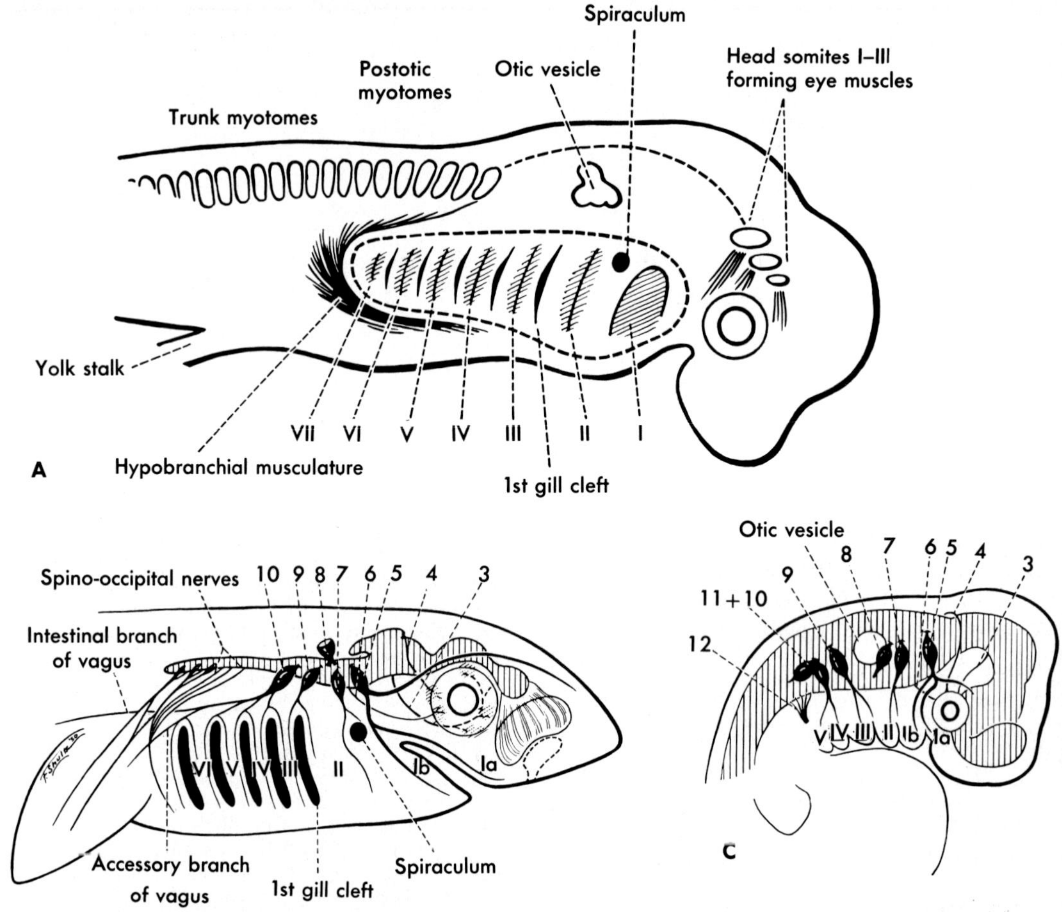

Fig. 11-1. A, The eye musculature, hypobranchial musculature, and branchial musculature in Selachian embryo. *I-VII,* Branchial arches with their musculature. **B,** The cranial nerves in a Selachian, and **C,** in a human embryo of about 5 weeks (8 to 10 mm. in length). The Arabic numerals refer to the cranial nerves, and the Roman to the branchial arches. In the Selachian there are five true gill clefts, the first of which is indicated. *Ia* and *Ib* refer to the maxillary and mandibular parts of the Ist, or maxillomandibular, branchial arch. (Diagrams prepared by Dr. H. Kuhlenbeck, Philadelphia; modified after Froriep, 1882, and Kuhlenbeck, 1927. Text on pages 145 through 148 was prepared in collaboration with Dr. H. Kuhlenbeck.)

as visceral arches. The doctrine of functional nerve components as used in this volume stresses function.

The basic achitectural plan of the brainstem has certain similarities to that of the spinal cord. Simply considered, both consist of ventral motor and dorsal sensory plates, divided by the sulcus limitans. The difference in configuration between the spinal cord and the brainstem is the result of dorsal flaring of the neural tube in the region of the brainstem, whereby the dorsal sensory plate is displaced laterally.

Motor plate and its derivatives (Fig. 11-2)

Somatic motor. The somatic motor component comprises the nuclei of origin of the twelfth, sixth, fourth, and third nerves. All four of these nuclei are located near the midline of the brainstem. They form an interrupted nuclear column homologous to the somatic motor part of the ventral horn of the spinal cord.

Branchial motor. The term *branchial motor* refers to the efferent fibers that supply the musculature derived from the branchial arch mesoderm. The nuclei originating from the branchial motor part of the basal plate are the eleventh, the nucleus ambiguus, the seventh, and the motor nucleus of the fifth nerve. Most of these nuclei have an intermediate ventrolateral position. The spinal nucleus of the eleventh nerve is situated in the

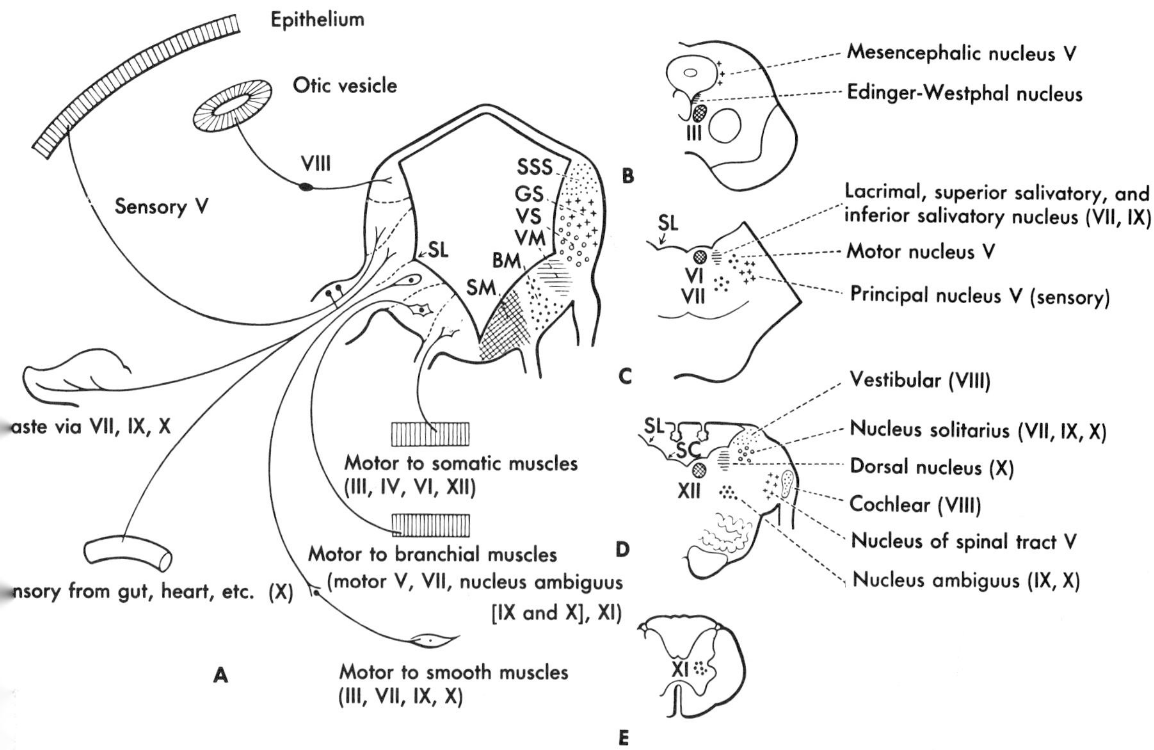

Fig. 11-2. The functional longitudinal zones of the human brainstem and their nuclear columns as seen (**A**) in a cross section of the embryonic human medulla oblongata and (**B-E**) at various levels of the adult brainstem. (Modified from His, 1904; Herrick, 1931; Kuhlenbeck, 1927; and Ranson, 1953.) In **A**, the alar (dorsal) plate is separated from the basal (ventral) plate by the sulcus limitans *(SL)*. Longitudinal zones: *SSS*, special somatic sensory; *GS*, general somatic sensory; *VS*, visceral sensory; *VM*, visceral motor; *BM*, branchial motor; *SM*, somatic motor.

Cross sections of the midbrain (**B**), pons (**C**), medulla oblongata (**D**), and upper cervical cord (**E**) illustrate the position of the brainstem nuclei. For example, the twelfth, third, fourth, and sixth nuclei, indicated by cross hatch, retain the same medial position occupied by the somatic motor column *(SM)* in the embryonic medulla oblongata. *SL*, Sulcus limitans; *SC*, sulcus intermedius ventralis. (Diagrams prepared in collaboration with Dr. H. Kuhlenbeck, Philadelphia.)

lateral part of the base of the ventral horn of the upper four cervical segments.

Visceral motor. The visceral motor component of the basal plate gives rise to the cranial parasympathetic nuclei. It is bounded laterally by the sulcus limitans. The continuity of this longitudinal zone is disrupted to a greater degree than that of any of the other zones. The derivatives comprise: the dorsal motor nucleus of the tenth nerve (which retains most clearly its primitive position with respect to the sulcus limitans), the inferior salivatory nucleus (the fibers of which join the ninth nerve), the superior salivatory and lacrimal nuclei (which send fibers into the seventh nerve), and the Edinger-Westphal nucleus (which is closely adjacent to the somatic motor elements of the third nucleus and in concert with them gives rise to the third nerve).

Sensory plate and its derivatives (Fig. 11-2)

Visceral sensory. In the most medial part of the sensory plate, immediately adjoining the sulcus limitans, is the visceral sensory longitudinal zone. This zone includes the nucleus of the tractus solitarius. Lying lateral and ventral to the dorsal motor nucleus of the vagus, it retains the relative position of the visceral sensory zone from which it arose. The pressoreceptor and chemoreceptor fibers of the ninth and tenth nerves, which originate in the carotid sinus, aortic arch, carotid glomus, and aortic glomus, may best be included with the visceral sensory.

General somatic sensory. If the sensory longitudinal zones conformed exactly to the motor longitudinal zones, the next two lateral zones would be the branchial sensory and the somatic sensory. However, the organization on the sensory side is such that these two are merged, and to designate them collectively the term *general somatic sensory* has been adopted. The derivatives of this portion of the sensory plate are the sensory nuclei of the fifth nerve—the mesencephalic nucleus, the principal sensory nucleus, and the nucleus of the spinal tract. The latter nucleus receives fibers also from the seventh, ninth, and tenth nerves, and is regarded as a serial homologue of the dorsal horns in the spinal cord. All the nuclei of the fifth nerve have strayed somewhat from the midlateral position that their cells of origin once occupied in the embryologic longitudinal zone, but they have retained the serial alignment (Fig. 10-3) they had during the embryonic stage.

Special somatic sensory. This longitudinal zone, originally the most dorsolateral, receives fibers from the vestibular apparatus and the cochlea, both of which are derived from the otic vesicle. In conformity with their primitive position, the vestibular and cochlear nuclei are situated dorsolaterally in the brainstem.

Intramedullary course of cranial nerve fibers

The fibers emerging from most of the cranial nerve nuclei course ventrally or ventrolaterally to the base of the brainstem. While most of them take a direct course, the fibers of the nucleus ambiguus follow a somewhat circuitous route, and the fibers of the facial nucleus much more so. The fourth nerve, in emerging from the brainstem through the superior medullary velum, is the only cranial nerve taking exit dorsally. Another exceptional feature of this nerve is that it undergoes complete decussation. All other nerves of the brainstem, except some fibers of the third (Fig. 13-6), emerge on the side on which they take origin.

Relation of the cranial nerve nuclei to the medial lemniscus and the spinothalamic tracts

Ventral or ventromedial to the cranial nerve nuclei of the medulla oblongata are the tracts that convey sensibility from the trunk and extremities. They are the medial lemniscus and the spinothalamic tracts, constituted as follows. (1) Long fibers of the posterior root system, carrying deep sensibility and a part of tactile sensibility, pass up the posterior column, synapse in the ipsilateral gracile and cuneate

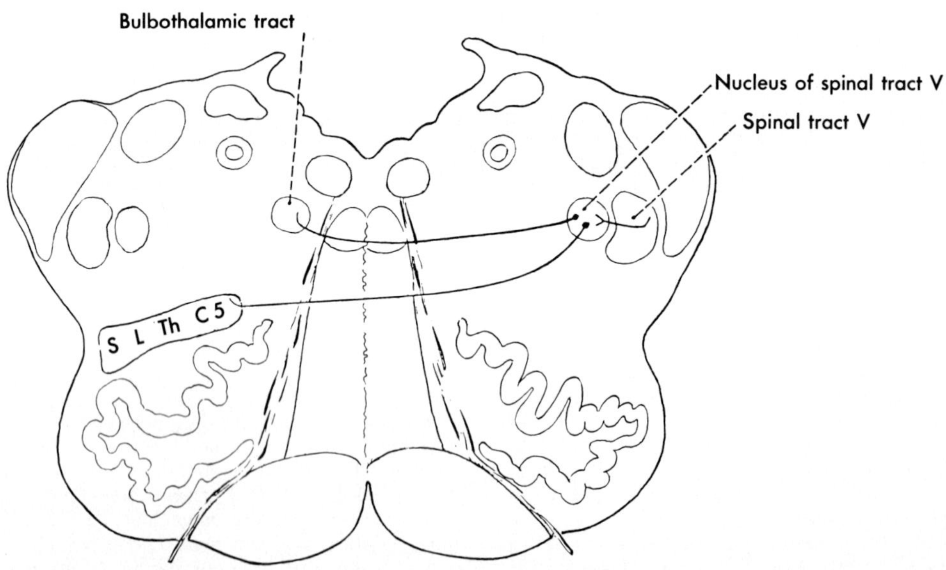

Fig. 11-3. The position in the medulla oblongata of the lateral spinothalamic tract and of pathways originating in the spinal nucleus of the fifth nerve. Shown to the left is the lateral spinothalamic tract and its components, the latter ascending from sacral *(S)*, lumbar *(L)*, thoracic *(Th)*, and cervical *(C)* levels. Indicated as lying most medial are fibers from the spinal nucleus of the fifth nerve *(5)* (the quintothalamic tract). Also shown is the bulbothalamic tract. Only decussating fibers are indicated; some also proceed upward in the corresponding position on the ipsilateral side. (From Rowbotham, 1938; Walker, 1940; White and Sweet, 1955.)

nuclei, cross the midline as internal arcuate fibers, and ascend in the medial lemniscus. (2) Short posterior root fibers, conveying pain, temperature, and a part of tactile sensibility, synapse in the posterior horn, decussate, then ascend in the lateral and anterior spinothalamic tracts.

On reaching the medulla oblongata, the lateral and anterior spinothalamic tracts intermingle to form a single group of fibers, generally referred to simply as the *spinothalamic tract.* At lowermost levels the spinothalamic tract lies next to the surface of the medulla oblongata in a position ventral to the spinal nucleus and tract of the fifth nerve (Fig. 10-7). At a somewhat higher level it is displaced, somewhat ventrally (Fig. 10-8), and at still higher levels of the medulla oblongata it lies just dorsal to the inferior olivary nucleus (Fig. 11-3) (Foerster and Gagel, 1932; Rasmussen and Peyton, 1941; Schwartz and O'Leary, 1942). Upon entering the pons, the spinothalamic tract is situated just lateral to the medial lemniscus. In the lower midbrain it merges with the lateral lemniscus and lies just ventral to the nucleus of the inferior colliculus (Fig. 10-14). At a slightly higher level the tract lies just medial to the medial geniculate body (Fig. 10-16). Ultimately the fibers terminate in the ventral posterolateral nucleus (VPL) of the thalamus (Walker, 1940).

Since the fibers conveying deep sensibility pass upward near the midline and those carrying pain and temperature sensibilities course upward in the reticular formation, a lesion must involve both areas in order to produce total anesthesia. Dissociated anesthesia occurs when these areas are involved singly. Thus, if the medial lemniscus is interrupted, there will be loss of deep sensibility and retention of pain and temperature sensibilities. Since most of the fibers carrying tactile impulses decussate to reach the contralateral anterior spinothalamic tract, destruction of the spinothalamic tracts is likely to cause hypesthesia as well as analgesia and thermoanesthesia.

At lower levels of the brainstem the two medial lemnisci are near the raphe, but from the middle of the pons upward they move laterally, thus becoming separated from each other.

Course of the pyramidal (corticospinal) fibers

The pyramidal fibers course in the ventral part of the midbrain and medulla oblongata. Within the pons they lie less superficially. Here they are split up into individual bundles by the transverse pontocerebellar fibers. The pyramidal tracts come closer and closer to the midline as they descend.

Course of the corticopontile and corticobulbar fibers

At the level of the basis pedunculi, the pyramidal fibers are segregated in corticospinal, corticopontile, and corticobulbar bundles (Fig. 10-14). As these bundles descend, they give off groups of fibers that take a somewhat oblique downward course, cross the midline, and terminate by synapsing in the motor nucleus of the fifth nerve, the nucleus ambiguus, and the nucleus of the twelfth nerve.

Course of the medial longitudinal fasciculus, spinal tract of the fifth nerve, and spinocerebellar tracts

These fiber systems maintain fairly constant spatial relations. The medial longitudinal fasciculus lies dorsally next to the raphe. The spinal tract of the fifth nerve is situated laterally from the middle third of the pons downward to spinal segment C2. The spinocerebellar tracts are also situated laterally, although only the ventral spinocerebellar tract is to be found above the level of the medulla oblongata.

LOCALIZATION OF BRAINSTEM LESIONS

Destruction of nuclei and interruption of ascending pathways

The caliber of the medulla oblongata is such that small lesions, especially when located dorsally, can give rise to marked disturbances of function, often bilateral in distribution. Thus, a small area of softening involving the twelfth nucleus on both sides will cause paralysis of the entire tongue. Since in the medulla oblongata and lower pons the medial lemnisci lie close to each other, a small lesion in the median plane at these levels may cause ataxia and loss of deep sensibility in all four limbs. Unilateral destruction of the medial lemniscus results in hemiataxia and loss of deep sensibility contralaterally. Moreover, lesions that interrupt the spinothalamic tract of one side give rise to contralateral analgesia and thermoanesthesia and, often, hypesthesia. At the level of the medulla oblongata and lower pons the fibers that convey pain impulses are located medially in the spinothalamic tract and those carrying thermal impulses are located laterally. Lesions involving this tract are thus likely to cause dissociated loss of sensibility in these realms. Moreover, a lesion of the tegmentum at the lower pontile level—for example, a glioma—may interrupt the seventh nerve, causing facial paralysis ipsilaterally and, in addition, interrupt the spinothalamic tract, giving rise to dissociated anesthesia of the body and limbs contralaterally. Interruption of the seventh nerve and of only the middle laminae of the spinothalamic tract will result in facial palsy and in loss of pain and thermal sensibility at a thoracic level—for example, Th4—so that multiple lesions may be suspected when only one exists.

Damage inflicted on the spinocerebellar tracts or the restiform body leads to ipsilateral hemiataxia of the cerebellar type.

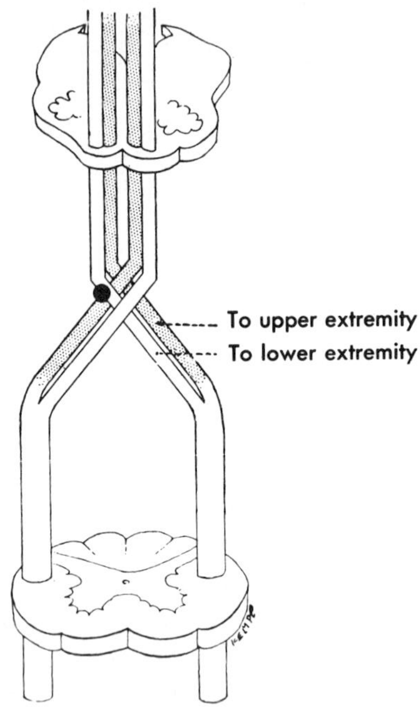

Fig. 11-4. The site of the lesion in the region of the pyramidal decussation (indicated by black spot) responsible for hemiplegia cruciata. The grouping of the pyramidal bundles is after Winkler (1927). The disorder is most often due to occlusion of paramedian branches of the anterior spinal artery.

Interruption at the level of the corticobulbar and corticospinal fibers

The pyramids, situated at the lowermost level of the medulla oblongata, are so close together that a small lesion can interrupt both pyramids and cause quadriplegia. A minute hemorrhage or lesion involving the lateral aspect of the pyramidal decussation, where crossed fibers to the leg and uncrossed fibers to the arm are passing, causes paresis of the ipsilateral leg and the contralateral arm (Fig. 11-4). This condition, known as *hemiplegia cruciata*, is rare. It is usually caused by occlusion of paramedian branches of the anterior spinal artery, and has been noted as a complication of trauma, such as a fall on the back of the head (Brun, 1952; Wallenberg, 1901, 1911).

In the pars basilaris pontis, where the pyramidal fibers are split into numerous individual bundles, a small lesion may remain without objective signs. This is explicable on the basis that relatively few pyramidal fibers have been damaged or that the lesion has affected only the transverse fibers of the pons. A subarachnoid mass compressing the ventral part of the pons may involve only the lower limbs (Crosby, 1953), an observation that has considerable localizing significance.

Lesions restricted to the pyramidal tract

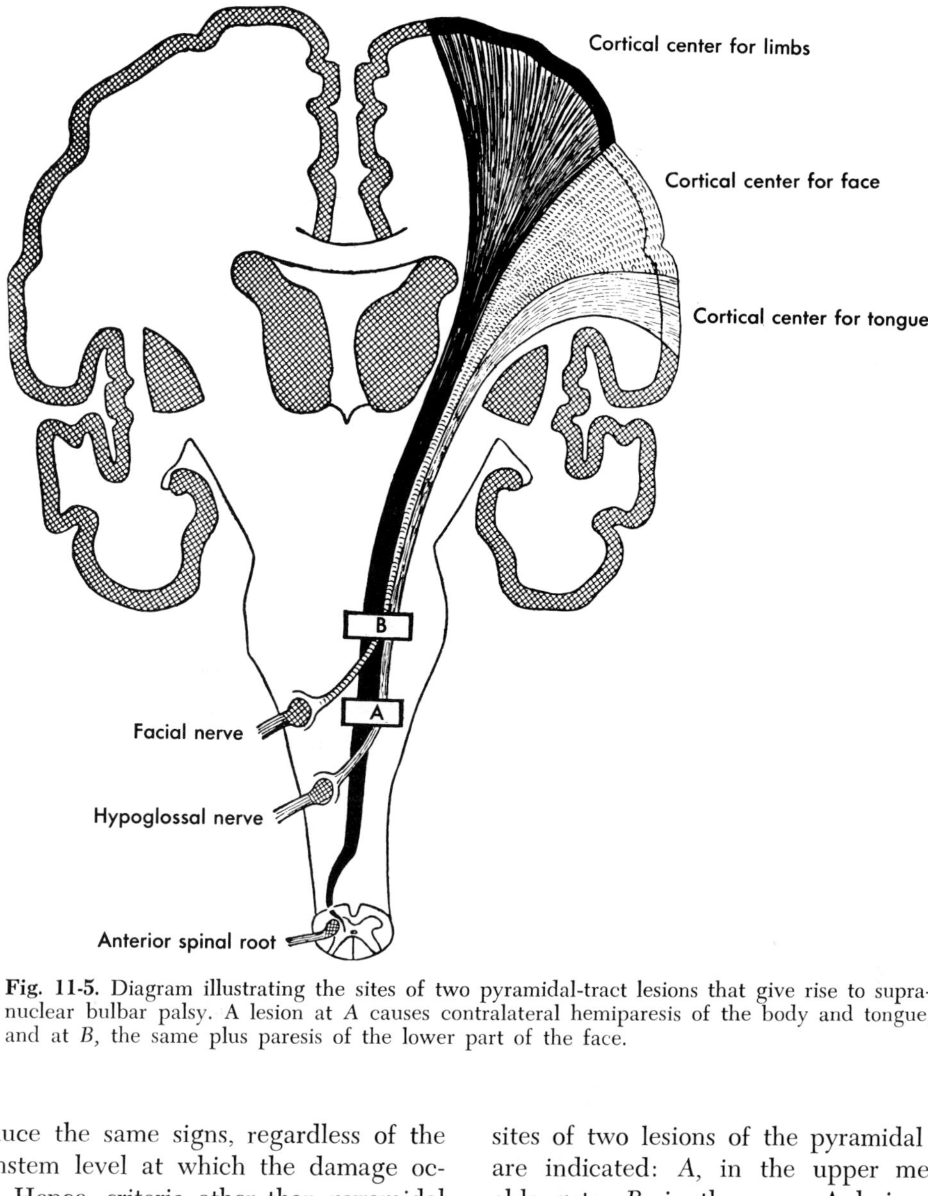

Fig. 11-5. Diagram illustrating the sites of two pyramidal-tract lesions that give rise to supranuclear bulbar palsy. A lesion at *A* causes contralateral hemiparesis of the body and tongue, and at *B*, the same plus paresis of the lower part of the face.

produce the same signs, regardless of the brainstem level at which the damage occurs. Hence, criteria other than pyramidal tract signs are needed if the level of a lesion is to be determined. Such criteria are furnished almost invariably in brainstem lesions by concomitant disturbances in cranial nerve function.

Isolated interruption of the corticospinal tract by a focal lesion is virtually impossible at brainstem levels (except the lowest), because this tract is accompanied by corticobulbar fibers that pass to the motor nuclei of cranial nerves. In Fig. 11-5, in which this relationship is illustrated, the sites of two lesions of the pyramidal tract are indicated: *A*, in the upper medulla oblongata; *B*, in the pons. A lesion at *A* causes paresis of the contralateral half of the tongue and the contralateral limbs and leaves unaltered the function of the facial muscles. With a lesion at *B* the tongue and limbs are affected as stated, and in addition there is paresis of muscles of the contralateral lower half of the face. When these changes are all unilateral and there is no muscular atrophy and no reaction of degeneration (R.D.), the site of the causative lesion must be supranuclear.

As a rule, a lesion interrupting the corticobulbar and corticospinal tracts also involves one or more of the cranial nerve nuclei. The level of such a lesion in the brainstem is indicated by the cranial nerve nuclei affected. The nuclei need not be directly damaged by the lesion, but may, instead, be compromised indirectly through pressure or circulatory disturbance induced by the lesion.

When a motor nucleus of the brainstem is destroyed, the resulting paralysis is of the peripheral type—atrophy and R.D. occur in the paralyzed muscles. Therefore, when the musculature of the face, tongue, or larynx or the muscles of mastication and of deglutition are atrophic and exhibit R.D., a purely supranuclear lesion can be excluded. It is not difficult to narrow down the site of a lesion once muscle atrophy in one region or another is established. A lesion in the tegmentum that causes atrophic paralysis of the face but does not involve the tongue, pharynx, larynx, or masseters must be situated at the level shown in Fig. 11-11 (at the caudal end of the pons—more specifically, in the region of the nucleus of the seventh nerve or along the course of the intramedullary fibers of this nerve).

A further guide, therefore, in determin-

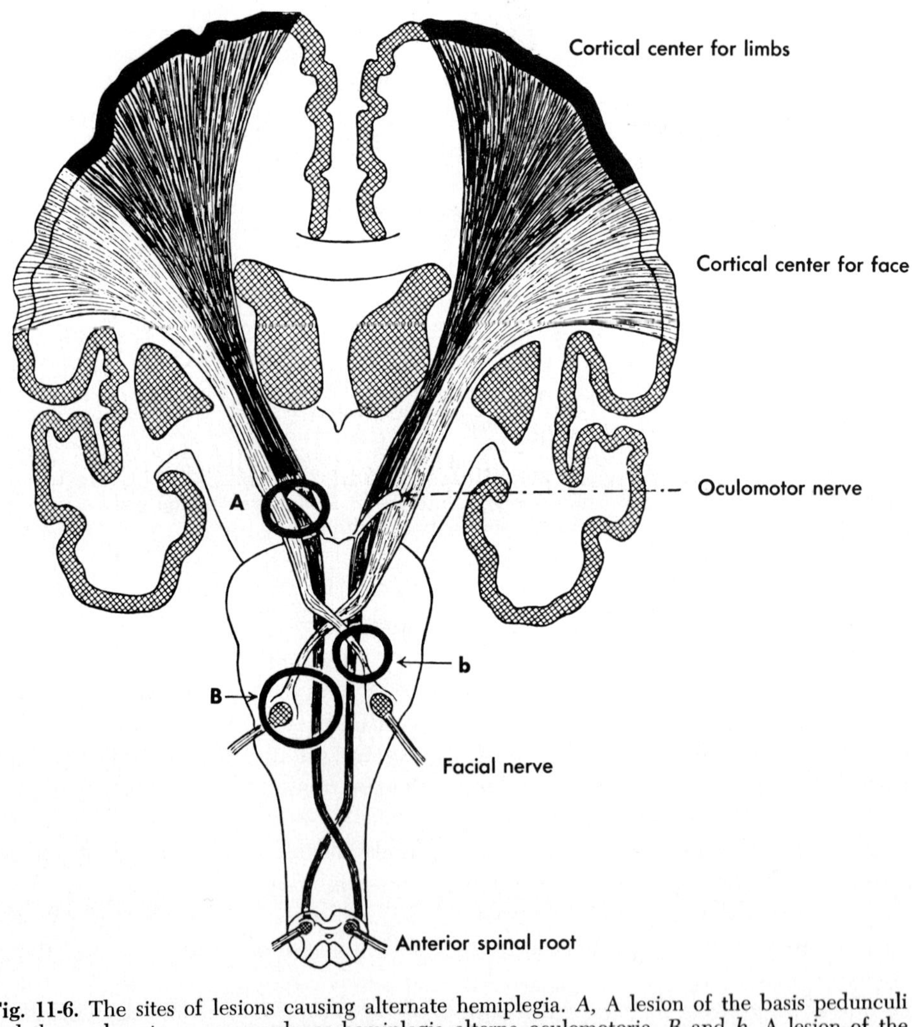

Fig. 11-6. The sites of lesions causing alternate hemiplegia. *A,* A lesion of the basis pedunculi and the oculomotor nerve produces hemiplegia alterna oculomotoria. *B* and *b,* A lesion of the tegmentum pontis produces hemiplegia alterna facialis; when at *B,* the lesion is accompanied by atrophy of the facial muscles, and when at *b,* there is no facial atrophy.

ing the level of a lesion in the brainstem is the site of atrophic muscle paralysis, for it tells which motor nuclei are affected by the lesion.

Atrophic paralysis of muscles supplied by cranial nerves may result from lesions situated not only in the region of the nuclei or their intramedullary fibers, but also in nerves in their course from the brainstem toward the periphery. Here another criterion as to the site of a brainstem lesion comes into consideration: atrophic cranial nerve paralysis combined with signs of interruption of tracts coursing longitudinally in the brainstem.

Hemiplegia alterna

Hemiplegia alterna is a common manifestation of brainstem lesions. On the side of the lesion there are disturbances of cranial nerve function and on the other side a loss of function of one or more of the long pathways (those concerned with motility or sensibility or both), as Fig. 11-6 illustrates.

Various patterns of *hemiplegia alterna* may be distinguished.

A lesion situated in the basis pedunculi at *A* in Fig. 11-6 (see also Fig. 10-15) produces (1) complete hemiplegia of the contralateral side by affecting fibers concerned in movements of the limbs, face, and tongue, and (2) paralysis of extraocular muscles of the ipsilateral side by interrupting the third cranial nerve *(hemiplegia alterna oculomotoria; Weber's syndrome).*

Foci that destroy fibers of the third nerve and the tegmentum through which they course, but that spare the pyramidal tracts, give rise to paralysis of ipsilateral extraocular muscles and to hyperkinesias (such as tremor, chorea, and athetosis) of the contralateral limbs. In some instances there is also contralateral hemiataxia *(Benedikt's syndrome).*

A lesion of the caudal part of the pons in the position indicated by *B* in Fig. 11-6 produces facial paralysis ipsilaterally and paresis of the tongue and limbs contralaterally *(the Millard-Gubler syndrome).* If the lesion involves the nucleus of the sixth nerve, there is also a paralysis of the lateral rectus *(Foville's syndrome)* and of conjugate ocular deviation to the side of the lesion. Both of these syndromes are most frequently observed in hemorrhage or tumor of the tegmentum at the more caudal levels of the pons. They are uncommon in lesions of vascular origin, such as in basilar artery occlusion.

In a lesion situated near the region indicated by *B* in Fig. 11-6, if the seventh nerve is not interrupted but only irritated, ipsilateral facial spasm may occur. A sufficiently extensive lesion, either intrapontile or extrapontile, may cause facial spasm and paralysis of the contralateral limbs *(syndrome of Brissaud-Sicard).*

Paralysis of the tongue on one side together with paresis of the contralateral limbs *(Jackson's syndrome)* is usually caused by a lesion in the pyramid that interrupts the fibers of the adjacent twelfth nerve. This syndrome is rare because a lesion in this location usually involves other structures as well.

Since the cranial nerve nuclei or their respective intramedullary nerve fibers are damaged in these various syndromes, the resultant paralyses are of the atrophic type. In some instances, however, the motor disability in the realm both of the cranial nerves and the limbs is of supranuclear origin. The site of the lesion causing a pattern of supranuclear paralysis is illustrated in Fig. 11-6, *b*. This lesion does not involve the facial nucleus or its respective fibers, but does affect the decussated supranuclear facial tract shortly before its fibers synapse in the nucleus.

The fifth nerve may also be implicated in hemiplegia alterna. This nerve enters the lateral aspect of the middle third of the pons and ends in the principal sensory nucleus at that level and in the nucleus of the spinal tract at lower levels. The efferent trigeminal fibers arise in the motor nucleus, situated just medial to the principal sensory nucleus (Fig. 10-12). Anesthesia or hypesthesia of the corresponding side of the face results from damage of the principal sensory nucleus, reduction in pain and temperature sensibility from involvement of the nucleus of the spinal tract, and disturbances in mastication from involvement of the motor nucleus. Thus the nature of the changes, or the lack of them, in the trigeminal realm will indicate the level of involvement of pyramidal fibers.

Loss of sensibility in parts of the body may be another feature of alternate syndromes. Thus, a lesion that results in hemiplegia may also affect the medial lemniscus, producing disturbances of deep sensibility on the hemiplegic side. Also a lesion may affect the medial lemniscus and the nuclei or intramedullary fibers of cranial nerves and spare the pyramidal tracts.

The following alternate syndromes are occasionally observed:

1. Contralateral hemiataxia with or without signs of ipsilateral cerebellar deficiency, paralysis of gaze (either upward or contralaterally), and variable ipsilateral internal and external ophthalmoplegia (due to involvement of the third nucleus) *(Nothnagel's syndrome).* The responsible lesion is in the more dorsal part of the midbrain, involving tegmentum and brachium conjunctivum as well as the region of the third nucleus; the lesion is either intrinsic or is secondarily induced, for example, through pressure exerted by a cerebellar vermis tumor. A rudimentary form of this syndrome is sometimes met with in occlusion of the superior cerebellar artery.
2. Contralateral anesthesia or hypesthesia with symmetrical or dissociated conjugate ocular paralysis on attempted ipsilateral gaze. Ocular nystagmus can sometimes be elicited. There may also be sensory deficit in the ipsilateral side of the face *(syndrome of Raymond-Cestan).* The responsible lesion involves the medial lemniscus, medial longitudinal fasciculus, and rostral pontile tegmentum.
3. Disturbances in the realm of nerves V through VIII ipsilateral to the lesion in association with sensory disturbances in the limbs of the opposite side, together with paralysis of conjugate ocular movement to the side of the affected cranial nerves *(Gasperini's syndrome).* The lesion is presumed to be in the caudal and more lateral part of the pontile tegmentum.

Another set of disturbances *(syndrome of Babinski-Nageotte)* includes cerebellar hemiataxia with lateropulsion, nystagmus, and Horner's syndrome on the same side as the lesion, and hemiparesis and sensory loss of variable nature on the contralateral side. The syndrome results from rather widespread damage of the transitional area between the medulla oblongata and pons. The damage involves ventromedial as well as dorsolateral structures and thus the syndrome, usually due to inflammatory lesions or tumor, is materially different from the syndrome of occlusion of the posterior inferior cerebellar artery. The main difference is that, in the latter, nausea, vomiting, and difficulty in swallowing and phonation occur, and, further, that crossed hemiparesis is very infrequent.

Making up another syndrome *(Vernet's syndrome)* is paralysis of the soft palate and the muscles of deglutition, paralysis of the sternocleidomastoid muscle, hemiageusia involving the posterior third of the tongue and hemianesthesia of the soft palate and upper part of the pharynx, all on the side of the lesion, and hemiplegia or hemiparesis on the opposite side. The causative lesion is situated in the medulla oblongata.

Thus one of the chief criteria in the

Table 11-1. Signs resulting from lesions illustrated in Figs. 11-7 to 11-12

		Left	*Right*
Fig. 11-7	Head	----------------	----------------
	Trunk and limbs	Spastic paralysis of all four limbs with intact sensibility	
Fig. 11-8	Head	Paralysis and atrophy of the tongue	----------------
	Trunk and limbs	----------------	Hemiplegia and reduction of deep sensibility
Fig 11-9	Head	Anesthesia, analgesia, and thermoanesthesia of face	----------------
	Trunk and limbs	Hemiataxia and hemiasynergia of cerebellar type	----------------
Fig. 11-10	Head	Bilateral paralysis and atrophy of the tongue	
	Trunk and limbs	Bilateral ataxia and loss of deep sensibility	
Fig. 11-11	Head	----------------	Paralysis of the face and lateral rectus, and of conjugate lateral ocular deviation to right
	Trunk and limbs	Reduction of superficial sensibility	----------------
Fig. 11-12	Head	----------------	Anesthesia of trigeminal distribution, paralysis of lateral ocular deviation to right, paralysis of face, probable hypacusis
	Trunk and limbs	Reduction of superficial sensibility	----------------

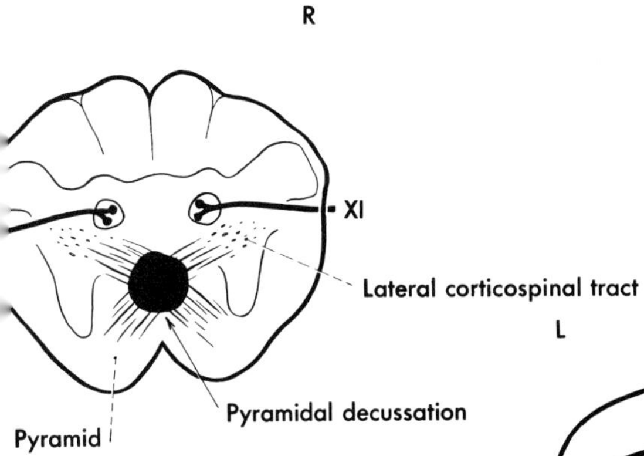

Fig. 11-7

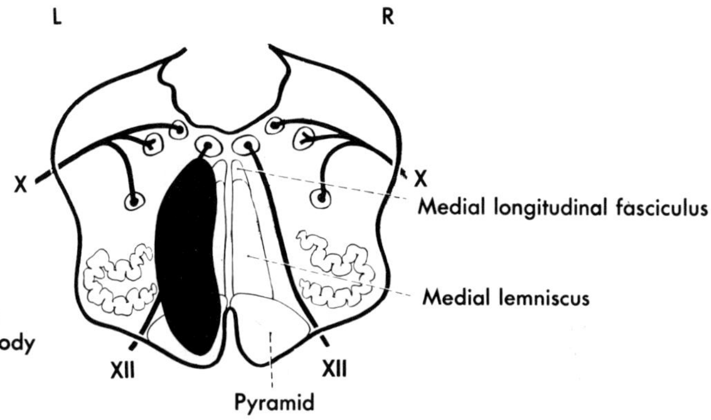

Fig. 11-8

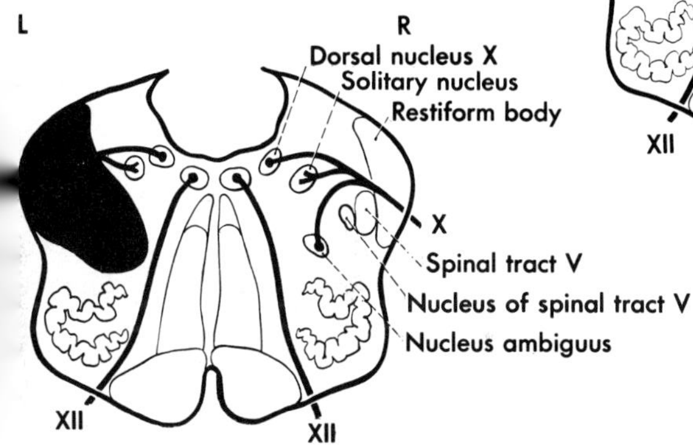

Fig. 11-9

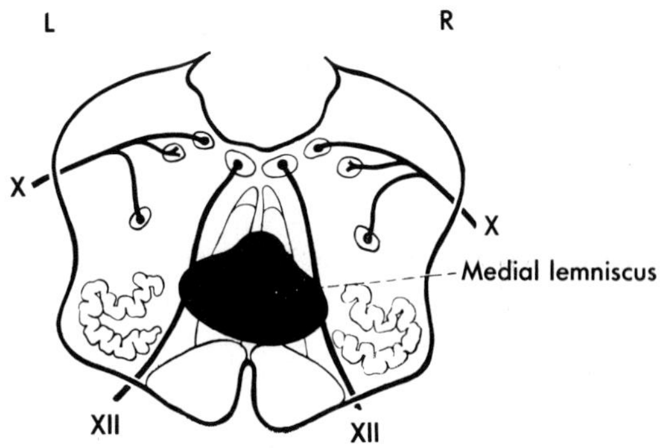

Fig. 11-10

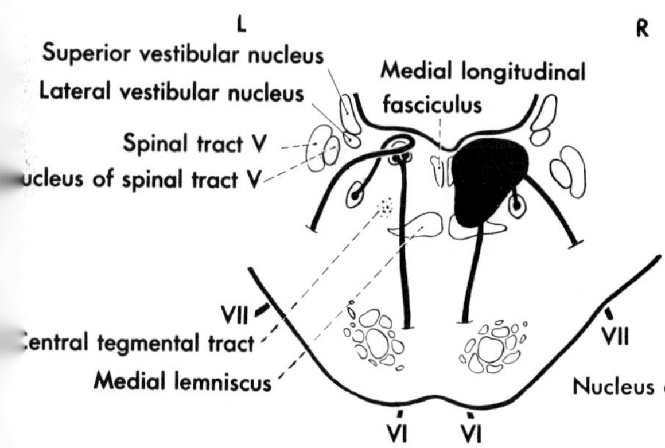

Fig. 11-11

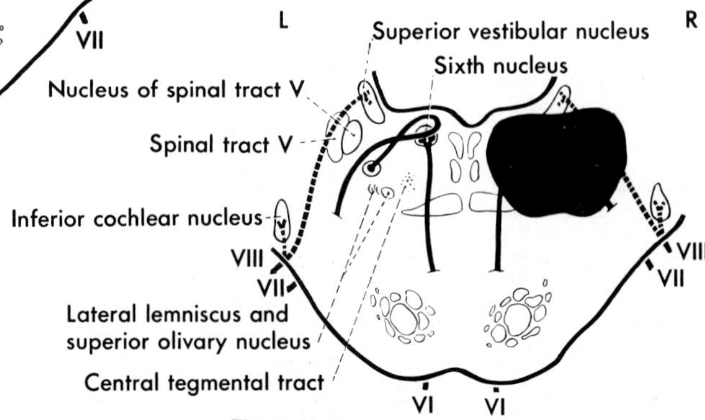

Fig. 11-12

Figs. 11-7 through **11-12.** Sites of lesions in the medulla oblongata and pons giving rise to various clinical syndromes (see text).

localization of the brainstem lesions is the "alternate" character of involvement. There can be no doubt as to the side, level, extent, or position (dorsal or ventral) of the lesion, when consideration is given the cranial nerves and the long tracts affected, whether the pyramidal tract or the medial lemniscus or both.

Interruption at the level of the midbrain

The clinical features of lesions involving the midbrain are numerous because of the many structures of differing function that lie within it, such as the nuclei of the third and fourth nerves, the medial and lateral lemnisci, fibers subserving pupillary reflexes, and the tegmentum together with the red nucleus it encloses. Since disorders involving these structures are described elsewhere in the text, only a few points will be mentioned here. An early manifestation of pressure on the tectum, for example by a pineal or a superior vermis tumor, is vertical nystagmus, usually in the upward direction. After continued pressure in this region there may be paralysis of conjugate vertical deviation of the eyes (a feature of *Parinaud's syndrome*). Moreover, under such conditions the paralysis of conjugate vertical gaze may be associated with weakness in ocular convergence. All these disturbances are probably caused by a lesion in the pretectal region, not in the tectum. Although the *colliculi* are sites of interaction of impulses concerned in vision, ocular movements, vestibular function, and so on, they appear to have little if any significance so far as *clinical* disturbances are concerned (Pasik, Pasik, and Bender, 1966).

In rostral midbrain lesions *attacks of tonic extensor spasm* are occasionally noted. In such attacks the entire bodily musculature suddenly becomes tonically rigid; the trunk is arched backward (opisthotonos) and the lower limbs are rigidly adducted and the hands pronated. Since the cerebellum seems to determine the posture assumed in decerebrate rigidity,

Table 11-2. Signs resulting from lesions illustrated in Figs. 11-13 to 11-18

		Left	*Right*
Fig. 11-13	Head	Trigeminal anesthesia and weakness and atrophy of the masticatory muscles	Weakness but no atrophy of face and tongue
	Trunk and limbs	----------------	Spastic hemiplegia
Fig. 11-14	Head	----------------	Trigeminal anesthesia and weakness and atrophy of the masticatory muscles
	Trunk and limbs	Hypacusis	----------------
Fig. 11-15	Head	Weakness but no atrophy of face and tongue	----------------
	Trunk and limbs	Spastic hemiplegia, reduction in deep sensibility	----------------
Fig. 11-16	Head	Trigeminal hypesthesia or anesthesia	Oculomotor nerve palsy
	Trunk and limbs	Hemianesthesia, choreoathetotic movements	----------------
Fig. 11-17	Head	Bilateral ophthalmoplegia	
	Trunk and limbs	----------------	----------------
Fig. 11-18	Head	Oculomotor nerve palsy	----------------
	Trunk and limbs	Weakness but no atrophy of face and tongue	Spastic hemiplegia

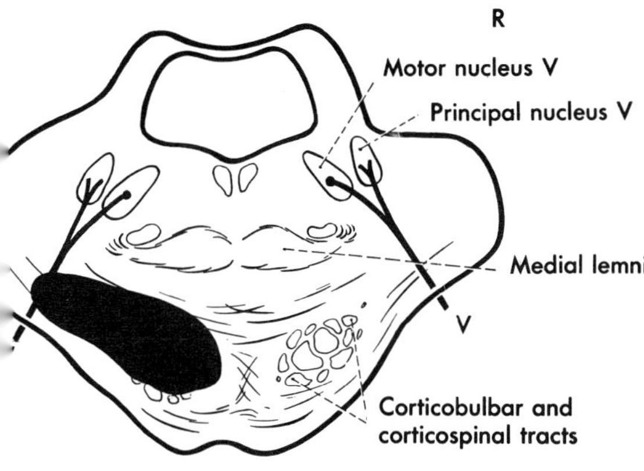

Fig. 11-13

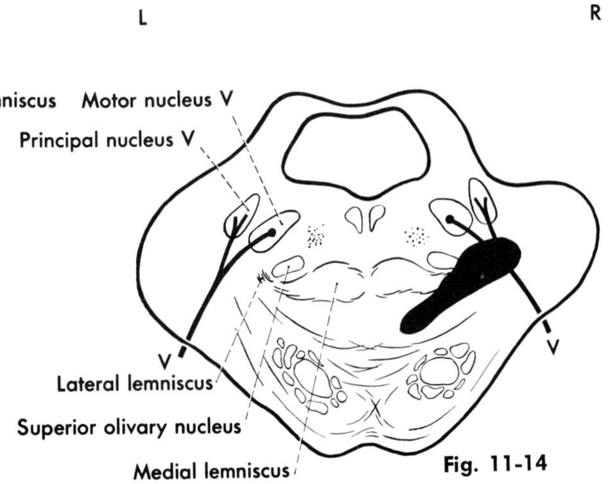

Fig. 11-14

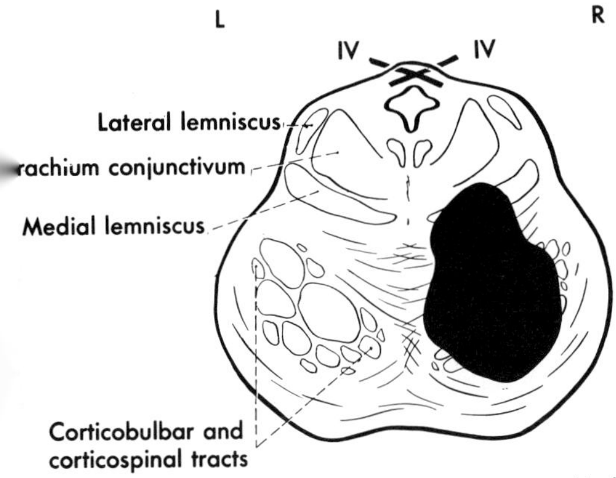

Fig. 11-15

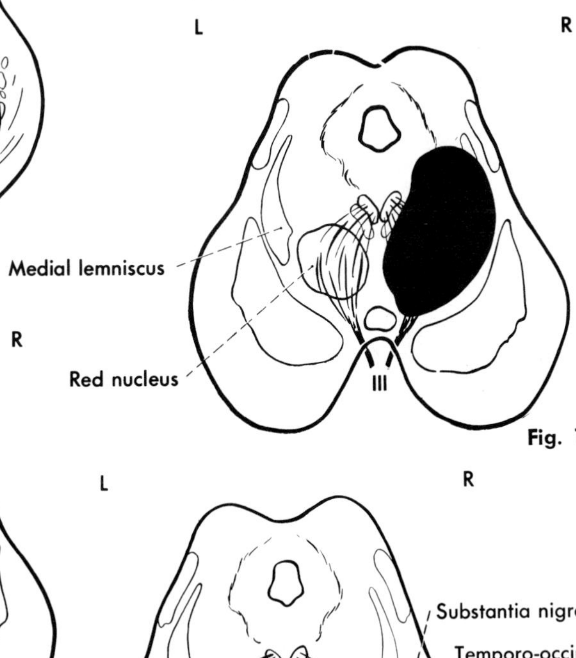

Fig. 11-16

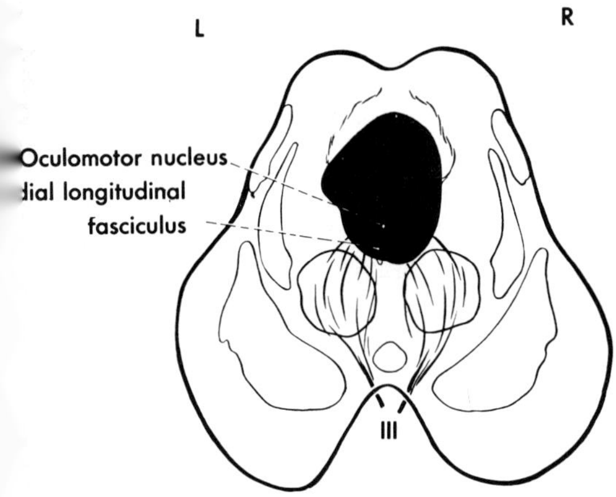

Fig. 11-17

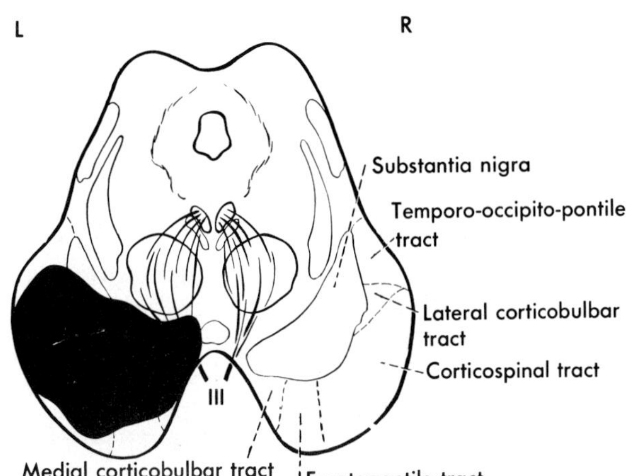

Fig. 11-18

Figs. 11-13 through 11-18. Sites of lesions in the pons and midbrain giving rise to various syndromes (see text).

the paroxysms have been referred to as *cerebellar fits*.

Progressive, partial extraocular muscle palsy without involvement of the intrinsic ocular muscles usually signifies damage of the third nucleus (Mauthner's rule). However, there are exceptions, for in damage of the third nerve itself the intrinsic ocular muscles may be spared (François and Neetens, 1968).

Occasionally in lesions at various levels of the brainstem, attacks of spasm are much more circumscribed. They may be limited, for instance, to the musculature of the neck (van Bogaert and Martin, 1928), or tumors situated in the immediate vicinity of the foramen magnum may give rise to spasms of the neck muscles, later complicated by contracture. Tumors within or near the fourth ventricle may also induce certain abnormal attitudes of the head (most often protracted flexion) and there may be vestibulocerebellar and cranial nerve disturbances, a Babinski reflex, and other signs of pyramidal tract involvement.

Interruption at the level of the pontile tegmentum

Functions mediated by the medial longitudinal fasciculus are likely to be affected. An irritative lesion (such as that brought about by hemorrhage) that involves the tegmentum of one side may cause conjugate lateral ocular deviation to the opposite side; a destructive lesion leads to paralysis of conjugate lateral gaze toward the side of the lesion, or, owing to the paralysis, a turning of the eyes away from the side of the lesion.

Involvement of *tegmental motor nuclei* is manifested by atrophic paralysis of the muscles supplied. If the lesion extends into the region of the medial lemniscus, sensory disturbances in the trunk and limbs will develop. Should the lesion spread ventrally, encroaching on the pyramids, there will also be paresis of the muscles at levels distal to the site of the lesion. The clinical features of lesions in these locations and elsewhere in the brainstem are indicated in Figs. 11-7 to 11-18 (see also corresponding Tables 11-1 and 11-2).

Disturbances in space perception (Pick's visions) are occasionally noted in lesions of the *tegmentum of the pons* situated near the floor of the fourth ventricle. A patient thus affected may see people in his room step through the wall into an adjacent room and still be visible as they walk about. The walls seem bent or otherwise distorted or they may seem to be collapsing. Such visual illusions (unaccompanied by diplopia or nystagmus) may result from a lesion in the general region of the medial longitudinal fasciculus that interferes with the blending of ophthalmostatic and vestibular impulses. A similar disturbance may occur in infarction of the lateral (retro-olivary) part of the medulla oblongata due to occlusion of the posterior inferior cerebellar artery: in such a case the patient stated that one wall of his room (the wall contralateral to the side of the infarction) became the floor; people appeared to enter the room through a door in the floor (Bjerver and Silfverskiöld, 1968). Likewise, visual illusions (faulty space perception) may be noted in lesions of the *midbrain*. Such have been produced by a lesion made in the upper midbrain for the relief of pain (Nashold and Gills, 1967). Disturbances of this kind are much more commonly observed in lesions of the temporo-occipital region than in the brainstem, as described in Chapter 21.

Interruption at the level of the nuclei and tracts of the fifth nerve

Because of the length of the nucleus and spinal tract of the fifth nerve, the exact level at which it is involved may be difficult to determine unless motor cranial nerves—usually the seventh or the twelfth—are also damaged. In lesions involving the principal sensory fifth nucleus, tactile sensibility of the entire contralateral side of face and the mucous membranes of the oral region may be lost; in lesions of the spinal nucleus or tract, the sensory loss (analgesia and thermoanesthesia) is not as extensive unless the lesion is at the zone of entry of the fifth nerve. Paralysis of the masticatory muscles points clearly to a lesion in the tegmentum pontis, in which the motor fifth nucleus is located.

Cranial nerve disturbances from basal lesions

The recognition of the *sequence* in which functions are lost helps greatly in the localization of lesions. This is especially true for aneurysms compressing the brainstem and for tumors invading the brainstem from without. *Compression* of the brainstem by basilar artery aneurysm may be manifested in early stages by pyramidal tract disturbances, which are bilateral and more or less symmetrical, and subsequently by evidence of damage of the tegmentum and cranial nerve nuclei. Since the sixth nerves gain exit from the brainstem near the midline, they may be the structures initially damaged by an aneurysm. In tumors at the base of the brainstem that originate from an emerging nerve or from the meninges, the neurological disturbances are often unilateral in distribution.

In basal lesions other than those due to compression, manifestations of pyramidal tract involvement, such as spasticity and the Babinski sign, are late in their appearance; the spasticity is slight at first, then increases progressively in severity. Only in the region of the basis pedunculi do noncompressive lesions involving the base of the brainstem have a tendency to interrupt pyramidal (corticospinal and corticobulbar) fibers in early stages of lesion development. The fibers in the basis pedunculi are somatotopically organized (representation of face, arm, and leg ventrodorsally, in that order, with a large representation for the arm; Martinez, Bertrand, and Botana-Lopez, 1967), and thus the resultant paresis may be unequal in intensity in the contralateral limbs. Moreover, lesions in this region have a tendency to affect both the basis pedunculi and the oculomotor nerve, giving rise to contralateral hemiplegia and ipsilateral oculomotor palsy *(Weber's syndrome).*

Various lesions situated at the base of the brainstem (neoplasm, tuberculoma, gumma, circumscribed meningitis) frequently affect the third, sixth, and seventh nerves. In regard to the third nerve, the fibers that innervate the levator palpebrae are often the most vulnerable, as mani-

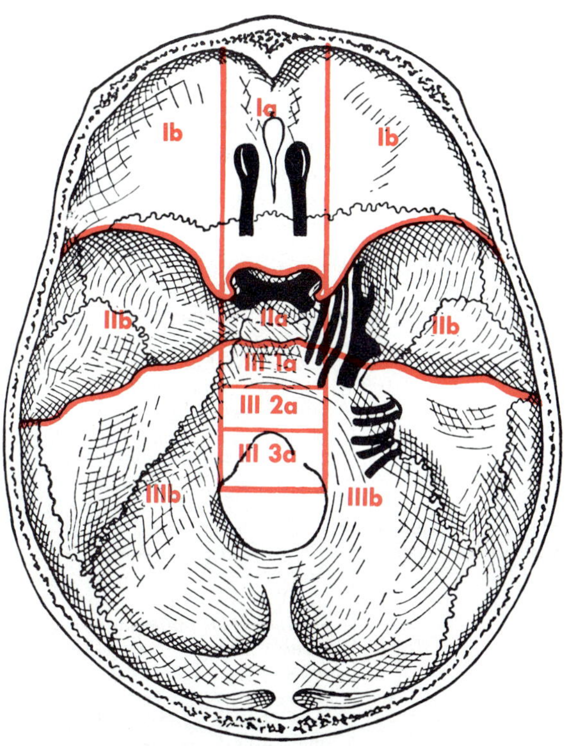

Fig. 11-19. Topographic subdivisions of the base of the skull. The three cranial fossae (I, anterior; II, middle; III, posterior) and their subdivisions; see Table 11-3 (p. 160) for localization of lesions in each fossa.

fested by the early appearance of ptosis. By contrast, in intramedullary lesions, these fibers appear less vulnerable. The reason for the difference is not evident.

Signs of *nerve irritation* are a common manifestation of basal lesions. Dysesthesias and neuralgiform pains of the face are characteristic of lesions compressing the root of the fifth nerve. Irritation of the motor trigeminal nucleus is manifested by *trismus,* a condition characterized by tonic spasm of the masseter muscle causing gnashing of the teeth. Irritation of the seventh nerve results in twitching of the facial musculature. Sensory irritative phenomena related to the eighth nerve, such as tinnitus, also occur. Although signs of irritation of cranial nerves (III through XII) are characteristic of basal lesions, they may also occur, in rare instances, in

Table 11-3. Manifestations of lesions of the base of the brain

	Lesions medially situated		*Lesions laterally situated*	
Cranial fossa	*Signs of irritation or destruction of cranial nerves*	*Other signs, and certain typical syndromes*	*Signs of irritation or destruction of certain cranial nerves*	*Other signs, including certain typical syndromes*
I. *Anterior*	*Olfactory nerve:* hemianosmia	Parosmia (piriform cortex)		Euphoria, etc. *(frontal lobe)*
II. *Middle*	*Optic nerve:* amaurosis or scotoma; *chiasm:* heteronymous binasal or bitemporal hemianopia; *optic tract:* homonymous lateral hemianopia with hemianopic pupillary rigidity	Adiposogenital dystrophy *(tuber cinereum);* diabetes insipidus *(supraoptico-hypophysial system;* hemiplegia, quadriplegia *(cerebral peduncle)*	*Oculomotor* *Trochlear* *Trigeminal* *Abducens*	
III. *Posterior*			*Facial, Acoustic, Glossopharyngeal* *Vagus* *Spinal accessory*	Ataxia Hypotonia Asynergia Adiadochokinesis etc. *(Cerebellum)*
1. Peduncular portion	*Oculomotor*	Weber's syndrome, Benedikt's syndrome *(oculomotor + cerebral peduncle)*		
2. Pontile portion	*Trigeminal, abducens, facial, acoustic*	Hemiplegia, quadriplegia *(pyramidal tracts);* Millard-Gubler's syndrome, Brissaud's syndrome *(pyramidal tracts + facial);* Foville's syndrome *(pyramidal tracts + facial + abducens)*		
3. Bulbar portion	*Facial, acoustic, glossopharyngeal, vagus, spinal accessory, hypoglossal*	Hemiplegia, quadriplegia *(pyramidal tracts);* syndrome of Avellis, Schmidt's syndrome *(glossopharyngeal + vagus + hypoglossal* [later] + spinal accessory [later]; Jackson's syndrome *(pyramidal tracts + hypoglossal);* hemianesthesia *(medial lemniscus)*		

lesions situated solely within the brainstem. Sudden hemorrhage in any one of several regions of the brainstem is the chief cause.

The *clinical features of basal lesions* are listed in Table 11-3. In making use of this table it is advisable to consult Fig. 11-19. Attention is also directed to the focal lesions illustrated in Figs. 11-16, 11-17, and 11-18, and to their clinical manifestations, listed in Tables 5-1 and 11-1. A study of these illustrations and tables will serve for recapitulation of the subjects discussed.

MYOCLONUS

Myoclonus occurs in a large and heterogenous group of disorders of the central nervous system, heredofamilial and otherwise. It is a sign, and occasionally a symptom, not a disease entity. In its simplest form, in which an isolated muscle or a part of a muscle is involved, myoclonus consists in a muscle twitch followed by relaxation. This characteristic distinguishes it from tremor, which is marked by alternate contractions of antagonistic muscles. When more widespread, myoclonus is characterized by persistent, repetitive, shock-like contractions of groups of muscles that are not synergically associated or mutually antagonistic. The contractions in myoclonus may be rhythmic or arrhythmic. They may be symmetrically synchronous at several sites or be asymmetrical and nonsynchronous. In larger muscles the contractions may leap and skip about like summer lightning. The rate at which the contractions occur varies: in palatal myoclonus the twitches ordinarily occur at the rate of 120 to 140 per minute, but they range from 30 to 300 per minute (Nehlil and others, 1966). Contraction of sufficient scope in a limb may cause movement of the limb. Despite all this, voluntary activity is not significantly interfered with. In myoclonus occurring at some sites (such as the soft palate) the contractions persist during sleep; at other sites, not. (Aigner and Mulder, 1960; Herrmann and Brown, 1967.)

As indicated, myoclonus may be an isolated phenomenon. For instance, myoclonus limited to the facial muscles has been known to complicate "geniculate" herpes zoster. The most familiar example of myoclonus is *hiccup* (singultus). It is characterized by sudden inspiration (due to clonic spasm of the diaphragm) that is abruptly terminated by an audible closure of the glottis. The phrenic nucleus and nerve are conceded to mediate the disorder. However, more is involved, for hiccup may persist after bilateral phrenicectomy. The vagus nerve (to the larynx and bronchi) and upper spinal nerves (to the intercostal muscles) share in the efferent limb of the arc. Involved also are the respiratory center, intercalated reticulospinal fibers, and the fasciculus gracilis and fasciculus cuneatus (Souadjian and Cain, 1968).

In a study of the etiology of persistent hiccup (lasting more than 48 hours) in 220 patients, Souadjian and Cain (1968) noted a sharp difference as to sex; the disorder was diagnosed as "psychogenic" in 92 percent of the women and in 7 percent of the men. Twenty-six percent of the men had diaphragmatic hernia, usually accompanied by some other disease, and in the others a wide range of organic disorders, including disturbances of the gastrointestinal tract, cerebrovascular insufficiency, or a metabolic disorder. The implication is that any one of numerous factors may "set off" hiccup. The disorder is commonly seen in uremia. In occasional instances, hiccup heralds intracranial tumor. Hiccup has been noted in tumor adjacent to or extending into the fourth ventricle (Baudouin, Bertrand, and Lereboullet, 1930; Brody and German, 1933). Lesions of the cervical cord, including tumor, can also bring it on. Intractable hiccup has also been attributed to sulphonamides when given to susceptible persons. Further, hiccup may occur in sustained form in encephalitis lethargica *(singultus epidemicus)*. Hiccup may also occur as a consequence of irritation of the phrenic nerve in its peripheral part by conditions such as aortic aneurysm, mediastinitis, pericarditis, or pleurisy. (Bing and Haymaker, 1939.)

In some instances myoclonus begins in one region—for example, the soft palate—then spreads, for example to the extraocular, cervical, intercostal, and diaphragmatic muscles. Or, as in lethargic encephalitis, myoclonus may commence in abdominal muscles, then spread. In *palatal myoclonus* the patient may first complain of a clicking or cracking in the ear, due to involvement of the musculature surrounding the eustachian tube, a noise produced by the tube snapping shut as the musculature relaxes. The myoclonus persists indefinitely. It may decrease or even cease during phonation or swallowing, but only temporarily. The disorder may appear shortly after development of an upper respiratory infection or following infarction in the brainstem; it may also occur in multiple sclerosis, in association with heredofamilial tremor, and so on (Hughes, 1965). Occasionally developing in association with palatal myoclonus is *ocular bobbing*, consisting in up-and-down movements of the eyes occurring synchronously with the palatal myoclonus (Yap, Mayo, and Barron, 1968).

Myorhythmia may be subdivided into three general classes, based on its common dissociation of frequency and differing response to voluntary innervation and to drugs: oculofaciocervical, velopharyngolaryngeal (or branchial), and skeletal. In the oculofacialcervical form, the abnormal ocular movements that occur may be any of numerous kinds (Mouren and others, 1962).

Circuits have been proposed as mechanisms for the mediation of the various forms of myoclonus. It has been suggested that myoclonus may result from interruption of any one fiber system in an olivocerebellorubrotegmento-(olivary) equipotential reverberating circuit (in any side of the *Guillain-Mollaret triangle*), and that dentatoreticular fibers can be part of this circuit. However, neither rubroolivary nor dentatoreticular connections have been established (Fig. 17-1). It appears that some disturbance of reticular modulation, however produced, not olivary discharge, may precipitate the myoclonus. In widespread myoclonus (velopharyngolaryngeal plus the extraocular muscles and the diaphragm), either the reticulo-olivary or the olivocerebellar pathway has been found interrupted. (Guillain and others, 1933a,b.) In some cases of myoclonus only the dentate nucleus has been degenerated (Hodskins and Yakovlev, 1930).

Degeneration of the central tegmental tract brought about by intrinsic lesions of the midbrain or upper pons is observed in a fair proportion of cases of myoclonus. A more common cause is infarction of the midbrain tegmentum resulting from occlusion of the superior cerebellar artery or related artery (Herrmann and Brown, 1967). Other responsible conditions (involving various levels of the brainstem) include neoplasms, multiple sclerosis, Schilder's disease, small pox, syringomyelia, lethargic encephalitis, subacute inclusion encephalitis, aneurysm of the vertebral artery, and a host of other disorders (Aigner and Mulder, 1960).

The extraordinarily pronounced gliosis that occurs in the inferior olivary nucleus (*pseudohypertrophy*) in association with nerve cell fallout has been regarded as resulting chiefly from circulatory disturbances in the nucleus rather than to degeneration of the central tegmental tract *per se* (Biemond, 1951). Pseudohypertrophy, though observed in myoclonus (such as in palatal myoclonus), can occur in the absence of myoclonus (Gautier and Blackwood, 1961; Girard and others, 1962).

Because of the wide extent of most of the causative lesions, the myoclonic movements are often associated with spastic paresis, dissociated cutaneous anesthesia, paralysis of conjugate ocular movement, and signs of cerebellar deficiency (van Bogaert and Bertrand, 1928; Sittig and Haskovec, 1939). Occasionally, amyotrophic lateral sclerosis complicates arrhythmic myoclonus involving pharynx, larynx, and abdomen (Nehlil and others, 1966).

Myoclonus, it should be mentioned, its most commonly encountered in association with generalized epileptic seizures—in 10 to 15 percent of cases according to Hodskins and Yakovlev (1930), with familial incidence frequent. Myoclonus may also occur between convulsive seizures. Moreover, jacksonian epilepsy is a form of intermittent myoclonic spasm.

The forms of myoclonus just described are distinguishable from *paramyoclonus multiplex*.

This disorder was so named because many muscles were simultaneously affected and because entire muscles underwent rhythmic contractions. In the case Friedreich (1881) described (in an adult), the myoclonus occurred spontaneously and doubtless belongs in a category described in previous paragraphs. However, other authors have described under the term *paramyoclonus multiplex* a relatively benign disorder occurring in families. Mahloudji and Pikielny (1967) proposed that this term be dropped and be supplanted by *hereditary essential myoclonus,* for a disorder characterized by (1) onset of the myoclonus in the first or second decade of life, with face, trunk, and proximal muscles of the limbs chiefly affected, either unilaterally or generalized, (2) equal sex incidence, (3) benign course compatible with an active life, (4) dominant mode of inheritance with variable severity, (5) absence of seizures, dementia, gross ataxia, and other neurological deficits, and (6) normal EEG.

Also to be distinguished is the *progressive myoclonus epilepsy of Unverricht and Lundborg.* This term embraces a heterogeneous group of genetic disorders of a progressive nature appearing in families and characterized by "diffuse intracellular neuronal disease." Onset is in early years—at ages from 6 to 15 years in the family reported by Unverricht (1891). The myoclonus, consisting in lightning-like twitches of muscle fibers or muscle bundles, occurs in the trunk, face, and limbs, and less commonly elsewhere. Generalized seizures set in when the myoclonus becomes severe, though in some cases seizures occur initially. Coordination, sensibility, and motility remained unaffected in Unverricht's cases. In other instances, motor disturbances in the form of pseudobulbar palsy and rigidity occur, ataxia is frequent, and quadriplegia-in-flexion may mark the late stage. Intellectual functions remained normal in Unverricht's series, while in Lundborg's series (1903) intellectual changes occurred from the outset and progressed to dementia. (Aigner and Mulder, 1960; Harriman and Millar, 1955; Watson and Denny-Brown, 1953.) In two familial cases (consanguinous) described by de Barsy and colleagues (1969) as instances of the degenerative type of progressive myoclonic epilepsy of Unverricht-Lundborg in which mental disturbances were absent, a myoclonic syndrome developed first and dominated the clinical picture, then epilepsy appeared. Postmortem study in one case revealed discrete involvement of the dentate nucleus with no alteration in the central tegmental tract. The gracile nuclei were also degenerated, the spinocerebellar and spinothalamic tracts slightly.

To be distinguished from the myoclonus epilepsy of Unverricht-Lundborg are *dyssynergia cerebellaris progressiva* of Hunt (1914) and *dyssynergia cerebellaris myoclonica* of Hunt (1921). The former was so named because of the coexistence of frank cerebellar signs, mainly chronic progressive intention tremor. Degeneration of the dentatofugal system was the main—and essential—finding. As emphasized by de Barsy and co-workers (1969), the dyssynergia cerebellaris myoclonica described by Hunt (1921) represented a heterogenous group made up of (1) some cases of myoclonic epilepsy with symptoms of dyssynergia cerebellaris progressiva, and (2) others having a combination of heredoataxia of Friedreich, dyssynergia cerebellaris progressiva, myoclonus, and epileptic attacks. Primary atrophy of the dentatofugal system was regarded by Hunt (1921) as responsible for both the cerebellar disturbances and the myoclonus. In two heredofamilial cases described by de Barsy and colleagues (1969), a cerebellar syndrome (hypotonia, assynergia, ataxia, intention tremor) ushered in the disorder and dominated the clinical picture, followed by arrhythmic myoclonus, then epilepsy. No mental disturbances occurred. Multisystem atrophies were encountered postmortem: dentatofugal, pallidoluysian, reticulospinal, and posterior spinal column. In essential points the sites affected were much the same as described by Hunt (1921).

Intracellular inclusions have been a feature of other disorders marked by myoclonus. Major seizures ushered in the progressive myoclonic epilepsy in a patient (a boy of 17) described by Lafora and Glück (1911). Dementia developed rapidly thereafter. Also noted were unsteady gait, ataxic speech, nystagmus, impaired vision (with papilledema), and signs of pyramidal tract disease. Death occurred in status epilepticus 2 years after onset. *Lafora bodies* (homogeneous or laminated structures, some with polycyclic outline, of "polysaccharide" nature) were found in the cytoplasm of nerve cells in much of the cerebral cortex. In subsequent cases in which the disease also became manifest in younger persons (usually in their teens), in whom the disease was apparently transmitted through an autosomal recessive mechanism, Lafora bodies were found in nerve cells, glial cells, and extracellularly in tissue in a wide variety of structures including the substantia nigra, certain basal ganglia, dentate nucleus, brainstem nuclei, retina, and axons of spinal nerves. The Lafora bodies stained like amyloid, and lipid inclusions resembling those observed in some of the lipidoses were found. (Allegranza, Canavini, and Strada, 1966; Harriman and Millar, 1955; Toga, Dubois, and Hassoun, 1968.) For the Lafora type of the disease, a genetically-determined enzyme error appears at fault (Yokoi and others, 1968). Further, in what was called *Unverricht-Lafora's disease,* no Lafora bodies were found in biopsy material from the cerebral cortex. However, there were intranuclear inclusions in nerve cells and astrocytes (and, rarely, in oligodendrocytes), and the cytoplasm of astrocytes contained huge balloon-like sacs filled with smaller saccules that were in association with dense, irregularly shaped lipid bodies. Lipid bodies were also found in perithelial cells. Other changes in all these cells were also noted. (Brown, Kotorii, and Riehl, 1968.)

In summary, myoclonus occurs under a variety of conditions and in association with lesions at various levels of the neuraxis. It may represent an isolated phenomenon (for example, in the form of hiccup); it may be the only manifestation of a nonprogressive disorder occurring in some families (essential myoclonus), or it may be one of a constellation of disturbances developing in certain progressive degenerative diseases. Progressive myoclonic epilepsy (Unverricht-Lundborg), dyssynergia cerebellaris progressiva (Hunt), and dyssynergia cerebellaris myoclonic (Hunt) are separable on nosological grounds. Mental disturbances mark the cases in which cellular inclusions develop. Success at localization of the responsible lesion in cases in which myoclonus occurs thus requires careful consideration from all standpoints.

BULBAR PARALYTIC DISTURBANCES

Bulbar poliomyelitis

This disorder frequently affects the nucleus ambiguus (resulting in dysphagia), less frequently the nuclei concerned in speech, and least, the twelfth nucleus (paresis of the tongue); the brainstem nucleus most commonly affected is the seventh.

Syringobulbia

The syrinx may be continuous upward into the brainstem from the cervical cord, or it may be situated solely in the brainstem. In either event, it usually consists of one or more narrow slits situated unilaterally in the more dorsal or (occasionally) the more ventral part of the medulla oblongata and commonly the pons as well, where it occupies the tegmentum. Occasionally the syrinx communicates with the fourth ventricle. Clinical syndromes encountered are diverse. When syringobulbia commences insidiously, phonation frequently suffers initially, signifying involvement of laryngeal muscles, which are innervated from the nucleus ambiguus. Deglutition, which is also dependent on the integrity of the nucleus ambiguus, may also be compromised early in the disorder. The tongue may become paralyzed and atrophic, particularly unilaterally. Nystagmus and ataxia are common. There also may be analgesia and thermoanesthesia of the ipsilateral side of the face and of the contralateral limbs. Horner's syndrome may develop; when present, miosis is conspicuous and constant, and ptosis and facial anhidrosis uncommon. Taste may suffer, persistent hiccup may occur, and there may be bouts of trigeminal neuralgia: all are, however, rare. In a minority of cases the onset is acute or apoplectiform, being characterized by headache, nausea, vomiting, vertigo, and even loss of consciousness. (Grossman, 1942; Sahu and Satapathy, 1962; Willis and Weaver, 1968.)

Bulbar form of amyotrophic lateral sclerosis

In later stages of the disease, amyotrophic lateral sclerosis may involve the bulb, or it may begin there. When the disorder is of the atrophic-paralytic type (in contrast to the spastic-paralytic type, next to be described) the outstanding disturbance is atrophy of muscles supplied by cranial nerves IX through XII, giving rise to labioglossolaryngeal paralysis. In general, the disturbances in phonation, articulation, mastication, and deglutition are much the same as observed in pseudobulbar palsy.

PSEUDOBULBAR PALSY

Pseudobulbar palsy—"pseudo" referring to the minor degree of bulbar muscle atrophy as contrasted with the severe atrophy observed in the "genuine" bulbar palsy just described—commonly occurs in the bulbar form of amyotrophic lateral sclerosis when the latter is of the spastic-paralytic form. Terms used to designate a kaleidoscopic disorder observed in other disease states include "pseudobulbar palsy," "striate pseudobulbar palsy," "supranuclear bulbar palsy," and "arteriosclerotic pseudoparalysis." Here the responsible lesions are situated mainly in the striatum and in corticobulbar systems. This form of the disorder is dealt with in the following.

The view has been put forward by Lewy (1942), and by others before his time, that pseudobulbar palsy represents essentially a striatal syndrome and that the lesions occurring in the internal capsule and other white matter are of incidental importance. The striatal lesions are characterized by infarctions or by *état lacunaire,* such as

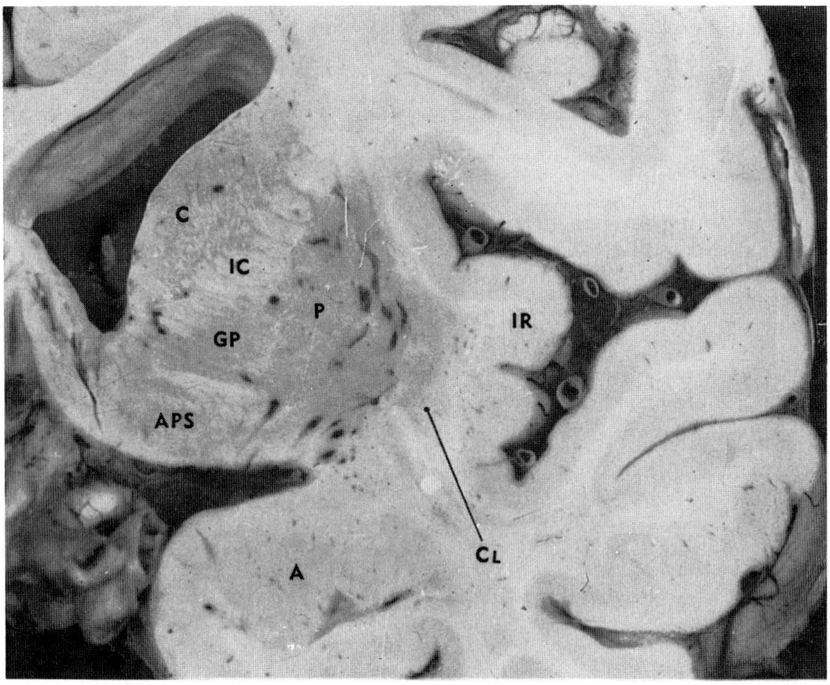

Fig. 11-20. *État lacunaire* involving chiefly the putamen *(P)*. Also affected is the anterior perforated substance *(APS)* in foci surrounding the lateral striate arteries. The septal region (to the left; unlabelled) is also affected. Arteries in the region of the lateral cerebral fissure are distended and have rigid walls. *A*, Amygdala; *C*, head of caudate nucleus; *CL*, claustrum; *GP*, globus pallidus; *IC*, anterior limb of internal capsule; *IR*, island of Reil. (From the Deutschen Forschungsanstalt für Psychiatrie, Max-Planck-Institut, München.)

illustrated in Fig. 11-20. Arteriosclerosis is dominant in such brains, and it is assumed that the lacunae are pathogenically related to the arteriosclerosis. However, some pathological process in the striatum other than the lacunae may be basically responsible for the manifestations of the syndrome. For instance, paralysis agitans resulting from pallidal degeneration may in later stages progress to pseudobulbar palsy if "arteriosclerotic" lacunae develop in the striatum (Denny-Brown, 1962).

Striatal lesions appear not to be a prerequisite to the development of pseudobulbar palsy of the type under discussion. Lesions at various levels that interrupt the corticobulbar pathways bilaterally have been observed in cases of pseudobulbar palsy in the region of the centrum semiovale or internal capsule or diencephalic-mesencephalic junctional area. Where there is a grossly visible lesion only on one side, microscopic examination will usually reveal multiple lesions of vascular origin on the other side as well. This is particularly true in the case of elderly persons. Lesions may interrupt the corticobulbar tracts of the two sides at different times: for some months or years a patient will have clear-cut hemiplegia, in which the functions of bulbar-innervated structures are in the realm of normal, and later on, following interruption of the opposite corticobulbar tract, pseudobulbar palsy supervenes. When interruption is at the midbrain or the upper pontile level, there may rather little associated involvement of the corticospinal pathway. (Bing and Haymaker, 1939.) Where lesions caused by basilar artery thrombosis occur bilaterally in the pars basilaris pontis in patients in whom pseudobulbar palsy subsequently develops, there may also be manifestations of cerebellar deficiency. However, these gradually recede as spastic contractures become dominant. (Lhermitte and Trelles, 1933, 1934.)

Conditions responsible for pseudobulbar palsy include, in addition to those already mentioned, multifocal cerebral softening secondary to hemorrhage or to vascular occlusion, embolic infarction secondary to mitral disease, syphilitic arterial disease, brain tumors, cerebral cysts, multiple sclerosis, tuberculous meningitis, and aneurysm of the basilar artery (Davison and Kelman, 1939; Tilney and Morrison, 1912).

Many of the clinical manifestations of pseudobulbar palsy, whether occurring in the disorders under discussion or in the bulbar form of amyotrophic lateral sclerosis, are related to disturbances in function of cranial nerves IX through XII as well as VII and V. The motor disability involves both sides of the pharynx, larynx, tongue, and face, and also the masticatory muscles.

Articulation and swallowing often suffer first. The speech is drawling and monotonous. The consonants are pronounced poorly and with difficulty, so that in severe cases speech becomes unintelligible. Use of vowels, on the other hand, is less interfered with. The breath is usually lost during speech, and therefore several attempts have to be made before a sentence can be completed. This results in interrupted and semi-explosive speech. If the lips are affected more than the other parts, the predominant change will consist in difficulty in forming labials; if the palatal paresis is the most pronounced, the predominant feature will be a nasal tone of the voice. Occasionally there is aphonia. Not only are the labial muscles involved but also other facial muscles. Spasticity of the facial muscles occurs and is betrayed by an increased abnormal spreading of the contraction of facial muscles on mechanical stimulation, and by their tendency to contract when stimuli are applied as far away as the shoulder.

The tongue may be so severely affected that it lies immobile on the floor of the mouth. Usually, however, it can be protruded somewhat, but lateral movements are weak, and the edges of the tongue cannot be raised to form a trough. Repeated protrusion of the tongue causes marked fatigue equivalent to paralysis. Saliva usually runs from the mouth. Palatal movements are either absent or sluggish and incomplete. The vocal cords are paretic, but seldom markedly so.

The muscles of mastication (fifth nerve) always suffer. There may be trismus of the masseter muscles, or the mouth may remain permanently half-open, with firm closure of the teeth impossible. In either state there is an exaggeration of the masseter reflex (abrupt upward movement of the jaw when the examiner's finger placed on the patient's chin is struck with a reflex hammer), and mandibular clonus is elicitable. Paralysis of the pterygoids, manifested by an inability to protrude the mandible and to perform lateral chewing movements, is frequently pronounced. In some few instances the patient cannot lower his jaw against resistance.

Because of weakness of the muscles of mastication and of tongue, lips, and cheeks, eating is difficult; not enough food can be brought between the teeth and as a result, the food, poorly chewed, often has to be pushed into the pharynx with a finger. If paralysis of the palate and pharynx also exists, particles of food may enter the nose or the larynx. Early paresis of the constrictor muscles of the pharynx can be detected by having the patient perform swallowing movements without anything in his mouth. The criterion for swallowing is the full up-and-down excursion of the laryngeal protuberance. A normal person is able to swallow three or four times in rapid succession, a patient with supranuclear bulbar palsy only once or not at all. Moreover, with caloric labyrinthine stimulation the quick phase of nystagmus may be absent. (Ford and Walsh, 1940; Holmes, 1921.)

Certain *reflexes,* some elicitable in normal infants, can be obtained in the region of the labial, palatal, and masticatory musculature. They may be obtained in the absence of pyramidal tract or cerebral signs and thus are of value in early diagnosis. They may also be easily elicited in well-advanced amyotrophic lateral sclerosis and in some forms of encephalopathy. The head retraction reflex (see the following) is helpful in distinguishing between upper cervical cord tumor and multiple sclerosis, for in the former the reflex is not elicitable.

Snout reflex. A brisk snout-like protrusion of the lips occurs when the center of the upper lip is tapped.

Mouth-opening reflex. The mouth opens when a lip or a corner of the mouth is stroked.

Mastication reflex. Chewing movements are elicited on stroking the tongue or lips.

Orbicularis oris reflex. Contraction of the orbicularis oris (downward and lateral displacement of the upper lip) occurs when the hard palate is stroked.

Head-retraction reflex. This is a deep muscle reflex that exists normally in latent form. With the patient sitting upright, the examiner bends the patient's head forward slightly (with the palm of the examiner's hand applied to the occiput), then with a percussion hammer, taps the chin in a downward direction, producing brisk stretching of the dorsal muscles of the neck. Abnormality is indicated by a sudden backward movement of the head. (Wilson, 1940.) The same occurs when the center of the upper lip or the bridge of the nose is tapped (Wartenberg, 1945).

PATHOLOGICAL LAUGHTER AND CRYING

Motiveless, unrestrained ("forced") laughing or crying, or both, occur in about half the cases of pseudobulbar palsy, and during these outbursts other bulbar manifestations are aggravated. Neural mechanisms involved are thus closely related with those already indicated in the previous section.

Emotional movements have been thought to be dependent on a neural mechanism arising in close association with telencephalic and diencephalic centers concerned in respiration, for in laughing or in crying a series of respiratory arrests and accelerations occur. Two *faciorespiratory pathways* have been postulated: a respiratory-arresting, originating in the inferior surface of the frontal lobe, and a respiratory-accelerating, arising in the parietal cortex and extending to the striatum, then to the globus pallidus, and downward. Evidence has suggested that they course rather close together in the region of the subthalamus, extend downward in the tegmentum medial to the red nucleus, and in the sagittal plane of the third nucleus, to reach the medulla oblongata. (Bailey and Sweet, 1940; Martin, 1950; Spencer, 1894; Wilson, 1929.) The temporal lobe and its efferent pathways may also be implicated, since temporal lobe seizures sometimes involve laughter (Daly and Mulder, 1957; Ironside, 1956). The same may be true for the globus pallidus, for a lesion here can result in emotional over-activity (Lewy, 1942).

The hypothalamus, in addition to structures such as the temporal lobe and globus pallidus, comes into consideration as having an influence on faciorespiratory synkinesis. Laughing seizures, occasionally succeeded by episodes of crying, have been known to occur in association with sexual precocity, sometimes under conditions in which a tumor was found in the region of the mamillary bodies (Money and Hosta, 1967). Swabbing of the floor of the third ventricle in the course of removal of a choroid plexus papilloma (under local anesthesia) gave rise in one patient to laughter with a verbal accompaniment (Ironside, 1956). Descending hypothalamic fibers reach the central gray of the midbrain, which appears to represent a multisynaptic station within the neuron paths for affective reactions (Hunsperger, 1956); extending downstream from this region are fibers that pass, in part at least, through central tegmental tract to the inferior olivary nucleus. Lesions almost anywhere in this general region, but particularly in the upper brainstem, may give rise to unilateral or bilateral amimia or to spasmodic avalanche-like outbursts of laughter or crying, sometimes in association with weakness or abolition of voluntary movements (Bender, Nathanson, and Gordon, 1952). Lesions observed in such cases, usually bilateral in distribution, include "primary" degenerative change in corticopontile and corticobulbar pathways, multiple sclerosis, neoplasm, and arteriosclerotic or syphilitic cerebral vascular thrombosis (Davison and Kelman, 1939; Tilney and Morrison, 1912; Wilson, 1929). Head trauma has occasionally been complicated by the disorder, with pathological crying occurring first in the convalescent stage, then pathological laughter, then both together in rapid succession (Poeck, Risso, and Pilleri, 1963).

Final common supranuclear pathways concerned in the performance of the faciorespiratory synkinesis just dealt with are considered to come into synaptic relation with the reticular core of the brainstem (Weinstein and Bender, 1943), from which fibers are funneled into the inferior olivary nucleus. It has been suggested that through the mediation of olivocerebellar fibers the cerebellum exerts a continuous, probably suppressive (feedback), modulatory influence on the rostral junction of the synkinesis mechanism, in the region of the confluence of emotive components in the upper midbrain reticular core. By this formulation, disinhibition at high brainstem levels could produce emotional display without a subjective accompaniment. (Herrmann and Brown, 1967.)

REFERENCES

Aigner, B. R., and Mulder, D. W. 1960. Myoclonus: clinical significance and an approach to classification. Arch. Neurol. **2**:600-615.

Allegranza, A., Canevini, P., and Strada, G. P. 1966. Progressive familial myoclonus epilepsy of Unverricht-Lundborg: histochemical and ultrastructural study of the S.C. Lafora's bodies. Proc. 5th Int. Cong. Neuropath. Zurich. Amsterdam, Excerpta Medica Foundation, pp. 99-1003.

Bailey, P., and Sweet, W. R. 1940. Effects of respiration, blood pressure and gastric motility of stimulation of orbital surface of frontal lobe. J. Neurophysiol. **3**:276-281.

Baudouin, A., Bertrand, I., and Lereboullet, J. 1930. Sur deux cas de syndrome de Babinski-Nageotte. Paris Méd. **77**:297-301.

Bender, M., Nathanson, M., and Gordon, G. 1952. Myoclonus of the eye, face and throat. Arch. Neurol. Psychiat. **67**:44-58.

Biemond, A. 1951. Thrombosis of the basilar artery and the vascularization of the brain stem. Brain **74**:300-317.

Bing, R., and Haymaker, W. 1939. Textbook of nervous diseases. St. Louis, The C. V. Mosby Co.

Bjerver, K., and Silfverskiöld, B. P. 1968. Lateropulsion and imbalance in Wallenberg's syndrome. Acta Neurol. Scand. **44**:91-100.

Brody, B. S., and German, W. J. 1933. Medulloblastoma of the cerebellum: a report of fifteen cases. Yale J. Biol. Med. **6**:19-29.

Brown, W. J., Kotorii, K., and Riehl, J.-L. 1968. Ultrastructural studies in myoclonus epilepsy (clinical Unverricht-Lafora's disease). Neurology **18**:427-438.

Brun, R. 1952. Drei Fälle von seltenen unterem Oblongata Syndrom. (Hemiplegia cruciata und hemiplegia alternans infima). Zugleich ein Beitrag zur Kenntnis des Faserverlaufs in der Pyramiden- und Schleifenkreuzung. Schweiz. Arch. Neurol. Psychiat. **68**:248-271.

Crosby, E. C. 1953. Relations of brain centers to normal and abnormal eye movements in the horizontal plane. J. Comp. Neurol. **99**:437-479.

Daly, D. D., and Mulder, D. W. 1957. Gelastic epilepsy. Neurology **7**:189-192.

Davison, C., and Kelman, H. 1939. Pathologic laughing and crying. Arch. Neurol. Psychiat. **42**:595-643.

de Barsy, T., Myle, G., Troch, C., Matthys, R., and Martin, J. J. 1969. La dyssynergie cerebelleuse myoclonique (R. Hunt): affection autonome ou variante du type degeneratif de l'epilepsie-myoclonie progressive (Unverricht-Lundborg): approche anatomo-clinique. J. Neurol. Sci. **8**:111-127.

Denny-Brown, D. 1962. The basal ganglia and their relation to disorders of movement. London, Oxford University Press.

Foerster, O., and Gagel, O. 1932. Die Vordenseitenstrangdurchschneidung beim Menschen. Z. Ges. Neurol. Psychiat. **138**:1-92.

Ford, F. R., and Walsh, F. B. 1940. Tonic deviation of the eyes produced by movements of head, with special reference to otolithic reflexes: clinical observations. Arch. Ophthal. **23**:1274-1284.

François, J., and Neetens, A. 1968. Oculomotor paralyses and tumors of the pituitary gland. Confin. Neurol. **30**:239-252.

Friedreich, N. 1881. Neuropathologische Beobachtungen. Arch. Path. Anat. **86**:421-434.

Froriep, A. 1882. Ueber ein Ganglion des Hypoglossus. Arch. Anat. Physiol., Anat. Abt., pp. 297-302.

Gautier, J., and Blackwood, W. 1961. Enlargement of the inferior olivary nucleus in association with lesions of the central tegmental tract or dentate nucleus. Brain **84**:341-362.

Girard, P., Gerest, F., Tommasi, M., and Rouves, L. 1962. Ramollissement géant du pied de la protubérance: modifications structurales des olives bulbaires: tableau clinique voison de celui du "mutisme akinétique de Cairns." Lyon Méd. **207**:877-892.

Grossman, M. 1942. Syringomyelia. J. Mt. Sinai Hosp. **9**:526-535.

Guillain, G., Bertrand, I., and Mollaret, P. 1933a. Sur la lésion responsable du syndrome myoclonique due tronc cérébral. Rev. Neurol. **2**: 666-675.

Guillain, G., Thurel, R., and Bertrand, I. 1933b. Examen anatomo-pathologique d'un cas de myoclonies vélo-pharyngo-oculo-diaphragmatiques associées à des myoclonies squelettiques synchrones. Rev. Neurol. **2**:801-812.

Harriman, D. G. F., and Millar, J. H. D. 1955. Progressive familial myoclonic epilepsy in 3 families; its clinical features and pathological basis, with appendix on genetic effects by A. C. Stevenson. Brain **78**:325-349.

Herrick, C. J. 1931. An introduction to neurology, ed. 3. Philadelphia, W. B. Saunders Company.

Herrmann, C., Jr., and Brown, J. W. 1967. Palatal myoclonus: a reappraisal. J. Neurol. Sci. **5**:473-492.

His, W. 1904. Die Entwickelung des menschlichen Gehirns während der ersten Monate. Leipzig, S. Hirzel.

Hodskins, M. B., and Yakovlev, P. I. 1930. Anatomico-clinical observations on myoclonus in epileptics and on related symptom complexes. Amer. J. Psychiat. **9**:827-848.

Holmes, G. 1921. Palsies of the conjugate ocular movements. Brit. J. Ophthal. **5**:241-350.

Hughes, J. 1965. Palatal myoclonus (a case report). Dis. Nerv. Syst. **26**:659-661.

Hunsperger, R. 1956. Affektreaktionen auf elektrische Reizung im Hirnstamm der Katze. Helv. Physiol. Pharmacol. Acta **14**:70-72.

Hunt, R. 1914. Dyssynergia cerebellaris progressiva: a chronic progressive form of cerebellar tumor. Brain **37**:247-268.

Hunt, J. R. 1921. Dyssynergia cerebellaris myoclonica—primary atrophy of the dentate system: a contribution to the pathology and symptomatology of the cerebellum. Brain **44**:490-538.

Ironside, R. 1956. Disorders of laughter due to brain lesions. Brain **79**:589-609.

Kuhlenbeck, H. 1927. Vorlesungen über das Zentralnervensystem der Wirbelthiere. Jena, Gustav Fischer, pp. 52, 354.

Lafora, G. R., and Glück, B. 1911. Beitrag zur Histologie der myoklonischen Epilepsie. Z. Neurol. Psychiat. **6**:1-14.

Lewy, F. H. 1942. Historical introduction: the basal ganglia and their diseases. Res. Publ. Ass. Res. Nerv. Ment. Dis., Proc. **21**:1-20.

Lhermitte, J., and Trelles, J. O. 1933. L'hypertrophie des olives bulbaires. Encéphale **28**:588-600.

Lhermitte, J., and Trelles, J. O. 1934. L'artériosclèrose du tronc basilaire et ses consequences anatomo-cliniques. Jahrb. Psychiat. Neurol. **51**: 91-107.

Lundborg, H. 1903. Die progressive Myoklonus-Epilepsie. Uppsala, Almqvist & Wiskell.

Mahloudji, M., and Pikielny, R. T. 1967. Hereditary essential myoclonus. Brain **90**:669-674.

Martin, J. P. 1950. Fits of laughter (sham mirth) in organic cerebral disease. Brain **73**:453-464.

Martinez, S. N., Bertrand, C., and Botana-Lopez, C. 1967. Motor fiber distribution within the cerebral peduncle: results of unipolar stimulation. Confin. Neurol. **29**:117-122.

Money, J., and Hosta, G. 1967. Laughing seizures with sexual precocity: report of two cases. Johns Hopk. Med. J. **120**:326-336.

Mouren, P. A., Tatossian, A., Giraud, F., Striglioni, L., Verne, P., and Poinso, Y. 1962. Le "nystagmus du voile du palais" (le syndrome myorhythmique du carrefour aéro-digestive). Rev. Otoneuroophtal. **34**:273-304.

Nashold, B. S., and Gills, J. P., Jr. 1967. Ocular signs from brain stimulation and lesions. Arch. Ophthal. **77**:609-618.

Nehlil, J., Thurel, R., Warnery, J., and Fabert, G. 1966. Le syndrome des clonies arythmiques pharyngo-laryngées. Rev. Neurol. **1**:235-241.

Pasik, T., Pasik, P., and Bender, M. B. 1966. The superior colliculi and eye movements: an experimental study in the monkey. Arch. Neurol. **15**:420-436.

Poeck, K., Risso, M., and Pilleri, G. 1963. Beitrag zur Pathophysiologie und klinischen Systematik des pathologischen Lachens und Weinens. Arch. Psychiat. Z. Ges. Neurol. **204**:181-198.

Ranson, S. W. 1953. The anatomy of the nervous system: its development and function, ed. 9. Revised by Clark, S. L. Philadelphia, W. B. Saunders Company, pp. 248-252.

Rasmussen, A. T., and Peyton, W. T. 1941. The location of the lateral spinothalamic tract in the brain stem of man. Surgery **10**:699-710.

Rowbotham, G. F. 1938. Treatment of pain in the face by intramedullary tractotomy. Brit. Med. J. **2**:1073-1076.

Sahu, R. N., and Satapathy, P. C. 1962. Syringobulbia. J. Indian Med. Ass. **39**:146-147.

Schwartz, H. C., and O'Leary, J. L. 1942. Section of the spinothalamic tract at the level of the inferior olive. Arch. Neurol. Psychiat. **47**: 293-304.

Sittig, O., and Haskovec, V. 1939. Palatal myoclonus. Arch. Neurol. Psychiat. **42**:413-424.

Souadjian, J. V., and Cain, J. C. 1968. Intractable hiccup: etiologic factors in 220 cases. Postgrad. Med. **43**:72-77.

Spencer, W. G. 1894. The effect produced upon respiration by faradic excitation of the cerebrum in the monkey, dog, cat, and rabbit. Philos. Tr., B **185**:609-657.

Tilney, F., and Morrison, J. F. 1912. Pseudobulbar palsy, clinically and pathologically considered, with the clinical report of five cases. J. Nerv. Ment. Dis. **39**:505-535.

Toga, M., Dubois, D., and Hassoun, J. 1968. Ultra-structure des corps de Lafora. Acta Neuropath. **10**:132-142.

Unverricht, H. 1891. Die Myoclonie. Leipzig, Franz Deuticke.

van Bogaert, L., and Bertrand, I. 1928. Sur les myoclonies associées synchrones et rythmiques par lésions en foyer du tronc cérébrale. Rev. Neurol. **1**:203-214.

van Bogaert, L., and Martin, P. 1928. Les tumeurs du quatrième ventricule et le syndrome cérébelleux de la ligne médiane. Rev. Neurol. **2**: 431-483.

Walker, A. E. 1940. The spinothalamic tract in man. Arch. Neurol. Psychiat. **43**:284-298.

Wallenberg, A. 1901. Anatomischer Befund in einem als "acute Bulbäraffection (Embolie der Art. cerebellar. post. inf. sinistr.?)" beschriebenen Falle. Arch. Psychiat. **34**:923-959.

Wallenberg, A. 1911. Neuere Fortschritte in der topischen Diagnostik des Pons und der Oblongata. Dtsch. Z. Nervenheilk. **41**:8-41.

Wartenberg, R. 1945. The examination of reflexes: a simplification. Chicago, Year Book Medical Publishers, Inc.

Watson, C. W., and Denny-Brown, D. 1953. Myoclonus epilepsy as a symptom of diffuse neuronal disease. Arch. Neurol. Psychiat. **70**:151-168.

Weinstein, E., and Bender, M. 1943. Integrated facial patterns elicited by stimulation of the brain stem. Arch. Neurol. Psychiat. **50**:34-42.

White, J. C., and Sweet, W. H. 1955. Pain: its mechanisms and neurosurgical control. Springfield, Illinois, Charles C Thomas, Publisher.

Willis, W. H., and Weaver, D. F. 1968. Syringomyelia with bilateral vocal cord paralysis: report of a case. Arch. Otolaryng. **87**:468-470.

Wilson, S. A. K. 1929. Modern problems in neurology. New York, William Wood and Company, pp. 260-296.

Wilson, S. A. K. 1940. Neurology, vol. 2. Baltimore, The Williams & Wilkins Co., p. 1020.

Winkler, C. 1927. Anatomie du système nerveux, vol. 3. Haarlem, E. F. Bohn.

Yap, C.-B., Mayo, C., and Barron, K. 1968. "Ocular bobbing" in palatal myoclonus. Arch. Neurol. **18**:304-310.

Yokoi, S., Austin, J., Witmer, F., and Sakai, M. 1968. Studies in myoclonus epilepsy (Lafora body form): isolation and preliminary characterization of Lafora bodies in two cases. Arch. Neurol. **19**:15-33.

Chapter 12

Localization of lesions involving cranial nerves IX through XII

Thus far the cranial nerves have been described from the standpoint of their nuclei of origin and their intramedullary course. This chapter and following chapters will deal with intramedullary and extramedullary involvement of these nerves. Not infrequently one or more cranial nerves are involved in their intraforaminal course. Fig. 12-1 illustrates the foramina.

The hypoglossal, spinal accessory, vagus, and glossopharyngeal nerves may be conveniently considered together as the *caudal nerve group* of the brainstem.

HYPOGLOSSAL NERVE

The nucleus of the hypoglossal, or twelfth cranial, nerve is situated in the lower third of the medulla oblongata (Figs. 10-3 and 10-9). The nerve leaves the skull by way of the hypoglossal canal, and in the inferior cervical region it joins the ansa hypoglossi. It supplies the ipsilateral intrinsic muscles of the tongue, hypoglossus, styloglossus, and genioglossus. From the clinical standpoint, the genioglossus (a muscle from chin [genio-] to tongue [glossus]) is the most important of the three, for it is mainly responsible for protrusion of the tongue.

Interruption of the twelfth nerve bilaterally produces total glossoplegia: the tongue lies immobile on the floor of the mouth, speech is indistinct, and there is difficulty in eating. Respiration is interfered with because the tongue tends to slip back into the throat, and as a result, tracheotomy may be necessary. In unilateral paralysis, by contrast, functional disturbances are minimal owing to the rich interlacing of muscle fibers of the tongue across the midline. However, when the tongue is protruded its tip deviates toward the side of the paralysis as a result of contraction of the genioglossus muscle of the sound side; moreover, the paralyzed side of the tongue is atrophic (Fig. 12-2). (Aldrich and Baker, 1948.)

SPINAL ACCESSORY NERVE

The spinal accessory nerve—the eleventh cranial nerve (Fig. 10-1)—arises in a group of cells in the ventrolateral part of the anterior horn of segments C1 through C4 (Fig. 10-7), a site to which they migrated from the motor nucleus of the tenth nerve during phylogenesis (Pearson, Sauter, and Herrin, 1964). The fibers exit from the lateral side of the cord both at the level of their origin (Fig. 10-7) and after ascending a segment or two in the region of the lateral horn; the two systems leave the spinal cord as separate roots (Truex, 1959). These roots unite with roots from successively higher cervical segments to form a common ascending trunk, which enters the intracranial cavity through the foramen magnum. Within the skull the trunk of the eleventh is joined by the bul-

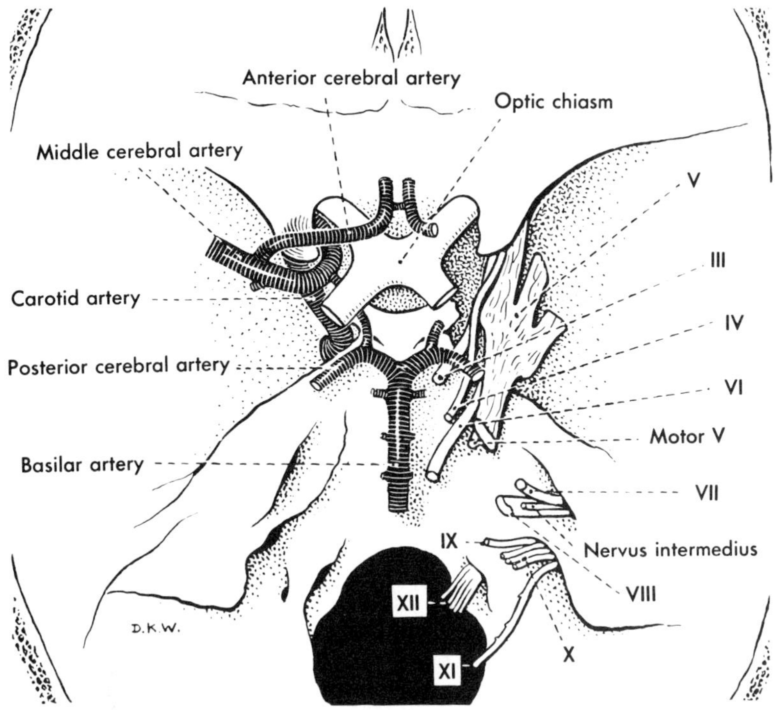

Fig. 12-1. The cranial nerves as seen dorsally. The optic nerve passes through the optic foramen. Nerves III, IV, and VI and the ophthalmic division of V pass through the *superior orbital fissure.* The maxillary division of V proceeds through the *foramen rotundum,* then the *inferior orbital fissure* to gain the orbit; and the mandibular division of V traverses the *foramen ovale.* Nerve VII passes through the *internal acoustic meatus,* and then the *facial canal.* Nerve VIII courses through the *internal acoustic meatus;* nerves IX, X, and XI, through the *jugular foramen,* though IX is enveloped in a separate sheath of dura mater. Nerve XII proceeds through the *hypoglossal canal.* The course of the internal carotid, which is S-shaped, is also indicated. The anterior cerebral artery passes over the dorsal aspect of the most proximal part of the optic nerve.

bar rootlets of the tenth nerve; on passing out of the intracranial cavity through the jugular foramen, the trunk loses its attachment with the tenth nerve and descends into the neck, where it supplies the sternocleidomastoid and trapezius muscles. En route it is joined by the primary rami of spinal segments C1 through C4. The sternocleidomastoid receives its innervation mainly from segment C2. The upper half

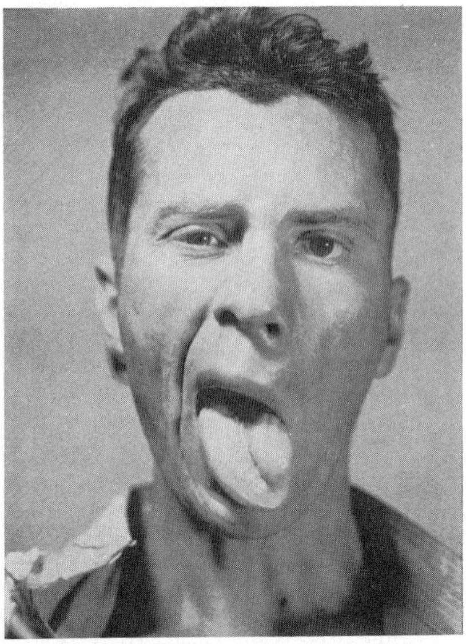

Fig. 12-2. Atrophy and paralysis of the left side of the tongue due to missile wound of the left side of the neck, with missile entrance in the region of the mastoid process (Fig. 12-3, *A*). The tip of the tongue deviates toward the paralyzed side. (From Walter Reed Army Hosp.; AFIP Neg. A45196-3.)

of the trapezius is supplied by the eleventh nerve, and the lower half by primary rami originating chiefly in spinal segments C3 and C4.

The eleventh nerve also possesses an *afferent* system of fibers. Cell bodies are found in ganglia situated along the course of the nerve. Fibers extending centralward take a course different from those of typical posterior root fibers; they pass into the cord ventral to the substantia gelatinosa, then turn dorsally to reach the posterior column and the caudal end of the fasciculus solitarius, in both of which they ascend (Pearson, Sauter, and Herrin, 1964).

Intramedullary lesions of sufficient magnitude to destroy the anterior gray column unilaterally at levels C1 through C4 usually cause total paralysis of the sternocleidomastoid and trapezius muscles of that side. *Interruption of the eleventh nerve* unilaterally after it emerges from the jugular foramen affects both these muscles, but in different degree. Paralysis occurs in the sternocleidomastoid, with subsequent atrophy (Fig. 12-3, *A*). The patient is able to turn his chin only to a limited degree away from the affected side, but can turn it satisfactorily toward the affected side (Fig. 12-3, *B*). In bilateral eleventh nerve palsy, the head tends to fall backward. The trapezius, by way of contrast, is usually involved only in its upper half because the lower half is most often innervated by nerves from spinal segments C3 and C4 (see Straus and Howell [1936] for variations). In subjects in whom the muscle is thus innervated, when the shoulder is at rest the scapula is displaced downward and laterally. The arm droops, as can be readily recognized by the lower level of the fingers of that side when the two arms hang loosely at the side of the legs. The inequality can be even better brought out by having the subject bring his arms out in front of him with palms together; the fingertips of the affected side project farther forward than those of the normal side.

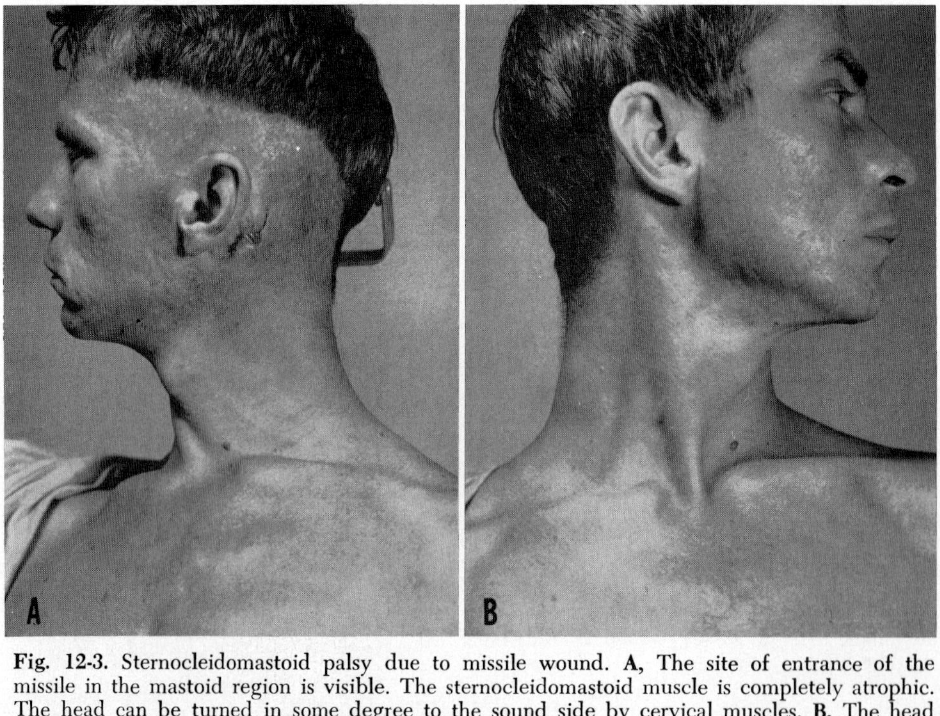

Fig. 12-3. Sternocleidomastoid palsy due to missile wound. **A,** The site of entrance of the missile in the mastoid region is visible. The sternocleidomastoid muscle is completely atrophic. The head can be turned in some degree to the sound side by cervical muscles. **B,** The head can be turned fully toward the affected side by the intact sternocleidomastoid muscle. (From Walter Reed Army Hosp.; AFIP Negs. A45196-4 and 5.)

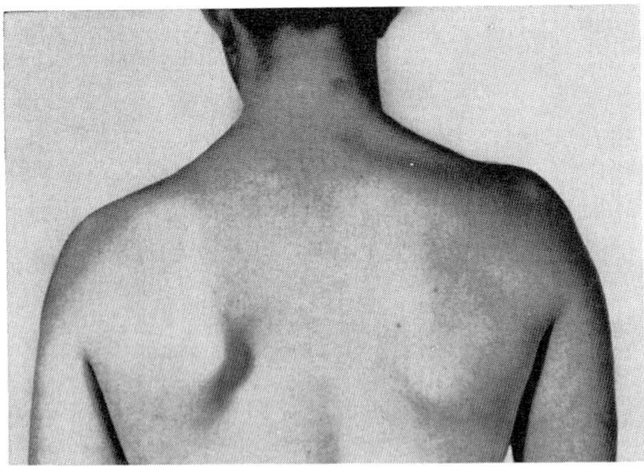

Fig. 12-4. Trapezius palsy, with the arm at rest. Seven months previously the patient sustained an oblique penetrating wound of the neck (see scar on right side of neck). There is upward and lateral displacement of the left scapula, atrophy of the superior third of the trapezius, and flaring of the vertebral border of the scapula. (From Haymaker and Woodhall, 1953.)

Moreover, in trapezius palsy following interruption of the nerve, there is flaring of the vertebral border of the scapula, with the flared superior angle displaced farther from the spine than the inferior angle (Fig. 12-4). This abnormal position is accentuated when the arm is moved laterally against resistance, but on forward flexion the flaring of the inferior angle almost disappears (Fig. 12-5, *A*). Only the upper part of the muscle becomes atrophied.

In *serratus magnus palsy* relatively little change is apparent when the arms are at rest at the sides of the body. The change consists in slight backward displacement of the shoulder girdle, slight winging of the lower part of the scapula, and slight medial rotation of the scapula so that its lower part is somewhat closer than normal to the vertebral column. However, on elevation of the arm, pronounced winging of the scapula occurs (Fig. 12-5, *B*).

VAGUS NERVE

The vagus nerve—the tenth cranial nerve—takes origin in the medulla oblon-

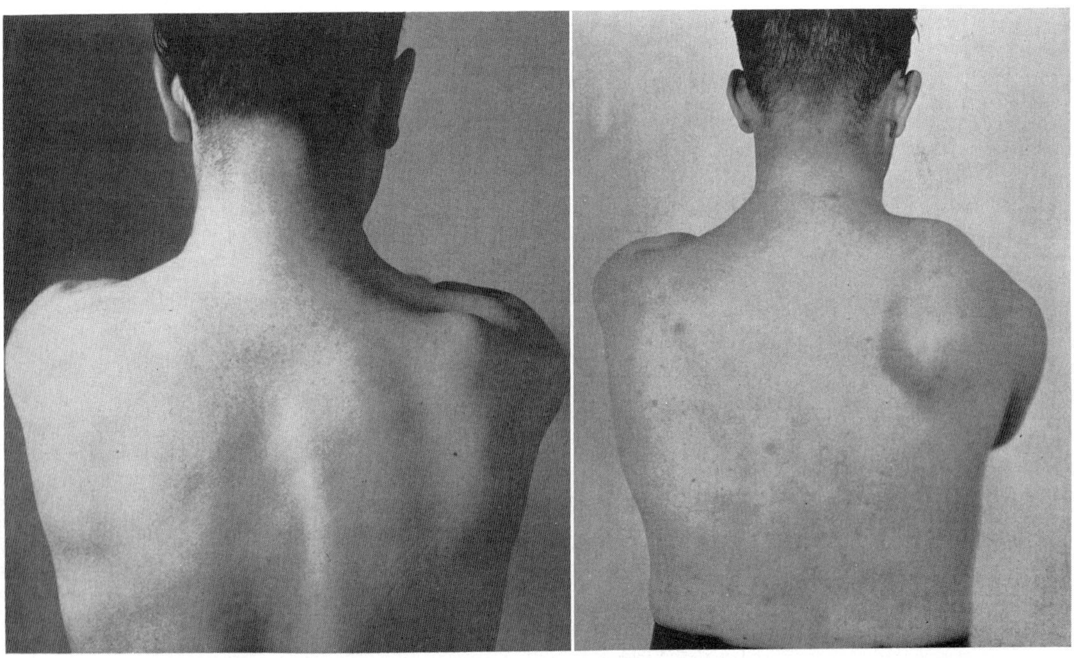

B

Fig. 12-5. **A,** Palsy of the right trapezius muscle. On forward flexion of the arms the flaring (such as is seen in Fig. 12-4) disappears and there is lateral displacement of the scapula. (From Bushnell General Hospital.) **B,** Palsy of the right serratus magnus muscle. On forward flexion of the arm the scapula becomes winged and moves upward and laterally. (From Haymaker and Woodhall, 1953.)

gata (Fig. 10-3) and emerges as a series of rootlets from the region of the restiform body at a level somewhat lateral to the olive (Figs. 10-1 and 10-9). The upper vagal rootlets are predominantly sensory, and the lower predominantly motor. The nerve leaves the skull by way of the jugular foramen to be distributed to structures in the neck, thorax, and abdomen.

A *motor* component of the tenth nerve originates in the nucleus ambiguus. This component supplies all muscles of the soft palate (except the tensor veli palatini), pharynx (except the stylopharyngeus), and the cricothyroid and all other intrinsic muscles of the larynx. As to the laryngeal muscles, the cricothyroid muscle is innervated from the rostral part of the nucleus ambiguus, the adductor muscle group from the caudal part, and the abductors from the intermediate part of the nucleus (Furstenberg and Magielski, 1955).

Another *motor* component arises in the dorsal nucleus of the vagus. It is motor to the smooth muscles of the trachea, bronchi, esophagus, and gastrointestinal tract (except the lower part of the large intestine) (Fig. 2-2). Functionally the fibers are inhibitory to heart muscle (they serve to reduce heart rate and the amplitude of the heartbeat) and to the sphincters of the upper gastrointestinal tract. They are coronary constrictors and pulmonary artery dilators. Moreover, they are secretory motor to the gastrointestinal tract, the liver, and the pancreas. Vagal activity potentiates both the release and the action of gastrin in the stomach (de Castella and Irvine, 1967). The cardia of the stomach is innervated not only by motor fibers but also by inhibitory fibers (Greenwood and others, 1962; Hwang, Essex, and Mann, 1947).

Sensory fibers of the tenth nerve carry impulses from the dura of the floor of the posterior cranial fossa (p. 234). An auricular branch (Arnold's nerve) conveys impulses from the inferior and posterior parts of the wall of the external auditory meatus, the posterior part of the tympanic membrane, and the boundary zone between the ear and the mastoid process (Fig. 12-6). Cell stations for these components are situated in the jugular ganglion. The fibers conveying pain impulses terminate in the spinal nucleus of the fifth nerve. Those carrying tactile impulses end in the principal nucleus of the fifth nerve and probably also in the (medial) cuneate nucleus after having descended in the spinal tract of the fifth nerve (Rhoton, 1968; Rhoton, O'Leary, and Ferguson, 1966).

Other *sensory* fibers are given off by the tenth nerve throughout much of its course. Some of the fibers convey taste impulses from the epiglottis. These terminate in the caudal part of the solitary nucleus (Rhoton, 1968). Fibers from the pharynx convey tactile impulses (pain fibers being carried by the ninth nerve; Ueihlein, Love, and Corbin, 1955). The tenth nerve carries pain fibers from the esophagus, trachea, and bronchi (White and Sweet, 1955), and apparently also from the larynx. Sensory fibers concerned with functions other than pain transmission come from the larynx, trachea, bronchi, esophagus, stomach, small intestine, and ascending colon. Afferent fibers come also from the heart. The cell bodies of all these sensory elements are situated in the jugular and nodose ganglia. The vagal fibers conveying pain impulses terminate in the nucleus of the spinal tract of the fifth nerve, while those carrying impulses concerned in cardiorespiratory and other visceral reflexes terminate in the caudal part of the solitary nucleus (Rhoton, O'Leary, and Ferguson, 1966).

Still other *sensory* fibers transmit chemoreceptor impulses from the aortic glomus and (with the ninth nerve) from the carotid glomus. Fibers also convey pressoreceptor impulses from the aortic arch and (with the ninth nerve) from the carotid sinus. The cell station is either in the nodose

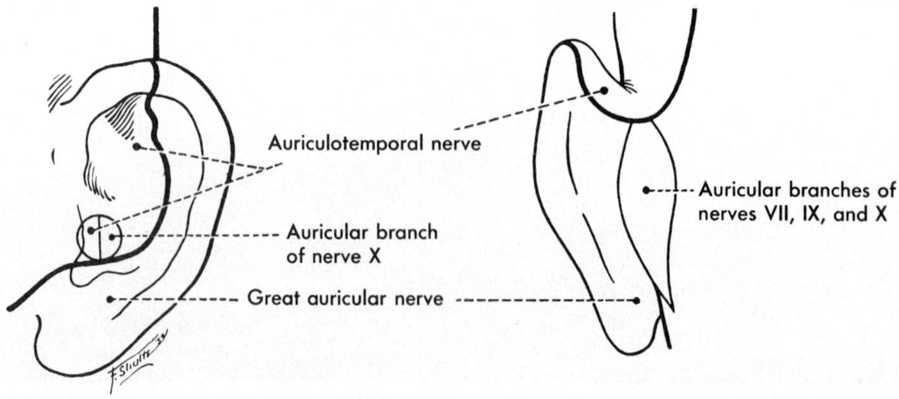

Fig. 12-6. Innervation of the ear, external auditory meatus, and tympanic membrane. The auriculotemporal nerve is a branch of the fifth cranial nerve. The great auricular nerve is derived from spinal segments C2 and C3. Its area of supply may be shared by branches of the small occipital nerve.

or the jugular ganglia, or in both. The fibers terminate chiefly in the solitary nucleus.

Reflexes dependent on the integrity of the tenth nerve include the pharyngeal and palatal reflexes.

The *pharyngeal (or gag) reflex* consists in elevation and constriction of the pharyngeal musculature accompanied by retraction of the tongue when a stimulus such as a tongue blade or applicator stick is applied to the posterior pharyngeal wall, faucial pillar, or tonsillar region. The afferent limb of the arc is through the ninth nerve and the efferent through the tenth; the afferent limb may, however, be in the tenth nerve and the efferent limb in the ninth. The *palatal and uvular reflexes* are elicited by stimulating the soft palate or the lateral or inferior surface of the uvula with an applicator stick or the like; normally the soft palate moves upward and the uvula retracts. The afferent part of the arc is through the ninth nerve (and possibly the tenth), and the efferent through the tenth (and possibly the ninth). Loss of the pharyngeal and palatal reflexes results from interruption of the appropriate branches of either the ninth or the tenth nerve. In this respect the ninth is the more important of the two. The fifth nerve may also serve the palatal reflex, and thus the reflex may be elicitable following interruption of the ninth nerve. Where the pharyngeal and palatal reflexes are exaggerated, as in supranuclear lesions, there is apt to be gagging or even retching and vomiting on swallowing.

Total bilateral interruption of the tenth nerve is rapidly fatal.

Total unilateral interruption intracranially or at the base of the skull results in widespread disturbances involving the palate, pharynx, and larynx of the ipsilateral side. The soft palate of that side hangs flaccid, and as a result, the voice has a nasal twang. Inspection of the pharynx when the patient talks with his mouth wide open may reveal a shift of the posterior pharyngeal wall to the normal side owing to paralysis of the superior constrictor muscle of the pharynx. The vocal cord of the affected side lies immobile in a position midway between abduction and adduction because neither the adductor nor the abductor of the glottis is able to function. Because of a compensatory shift of the opposite vocal cord across the midline, the voice may remain normal except for the nasal twang imparted by the palatopharyngeal palsy; however, as a rule, the voice is hoarse and brassy and may break into falsetto. Difficulty in swallowing occurs, and it may or may not be pronounced. Respiratory disturbances, such as slowing and irregularity of breathing, seldom occur, but cardiac arrhythmia and tachycardia are common. (Harris, 1926; Sicard and Bollack, 1912.)

Progressive damage of the tenth nerve results first in paralysis of the abductors of the vocal cords (the cords lie in midline position), then paralysis of the tensor, and, finally, paralysis of the adductors (the cord lies in the cadaveric position) (Semon's law). In psychogenic disorders, by way of contrast, only the adductors are affected.

Disturbances following damage of the tenth nerve intracranially or in its early course in the cervical region may be less widespread and less severe than just indicated. Thus, in isolated injury of the tenth nerve caused by unilateral fracture of the basis of the skull, difficulty in swallowing may be the outstanding symptom. The striking disturbance in swallowing resulting from severance of the tenth nerve by missiles is due largely to bulging of the paralyzed pharyngeal constrictors and to failure of the epiglottis to occlude the laryngeal opening during the swallowing effort (Naffziger, Davis, and Bell, 1948). Also, instead of total vocal cord paralysis such as is noted in proven tenth nerve interruption, the paralysis occurring as the result of trauma may be limited to the cricoarytenoideus posterior. This muscle has the function of opening the glottis on inspiration. The abductor paralysis, when occurring unilaterally, usually is manifested by hoarseness; when bilateral, inspiration is embarrassed and the voice little affected. The converse—aphonia together with normal respiration—probably occurs only in hysteria.

The *recurrent laryngeal nerve* enters the larynx from below (through its branch, the inferior laryngeal nerve). It supplies all the intrinsic muscles of the larynx except the cricothyroid. The paralysis occurring as a result of interruption of the recurrent laryngeal nerve unilaterally may in some instances be nonsymptomatic. Usually, however, the voice is reduced to a whisper or has a hoarse quality. Explosive cough is no longer possible. There is seldom if ever any respiratory problem. Bilateral recurrent laryngeal nerve paralysis is manifested by hoarseness, usually combined with severe inspiratory stridor. (Clerf, 1955; Harris, 1926; Morrison, 1945.)

The recurrent laryngeal nerve tends to be affected bilaterally in *chronic lead poisoning.* Aphonia occurs, and there may be such severe dyspnea and stridor that tracheotomy may be necessary. Only in exceptional cases are the vocal cords in cadaveric position, and then temporarily, for the cords gradually return to the median position over a period of weeks or months. Lead has an affinity for motor fibers, and hence in chronic lead poisoning, pain, paresthesias, and sensory deficit are slight or nonexistent. Nerves are demyelinated and it is possible that the primary site of involvement is in Schwann cells. Other nerves involved are the radial (wrist drop), peroneal (foot drop), and facial (tremor, fibrillary twitchings, and, occasionally, palsy of facial muscles) (Legge and Goadby, 1912; Myerson, 1934). The recurrent laryngeal nerve may also be damaged in *mitral valvular disease,* owing probably to squeezing of the nerve in the region where it passes between the left pulmonary artery and the aorta at the ligamentum arteriosum (Camishion and others, 1966). In this general area the recurrent laryngeal nerve may also be damaged through compression by *tumor* or by *hypertrophic (neoplastic) lymph nodes.* Dysphagia occurring in the presence of *bronchogenic carcinoma*—occasionally dysphagia is the presenting symptom—is probably due to pressure exerted by tumor-bearing inferior tracheobronchial and periesophageal lymph nodes on the esophagus, not primarily on a branch of the vagus nerve; the dysphagia indicates advanced disease and usually forecasts inoperability (Stankey, Roshe, and Sogocio, 1969).

Damage of the recurrent laryngeal nerve resulting in vocal cord paralysis may also occur in *benign and malignant disease of the thyroid gland,* but the incidence is very low. Usually the damage is inflicted in the vicinity of a solitary thyroid nodule, with the vocal cord paralysis usually ipsilateral and occasionally contralateral to the nodule. Compression of the nerve, or complicating intense fibrosis of the nerve, may be responsible. Other explanations have been offered (Holl-Allen, 1967).

About 30 percent of the branches of the inferior laryngeal nerve are located in the thyroid area. In *thyroidectomy,* some or all of these branches may be severed bilaterally. Severance bilaterally does not leave the vocal cords in a cadaveric position, for interruption of both the inferior laryngeal and superior laryngeal nerves is necessary to bring this about. Instead, the vocal cords assume various positions, depending on the branches severed. Stridor occurs immediately as the result of laryngeal obstruction, and in some cases requires emergency tracheotomy. At later stages breathlessness, which can be very distressing, is the chief disturbance. Hoarseness may also occur postoperatively, but it gradually disappears. (Gorman and Woodward, 1965.)

In about a third of all cases of recurrent laryngeal nerve paralysis, no cause whatsoever for the paralysis has been found (Williams, 1959).

Spastic dysphonia is a disorder now and then encountered in auctioneers or in others who habitually abuse their voices. Great effort is expended in speaking, with the larynx usually being displaced far upwards. The voice is choked, with momentary interruptions of phonation during initial or stressed vowel sounds. Variations occur in intensity, pitch, and timber of the words spoken, and there are fluctuations in emphasis of words in a sentence. Phonation is sometimes painful. Synkinetic movements of the face are often exaggerated. Thus, "a conflicting and inappropriate simultaneous activation occurs in many muscles." Inspection of the larynx usually reveals no local lesion; spasms and irregular contractions occur in vocal cord tensors, adduction is strong, and opposition of the ventricular bands may be seen. Usually the disorder cannot be tied to a neurological lesion. However, there are instances in which spastic dysphonia is observed in association with cerebellar, pyramidal tract, and extrapyramidal disease. (Bicknell, Greenhouse, and Pesch, 1968.)

Vagotomy for the treatment of duodenal and gastric ulceration is complicated occasionally by dysphagia from esophageal disturbances, more commonly following transthoracic than after transabdominal vagotomy. The dysphagia may result directly from vagal denervation, or occasionally from complicating periesophageal inflammation and fibrosis or from postoperative esophagitis brought about, for example, by prolonged nasogastric intubation. Diagnosis is established by esophageal motility studies; in vagal denervation the esophageal sphincter fails to relax after deglutition. (Guillory and Clagett, 1967.) Reflux at the gastroesophageal junction is common after transabdominal vagotomy, but only rarely is it clinically significant. Since the vagus is both inhibitory and motor to the sphincter in this region, it is not surprising that cardiospasm (achalasia) may also follow vagotomy. Hiatal hernia may also be a complication. (Clarke, Penry, and Ward, 1965; Postlethwait, Kim, and Dillon, 1969.)

The tenth nerve may be affected by conditions other than those already mentioned. In the early stages of diphtheria when the infection is faucial, palatal and laryngeal palsy are common, while pharyngeal palsy is much less common. There may also be anesthesia of the palate and pharynx and loss of the palatal reflex. The cardiac disturbances that occur in diphtheria are consonant with the lesions found in the region of sinus and atrioventricular nodes (James, 1967). The tenth nerve may be involved in tabes dorsalis (Léri and Boudet, 1910) or in cerebellopontile angle tumor. Dysphagia is common in aneurysm of the internal carotid artery situated in the cervical region (Alexander, Wigser, and Davis, 1966). Dysphonia occurring in association with abductor paralysis is occasionally encountered as a leading symptom in myasthenia gravis (Friedman and Goffin, 1966).

GLOSSOPHARYNGEAL NERVE

The glossopharyngeal, or ninth cranial, nerve originates in the medulla oblongata and emerges as a series of one to three rootlets just above the vagal rootlets (Figs. 10-1 and 10-3). In company with the tenth and eleventh nerves, it leaves the skull by way of the jugular foramen. After giving off branches to the tympanic plexus and otic ganglion, the ninth nerve extends to the side of the pharynx at the level of the hyoid bone, where it enters into the formation of the pharyngeal plexus.

The only muscles supplied by the ninth nerve are the stylopharyngeus (an elevator of the upper pharynx) and the muscles of the anterior and posterior pillars of the fauces (concerned in deglutition). Deviation of the pharynx, lowering of the palatal arch, and difficulty in swallowing may result from interruption of this nerve.

The ninth nerve is largely sensory, its cell bodies lying in the superior and petrosal ganglia. Its tympanic branch (Jacobson's nerve) emerges from the petrosal ganglion and passes through a foramen in the ridge of bone between the carotid canal and the jugular fossa. This nerve transmits impulses from the lining of the tympanic cavity, the inner aspect of the tympanic membrane, the mastoid air cells, and the eustachian tube. The ninth nerve also carries impulses from the posterior part of the soft palate, the uvula, the epiglottis, the posterior and lateral wall of the pharynx in the region between the eustachian tube and the epiglottis, and the tonsillar region up to the anterior pillar (Fig. 12-7) (Erickson, 1936; Reichert and Poth, 1933). Taste impulses and impulses of general sensibility from the posterior third of the tongue are carried by this nerve, and it joins with the tenth nerve in supplying the region of the angle between the ear and mastoid through its auricular branch (Fig. 12-6). Moreover, as indicated in the description of the tenth nerve, the ninth nerve conveys chemoreceptor impulses from the carotid glomus and pressoreceptor (or baroreceptor) impulses from the carotid sinus. Pain fibers from the tympanic membrane and adjoining part of the external auditory meatus, and from the tympanic cavity and the region between ear and mastoid, terminate in the nucleus of the spinal tract of the fifth nerve. Fibers

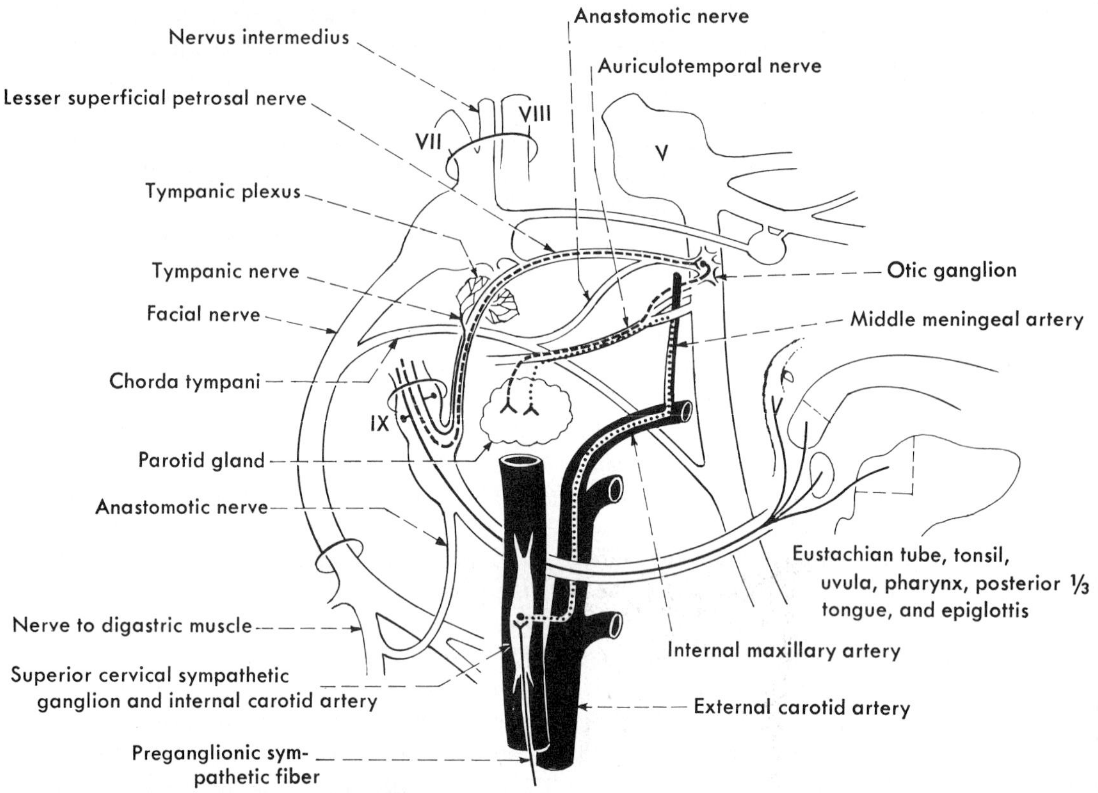

Fig. 12-7. Major components of the ninth nerve, as viewed from the medial aspect. *Solid lines:* (1) sensibility from the tympanic cavity, medial aspect of tympanum, and mastoid air cells and (2) taste sensation from the posterior third of the tongue and general sensation from the posterior part of the soft palate, uvula, eustachian tube, epiglottis and intervening pharyngeal wall, and fauces, including the tonsillar region. *Dashed line:* parasympathetic fibers to the parotid gland. Also indicated is the sympathetic supply of the parotid gland.

conveying tactile impulses from these various regions terminate partly in the principal nucleus of the fifth nerve and partly in the (medial) cuneate nucleus (Rhoton, O'Leary, and Ferguson, 1966). The fibers conveying the sensation of taste end in the caudal part of the solitary nucleus.

Studies following surgical section of the ninth and tenth nerves have revealed further information in regard to nerve supply. On sectioning the ninth nerve, pain in the pharynx was abolished but tactile sensibility persisted, from which it was concluded that pain fibers from the pharynx are carried by the ninth nerve and tactile fibers by the tenth (Uihlein, Love, and Corbin, 1955). Section of the ninth nerve does not result in loss of sensation of the tympanic membrane (Dandy, 1927, 1945).

With respect to *baroceptive function,* Wycis (1945) found that following section of the ninth nerve bilaterally the blood pressure rose immediately and remained elevated for 4 weeks, then reverted to the previous state. In another case of bilateral section of the ninth nerve, increase in blood pressure occurred and lasted 2 weeks (Whisler and Voris, 1965). Combined baroreceptor and chemoreceptor block (produced by ninth and tenth nerve denervation through the use of 1 percent lignocaine) not only leads to marked hypertension but also to almost complete abolition of the hyperventilation that occurs when breathing a hypoxic gas mixture. Further, such block results in a prolongation of maximum breath-holding time at all lung volumes with alleviation of the associated distress. Other studies have shown that respiratory distress can be considered as being of vagal origin only when it occurs on lung deflation. (Guz and others, 1966a, b.)

Parasympathetic fibers carried in the ninth nerve arise in the inferior salivatory nucleus in the caudalmost pons (Fig. 10-3) and take a circuitous course in reaching the parotid gland (Fig. 12-7). The prevalent view is that the fibers emerge from the petrosal ganglion, course in the tympanic nerve to the tympanic plexus, then through the lesser superficial petrosal nerve to the otic ganglion, from which postganglionic fibers proceed via the auriculotemporal nerve to the parotid (Wallenborn, 1968). However, according to Reichert and Poth (1933), the fibers leave the ninth nerve in the region of petrosal ganglion, traverse an anastomotic branch to reach the nerve to the digastric muscle, and course up this nerve into the facial nerve trunk, then into the chorda tympani. Some fibers pass from the chorda tympani into an anastomotic branch to reach the otic ganglion, from which postganglionic fibers extend down the auriculotemporal nerve to the parotid gland, in which they terminate. Other fibers are said to supply the submaxillary and sublingual glands, taking the same route in the nervus intermedius and lingual nerve as the parasympathetic fibers running from the seventh nerve. Innervation in this manner is in accord with Reichert and Poth's (1933) observation that secretion from these glands is reduced for a significant period of time after section of the ninth nerve and that salivary secretion is also markedly and permanently diminished following section of the chorda tympani. Erickson (1936) found that only parotid secretion was affected after ninth nerve section. The postganglionic *sympathetic fibers* for the parotid gland pass from the superior cervical sympathetic ganglion to the external carotid artery, then the middle meningeal artery, to reach the otic ganglion, and then the gland (Fig. 12-7).

Loss of taste (ageusia) in the posterior third of the tongue is a highly important symptom of interruption of the ninth nerve. Taste may be tested by applying a galvanic current of ¼ to ½ ma. to the tongue; lack of the acid taste normally induced by the current indicates ageusia. Interruption of the nerve is also manifested by *anesthesia of the upper pharynx* and by *loss of the pharyngeal and palatal reflexes.* These reflexes (p. 175) are of localizing significance only when they are absent unilaterally, for they are frequently absent bilaterally under normal conditions. Since the stylopharyngeus and the pharyngopalatinus muscles (the latter supplied by the tenth nerve) participate in elevating the pharynx, paralysis is limited to the stylopharyngeus and does not become clinically manifest. With ninth nerve palsy, a reduction in salivary secretion may occur.

Isolated palsy of the ninth nerve is decidedly uncommon. As a rule, other nerves, particularly the tenth, are jointly affected, for example in fracture of the base of the skull, thrombosis of the sigmoid sinus, neoplasm situated in the lower part of the posterior cranial fossa, and aneurysm of the vertebral or basilar artery.

NEURALGIA AND OTHER IRRITATIVE PHENOMENA

Glossopharyngeal neuralgia combined or not with *vagal neuralgia* is a rare disorder occurring in persons past 30 years of age but not sharing with trigeminal neuralgia a predilection for the aged. The onset is sudden and unexpected. The first attack may not be followed by the next one until a few weeks or a few months have passed. The attacks are characterized by unilateral stabbing, shooting, or intense burning pain lasting several seconds (and in chronic stages, much longer). Successive attacks may come only after intervals of minutes, hours, or longer. Sudden cessation of the pain is as characteristic as sudden onset. The pain occurs in the base of the tongue, the soft palate, the side of the pharynx, or in the tonsillar region; it may radiate into the internal ear or, less frequently, into the back of the mandible, the upper cervical region, or even the teeth. In occasional instances the pain originates in the region of the external auditory meatus or deep in the ear, or beneath the angle of the jaw, and radiates into the pharynx, thus encompassing the territory of supply of both the ninth and tenth nerves (the auricular and pharyngeal branches of the latter). In contrast to trigeminal neuralgia, a trigger zone can only occasionally be located; usually it is found in a sharply localized area at the base of the tongue; other sites are the fauces, pharynx, and tragus of the ear. The attacks are most readily provoked by swallowing, but may be brought on by chewing, protrusion of the tongue, talking, blowing the nose, or coughing. Sometimes the ninth nerve has to be sectioned to allow the patient to swallow. Remissions can last as long as 4 years. A characteristic of this disorder is that sensory loss in the region of distribution of the pain is lacking. Glossopharyngeal-vagal neuralgia occasionally develops in the presence of a tumor of the tonsillar region or pharynx, usually a malignant tumor. The neuralgia may also be a symptom of cerebellopontile angle tumor, in which case sensory loss can usually be detected in the region of supply of the ninth and tenth nerves. Under all these conditions the neuralgia may at first be indistinguishable from that described above, but it soon tends to be continuous though interrupted by paroxysms. Spread of disturbances to the territories of adjacent nerves tends also to occur. (Bohm and Strang, 1962; Chawla and Falconer, 1967; Deparis, 1968; Peet, 1935.)

Because of involvement of the pressor nerve fibers from the carotid sinus, hypotension alone or cardiac arrest with syncope may occasionally be associated with glossopharyngeal neuralgia. Generalized convulsions occur in some attacks. In such cases, pressure on the neck in the region of the carotid sinus may induce pain at the base of the tongue and in the tonsillar region. (Ray and Stewart, 1948; White, Smithwick, and Simeone, 1952; White and Sweet, 1955.)

Glossopharyngeal and trigeminal neuralgia occasionally occur together (Brzustowicz, 1955).

Neuralgia involving a branch of the vagus, the *superior laryngeal nerve,* has also been identified. The sensory components of this nerve supply the epiglottis, the base of the tongue, and the supraglottal portion of the larynx. The initial site of the pain during attacks is in the throat in the general region of the hyoid bone and upper part of the superior thyroid cartilage (Harris, 1926; White and Sweet, 1955).

Irritative phenomena in the domain of nerves IX to XII are noted in tumor situated in the region of the foramen magnum, in which blockage in the flow of fluid into the spinal subarachnoid space is at least partly responsible. The syndrome is characterized by attacks consisting in suboccipital headache, spasm or contracture of neck muscles, increasing tachypnea, vasomotor disturbances in the face and neck, and pharyngeal spasms on swallowing. Moreover, tumors of the lower brainstem involving the floor of the fourth ventricle may give rise to persistent hiccup and be associated with pains referable to the heart, stomach, gallbladder, and so on.

The *tongue* is subject to spasm and to tonic and clonic contractions, and the neck muscles to spasm, but the origin of these disturbances is usually obscure. As a rule, motor hyperactivity of the *pharynx, larynx, and esophagus* is not traceable to lesions involving the tenth nerve. Now and then these conditions are part and parcel of an extrapyramidal disorder. Frequently they are reflexive in origin, with the lesion in the respiratory or the gastrointestinal tract. They are also occasionally observed in tetany, tabes dorsalis, rabies, and tetanus.

DISTINCTION BETWEEN LESIONS AT SUPRANUCLEAR, NUCLEAR, AND INFRANUCLEAR LEVELS

Since irritative symptoms and signs originating in nerves IX through XII are often to be discounted as being of little value in the localization of lesions, one has to depend, in localization, upon evidence of a reduction in their functions. When confronted with a patient who has manifestations of a bulbar disorder, it is necessary to ascertain the level at which the pathways from the cerebral cortex to the periphery have been interrupted—whether between the cerebral cortex and medulla oblongata *(supranuclear),* in the region of the brainstem nuclei *(nuclear),* or in the nerves as they pursue their intramedullary and peripheral courses *(infranuclear),* and in the latter whether intracranial or extracranial.

Unilateral supranuclear lesions

As far as motor function is concerned, lesions of supranuclear location are characterized by paresis and by lack of atrophy in the affected muscles. Moreover, the reaction of degeneration (R.D.) is absent. In later stages the involved muscles may exhibit increased mechanical irritability.

A special feature of nerves IX through XII is that they have bilateral supranuclear innervation, that is, both cerebral hemispheres participate in the innervation of each nucleus. The tenth nerve is an outstanding example. Because of bilateral supranuclear innervation, unilateral interruption of the fibers to the nucleus ambiguus does not cause clinically detectable disturbances: one hemisphere remains in unbroken communication with the nucleus ambiguus of each side, which suffices to maintain the functions of the pharyngeal and laryngeal muscles of both sides (Fig. 12-8). In unilateral pharyngoplegia and laryngoplegia, one can therefore be certain that the site of the lesion is nuclear or infranuclear.

The same applies in part to the eleventh and twelfth nerves. In supranuclear lesions (such as cerebral infarct), the function of the eleventh nerve in supplying the sternocleidomastoid is not appreciably altered. The assumption thus is warranted that this muscle receives adequate bilateral cortical innervation. By contrast, the tra-

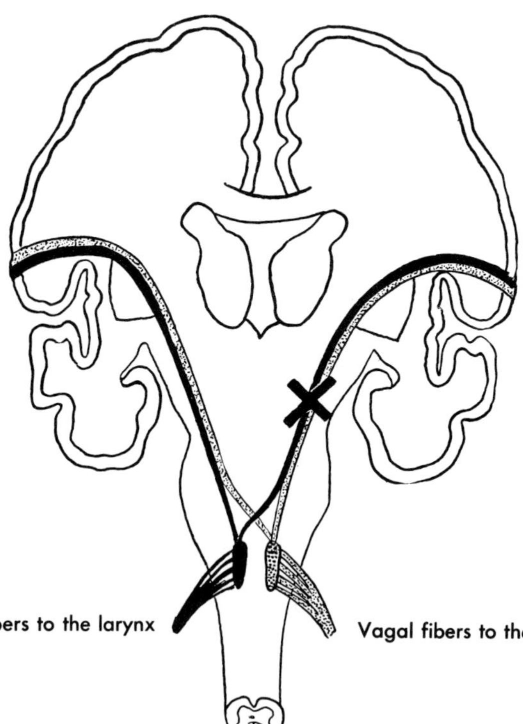

Fig. 12-8. The supranuclear and infranuclear fibers concerned in innervation of the larynx. The infranuclear fibers originate in the nucleus ambiguus. Since each of these nuclei receives fibers from the cortex bilaterally, a supranuclear lesion involving one side (at X) does not produce laryngeal paralysis.

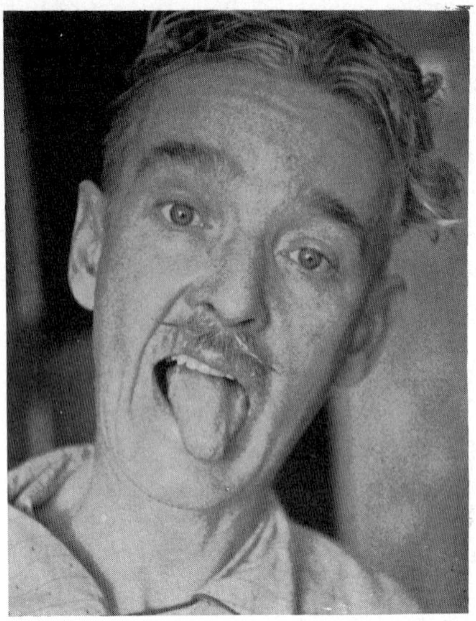

Fig. 12-9. Deviation of the tongue to the left (the paretic side) in the presence of a tumor of the right frontal lobe. The lower part of the left side of the face is also paretic. (Courtesy Dr. A. Ornsteen, Philadelphia.)

pezius muscle retains normal function only in its lower half, because only this part of the muscle derives a supply from both hemispheres and then by way of the upper cervical roots. Involvement of supranuclear fibers passing to the nucleus of the twelfth nerve of one side is also not of much import functionally. Even nuclear or infranuclear paralysis does not seriously affect motility of the tongue because the palsied side is so closely linked with the normal side by interlacing fibers. In supranuclear lesions there is merely a deviation of the protruded tongue toward the paralyzed side (Fig. 12-9).

Only certain of the cranial nerves—the twelfth and the seventh—are implicated by unilateral pyramidal tract lesions. On the other hand, the nucleus ambiguus of the tenth nerve and the motor nucleus of the fifth have a bilateral cortical innervation and are therefore involved only by lesions of the corticobulbar tracts of the two sides. Interruption of the corticobulbar tracts must be bilateral in order to interfere with the lips as instruments of speech.

Disturbances of nuclear origin

From a clinical standpoint, nuclear lesions of cranial nerves IX to XII can be easily distinguished from those of supranuclear origin. R.D. is readily demonstrable in the tongue, sternocleidomastoid, and upper trapezius, but is somewhat more difficult to detect in the palate and pharynx. Paralysis of the larynx may be demonstrated by electrically stimulating the neck over the region of the recurrent laryngeal nerve. Interruption of the tenth nerve can be assumed if the stimulation (which should be strong) fails to adduct the vocal cords. In lesions involving the nucleus of the twelfth nerve, the tongue is small, deeply furrowed, soft, and flabby, and is beset by fascicular contractions.

Disturbances of infranuclear origin

Nuclear and infranuclear paralyses are less easily distinguished. Where difficulty exists in determining whether the lesion is in the nucleus or in the intramedullary or extramedullary course of a nerve, the presence or the absence of indications of involvement of other structures provides the clue. The medulla oblongata is so small that a lesion rarely damages only the nucleus or the intramedullary fibers of the respective nerves. Even if only one of these nuclei is damaged, disturbances of sensibility and motility usually occur, with the paralysis most commonly of the alternating type (paralysis alterna). The twelfth nuclei of the two sides are so close together that a lesion that affects one often encroaches on the other, causing bilateral paralysis of the tongue. A lesion involving the twelfth nucleus produces not only lingual paralysis but also ipsilateral paresis of the orbicularis oris muscle, or even atrophy, a point of considerable localizing value in view of the absence of orbicularis oris involvement in infranuclear twelfth nerve lesions.

Because of this observation it seems logical to assume that the twelfth nucleus participates with the seventh nucleus in supplying the orbicularis oris. It is possible that the fibers in question pass from the twelfth nucleus to the seventh nerve, as illustrated in Fig. 14-5, but it is just as possible that the connection is affected through anastomoses between the twelfth and seventh nerves at the periphery.

Combined paralyses of cranial nerves IX through XII may be brought about by pathological processes in the posterior cranial fossa, such as meningitis, tumor, or aneurysm. The resultant syndromes include paralysis of the palate, larynx, tongue, and sternocleidomastoid and trapezius muscles in various combinations. The orbicularis oris is usually spared. The sequence in which the symptoms and signs develop often provides the clue to the precise site of the lesion and sometimes its nature.

Simultaneous interruption of three or all four of these nerves as they pursue their *extracranial* courses is of rare occurrence, and then usually results from a lesion in the most superior side of the neck, where inspection, palpation, and x-ray studies will usually reveal the cause of the disorder. Trauma due to the penetration of missiles is a common cause (Aldrich and Baker, 1948; Purves-Stewart and Evans, 1919). Interruption of the tenth nerve rarely affects deglutition because the branches to the muscles in question are given off from the uppermost part of this nerve. If the tenth nerve is damaged in its course through the mediastinum (for example, by a neoplasm or an aneurysm of the aorta), the only branch affected is the recurrent laryngeal, which supplies the ipsilateral vocal cord. If the twelfth nerve is interrupted in the region where it joins the upper cervical nerves to form the ansa hypoglossi, not only will there be glossoplegia on that side but also paralysis of the ansa-innervated external laryngeal muscles (sternohyoid, sternothyroid, omohyoid), as manifested by atrophy of the muscles overlying the thyroid cartilage and by lateral displacement of the larynx on swallowing. Tumor (neurinoma) of the ninth nerve intracranially resembles acoustic neuroma symptomatically (Naunton, Proctor, and Elpern, 1968).

Some of the better known syndromes of involvement of cranial nerves IX to XII are the following:

Involvement of all four nerves, as manifested by loss of taste in the posterior third of the tongue (IX), paralysis of the soft palate and vocal cord (X), paralysis of the sternocleidomastoid and trapezius (XI), and hemianesthesia of the soft palate, pharynx, and larynx (IX and X) *(syndrome of Collet-Sicard)*. This syndrome is most frequently caused by missile wounds deep in the retroparotid region. Such a case is illustrated in part in Figs. 12-2 and 12-3; in addition, the missile interrupted cranial nerves VII (Fig. 14-3) and VIII. Involvement of cranial nerves X and XI in their intracranial course is usually known as *Schmidt's syndrome;* but in the case Schmidt (1897) described, the twelfth was also affected (vertebral artery aneurysm was suspected). If nerves X and XI plus the cervical sympathetic trunk are affected, the disorder is called *Tapia's syndrome;* tachycardia may be an added feature. Involvement of cranial nerves X, XI, and XII is usually referred to as *Jackson's syndrome;* but in the cases which Jackson (1886) and Jackson and Mackenzie (1870) described, emphasis was placed on paralysis of the tongue, soft palate, and vocal cords, although in some instances there was evidence of involvement of other cranial nerves as well. Signs of pyramidal tract injury were also occasionally noted.

Skull fracture involving the region of the *jugular foramen,* whether resulting from the penetration of a missile or from some other form of trauma, tends to damage nerves IX and XI and sometimes X as well (*Vernet's syndrome* or *jugular foramen syndrome;* see Rivers, Svien, and Baker, 1963). Tumor occupying the jugular foramen may have the same effect; if the pericarotid sympathetic fibers are involved, Horner's syndrome will also be evident. A variation, observed in tumor (meningioma) attached to the lateral wall of the posterior cranial fossa, consisted in palsy of nerve X (dysphagia, hoarseness) and nerve XI, also hearing deficit and diplopia on looking toward the ipsilateral side (Cherington, 1968).

In basal meningitis, tabes dorsalis, spread of an inflammatory process from the mastoid (Fox and West, 1947), or prolonged lowering of the shoulder due to holding a heavy weight, there may be paralysis of the laryngeal and palatal branches of the tenth nerve *(Avellis' syndrome)*. To the syndrome of Avellis may be added miosis *(Cestan-Chenais' syndrome)*. Paralysis of the twelfth, the tenth (either above or below the level at which branches are given off to the soft palate and pharynx), and the cervical sympathetic, is known as *Villaret's syndrome;* the seventh nerve is sometimes affected also. This syndrome commonly occurs following the lodgement of a missile between the mastoid process and the neck of the mandible. It may also be due to parotid tumor, carotid aneurysm, or abscess of the cervical region secondary to suppurative mastoiditis.

REFERENCES

Aldrich, E. M., and Baker, G. S. 1948. Injuries of the hypoglossal nerve: report of ten cases. Mil. Surgeon **103**:20-25.

Alexander, E., Jr., Wigser, S. M., and Davis, C. H. 1966. Bilateral extracranial aneurysms of the internal carotid artery: case report. J. Neurosurg. **25**:437-442.

Bicknell, J. M., Greenhouse, A. H., and Pesch, R. N. 1968. Spastic dysphonia. J. Neurol. Neurosurg. Psychiat. **31**:158-161.

Bohm, E., and Strang, R. R. 1962. Glossopharyngeal neuralgia. Brain **85**:371-388.

Brzustowicz, R. J. 1955. Combined trigeminal and glossopharyngeal neuralgia. Neurology **5**: 1-10.

Camishion, R. C., Gibbon, J. H., Jr., Pierucci, L., Jr., and Iida, J. 1966. Paralysis of the left recurrent laryngeal nerve secondary to mitral valvular disease: report of two cases and literature review. Ann. Surg. **163**:818-828.

Chawla, J. C., and Falconer, M. A. 1967. Glossopharyngeal and vagal neuralgia. Brit. Med. J. **3**: 529-531.

Cherington, M. 1968. Accessory nerve: conduction studies. Arch. Neurol. **18**:708-709.

Clarke, S. D., Penry, J. B., and Ward, P. 1965. Oesophageal reflux after vagotomy. Lancet **2**: 824-826.

Clerf, L. H. 1955. Bilateral abductor paralysis of the larynx; results of treatment by modified King operation. Ann. Otol. **64**:38-46.

Dandy, W. E. 1927. Glossopharyngeal neuralgia (tic douloureux): its diagnosis and treatment. Arch. Surg. **15**:198-214.

Dandy, W. E. 1945. Surgery of the brain. In Lewis, D., editor: Practice of surgery, vol. 12. Hagerstown, Maryland, W. F. Prior Company, Inc.

de Castella, H., and Irvine, W. T. 1967. The role of the vagus in the antral response to food. Brit. J. Surg. **54**:828-831.

Deparis, M. 1968. Glossopharyngeal neuralgia. In Vinken, P. J., and Bruyn, G. W., editors: Handbook of neurology, vol. 5. Amsterdam, North-Holland Publishing Company, pp. 350-361.

Erickson, T. C. 1936. Paroxysmal neuralgia of tympanic branch of the glossopharyngeal nerve; report of a case in which relief was obtained by intracranial section of the glossopharyngeal nerve. Arch. Neurol. Psychiat. **35**:1070-1074.

Fox, S. L., and West, G. B., Jr. 1947. Syndrome of Avellis: a review of the literature and report of one case. Arch. Otolaryng. **46**:773-778.

Friedman, S., and Goffin, F. B. 1966. Abductor vocal weakness in myasthenia gravis: report of a case. Laryngoscope **76**:1520-1523.

Furstenberg, A. C., and Magielski, J. E. 1955. A motor pattern in the nucleus ambiguus: its clinical significance. Ann. Otol. **64**:788-793.

Gorman, J. B., and Woodward, F. D. 1965. Bilateral paralysis of the vocal cords: management of twenty-five cases. Southern Med. J. **58**: 34-38.

Greenwood, R. K., Schlegel, J. F., Code, C. F., and Ellis, F. H., Jr. 1962. The effect of sympathectomy, vagotomy, and oesophageal interruption on the canine gastro-oesophageal sphincter. Thorax **17**:310-319.

Guillory, J. R., and Clagett, O. T. 1967. Postvagotomy dysphagia. Surg. Clin. N. Amer. **47**: 833-839.

Guz, A., Noble, M. I. M., Widdicombe, J. G., Trenchard, D., and Mushin, W. W. 1966a. Peripheral chemoreceptor block in man. Resp. Physiol. **1**:38-40.

Guz, A., Noble, M. I. M., Widdicombe, J. G., Trenchard, D., Mushin, W. W., and Makey, A. R. 1966b. The role of the vagal and glossopharyngeal afferent nerves in respiratory sensation, control of breathing and arterial pressure regulation in conscious man. Clin. Sci. **30**: 161-170.

Harris, W. 1926. Neuritis and neuralgia. London, Oxford University Press, pp. 375-377.

Haymaker, W., and Woodhall, B. 1953. Peripheral nerve injuries: principles of diagnosis, ed. 2. Philadelphia, W. B. Saunders Company.

Holl-Allen, R. T. J. 1967. Laryngeal nerve paralysis and benign thyroid disease. Arch. Otolaryng. **85**:335-337.

Hwang, K., Essex, H. E., and Mann. F. C. 1947. Study of certain problems resulting from vagotomy in dogs with special reference to emesis. Amer. J. Physiol. **149**:429-448.

Jackson, J. H. 1886. Paralysis and wasting of the right side of the tongue, and paralysis of the right side of the palate and the right side of the vocal cord. Lancet **1**:689-690.

Jackson, J. H., and Mackenzie, M. 1870. Cases of palsies of several cranial nerves, including the nerves of the larynx, all on the left side—weakness of the limbs of the right side. Med. Times Gaz. **1**:34-35.

James, T. N. 1967. Cardiac innervation: anatomic and pharmacologic relations. Bull. N. Y. Acad. Med. **43**:1041-1086.

Legge, T. M., and Goadby, K. W. 1912. Lead poisoning and lead absorption. New York, Longmans, Green & Co.

Léri, A., and Boudet, G. 1910. Hémiplégie d'origine bulbo-médullaire chez un tabétique. (Contribution à l'étude des paralyses du spinal dans le tabes.) Rev. Neurol. **19**:561-564.

Lewis, D., and Dandy, W. E. 1930. The course of the nerve fibers transmitting sensation of taste. Arch. Surg. **21**:249-288.

Morrison, L. F. 1945. Further observations on the King operation for bilateral abductor paralysis. Ann. Otol. **54**:390-408.

Myerson, M. C. 1934. Paralysis of the larynx due to lead poisoning; including a contradiction to "Semon's law." Arch. Otolaryng. **20**:659-664.

Naffziger, H. C., Davis, C., and Bell, H. G. 1948. Paralysis of deglutition: surgical correction. Ann. Surg. **128**:732-742.

Naunton, R. F., Proctor, L., and Elpern, B. S. 1968. The audiologic signs of ninth nerve neuroma. Acta Otolaryng. **87**:222-227.

Pearson, A. A., Sauter, R. W., and Herrin, G. R. 1964. The accessory nerve and its relation to the upper spinal nerves. Amer. J. Anat. **114**: 371-392.

Peet, M. M. 1935. Glossopharyngeal neuralgia. Arch. Surg. **101**:256-268.

Postlethwait, R. W., Kim, S. K., and Dillon, M. L.

1969. Esophageal complications of vagotomy. Surg. Gynec. Obstet. **128**:481-488.

Purves-Stewart, J., and Evans, A. 1919. Nerve injuries and their treatment, ed. 2. London, Frowde, pp. 108-128.

Ray, B. S., and Stewart, H. J. 1948. Glossopharyngeal neuralgia: a cause of cardiac arrest. Amer. Heart J. **35**:458-462.

Reichert, F. L. 1934. Neuralgias of the glossopharyngeal nerve with particular reference to the sensory, gustatory and secretory functions of the nerve. Arch. Neurol. Psychiat. **32**:1030-1037.

Reichert, F. L., and Poth, E. J. 1933. Recent knowledge regarding the physiology of the glossopharyngeal nerve in man with an analysis of its sensory, motor, gustatory and secretory functions. Bull. Johns Hopk. Hosp. **53**:131-139.

Rhoton, A. L., Jr. 1968. Afferent connections of the facial nerve. J. Comp. Neurol. **133**:89-100.

Rhoton, A. L., Jr., O'Leary, J. L., and Ferguson, J. P. 1966. The trigeminal, facial, vagal, and glossopharyngeal nerves in the monkey: afferent connections. Arch. Neurol. **14**:530-540.

Rivers, M. H., Svien, H. J., and Baker, H. L. 1963. Diagnostic principles in the jugular foramen syndrome. Surg. Clin. N. Amer. **132**:1129-1133.

Schmidt, M. 1897. Die Krankheiten der oberen Luftwege, ed. 2. Berlin, Springer-Verlag, p. 48.

Sicard and Bollack. 1912. Hémiplégie linguale, laryngo-pharyngienne et cléido-trapézienne avec tachycardie. Rev. Neurol. **2**:743-744.

Stankey, R. M., Roshe, J., and Sogocio, R. M. 1969. Carcinoma of the lung and dysphagia. Dis. Chest **55**:13-17.

Straus, W. L., Jr., and Howell, A. B. 1936. The spinal accessory nerve and its musculature. Quart. Rev. Biol. **11**:387-402.

Truex, R. C. 1959. Strong and Elwin's human neuroanatomy, ed. 4. Baltimore, The Williams & Wilkins Co.

Uihlein, A., Love, J. G., and Corbin, K. B. 1955. Intracranial section of the glossopharyngeal nerve: sensory changes observed postoperatively. Arch. Neurol. Psychiat. **74**:320-324.

Wallenborn, W. McK. 1968. Parotid gland atrophy produced by transtympanic destruction of the tympanic plexus. Laryngoscope **78**:132-144.

Whisler, W. W., and Voris, H. C. 1965. Effect of bilateral glossopharyngeal nerve section on blood pressure: a case report. J. Neurosurg. **23**:78-81.

White, J. C., Smithwick, R. H., and Simeone, F. A. 1952. The autonomic nervous system: anatomy, physiology and surgical application, ed. 3. New York, The Macmillan Company.

White, J. C., and Sweet, W. H. 1955. Pain: its mechanisms and neurosurgical control. Springfield, Illinois, Charles C Thomas, Publisher.

Williams, R. G. 1959. Idiopathic recurrent laryngeal nerve paralysis. J. Laryng. **73**:161-166.

Wycis, H. 1945. Bilateral intracranial section of the glossopharyngeal nerve. Arch. Neurol. Psychiat. **54**:344-347.

Chapter 13

Localization of lesions involving the statoacoustic nerve

Jorge Huertas
Webb Haymaker

The statoacoustic nerve, or eighth cranial nerve, consists of two parts. One is the vestibular nerve, which transmits impulses concerned in orientation of the body in space (static), and the other is the cochlear nerve, which subserves hearing (acoustic). United in a common trunk, though separated in some degree by a connective tissue septum (Rasmussen, 1940), the two nerves pass centrally through the internal auditory meatus in company with the facial nerve and the nervus intermedius, and after traversing the region of the cerebellopontile angle they enter the brainstem and run separate courses.

The specialized function of the statoacoustic nerve is reflected in the structure of its receptor organs. These organs are located in relation to the membranous labyrinth in the inner ear and are of three different types: *cristae,* situated in the ampullae of the semicircular canals (concerned in perception of rotation of the head), *otoliths,* in the utricle and saccule (concerned in the perception of linear displacements and gravity), and the *organ of Corti,* in the cochlea (concerned in the perception of sound). In spite of the differences in form of these three types of sensory complex, their basic structure is quite stereotyped. The functional unit is a rather large colony of sensory, or hair, cells typically arranged. One surface of these cells has a series of cilia, or hairs, which are embedded in a matrix (gelatinous in the case of the vestibular end-organs, and collagenous in the case of the tectorial membrane of the organ of Corti). The lower pole of each hair cell is in relation to nerve endings.

The membranous labyrinth (the three semicircular canals with their ampullae, the utricle, the saccule, and the cochlear duct) is a closed system filled with fluid, the endolymph. The vestibular and cochlear end-organs lie in contact with the endolymph situated in the cochlear duct, but they do not contain endolymph. The endo-

Table 13-1. Electrolyte content of endolymph and perilymph (in the cat)*

Constituent	*Utricular endolymph*	*Perilymph*
Sodium (mEq./L.)	26 (8)†	148 (12)†
Potassium (mEq./L.)	142 (9)	5 (12)
Chloride (mEq./L.)	110 (3)	120 (9)
Protein (mg./100 g.)	25 (6)	75 (6)
Nonprotein nitrogen (mg./100 g.)	21.5 (6)	20 (6)

*From Citron, Exley, and Hallpike, 1956.
†Values in parentheses refer to the number of analyses made.

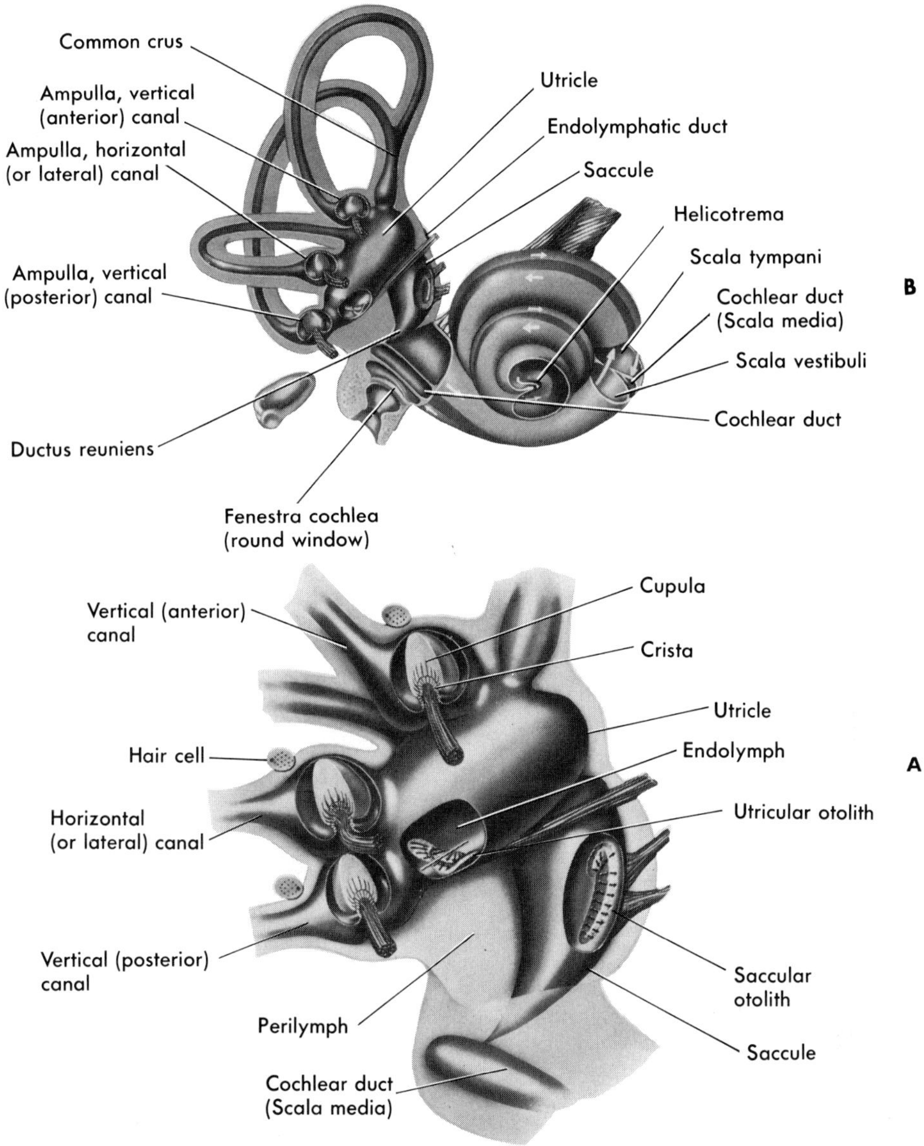

Fig. 13-1. A, View of the right labyrinth as seen from in front. The bony labyrinth has been removed. Light gray represents the perilymphatic space, in which the membranous labyrinth (in black) is bathed. The membranous semicircular canals occupy about one-fourth the diameter of the bony labyrinth and "float" in the perilymph (they are held in place by delicate connective tissue strands). Endolymph fills the four compartments of the membranous labyrinth: (1) the *semicircular canals,* communicating with the utricle through an aperture; (2) the *utricle,* communicating on one side with the semicircular canals and on the other side with the saccule by means of a duct; (3) the *saccule,* communicating with the utricle and also with the cochlear duct through the ductus reuniens; and (4) the *cochlear duct* (or scala media), communicating with the saccule as indicated. The helicotrema is a small passage that connects the scala tympani with the scala vestibuli at the apex of the cochlea. The stapes has been removed. Its base fits into the oval window (not illustrated).

B, Enlarged view of the vestibular compartment. The hair cells in cross section are indicated to the left side of each ampulla. Polarity (orientation) of the stereocilia to the kinocilium (the heavy dot) is indicated. (Polarity refers to the direction of flow of endolymph from stereocilia toward the kinocilium that will bend the cupula and its hair cells and thus initiate a neural response.) Polarity of the hair cells of the utricular otolith and the saccular otolith is indicated by arrows. The utricular otolith has a concave surface, the saccular otolith a convex surface. The white line crossing the middle of the utricular otolith indicates the level at which polarity of the hair cells is reversed. (Courtesy NASA, Ames Research Center, Moffett Field, California.)

lymph is partly a plasma filtrate originating from the vestibular and cochlear stria vascularis and partly a secretion originating from specialized cells located alongside the cristae (Fig. 13-1). Endolymph outflow takes place mainly from the endolymphatic sac, the endolymph then entering the venous system surrounding the sac. (Dohlman, 1968.) All the membranous system is suspended from the surrounding bony labyrinth by loose connective tissue bathed in perilymph, the latter probably a filtrate of cerebrospinal fluid (Palva and Raunio, 1968). Perilymph filters through the basilar membrane of the cochlear duct into the spaces within the organ of Corti but not into the vestibular end-organs. The electrolyte content of the endolymph and perilymph is indicated in Table 13-1. The values signify that the differences in electrolyte content between endolymph and intracellular fluids are very small, also that potassium is in far higher concentration in the endolymph than in the perilymph. Possibly, Reissner's membrane functions as a simple isolator, allowing the passage of sodium but not potassium from the cochlear duct (scala media) to the scala vestibuli.

The membranous labyrinth is divided into two parts: the vestibular labyrinth and the auditory labyrinth. Considered phylogenetically, the pars inferior of the system—the cochlea and the saccule—is the newer part (Schuknecht, Igarashi, and Gacek, 1965).

End-organs in both parts of the labyrinth receive *efferent* fibers from the brainstem. The fibers reaching the vestibular labyrinth terminate in the vestibular epithelium in the form of vesiculated nerve endings. They originate in the ipsilateral vestibular nuclear complex (mainly, if not entirely, in the lateral and spinal vestibular nuclei), and travel distally in the vestibular nerve as a compact bundle dorsal to the efferent cochlear bundle. In the cat there are about 300 efferent fibers as compared with 1,200 afferent fibers in the vestibular nerve. As to the efferent fibers reaching the organ of Corti, they originate in the superior olivary nucleus in the pons, and they represent the final link in the neuron chains arising in the auditory cortex and coursing downward, parallel with the upgoing auditory pathway. Apparently the fibers terminating in the vestibular and auditory labyrinths have an inhibitory action on nerve elements in the respective end-organs, and apparently the fibers also serve in vestibular and cochlear adaptation and habituation. (Gacek, 1968a, b; Galambos, 1956; Iurato, 1962; Nomura and Kirikae, 1967; Rasmussen, 1960.)

Blood supply is from various sources. The bony otic capsule receives its supply from a branch of the basilar artery (arteria subarcuata) and from

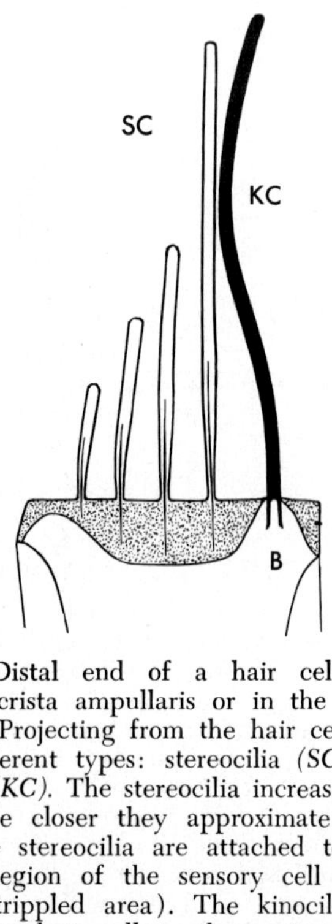

Fig. 13-2. Distal end of a hair cell (sensory cell) in a crista ampullaris or in the macula of an otolith. Projecting from the hair cell are cilia of two different types: stereocilia *(SC)* and the kinocilium *(KC)*. The stereocilia increase in length stepwise the closer they approximate the kinocilium. The stereocilia are attached to the hair cell in a region of the sensory cell called the cuticule (strippled area). The kinocilium is attached to its hair cell in the region called the centriole *(B)*. The base of the hair cell, with which nerve endings come into relation, is not illustrated. When fluid circulates from *SC* toward *KC* a shearing effect is produced which bends the hairs, inducing a facilitatory response. If the fluid circulates in the opposite direction the response by the hair cell is inhibitory. Because of this peculiarity, the hair cell is said to have a *polarity* determined by the orientation of the kinocilium to the stereocilia or vice versa.

branches of the external carotid and ascending pharyngeal arteries (arteriae tympanica inferior, meningea media, mastoidea recurrens, stylomastoidea, stylomastoidea accessorius). The membranous otic labyrinth is supplied by the internal auditory artery through its three branches: the vestibular artery, the vestibulocochlear artery (which supplies the basal turn of the cochlea and parts of the vestibular system), and the cochlear artery (which enters the modiolus and gives rise to spiral arteries). (Bast and Anson, 1949; Rüedi, 1965.)

VESTIBULAR END-ORGANS AND NERVE

Anatomy and functions

The vestibular end-organs are of two types: the cristae ampullares and the maculae of the utricle and the saccule (Fig. 13-1).

1. A crista ampullaris is situated in the widened (ampullated) end of each of the three semicircular canals. Three semicircular canals representing the three dimensions of space in the labyrinth are present on each side of the skull, one horizontal and two vertical canals: anterior and posterior (six altogether).

The sensory epithelium of each crista ampullaris is composed of hair cells (sensory cells) and supporting cells. Projecting from each hair cell are many stereocilia (75 to 100) and a single kinocilium. All the cilia are embedded in a gelatinous cupula that reaches the roof of the ampulla (Fig. 13-1). In the crista ampullaris all the hair cells are arranged in the same fashion. All kinocilia in the same ampulla are polarized toward the same side. The stereocilia vary in length; the longest bristles are closest to the kinocilium, and the shortest the farthest away (Fig. 13-2). In the horizontal canals the polarization of the kinocilium is toward the utricle (utriculopetal); in the vertical canals the polarization of the kinocilium is away from the utricle (utriculofugal). Flow of endolymph will stimulate (facilitate) the hair cells only when it occurs in the direction from the stereocilia toward the kinocilium. Flow in the opposite direction will inhibit the formation of a generator potential. A hair cell responds with facilitation or inhibition most forcefully when a stimulus is applied at a 90 degree angle to the hair (shearing force). (The common belief that the cells are pressed like a spring is not valid.) The impedance for ventriculopetal flow (in the horizontal canals) is less than the impedance produced by the ventriculofugal flow (in the vertical canals). Less energy is therefore required to stimulate the horizontal canals during lateral motion (Trincker, 1957).

The six semicircular canals are illustrated in Fig. 13-3. The canals are located in the temporal bone at the lateral pole of the vestibular apparatus. They are arranged in pairs having complementary functions. The two horizontal canals form one unit, the anterior vertical canal of one side together with the posterior vertical canal of the other side constitute another unit, and the two remaining canals form the third unit.

The *two horizontal canals,* right and left, are each shaped like a horseshoe, with the opening facing forward. Viewed from the side, the plane of the horizontal canals is tilted 30 degrees over the

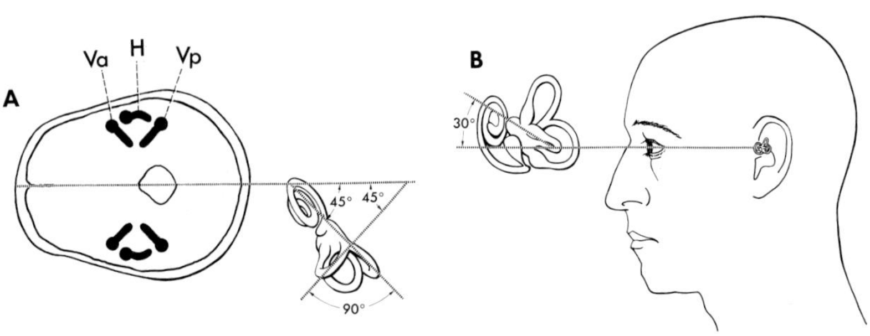

Fig. 13-3. Orientation of the semicircular canals. **A,** Base of the skull as seen from above. The horizontal *(H),* vertical anterior *(Va),* and vertical posterior *(Vp)* semicircular canals are indicated. The enlargements represent the ampullae of the semicircular canals. The horizontal semicircular canals of the two sides are located in such a way that rotation of the head produces a displacement of the endolymph in different directions with respect to the ampullae. The vertical semicircular canals are oriented at a 45-degree angle to the horizontal. The left anterior semicircular canal is parallel with the right posterior semicircular canal. The mechanism of action in these canals is similar to that in the horizontal canals. Bending the head to the right will stimulate the anterior semicircular canal in a direction away from the ampulla (ampullofugal), and the left posterior semicircular canal in a direction toward the ampulla (ampullopetal), thus establishing a reciprocal interaction between the right and the left semicircular canal systems.

B, The relative position of the horizontal semicircular canal within the head and in relation to the equator of the eye. On forward gaze the horizontal canal is 30 degrees above the horizontal. Therefore, the normal position for maximal stimulation of the horizontal canal is with the head inclined downward, as in reading.

horizontal (Fig. 13-3, *B*). The lowest part of the canals is the posterior arch. The ampullary part is located in the outer arm. The endolymph must flow from the canal into the utricle (utriculopetal) in order to stimulate the hair cells at the crista (by deflecting the cupula). Lateral rotation of the head, with the odontoid process the axis, will therefore stimulate the horizontal semicircular canal of the side toward which the rotation is performed, whereas the opposite side is inhibited.

In the case of the *vertical* canals the situation differs slightly. Both vertical canals have one common limb, and the two free circlings contain the ampullae and cristae. The plane of the anterior vertical canal is at an angle of 45 degrees (supplementary angle) to the sagittal plane, and the posterior vertical is at an angle of 45 degrees (supplementary angle) to the sagittal plane (Fig. 13-3, *A*). The flow of endolymph that stimulates the hair cells of the vertical canals, in contrast to the horizontal, is ampullofugal; the endolymph has to be "funneled" into the ampulla and semicircular canal. Inclination of the head forward and laterally will therefore stimulate the anterior canal of the same side and inhibit of posterior canal of the opposite side. Lifting the head in the same angle will produce the inverse action.

2. The utricle and the saccule each contain a *macula*. The sensory epithelium of each of the maculae consists of hair cells and supporting cells, the hair cells having stereocilia and a kinocilium; all these cells are embedded in a gelatinous matrix that contains statoconia (otoconia, or statoliths) (calcium carbonate crystals having a specific gravity of 2.7). The whole unit—the macula, the gelatinous matrix, and the crystals (statoconia)—is called the *otolith* (Fig. 13-1). The hair cells are arranged in groups in accordance with orientation of the cilia, which reach out in many different directions.

The *macula of the utricle* is located on the floor of the utricle (Fig. 13-1). When the head is upright, the macula is oriented, in general, parallel with the ground (the posterior end is horizontal, while the anterior end is elevated, forming with the horizontal an inclined plane of about 45 degrees). The shape and relative position of the macula is that of the hands of a person who extends them in front of him, with palms up, to catch a falling object. As in the cristae in the ampulla of the semicircular canals, the hair cells in the utricular macula are polarized, but the polarization is not as simple as in the cristae. "The direction of polarization spreads fan-like from the medial and anterior part of the macula up to a curved boundary line beyond which the polarization of the sensory hairs is reversed" (Spoendlin, 1965). Hence, half of the macula is stimulated by displacement of the otoliths in one direction, whereas the other half is inhibited, and vice versa. Tilting of the head produces a shearing effect, which will stimulate the hair cells. The utricular macula is the organ stimulated by the force of gravity. Fig. 13-4 shows the sites of the two maculae, one on each side, and indicates that the interplay of surfaces by tilting is similar to the reciprocal interplay described for heterolateral semicircular canals by rotation.

The *macula of the saccule* is an elongated structure that lies vertical to the ground when the head is upright. It has a different polarization than that described for the crista ampullaris or for the macula utriculi. As seen from above, it has a curved ridge down its center. The top of the ridge divides the macula into two slopes. Polarization of all the cells of each slope is *away from* the polarization of the other slope (Fig. 13-1). The vertical orientation of the macula and the "roof-like arrangement in which the cells are polarized" suggest that the statoconia (the crystals) are displaced by linear accelerations in the forward direction.

To summarize: The utricular macula and the saccular macula have surface orientation in different planes (Fig. 13-1). The surface of the utricular macula is essentially horizontal though somewhat concave, while the surface of the saccular macula is essentially vertical, having slopes on either side. Consequently, in the case of the utricle, acceleratory forces coming in one direction will excite the hair cells

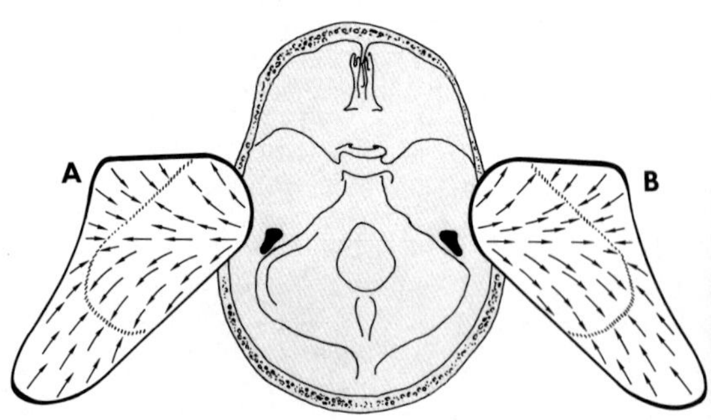

Fig. 13-4. Schematic representation of the position of the utricular maculae in the cranium. Note their relation to the foramen magnum. The dotted lines represent the striole of the maculae, that is, the anatomical boundary at which polarity of the hair cells is changed by 180 degrees. The arrows show the direction of the acceleratory force on the otoconia which will stimulate the hair cells. It is important to keep in mind that from the coronal axis forward the maculae are curled up (Fig. 13-1). For each direction of motion two components of the same macula become activated: facilitation on one side of the macula (up to the striole) and inhibition on the other side. By tilting this figure the reader can get an idea as to the parts of the maculae that will be stimulated with each motion, whether that motion is, for example, lateral or anterior-posterior. For instance, if the head is tilted to the right the hair cells to the left of the striole in *A* will be stimulated, while the hair cells to the right in *A* will be inhibited. (Modified from Spoendlin, 1965.)

of one population and an acceleratory force from the opposite direction will excite another population. These two populations are separated by a boundary line reaching along the axis of the macula. By contrast, in the case of the saccule the acceleratory forces excite an anatomical system that diverges from a central boundary line, and so produce a stimulatory effect. To put it in another way, the utricular macula is comparable to a funnel in which the stimulatory acceleratory forces converge, while the saccular macula is comparable to an arched roof in that the stimulatory forces diverge from a central line.

It is accepted that the utricular macula is stimulated by vertically directed acceleratory forces, particularly by the acceleratory forces of gravity. This happens mainly during the tilting of the head. But because of the special arrangement of the hair cells, not all the acceleratory forces have to be directed in the vertical direction in order to stimulate the macula; the utricular macula can be stimulated even by horizontally directed acceleration. In the case of the saccule, anatomical characteristics suggest that it is stimulated particularly by acceleratory forces directed in the anteroposterior plane, as when the face is displaced forward. In general, the maculae of the utricle and the saccule have an arrangement by which acceleration in any direction will stimulate or inhibit a specific population of hair cells.

The vestibular end-organs act in two spheres: (1) they reinforce muscular tonus while a person is in any stationary position, and (2) they trigger the central mechanisms that produce an appropriate muscular contraction in response to changes in head and body position.

The cell station of the vestibular nerve is in Scarpa's ganglion, situated within the internal auditory canal. Cell bodies in this ganglion form a superior and an inferior division. Their respective dendrites make up the superior and inferior branches of the vestibular nerve. The superior division innervates the cristae of the superior and horizontal canals and the maculae of the utricle and of part of the saccule; the inferior division innervates the cristae of the posterior canal and most of the saccular macula (Wersäll, 1960).

Axons of the vestibular nerve terminate in four vestibular nuclei: *superior, lateral, medial,* and *spinal* (or *inferior*) (Fig. 13-5).

Vestibular pathways in the central nervous system

To be considered in the following are: (1) the pathways from the utricular and the saccular maculae and from the cristae of the semicircular canals, (2) the vestibulospinal tract, (3) the components of the medial longitudinal fasciculus, and (4) the vestibulothalamocortical pathway.

(1) Fibers originating from the *utricular macula* bifurcate on reaching the vestibular complex. The ascending ramus terminates in the lateral vestibular nucleus and the medial vestibular nucleus, while the descending ramus terminates in the spinal vestibular nucleus. From the *saccular macula* some fibers proceed to the lateral vestibular nucleus. Neither utricular nor saccular fibers proceed to the cerebellum (Fig. 13-5). The main connection of the utricular fibers is with the lateral vestibular nucleus, whose fibers pass downward in the vestibulospinal tract. Another important connection is with the spinal vestibular nucleus, in areas of the nucleus where fibers from the semicircular canals also terminate. The spinal nucleus is the one most closely connected with the cerebellum.

Semicircular canal afferents bifurcate and terminate in the lateral, medial, and spinal vestibular nuclei, while others proceed to the superior vestibular nucleus. The key vestibular nuclei giving rise to fibers for the medial longitudinal fasciculus are the superior and medial nuclei (Fig. 13-6). In addition, some semicircular canal fibers course into the juxtarestiform body, in which they ascend to the cerebellum, terminating in the cortex of the flocculonodular lobe (and adjacent cortex) and also in the fastigial nucleus bilaterally. En route, they are joined by fibers originating mainly in the spinal vestibular nucleus and, in less degree, by fibers from the medial vestibular nucleus. Fibers originating in the cerebellar cortex from sites at which the fibers just mentioned terminate proceed to the ipsilateral fastigial nucleus. *Cerebellofugal fibers* from the fastigial nucleus of both sides pass via the juxtarestiform body of one side, and terminate in all four vestibular nuclei. In this manner the cerebellum can exert an influence on all the

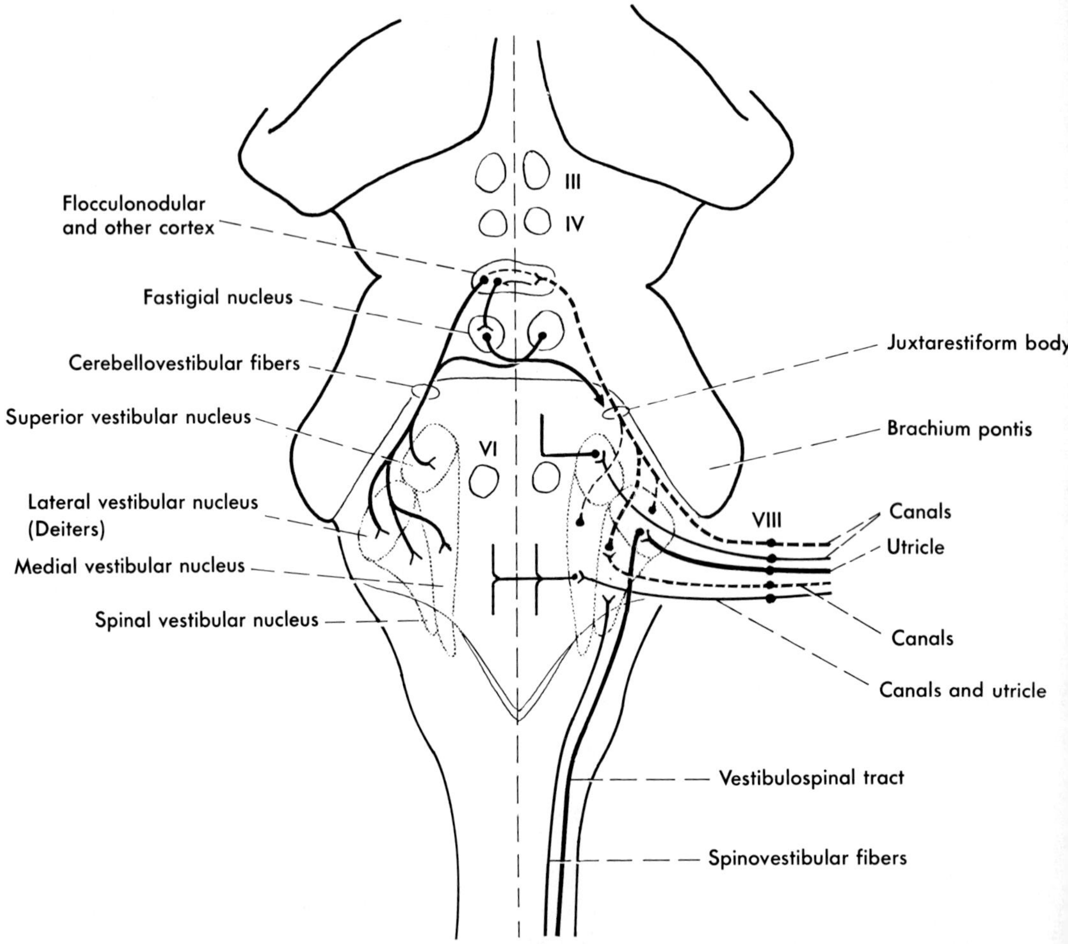

Fig. 13-5. Semicircular-canal and utricular connections with the vestibular nuclei. Fastigiofugal fibers extending to the vestibular nuclei are also shown. Semicircular canal fibers project (1) to the flocculonodular and adjoining cerebellar cortex and (2) to the spinal vestibular nucleus (and the other nuclei indicated), from which secondary fibers proceed to the flocculonodular and adjoining cortex; (3) other canal fibers pass to the superior vestibular and medial vestibular nuclei, from which secondary fibers proceed to the medial longitudinal fasciculus. Utricular fibers extend (1) to the medial vestibular nucleus, in a region whence fibers for the medial longitudinal fasciculus spring, and also (2) to the lateral vestibular nucleus, from a region in which the vestibulospinal tract arises; (3) some also proceed to the spinal vestibular nucleus, which sends a strong contingent of secondary fibers to the flocculonodular and adjoining cerebellar cortex. Fibers from the saccule (not illustrated) proceed to the spinal vestibular and lateral vestibular nuclei. The main orientation of the fibers originating in the spinal vestibular nucleus is with the cerebellar cortex (via the juxtarestiform nucleus), while the main orientation of the secondary fibers from the lateral vestibular nucleus is to the cervical segments of the spinal cord. (Gacek, 1968a, b.)

vestibular complex. This influence is generally thought to be of an inhibitory nature, involving ocular movements, for example, through connections with the superior and medial vestibular nuclei, and also spinal muscle reflexes, through the medium of the lateral vestibular nucleus. (Brodal and Hoivik, 1964; Carpenter, 1959; Fulton and Dow, 1937; Gacek, 1968 a, b; Larsell, 1951.)

(2) From the lateral vestibular nucleus, fibers descend in the anterior column of the spinal cord as the *vestibulospinal tract* (Figs. 1-2 and 13-5) and terminate on ipsilateral interneurons and motoneurons at all spinal levels. Through these fibers the labyrinth exerts an influence on posture by aiding in the maintenance of muscle tonus, particularly that of the extensor muscles. The vestibulospinal fibers are necessary to the development of the decerebrate rigidity induced by rostral midbrain transection, for the rigidity disappears when the lateral vestibular nucleus is destroyed or the vestibulospinal tract interrupted. Decere-

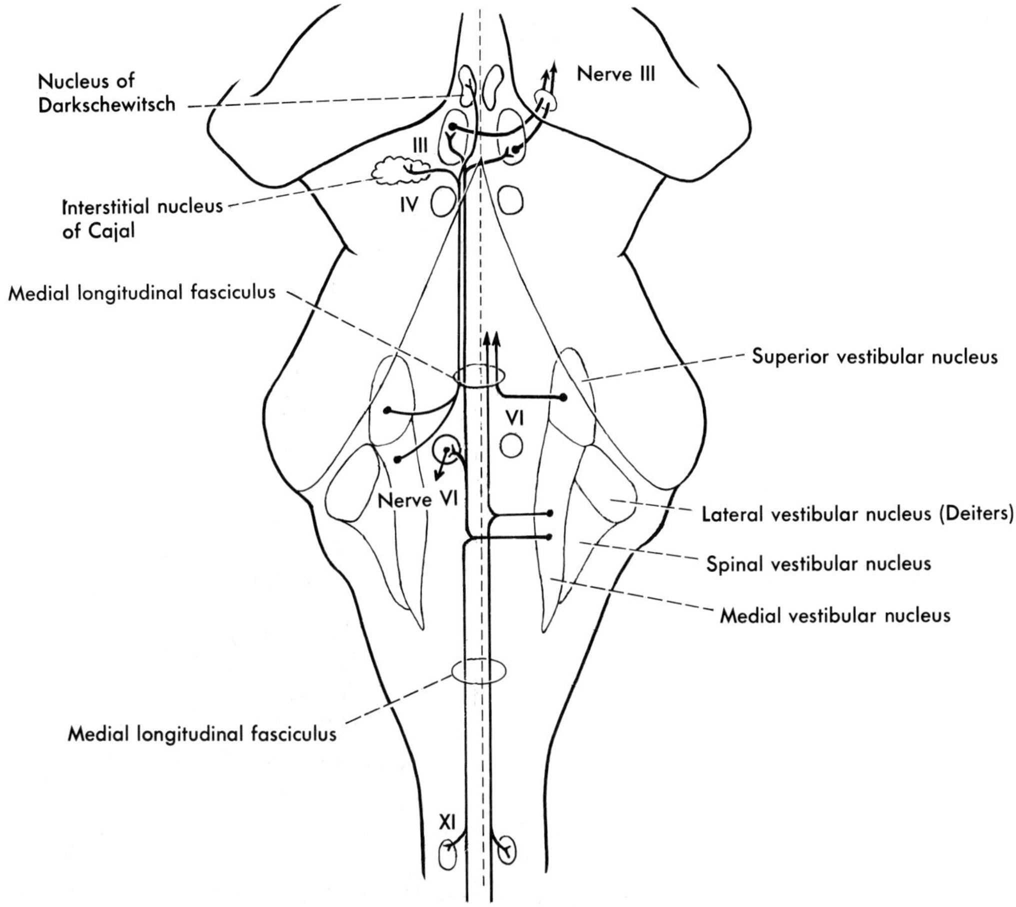

Fig. 13-6. Fiber systems extending from vestibular nuclei to nuclei III, VI, and XI by way of the medial longitudinal fasciculus. A mechanism is indicated whereby activation of the semicircular canals on the right side results in conjugate lateral ocular deviation to the left (through nerve VI, which supplies the abductor of the eye, and nerve III, which supplies the adductor). The decussating third nerve fibers shown in this diagram have been established electrophysiologically (Bender and Weinstein, 1943; Warwick, 1953), not anatomically.

brate rigidity is strictly an antigravity reaction attributable to interruption of the fibers extending from the otoliths to the lateral vestibular nucleus, and mediated by the lateral vestibular tract.

(3) As indicated in the foregoing, the superior vestibular nucleus and the medial vestibular nucleus are the main sources of the fibers that make up the *medial longitudinal fasciculus*. Through this fasciculus, fibers are distributed to cranial nerve nuclei III, IV, VI, and XI (Fig. 13-6). The fibers originating in the superior vestibular nucleus course to the ipsilateral fasciculus, in which they ascend to reach nuclei III and IV. On the other hand, the fibers arising in the medial vestibular nucleus pass to the fasciculus of both sides, and descend as well as ascend in the fasciculi.

These fasciculi are concerned in two general spheres: (a) in maintained postural deviation of the eyes, which is under the control of the maculae of the utricle and saccule, and (b) in postural adjustments of the eyes and the head and neck in response (i) to stimulation of the cristae in the ampullae of the semicircular canals brought about by rotation of the head, and (ii) to proprioceptive impulses arising in the neck muscles. Fibers conveying the latter proceed upward in the spinal cord to the spinal vestibular nucleus, thence via neurons (not illustrated in Fig. 13-6) that proceed to the medial longitudinal fasciculus, in which they course to nuclei III, IV, and VI.

The pathways indicated as originating in vestibular nuclei and proceeding to contralateral nuclei III, IV, and VI are concerned in the contraction of some extraocular muscles and the reciprocal relaxation of others in the performance of conjugate ocular movements.

Also associated with the medial longitudinal fasciculus as well as with the posterior commissure are the nucleus of Darkschewitsch and the interstitial nucleus of Cajal. The *nucleus of Darkschewitsch* is situated along the edge of central gray at the level of the caudal part of the third ventricle and the rostral part of the aqueduct, on a line with the dorsal border of the red nucleus; the *interstitial nucleus of Cajal* also lies close to the central gray, but is located somewhat ventral to the nucleus of Darkschewitsch. Both nuclei receive connections from the premotor cortex (areas 6 and 8), motor cortex (area 4), and striate cortex (area 17), also from the globus pallidus by way of the fasciculus lenticularis. Other connections are received from the cerebellum (p. 280). Further, the two nuclei of one side receive fibers from the superior and medial vestibular nuclei of both sides, of which only those ascending ipsilaterally are shown in Fig. 13-6. *Efferent* fibers of the nucleus of Darkschewitsch appear related functionally to nuclei III and IV. Electrical stimulation of the nucleus of Darkschewitsch (in cats) results in relaxation of all extraocular muscles and in inhibition of vestibulum-induced ocular movements. The nucleus of Darkschewitsch may thus have the function of exerting an inhibitory action on oculomotor nuclei. Clinically, the nucleus of Darkschewitsch appears to be concerned in conjugate upward gaze (p. 270). As to the interstitial nucleus of Cajal, some of the fibers passing from this nucleus as well as from the nucleus of Darkschewitsch are described as coursing down the medial longitudinal fasciculus ipsilaterally and contralaterally to motor centers of the brainstem and spinal cord (the fasciculus interstitiospinalis of Muskens). Other fibers originating in the interstitial nucleus of Cajal proceed downward in the ipsilateral medial longitudinal fasciculus and terminate in the medial vestibular nucleus. Electrical stimulation of the interstitial nucleus (in cats) produces, ipsilaterally, both activation and inhibition of vestibular units; stimulation also produces conjugate vertical and rotatory movement of the eyes and rotatory movement of the head in the frontal plane. The interstitial nucleus thus appears to be a substation for the transmission of pyramidal and extrapyramidal influences to the brainstem and spinal cord motor nuclei and to exert an action on extraocular nuclei through the medium of the vestibular nuclei. (Crosby, Humphrey, and Lauer, 1962; Hyde and Toczek, 1962; Markham, Precht, and Shimazu, 1966.)

(4) The presence of a *vestibulothalamocortical pathway* is well established, but there is no consensus as to its course (Brodal, Pompeiano, and Walberg, 1962). A recent review cites the results of various workers in the field—from Spitzer to current authors (Schäfer, 1966). In man, some of the fibers originating from the vestibular nuclei cross to the opposite side of the pons to the region of the cerebellopontile angle before ascending, judging from the results of testing of semicircular canal function (p. 200). As based on studies of cerebral and cerebellar cortical action potentials following stimulation of the labyrinth by rotation (in cats), and from anatomical connections cited in the literature, Price and Spiegel (1937) inferred that vestibular pathways course cephalad via the cerebellum and medial longitudinal fasciculus and also via a reticulothalamic pathway. In man, with the usual Grass scalp electrodes in place, rotation carried out in a Bárány chair induced EEG responses limited to or prevalent in preoccipital areas, and occasionally in frontal areas. The assumption was that the preoccipital response may be part of the reaction of the diffuse thalamic projection system, particularly of a system synapsing in the pulvinar, or may be due to responses propagated from the second somatic sensory area, situated in or around the upper bank of the sylvian fissure adjacent to area 4 of the cortex (Spiegel and others, 1965). Clinical data are given on pp. 381 and 382.

Factors concerned in conjugate ocular movements and the occurrence of nystagmus

Basically, three mechanisms are concerned in the maintenance of ocular posture: labyrinthine, gaze, and fixation mechanisms.

In some animals, for example, the rabbit, a fourth mechanism can be added, namely *tonic neck reflexes*. In such animals, rotation of the head following removal of the vestibular apparatus results in conjugate ocular movement in the direction opposite to the head movement and represents an attempt by the animal to maintain the position of regard. In man, tonic neck reflexes as they relate to the labyrinthine apparatus have been submerged in favor of activity by the pyramidal and extrapyramidal systems. These reflexes may be obtained in the presence of unilateral or bi-

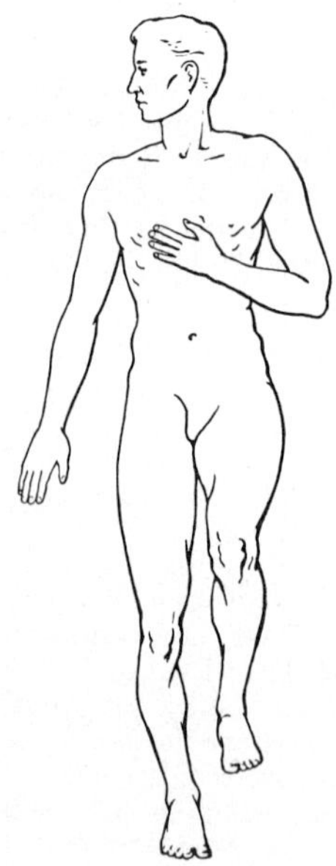

Fig. 13-7. The tonic neck reflex. Turning of the head to the right in the presence of hemiplegia of the right side induces increased extensor tonus of the right limbs and flexion of the left arm and leg. (Redrawn from Holmes, 1952.)

lateral lesions that involve pyramidal and extrapyramidal pathways jointly. When the examiner turns the head of a patient with right-sided hemiplegia to the right, the limbs of that side may exhibit increased extensor tonus or tonic extension, while the limbs on the left may become tonically flexed (Fig. 13-7). The same occurs when the head is bent forward. When, however, the head is moved toward the normal side or moved backward, the limbs of the paretic side undergo tonic flexion. In traumatic cord transection, especially at upper thoracic levels, a change in the position of the limbs occurs following a change of body posture, indicating that the spinal cord as a whole shares in the function of body reflex adjustment (Pollock and others, 1955). These responses may be even better brought out when the patient himself induces these movements as forcibly as possible.

Labyrinthine activation. The vestibular labyrinth exerts influence on ocular movements through two mechanisms. One is *ophthalmostatic,* that is, the maintenance of gaze when the head is still. Tilting of the head will produce a slight rotation of the eyes to adapt the gaze to the new perspective. This is a reflection of otolithic function. The other mechanism is *ophthalmokinetic,* that is, motion of the eyes in response to acceleratory movements of the head, particularly rotation. Under such conditions the end-organs of the semicircular canals are stimulated. The end-organ of each of the three semicircular canals of the labyrinth may be activated independently. In accordance with Flourens' law, stimulation of each semicircular canal end-organ causes rhythmic ocular movements that are in the same plane as the canal (Fig. 13-8)—*horizontal* nystagmus from the horizontal semicircular canals and *vertical* nystagmus from the vertical semicircular canals. The ocular movements are in the same direction as the convection hydraulic current set up in the semicircular canals. The nystagmus consists in a slow (pursuit) and a fast (saccadic) movement, and is named in accordance with the direction of the fast movement. The slow movement, which is toward the side stimulated, is in response to the hallucination of movement produced by the endolymph current. (Goto, Tokumasu, and Cohen, 1968.)

Gaze mechanisms. These mechanisms are discussed in Chapter 16. Pathways ex-

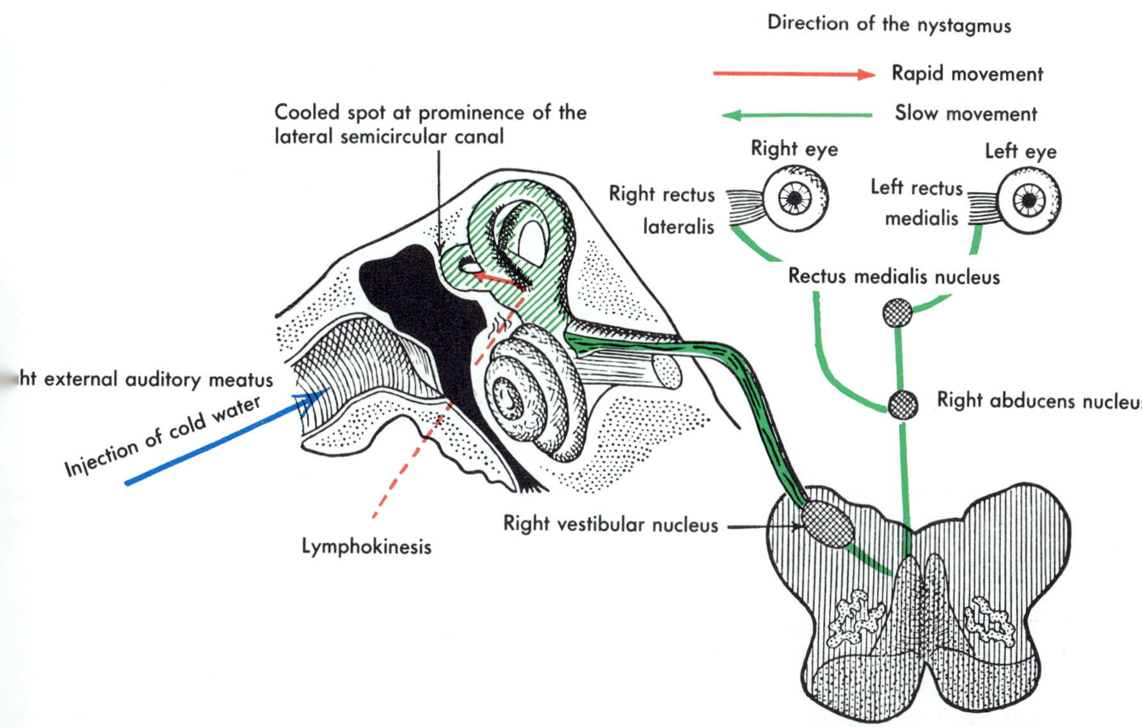

Fig. 13-8. Mechanism by which caloric nystagmus in induced.

tend from the cerebral cortex and subcortical structures to brainstem mechanisms concerned in the carrying out of conjugate vertical and horizontal gaze, with transferral of the impulses to the nuclei of the extraocular muscles.

Fixation mechanisms. Concerned here are neural mechanisms that convert ocular movements to steady, precise, integrative activities for the viewing of an object. Pathways run from the retina, visual cortex, visual associative cortex, and so on (Chapter 16).

Pathological ocular nystagmus

Nystagmus may be defined as rhythmic, oscillatory, involuntary movements occurring in one or both eyes in any or all fields of gaze. It is always abnormal if sustained. Direction of nystagmus has been arbitrarily set as the direction of the fast component. When there is a fast and a slow component the nystagmus is said to be *jerky,* and when the speed is equal in all directions it is said to be *pendular.* Nystagmus may be horizontal, vertical, oblique, rotatory, circular, or mixed; its direction may change in the various fields of gaze. *Rotary nystagmus* is designated by the direction of movement of the 12 o'clock point on the limbus. *Vertical nystagmus* may be in the upward, downward, or forward plane of gaze. Nystagmus is usually conjugate, although it may be disjunctive or even unilateral.

Spontaneous nystagmus is defined as a rhythmic nystagmus present when the patient's head is in the erect position. It is designated as of the first degree only when it occurs following turning of the eyes 30 degrees in the direction of the fast movement. Second degree nystagmus occurs when the eyes are directed straight ahead, and third degree when the eyes are turned 30 degrees in the direction opposite the fast movement. *Positional nystagmus* is that evoked or modified following a change in the position of the head. *Induced nystagmus* is a nystagmus that occurs in response to a stimulus such as rotation. *Provoked nystagmus* is the term used when the nystagmus is present only after the time of its expected cessation following vestibular stimulation employed in testing.

Ocular nystagmus occurring under pathological conditions is considered in the following under the following headings: (1) vestibular nystagmus, (2) nystagmus related to fixation mechanisms, and (3) gaze nystagmus (Norton, 1964).

Vestibular nystagmus. This form of nystagmus is characterized by horizontal-rotary, jerky eye movements and is due to damage either of (a) the labyrinth or the vestibular nerve, or (b) some central mechanism—probably a portion of the vestibular nuclei. In the former the nystagmus remains in the same direction in all fields of gaze; in the latter the nystagmus may change its direction on right and left lateral gaze, and it may become vertical on upward or downward gaze.

Fixation nystagmus. Nystagmus when due to disturbances in fixation mechanisms almost invariably occurs on forward gaze. Examples are: (a) congenital pendular nystagmus associated with ocular disease (jerky nystagmus occurs on right or left lateral gaze, with the fast component in the direction of gaze); (b) acquired pendular nystagmus (usually horizontal, and sometimes vertical) due to brainstem disease in which the outside environment may appear to move *(oscillopia)*—here the nystagmus is directional, horizontal nystagmus occurring on lateral gaze and vertical nystagmus on upward and, sometimes, downward gaze; (c) convergence nystagmus due to upper brainstem disease, characterized by intermittent convergence movements of the eyes brought out on horizontal gaze. When severe, it may merge into a combination of convergence and retraction movements *(nystagmus retractorius).* Belonging in the category of fixation nystagmus are postural nystagmus and see-saw nystagmus, to be described later.

Gaze nystagmus. This is perhaps the most common form of nystagmus. It occurs not when gaze is directed forward, but does develop when the subject directs his gaze to the right or the left or in another direction. The fast component is always in the direction of the gaze. In general, the responsible lesion is usually situated in the brainstem. *Dissociated gaze nystagmus,* consisting in monocular horizontal nystagmus in the abducting eye signifies involvement of the medial longitudinal fasciculus (pp. 272-273).

Observation of nystagmus is greatly facilitated by the use of Frenzel's eyeglasses, which carry internal illumination. When the subject wears these glasses (+20 diopters), refraction is distorted, and since he cannot focus he is unable to fix his gaze on an external object and thus inhibit nystagmus. The short focal point of the lenses makes it easy for the examiner to observe even small movements of the eyes. *Electronystagmography* offers a means of electronically recording the amplitude, frequency, and speed of nystagmus in a subject with eyes closed, thus eliminating the factor of fixation. Each motion of the eyeball is accompanied by a change in a dipole electric field (D.C.). The differences in potentials are picked up by electrodes located in the same axis in which nystagmus is expected (usually horizontal) (Reddy and Liu, 1966).

Tests of semicircular canal function

Caloric test. The subject sits erect, with his head tilted backward at an angle of 60 degrees in order to bring the horizontal canal into the vertical position, where it will be maximally influenced by the convection currents set up in the endolymph by the water to be used. Douching of the ear with cool water (30° C.) lowers the temperature of the prominence of the lateral semicircular canal, condenses the endolymph, and thus induces a convection current in the direction of the cooling (ampullofugal lymphokinesis) (inhibition of the hair cells). Three points need emphasis. (a) The endolymph is set in circulation by differences in temperature, the warmer endolymph migrating upward. (b) The canal to be examined must, therefore, be in vertical position. In order to have an effective fluid current the direction of the current must be in the same direction as that in which the hair cells are polarized. (c) If irrigation is carried out for too long a time, a temperature equilibrium might be reached. The fact that a semicircular canal normally responds to both warm and cold water is not fully understood. If the cupula is malfunctioning, the semicircular canal will not respond when the fluid circulates in the direction facilitatory to the cells, while it might respond when it circulates in the direction inhibitory to the cells, when no reaction is expected (due to response of the other canals?). The change in direction of the endolymph current causes the eyes to be turned slowly toward the side of the irrigated ear, the movement being interrupted alternately by a fast return movement toward the opposite side (Fig. 13-8). If the ear is douched with warm water (40° C.), the endolymph expands, and the resulting ampullopetal convection current (facilitation of the hair cells) produces the reverse; the eyes turn away from the side of the irrigated ear, with the fast return movement toward the side irrigated (direction of the quick movement can be remembered by recalling the word "cows"—cold, opposite; warm, same). If the fast movement is toward the side opposite to that expected, or if the fast movement is vertical rather than horizontal (perverted nystagmus), the responsible lesion can be assumed to be situated in the brainstem. The same conclusion is warranted when one eye lies motionless while the other moves or when it moves sluggishly or in an opposing direction (dissociated nystagmus).

When the test is carried out on a standing person with his arms stretched out in front of him, certain body deviations occur through the mediation of the vestibulospinal tract. As nystagmus appears, his trunk and limbs deviate toward the side of the slow phase of the nystagmus, and he tends to fall in that direction. There is also past-pointing in that direction and vertigo.

Directional preponderance of nystagmus induced calorically in patients with vertigo provides information as to whether the vertigo is due to hypofunctioning labyrinth or to a central lesion. The end-point here is the side to which nystagmus lasts the longest. Usually the directional preponderance of the nystagmus is away from the side of labyrinthine involvement, toward the side of central involvement.

Rotation test. When a seated person is whirled rapidly around and around at the rate of ten times in 20 seconds, and then is suddenly brought to a standstill, nystagmus occurs. Its fast phase is toward the side opposite the direction of the rotation. When the rotation is carried out in the direction toward a damaged labyrinth (facilitation of the hair cells)—clockwise in case the right labyrinth is damaged—the response is lessened. The response will be more marked when the rotation is carried out in the reverse direction. This is because at this point the affected labyrinth is excited with a positive stimulus to which it cannot respond.

In a refinement of the rotation test, *cupulometry,* rotation of the chair is started so slowly that the subject is not aware that the motion has been initiated. He is accelerated at a constant rate, then rotation is continued at a constant speed, then the chair is suddenly stopped. The speeds usually employed are 6 degrees, 12 degrees, 18 degrees, or 30 degrees per second^2. Duration of the nystagmus is measured with a stop watch or, even better, by means of electronystagmography. Simultaneously the patient is asked how long the sensation of rotation persisted. The plot on logarithmic paper of these two variables, which is a straight line, is called the *cupulogram.*

Galvanic nystagmus. The nystagmus induced by

galvanic current is not of much diagnostic importance because it can be obtained despite a negative caloric test and after extirpation of the labyrinth. The current stimulates both the otoliths and the ampullary cristae. Stimulation of the left ear with a 10 to 25 ma. current produces nystagmus to the left if the negative pole is used.

Tests of otolithic function

Parallel swing test. The parallel swing consists of a solid platform that hangs from the ceiling by four ropes. The ropes should be as long as possible in order to lessen the lifting effect of the swinging radius of the rope (Fig. 13-9). The excursion of the parallel swing should not be excessive. This is in order to balance the horizontal and vertical forces and to obtain a motion as close to horizontal as possible (linear acceleration). Both the objective and the subjective components of the parallel swing test are of localizing value. Objectively, the eyes will deviate in the direction opposite the swinging motion (head ➔ foot ➔ head, and so on). Absence of this motion indicates loss of otolithic function bilaterally. Subjectively, the patient experiences a "sinking" sensation in the cephalad swinging motion and a "lifting" sensation in the caudally directed swinging motion. Exaggeration of this sensation indicates hypersensitivity of the otolithic mechanism. Absence indicates no otolith function at all.

Weighing, walking, and standing tests. These are a measure of otolithic function. (a) On weighing a normal person on two balances, with one foot on each balance, he weighs the same on each balance. However, if there are disturbances in static equilibrium (of otolithic origin), one side—the abnormal side—will weigh more than the other. (b) On walking with eyes closed, a person with vestibular damage involving otolithic function (possibly a saccular function) does not walk in a straight line. Instead, his trunk deviates toward the side opposite the hypersensitive organ or to the same side as the hyposensitive organ. The results of the test are obscured in chronic illnesses through adaptive mechanisms. To avoid this, the examiner should ask the subject to perform motions in the direction to which he has not adapted—for example, to walk backwards. The examiner should also watch him stand next to a vertical line. A door frame will do. He has his eyes closed and the hands fixed. In vestibular affections he will deviate from the vertical. (c) A standing person with a diseased otolith macular system, on lifting a knee high up and looking at a fixed spot, will slowly rotate to the affected side.

Positional nystagmus and positional vertigo

By "positional" nystagmus is meant nystagmus that appears paroxysmally only when the head is in a certain position, or nystagmus that is greatly aggravated by a certain position of the head. Positioning that produces nystagmus may or may not be accompanied by vertigo and often is not. Conversely, only in about 25 percent of patients with vertigo does positional nystagmus occur.

Method of testing has varied considerably, and the results have varied accordingly. A commonly used method is the following: the subject reclines on the examining table with his trunk horizontal, either in a supine position or on the lateral side; the subject moves his head into one of three positions—right lateral, left lateral, or in hyperextension by letting his head hang over the edge of the table. Observations with respect to nystagmus are made after the head has become still. While the head is in each of these positions the subject is asked to follow with his eyes the movement of the examiner's finger into the right and the left end-positions of conjugate ocular deviation, as is ordinarily done in testing for nystagmus. Electronystagmography may be carried out as an alternative.

The nystagmus that occurs during the testing is essentially of two types.

Direction-changing. In this type, irregularity in

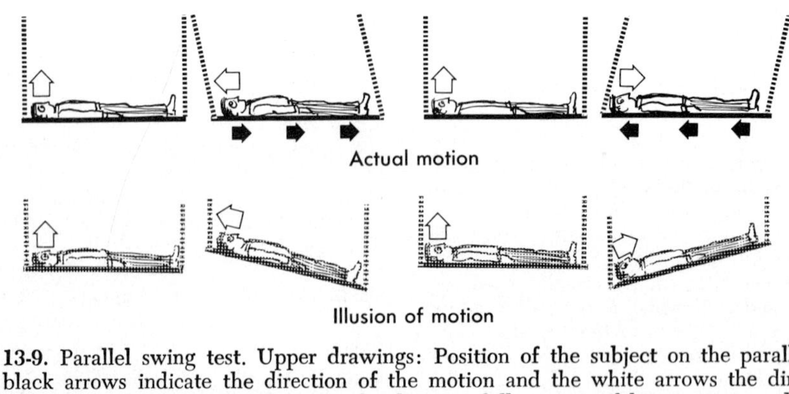

Fig. 13-9. Parallel swing test. Upper drawings: Position of the subject on the parallel swing. The black arrows indicate the direction of the motion and the white arrows the direction of gaze. When no motion occurs the normal subject is fully aware of his position, and his gaze is directed to the ceiling. Motion in the direction of the feet causes the eyes to be directed cephalad; the subject has the feeling that his lower limbs are sinking. Movement in the direction of the head in the normal subject produces the opposite phenomenon: the eyes are turned caudalward, and the subject feels as though his head were sinking below the horizontal.

the direction of the nystagmus or a change in the direction of the nystagmus occurs during and after alteration in the position of the head. The position of the eyes undergoing nystagmus may, for example, change from right to left as the head alters its position, or the nystagmus may occur in all positions that the eyes and head assume. Nystagmus with these characteristics is seen mostly in lesions involving structures in the posterior cranial fossa—for example, in multiple sclerosis, brainstem damage from vascular disease, and posterior fossa tumor, the latter apparently producing its effect either through pressure exerted on the brainstem or through traction on blood vessels. The nystagmus may also occur in the presence of cerebral cortical lesions and in diffuse processes—for example, in chronic alcoholism and traumatic brain injury. Occasionally, nystagmus with these characteristics is also seen in ear disease—for example, Ménière's disease.

When the (direction-changing) nystagmus is paroxysmal and has a short latency period and is transient and fatigable on repeated testing, it is seldom if ever associated with intracranial disease.

Direction-fixed. This type is characterized by constancy in the direction of the nystagmus after the position of the head is changed. Two possible variants may occur within this type: when the head is in the right lateral, left lateral, or hyperextended position, the nystagmus is to the right; when the head is in the same positions, the nystagmus is to the left. Nystagmus occurring under these conditions may sometimes be found in central lesions, but more commonly it denotes a lesion involving the peripheral vestibular apparatus or nerve (Schiller and Hedberg, 1960). Positional nystagmus of this type has been attributed to otolithic disorders, pathological lymphokinesis of the internal ear, sudden partial loss of labyrinthine function, and vascular disorders involving the internal ear. (Lindsay, 1945; Nylén, 1950; Stahle and Terins, 1965; Stenger, 1955.) Head trauma, usually with petrous bone fracture, is a frequent basis of direction-fixed positional nystagmus, occurring, according to Barber (1964), in 25 percent of all cases of head injury. In unilateral fracture the nystagmus occurs only when the ear of the affected side is undermost during testing (Dix and Hallpike, 1952). Incidence of the positional nystagmus is far higher in longitudinal then in transverse fracture of the petrous pyramid, for the reason that in transverse fracture the vestibular nerve is usually interrupted, rendering the brainstem vestibular mechanisms functionless (McHugh, 1966).

Positional vertigo is that which occurs only when the head is turned in a particular manner or assumes a certain position. Vertigo may appear upon lying down, turning over in bed, or turning the head backward to look up. Usually the vertigo is momentary. In the vertigo that occurs on assuming a certain "critical" position, the responses are of two types, one suggesting a disorder of peripheral origin, and the other a disorder of central origin. In the peripheral variety, when the head is placed in the critical position, latency of a few seconds is followed by nystagmus and vertigo. The nystagmus is usually of the rotary type, is directed toward the undermost ear, increases in rapidity for a period of a few seconds, then declines. In the central type, nystagmus appears as soon as the critical position is assumed, there being no latency. Moreover, the nystagmus continues as long as the head is maintained in that position. Vertigo seldom accompanies the nystagmus; if it does, it is mild. Further, the direction of the nystagmus may change with different positions of the head. Occasionally the peripheral type of response is observed in central lesions, particularly in tumor. Nature of the lesions giving rise to the two types of response is much the same as indicated in the previous paragraph. (Wolfson and others, 1965.)

Nystagmus and related disorders from lesions involving the labyrinth and various levels of the neuraxis

In acute hyperexcitatory labyrinthine states—for example, in Ménière's disease—the nystagmus is usually rotary and toward the opposite side. Its amplitude is increased on looking to the side of the rapid movement, and decreased on looking in the reverse direction.

Nystagmus due to a lesion involving not only the peripheral vestibular apparatus, but also the eighth nerve trunk, is always horizontal or rotary or a combination of the two; further, it is pendular, the initial deviation being slow in relation to the quick recoil. The nystagmus is always accompanied by the sensation of vertigo or dizziness. By contrast, nystagmus due to disruption of vestibular connections in the central nervous system may be in any direction: horizontal, vertical, rotary, or oblique. The nystagmus may be sustained indefinitely. It is seldom accompanied by vertigo.

In head trauma resulting in fractures of the petrous pyramid of one side, horizontal nystagmus occurs immediately. The quick component beats to the opposite side, and the slow component to the side of the injury. If the injury is severe, the nystagmus will be present in all three positions (third degree). It lasts three weeks at most. (McHugh, 1966.)

In subacute or chronic damage of the vestibular labyrinth, the initial direction of the nystagmus may be toward the side of the lesion, but when the vestibular labyrinth becomes functionless, the direction of the nystagmus will change, and be toward the normal ear. At this stage, caloric nystagmus cannot be induced; nor is there past-pointing, tendency to fall to one side, or vertigo. In partial destruction of either of these structures the responses appear only after longer stimulation and are of shorter duration than normal.

Some lesions in the region of the cerebellopontile angle, particularly lesions produced by acoustic neuroma, are characterized by a reduction or loss in excitability of the labyrinth on the same side as the lesion and sometimes by a lack of response from the vertical semicircular canal on the opposite side (Nylén, 1939).

In severe damage of the vestibular nuclei the caloric stimulus fails to induce nystagmus. Instead, the eyes usually deviate toward the side of the lesion, in the direction in which voluntary movement is not possible. Furthermore, neither past-pointing nor vertigo occurs on caloric stimulation (Jones and Spiller, 1925). By contrast, a strongly irritative lesion involving the lateral and medial vestibular nuclei causes deviation of the eyes to the side opposite the lesion. If the irritation is less pronounced, or if the lesion is smaller, the eyes may turn slowly toward the opposite side, then quickly return to center, then undergo a series of successive slow deviations and quick returns (horizontal nystagmus, with its direction named in accordance with the quick movement). If a lesion progresses from irritative to destructive, the direction of the nystagmus reverses. A lesion involving the superior vestibular nucleus may give rise to vertical or oblique nystagmus, and if all four of the vestibular nuclei are affected, the nystagmus may be rotary or of irregular form (Cranmer, 1951; Crosby, 1953).

Lesions within the *cerebellum,* on the other hand, have almost no influence on caloric nystagmus; however, when the arms are outstretched, the arm on the same side as the lesion has the tendency to undergo lateral deviation. Nystagmus of cerebellar origin is usually horizontal, but it may be vertical or rotary or of combined type. The nystagmus occurs on fixing the gaze in any direction, with the slow movement toward the position of rest (10 to 30 degrees from the point of fixation) and the rapid movement toward the periphery. Covering the eyes accentuates the nystagmus. In unilateral lesions of the cerebellum, the nystagmus is slower and coarser when the eyes are directed toward the side of the lesion than toward the opposite side. Nystagmus of cerebellar origin usually disappears in a few weeks. If, in the presence of a cerebellar tumor, nystagmus persists, it is to be regarded as a consequence of pressure on, or invasion of, the vestibular nuclei. In lesions involving cerebellar and vestibular connections with the brainstem, the same forms of nystagmus as just described may occur.

Nystagmus may result from lesions involving the *upper cervical cord.* In testing for nystagmus the subject should be seated in an armchair that can be rotated, with his head turned half-way to the right and his head held in this position by the examiner. The nystagmus, of feeble amplitude, occurs in the horizontal plane to the left if the body is turned to the right, and the reverse if the body is turned to the left. The response may be unilateral or bilateral. If spontaneous nystagmus exists, it will be accelerated or slowed by the rotation of the body; should no difference in the nystagmus occur, then the nystagmus is not of cervical origin. Nystagmus of cervical origin is induced, presumably, by an abnormal flow of proprioceptive impulses upward in the spinovestibular pathways. Lesions responsible may originate from cervical trauma (for example, in "whiplash" injury), circulatory disturbances in the cervical region (from arterial disease), cervicoarthrosis, and certain intrinsic disorders such as multiple sclerosis and cervical myelopathy. (Collard and others, 1967.)

Lesions presumed to involve a diencephalic-mesencephalic mechanism may be responsible for *see-saw nystagmus*, which is of rare occurrence. This kind of nystagmus has been observed in chiasmatic-diencephalic tumor, in chromophobe adenoma of the pituitary, in presumed midbrain lesions originating from vascular disorders, and in undiagnosed febrile illness. The nystagmus was also noted by Drachman (1966) in a case in which a vestibular abnormality occurred in combination with bitemporal hemianopia. He suggested that see-saw nystagmus may be due to several possible combinations of lesions involving visual, vestibular, or other structures, rather than to a lesion in a single system.

The characteristic feature of the nystagmus is that one eye rises while the other eye falls. In most instances, however, the nystagmus is basically rotary (torsional) in type with superimposed dissociated vertical movements. The eyes move conjugately clockwise, then counterclockwise; during the torsional movements, the intorting eye rises, while the other eye, which is extorting, falls. The vertical components of the nystagmus are sometimes exaggerated on downward gaze. Apparently the oblique muscles are underactive, allowing their synergists, the vertical recti, to dominate the eye movements, the superior rectus both elevating and intorting, while the inferior rectus depresses and extorts. (Daroff, 1965; Druckman and others, 1966.)

Vertigo

A patient with vertigo has an hallucination of motion. Either he feels himself stationary, with the objects about him moving (objective vertigo), or he feels that he himself is turning in a stationary environment (subjective vertigo). In either instance the movement is always in the same direction (systematic). This sensation leads reflexly to a feeling of listlessness and nausea that sometimes culminates in vomiting. Dizziness or giddiness, by way of contrast, represents a nonsystematic disturbance in perception relating to the position of the body in space. The person feels light-headed, unsteady, or faint.

Vertigo may be explained as follows. The labyrinth subserves spatial orientation by means of variations in hydrostatic and/or inertial forces. These forces, operating in three dimensions, excite neural impulses that pass to the vestibular nuclei and then to other parts of the central nervous system. If a condition is brought about whereby the stimulation of the epithelium of the semicircular canals is not that which arises normally in response to that particular situation, the hair cells will respond, conveying information that is not in agreement with the physical reality of the environment. The subjective discrepancy is manifested by the sensation of vertigo. In the case of a diseased labyrinth, one labyrinth fires out of rhythym with its fellow; what previously functioned as a paired unit now is unsynchronized and not superimposable on the other. Impulses reaching the cerebrum thus create the impression that the body is in motion. A sensation of vertigo results. (Leivers, 1968.)

Vestibular vertigo may be induced in a normal person by whirling him around in a revolving chair. It may also be brought about by passing a galvanic current through the head at the level of the ears. The current produces a sensation of vertigo and causes the head to incline toward the side on which the anode is applied. If both labyrinths and both vestibular nerves are destroyed, these reactions do not occur. If, however, one of these structures is sufficiently damaged the head always inclines toward the injured side regardless of the side on which the anode is applied.

Vertigo may be *sustained* or *paroxysmal.* Normally the vestibular system in the brainstem receives an equal input from the labyrinths of the two sides, and this serves to maintain symmetrical reflex activity. However, when the balance is disturbed by acute loss of function of one labyrinth, resulting in unequal input from the two sides, sustained vertigo occurs and persists until central reflexes can compensate for the labyrinthine deficit. Paroxysms characterize positional vertigo; they are observed, for example, in chronic otitis media, intermittent vertebral-basilar arterial insufficiency, and head injury. Paroxysmal vertigo also occurs in Ménière's disease.

Vestibular vertigo is of greatest intensity when the causative disorder is acute and affects the vestibular labyrinth or the vestibular nerve. The conditions under which vertigo occurs include the following:

1. *Lesions involving end-organs in the vestibular labyrinth.* These are discussed at the end of the chapter.
2. In regard to *lesions of the vestibular nerve and the vestibular nuclei,* intermittent vertebral-basilar arterial insufficiency is among the commoner

causes of vertigo (Bergan and others, 1967). Vertigo also occurs in occlusion of medullary branches of the posterior inferior cerebellar artery and in occlusion of the internal auditory artery. Acute abscess of the pons and suddenly spreading syringobulbia may also be responsible. Multiple sclerosis is also to be included; in a small percentage of cases, vertigo is the initial symptom (Carter, Sciarra, and Merritt, 1950). Tumors in the cerebellopontile angle may induce vertigo by compressing or invading the vestibular nerve or nuclei (Weisenburg, 1922). Vertigo may be induced by increased intracranial pressure, especially in posterior fossa tumor; here the important factors are compression of the endolymphatic sac (situated in the dura mater) and/or the vestibular nerve.

3. *Vertigo induced by a cerebellar lesion* is closely related to, if not identical with, vestibular vertigo. Vertigo causes nystagmus, and nystagmus causes vertigo, making it notoriously difficult to distinguish lesions in the two locations on the basis solely of the vertigo and nystagmus. Even when the lesion is strictly intracerebellar, the vertigo is to be regarded as a symptom of irritation of the vestibular fibers coursing in the cerebellum. Vertigo of cerebellar origin is most likely to occur in acute lesions of the flocculonodular lobe—for example, in posterior inferior cerebellar artery thrombosis.
4. An undue accumulation of wax in the ear may cause vertigo, although dizziness, difficulty in hearing, and "full head" are the usual complaints. Vertigo in migraine is ascribed to circulatory disturbances in the bed of the internal auditory artery. Blood dyscrasias and various states of severe anemia may also be responsible. The vertigo occurring in tabes dorsalis may be attributed to the lack of proprioceptive impulses that are normally transmitted from the limbs to the cerebellum. The same is true for Friedreich's and other forms of ataxia. The vertiginous sensation occurring in association with extraocular muscle palsies is due to disturbed spatial orientation brought about by the projection of altered visual images impinging on the retinae, and may be abolished by closing one eye.
5. Head injury involving the vestibular apparatus, usually due to fracture of the petrous pyramid, is another cause of vertigo. However, the vertigo occurs in only a small percentage of these fractures (10 to 15 percent), and it usually vanishes within three weeks. (Hough and Stuart, 1968.) The vertigo is usually severe in transverse fracture of the petrous bone, and mild in longitudinal fracture (McGovern, 1968). Nystagmus is a more tell-tale manifestation of petrous pyramid fracture (p. 199).

Differential diagnosis between these disorders is usually not difficult if one takes into consideration the other symptoms and signs that lesions at these three sites induce. Damage of the vestibular nerve in the region between labyrinth and nucleus gives rise not only to vestibular nerve symptoms but also to disturbances referable to the adjacent pons and medulla oblongata. Moreover, consideration needs to be given to the fact that cerebellar tumors tend to infiltrate or compress pontile or midbrain structures just as, conversely, tumors of the pons and of the acoustic nerve may damage the cerebellum. As a rule, destructive processes at cerebellar and at pontile levels decrease labyrinthine excitability (as revealed in caloric and other tests), whereas with destructive processes at lower midbrain levels labyrinthine excitability tends to be increased.

Another point is that labyrinthine and vestibular nerve lesions are usually characterized either by loss of function or by irritation of the cochlear nerve (by hearing deficit or tinnitus); this is not true for strictly intracerebellar lesions. Furthermore, in labyrinthine and vestibular nerve lesions the vertigo is usually proportional to the associated nystagmus and disturbed equilibrium. Ataxia may occur in either, but if present after the attack of vertigo has subsided, a cerebellar lesion is to be suspected; the central nervous system is always to be favored over the labyrinth or vestibular nerve as the site of the lesion when, for reasons already presented, there is intense nystagmus in the absence of vertigo.

Position and movement influence the development and the intensity of the vertigo. At the beginning of an attack, the vertigo is aggravated with each change in position. As the attack is lessening, vertigo can be precipitated only when certain positions are assumed. During some attacks, the vertigo is of postural origin from the onset. Localization of the site of the lesion is based on the nature of the accompanying positional nystagmus. In most cases the nystagmus indicates the presence of a lesion of the central nervous system. In Ménière's disease positional vertigo is often absent. (Lindsay, 1945; Nylén, 1939, 1950.) While vertigo of labyrinthine origin is characteristically aggravated by any sudden movement of the head, vertigo of vestibular nerve, brainstem, or cerebellar origin may occur only when the position of the head is changed *(Bruns' sign)*. In progressively enlarging tumors of the posterior cranial fossa, "cerebellar" (or "vestibular") attacks may occasionally occur. Such attacks develop paroxysmally and are characterized not only by vertigo but also by severe ataxia, headache, protracted vomiting, tinnitus, syncope, and nystagmus. Positional nystagmus will usually tip the scale in favor of organic versus psychogenic dizziness.

Among the disorders that have their inception in labyrinthine stimulation are seasickness and airsickness. The symptoms of motion sickness, in their order of appearance, are drowsiness, pallor (chiefly facial), cold sweating, increased salivation with swallowing movements, the sensation of nausea, and finally vomiting. Dizziness frequently occurs, but nystagmus and vertigo are rare (Tyler and Bard, 1949). Moreover, blockage of the eustachian tube or failure of the tube to open during quick ascent or descent in airplanes may lead to aero-otitis media, in which vertigo may be a feature.

Further causes of vertigo are discussed at the end of the chapter.

COCHLEAR END-ORGAN AND NERVE

Anatomy and functions

The end-organ of hearing is the organ of Corti, which rests on the basilar membrane. It is made up of hair cells and supporting (and other) elements and, above, by the tectorial membrane, a fairly rigid collagenous structure. The tips of the hairs are embedded in the tectorial membrane. The organ of Corti runs along the entire length of the cochlea, which has two and a half turns. It is situated in the lower wall of the cochlear duct (or scala media), and contains perilymph, not endolymph. This duct, a membranous structure of prismatic shape, is coiled around the axis (modiolus) of the cochlea; when viewed in cross section it is limited above by the scala vestibuli, below by the scala tympani, and laterally by the spiral ligament, the latter composed of modified periosteum. Perilymph occupies the scala tympani and scala vestibuli. (Anson and others, 1965; Anson, Warpeha, and Rensink, 1968; Davis, 1968.)

The hair cells, numbering about 32,000 in each organ of Corti, are aligned in rows: the inner hair cells form a single row, and the outer hair cells form three or four rows. From each hair cell, about 140 orderly arranged stereocilia together with remnants of a kinocilium (situated on the spiral ligament side of the stereocilia) protrude into the tectorial membrane. This arrangement is such that stimulation of the stereocilia occurs only when they are bent toward the remnant of the kinocilium. (Smith, 1961.)

When the cilia are bent toward the spiral ligament by movement of the basilar membrane, which separates the ductus cochlearis from the scala tympani, a shearing force between the tectorial membrane and the hair cells comes into play. The cilia are thus stimulated, and this causes an impulse to originate in the hair cell, from which it is transmitted to the nerve endings at the base of the hair cells.

Up-and-down movement of the organ of Corti (together with the basilar membrane) originates from movements of the perilymph of the cochlea in the form of a traveling wave initiated by the piston-like action of the stapes in the fenestra ovale. In accordance with the frequency of the sound stimulus transmitted through the ossicular chain the wave will have its greatest amplitude at different points along the basilar membrane from basal turn to apex. Physical properties of the cochlea and of the basilar membrane determine the point of maximal amplitude (the point of maximal displacement of the organ of Corti), which is the point of maximal stimulation of hair cells. Tones of higher pitch are picked up in the most basal end of the cochlea, those of lower pitch in the apex, and those of intermediate pitch in an orderly manner in between. (Bredberg, Engström, and Ades, 1965; Davis, 1957; Engström, Ades, and Andersson, 1966; Smith and Sjostrand, 1961; von Békésy, 1960.)

The cell station of the cochlear nerve is in the spiral ganglion, situated in the spiral canal of the modiolus (Rosenthal's canal). The cells in this ganglion are bipolar. Their dendrites extend to the base of the hair cells of the organ of Corti. The dendrites innervating the inner hair cells have a relatively simple pattern: each dendrite terminates on one or two of the hair cells by means of fairly large endings. Innervation of the outer hair cells is more complicated. Suffice it to say that each dendrite ends on many hair cells over a considerable length of the basilar membrane. Moreover, the organ of Corti receives an efferent nerve supply coming from the pons (p. 188). Cochlear nerve potentials are reduced when these efferent fibers are stimulated (Fex, 1959). Presumably this system is part of a mechanism by which central structures control sensory input (Campbell, 1965).

The central processes (axons) of the cochlear nerve, on gaining the border zone between medulla oblongata and pons, undergo bifurcation, some terminals reaching the ventral cochlear nucleus and the others the dorsal cochlear nucleus (Fig. 13-10). Fibers from the ventral cochlear nucleus enter the corpus trapezoideum, cross the midline, and turn upward in the lateral lemniscus to reach the inferior colliculus and, through the brachium of the inferior colliculus, the medial geniculate body, synapsing en route in the corpus trapezoideum (not indicated in Fig. 13-10), the superior olivary, and the other nuclei indicated in Fig. 13-10. Fibers arising in the dorsal cochlear nucleus take a course dorsal to the restiform body and run subjacent to the ventricular floor (not in the striae medullares); they then bend ventrally beneath the medial longitudinal fasciculus, cross the midline, gain the region of the superior olivary nucleus, in which they synapse, and in union with the fibers from the ventral cochlear nucleus turn upward to end in the inferior colliculus and the medial geniculate body. Fibers traversing the commissure of the inferior colliculus (Fig. 13-10) provide a means by which impulses originating in one ear reach the inferior colliculus of the contralateral side, thence the cortex. (Barnes, Magoun, and Ranson, 1943; Lewy and Kobrak, 1936; Polyak, 1932.)

From the medial geniculate body, fibers pass laterally via the auditory radiation (in the sublenticular part of the internal capsule; Fig. 19-11) to the auditory cortex situated in the transverse gyri of Heschl, the latter situated in the upper aspect of the temporal lobe (Fig. 19-8). (For details on distribution, see Campbell, 1965.) The auditory cortex of one side is brought into communication with the other side via the corpus callosum.

Functionally, at the level of the organ

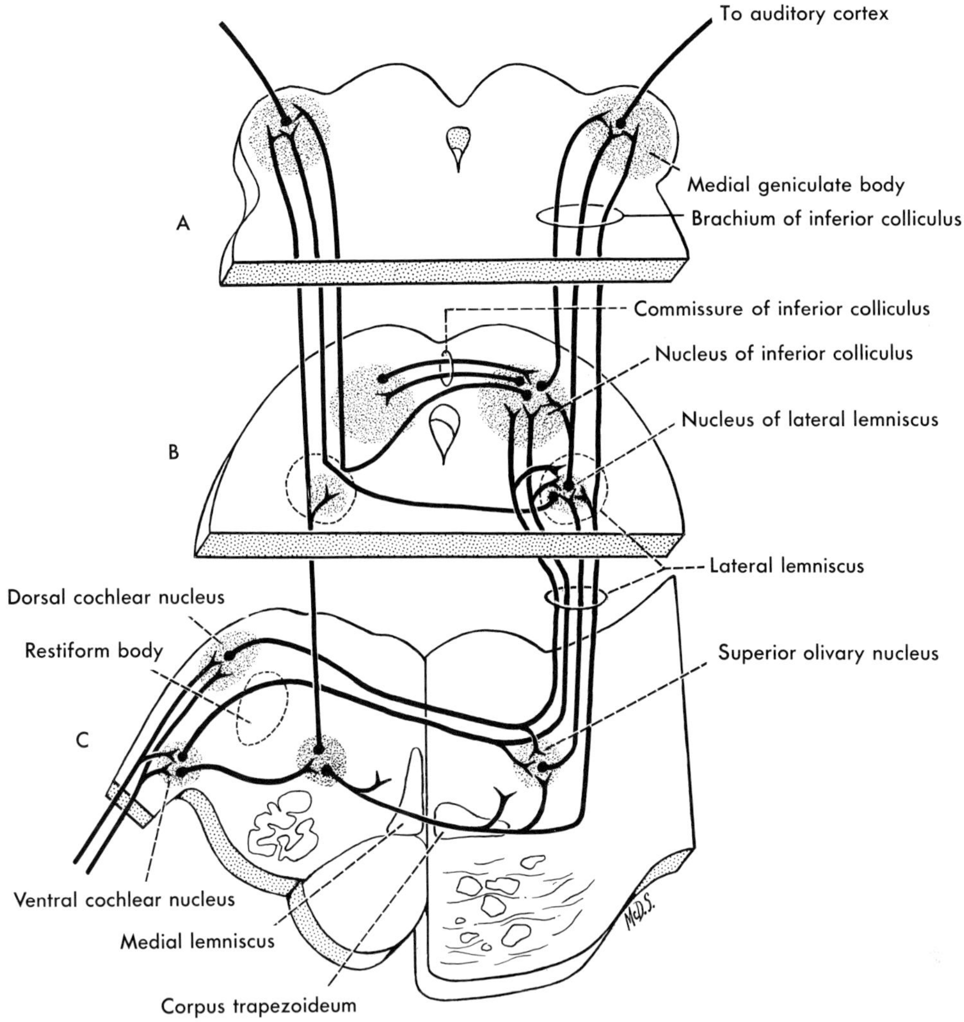

Fig. 13-10. Levels of superior colliculus *(A)*, inferior colliculus *(B)*, and pons and medulla oblongata *(C)*. Main cochlear pathways. Some cross the midline as "trapezoid fibers," others (more dorsally) as "secondary auditory fibers." Branches given off from decussating fibers extend into the reticular core of the medulla oblongata and pons.

of Corti the afferent fibers of the vestibular nerve, together with their 30,000 ganglion cells, are concerned in the coding of sound signals into the correct number and sequence of nerve impulses to be transmitted into the central auditory pathways. At the level of the ventral and dorsal cochlear nuclei, incoming nerve fibers and their recipient cells are sound-frequency oriented. The superior olivary nuclei appear to serve in the analysis of binaural time disparity, and evidence suggests that the medial geniculate bodies are heavily concerned in the realm of pitch and intensity of sound, as these qualities can still be appreciated after destruction of the auditory cortex bilaterally. The auditory cortex functions in integrating sounds into an organized auditory space, also in the integration of analyzed sound. (Katsuki, Watanabe, and Masuyama, 1959; Masterton, Jane, and Diamond, 1967.)

Reduction of auditory threshold

Magnitude of reduction in auditory threshold in end-organ injury is dependent on two factors: degree of damage of the end-organ per se, and the physical properties of the basilar membrane in the different turns in the cochlea. The first is of paramount importance.

In *end-organ damage,* the hair cells are the most vulnerable in most forms of cochlear injury. Partial loss of hair cells results, apparently, in hearing losses for the involved frequencies of less than 50 decibels (db.), and greater loss of these cells in hearing deficits for frequencies greater than 50 db.; if the cell loss is complete, deafness is total. This is true even if the cochlear nerve remains unaltered.

The *physical properties* of the basilar membrane are such that the membrane vibrates in the form of a traveling wave in response to sound stimulation, with the maximum amplitude in the areas corresponding to the frequency involved. With increase in stimulus intensity for that particular frequency, a spread of the field of excitation on the basilar membrane (and organ of Corti) occurs almost exclusively in a basal direction. For basal-turn lesions the magnitude of the threshold loss is therefore always greater, and the gradient of loss always steeper, than for apical and middle-turn lesions of comparable severity. Total loss of hair cells in the basal end of the turn results in an abrupt loss of 50 db. for the high frequency concerned (because there can be no upward spread of the excitation wave with increasing stimulus intensity), while with total loss of hair cells in the apical turn the threshold loss for low frequences (125 to 250 c.p.s.) will be less than 50 db. (because as the stimulus intensity increases above normal threshold the excitation wave spreads basalward to excite the normal organ of Corti in the middle and basal turns and gives a response before the intensity reaches 50 db.). (Iinuma and others, 1967; Schuknecht and Neff, 1952.)

Clinical disturbances

Hearing loss. Interruption of the cochlear nerve results in diminution or loss of hearing *(hypacusis* or *anacusis).* The degree of deafness can be assessed by the whispering test. Whispered words can normally be heard at a distance of 20 feet (6 meters). A shortening of this distance to 15 feet indicates slight deafness, to 4 feet moderate deafness, and to less than 4 feet severe to total deafness.

The two chief characteristics of *sensorineural deafness* ("nerve deafness," "perceptive deafness") are diminution or loss of hearing of sound conducted through the bones of the skull, and partial loss of perception of high-pitched sounds.

Partial deafness due to lesions of the sound-conducting apparatus (tympanum, ossicles), known as *middle-ear deafness* (conductive deafness) is characterized by (a) intensification and prolongation of hearing of bone-conducted sound, and (b) partial loss of perception of low-pitched sound.

The acuity of hearing through bone is easily determined by placing a vibrating tuning fork on the mastoid process and establishing the length of time over which the sound is appreciated, and then comparing this value with that obtained when the examiner (with normal hearing) places the vibrating fork on his own mastoid process (Schwabach's test). In partial sensorineural deafness there is a decrease in the length of time the tuning fork is heard through bone, and in complete sensorineural deafness no bone-conducted sound is heard. In middle-ear deafness the sound of the tuning fork applied over the mastoid is heard longer than normally. Schwabach's test is of diagnostic value only when the diminished acuity of hearing is bilateral. A tuning fork having a frequency of 516 c.p.s. is most satisfactory for use in this test, and a fork with a frequency of 2,000 c.p.s. when sensorineural loss in connection with perception of speech is suspected.

Rinne's test is also employed to detect impairment of hearing. A vibrating tuning fork is placed on the mastoid process of the patient, and when he ceases to hear the sound, the fork is removed from the bone and placed before the external canal of the ear. A person with normal hearing perceives the sound anew, and he hears it about twice as long as he did when it was placed on the bone. Under such conditions the Rinne test is "positive." In involvement of the sound-conduction apparatus, in which perception of air-conducted sound is decreased and that of bone-conducted sound is unaltered, the tuning fork is not heard in the latter phase of the test and the Rinne test is thus "negative." In sensorineural hypacusis of moderate severity the Rinne test is positive. In complete sensorineural deafness neither bone-conducted nor air-conducted sound is heard.

Dependable data are obtained by Rinne's test

only when acuity of hearing is diminished on both sides, for in unilateral sensorineural deafness the vibrations may be transmitted to the normal ear and may be perceived in that ear for a longer time than the vibrations conveyed by air conduction to the affected ear. The Rinne test is thus "falsely negative."

Weber's test gives more clear-cut information with respect to acuity of hearing. If a vibrating tuning fork is placed on the middle of the forehead or on the vertex of the skull of a normal person, it can be heard equally in both ears. If the canal of one ear is plugged—for example, by a finger—thus eliminating air conduction, the sound is "lateralized," heard loudest on that side. The sound is likewise lateralized to the affected ear in patients with unilateral disease of the conduction apparatus ("positive Weber"). The opposite holds true in unilateral sensorineural deafness; the sound is lateralized to the normal side ("negative Weber"). In bilateral deafness Weber's test is of no value, nor does it give any information when there is both sensorineural deafness and middle ear disease unilaterally.

To avoid incorrect answers one should be on his guard lest the patient lateralize the sound to the normal ear, for he may be convinced that it cannot be otherwise.

In sensorineural deafness the words hardest to hear are those with sibilants and bright vowels (*e* and *i*), such as vessel, fish, sister, and stillness. The patient has no difficulty in hearing flat consonants and vowels *(a, o, u)*, such as warm, book, hundred, and vanguard. In hypacusis of non-neural origin the reverse is the case, sibilants and bright vowels being best heard.

Complete deafness always denotes nerve involvement. As mentioned, in severe hearing deficit due to disease of the middle ear some perception of higher notes persists. Audimetry furnishes a means for determining whether unilateral hypacusis is of neural or non-neural origin; the hypacusis can be of neural origin only if the sound reaching both ears equally is loudest in the affected ear.

Speech discrimination. Speech reception threshold is determined on the basis of the subject's ability to hear familiar two-syllable words, such as "bullfrog" or "football," that depend for their recognition on vowel sounds. Then at greater sound intensity—25 to 30 db.—one-syllable words recognizable by their higher-pitched consonants—"slim" or "pin"—are repeated to him. Fifty words of these kinds are read off to the subject, with each word given a value of 2 percent. A very low score (0 to 10 percent) indicates eighth nerve damage (usually acoustic neuroma); a score of 40 to 80 percent indicates cochlear damage.

Loudness recruitment. This is a phenomenon elicitable from a partially deaf ear. A person who may not hear a tone of 50 db. will, by the time it is increased by 2 or 3 db., hear it normally. When intensity is further increased slightly, the tone may become painful. Occurrence of this phenomenon, when due to cochlear damage, presupposes a less than normal complement of external hair cells and a normal nerve fiber population. Despite threshold hearing loss owing to the hair cell loss, the potentials generated by stimulation of the remaining hair cells by the higher stimulus intensities activate a sufficient number of neurons to allow the person to hear. In testing loudness recruitment both ears should be examined, and a comparison made. (Menzel, 1966.) The loudness recruitment phenomenon has generally been thought to signify only peripheral sensorineural hearing loss, but there is strong evidence for its occurrence in pontile lesions, for example, in multiple sclerosis, vertebral-basilar arterial insufficiency, and infarct (Parker, Decker, and Richards, 1968).

Paracusis. A difference of opinion still exists as to the nature of the phenomenon known as paracusis Willisiana, characterized by the ability to hear better in a noisy place, such as in a moving train, than in quiet surroundings. The disorder is found only in people having some form of middle-ear deafness. Some otologists believe that the paracusic can hear better in noisy surroundings because the loud extraneous noise shakes the ossicular chain, thereby lessening its rigidity or, alternatively, that the ambient noise increases sensitivity of the organ of Corti. Others believe that the internal ear responds to intense stimuli in a different fashion than at threshold intensity, possibly due to a special function of the inner rods of Corti, which stretch across the tunnel of Corti. Findings in the paracusic are as follows: (1) the sensitivity of the normal ear to ambient noise is reduced considerably for all frequencies but especially for frequencies higher than 1,500 c.p.s. and (2) to intense ambient noise the conduction-impaired ear responds as well as, if not better than, the normal ear, especially for tones above 1,500 c.p.s. The rate of change of sensitivity of the abnormal conduction deafened ear relative to the normal ear is large. (Shapiro, 1967.)

Tinnitus. An irritative lesion involving the labyrinth or cochlear nerve manifests itself subjectively by noises that may be roaring, humming, whistling, or hissing (like escaping steam) in character. The tinnitus may seem to be originating within the ear or coming from the surroundings. The responsible lesion is difficult for the examiner to localize, for tinnitus may occur in affections of the labyrinth, cochlear nerve, or middle ear. Of middle ear disorders, only *otosclerosis* need be mentioned as a cause of tinnitus; the tinnitus has been attributed variously to (a) pathological disturbances in cochlear hair cells or ganglion cells from toxic substances or impaired blood supply, and (b) an unmasking of visceral tinnitus, the usually subaudible vascular and muscular noises now acting as auditory stimuli due to the removal of the normal masking effect of ambient noise. The tinnitus is particularly intense in patients having active foci in middle ear structures and when otosclerosis is associated with internal ear involvement (as indicated by decreasing hearing). Complicating internal ear involvement is common and in some instances may be related to drainage of material from otosclerotic foci into the venous system of the membranous labyrinth via a "venous shunt" occurring as a consequence of new vessel formation in the otosclerotic foci. (Glasgold and Altmann, 1966; Jørgensen and Kristensen, 1967; Rüedi, 1965; Spiegel and Sommer, 1944.)

Tinnitus is such a constant symptom of nerve lesions that it may be said a priori that if the patient has (or has had) no tinnitus, he has no sensorineural deafness. Localization of the responsible lesion may be made on the basis of certain qualitative peculiarities of the tinnitus. Thus, the tinnitus of middle ear origin (as in otosclerosis) is constant, while in sensorineural deafness the intensity of the tinnitus varies markedly from time to time. In both conditions, pitch of the tinnitus varies from low to high.

In cases of obvious sensorineural deafness in which tinnitus occurs, the responsible lesion cannot be localized with any degree of certainty to the cochlear nerve unless there is evidence that neighboring structures are also affected. The structure most likely to be simultaneously involved is the adjoining vestibular nerve, as manifested chiefly by vertigo. The seventh and sixth nerves may also be affected. That the tinnitus may be due to an extrinsic lesion is also indicated by symptoms and signs referable to the medulla oblongata, the pons, or even the cerebellum.

Deafness and/or tinnitus of peripheral origin. The responsible lesions are diverse. They include acute labyrinthitis, chronic otitis interna, and arterial or venous disease. Chronic otitis media may also be a basis (of deafness) owing to postinflammatory fixation of the malleus (Hilding, 1965). Deafness and/or tinnitus may be due to tumor involving the intrapetrous part of the nerve (Jefferson and Smalley, 1938; Love, 1950). In osteitis deformans the internal auditory meatus may become hyperplastic and thus lead to compression of the eighth nerve, with deafness associated or not with tinnitus. Deafness in congenital syphilis is usually due to involvement of the internal ear; deafness in tabes is attributable to syphilitic damage of the trunk of the eighth nerve.

Severe hearing loss commonly occurs following fracture of the petrous pyramid. If the fracture is in the longitudinal plane (lengthwise through the petrous pyramid), the hearing loss may, according to McHugh (1959), be of the sensorineural or the middle-ear type and be permanent in 70 percent of cases; deafness of the middle-ear type is partly reversible. McGovern (1968), on the other hand, found that hearing loss following longitudinal fracture was usually reversible. In transverse fracture the deafness is usually of the sensorineural type, and is often permanent (McGovern, 1968).

Ways exist for distinguishing between damage of the cochlear nerve alone and damage of both cochlear nerve and organ of Corti. A loss of speech discrimination in the involved ear out of proportion to pure tone thresholds for that ear usually signifies damage of the cochlear nerve (and integrity of the organ of Corti). Under these conditions, loudness recruitment does not occur. Where, by contrast, the cochlear nerve lesion occludes the blood supply to the cochlea, damaging the organ of Corti, loudness recruitment *does* occur. (Schuknecht and Woellner, 1955.)

Deafness and/or tinnitus due to pathological processes in the region of the cerebellopontile angle. Damage of the eighth nerve in the region between the porus acusticus and the edge of the lowermost pons gives rise to a variety of clinical disturbances referred to as the *cerebellopontile angle syndrome.* Responsible inflammatory processes include syphilitic meningovasculitis (Friedman, Brock, and Denker, 1933) and tuberculous and other forms of meningitis. Cholesteatomas and hemangiomatous malformations are sometimes found in this region. Neoplasms found here include papillary ependymoma (Kernohan, Woltman, and Adson, 1948), meningioma, hemangioendothelioma, ninth nerve neurinoma (Naunton, Proctor, and Elpern, 1968), and seventh nerve neurinoma (Johnson, 1966). Neoplasms invading the region of the angle include hemangioendothelioma (Johnson, 1966), medulloblastoma (Alexander, 1937), and carcinoma and other neoplasms situated in the region of the gasserian ganglion. But by far the most common tumor in this region is *acoustic neuroma.*

Acoustic neuroma is usually located in the porus acusticus but may occasionally be found within the internal auditory canal. When located in the porus, the tumor usually grows slowly into the cerebellopontile angle, and may reach considerable size (Fig. 13-11). It originates from neurilemmal cells of the vestibular part of the eighth nerve. Nerve fibers un-

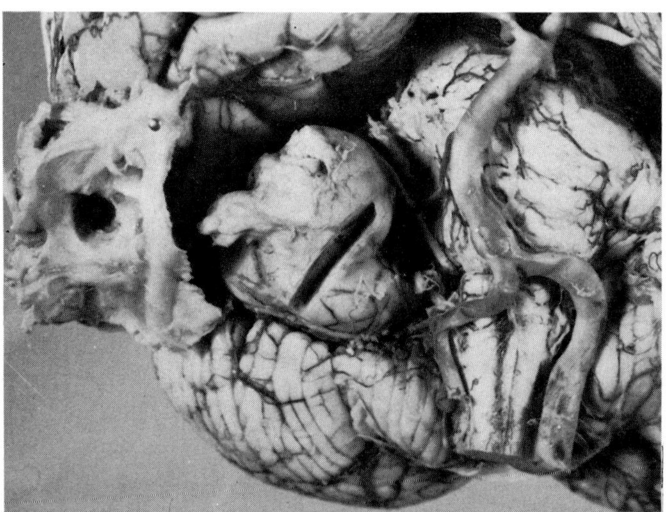

Fig. 13-11. Acoustic neuroma in the region of the porus acusticus, with great enlargement of the porus. Complicating hypertensive internal hydrocephalus occurred as a result of chronic herniation of the cerebellar tonsils into the foramen magnum and obstruction of the foramen of Magendie. The patient was admitted to a mental hospital, where he was found confused and forgetful. The tumor went undiagnosed. (Courtesy Dr. Richard Lindenberg, Baltimore.)

dergo degeneration, but unless labyrinthine blood vessels are compressed, the vestibular end-organs and the organ of Corti remain unaltered. Growth of the tumor usually becomes clinically evident in the fifth decade of life. Tinnitus is usually the initial symptom. Should the first complaints be referable to any other nerve or to some other neighboring structure, it is improbable that the responsible lesion is an acoustic neuroma. Impairment of labyrinthine function is usually detectable early in the clinical course. Characteristically there is a tilting and rotation of the head so that the chin is directed toward the side of the tumor. Lack of response from the vertical semicircular canals and a normal response from the contralateral horizontal canal, sometimes observed, may be interpreted as an indication that pressure is being exerted on the side of the lower pons and implicating only the fibers from the opposite vertical canals, which are presumed to course superficially in this region (p. 200). Vertigo occurs in some 25 percent of patients. A sensorineural type of hearing loss is noted in practically all patients, and sometimes the deafness is so advanced that only pure tone thresholds or pure tone and speech thresholds can be elicited (Johnson, 1966). Occasionally the hearing loss is of the middle-ear type, strongly suggestive of that observed in otosclerosis (Halperin, 1965).

Three syndromes in accordance with location of the acoustic neuroma have been distinguished by Hitselberger and House (1966): (1) intracanalicular neuroma, associated with cochlear, vestibular, and/or sensory facial involvement; (2) neuroma outside the internal auditory canal, associated or not with fifth or other cranial nerve involvement; and (3) neuroma outside the internal auditory canal, associated with elevated intracranial pressure, tonsillar herniation, and disturbances of cerebellar origin such as incoordination and staggering gait and diminution of pendular movement of the upper limb of the affected side. Early in the course of growth of the tumor there may be suboccipital discomfort or headache limited to or predominant on the side of the neuroma. Dysarthria, dysphagia, respiratory embarrassment, and tonic seizures may occur. There may be dysesthesias, pain, or hypalgesia in parts of the face as a result of compression of the spinal nucleus and tract of the fifth nerve, or of the fifth nerve itself. The corneal reflex is commonly reduced or abolished. Another nerve subject to involvement is the seventh; if involved there may be facial weakness and muscle twitching, and, less commonly, intermittent facial spasm. Diplopia due to implication of the sixth nerve nucleus may also develop. Furthermore, there may be conjugate ocular paresis and nystagmus toward the side of the lesion, from pressure exerted on the pontile mechanism for conjugate ocular movement. Positional nystagmus may also occur. (Cushing, 1917; Johnson, 1966; Pool and Pava, 1957; Revilla, 1947.)

Increased intracranial pressure does not, per se, appear to cause hearing deficit (Hansen, 1968).

Brainstem deafness. Deafness due to intrinsic lesions of the brainstem is not uncommon. Thrombosis involving the quadrigeminal branch of the superior cerebellar artery may result in partial deafness, which is of sudden occurrence. Hearing loss may also be a symptom of circulatory deficit in the pons; the hearing loss usually vanishes during the asymptomatic intervals. In multiple sclerosis a loss of more than 25 db. in one or both ears, due presumably to involvement of cochlear nuclei or nerve, has been observed in 40 percent of cases (von Leden and Horton, 1947). In pontile tumors the hearing deficit tends to be on one side, usually contralateral to the lesion. Consistent with the wide extent of the corpus trapezoideum and the high margin of physiological safety of the cochlear system in general, hearing loss due to its involvement is likely to be predominantly unilateral and partial. Tumors at higher brainstem levels having a tendency to cause deafness are gliomas of the tegmentum or tectum or the midbrain-diencephalic transitional area, also pineal tumors and, rarely, suprasellar tumors. At the level of the lower midbrain, where the cross-sectional area is smaller than in the pons, deafness due to neoplastic and inflammatory lesions is fairly common. Although occurring, as a rule, late in the clinical course, deafness due to a lesion in this region tends to develop with almost apoplectiform suddenness. Objective testing reveals decrease in bone conduction time. Tumors in the midbrain are likely to be associated with labyrinthine hyperexcitability, which distinguishes them from pontile and cerebellar tumors, in which a decrease in labyrinthine excitability is the rule. (Glaser, 1929; Sloane, Persky, and Saltzman, 1943.)

Study of auditory function in patients having lesions of various kinds in the pons (in multiple sclerosis, infarction, vertebral-basilar arterial insufficiency) has revealed average results reasonably distinct from average results obtained from a like number of cases in which lesions involved the eighth nerve or other structures in the cerebellopontile angle. Pontile lesions were characterized by severe pathological adaptation or tone perversion commonly associated with relatively good pure tone threshold, relatively good discrimination scores, complete recruitment, bilaterality of adaptation or tone perversion, and active caloric response. (Parker, Decker, and Richards, 1968.)

Hearing loss in hemiplegic patients. In about 50 percent of patients with hemiplegia, auditory threshold (to a pure tone at a frequency of 512 Hz. for 1 second) is significantly higher in the contralateral ear than in the other ear or in nonbrain-damaged control patients (Karp, Belmont, and Birch, 1969).

Cortical deafness. See page 380.

SITES OF END-ORGAN DAMAGE, AND SYMPTOMATOLOGY

Of *viral infections*, mumps and measles are prone to affect only the cochlea—its hair cells—particularly the hair cells in the basal turn. The saccular macula may, however, share in the damage. Usually, the cochlear involvement is unilateral. The hearing loss can be of any degree and can be reversible or irreversible. Maternal prenatal rubella involves both ears. In this disorder, stria vascularis, tectorial membrane and other components of the organ of Corti, and the saccule have been found degenerated. (Ward, Honrubia, and Moore, 1968.)

Bacterial infections can involve the labyrinths secondarily in acute otitis media or as a consequence of fracture of the petrous bone, in which case sensory cells may suffer, leading to vertigo and hearing loss. Total deafness may result from suppurative labyrinthitis (Carmichael, Dix, and Hallpike, 1956).

In *congenital syphilis*, endolymphatic hydrops, perilabyrinthitis, and labyrinthitis are key pathological features. The hearing disturbances are similar to those occurring in Ménière's disease.

Among agents toxic to the internal ear are *antibiotics* derived from the streptomyces strain. Streptomycin and dihydrostreptomycin when given over a prolonged period of time in effective dosage selectively destroy hair cells of the cristae of the semicircular canals (Berg, 1949; Christensen and others, 1951; McGee and Olszewski, 1962). Both these antibiotics also cause degenerative changes in the hair cells of the basal turn of the organ of Corti, the first row of outer hair cells suffering the most. With the use of streptomycin sulfate, the degeneration may occur only after the caloric response of the semicircular canals has been eliminated in the course of the therapy. Dihydrostreptomycin action is not nearly as predictable; dosage large enough to destroy only the hair cells of the cristae may lead to hearing loss within a few months (Hawkins, 1950). Neomycin has a severe ototoxic effect, which may be disastrous so far as the cochlea is concerned. Kanamycin, also potentially disastrous, leads first to hearing loss in the high frequency range, consonant with the observation that degeneration of the organ of Corti begins in the basal coil, involving the outer hair cells almost selectively. (Engström, Ades, and Andersson, 1966.)

In fracture of the petrous pyramid, erythrocytes and an increase in protein have been noted in endolymph and perilymph and, subsequently, degenerative changes in the organ of Corti and collapse of Reissner's membrane (Videbech, 1935).

Concussion, as from blows on the head, may induce hearing loss, which is maximum for the 4,000 c.p.s. tone (Schuknecht and Davison, 1956). The nature of the hearing loss is similar to that now to be discussed.

Exposure to *intense noise* results in hearing losses that are usually most severe for the high frequencies. These include continuous high-intensity noise, gunfire, and explosions. It is often stated that hair cells in basal part of the coil, representing the 4,000 c.p.s. frequency, suffer the most damage. However, in one study (Engström, Ades, and Andersson, 1966), hair cells at levels one and a half to two and a half coils from the base were the most severely affected. Under extreme exposure conditions supporting cells in the organ of Corti together with neuronal elements may also undergo degeneration (Covell, 1953).

Ménière's disease, occurring in middle-aged persons, somewhat more frequently in men than in women, is a disorder resulting from progressive hydrops involving both the cochlear and the vestibular part of the labyrinth (Hallpike and Cairns, 1938; Lindsay, 1944). Tinnitus may be the initial symptom. Usually only one ear is affected. Cochlea and saccule tend to be affected first, then the semicircular canals and the utricle. Accordingly, in the preparoxysmal stage of the disease, hearing loss for low frequency tones may be complained of. Attacks of vertigo together with tinnitus and nystagmus then occur. Progressive hearing loss occurs as the pathological process advances. Frequently added to this triad (tinnitus, vertigo, deafness) is headache, either occipital or generalized, and either intermittent or constant. Nausea and vomiting also occur during attacks. It has been postulated that the attacks coincide with rupture(s) of the vestibular endolymphatic system, an attack continuing as long as endolymph circulation is abnormal and ceasing when the site of rupture(s) is sealed over (Schuknecht, Benitez, and Beekhuis, 1962). Sensitivity of the cristae ampullares, as brought out by caloric testing, may be entirely normal.

Vestibular neuronitis is a term given a disorder characterized by acute vertigo accompanied by nystagmus (toward the sound ear) and unilaterally decreased caloric and galvanic reactions. Nausea and vomiting commonly occur during attacks, and the symptoms are made worse by rapid change in the position of the head. The disorder occurs in persons in a wide age range (17 to 65 years). Absence of tinnitus and impaired hearing distinguish the disorder from Ménière's disease. An infection, frequently involving the nose or pharynx—for example, common cold or sinusitis—usually immediately precedes the acute symptomatic stage. Caloric testing reveals evidence of interruption of the nerve (in its intracanalicular course) in most patients, and directional preponderance of the nystagmus in others. Disability usually lasts 3 to 12 weeks. A lesion of the vestibular nerve in a region central to the labyrinth is considered responsible for the disorder. (Lumio and Aho, 1965.)

Hearing loss in the course of an *aging process* in the cochlear epithelium and cochlear nerve first appears in some persons in their forties. It generally consists in a slight high-tone sensorineural hearing loss. At this stage and subsequently, the hearing loss varies in nature in accordance with the sites at which the aging process occurs. Tests for recruitment can serve to distinguish the various types. One type is called *sensory presbycusis.* It begins during middle age. Hearing loss of high-frequency tones occurs abruptly, and the condition gradually worsens over the years as hearing of lower tones also decreases. Speech discrimination also suffers. The disorder is due to atrophy of the organ of Corti and the spiral ganglion of the auditory nerve along the first few millimeters of the basal coil of the cochlea. A second type (*metabolic presbycusis*), also with onset in middle age, is characterized by "flat" sensorineural hearing loss (in contrast to the descending loss just mentioned). Atrophy of the stria vascularis, particularly in the middle and apical turns of the cochlea, has been noted. Speech discrimination remains normal. A further type (*neural presbycusis*), which becomes evident in later life, is due to neuron loss in the cochlear nerves and in the respective pathways in the central nervous system. The end-organs, by contrast, show little evidence of change. Hearing, chiefly of high tones, suffers, and there is a marked inability to hear or understand words. However, there may be relatively mild high-tone hearing loss for pure tones in association with rather severe speech discrimination loss ("phonemic regression"). (Bredberg, 1967; Campanelli, 1968; Myers and Carmel, 1967; Schuknecht, 1955, 1964.)

OTALGIA

Intrinsic causes aside, pain in the ear may develop as a consequence of painful or nonpainful disease states involving structures at distant sites. Exposed dentin or tooth caries may give rise to otalgia, as may an unerupted or impacted tooth or malocclusion. Temporomandibular joint disease, tonsillitis, nasopharyngitis, tracheal disease, eustachian tube blockage, and ulceration of the posterior third of the tongue are additional causes. To be included are trapezius spasm (torticollis) and tuberculous caries of cervical vertebrae. Aneurysm of the thoracic aorta or of the innominate artery, angina pectoris, and gastric lesions are other disorders in which pain may develop in the ear. Under these conditions the pain is felt deep in the ear and it is often of a throbbing character. (Hubert, 1923; Tremble, 1965; Yules, 1967.)

Pain referred to the ear from many sources is consistent with the diversity of origin of the ear's sensory nerve supply. The ear receives branches from the fifth, seventh, ninth, and tenth nerves. Innervation is illustrated in part in Fig. 12-6. Where pain is referred to the ear from a lesion elsewhere, it is likely that both the ear and the area containing the lesion receive their sensory innervation from the *same* cranial nerve, with spread of the pain impulses in the gray matter of the brainstem via connections between cell groups in the recipient nucleus. The maxillary division of the fifth nerve provides sensory innervation both for the ear and the region of the mandible and the tongue, the ninth nerve both for the ear and the tonsil, and the tenth both for the ear and the larynx. In the first instance, impulses from a diseased third molar or from a diseased temporomandibular joint would reach the nucleus of the spinal tract of the fifth nerve, spread to adjacent cell groups receiving impulses from the ear (wall of the external auditory meatus and tympanic membrane), and be interpreted as actually coming from the ear. To cite another example: somatic afferent fibers from a painful larynx travelling in the tenth nerve would reach the nucleus of the spinal tract of the fifth nerve and, as before, be transferred to the cell group receiving impulses from the ear. (Tremble, 1965.) As an alternative, the pain impulses could overflow via interconnections at the level of the sensory ganglia (Sinclair, Weddell, and Feindel, 1948).

REFERENCES

Alexander, L. 1937. Tumors and cysts of the cerebellopontine angle and their relation to the lateral recesses of the fourth ventricle. Res. Publ. Ass. Res. Nerv. Ment. Dis., Proc. **16**: 266-314.

Anson, B. A., Donaldson, J. A., Warpeha, R. L., and Winch, T. R. 1965. II. Anatomic considerations. Laryngoscope **75**:1497-1517.

Anson, B. J., Warpeha, R. L., and Rensink, M. J. 1968. The gross and macroscopic anatomy of the labyrinths. Ann. Otol. Rhin. Laryng. **77**: 583-608.

Barber, H. O. 1964. Positional nystagmus, especially after head injury. Laryngoscope **74**:891-944.

Barnes, W. T., Magoun, H. W., and Ranson, S. W. 1943. The ascending auditory pathway in the brain stem of the monkey. J. Comp. Neurol. **79**:129-152.

Bast, T. H., and Anson, B. 1949. The temporal bone and the ear. Springfield, Illinois, Charles C Thomas, Publisher.

Bender, M. B., and Weinstein, E. A. 1943. Functional representation in the oculomotor and trochlear nuclei. Arch. Neurol. Psychiat. **49**: 98-106.

Berg, K. 1949. The toxic effect of streptomycin on the eighth cranial nerve. Ann. Otol. Rhin. Laryng. **58**:448-456.

Bergan, J. J., Levy, J. S., Trippel, O. H., and Jurayj, M. 1967. Vascular implications of vertigo. Arch. Otolaryng. **85**:292-297.

Bredberg, G. 1967. The human cochlea during

development and ageing. J. Laryng. Otol. **81**: 739-758.

Bredberg, G., Engström, H., and Ades, H. W. 1965. Cellular pattern and nerve supply of the human organ of Corti: a preliminary report. Arch. Otolaryng. **82**:462-469.

Brodal, A., and Hoivik, B. 1964. Site and mode of termination of primary vestibulocerebellar fibers in the cat. Arch. Ital. Biol. **102**:1-21.

Brodal, A., Pompeiano, O., and Walberg, F. 1962. The vestibular nuclei and their connections, anatomy and functional correlations. Springfield, Illinois, Charles C Thomas, Publisher.

Campanelli, P. A. 1968. Audiological perspectives in presbycusis. Eye, Ear, Nose, Throat Mthly. **47**:1-9, 81-86.

Campbell, H. J. 1965. Correlative physiology of the nervous system. New York, Academic Press, Inc.

Carmichael, E. A., Dix, M. R., and Hallpike, C. S. 1956. Pathology, symptomatology and diagnosis of organic affections of eighth nerve system. Brit. Med. Bull. **12**:146-152.

Carpenter, W. B. 1959. Lesions of the fastigial nuclei in the rhesus monkey. Amer. J. Anat. **104**:1-33.

Carter, S, Sciarra, D., and Merritt, H. H. 1950. The course of multiple sclerosis as determined by autopsy proven cases. Res. Publ. Ass. Res. Nerv. Ment. Dis., Proc. **28**:471-511.

Christensen, E., Hertz, H., Riskaer, N., and Vra-Jensen, G. 1951. Histological investigations in chronic streptomycin poisoning in guinea pigs. Ann. Otol. Rhin. Laryng. **60**:343-347.

Citron, L., Exley, D., and Hallpike, C. S. 1956. Formation, circulation and chemical properties of the labyrinthine fluids. Brit. Med. Bull. **12**: 101-104.

Collard, M., Conraux, C., Thiébaut, M.-S., and Thiébaut, F. 1967. Le nystagmus d'origine cervicale. Rev. Neurol. **2**:677-688.

Covell, W. P. 1953. Histologic changes in the organ of Corti with intense sound. J. Comp. Anat. **99**:43-59.

Cranmer, R. 1951. Nystagmus related to lesions of the central vestibular apparatus and the cerebellum. Ann. Otol. Rhin. Laryng. **60**:186-196.

Crosby, E. C. 1953. Relations of brain centers to normal and abnormal eye movements in the horizontal plane. J. Comp. Neurol. **99**:437-479.

Crosby, E. C., Humphrey, T., and Lauer, E. W. 1962. Correlative anatomy of central nervous system. New York, The Macmillan Company.

Cushing, H. 1917. Tumors of the nervus acusticus and the syndrome of the cerebellopontile angle. Philadelphia, W. B. Saunders Co.

Daroff, R. B. 1965. See-saw nystagmus. Neurology **15**:874-877.

Davis, H. 1957. Biophysics and physiology of the inner ear. Physiol. Rev. **37**:1-49.

Davis, H. 1968. Mechanisms of the inner ear. Ann. Otol. Rhin. Laryng. **77**:644-656.

Dix, M. R., and Hallpike, C. S. 1952. The pathology, symptomatology and diagnosis of certain common disorders of the vestibular system. Proc. Roy. Soc. Med. **45**:341-354.

Dohlman, G. F. 1968. Secretion and absorption of the endolymph. Third symposium of the role of the vestibular organs in space exploration. NASA SP-152. Washington, D. C., Government Printing Office, pp. 101-123.

Drachman, D. A. 1966. See-saw nystagmus. J. Neurol. Neurosurg. Psychiat. **29**:356-361.

Druckman, R., Ellis, P., Kleinfeld, J., and Waldman, M. 1966. Seesaw nystagmus. Arch. Ophthal. **76**:668-675.

Engström, H., Ades, H. W., and Andersson, A. 1966. Structural pattern of the organ of Corti: a systematic mapping of sensory cells and neural elements. Baltimore, The Williams & Wilkins Co.

Fex, J. 1959. Augmentation of cochlear microphonic by stimulation of efferent fibers of the cochlea. Acta Otolaryng. **50**:540-541.

Friedman, E. D., Brock, S., and Denker, P. 1933. Syphilis of the cerebellopontine angle. J. Syph. **17**:330-338.

Fulton, J. F., and Dow, R. S. 1937. The cerebellum: a summary of functional localization. Yale J. Biol. Med. **10**:85-119.

Gacek, R. R. 1968a. Neuroanatomical pathways of the vestibular system. Ann. Otol. Rhin. Laryng. **77**:210-215.

Gacek, R. R. 1968b. The innervation of the vestibular labyrinth. Ann. Otol. Rhin. Laryng. **77**: 676-686.

Galambos, R. 1956. Suppression of the auditory nerve activity by stimulation of efferent fibers to the cochlea. J. Neurophysiol. **19**:424-437.

Glaser, M. A. 1929. Tumors of the pineal, corpora quadrigemina and third ventricle: the interrelationship of their syndromes and their surgical treatment. Brain **52**:226-261.

Glasgold, A., and Altmann, F. 1966. The effect of stapes surgery on tinnitus in otosclerosis. Laryngoscope **76**:1524-1532.

Goto, K., Tokumasu, K., and Cohen, B. 1968. Return eye movements, saccadic movements, and the quick phase of nystagmus. Acta Otolaryng. **65**:426-440.

Hallpike, C. S., and Cairns, H. 1938. Observations on the pathology of Ménière's syndrome. J. Laryng. Otol. **53**:625-655.

Halperin, D. 1965. VIII nerve tumor. Report of a case. Ann. Otol. Rhin. Laryng. **74**:669-672.

Hansen, C. C. 1968. Perceptive hearing loss and increased intracranial pressure. Arch. Otolaryng. **87**:45-47.

Hawkins, J. E., Jr. 1950. Cochlear signs of streptomycin intoxication. J. Pharmacol. Exp. Ther. **100**:38-44.

Hilding, D. A. 1965. Postinflammatory fixation of the malleus. Arch. Otolaryng. **81**:17-19.

Hitselberger, W. E., and House, W. F. 1966. Classification of acoustic neuromas. Arch. Otolaryng. **84**:245-246.

Holmes, G. 1952. Introduction to clinical neurology, ed. 2. Baltimore, The Williams & Wilkins Co.

Hough, J. V. D., and Stuart, W. D. 1968. Middle ear injuries in skull trauma. Laryngoscope **78**: 899-937.

Hubert, L. 1923. Study of mechanism of pain as

seen in otological cases. Laryngoscope 33:596-608.

Hyde, J. E., and Toczek, S. 1962. Functional relation of interstitial nucleus to rotary movements evoked by zona incerta stimulation. J. Neurophysiol. **25**:455-466.

Iinuma, T., Shitara, T., Hoshino, T., and Kirikae, I. 1967. Sensorineural hearing loss for low tones. Arch. Otolaryng. **86**:136-142.

Iurato, S. 1962. Efferent fibers to the sensory cells of Corti's organ. Exp. Cell Res. **27**:162-164.

Jefferson, G., and Smalley, A. A. 1938. Progressive facial palsy produced by intratemporal epidermoids. J. Laryng. Otol. **53**:417-443.

Johnson, E. W. 1966. Confirmed retrocochlear lesions: auditory test results in 163 patients. Arch. Otolaryng. **84**:245-291.

Jones, I. H., and Spiller, W. G. 1925. The central tracts of the nervus vestibularis. Brain **48**:334-361.

Jørgensen, M. B., and Kristensen, H. K. 1967. Frequency of histological otosclerosis. Ann. Otol. Rhin. Laryng. **76**:83-88.

Karp, E., Belmont, I., and Birch, H. G. 1969. Unilateral hearing loss in hemiplegic patients. J. Nerv. Ment. Dis. **148**:83-86.

Katsuki, Y., Watanabe, T., and Masuyama, N. 1959. Activity of auditory neurons in upper levels of brain of cat. J. Neurophysiol. **22**:343-359.

Kernohan, J. W., Woltman, H. W., and Adson, A. W. 1948. Gliomas of the cerebellopontine angle. J. Neuropath. Exp. Neurol. **7**:349-367.

Larsell, O. 1951. Anatomy of the nervous system, ed. 2. New York, Appleton-Century-Crofts.

Leivers, E. 1968. Vertigo: an explanation—labyrinthine arrhythmia. Arch. Otolaryng. **88**:373-376.

Lewy, F. H., and Kobrak, H. 1936. The neural projection of the cochlear spirals on the primary acoustic centers. A.M.A. Arch. Neurol. Psychiat. **35**:839-852.

Lindsay, J. R. 1944. Ménière's disease: histopathological observations. Arch. Otolaryng. **39**: 313-318.

Lindsay, J. R. 1945. The significance of a positional nystagmus in otoneurological diagnosis. Laryngoscope **55**:527-551.

Love, J. G. 1950. Unilateral deafness and progressive facial palsy due to intrapetrous neurofibroma: surgical treatment. Proc. Staff Meet. Mayo Clin. **25**:228-232.

Lumio, J. S., and Aho, J. 1965. Vestibular neuronitis. Ann. Otol. Rhin. Laryng. **74**:264-271.

Markham, C. H., Precht, W., and Shimazu, H. 1966. Effect of stimulation of interstitial nucleus of Cajal on vestibular unit activity in the cat. J. Neurophysiol. **29**:493-507.

Masterton, B., Jane, J. A., and Diamond, I. T. 1967. Role of the brainstem auditory structures in sound localization: trapezoid body, superior olive, and lateral lemniscus. J. Neurophysiol. **30**:341-359.

McGee, T. M., and Olszewski, J. 1962. Streptomycin sulfate and dihydrostreptomycin toxicity: behavioral and histopathologic studies. Arch. Otolaryng. **75**:295-311.

McGovern, F. H. 1968. Facial nerve injuries in skull fractures: recent advances in management. Arch. Otolaryng. **88**:536-542.

McHugh, H. E. 1959. The surgical treatment of facial paralysis and traumatic conductive deafness in fractures of the temporal bone. Ann. Otol. Rhin. Laryng. **68**:855-889.

McHugh, H. E. 1966. Auditory and vestibular disorders in head injury. In Caveness, W. F., and Walker, A. E., editors: Head injury. Philadelphia, J. B. Lippincott Company, pp. 97-105.

Menzel, O. J. 1966. The short increment sensitivity index (SISI). Eye, Ear, Nose, Throat Mthly. **45**:102-103.

Myers, D., and Carmel, N. 1967. Hearing disabilities in the geriatric patient. Eye, Ear, Nose, Throat Mthly. **46**:1385-1391.

Naunton, R. F., Proctor, L., and Elpern, B. S. 1968. The audiologic signs of ninth nerve neurinoma. Acta Otolaryng. **87**:222-227.

Nomura, Y., and Kirikae, I. 1967. Innervation of the human cochlea. Ann. Otol. Rhin. Laryng. **76**:57-68.

Norton, E. W. D. 1964. Nystagmus. In Smith, J. L., editor. University of Miami Neuro-Ophthalmology Symposium. Springfield, Illinois, Charles C Thomas, Publisher, pp. 288-305.

Nylén, C. O. 1939. The oto-neurological diagnosis of tumours of the brain. Acta Otolaryng., suppl. 33, pp. 1-151.

Nylén, C. O. 1950. Positional nystagmus: a review and future prospects. J. Laryng. Otol. **64**: 295-318.

Palva, T., and Raunio, V. 1968. The origin of perilymph albumin. Acta Otolaryng. **66**:136-144.

Parker, W., Decker, R. L., and Richards, N. G. 1968. Auditory function and lesions of the pons. Arch. Otolaryng. **87**:228-240.

Pollock, L. J., Boshes, B., Zivin, I., and others. 1955. Body reflexes acting on the body. A.M.A. Arch. Neurol. Psychiat. **74**:527-533.

Polyak, S. 1932. The main afferent fiber systems of the cerebral cortex in primates: an investigation of the central portions of the somatosensory, auditory, and visual paths of the cerebral cortex, with consideration of their normal and pathologic function, based on experiments with monkeys. Berkeley, University of California Press.

Pool, J. L., and Pava, A. A. 1957. The early diagnosis and treatment of acoustic nerve tumors. Springfield, Illinois, Charles C Thomas, Publisher.

Price, J. B., and Spiegel, E. A. 1937. Vestibulocerebral pathways: a contribution to the central mechanism of vertigo. Arch. Otolaryng. **26**: 658-667.

Rasmussen, A. T. 1940. Studies of eighth cranial nerve of man. Laryngoscope **50**:67-83.

Rasmussen, G. L. 1960. Efferent fibers of the cochlear nerve and cochlear nucleus. In Rasmussen, G. T., and Windle, W. F., editors: Neural mechanisms of the auditory and vestibular systems. Springfield, Illinois, Charles C Thomas, Publisher, pp. 105-115.

Reddy, J. B., and Liu, J.-C. 1966. Clinical nystagmography. Eye, Ear, Nose, Throat Mthly. **45**:48-57.

Revilla, A. G. 1947. Neurinomas of the cerebellopontile recess: a clinical study of one hundred and sixty cases including operative mortality and end results. Bull. Johns Hopk. Hosp. **80**:254-296.

Rüedi, L. 1965. Histopathologic confirmation of labyrinthine otosclerosis. Laryngoscope **75**:1582-1609.

Schäfer, J.-H. 1966. Über die Veränderungen der Vestibularisfunktion bei stereotaktischen Thalamus-Eingriffen am Menschen. Confin. Neurol. **28**:117-156.

Schiller, F., and Hedberg, W. C. 1960. An appraisal of positional nystagmus. A.M.A. Arch. Neurol. **2**:309-316.

Schuknecht, H. 1955. Presbycusis. Laryngoscope **65**:402-419.

Schuknecht, H. 1964. Further observations on the pathology of presbycusis. Acta Otolaryng. **80**: 369-382.

Schuknecht, H. F., Benitez, J. T., and Beekhuis, J. 1962. Further observations on the pathology of Ménière's disease. Ann. Otol. Rhin. Laryng. **71**: 1039-1053.

Schuknecht, H. F., and Davison, R. C. 1956. Deafness and vertigo from head injury. Arch. Otolaryng. **63**:513-518.

Schuknecht, H. F., Igarashi, M., and Gacek, R. R. 1965. The pathological types of cochleo-saccular degeneration. Acta Otolaryng. **59**:154-170.

Schuknecht, H. F., and Neff, W. D. 1952. Hearing losses after apical lesions in the cochlea. Acta Otolaryng. **42**:263-274.

Schuknecht, H. F., and Woellner, R. C. 1955. An experimental and clinical study of deafness from lesions of the cochlear nerve. J. Laryng. Otol. **69**:75-97.

Shapiro, S. L. 1967. Paracusis Willisiana. Eye, Ear, Nose, Throat Mthly. **46**:622-625.

Sinclair, D. C., Weddell, G., and Feindel, W. H. 1948. Referred pain and associated phenomena. Brain **71**:184-211.

Sloane, P., Persky, A. H., and Saltzman, M. 1943. Midbrain deafness: tumor of the midbrain producing sudden and complete deafness. Arch. Neurol. Psychiat. **49**:237-243.

Smith, C. A. 1961. Innervation pattern of the cochlea: the internal hair cell. Ann. Otol. Rhin. Laryng. **70**:504-527.

Smith, C. A., and Sjostrand, F. S. 1961. Structure of the nerve endings on the external hair cells of the guinea pig cochlea as studied by serial sections. J. Ultrastr. Res. **5**:523-556.

Spiegel, E. A., and Sommer, I. 1944. Neurology of the eye, ear, nose and throat. New York, Grune & Stratton, Inc.

Spiegel, E. A., Szekely, E. G., Moffet, R., Gildenberg, P., Lehman, R., and Robbins, A. 1965. Cortical projections of the labyrinth. In Kirikae, I., editor: International symposium on vestibular and oculomotor problems. University of Tokyo, Japan Society for Vestibular Research, pp. 9-14.

Spoendlin, H. H. 1965. The role of the vestibular organs in the exploration of space. NASA SP-77. Washington, D.C., Government Printing Office.

Stahle, J., and Terins, J. 1965. Paroxysmal positional nystagmus. An electronystagmographic and clinical study. Ann. Otol. Rhin. Laryng. **74**: 69-83.

Stenger, H. H. 1955. Über Lagerungsnystagmus unter besonderer Berücksichtigung des gegenläufigen transitorischen Provokationsnystagmus bei Lagewechsel in der Sagittalebene. Arch. Ohr.-Nas.-Kehlkopfheilk. **168**:220-268.

Tremble, G. E. 1965. Referred pain in the ear: causes and probable nerve pathways. Arch. Otolaryng. **81**:57-63.

Trincker, D. 1957. Bestandspotentiale im Bogengangssystem des Meerschweinchens und ihre Änderungen bei experimentellen Cupula-Ablenkungen. Pflügers Arch. Ges. Physiol. **264**: 351-382.

Tyler, D. B., and Bard, P. 1949. Motion sickness. Physiol. Rev. **29**:311-369.

Videbech, H. 1935. Affection du labyrinthe se présentant sous les traits du syndrome de Ménière. (Exploration fonctionelle et examen microscopique du labyrinthe.) Acta Otolaryng. **22**:51-65.

von Békésy, G. 1960. Experimental models of the cochlea with and without nerve supply. In Rasmussen, G. L., and Windle, W. F., editors: Neural mechanisms of the auditory and vestibular systems. Springfield, Illinois, Charles C Thomas, Publisher, pp. 3-20.

von Leden, H., and Horton, B. T. 1947. The auditory nerve in multiple sclerosis. Proc. Staff Meet., Mayo Clin. **22**:279-280.

Ward, P. H., Honrubia, V., and Moore, B. S. 1968. Inner ear pathology in deafness due to maternal rubella. Arch. Otolaryng. **87**:22-28.

Warwick, R. 1953. Representation of the extraocular muscles with oculomotor nuclei of the monkey. J. Comp. Neurol. **84**:449-504.

Weisenburg, T. H. 1922. Equilibration and the vestibular apparatus. Arch. Neurol. Psychiat. **7**: 210-219.

Wersäll, J. 1960. Electron micrographic studies of vestibular hair cell innervation. In Rasmussen, G. T., and Windle, W. F., editors: Neural mechanisms of the auditory and vestibular systems. Springfield, Illinois, Charles C Thomas, Publisher, pp. 247-257.

Wolfson, R. J., Myers, D., Schlosser, W. D., and Winchester, R. A. 1965. Vertigo. CIBA Clin. Sympos. **17**:99-133.

Yules, R. B. 1967. Differential diagnosis of referred otalgia. Ear, Nose, Throat Mthly. **46**: 587-588.

Chapter 14

Localization of lesions involving the facial nerve

ANATOMY AND FUNCTIONS

The facial or seventh cranial nerve, together with its sensory-parasympathetic component, the nervus intermedius (pars-intermedia of the facial nerve), emerges from the brainstem in the region of the cerebellopontile angle (Fig. 10-1). In company with the eighth nerve, the seventh nerve and the nervus intermedius pass distally to enter the internal auditory meatus. En route distalward through the posterior cranial fossa the nervus intermedius may run a course separate from the seventh and eighth nerves (Fig. 14-1) or be incorporated in the seventh nerve or be adherent to the vestibular nerve (in 20 percent of cases); or rootlets may leave the nervus intermedius or seventh nerve and join the vestibular nerve prior to entrance of the latter into the internal auditory meatus. Still farther distally the seventh nerve and the nervus intermedius continue in their own bony canal, the facial canal (or fallopian canal), giving off branches en route (Fig. 14-1). (Rhoton, Kobayashi, and Hollinshead, 1968; Sachs, 1968.)

The seventh nerve takes origin in a nucleus (the facial nucleus) situated deep in the tegmentum of the pons (Fig. 10-11). After traversing the facial canal it leaves the skull by way of the stylomastoid foramen. Having emerged from this foramen, the nerve separates into a large temporofacial and a small cervicofacial division, the bifurcation occurring in the cleft between the superficial and deep lobes of the parotid gland (Hoyt and Loeffler, 1965). Further branching occurs in the parotid gland within this plane of connective tissue. The branches supply all muscles of the face, from the frontalis above to the platysma below (including the orbicularis oculi and the buccinator), except the levator palpebrae superioris, which is supplied by the third nerve. The seventh nerve also supplies the stylohyoid muscle and the posterior belly of the digastric; further, it both innervates and receives fibers from the stapedius muscle (Blevins, 1967).

The seventh nerve in its infratemporal and intracanalicular course receives its *blood supply* from five sources: stylomastoid branch of the posterior auricular artery, petrosal branch of the middle meningeal artery, and branches from the internal auditory, anterior inferior cerebellar, and basilar arteries. The distribution of the vasa nervorum is such that the nerve is supplied by a series of overlapping arterial systems so that at any level the nerve contains vessels which reach it from two separate sources. (Sunderland and Cossar, 1953.) Other studies of the blood supply of this nerve have been reviewed by McGovern (1968b).

An imposing branch given off by the seventh nerve is the *chorda tympani* (Fig. 14-1). This branch usually leaves the seventh nerve just prior to emergence of the latter from the stylomastoid foramen. Considerable variation exists, however, with respect to the point of junction of the

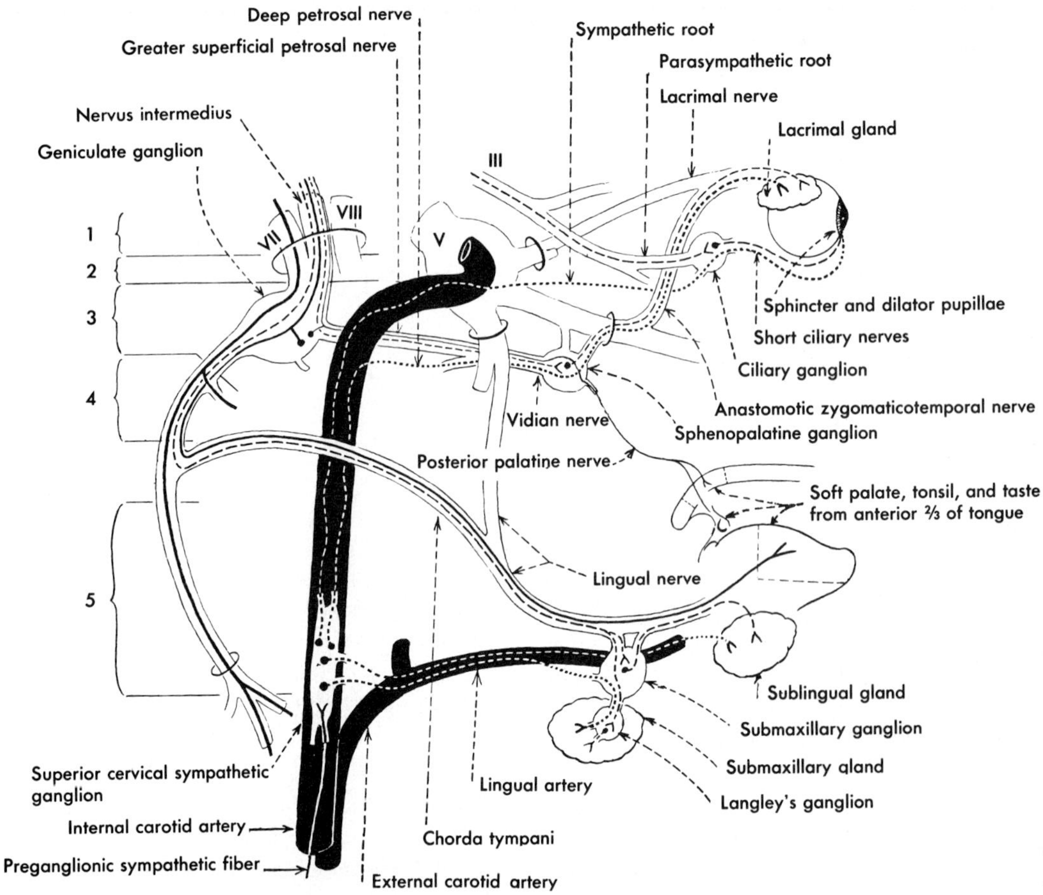

Fig. 14-1. The distribution of the components of the facial nerve and its sensory-parasympathetic component, the nervus intermedius, as seen from the medial aspect. *Heavy solid lines,* branchial motor fibers to the facial muscles and taste (visceral sensory) fibers from the anterior two-thirds of the tongue. *Broken lines,* parasympathetic fibers to the lacrimal, submaxillary, and sublingual glands. *Dotted lines,* postganglionic sympathetic fibers to the lacrimal, submaxillary, and sublingual glands and to the dilator pupillae. Also illustrated is the third nerve and the course of its parasympathetic fibers to the sphincter pupillae. The manifestations of lesions of the facial nerve in the bracketed regions are given in Table 14-1.

chorda tympani with the facial nerve. This point can lie in any region from the level of the lateral semicircular canal to just outside the stylomastoid foramen (Haynes, 1955). Soon after the chorda tympani leaves the facial nerve it enters the tympanic cavity through the iter chordae posterius, where it becomes invested in mucous membrane. It then courses within the middle ear; here it is in relation medially to the long process of the incus and laterally to the upper part of the handle of the malleus. It exits through the anterior wall of the middle ear via the iter chordae anterius (canal of Huguier). (Durcan, Shea, and Sleeckx, 1967.)

Fibers conveying sensibility

Fibers carrying general sensibility from the soft palate and tonsillar region course centralward via the posterior palatine nerve (maxillary division of the fifth nerve), the sphenopalatine ganglion, the greater superficial petrosal nerve, the geniculate ganglion (where the cell station is situated), then the nervus intermedius (Fig. 14-1) (Rasmussen, 1941). However, in some brains the fibers conveying pain impulses bypass the most proximal part of the nervus intermedius (they proceed through an anastomotic branch of the seventh nerve to the vestibular division of the eighth nerve, in which they reach the brainstem) (Sachs, 1968). Further, the auricular branch of the seventh nerve transmits sensory impulses from the cutaneous region in the angle between the ear and mastoid process (Fig. 12-6) (Rhoton, 1968). This branch probably shares with the ninth and tenth nerves the supply of the tympanic membrane and the external auditory meatus. Support for auricular nerve supply of these structures comes from the observation that on electrical stimulation of the nervus intermedius pain occurs in the ear, and that following section of this nerve the sensitivity of the auricular zone is decreased (Clark and Taylor, 1909; Furlow, 1942). Upon entering the brainstem, the fibers conveying pain sensation from the regions indicated course downward in the dorsal part of the spinal tract of the fifth nerve and end in the part of the fifth nucleus situated in the posterior horn of the upper three spinal segments (Foley, 1960; Rhoton, 1968; Taren, 1964); the fibers conveying tactile sensation are assumed to end in the principal nucleus of the fifth nerve (Rhoton, 1968). In regard to deep pressure sensibility and proprioceptive sensibility of the facial muscles (exclusive of the masticatory muscles), possibly they are transmitted via the nervus intermedius to the principal nucleus of the fifth nerve but this appears unlikely (Rhoton, 1968; Rhoton, Kobayashi, and Hollinshead, 1968). The alternative is that they are carried by the fifth nerve (p. 237).

Fibers conveying the sensation of taste from the anterior two-thirds of the tongue; autonomic innervation

After coursing for a distance centralward in the lingual nerve, the fibers carrying taste impulses from the anterior two-thirds of the tongue traverse the chorda tympani and, in turn, the trunk of the seventh nerve as far as the geniculate ganglion, where they have their cell stations (Fig. 14-1). From this ganglion the fibers may course centrally via the nervus intermedius (Reichert and Poth, 1933; Rowbotham, 1938a, b) or via the vestibular nerve (p. 217). Passage of fibers by the latter route would explain the persistence of taste following resection of the nervus intermedius in the region near the porus acusticus (Gardner, Stowall, and Dutlinger, 1947; Sachs, 1968; White and Sweet, 1955). The taste fibers terminate in the rostral part of the solitary nucleus (Rhoton, 1968; Rhoton, O'Leary, and Ferguson, 1966).

Parasympathetic (vasodilator) fibers reach the anterior two-thirds of the tongue by way of the lingual nerve, and *sympathetic (vasoconstrictor) fibers* by way of the cervical sympathetic trunk through the twelfth nerve (Chorobski and Penfield, 1932).

Autonomic pathways

In addition to the pathways just mentioned, autonomic fibers proceed to the lacrimal and other glands and also to mucous membranes. Moreover, they innervate vessels. From all the structures to be mentioned, including vessels, visceral afferent fibers proceed centralward and terminate in the nucleus of the tractus solitarius. Their cell bodies are in the geniculate ganglion. (Chorobski and Penfield, 1932.)

Fibers concerned in tear secretion. *Parasympathetic fibers* originate in the lacrimal nucleus in the floor of the fourth ventricle (Fig. 10-5) and pass down the nervus intermedius to reach the level of the geniculate ganglion (Fig. 14-1). From here they course in the greater superficial petrosal nerve and the vidian nerve and terminate in the sphenopalatine ganglion about postganglionic cells. The fibers of these postganglionic cells extend to the lacrimal gland by traversing, in turn, the maxillary division of the fifth nerve, the anastomotic zygomaticotemporal nerve, and the lacrimal nerve (Crosby and De-

Jonge, 1963). Sympathetic fibers to the lacrimal gland run a double course. Preganglionic fibers terminate in the superior cervical sympathetic ganglion. Postganglionic fibers gain the internal carotid artery and course in its plexus. Some fibers pass in the carotid plexus to the ophthalmic artery and extend along this artery to reach the lacrimal gland (not illustrated in Fig. 14-1); others leave the internal carotid and traverse, in turn, the deep petrosal nerve, the vidian nerve, the sphenopalatine ganglion, the maxillary division of the fifth nerve, the anastomotic zygomaticotemporal nerve, and finally the lacrimal nerve, through which they reach the lacrimal gland. Both the parasympathetic and the sympathetic fibers are concerned in tear secretion, and the parasympathetic alone in the dilation of vessels in the lacrimal gland. Section of the nervus intermedius usually results in loss of tear secretion, though in some cases no such loss occurs, presumably because the fibers reach the eighth nerve through an anastomotic bundle issuing from the seventh nerve (Sachs, 1968).

Fibers reaching the mucous membrane of the nasal cavity and region of the mouth and throat. The origin and the early course of *parasympathetic fibers* reaching the mucous membrane in these regions is much the same as that just mentioned. The fibers synapse in the sphenopalatine ganglion. Postsynaptic fibers (not shown in Fig. 14-1) proceed by way of palatine nerves to the mucous membrane of the nasal cavity, upper pharynx, soft palate, uvula, tonsillar region, roof of the mouth, and upper lip. Both secretory and vasodilatory fibers are carried to these regions by way of the palatine nerves. *Sympathetic fibers* also course in the manner indicated; they function in a vasoconstrictor capacity (Chorobski and Penfield, 1932).

Fibers concerned in salivary gland secretion. Arising from the superior salivatory nucleus in the floor of the fourth ventricle (Fig. 10-5), *parasympathetic fibers* pass peripherally in the nervus intermedius, enter the seventh nerve at the level of the geniculate ganglion, traverse this nerve, and exit from it a short distance above the stylomastoid foramen to become a component of the chorda tympani; they leave the chorda tympani, join the lingual branch of the fifth nerve, and ultimately synapse in the submaxillary ganglion and in Langley's ganglion (Fig. 14-1). Postganglionic neurons arising in the submaxillary ganglion pass by way of the lingual nerve to the sublingual gland, and those originating in Langley's ganglion extend to the submaxillary gland. *Sympathetic fibers* arise in the superior cervical sympathetic ganglion, course upward along the external carotid artery, then along the lingual artery and its branches. Some pass through the submaxillary ganglion and Langley's ganglion to gain the submaxillary gland, while others course to the sublingual gland. Parasympathetic fibers convey impulses concerned in vasodilatation and in the secretion of copious watery secretion high in enzyme content, whereas the sympathetic fibers are responsible for vasoconstriction and the secretion of mucus, which is thick, scanty, and low in enzyme content. (Crosby and DeJonge, 1963; Kuntz and Richins, 1946.)

Fibers extending to arteries. *Parasympathetic fibers* originate in the floor of the fourth ventricle in the region of the dorsal nucleus of the tenth nerve, and proceed by way of the nervus intermedius component of the seventh nerve to the region of the geniculate ganglion. From here they course by way of the greater superficial petrosal nerve, near the proximal part of which they appear to synapse. Postganglionic fibers proceed to the internal carotid artery, where they join the carotid plexus and then gain the carotid nerve, which runs along the carotid artery. In this nerve and in the plexus the fibers pass both centralward and peripheralward. The fibers proceed to cerebral arteries and to pial arteries in certain locations. On the basis of electrical stimulation at various sites, these fibers were found to be vasodilators. *Sym-*

Table 14-1. Disorders of conductivity of the facial nerve

A: Lesions of the nuclear and infranuclear portions of the facial	*B: Lesions of the supranuclear portion of the facial*
General characteristics 1. Usually unilateral. 2. Diminution of electrical irritability, R. D. 3. As a rule an involvement of the entire facial musculature. Keratitis may be a complication.	*General characteristics* 1. Practically always unilateral. 2. No diminution of electrical irritability. 3. Little involvement of the upper part of the face (bilat. innervation, see pp. 151 and 230 and Fig. 15-1).
Special characteristics I. Infranuclear lesions a. *Those of Extracranial Origin* Almost always a facial monoplegia. 1. *Distal to the branching off of the chorda tympani* (see Fig. 14-1, *5*). *Signs:* Paralysis of the facial muscles alone; if the lesion is more peripheral, i.e., distal to terminal radiation of the facial nerve (pes anserinus), some of the branches of the facial will escape. 2. *In the canal of the facial nerve between the branching off of the chorda tympani and the stapedius* (see Fig. 14-1, *4*). *Signs:* Facial paralysis; loss of appreciation of taste in the anterior two-thirds of the tongue; impairment of salivary secretion. 3. *In the canal of the facial nerve between the branching off of the stapedius and the ganglion of the facial nerve* (ganglion geniculi) (see Fig. 14-1, *3*). *Signs:* Facial paralysis; loss of appreciation of taste in the anterior two-thirds of the tongue; impairment of salivary secretion; hyperacusis. 4. *Between the internal auditory meatus and the geniculate ganglion of the facial nerve* (see Fig. 14-1, *2*). *Signs:* Facial paralysis; no disturbance of taste; impairment of salivary secretion; sensorineural deafness when there is accompanying involvement of the acoustic nerve (see below); in the absence of acoustic nerve involvement—hyperacusis, loss of affective and reflex tear secretion. b. *Those of Intracranial Origin—Basal Lesions* (see Fig. 14-1, *1*) Not infrequently facial diplegia (chronic basal meningitis). *Signs:* Those described above, in a, 4; usually an accompanying involvement of other basal nerves (acoustic, abducens, glossopharyngeal, vagus, spinal accessory, hypoglossal); evidence of increased intracranial pressure, such as headache, papilledema, vertigo, and vomiting. II. Nuclear lesions In a high percentage of cases the upper part of the face is spared. *Other Structures Involved:* The abducens is practically always involved. A medial lemniscus (hemianesthesia alterna) or a pyramid (Millard-Gubler syndrome; see p. 20 and B in Fig. 11-6) may also be affected.	*Special characteristics* I. Lesions in the region of the cerebrum, cerebral peduncles and upper pons. Facial palsy is associated with paralysis of the ipsilateral limbs because the central facial neurons and the pyramidal tracts course together. II. Lesions in the region of the lower pons, prenuclear lesions. Facial palsy is associated with paralysis of the contralateral limbs (see p. 151 and *b* in Fig. 11-6).

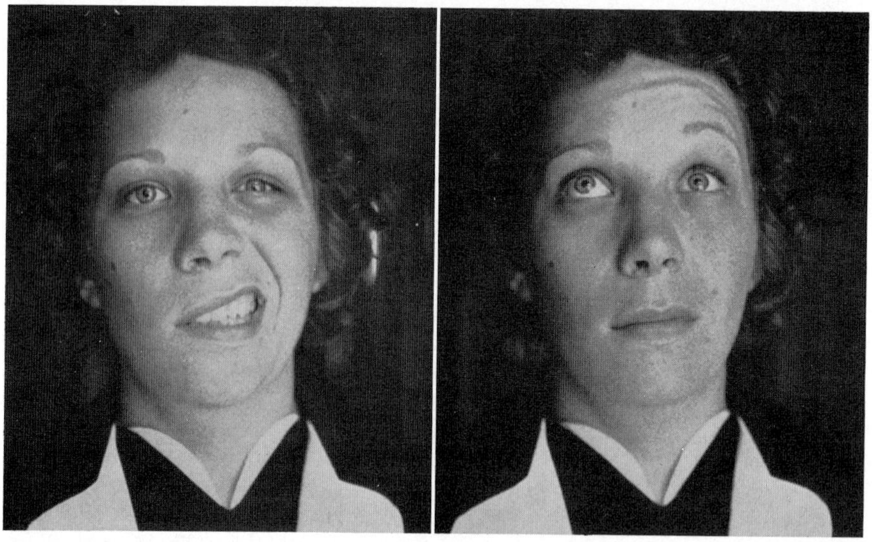

Fig. 14-2. Slight Bell's palsy. *Left,* Weakness of all the muscles on the right side of the face becomes evident when the patient tries to smile; *right,* weakness of the muscles of the right side of the forehead on looking upward. The upward-outward movement of the right eye is unexplained. (Courtesy Dr. A. Ornsteen, Philadelphia.)

pathetic fibers, originating mostly in the superior sympathetic ganglion, run in the carotid plexus and continue as periarterial nerves along the walls of all major cerebral arteries. Some presynaptic fibers appear to traverse the superior cervical sympathetic ganglion and to course along the carotid for a distance prior to joining with postsynaptic fibers; still others may find their postsynaptic stations on the walls of more distal cerebral arteries. Sympathetic fibers also find their way to major intracranial arteries by other routes. (Chorobski and Penfield, 1932.)

The course of the fibers just outlined enables one to determine with considerable precision the level at which the facial nerve complex has been interrupted. Correlation of the site of the lesion (1 through 5 in Fig. 14-1) with the signs and symptoms provoked is indicated in Table 14-1.

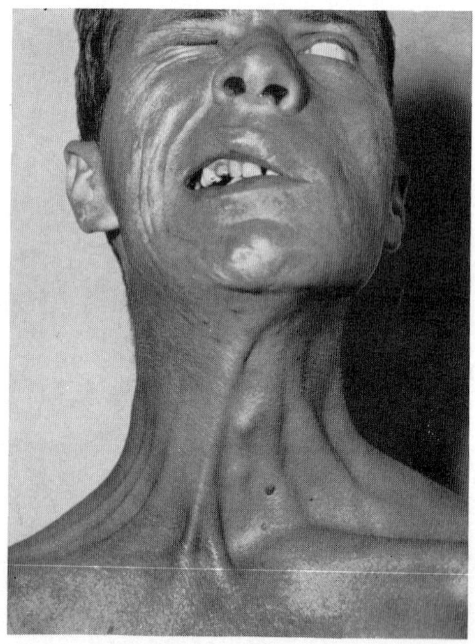

Fig. 14-3. Facial nerve palsy due to missile wound in the region of the mastoid process, as is to be seen in Fig. 12-3, *A*, from the same patient. On attempted closure of both eyes, the right eye closes satisfactorily, whereas the left remains open *(lagophthalmos)* and, as under normal conditions, the eyeball moves upward *(Bell's phenomenon).* The left side of the face is masklike and the angle of the mouth immobile. (From Walter Reed Army Hosp.; AFIP Neg. A 45196-6.)

INFRANUCLEAR AND NUCLEAR PALSIES

Manifestations of interruption of the seventh nerve

Interruption of the motor part of the seventh nerve results in facial paralysis. When paralysis is total, the affected side of the face is mask-like and immobile, the forehead cannot be wrinkled, the nasolabial fold is smoothed out, the corner of the mouth sags and is drawn toward the normal side, and the palpebral fissure is widened. When an effort is made to close the eyes, the lids of the affected side remain open (*lagophthalmos*) and the eyeballs turn upward and slightly outward (*Bell's phenomenon*) (Figs. 14-2 and 14-3). Blinking no longer occurs. Because of palsy of the lower lid, tears collect and commonly flow down the side of the face (*epiphora*); lack of epiphora may indicate interruption of nervus intermedius fibers in the trunk of the seventh nerve. Further, in seventh nerve paralysis the base of the tongue is lowered because of paralysis of the stylohyoid muscle and the posterior belly of the digastric. The cheek puffs out with expiration because of buccinator paralysis. Increased acuity of hearing and undue sensitivity to low tones (*hyperacusis*) occur as the result of paralysis of the stapedius, the function of which is to reduce the amplitude of vibratory excursions of the stapes in the oval window.

Fibers from the twelfth nucleus appear to participate with fibers in the seventh nerve in supplying the *orbicularis oris* (Fig. 14-5). If, then, there is paresis of the lips together with paralysis of the tongue (of the nuclear type) it may be concluded, in the absence of other seventh nerve signs, that the seventh nerve is not involved. Moreover, from the observation that the *orbicularis oculi* is weakened in damage to the third nucleus it would follow that this muscle receives part of its supply from the third nucleus. The pathway of fibers from the third nucleus to the orbicularis oculi is presumed to be through the upper part of the seventh nucleus, then through the seventh nerve.

There are circumstances in which only certain fascicles or branches of the seventh nerve are interrupted. The orbicularis oculi comes particularly into consideration. Its upper half as well as the accessory muscles of lid closure (frontalis, corrugator supercilii, and pyramidalis) are supplied by the *temporal branch* of the upper temporofacial division of the seventh nerve, and its lower half is supplied by the *zygomatic branch*. By running rostrally and upward, both the temporal and the zygomatic branches cross or lie along the zygoma somewhere between the mandibular condyle and the anterior edge of the temporal fossa. Both may be damaged in facial fracture or in injury to soft tissue, as manifested by *weakness in lid closure*. More specifically, laceration over the zygoma or temple or along the lateral margin of the orbit may selectively paralyze the orbicularis muscle of the lower lid or of the upper lid, brow, and forehead. The same may be brought about in the course of surgery on the parotid gland. Further, during frontotemporal craniotomy the temporal branch may be contused or incised where it crosses the zygoma (1 cm. anterior to the ear), resulting in an immobile forehead ipsilaterally, a lowered brow, a paralyzed corrugator supercilii, and a weakened orbicularis in the upper lid. *Partial weakness of the orbicularis oculi* causes incomplete reflex blinking without altering the rate of blinking. (Hoyt and Loeffler, 1965.)

Lack of eyelid vibration on testing eyelid closure is a sensitive sign of weakness of the orbicularis oculi and is of special value when interruption of the seventh nerve is in doubt. In the presence of orbicularis palsy, the amplitude and rate of vibration of the upper lid are found reduced when the patient tries to close his eye while the examiner tries to open it by exerting slight upward pressure on the upper lid with the ball of his thumb. Normally the vibration can best be felt when the patient resists slightly the examiner's attempt to raise the eyelid (Wartenberg, 1939). Moreover, with complete seventh nerve interruption the *orbicularis oculi reflex* is lost on the affected side. Normally when the glabella is tapped with a percussion hammer the orbicularis of both eyes contracts—the subject blinks. With weakness of the facial muscles unilaterally, the orbicularis oculi reflex on that side is reduced in strength. In early facial weakness, diminution of the reflex may be the earliest sign of ensuing facial palsy. Another is the *orbicularis oculi stretch reflex*. This is elicited by grasping the lateral part of the orbital fibers between the thumb and index fingers, then tapping the thumb with a percussion hammer (Wartenberg, 1945). The afferent impulses for this reflex apparently arise from stretch receptors in the muscle and proceed centrally by way of sensory dendrites to cell bodies in the geniculate ganglion or mesencephalic nucleus (Rushworth, 1962), then by way of the axons to the nucleus of the seventh nerve to form a monosynaptic arc (Crosby, Humphrey, and Lauer, 1962).

The orbicularis oculi (blink) reflex has two components—a rapid, monosynaptic *proprioceptive* component (as already described, elicited by a tap on the glabella or periorbital region) and a slow, bisynaptic or polysynaptic, *nociceptive* component (elicited by electrical stimulation of the supraorbital nerve). Impulses in the nociceptive component are conveyed centrally by way of the fifth cranial nerve (Kugelberg, 1952). Sometimes only the early response is absent in Bell's palsy (Gandiglio and Fra, 1967; Rushworth, 1962). From the observation that the trigeminofacial reflex (blink reflex) does not normally appear in infants until they are nine months old, it has been suggested that reflex may serve as an index of motor maturation (Hopf, Hufschmidt, and Ströder, 1965).

Loss of the sense of taste is noted in Bell's palsy in 10 percent of patients (Miller, 1967) or in 60 percent if perverted taste is included in loss of taste (Kettel, 1959). Lacrimation is commonly defective, indicating involvement of the parasympathetic outflow at the level of the geniculate ganglion (Cawthorne, 1965a).

When in the course of Bell's palsy functional restoration is incomplete, contracture of the facial muscles may develop. The contracture becomes more evident when the face is animated, as manifested by deepening of the labiofacial fold and lowering of the affected eyebrow. Abnormal associated movements may also occur. When the patient closes his eyes there may be an involuntary elevation of the corner of the mouth on the affected side or a wrinkling of the forehead; on baring the teeth, the patient's eye on the affected side may close; when the patient moves any part of his face every muscle of the palsied side may contract (Ford and Woodhall, 1938; Ornsteen, 1935; Spiller, 1919; Wartenberg, 1946). The associated movements are presumed to be caused by faulty innervation, regenerating fibers having travelled to the "wrong" muscle fibers (Taverner, 1955).

Another occasional complication of lingering Bell's palsy is lacrimation when the patient takes food, particularly when it is highly seasoned (*crocodile tear phenomenon*). Ford (1933) suggested that regenerating seventh nerve fibers become misdirected so that they grow at random in various nerve trunks, some of which should have returned to salivary glands but were directed instead to the lacrimal glands. This view has been supported by the results of electromyographic studies (Taverner, 1955).

A certain parallelism exists between the crocodile tear phenomenon and *gustatory hyperhidrosis.* This disorder is characterized by reddening and profuse sweating in the region of distribution of various nerves during eating. When occurring on the side of the face, the disturbance is referred to as the *auriculotemporal syndrome.* A *chorda tympani syndrome* has also been described. The reddening and sweating during eating may be widespread, involving one side of the face, the neck, upper back, and chest. A subjective feeling of warmth in the involved area is a common complaint. Also, there may be objective sensory deficit and a decrease or loss of thermal sweating in the area. The auriculotemporal syndrome is exceedingly common following suppurative parotitis, trauma of the parotid, or parotid tumor extirpation. The syndrome usually develops after a lapse of a few months. (Daly, 1967; Gardner and McCubbin, 1956; Laage-Hellman, 1957; Schulze, 1955.) Gustatory hyperhidrosis has also been observed in encephalitis, syringobulbia, osteoma of the cervical spine, bronchial carcinoma, and after cervical sympathectomy or thyroidectomy (Cunliffe and Johnson, 1967).

In explanation of the development of the gustatory hyperhidrosis, it has been suggested that parasympathetic fibers (cholinergic) sprout new axons that proceed along sympathetic pathways, which are also cholinergic. The afferent pathway of the arc normally mediating gustatory sweating is by way of the ninth nerve (Fig. 12-7) and probably also by way of the tenth nerve. Second order neurons originating in the nucleus solitarius course cephalad, probably to the hypothalamus. The efferent part of the arc is via sudomotor sympathetic fibers. The hyperhidrosis is presumed to originate from hypothalamic discharge.

Sweating in the involved area is inhibited by atropine and is provoked by pilocarpine (both given parenterally) and by acetylcholine injected locally in a dose that is ineffective on the other (sound) side. Moreover, there is no local hypersensitivity of the sweat glands to beta-methylcholine. Gustatory hyperhidrosis thus appears to represent a reaction to re-innervation (Cunliffe and Johnson, 1967; Daly, 1967).

Causes of interruption and irritation of the facial nerve in its intracanalicular or more peripheral course

Where facial paralysis occurs acutely without known cause, the condition is referred to as *Bell's palsy.*

Pleocytosis and increase in protein in the cerebrospinal fluid have been observed in some cases (Park and Watkins, 1949), suggesting an inflammatory state involving the seventh nerve, but no organism has been recovered in such cases. An hereditary factor has been invoked: Alter (1963) found that 30 percent of patients with Bell's palsy had a close relative with the same condition. The nature of the hereditary defect needs yet to be ascertained. In other cases, overexposure of the face to cold has been blamed. Nerve edema, leading to strangulation of the nerve through the space limitations imposed by its perineurium and epineurium, has often been suggested as a basis. Prominent "bulging" of nerve contents following incision of the epineurium and perineurium in cases of Bell's palsy has been taken as evidence in support for this view (Cawthorne and Wilson, 1963; Kettel, 1947). However, there are other cases in which undue bulging following incision did not occur. Entrapment of the facial nerve in the fallopian canal owing to nerve swelling—and so leading to functional interruption of the nerve—has also been regarded as a basis of Bell's palsy (Kettel, 1966b; Langworth and Taverner, 1963), but there is the opposing argument that the nerve normally fills no more than 30 to 50 percent of the cross-sectional diameter of the canal (Sunderland and Cossar, 1953). The primary site of the lesion in Bell's palsy is frequently found (at operation) to be at or near the stylomastoid foramen, from which it has been concluded that denseness and a constricting effect on the stylomastoid collar may be responsible (McGovern, 1968a). Biopsied epineurium from the intracanalicular part of the nerve has shown no pathological changes, but wallerian degeneration and other changes in the nerve have been observed postmortem (Sade, Levy, and Chaco, 1965). Ischemia of the nerve has been suggested as the initial event in Bell's palsy. However, according to Drachman (1969), palsy from ischemia may occur only under exceptional conditions: in occlusion of large vessels (for example, in Leriche's syndrome), in multiple small vessel disease, and possibly in diabetes mellitus.

Facial palsy may occur as a consequence of spread of a neighboring infection. Extreme degenerative atrophy of the facial nerve has been noted as a complication of otitis media; interference with the nerve's blood supply has been considered the basis (Kettel, 1966a). Spread of infection from the mastoid to the facial nerve can also result in facial palsy. The nerve may also be damaged as a complication of mastoidectomy (Stricker, 1963). Moreover, otitis externa with myringitis may be complicated by facial palsy; in such cases the palsy appears to be due to extension of the infection by way of the tympanic membrane to the chorda tympani, then along the chorda to the facial canal, where the infective process involves the facial nerve (Sadé, 1965). Hemorrhage into the facial nerve or in the facial canal in hypertensive cardiovascular disease is another cause of facial palsy, both in adults (Clarke and Murphy, 1956) and in children (Lloyd, Jewitt, and Still, 1966). In this condition the auricular pain and the perverted sense of taste characteristic of classical Bell's palsy are usually absent (Merwarth, 1942).

The facial nerve is also apt to be affected in certain systemic disorders such as disseminated polyradiculoneuritis (Landry-Guillain-Barré syndrome) (Matsuyama and Haymaker, 1967). Involving the facial nerve less commonly are sarcoid, uveoparotid fever (Levin, 1935), leukemic deposits, mumps, porphyria, osteitis fibrosa involving the facial canal, and thiamine deficiency (de Wardener and Lennox, 1947). Leprosy also involves the facial nerve and is reputed to be the only cause of bilateral facial paralysis in which the upper face is more often affected than the lower (Miller, 1967). In one series of Bell's palsy, at least 5 percent of the patients were diabetic (Leibowitz, 1966). Syphilis as a cause (Drachman, 1969) is negligible.

The *Ramsay Hunt syndrome* (Hunt, 1907, 1937) also comes into consideration. This is a viral disorder (herpes zoster), presumably having its seat in the geniculate ganglion—hence called *geniculate herpes zoster;* however, in the one case thus far studied histologically (the ganglion in Hunt's case was lost), an inflammatory reaction was found limited to the seventh nerve (Denny-Brown, Adams, and Fitzgerald, 1944).

The herpetic eruption occurs in various regions: tympanic membrane (rarely), external auditory canal, outer surface of the ear, junctional zone between ear and mastoid (the area illustrated in Fig. 12-6), and the anterior pillar of the fauces. Some cases are characterized by vesicle eruption alone, others by aural herpes and facial palsy, and still others by eighth nerve disturbances as well, such as tinnitus, hypacusis, and vertigo mimicking Ménière's disease. After the vesicles have dried, neuralgia may develop *(postherpetic neuralgia).* The pain, which is sharp and steady and lasts a half-hour or more, occurs spontaneously; it is not reflexly induced. It occurs within the ear, behind the ear, and deep in the face, particularly in the nasal and zygomatic regions. There may also be pain in the region of the palate. Sleep is fairly often disturbed by the pain. Clonic spasms of the facial muscles may also occur. Curiously, loss of taste perception in the anterior two-thirds of the tongue is infrequent. The attacks of pain usually decrease in duration and intensity over a period of 6 to 18 months. (McGovern and Fitz-Hugh, 1952; Miller, 1968.)

The facial nerve is especially prone to traumatic injury in the region of its emergence from the stylomastoid foramen: by missiles (Purves-Stewart and Evans, 1919), by stab wounds, through the application of blunt force, by compression during operations under anesthesia, or through application of forceps to the head during birth. Stretching of the nerve as a consequence of prolonged instrumental opening of the mouth is another cause.

Closed head injury may also lead to facial palsy, immediate or delayed. The palsy thus caused is almost always due to fracture of the petrous part of the temporal bone. In longitudinal fracture (that is, fracture running lengthwise through the petrous bone), the facial nerve is usually involved in its tympanic course; the palsy, due mostly to edema of the nerve, comes on after some delay and is usually temporary. Transverse fracture, less frequent than longitudinal fracture, is more serious; the nerve may be contused, lacerated, or severed; paralysis often occurs immediately. Bleeding from the ear and rupture of the tympanum occur most commonly following longitudinal fracture, and cerebrospinal fluid otorrhea most commonly after transverse fracture. Coincident permanent deafness is far more frequent in transverse than in horizontal fracture. The sensation of taste may be involved in either form. (Briggs and Potter, 1967; Kettel, 1966a, b; McGovern, 1968b; Miller, 1967; Potter, 1964; Turner, 1944.)

Progressive facial palsy may occur under various conditions but not as a complication of Bell's palsy. Tumor is a fairly common cause; the tumor can involve the nerve almost anywhere in its intracanalicular course. These include neurofibroma or neurinoma (Curtin and Lanigan, 1964; Lavoie, Gauthier, and Lavoie, 1967), epidermoid tumor (Jefferson and Smalley, 1938), tumor of the greater superficial petrosal nerve (Tremble and Penfield, 1936), squamous cell carcinoma in the temporal bone in association with chronic suppurative otitis media (Maddox, 1967), metastatic tumor—particularly breast tumor and hypernephroma—lodging in the temporal bone (Maddox, 1967), and parotid tumor invading the facial canal (van der Borden and Snijder, 1968). Sensorineural deafness may be an associated finding if the tumor is in the region of the internal auditory meatus, and the conductive type of deafness if in the middle ear.

Pontile lesions involving the seventh nucleus and its intramedullary fibers

The seventh nucleus itself and/or the intrapontile fibers of the seventh nerve may be compromised by a number of pathological processes. The nucleus may be affected in poliomyelitis; facial paralysis may, in fact, be the only sign of an acute attack of paralytic poliomyelitis (Miller, 1967). Fever, stiffness of the neck, and headache commonly precede such an attack.

Multiple sclerosis also comes into consideration. The facial palsy appears "out of the blue" (without prior pain) and is perhaps the only lower motoneuron manifestation of the disease. Facial paralysis occasionally heralds multiple sclerosis (Carter, Sciarra, and Merritt, 1950). Taste disturbances are not known to occur in this disease (Miller, 1967).

Facial palsy may be observed in other pathological processes involving the pons, for example, in progressive bulbar palsy, pontile-artery thrombosis, and syringobulbia. Of causative neoplasms the most common is pontile glioma (Alpers and Yaskin, 1937; Bucy and Keplinger, 1959). In pontile neoplasm facial paralysis is seldom as complete as in interruption of the nerve in its peripheral course. This is illustrated in Fig. 14-4, in a patient with hemangioma of the pons in whom facial paralysis was slight. Sensory changes in the face predominated in this patient.

Lesions of the seventh nucleus frequently give rise to *fasciculation* of facial muscles. This occurs, for example, in facial paralysis resulting from an attack of poliomyelitis. Fasciculation may also occur in involvement of intramedullary fibers of the seventh nerve, but not nearly as commonly as when the nucleus is affected.

Facial *myokymia,* another disorder to be considered, is characterized by unilateral, involuntary, fine, continuous, undulating movements of facial muscles. The disorder occurs in persons of almost any age, and it may persist for months or years. The myokymia has been observed in multiple sclerosis, brainstem tumor, and extramedullary neoplasms occupying the posterior cranial fossa (Andermann and others, 1961; Espinosa, Lambert, and Klass, 1967). In some instances in which apparently no central lesion exists, the myokymia in-

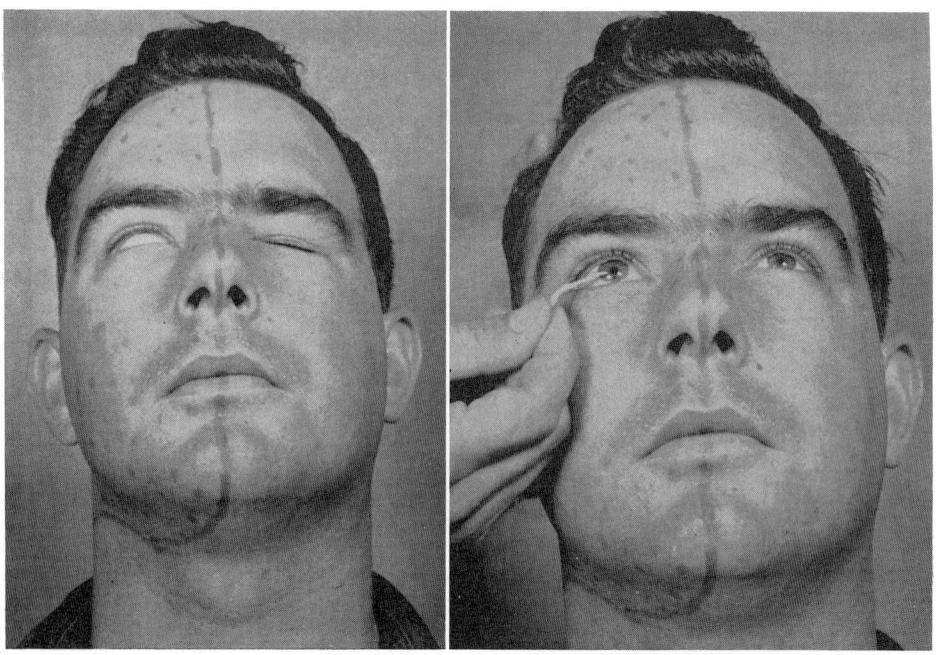

A B

Fig. 14-4. Paralysis of the seventh and fifth nerves. The area of trigeminal anesthesia (on the right side of the face) is indicated by dots. **A,** The right side of the face is slightly palsied. This becomes more evident by the occurrence of lagophthalmos when the patient attempts to close his eyes. **B,** The corneal reflex is absent, and no consensual eye closure occurs. A hemangioma was found in the pons at operation. (Courtesy Dr. A. G. Bingel, San Antonio, Texas.)

volves not only the muscles of the face but also those of the tongue, limbs, and trunk bilaterally; thyrotoxicosis was suspected in such a case (Harman and Richardson, 1954).

Less commonly observed is *persistent tonic facial spasm,* which has been noted only in pontile tumors. Facial paresis of gradual evolution appears subsequently. By contrast, *intermittent* facial spasm, at times reduced to simple fascicular twitchings of the lower eyelid and upper lip muscles, is seen in acoustic neuroma and other pathological processes in the region of the cerebellopontile angle and is also observed in intracranial vascular malformations, in lesions in the brainstem of vascular origin, and in multiple sclerosis. Offered as an explanation of *persistent* tonic facial spasm is lack of suppression of the facial nucleus resulting from a lesion involving certain inhibitory mechanisms, such as Henshaw's circuit. The motoneurons would thus be deprived of their natural frequency limiters and would discharge continuously. (Arseni and Petrovici, 1968.)

Spastic contracture of the face is a rare manifestation of a pontile lesion. In such a case, in which glioma occupied one side of the tegmentum of the pons, the contracture developed gradually in the ipsilateral side of the face in association with facial weakness on that side. Other disturbances of pontile origin included nystagmus, sixth nerve palsy, and staggering gait. Deafness and tinnitus also occurred, suggesting the diagnosis of acoustic neuroma or other cerebellopontile angle tumor. However, these conditions were ruled out by the absence of papilledema and the lack of roentgenographic changes in the porus acusticus. Bell's palsy could also be ruled out, on the basis of lack of associated facial movements. (Sogg, Hoyt, and Boldrey, 1963.)

"Dry eye," loss of salivary flow from the submaxillary gland, and facial paralysis are components of a syndrome resulting from thrombosis of vessels in the region of the pontile tegmentum in which the lacrimal, the superior salivatory, and the facial nuclei are located. Vertical (or, occasionally, rotatory) nystagmus occurs when vestibular nuclei are also affected. (Crosby, 1953.)

Involvement of the seventh nerve in the region of the cerebellopontile angle

In the region in which the seventh nerve traverses the cerebellopontile angle, it is apt to be affected by any one of a number of pathological processes. Pressure exerted on the seventh nerve by acoustic neuroma heads the list of causes of *unilateral* facial palsy originating in this region. Other nerves may also be affected (p. 210). Meningioma, chordoma, and other neoplasms may occasionally be responsible (p. 209). Basilar artery aneurysm also needs mention. Bilateral facial palsy of "angle" origin occurs most commonly in pathological processes involving the meninges (in meningeal carcinomatosis and granulomatous meningitis, including syphilitic meningitis).

Clonic facial spasms

Clonic facial spasms constitute a distressing disorder occurring most frequently in middle-aged women. No weakness of the affected muscles is encountered. Each muscle twitch is over in a flash and may be rapidly repeated for as long as a minute before gradually dissipating. The contractions usually involve one side of the face only, but sooner or later may develop on the opposite side as well. They have been considered as the motor counterpart of trigeminal neuralgia. However, the paroxysms differ in that they are not self-limited or followed by a refractory period such as occurs in trigeminal neuralgia. The contractions often begin as intermittent twitching of the orbicularis oculi, and may gradually come to include the muscles of the lower part of the face, especially those at the angle of the mouth; they may then spread to the remainder of the facial muscles. When developing subsequently on the opposite side of the face the paroxysms are neither synchronous nor symmetric on the two sides. Paroxysms may be precipitated by facial movement, even during sleep. (Cawthorne, 1965b; Gardner and Dohn, 1966.)

The disorder has been shown in some cases to have an organic basis. Thus, clonic facial spasms may be reflexly induced by painful lesions of the face or the buccal cavity, and sometimes are noted in association with geniculate zoster. Pathological changes in the region of the cerebellopontile angle—for example, from neoplasm or aneurysm—may occasionally be responsible (Gardner and Dohn, 1966). The contractions may also develop as the consequence of scarring of the seventh nerve in its peripheral course, or in neurofibroma or epidermoid tumor (primary cholesteatoma) involving the nerve in its course in the facial canal (Cawthorne, 1965b). Only exceptionally in such lesions is there increased mechanical irritability of the seventh nerve, manifested by twitching of the facial muscles when the skin over the pes anserinus is tapped or stroked (*Chvostek's phenomenon*). The clonic facial spasms under discussion are altogether different from the tonic facial spasm of Bell's palsy (facial contracture); moreover, Bell's palsy can be ruled out by the lack of facial paresis.

Wartenberg (1952) suggested as a basis of "cryptogenic" clonic facial spasm an upper motoneuron "release phenomenon" involving the cells of the facial nucleus. Gardner and Sava (1962) expressed the belief that "squeezing together of nerve fibers and the resulting reduction in thickness of their insulating myelin sheaths, permit transaxonal 'short circuiting' of the action current" (between the afferent [proprioceptive] and efferent [motor] fibers of the nerve, thus setting up a reverberating circuit).

Facial tic, by contrast, consists in bilateral repetitive movements (for example, blinking) usually initiated automatically as a result of some extrinsic inciting factor or intrinsic stimulus (for example, conjunctivitis), and perpetuated as a compulsion after the originating stimulus has ceased to operate.

DISTURBANCES IN SUPRANUCLEAR INNERVATION OF FACIAL MOVEMENTS

Voluntary movements of the face and *voluntary eyelid closure* are under the control of the lower third of the precentral gyrus, through fibers that course downward in the genu of the internal capsule (as the corticopontile tract) and the basis pedunculi to end in the nucleus of the seventh nerve (Fig. 14-5). The component of the seventh nucleus that supplies the upper part of the face is innervated from the cortex of both sides (Dandy, 1933; Lauer, 1952).

Additional innervation, through which movements of other kinds may be influenced (for example, periodic and emotional blinking; Hoyt and Loeffler, 1965), is received from varied sources. Ipsilateral innervation may originate in the "second motor area" situated in the temporal lobe (Schneider and Crosby, 1954). Other structures concerned in facial movements as well as in eyelid closure include the cingulate gyrus, insula, and amygdala, judging from the results of electrical stimulation in monkeys (Hoyt and Loeffler, 1965). Moreover, innervation is mediated from the cortex by way of COEPS (p. 318) to basal ganglia, mainly the putamen (Crosby and DeJonge, 1963), thence via extrapyramidal fibers to tegmental nuclei, then the facial nucleus. The neuronal mechanism controlling periodic blinking is thought to be centrally located, probably in the brainstem reticular substance, the basal ganglia, or both (Hoyt and Loeffler, 1965).

The bilaterality of cortical innervation provides the frontal and eyelid muscles with the means for bilateral synergic action and accounts for the fact that, in normal persons, the orbiculares oculi always contract simultaneously. Unilateral winking, on the other hand, must be learned. By contrast, the lower part of the face (the mouth and cheek muscles) derives its supranuclear innervation from the contralateral cortex only; in eating, in mimicry, and in other actions the muscles of the two sides are often used asymmetrically.

In lesions involving the area of representation of facial movements in the cortex, little of an abnormal nature is noted in the face when it is at rest; nothing more may

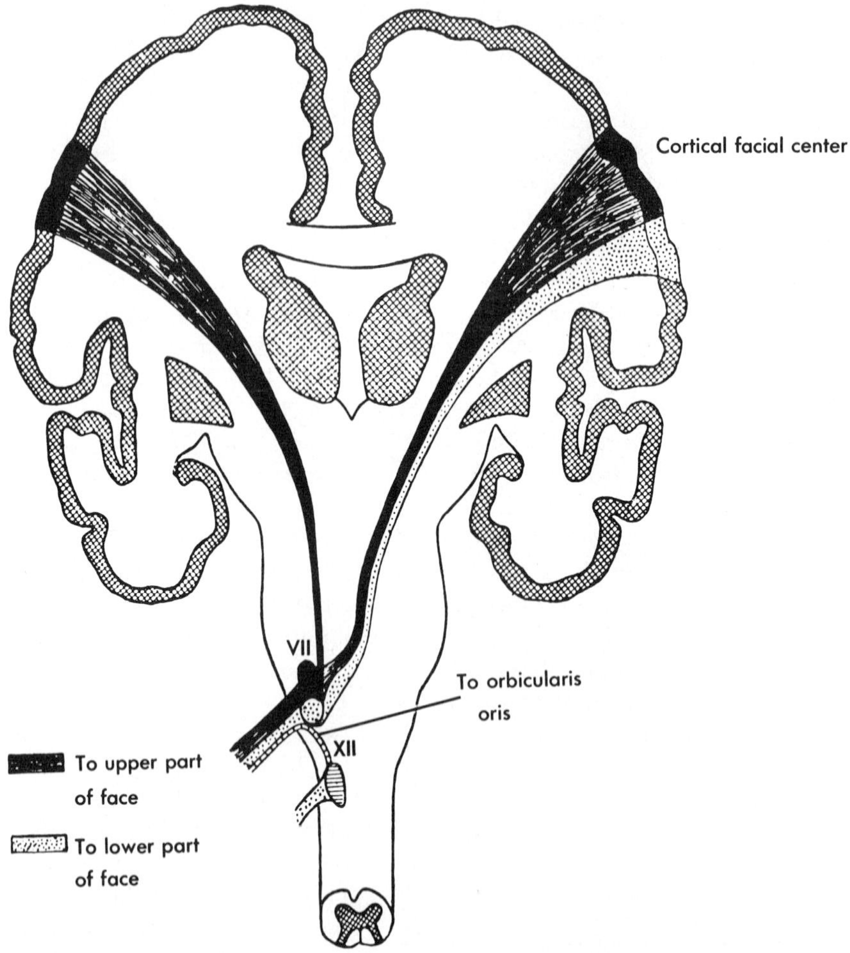

Fig. 14-5. Innervation of the facial movements by way of supranuclear fibers, and of the muscles of the face by nerve VII. Also indicated are postulated fibers running from nucleus XII to the facial nerve for the supply of the orbicularis oris.

be seen than a flattening of the nasolabial fold and a drooping of the corner of the mouth on the side contralateral to the lesion. Voluntary facial movement accentuates these deficits. Usually in cortical lesions that compromise facial movements, the tongue on the same side as the facial involvement is paretic because of the proximity of the cortical representation of tongue and facial movements. Further, facial palsy is occasionally encountered in temporal lobe lesions (Miller, 1967).

In lesions involving the corticopontile tract in its deeper course, the muscles of the contralateral lower half of the face are also paretic. Muscles of the upper part of the face are weakened, but much less obviously. The weakness is most evident in the orbicularis oculi muscles of that side. This the examiner brings out by elevating the upper lid of the two eyes with the ball of his thumb; on the paretic side the eyelid can be easily raised, while on the sound side the attempt meets with resistance so that eye remains closed. Power of reflex closure of the eye is also compromised on the affected side. (Cole, 1968.)

Unilateral loss of the ability to wink one eye is a sensitive sign of early corticopontile tract involvement and may be noted when the bilateral actions such as blinking are intact (Berlin, 1955).

In corticopontile tract involvement, emotional and associated movements can still be carried out on the paretic side of the face, but they are often accelerated and exaggerated (Monrad-Krohn, 1924). This never occurs in interruption of the seventh nerve.

Quite another problem in localization is posed when there is deficit of emotional facial expression in association with intact volitional movements. The deficit is almost always unilateral. The disorder occurs in lesions involving the caudolateral part of the thalamus or the globus pallidus. Under such conditions the lower part of the contralateral side of the face may be totally incapable of emotional expression. Deficit in emotional expression is also noted in lesions involving the region supplied by the posterior communicating artery—namely, hypothalamus, medial thalamus, subthalamus, and base and adjoining tegmentum of the midbrain. (Freeman and Jaffe, 1941; Mills, 1912; Russel, 1931; Wilson, 1929.) Details are given on pp. 167-168.

REFERENCES

Alpers, B. J., and Yaskin, J. C. 1939. Gliomas of the pons: clinical and pathologic characteristics. Arch. Neurol. Psychiat. **41**:435-459.

Alter, M. 1963. Familial aggregation of Bell's palsy. Arch. Neurol. **8**:557-564.

Andermann, F., Cosgrove, J. B. R., Lloyd-Smith, D. L., Gloor, P., and McNaughton, F. L. 1961. Facial myokymia in multiple sclerosis. Brain **84**:31-44.

Arseni, C., and Petrovici, I. 1968. Persistent tonic facial spasm in brain stem tumours. J. Neurol. Sci. **7**:107-114.

Berlin, L. 1955. Compulsive eye opening and associated phenomena. Arch. Neurol. Psychiat. **73**:597-601.

Blevins, C. E. 1967. Innervation patterns of the human stapedius muscle. Arch. Otolaryng. **86**: 30-36.

Briggs, M., and Potter, J. M. 1967. Prevention of delayed traumatic facial palsy. Brit. Med. J. **4**:464-465.

Bucy, P. C., and Keplinger, J. E. 1959. Tumors of the brain stem with special reference to ocular manifestations. Arch. Ophthal. **62**:541-554.

Carter, S., Sciarra, D., and Merritt, H. H. 1950. The course of multiple sclerosis as determined by autopsy proven cases. Res. Publ. Ass. Ment. Dis., Proc. **28**:471-511.

Cawthorne, T. 1965a. Idiopathic facial palsy. Arch. Otolaryng. **81**:494-496.

Cawthorne, T. 1965b. Clonic facial spasm. Arch. Otolaryng. **81**:504-505.

Cawthorne, T., and Wilson, T. 1963. Indications for intratemporal facial nerve surgery. Arch. Otolaryng. **78**:429-434.

Chorobski, J., and Penfield, W. 1932. Cerebral vasodilator nerves and their pathway from the medulla oblongata: with observations on the pial and intracerebral vascular plexus. Arch. Neurol. Psychiat. **28**:1257-1289.

Clark, L. P., and Taylor, A. S. 1909. True tic douloureux of the sensory filaments of the facial nerve: clinical report of a case in which cure was effected by physiologic extirpation of the geniculate ganglion: report of surgical treatment. J.A.M.A. **53**:2144-2146.

Clarke, E., and Murphy, E. A. 1956. Neurological manifestations of malignant hypertension. Brit. Med. J. **2**:1319-1326.

Cole, M. 1968. Eyelid tone: a sign of facial paresis. Neurology **18**:413-414.

Crosby, E. C. 1953. Relations of brain centers to normal and abnormal eye movements in the horizontal plane. J. Comp. Neurol. **99**:437-480.

Crosby, E. C., and DeJonge, B. R. 1963. Experimental and clinical studies of the central connections and central relations of the facial nerve. Ann. Otol. Rhin. Laryng. **72**:735-755.

Crosby, E. C., Humphrey, T., and Lauer, E. W. 1962. Correlative anatomy of the nervous system. New York, The Macmillan Company.

Cunliffe, W. J., and Johnson, C. E. 1967. Gustatory hyperhidrosis: a complication of thyroidectomy. Brit. J. Dermatol. **79**:519-526.

Curtin, J. M., and Lanigan, G. P. 1964. Neurilemmoma of the seventh nerve with intracranial extension. J. Laryng. Otol. **78**:212-219.

Daly, R. F. 1967. New observations regarding the auriculotemporal syndrome. Neurology **17**: 1159-1168.

Dandy, W. E. 1933. Physiological studies following extirpation of the right cerebral hemisphere in man. Bull. Johns Hopk. Hosp. **53**:31-51.

Denny-Brown, D., Adams, R. D., and Fitzgerald, P. J. 1944. Pathologic features of herpes zoster; note on "geniculate herpes." Arch. Neurol. Psychiat. **51**:216-231.

de Wardener, H. E., and Lennox, B. 1947. Cerebral beriberi (Wernicke's encephalopathy): review of 52 cases in a Singapore prisoner-of-war hospital. Lancet **1**:11-17.

Drachman, D. A. 1969. Bell's palsy: a neurological point of view. Arch. Otolaryng. **89**: 147-151.

Durcan, D. J., Shea, J. J., and Sleeckx, J. P. 1967. Bifurcation of the facial nerve. Arch. Otolaryng. **86**:619-631.

Espinosa, R. E., Lambert, E. H., and Klass, D. W. 1967. Facial myokymia affecting the electroencephalogram. Mayo Clin. Proc. **42**:258-270.

Foley, J. D. 1960. A quantitative study of the functional components of the facial nerve. Amer. J. Anat. **107**:237-244.

Ford, R. F. 1933. Paroxysmal lacrimation during eating as a sequel of facial palsy (syndrome of crocodile tears): report of four cases with a possible interpretation and comparison with the auriculotemporal syndrome. Arch. Neurol. Psychiat. **29**:1279-1288.

Ford, F. R., and Woodhall, B. 1938. Phenomena due to misdirection of regenerating fibers of cranial, spinal and autonomic nerves. Arch. Surg. **36**:480-496.

Freeman, W., and Jaffe, D. 1941. Occlusion of the superior cerebellar artery: report of a case with necropsy. Arch. Neurol. Psychiat. **46**: 115-126.

Furlow, L. T. 1942. Tic douloureux of the nervus intermedius (so-called idiopathic geniculate neuralgia). J.A.M.A. **119**:255-259.

Gandiglio, G., and Fra, L. 1967. Further observations on facial reflexes. J. Neurol. Sci. **5**: 273-285.

Gardner, W. J., and Dohn, D. F. 1966. Trigeminal neuralgia—hemifacial spasm—Paget's disease: significance of this association. Brain **89**: 555-562.

Gardner, W. J., and McCubbin, J. W. 1956. Auriculotemporal syndrome, gustatory sweating due to misdirection of regenerated nerve fibers. J.A.M.A. **160**:272-277.

Gardner, W. J., and Sava, G. A. 1962. Hemifacial spasm—a reversible pathophysiologic state. J. Neurosurg. **19**:240-247.

Gardner, W. J., Stowall, A., and Dutlinger, R. 1947. Resection of the greater superficial petrosal nerve in the treatment of unilateral headache. J. Neurosurg. **4**:105-114.

Harman, J. B., and Richardson, A. T. 1954. Generalised myokymia in thyrotoxicosis: report of case. Lancet **2**:473-474.

Haynes, D. R. 1955. The relations of the facial nerve in the temporal bone. Ann. Roy. Coll. Surg. Engl. **16**:175-185.

Hopf, H. C., Hufschmidt, H.-J., and Ströder, J. 1965. Development of the "trigemino-facial" reflex in infants and children. Ann. Paediat. **204**: 52-64.

Hoyt, W. F., and Loeffler, J. D. 1965. Neurology of the orbicularis oculi: anatomic, physiologic, and clinical aspects of lid closure. In Smith, J. L., editor: Neuro-ophthalmology, Symposium of the University of Miami, vol. 2. St. Louis, The C. V. Mosby Co.

Hunt, J. R. 1907. On herpetic inflammations of the geniculate ganglion: a new syndrome and its complications. J. Nerv. Ment. Dis. **34**:73-96.

Hunt, J. R. 1937. Geniculate neuralgia (neuralgia of the nervus facialis): a further contribution to the sensory system of the facial nerve and its neuralgic conditions. Arch. Neurol. Psychiat. **37**:253-285.

Jefferson, G., and Smalley, A. A. 1938. Progressive facial palsy produced by intratemporal epidermoids. J. Laryng. Otol. **53**:417-443.

Kettel, K. 1947. Bell's palsy. Arch. Otolaryng. **46**: 427-472.

Kettel, K. 1959. Peripheral facial palsy. Copenhagen, Ejnar Munksgaard.

Kettel, K. 1966a. Degeneration of the facial nerve. Arch. Otolaryng. **83**:27-29.

Kettel, K. 1966b. Surgery of the facial nerve. Arch. Otolaryng. **84**:99-109.

Kugelberg, E. 1952. Facial reflexes. Brain **75**: 385-396.

Kuntz, A., and Richins, C. A. 1946. Components and distribution of the nerves of the parotid and submaxillary glands. J. Comp. Neurol. **85**: 21-32.

Laage-Hellman, J. E. 1957. Gustatory sweating and flushing after conservative parotidectomy. Acta Otolaryng. **48**:234-252.

Langworth, E. P., and Taverner, D. 1963. The prognosis in facial palsy. Brain **86**:463-480.

Lauer, E. W. 1952. Ipsilateral facial representation in motor cortex of macaque. J. Neurophysiol. **15**:1-4.

Lavoie, R., Gauthier, G-T., and Lavoie, J.-C. 1967. Neurinoma of the facial nerve. Arch. Otolaryng. **86**:374-376.

Levin, P. M. 1935. The neurological aspects of uveo-parotid fever. J. Nerv. Ment. Dis. **81**: 176-191.

Leibowitz, U. 1966. Bell's palsy—two disease entities? Neurology **16**:1105-1109.

Lloyd, A. V. C., Jewitt, D. E., and Still, J. D. L. 1966. Facial paralysis in children with hypertension. Arch. Dis. Childh. **41**:292-294.

Maddox, H. E. 1967. Metastatic tumors of the temporal bone. Ann. Otol. Rhin. Laryng. **76**: 149-166.

Matsuyama, H., and Haymaker, W. 1967. Distribution of lesions in the Landry-Guillain-Barré syndrome, with emphasis on involvement of the sympathetic system. Acta Neuropath. **8**:230-241.

McGovern, F. H. 1968a. A review of the experimental aspects of Bell's palsy. Laryngoscope **78**:324-333.

McGovern, F. H. 1968b. Facial nerve injuries in skull fractures: recent advances in management. Arch. Otolaryng. **88**:538-542.

McGovern, F. H., and Fitz-Hugh, G. S. 1952. Herpes zoster of the cephalic extremity. Arch. Otolaryng. **55**:307-320.

Merwarth, H. R. 1942. The occurrence of peripheral facial paralysis in hypertensive vascular disease. Ann. Int. Med. **17**:298-307.

Miller, H. 1967. Facial paralysis. Brit. Med. Bull. **3**:815-819.

Miller, H. 1968. Pain in the face. Brit. Med. J. **2**:577-580.

Mills, C. K. 1912. Preliminary note on a new symptom complex due to lesion of the cerebellum and cerebello-rubro-thalamic system, etc. J. Nerv. Ment. Dis. **39**:73-76.

Monrad-Krohn, G. H. 1924. On the dissociation of voluntary and emotional innervation in facial paresis of central origin. Brain **47**:22-35.

Ornsteen, A. M. 1929. Incipient parkinsonism: a diagnostic triad for its early recognition. Arch. Neurol. Psychiat. **22**:709-713.

Park, H. W., and Watkins, A. L. 1949. Facial paralysis: analysis of 500 cases. Arch. Phys. Med. **30**:749-762.

Potter, J. M. 1964. Facial palsy following head injury. J. Laryng. **78**:654-657.

Purves-Stewart, J., and Evans, A. 1919. Nerve injuries and their treatment, ed. 2. London, Frowde, pp. 108-128.

Rasmussen, A. T. 1941. The principal nervous pathways: neurological charts and schemas with explanatory notes, ed. 2. New York, The Macmillan Company.

Reichert, F. L., and Poth, E. J. 1933. Recent knowledge regarding the physiology of the glosso-pharyngeal nerve in man with an analysis of its sensory, motor, gustatory and secretory functions. Bull. Johns Hopk. Hosp. **53**:131-139.

Rhoton, A. L., Jr. 1968. Afferent connections of the facial nerve. J. Comp. Neurol. **133**:89-100.

Rhoton, A. L., Jr., Kobayashi, S., and Hollinshead, W. H. 1968. Nervus intermedius. J. Neurosurg. **29**:609-618.

Rhoton, A. L., Jr., O'Leary, J. L., and Ferguson, J. P. 1966. The trigeminal, facial, vagal, and glossopharyngeal nerves in the monkey: afferent connections. Arch. Neurol. **14**:530-540.

Rowbotham, G. F. 1938a. Observations on the effects of trigeminal denervation. Brain **62**: 364-380.

Rowbotham, G. F. 1938b. Treatment of pain in the face by intramedullary tractotomy. Brit. Med. J. **2**:1073-1076.

Rushworth, G. 1962. Observations on blink reflexes. J. Neurol. Neurosurg. Psychiat. **25**:93-108.

Russel, C. K. 1931. The syndrome of the brachium conjunctivum and the tractus spinothalamicus. Arch. Neurol. Psychiat. **25**:1003-1010.

Sachs, E., Jr. 1968. The role of the nervus intermedius in facial neuralgia: report of four cases with observations on the pathways for taste, lacrimation, and pain in the face. J. Neurosurg. **28**:54-60.

Sadé, J. 1965. Retrograde facial paralysis. Ann. Otol. Rhin. Laryng. **74**:94-109.

Sade, J., Levy, E., and Chaco, J. 1965. Surgery and pathology of Bell's palsy. Arch. Otolaryng. **82**:594-602.

Schneider, R. C., and Crosby, E. C. 1954. Stimulation of "second" motor areas in the macaque temporal lobe. Neurology **4**:612-622.

Schulze, E. 1955. Das auriculotemporale Syndrome. Dtsch. Med. Wschr. **80**:900.

Sogg, R. L., Hoyt, W. F., and Boldrey, E. 1963. Spastic paretic facial contracture: a rare sign of brain stem tumor. Neurology **13**:607-612.

Spiller, W. G. 1919. Contracture occurring in partial recovery from paralysis of the facial nerve and other nerves. Arch. Neurol. Psychiat. **1**:564-566.

Stricker, G. 1963. Die Fazialparese als Komplikation von Ohrenkrankungen. Wschr. Ohrenheilk. **97**:115-121.

Sunderland, S., and Cossar, D. F. 1953. The structure of the facial nerve. Anat. Rec. **116**:147-165.

Taren, J. A. 1964. The positions of the cutaneous components of the facial, glossopharyngeal and vagal nerves in the spinal tract of V. J. Comp. Neurol. **122**:389-397.

Taverner, D. 1955. Bell's palsy: a clinical and electromyographic study. Brain **78**:209-228.

Tremble, G. E., and Penfield, W. 1936. Operative exposure of the facial canal, with removal of a tumor of the greater superficial petrosal nerve. Arch. Otolaryng. **23**:573-579.

Turner, J. W. A. 1944. Facial palsy in closed head injuries: the prognosis. Lancet **1**:756-757.

van der Borden, J., and Snijder, J. 1968. Paralysis of the facial nerve caused by acinic cell carcinoma. Arch. Otolaryng. **87**:41-44.

Wartenberg, R. 1939. A sign of facial palsy. Arch. Neurol. Psychiat. **41**:586-588.

Wartenberg, R. 1945. The examination of reflexes: a simplification. Chicago, Year Book Medical Publishers, Inc.

Wartenberg, R. 1946. Associated movements in the oculomotor and facial muscles. Arch. Neurol. Psychiat. **55**:439-488.

Wartenberg, R. 1952. Hemifacial spasm: a clinical and pathophysiological study. New York, Oxford University Press.

White, J. C., and Sweet, W. H. 1955. Pain: its mechanisms and neurosurgical control. Springfield, Illinois, Charles C Thomas, Publisher.

Wilson, S. A. K. 1929. Modern problems in neurology. New York, William Wood & Company, pp. 260-296.

Chapter 15

Localization of lesions involving the trigeminal nerve

ANATOMY

William R. Mehler

Peripheral distribution

The trigeminal nerve, or fifth cranial nerve, emerges from the ventrolateral aspect of the midpontile region as two closely approximated roots; one motor, which is comparatively small, and the other sensory, which is large (Fig. 10-1). The two roots extend forward through the pontile cistern and pierce the dura mater in the region just below the region where the tentorium cerebelli attaches to the tip of the temporal bone. The gasserian (or semilunar) ganglion is situated in a depression in the petrous part of the temporal bone, where it is enclosed in a "pouch" of dura. The motor root runs along the inferior surface of the ganglion and becomes incorporated in the mandibular division. The sensory root, surrounded by dura, unites with the gasserian ganglion. Three divisions are given off from the region of the gasserian ganglion.

The *ophthalmic division* extends forward through the middle cranial fossa to the orbit. It traverses the superior orbital fissure to enter the orbit, and while within the fissure the division gives off three main branches: lacrimal, frontal, and nasociliary. En route, the ophthalmic division passes through the lateral wall or part of the cavernous sinus. Here it is situated below the fourth nerve and lateral to the third and sixth nerves (Fig. 16-1). At this level a branch of the division (n. tentorii) extends (1) to the tentorium cerebelli, (2) to much of the falx—in which it runs in a rostral direction—(3) to adjacent dural venous sinuses and the veins running to them, and (4) to the dura of the parieto-occipital region. Dural venous sinuses supplied include the superior sagittal (posterior and middle thirds), transverse, and inferior sagittal. Supplied also by the ophthalmic division, through its anterior and posterior ethmoid nerves, is the dura of the anteromedial part of the anterior cranial fossa, including the anterior leaf of the falx and the neighboring part of the superior sagittal sinus. (Feindel, Penfield, and McNaughton, 1960; McNaughton, 1938; Penfield and McNaughton, 1940.)

The more superior part of the dura of the posterior cranial fossa is supplied by occipital branches of the tentorial nerve. The dura of the anterior part of the floor of the fossa receives ascending branches of meningeal rami of the upper three cervical levels, but mostly from the ramus of C2. The nerves reaching the dura of the lateral and posterior walls of the fossa are branches of cervical nerves I and II and the superior cervical ganglion, also branches of cranial nerves X and XII, all entering the fossa through the jugular foramen and the hypoglossal canal. (Kimmel, 1961.)

Through these sources—the ophthalmic division of the fifth nerve, on the one hand, and the upper cervical nerves and nerves X and XII on the other hand—sensory fibers also reach the intracranial arteries in certain parts of their course: the intracranial part of the internal carotid artery, the middle cerebral artery (the proximal 1 to 2 cm. of its stem), the anterior cerebral artery (from its origin to 1 cm. beyond the genu of the corpus callosum), and the vertebral-basilar arterial system (the vertebral and the basilar arteries themselves and 1 to 2 cm. of the proximal parts of their branches). (Fisher, 1968; Wolff, 1963.)

The *maxillary division* courses forward in close relation to the inferior aspect of the cavernous sinus. It traverses the foramen rotundum and courses through the pterygopalatine (sphenopalatine) fossa. It then enters the orbit via the inferior orbital fissure, from which it continues forward as the infraorbital nerve. This nerve reaches the face after passing through the infraorbital foramen.

In the cavity of the cranium the division gives off a minute nerve (n. meningeus medius) to the adjoining dura of the middle cranial fossa.

The *mandibular division* and its motor root leave the skull by traversing the foramen ovale, which has a smooth border. The division enters the infratemporal fossa, and as it does so its sensory and motor components fuse. Branches of the division include the inferior alveolar nerve, which runs within the mandible, and the lingual nerve, which extends to the tongue (Fig. 14-1). After coursing through the foramen ovale and reaching the outer surface of the skull, the mandibular division gives off the nervus spinosus, which reenters the skull by passing through the foramen spinosum with the middle meningeal artery. This nerve supplies most of the dura of the middle cranial fossa and the dura of the lateral part of the anterior cranial fossa; it also supplies mastoid cells. The auriculotemporal branch of the mandibular division supplies the superior and anterior walls of the external auditory meatus, the anterior part of the tympanic membrane, and a fairly small part of the auricle (Fig. 12-6). Another branch innervates the internal pterygoid muscle; that branch also provides a connection with the otic ganglion, through which fibers extend to the tensor tympani and tensor veli palatini muscles.

Proximal to the gasserian ganglion the dorsally situated ophthalmic division and the ventrally situated mandibular division undergo inversion. Consequently, in the region next to the pons the fibers of the sensory root exhibit a new topological arrangement (not shown in Fig. 15-1). Fibers of the mandibular division are situated dorsally, those of the maxillary division next, while the fibers of the ophthalmic division lie ventrally (Kerr, 1963a, b).

Central distribution

The sensory and motor roots of the fifth nerve are strict analogues of the posterior and anterior spinal roots. As the posterior spinal root enters the spinal cord it bifurcates into a long ascending division and a shorter descending division. Analogously, incoming nerve fibers of the fifth nerve bifurcate on entering the brainstem. However, the ascending division is the shorter limb, and it terminates in the principal trigeminal nucleus, situated at the midpontile level.

The longer, descending division, which constitutes the spinal tract of the trigeminus, terminates as collaterals throughout the length of the nucleus of the spinal tract, which extends into segment C3 of the spinal cord and possibly as far down as C4 (Taren, 1964; Taren and Kahn, 1962) (Fig. 15-1). Here the nucleus occupies the posterior horn, where it is continuous with the substantia gelatinosa, the latter forming a cuff around the lateral half of the spinal tract (Rhoton, 1968; Rhoton, O'Leary, and Ferguson, 1966). The remaining sensory neurons have their cell stations in the mesencephalic nucleus, situated at the edge of the periaqueductal gray matter.

The *principal sensory nucleus* is no different from the trigeminal sensory root in its organization: fibers of the mandibular division extend into the dorsal part of the nucleus, those of the maxillary division into the middle part, and those of the ophthalmic division into the ventral part.

In the *spinal tract*, lamination is also recognizable, the fibers of the ophthalmic division lying ventrolateral in the tract, those of the mandibular division dorsomedial, and the fibers of the maxillary division lying in between the two. According to Kunc (1960), fibers of the ophthalmic and mandibular divisions descend all the way into the cervical region, while most of the fibers of the maxillary division terminate in more rostral levels of the spinal nucleus. This is as based on the observation that the perioral-nasal region showed little or no analgesia following tractotomy at more caudal levels. Kerr (1963a, b), on the other hand, contends that a sizable proportion of fibers of all three divisions reaches caudal levels, with the fibers of each division giving off collaterals to the nucleus en route (Fig. 15-1).

The sensory trigeminal neurons of the second order take diverse courses.

1. From the *principal sensory nucleus*, the fibers course cephalad ipsilaterally in the mid-dorsal tegmentum of the pons to levels of the lower midbrain, where most of them cross to the contralateral side (others remaining ipsilateral), then con-

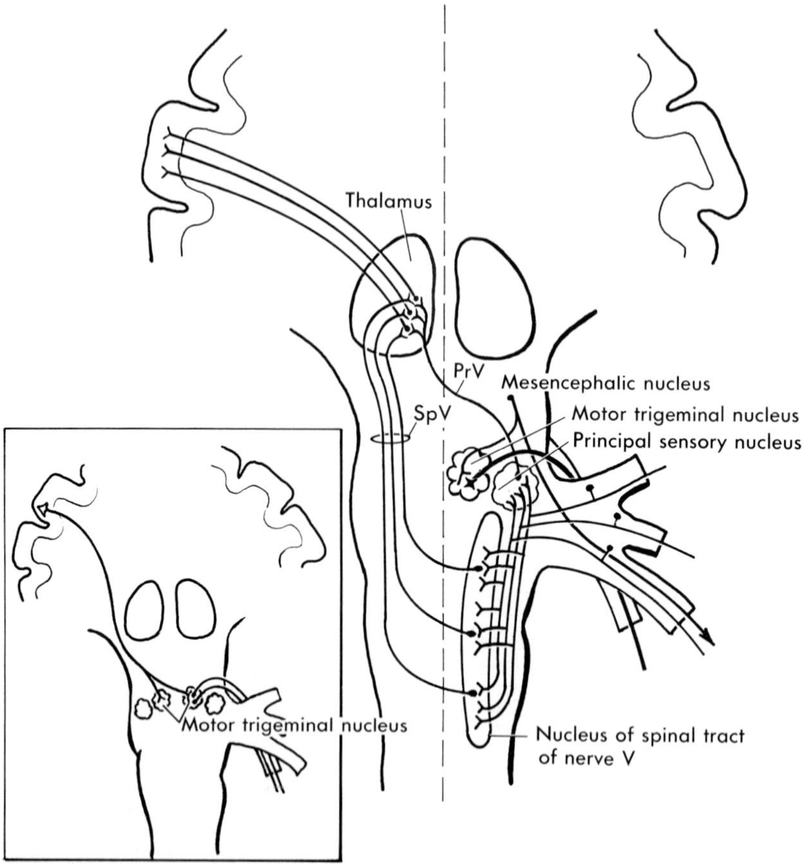

Fig. 15-1. Trigeminal nuclei and pathways. The sensory nuclei are the mesencephalic, the principal sensory, and the spinal sensory (or the nucleus of the spinal tract of the fifth nerve). Neurons of the second order (*PrV* and *SpV*) proceed to the thalamus to end in its ventral posteromedial nucleus (VPM). The course of the motor components of the fifth nerve, supranuclear and infranuclear, is indicated in the inset.

tinue their ascent through the dorsal midbrain tegmentum to terminate in the ventral posteromedial nucleus (VPM) of the thalamus (Fig. 15-1). In their course through the upper midbrain the fibers lie dorsal to the red nucleus and on the medial side of the medial lemniscus. These fibers carry tactile and discriminatory tactile impulses from the face. (Walker, 1938, 1939.)

2. From the *nucleus of the spinal tract*, the courses the fibers pursue are widespread (Figs. 11-3 and 15-1). Some fibers conveying pain impulses decussate (as internal arcuate fibers) and attain a position medial to the lateral spinothalamic tract (5 in Fig. 11-3), then pass upward as the *quintothalamic tract* (Sheehan and Smyth, 1937; Stopford, 1925). At upper pontile levels this tract merges with the more lateral part of the medial lemniscus. At higher levels its fibers course along the medial surface of the medial geniculate body, and still higher, they lie along the dorsal and medial aspects of the medial lemniscus. They then turn laterally to terminate in VPM (of the thalamus) (Walker, 1940).

Other fibers reportedly arising in the nucleus of the spinal tract of the fifth nerve, decussate at a more dorsal level and, on reaching a position just ventrolateral to the twelfth nucleus, turn upward. These comprise the so-called *bulbothalamic tract* (Fig. 11-3). At higher levels this tract lies in the more dorsal part of the tegmentum (Figs. 10-14 and 10-16) (Glees and Bailey, 1951; Wallenberg, 1896, 1901). Fibers carrying temperature impulses are assumed to travel the same route as the pain fibers. Existence of this "Wallenberg tract" has not been experimentally confirmed.

There appears to be another central pathway that conveys pain impulses from the face. Evidence exists that it extends cephalad in the midbrain in the medial part of the dorsal tegmentum and the adjoining periaqueductal gray, in close association with the "medial" pain pathway from spinal levels (pp. 8 and 9). The pathway ascends both ipsilaterally and contralaterally. Possibly it is a component of the bulbothalamic tract or of the quintothalamic tract or both. Or it may be a multisynaptic pathway. Electrical stimulation of this medial area in human patients induced sensations in central parts of the face (including the oral and nasal cavities) and body, on both sides of the midline: "fearful" pain, burning, heat, or cold. Different qualities of sensation in the face were elicited by stimulation lateral to this "medial" area (in the lateral spinothalamic tract). (Nashold, Wilson, and Slaughter, 1969.) Site of termination of this pathway in the thalamus needs yet to be ascertained.

3. Neurons comprising the *mesencephalic nucleus* are unique in their composition. From a given cell body in the nucleus (a) a collateral extends to the motor nucleus of the fifth nerve, synapsing with neurons, the fibers of which proceed to the muscles of mastication; (b) an axon passes, without interruption, via the mandibular division to the muscles of mastication; and (c) a collateral courses downward, medial to the spinal nucleus of the fifth nerve, and synapses with neurons in the reticular formation. These reticular neurons apparently serve as internuncial connections with the spinal nucleus of the fifth nerve and the twelfth nucleus (Mehler, 1963; Szentágothai, 1948) (Fig. 15-1). Some cells similar in type to those of the mesencephalic nucleus, together with a fiber bundle originating from the mesencephalic nucleus, are situated in the cerebellum (Pearson, 1949). The mesencephalic nucleus receives proprioceptive impulses from the masticatory muscles (Corbin, 1940; Smith, Marcarian, and Niemer, 1967). Whether fibers carrying deep sensibility and proprioceptive impulses from the muscles of the face belong to this system, or whether they run in the nervus intermedius to the principal nucleus of the fifth nerve, or elsewhere, has not been decided (Rhoton, 1968).

The *motor nucleus of the fifth nerve* derives its supranuclear innervation from the lower part of the precentral gyrus of both sides, with the contralateral connection by far the stronger (Dandy, 1933). Similarly, the nucleus of the spinal tract of the fifth nerve receives multiple corticobulbar feedback connections from corresponding regions of the postcentral gyri (Kuypers, 1958a, b).

The three trigeminal divisions have the distribution indicated in Fig. 15-2 and Table 15-1.

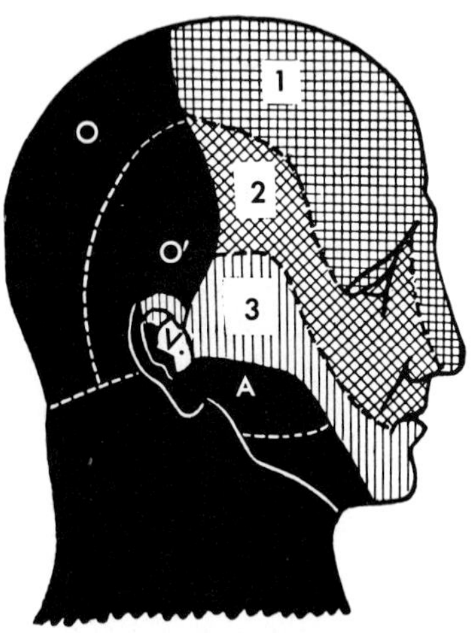

Fig. 15-2. Sensory innervation of the head.

Shaded areas: Trigeminal nerve
1, Ophthalmic division
2, Maxillary division
3, Mandibular division
White area: Auricular branch of vagus nerve *(V)*
Black areas: Cervical nerves
O, Greater occipital nerve
O′, Lesser occipital nerve
A, Great auricular nerve

Table 15-1. Distribution of the trigeminal nerve (for supply of the dura and trunks of blood vessels, see text)

Ophthalmic division

- Area of skin labeled *1* in Fig. 15-2
- Cornea, conjunctiva and intraocular structures (the sclera is innervated by fibers of the anterior branches of the ciliary plexus; Teng, 1962)
- Mucosa of paranasal sinuses (frontal, sphenoid and ethmoid)
- Mucosa of upper and anterior nasal septum and lateral wall of nasal cavity
- Lacrimal duct

Maxillary division

- Area of skin labeled *2* in Fig. 15-2
- Mucosa of maxillary sinus
- Mucosa of posterior part of nasal septum and lower part of nasal cavity
- Upper teeth and gum
- Hard palate
- Soft palate and tonsil (via sphenopalatine ganglion, greater petrosal nerve, and nervus intermedius)

Mandibular division

- Area of skin labeled *3* in Fig. 15-2
- Mucosa of the cheek, lower jaw, floor of the mouth, tongue
- Proprioception from jaw muscles
- Lower teeth and gum
- Mastoid cells
- Muscles of mastication

MANIFESTATIONS OF INTERRUPTION OF THE TRIGEMINAL NERVE

Sensory and reflex changes

Interruption of any one of the divisions of the fifth nerve results in anesthesia or hypesthesia of the parts it supplies. Under such conditions changes occur in reflexes. Interruption of the ophthalmic division leads to reduction or loss of the *corneal reflex:* application of a wisp of cotton to the edge of the cornea of the affected side fails to elicit winking on either side, but if applied on the sound side will cause bilateral winking. The afferent limb is in the fifth nerve, the efferent in the seventh. The reflex arc includes supranuclear fibers; interruption of these fibers may cause impairment of the corneal reflex of the opposite side. Another reflex abolished by interruption of the ophthalmic division is the *orbicularis oculi reflex;* the afferent limb of this reflex is dependent on the integrity of the fifth nerve, and the efferent on the seventh nerve (p. 223). The *sneeze reflex,* which under normal conditions can be produced by tickling the nasal mucosa, may also be affected by lesions of the fifth nerve: tickling of the *upper* nasal mucosa no longer induces the sneeze reflex if the ophthalmic division is interrupted, and the same applies to tickling the *lower* nasal mucosa if the maxillary division is interrupted. The *palatal reflex* (elevation of the soft palate when its lateral edge is stroked), although largely dependent on the integrity of the ninth and tenth nerves, may be lost ipsilaterally in lesions involving the posterior palatine nerve or the sphenopalatine ganglion (see Fig. 14-1 for the pathways involved). Furthermore, the smarting effect normally experienced upon inhalation of ammonia or acetic acid as the result of irritation of sensory trigeminal terminals in the nasal mucosa is lost when the fifth nerve is interrupted. Also lost are the various reflex responses that inhalation of these substances brings about: lacrimation, changes in pulse rate, and momentary cessation of respiration. These reflexes, especially the palatal, are subject to individual variation and thus are of localizing importance only when they are absent unilaterally.

The fifth nerve also carries fibers concerned in the transmission of *proprioceptive sensibility* of the muscles of the jaw. Interruption of these fibers may lead to disturbances in the coordination of mimetic movements of the lower part of the face; because of the elimination of centripetal impulses necessary to the maintenance of tonus of the muscles in this part of the face, relaxation of these muscles occurs, giving the visage in this region an "ironed-out" appearance. Moreover, *pressure pain,* conveyed from the face by way of the fifth nerve, may be lost as a result of severe damage of the mandibular division or of the gasserian ganglion or root (Carmichael and Woollard, 1933).

Motor changes

The muscles innervated by the *mandibular division* of the fifth nerve are the masticatory muscles, the mylohyoid and the anterior belly of the digastric, and the tensor tympani and the tensor veli palatini.

In *unilateral paralysis of the masticatory muscles* (masseter, temporal, pterygoids, digastric), lateral movement of the lower jaw can occur only toward the paralyzed side, a movement made possible mainly by the pterygoids of the normal side. Paralysis of the temporal and masseter muscles may also be detected by having the patient bite firmly and then having him relax his bite without separating the teeth; simultaneously the examiner palpates the muscles, noting their volume and their degree of hardness. In temporal and masseter paralysis, all three muscles suffer. When teeth are absent or when the patient wears dentures, it may be difficult to decide whether the muscles are contracting normally. Under such conditions the patient should be asked to bite on several thicknesses of a folded cloth.

In *bilateral paralysis of the masticatory muscles* the lower jaw drops and active jaw movement cannot be performed. The *masseter ("jaw") reflex,* dependent upon the integrity of the mandibular division of the fifth nerve, is not elicitable. In this reflex the masseters contract when the examiner's finger, placed on the patient's chin, is tapped with a percussion hammer. The reflex is most easily elicited when the mouth is slightly open and the muscles of the jaw are relaxed. Now and then the reflex is absent in normal persons. In supranuclear lesions the masseter reflex is exaggerated and its elicitation may be associated either with clonus or trismus.

Paralysis of the mylohyoid muscle and of the anterior belly of the digastric is manifested by flaccidity of the floor of the mouth of that side. Palpation of the floor of the mouth while the patient attempts to swallow a bolus placed in the anterior part of the mouth will reveal that the muscles of the paralyzed side remain soft. In *paralysis of the tensor tympani muscle* there may be partial deafness for low-pitched sounds, and in *paralysis of the tensor veli palatini,* a slight descent of the palatopharyngeal arch.

INVOLVEMENT OF MORE DISTAL LEVELS OF THE TRIGEMINAL NERVE

Either loss of function or irritative phenomena may occur as a result of involvement of more distal levels of the fifth nerve.

In *head injuries* the supraorbital is the nerve most frequently affected, the damage being inflicted either by blunt injury or by fracture of the upper margin of the orbit. The infraorbital nerve may be involved in fracture of the maxilla. The ophthalmic division in general is particularly subject to injury in fracture of the wall of the orbit involving the superior orbital fissure. Occasionally, the nasociliary nerve is interrupted in fracture of the orbit. Injury of any of these nerves may be complicated by severe neuralgia when only partial regeneration of the nerves has occurred. (Russell, 1945.)

Vitamin B deficiency is a cause of numbness in the region of distribution of the trigeminus (de Wardener and Lennox, 1947). *Trichlorethylene* sometimes damages sensory fibers of the fifth nerve, causing numbness of the face. Later, anesthesia and, occasionally, psychosis may occur. (Glaser, 1931.)

Pain originating in teeth, in the temporomandibular joint, or in the paranasal sinuses is usually localizable on the basis of the local signs and symptoms and also on the site to which the pain is projected.

Odontogenic pain is revealed by its aggravation on exposure of the tooth to cold or heat. The pain is usually throbbing. The pain is referred to diverse areas, depending on the tooth involved; for instance, pain from infected maxillary central and lateral incisors is referred to the frontal area (Glick, 1962). Pain from *malocclusion of the teeth* radiates, for example, from the ala of the nose around the mouth to the chin of one or both sides. *Temporomandibular joint or muscle pain* is usually dull, constant, and limited to the region of supply of the fifth nerve, though it may be felt in the neck and shoulder as well. Commonly the pain occurs in the condylar, auricular, and temporal regions, and radiates forward over the cheek and face. Now and then, tic-like sensations are felt in the lips, cheek, and gingiva. The pain is almost always unilateral. It is brought on or aggravated by chewing. Deviation of the jaw may occur on opening the mouth and there may be hypermobility of the jaw or a painful trismus which drastically limits mandibular movements. In some patients the temporomandibular joint is tender to pressure, while in others it is not. Muscles involved in mastication are themselves commonly tender and in numerous patients there is evidence of a self-perpetuating spasm of these muscles. Mandibular hyperextension or habitual clenching or grinding of the teeth may be initiating factors. Rheumatic disease is one of the many disorders that may involve the temporomandibular joint. (Brussell, 1949; Kawamura, 1968; Schwartz and Chayes, 1968.) *Paranasal sinus pain* is deep, dull, aching, and persistent. When originating from the posterior group of sinuses, pain is felt behind and between the eyes and over the parietal region; the pain tends to radiate to the vertex of the skull. With involvement of the anterior group of sinuses the pain occurs in the region of the forehead and between the eyes. In maxillary sinusitis, pain and tenderness are noted over the cheek. Seldom if ever in sinus disease is pain referred to the ear, except rarely in infective states involving posterior ethmoid cells or the sphenoid sinus (Couch, 1956). Pain due to expansion of air trapped in the maxillary sinus during high altitude flying may in some instances be referred to the teeth *(aerodontalgia).* Such pain is almost always referred to teeth on which traumatic dental work has been carried out, illustrating the commonly observed habit reference of pain. (Reynolds and Hutchins, 1948.) The *anterior ethmoid nerve syndrome* ("nasociliary neuralgia") is thought to be due to injury of the nerve consequent to pressure from prolonged swelling of the nasal mucosa. The disorder is characterized by pain, usually unilateral, involving the medial part of the eyebrow and having a tendency to extend to the face, vertex of the skull, or even the neck. The headache, although usually dull, may be severe and last from half an hour to several days. The headaches may occur off and on for years; their intensity does not fluctuate. For the diagnosis to be sustained, probing of the area supplied by the anterior ethmoid nerve must reproduce the headache. Cocainization of the nerve relieves the headache. The disorder may masquerade under the diagnosis of "migraine." (Shalom, 1966.)

Pain may be referred to the face and head and adjacent regions from *affections of the dura mater and dural venous sinuses,* as gathered from the results of electrical stimulation or digital pressure exerted at various sites: stimulation in the *region of most rostral falx,* pain in the midline of forehead or nose; *posterior third of falx,* pain on the same side of the head; *region of rostral two-thirds of the superior sagittal sinus,* pain in the ipsilateral forehead, temple, face, or ear, radiating down into the neck; *more caudal part of superior sagittal sinus,* pain behind the ipsilateral eye or in the forehead; *region of basal venous sinuses,* pain in the ipsilateral eye or forehead; *lateral sinus,* pain in the ipsilateral mastoid region; *floor of posterior cranial fossa,* pain in the ipsilateral eye or forehead; *pressure in vicinity of the jugular foramen,* pain in the ipsilateral mastoid and cervical regions; *pressure upward on tentorium,* pain in the ipsilateral frontal region, and *pressure downward,* apparently pain in suboccipital region and down the back of the neck; *middle cranial fossa,* pain in the ipsilateral temple; *middle meningeal artery and its branches,* sharp pain frequently in ipsilateral temporal region; *middle cerebral artery near the circle of Willis,* occasionally pain in the ipsilateral temporal region or above the ipsilateral eye. (Feindel, Penfield, and McNaughton, 1960; Penfield and McNaughton, 1940.)

Further, pain may be referred from *occluded cerebral arteries,* particularly when stroke is imminent: pain over the ipsilateral eye in occlusion of the internal carotid, middle cerebral, or posterior cerebral artery, and pain over the occiput, often lateralized, in occlusion of the vertebral, basilar, posterior inferior cerebellar, or superior cerebellar artery (Fisher, 1954).

Neuralgias (or headaches) other than those already mentioned that involve the face and adjacent regions have been given various designations, in accordance with the presumed nerve(s) or presumed vessel(s) involved. A classification provided by Friedman, Finley, and others (1968), slightly modified, will serve as a guide to the descriptions that follow:

1. *Cranial neuralgias.* Included here are trigeminal neuralgia, dealt with in the following text, and glossopharyngeal neuralgia (pp. 179 and 180).
2. *Vascular headaches of migraine type.* These are characterized by recurrent attacks of headache, widely varied in intensity, frequency, and duration.

Trigeminal neuralgia

In trigeminal neuralgia, paroxysmal attacks of sharp, lancinating, agonizing pain occur and are accompanied by vasomotor and secretory disturbances. Muscle twitching occurs during attacks (hence *tic* douloureux). Practically all the patients are past age 40, and most are elderly; only rarely is the disorder noted in younger persons (in which case multiple sclerosis may be the cause). Women are affected twice as often as men. The pain radiates like an electric shock, and involves the region of distribution of the maxillary division, less commonly the mandibular, and seldom (in 1 to 5 percent of cases) the ophthalmic division. Seldom if ever do the pains commence in the region of the eye. Only one side of the face is affected, most often the right; this is with exception of about 3 percent of cases, in which the attacks run independently on the two sides of the face. The pain is felt superficially in the skin. Initially the attacks last from a few seconds to a minute or two, but subsequently they may be of longer duration; the attacks tend to occur on a daily basis for a few weeks; during sleep, attacks are rare. Remission then occurs; paroxysms invariably recur. An attack may be provoked by a variety of stimuli, such as exposure of the face to a draft of cold air, chewing, yawning, talking, or swallowing. Light tactile stimuli applied to circumscribed areas can set off the pain. These "trigger zones" may be only punctate in size. They may be situated on the upper lip or at the angle of the mouth, side of the tongue, supraorbital notch, or elsewhere. The affected area of the face usually appears hyperesthetic and hyperalgesic, though mild hypesthesia and hypalgesia and a reduction in the number of tactile pain points have been noted in 25 percent of patients—suggesting, according to Lewy and Grant (1938), not a true hyperesthesia, but rather a central over-response. Function of the masticatory muscles is unaltered. (Harris, 1940; Kerr, 1963b; Miller, 1968; Sperling and Stender, 1955.) Proposed causes of trigeminal neuralgia are many; emphasis has, however, been given to mechanical factors as instrumental. A current hypothesis is that the disorder is due to traction of the mandibular division as a consequence of asymmetrical jaw protrusion, with ipsilateral involvement of the other two divisions the result of displacement of these structures against bony and dural edges. Overcorrection of the mandibular deficit through manual retraction of the jaw is reported to bring about a progressive decline in frequency and severity of tic douloureux (Carney, 1967). Another view along this line is that trigeminal neuralgia is due to occlusal displacement and mandibular overclosure occurring in association with temporomandibular joint dysfunction; "cure" has been achieved by the establishment of correct vertical dimension of the occlusion with molar support (Lindsay, 1969). Electron microscopic examination of the gasserian ganglion and trigeminal sensory root has revealed, in rather numerous cases, pronounced proliferative degenerative changes in myelin sheaths at both sites, of a nature suggesting that the primary site of involvement may be in the myelin (Kerr and Miller, 1966).

Vascular headaches of migraine type

"Lower-half" headache. One variety of lower-half headache is called *buccal neuralgia.* The pain occurs in the region of the nose, cheeks, lips, gingiva, tongue, and upper and lower jaw, and is of a burning, aching, boring, or throbbing character. The pain may last from a few minutes to several days. It may be precipitated by talking, chewing, or by local temperature change. No true trigger zones are found. In occasional instances the pain has been relieved by stripping the external carotid artery of nerve fibers or by removing a segment of facial artery in the region of the inferior border of the jaw. (Adson, 1948; Shanasy, 1949.)

Sluder's (1927) *sphenopalatine neuralgia* and Vail's (1932) *vidian neuralgia* have been discredited by some authors as far as proposed neural origin is concerned. The pain originates in the base of the nose and region of the orbit and radiates ipsilaterally into the upper jaw and teeth, also in some instances over the side of the head, into the occiput and neck, and even into the arm. The pain may be more or less constant, or it may be throbbing and paroxysmal. There may also be tinnitus and vertigo. Cocainization of the nasal mucosa in the region just posterior to the middle turbinate will relieve the pain. This disorder has been included among the *sympathalgies faciales* (Bing and Haymaker, 1939). Harris (1936) also considers the disturbance as of sympathetic origin. Aubry and Pialoux (1968) are of the opinion that Sluder's syndrome represents a disorder of both the sphenopalatine ganglion and the perivascular plexus of the internal maxillary artery and its branches.

"Cluster" headache. "Cluster" headache refers to the periodic occurrence of bouts of headache followed by complete remission for months. This type of headache has been described under a number of designations.

Erythroprosopalgia, according to Bing's (1952) account, occurs most commonly in men in their thirties or forties. Attacks of pain appear on one side of the face, though occasionally on both sides, either abruptly without warning or after a brief prodrome of prickling paresthesias. The pain is severe, and of burning, boring, or stabbing quality. It lasts from a few minutes to a few hours. Circumscribed areas of reddening and swelling and, sometimes, hyperhidrosis appear in the cheek or periorbital region. The nasal mucosa may also be involved, in which case rhinorrhea occurs. Another manifestation, which is uncommon, is conjunctival congestion. During attacks, a pressure-sensitive area can usually be found in the infraorbital region. Pulsations of the superficial temporal artery or transverse facial artery are remarkably strong and can be easily detected. Horner's syndrome ipsilateral to the facial pain is sometimes encountered.

Ciliary (migrainous) neuralgia, described by Harris (1936), carries a long history of intermittent attacks of pain referred anteriorly (and usually ipsilaterally) to the temple, eye, cheek, and jaws. Commonly the paroxysms last for as short as 10 or 15 minutes, and there may be four to six attacks in 24 hours; they may last as long as 30 hours. They commonly occur in the early hours after midnight. In about 50 percent of cases the attack culminates in conjunctival congestion and in lacrimation—a veritable ocular crisis. The term "ciliary" does not necessarily imply that the responsible pathological change resides in the ciliary ganglion, but rather that the disorder involves its area of innervation, the eye. Spasm of recurrent meningeal vessels resulting in the transmission of abnormal impulses through branches of the fifth nerve is considered the basis. Teichopsia and hemianopia, such as are observed in migraine in which spasm of the posterior cerebral artery is presumed, do not occur. Alcohol injection into the gasserian ganglion or into the infraorbital or supraorbital branches of the fifth nerve proved effective. Congestive glaucoma has been known to masquerade under the diagnosis, "ciliary neuralgia" (Hobbs, 1964).

A particular variety of headache was the title used by Symonds (1956) in describing a series of cases which, as he stated, fell in the domain of Harris's "ciliary (migrainous) neuralgia." Noted in his patients, aged 14 to 43 years, were paroxysms of intense unilateral pain of sudden onset, 10 minutes to 2 hours or somewhat longer in duration, which occurred in bouts lasting several weeks. The paroxysms came on either in the day or night. Emphasis was placed on the complete freedom from pain over long intervals of 6 months to a few years. During the paroxysm the pain was felt mainly on the supraorbital region or in or behind the eyes; it usually spread beyond this region, occasionally even into the neck. Ergotamine tartrate (a vasoconstrictor) effectively prevented attacks. The disorder was considered a migrainous variant.

In the *histaminic cephalgia* of Horton (Horton, 1941, 1956; Horton, MacLean, and Craig, 1939), the pain, which was severe, was situated mainly in and around the eye and was commonly succeeded by congestion and wateriness of the eye and stuffiness of the nose. The distribution of the pain tended to coincide with that of the ramifications of the external carotid artery. Attacks usually lasted less than an hour, and they tended to occur at night. In about 30 percent of cases attacks could be reproduced by an injection of histamine. Treatment consisted in histamine desensitization. Relief was obtained in most of the patients for periods from 2 weeks to 18 months. Bing (1952) considered the disorder the same as his "erythroprosopalgia." In Kunkle's view (1959), this form of headache may be evoked by discharge of parasympathetic components of the seventh nerve or, more rarely, the tenth nerve, a view suggested by the finding of an acetylcholine-like substance in the cerebrospinal fluid during attacks. However, the presence of such a substance in sizable quantity in the CSF has not been confirmed. Acetylcholine, according to Ikonomoff (1968), appears incapable of provoking an attack of migraine on the basis that galantamine (Nivaline) and neostigmin (Syntostigmin) intensify the effect of acetylcholine by inhibiting cholinesterase, and yet are effective as therapy for migraine. Both drugs also have antiserotinin-like effect and apparently improve blood vessel tonus.

Petrosal neuralgia, described by Gardner, Stowell, and Dutlinger (1947), is also marked by lacrimation and nasal congestion during paroxysms, as well as by other features already mentioned. The postulate was that the disorder was due to involvement of the greater superficial petrosal nerve. Accordingly, section of the nerve was undertaken. This was more or less effective for various periods in 75 percent of the cases; in three patients there was no recurrence until 18 to 30 months later. White and Sweet (1955) performed petrosal neurectomy in six cases designated as "Horton's neuralgia," with success in four; in the other two, relief was transitory.

Nervus intermedius (Hunt's) neuralgia occurring in association with herpes zoster is described on pages 225 and 226. The neuralgia may, however, occur independently of vesiculation. One form is spoken of as *prosopalgic*. It is characterized by pain deep in the face on one side, with radiation of the pain to the ear in some cases; the pain is often accompanied by lacrimation and nasal congestion on that side, and, in some instances, by salivation as well. The pain frequently comes on at night within an hour or so after the subject has fallen asleep, and lasts from half an hour to several hours. Trigger points may be found in the external auditory canal. Men tend to be affected more than women. Complete relief has been obtained by section of the nervus intermedius (Sachs, 1968). The other form is called *otalgic*. The most notable feature is the occurrence of paroxysmal attacks of pain, usually in the region of the external auditory canal but sometimes just in front of the ear or behind it. With the passage of time, the pain during a paroxysm may spread to the eye, lips, nose, or lower jaw. (Wegner, 1968.)

Atypical neuralgia is a term given facial, head, and neck pain, not conforming to cranial nerve distribution, but instead to the area of supply of the external carotid artery, particularly the internal maxillary artery or any one or more of its major branches. In some instances, the propagation of the disturbances may be along the internal carotid artery and its branches. In pathological processes involving, for example, sympathetic nerves in the sheath of the external carotid artery the clinical disturbances are located below eye level, and when irritation is propagated in sympathetic nerves coursing along the ophthalmic artery the disturbances are at eye level and above

Table 15-2. Differentiation of typical and atypical neuralgia (from Friedman, 1964)

Factors involved	*Typical*	*Atypical*
Distribution of pain	Limited in the field of one of the cranial nerves	Does not follow nerve distribution
Character of pain	Paroxysmal, sharp, localized	Diffuse, deep-seated, poorly localized; described as pulling, gripping, etc.
Duration of pain	Seconds to minutes	Hours or days
Autonomic nervous system signs	None	Lacrimation, flushing, nasal congestion, other symptoms
Precipitation by external stimuli	Yes	No
Trigger zone	Present	Absent
Age	Older age group	Younger age group
Pharmacology		
Vasoconstrictor	No relief	Frequent relief
Vasodilator	Inadequate relief	No relief
Narcotics	Inadequate relief	Frequent relief
Relief by surgical or chemical interruption of cranial nerve	Relief	No relief
Personality	Neurotic traits not prominent	Neurotic traits prominent

(Weisengreen and Winters, 1952). Atypical neuralgia embraces some of the neuralgias dealt with in the foregoing discussion. To be included as responsible for atypical neuralgia is an *elongated styloid process,* or a styloid process of normal length so turned inward that its tip lies against the external or internal carotid. Where such a process exists, tonsillectomy is likely to set off a neuralgic disturbance, including referral of pain to the ear. Fracture of the styloid process can have much the same consequence (Douglas and Huebsch, 1953). *Dural scar* may also be responsible (Penfield and McNaughton, 1940). Further, *thyroid hormone deficiency* may be associated with recurring headaches and with recurring dull or aching or throbbing pains in the face and neck; relief has been obtained by administering thyroid extract (Watts, 1951).

In atypical neuralgia the pain is deep seated and pulling or aching; it is usually continuous, but paroxysmal pain of greater or lesser intensity may be superimposed on it. Most commonly affected is the region of distribution of the maxillary division of nerve V. In most patients the pain is unilateral, and in about half there are manifestations of autonomic disturbances: flushing of the face, nasal discharge, salivation, puffiness of the face, and ocular disturbances. Some distinguishing features between typical and atypical neuralgias are indicated in Table 15-2.

DISTURBANCES FROM LESIONS AT MORE PROXIMAL LEVELS OF THE TRIGEMINUS

When pain is encountered in association with *intramedullary lesions* the cause is to be sought in some extramedullary structure. For instance, the occurrence of trigeminal neuralgia in multiple sclerosis (Rushton and Olafson, 1965) may be due to some mechanical factor incident to multiple sclerosis in which the mandibular division is involved.

A sign, too often encountered in comatose patients to go unmentioned, is the *tendency to rub, pull, or finger the nose or lips.* This is observed particularly in expanding temporal lobe tumor or abscess (de Crinis, 1942), also in increased intracranial pressure generally. It is probably attributable to an excitatory (pressure) effect exerted by the swollen temporal lobe on sensory fibers of the fifth nerve.

Irritation of the *motor root of the fifth nerve* may induce tonic and clonic spasms of the muscles of mastication; the tonic spasms are referred to as trismus, and the clonic spasms as *masticatory spasms.* Both (or one or the other) may occasionally be noted in acute lesions involving the pons, as in meningitis, encephalitis, rabies, tetany, multiple sclerosis, and strychnine poisoning (also in hysteria). Trismus from compression of the cerebral cortex by subdural hematoma may occasionally be so pronounced that tetanus is suspected; this is because the patient is unable to move his jaws or to speak (Foerster, 1931).

Trismus is a classical manifestation of the cephalic form of *tetanus;* the trismus is usually accompanied by tetanic spasms of the facial, pharyngeal, and cervical muscles, and by extraocular nerve palsy, particularly sixth nerve palsy (Sanchez-Longo and Schlezinger, 1955). Besides bringing about overactivity of somatic motoneurons, the neurotoxin of *Clostridium tetani* produces widespread effects indicative of overaction of the sympathetic system; the disturbances are much the same as those observed following an injection of epinephrine (Kerr and others, 1968).

Pain in the face from *trigeminal root* involvement is encountered under a number of conditions. Among them is syphilis, particularly in the tabes dorsalis phase of the disease. The pain is dull, though shooting pain is at times superimposed. At night the pain commonly increases; in some cases it is paroxysmal and thus simulates tic douloureux. A trigger zone is, however, lacking. As in other systemic disorders involving the fifth nerve, the pain in syphilis is usually bilateral. Paroxysms of trismus may also occur. (Shanasy, 1949.) In suppurative petrositis complicating otitis media, facial neuralgia can result from spread of an infective process to the region of the trigeminal root. When combined with palsy of the lateral rectus, the disorder is known as *Gradenigo's syndrome.* Tumor occupying the cerebellopontile angle, including trigeminal root neurinoma and acoustic neuroma, may be manifested in initial stages by paroxysmal facial pain, though paresthesia as a presenting symptom is far more common. Such tumors may also induce signs and symptoms referable to pressure on the brainstem and superior cerebellar peduncle (pyramidal tract and "cerebellar" signs). Objective loss of facial sensibility characterizes these cases; the loss usually overshadows any pain that may be present. Another feature of tumor in this location is the absence of the corneal reflex. (Glaser, 1935; Jefferson, 1955; Krayenbühl, 1936.) Facial neuralgia (later, anesthesia dolorosa) is now and then encountered in the presence of increased intracranial pressure resulting from glioma or meningioma in the occipital region; stretching of the root of the fifth nerve may be the basis.

Another level of the trigeminus from which pain can be induced is the *gasserian ganglion.* Extrinsic tumors that encroach upon or invade the gasserian ganglion may lead to severe facial pain. Tumors usually reach the ganglion through invasion along transbasal routes. They include tumor of the roof of the nasopharynx (which extends on to the floor of the skull by passing through the foramen lacerum), pituitary tumor (adenoma in particular), and tumor of the sphenoid sinus. Carcinoma may also reach the ganglion in the form of metastases. Spreading carcinoma usually involves the sixth nerve before reaching the ganglion. Whether reaching the ganglion directly or metastatically, carcinoma induces nonparoxysmal, unremitting, intolerable, deep-seated pain, followed by anesthesia dolorosa in part or all of the region of trigeminal distribution. Now and then the temporal and masseter muscles undergo atrophy. Dissociated loss of sensibility may occur. (Godtfredsen, 1947; Rosenbaum and Seaman, 1955.)

Meningioma adherent to the *gasserian ganglion* gives rise at first to dysesthesias of the face and later to anesthesia dolorosa. As the tumor enlarges, the third nerve may be encroached upon, causing ptosis that fluctuates in severity. Slight exophthalmos usually occurs. The pupils may be dilated or small, depending on the site of predominant pressure—whether on the third nerve or on adjacent sympathetic fibers (the location of which is indicated in Fig. 14-1). (Cushing and Eisenhardt, 1938.) Meningioma or other tumor involving the gasserian ganglion may eventually grow downward over the petrous ridge producing facial paralysis, deafness, and nystagmus.

Other causes of damage of *trigeminal root and/or gasserian ganglion* are aneurysm of the internal carotid, transverse basal fractures at levels behind the sella turcica, and granulomatous meningitis. Instead of pain, one commonly finds anesthesia of the entire ipsilateral region of trigeminal distribution and paralysis of the ipsilateral masticatory muscles.

In *herpes zoster* involving the region supplied by the trigeminal nerve the primary lesion is situated in the *gasserian ganglion.* Redness and pain occur in the involved part of the face, and vesicular eruption develops two or three days later. The vesicles are always limited to one side of the face. They may predominate in the field of any of the trigeminal divisions. However, the ophthalmic division is usually implicated alone *(ophthalmic zoster).* Vesicles appear on the conjunctiva and cornea, also on the forehead, and along the bridge of the nose in the territory supplied by the nasociliary nerve. The sclera or cornea (or both) may undergo ulceration; occasionally, panophthalmitis with or without primary optic atrophy and glaucoma results. In the absence of these complications the pupil on the affected side may not constrict on exposure to light but reacts well in accommodation. Partial third nerve palsy may also occur. Much less frequent is palsy of the sixth and/or fourth nerves (Chance, 1915), and there may be an associated seventh nerve palsy. At about the time the vesicular lesions dry, the pain in the face usually recedes. However, *postzoster neuralgia* may develop. The pain is persistent and has a burning, tearing quality sometimes reminiscent of causalgia. Instead of pain there may be anesthesia over the whole area of supply of the ophthalmic division. Ophthalmic zoster may be mimicked by gasserian ganglion involvement by tumor.

In differential diagnosis, *herpes simplex keratitis* (herpetic keratitis) also needs to be considered. This is a disorder in which small vesicles form on the cornea and in which the corneal nerves are usually destroyed. The infection, usually unilateral, complicates febrile disorders—for example, epidemic influenza, bronchitis, pneumonia, and pertussis. Scrapings from the conjunctival sac often reveal multinucleated epithelial cells and intranuclear inclusion bodies characteristic of the disease (Kimura and Thygeson, 1955).

Neuroparalytic or *neurotrophic keratopathy* is a nonspecific disorder resulting from interruption of the ophthalmic division of the fifth nerve at any level from the gasserian ganglion peripheralward (for example, from skull fracture, granulomatous meningitis, or intracranial tumor in the region of the fifth nerve). Characteristic are bullous changes in the epithelium of the sclera and edema of the scleral stroma. Decrease in the lid reflex and diminished tear secretion are accompaniments. While neuroparalytic keratopathy may not occur in unilateral interruption of the ophthalmic division—the consensual reflex according adequate protection—it always develops in bilateral interruption of the division. The keratopathy is most severe when both the fifth and the seventh nerve are affected. In seventh nerve palsy the involvement of the cornea represents an "exposure" keratitis, such as may occur also in exophthalmos and in deep coma.

DISORDERS OF AUTONOMIC COMPONENTS OF THE TRIGEMINAL NERVE

Parasympathetic fibers arise from the superior salivatory, lacrimal, and inferior salivatory nuclei, course in the seventh and ninth nerves, and traverse certain branches of all three division of the fifth nerve (Fig. 14-1). *Sympathetic fibers* for the supply of sweat glands and arterioles of the face are derived from the intermediolateral horns of spinal segments Th1 and Th2. They pass through the corresponding anterior roots and white sympathetic rami, ascend in the cervical sympathetic chain, and synapse in the superior cervical sympathetic ganglion. From here the postganglionic fibers pass upward in the sheath of the external and internal carotid arteries. The fibers join all three divisions of the fifth nerve in the region of their emergence from the skull or more distally. Lesions of peripheral branches may lead, therefore, to sympathetic paralysis in corresponding regions of the face. Damage to the nasociliary nerve (a branch of the ophthalmic division that traverses the orbit) causes *Horner's syndrome.*

Some autonomic fibers contained in the ophthalmic and maxillary divisions of the fifth nerve have the function of secreting nasal mucus. Interruption of either of these divisions leads not only to anesthesia of the corresponding part of the face but also to an abnormal dryness of the nasal mucosa followed by impairment in the sense of smell.

Lacrimal fibers pass by way of the zygomatic nerve to reach the ophthalmic division of the fifth nerve (Fig. 14-1). Interruption of the ophthalmic division proximal to this site (for example, as the fibers traverse the gasserian ganglion) does not interfere with tear secretion. *Reduction or abolition of lacrimation* may occur only when conduction is interrupted in the sphenopalatine ganglion, the more proximal part of the maxillary division, the zygomatic nerve, or the lacrimal nerve.

By contrast, *impairment of salivary secretion* by a trigeminal lesion can occur only when a lesion interrupts the lingual nerve in the region distal to the point where it receives the chorda tympani (Fig. 14-1).

Disturbances of taste in the anterior two-thirds of the tongue occur as a result of interruption of the lingual nerve distal to its junction with the chorda tympani (Fig. 14-1). If loss of taste occurs in the anterior two-thirds of the tongue and there is a reduction of salivary secretion but no anesthesia in the region of trigeminal innervation and no paralysis of structures supplied by the seventh nerve, the chorda tympani must be the site of the lesion. Chorda tympani involvement is often due to infectious processes in the tympanic cavity.

LOCALIZATION OF LESIONS OF THE NUCLEUS OF THE SPINAL TRACT OF THE TRIGEMINAL NERVE

Because of its length, the nucleus of the spinal tract of the fifth nerve may readily be affected by lesions in the lateral part of the medulla oblongata and/or the uppermost cervical cord—for example, from syringobulbia, a thrombosed posterior inferior cerebellar artery, tumor, inflammatory state, or multiple sclerosis. In these disorders clinical evidence of co-involvement of structures in the vicinity of the nucleus can usually be found. The level of the nuclear lesion is indicated by the nature of the resulting syndrome alternans (pp. 153 and 154).

Clinical studies occasionally indicate that an "onion peel" layering of disturbed sensibility (dysesthesias and hypesthesia) involves the face (Fig. 15-3), especially the perioral-nasal region, in patients having lesions in the medulla oblongata or vicinity (Kraus, 1935; Richter and Woodruff, 1942; Sjöqvist, 1938). It has been contended that this layering signifies that the spinal nucleus of the fifth nerve has a segmental as well as a divisional representation. However, there is nothing in the organization of this nucleus (Fig. 15-1) to support this view. Lesions crossing divisional boundaries at certain levels in the spinal tract of the fifth nerve could, theoretically, give rise to sensory disturbances having "onion peel" distribution. However, it is more likely that interruption of a system ascending in the periventricular and periaqueductal gray could be responsible. Evidence in support is the observation by Nashold, Wilson, and Slaughter (1969) that electrical stimulation unilaterally in the periaqueductal gray in man can give rise to sensations bilaterally in the region of face and the perioral and buccal regions, straddling the midline. Tactile impulses alone appear to be carried by this pathway.

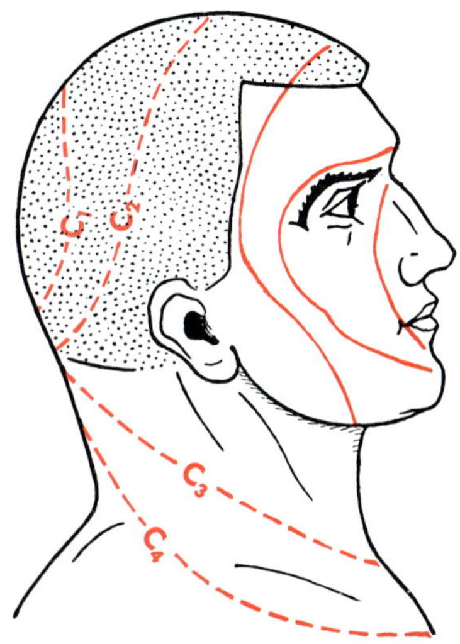

Fig. 15-3. "Onion peel" sensory distribution in the head and neck. The lines on the face represent lateral boundaries at which dysesthesia or hypesthesia may occur. C_1 through C_4 traverse the midzone of the cutaneous areas supplied from the respective cervical segments.

MANIFESTATIONS OF SUPRANUCLEAR LESIONS

Interruption of the supranuclear fibers passing from the cortex to the motor fifth nucleus of one side does not result in functional disturbances of trigeminal innervated muscles because the nucleus of one side receives fibers from the cortex of both sides (Fig. 15-1). If, however, the supranuclear tracts of both sides are destroyed, there will be masticatory diplegia.

REFERENCES

Adson, A. W. 1948. Neuralgia of face; diagnosis and treatment. J. Int. Coll. Surg. **11**:1-8.

Aubry, M., and Pialoux, P. 1968. Sluder's syndrome. In Vinken, P. J., and Bruyn, G. W., editors: Handbook of clinical neurology, vol. 5. Amsterdam, North-Holland Publishing Company, pp. 326-332.

Bing, R. 1952. Histamin-Kopfschmerz oder Erythroprosopalgie? J. Nerv. Ment. Dis. **116**:862-873.

Bing, R., and Haymaker, W. 1939. Textbook of nervous diseases. St. Louis, The C. V. Mosby Co.

Brussell, I. J. 1949. Temporomandibular joint disease; differential diagnosis and treatment. J.A.D.A. **39**:532-554.

Carmichael, E. A., and Woollard, H. H. 1933. Some observations on the fifth and seventh nerves. Brain **56**:109-125.

Carney, L. R. 1967. Considerations on the cause and treatment of trigeminal neuralgia. Neurology **17**:1143-1151.

Chance, B. 1915. Herpes zoster ophthalmicus. Ann. Ophthal. **24**:693-717.

Corbin, K. B. 1940. Observations of the peripheral distribution of the fibers arising in the mesencephalic nucleus of the fifth cranial nerve. J. Comp. Neurol. **73**:153-177.

Couch, C. D., Jr. 1956. Facial pain. J. Oral Surg. **14**:216-227.

Cushing, H., and Eisenhardt, L. 1938. Meningiomas: their classification, regional behavior, life history and surgical end results. Springfield, Illinois, Charles C Thomas, Publisher.

Dandy, W. E. 1933. Physiological studies following extirpation of the right cerebral hemisphere in man. Bull. Johns Hopk. Hosp. **53**:31-51.

de Crinis, A. 1942. Zur Symptomatologie der Schläfenlappentumoren. Z. Ges. Neurol. Psychiat. **174**:166-193.

de Wardener, H. E., and Lennox, B. 1947. Cerebral beriberi (Wernicke's encephalopathy): review of 52 cases in a Singapore prisoner-of-war hospital. Lancet **1**:11-17.

Douglas, B. L., and Huebsch, R. F. 1953. Atypical facial neuralgia resulting from fractured styloid process of the temporal bone. Oral Surg. **6**:1199-1201.

Feindel, W., Penfield, W., and McNaughton, F. 1960. The tentorial nerves and localization of intracranial pain in man. Neurology **10**:555-563.

Fisher, C. M. 1968. Headache in cerebrovascular disease. In Vinken, P. J., and Bruyn, G. W., editors: Handbook of clinical neurology, vol. 5. Amsterdam, North-Holland Publishing Company, pp. 124-156.

Fisher, M. 1954. Concerning cerebral arteriosclerosis. J. Amer. Geriat. Soc. **2**:1-18.

Foerster, O. 1931. The cerebral cortex in man. Lancet **2**:309-312.

Friedman, A. P. 1964. Facial pain. Oral Surg. **18**:730-736.

Friedman, A. P., Finley, K. H., and others. 1968. Drug trials for headache: principles and methods. NINDB Monogr. No. 6.

Gardner, W. J., Stowell, A., and Dutlinger, R. 1947. Resection of the greater superficial petrosal nerve in the treatment of unilateral headache. J. Neurosurg. **4**:105-114.

Glaser, M. A. 1931. Treatment of trigeminal neuralgia with trichlorethylene. J.A.M.A. **96**:916-920.

Glaser, M. A. 1935. Tumors arising from sensory root of trigeminal nerve in posterior fossa; perineural fibroblastoma. Ann. Surg. **101**:146-155.

Glees, P., and Bailey, R. A. 1951. Schichtung und Fasergrösse des Tractus spinothalamicus des Menschen. Mschr. Psychiat. Neurol. **122**:129-141.

Glick, D. H. 1962. Locating referred pulpal pains. Oral Surg. **15**:613-623.

Godtfredsen, E. 1947. Ophthalmo-neurological symptoms in malignant nasopharyngeal tumors. Proc. Roy. Soc. Med. **40**:131-135.

Harris, W. 1936. Ciliary (migrainous) neuralgia and its treatment. Brit. Med. J. **1**:457-460.

Harris, W. 1940. An analysis of 1,433 cases of paroxysmal trigeminal neuralgia (trigeminal-tic) and the end-results of gasserian alcohol injection. Brain **63**:209-224.

Hobbs, H. E. 1964. Headache. Trans. Ophthal. Soc. U. K. **84**:637-662.

Horton, B. T. 1941. Use of histamine in the treatment of specific types of headache. J.A.M.A. **116**:377-383.

Horton, B. T. 1956. Histaminic cephalgia: differential diagnosis and treatment. Proc. Staff Meet., Mayo Clin. **31**:325-333.

Horton, B. T., MacLean, A. R., and Craig, W. McK. 1939. A new syndrome of vascular headache: results of treatment with histamine: preliminary report. Proc. Staff Meet., Mayo Clin. **14**:257-260.

Ikonomoff, S. I. 1968. Nouvelle méthod de traitement de la migraine au moyen de médicaments anticholinésterasiques. (Observations cliniques.) Arch. Suiss. Neurol. Psychiat. **102**:299-312.

Jefferson, G. 1955. The trigeminal neurinomas with some remarks on malignant invasion of the gasserian ganglion. In Clinical neurosurgery, Congress of Neurological Surgeons, Proceedings, vol. 1. Baltimore, The Williams & Wilkins Co., pp. 11-45.

Kawamura, Y. 1968. Mandibular movement: normal anatomy and physiology and clinical dysfunction. In Schwartz, L., and Chayes, C. M.: Facial pain and mandibular movement. Philadelphia, W. B. Saunders Co., pp. 37-82.

Kerr, F. W. L. 1963a. The divisional organization of afferent fibres of the trigeminal nerve. Brain **86**:721-732.

Kerr, F. W. L. 1936b. The etiology of trigeminal neuralgia. Arch. Neurol. **8**:15-25.

Kerr, F. W. L., and Miller, R. H. 1966. The pathology of trigeminal neuralgia: electron microscopic study. Arch. Neurol. **15**:308-319.

Kerr, J. H., Corbett, J. L., Prys-Roberts, C., Smith, A. C., and Spalding, J. M. K. 1968. Involvement of the sympathetic system in tetanus: studies on 82 cases. Lancet **2**:236-241.

Kimmel, D. L. 1961. Innervation of spinal dura mater and dura mater of the posterior cranial fossa. Neurology **11**:800-809.

Kimura, S. J., and Thygeson, P. 1955. The cytology of external ocular disease. Amer. J. Ophthal. **39**:137-145.

Kraus, W. M. 1935. The cutaneous distribution of the trigeminal nerve. Ann. Surg. **101**:212-221.

Krayenbühl, H. 1936. Primary tumours of the root of the fifth cranial nerve: their distinction from tumours of the gasserian ganglion. Brain **59**:337-352.

Kunc, Z. 1960. La localisation des trajects de la douleur des nerfs IX, X et VII dans la moelle allongonée et la possibilité de leur tractotomie sélective. Acta Neurochir. **8**:327-334.

Kunkle, E. C. 1959. Acetylcholine in the mecha-

nisms of headache of the migraine type. Arch. Neurol. Psychiat. **81**:135-141.
Kuypers, H. G. J. M. 1958a. Some projections from the peri-central cortex to pons and lower brain stem in monkey and chimpanzee. J. Comp. Neurol. **110**:221-255.
Kuypers, H. G. J. M. 1958b. Corticobulbar connections to the pons and lower brain stem in man. Brain **81**:364-388.
Lewy, F. H., and Grant, F. C. 1938. Physiopathologic and pathoanatomic aspects of major trigeminal neuralgia. Arch. Neurol. Psychiat. **40**:1126-1134.
Lindsay, B. 1969. Trigeminal neuralgia: a new approach. Med. J. Austr. **1**:8-13.
McNaughton, F. 1938. The innervation of the intracranial blood vessels and dural sinuses. Res. Publ. Ass. Res. Nerv. Ment. Dis., Proc. **18**:178-200.
Mehler, W. R. 1963. Some observations on the connections of the mesencephalic root of the trigeminus. Anat. Rec. **145**:260.
Miller, H. 1968. Pain in the face. Brit. Med. J. **2**:577-580.
Nashold, B. S., Jr., Wilson, W. P., and Slaughter, D. G. 1969. Sensations evoked by stimulation in the midbrain of man. J. Neurosurg. **30**:14-24.
Pearson, A. A. 1949. The development and connections of the mesencephalic root of the trigeminal nerve in man. J. Comp. Neurol. **90**:1-46.
Penfield, W., and McNaughton, F. 1940. Dural headache and innervation of the dura mater. Arch. Neurol. Psychiat. **44**:43-75.
Reynolds, O. E., and Hutchins, H. C. 1948. Reduction of central hyperirritability following block anesthesia of peripheral nerve. Amer. J. Physiol. **152**:658-662.
Rhoton, A. L., Jr. 1968. Afferent connections of the facial nerve. J. Comp. Neurol. **133**:89-100.
Rhoton, A. L., Jr., O'Leary, J. L., and Ferguson, J. P. 1966. The trigeminal, facial, vagal, and glossopharyngeal nerves in the monkey: afferent connections. Arch. Neurol. **14**:530-540.
Richter, C. P., and Woodruff, B. G. 1942. Facial patterns of electrical skin resistance: their relation to sleep, external temperature, hair distribution, sensory dermatome and skin disease. Bull. Johns Hopk. Hosp. **70**:442-459.
Rosenbaum, H. E., and Seaman, W. B. 1955. Neurologic manifestations of nasopharyngeal tumors. Neurology **5**:863-874.
Rushton, J. C., and Olafson, R. A. 1965. Trigeminal neuralgia associated with multiple sclerosis: report of 35 cases. Arch. Neurol. **13**:383-386.
Russell, W. R. 1945. Transient disturbances following gunshot wounds of head. Brain **68**:79-97.
Sachs, E., Jr. 1968. The role of the nervus intermedius in facial neuralgia: report of four cases with observations on the pathways for taste, lacrimation, and pain in the face. J. Neurosurg. **28**:54-60.
Sanchez-Longo, L. P., and Schlezinger, N. S. 1955. Cephalic tetanus. Neurology **5**:381-389.
Schwartz, L., and Chayes, C. M. 1968. Facial pain and mandibular dysfunction. Philadelphia, W. B. Saunders Co.
Shalom, A. S. 1966. The diagnosis and treatment of the anterior ethmoid nerve syndrome. Geriatrics **21**:166-172.
Shanasy, F. 1949. Headache and facial pain. Oral Surg. **2**:752-759.
Sheehan, D., and Smyth, G. E. 1937. A study of the anatomy of vertebral thrombosis, with reports on two cases. Lancet **2**:614-618.
Sjöqvist, O. 1938. Studies on pain conduction in the trigeminal nerve. Acta Psychiat. Neurol., suppl. 17.
Sluder, G. 1927. Nasal neurology, headaches and eye disorders. St. Louis, The C. V. Mosby Co.
Smith, R. D., Marcarian, H. Q., and Niemer, W. T. 1967. Bilateral relationship of the trigeminal mesencephalic nuclei and mastication. J. Comp. Neurol. **131**:79-92.
Sperling, E., and Stender, A. 1955. "Tic douloureux" und Gesichtschmerz (therapeutische und pathogenetische Betrachtungen). Deutsch. Z. Nervenheilk. **173**:161-183.
Stopford, J. S. B. 1925. The function of the spinal nucleus of the trigeminal nerve. J. Anat. **59**:120-128.
Symonds, C. P. 1956. A particular variety of headache. Brain **79**:217-232.
Szentágothai, J. 1948. Anatomical consideration of monosynaptic reflex arcs. J. Physiol. **2**:445-454.
Taren, J. A. 1964. The positions of the cutaneous components of the facial, glossopharyngeal, and vagal nerves in the spinal tract of V. J. Comp. Neurol. **122**:389-397.
Taren, J. A., and Kahn, E. A. 1962. Anatomic pathways related to pain in face and neck. J. Neurosurg. **19**:116-122.
Teng, C. C. 1962. Fine structure of the human cornea: epithelium and stroma. Amer. J. Ophthal. **54**:969-1002.
Vail, H. H. 1932. Vidian neuralgia. Ann. Otol. **41**:837-856.
Walker, A. E. 1938. The primate thalamus. Chicago, University of Chicago Press.
Walker, A. E. 1939. The origin, course and terminations of the secondary pathways of the trigeminal nerve in primates. J. Comp. Neurol. **71**:59-89.
Walker, A. E. 1940. The spinothalamic tract in man. Arch. Neurol. Psychiat. **43**:284-298.
Wallenberg, A. 1896. Die secundäre Bahn des sensiblen Trigeminus. Anat. Anz. **12**:95-110.
Wallenberg, A. 1901. Anatomischer Befund in einem als "acute Bulbäraffection (Embolie der Art. cerebellar, post. inf. sinistr.?)" beschriebenen Falle. Arch. Psychiat. **34**:923-959.
Watts, F. B. 1951. Atypical facial neuralgia in hypothyroid state. Ann. Intern. Med. **35**:186-193.
Wegner, W. 1968. Nervus intermedius (Hunt's) syndrome. In Vinken, P. J., and Bruyn, G. W., editors: Handbook of clinical neurology, vol. 5. Amsterdam, North-Holland Publishing Company, pp. 337-344.

Weisengreen, H. H., and Winters, S. E. 1952. Pathways of referred pain with special reference to head and neck; a neuroanatomic study. Oral Surg. **5**:500-512.

White, J. C., and Sweet, W. H. 1955. Pain: its mechanisms and neurosurgical control. Springfield, Illinois, Charles C Thomas, Publisher.

Wolff, H. G. 1963. Headache and other head pain. New York, Oxford University Press.

Chapter 16

Localization of lesions involving the extraocular nerves

The movement of each eye is brought about by the combined action of its six muscles, the latter supplied by the oculomotor, trochlear, and abducens nerves. Conjugate movements of the eyes are controlled by supranuclear mechanisms. Consideration will be given first to the innervation of individual extraocular and intraocular muscles, and then to innervation of a further muscle, the levator palpebrae superioris.

INNERVATION OF THE OCULAR MUSCLES

Oculomotor, or third cranial, nerve

The nucleus of the third nerve is situated in the ventral periaqueductal gray at the level of the superior colliculus (Figs. 10-5 and 10-16). From this nucleus the nerve fibers sweep ventrally through the medial longitudinal fasciculus, red nucleus, and substantia nigra and emerge on the medial aspect of the basis pedunculi. The nerve then extends forward through the interpeduncular cistern in close relation to the posterior communicating artery. Proceeding through a smaller triangular dural space lateral to the posterior clinoid process, the nerve courses in the lateral wall of the cavernous sinus (Fig. 16-1); upon emerging, it lies in close relation to the upper part of the lateral wall of the sphenoid sinus and the upper part of the wall of the ethmoid sinus. It then passes through the superior orbital fissure to enter the orbit. Here it divides into two branches—the upper extends to the levator palpebrae superioris and superior rectus, and the lower passes to the inferior oblique muscle and the medial and inferior recti.

Most of the fibers coursing peripherally in the third nerve arise in the ipsilateral oculomotor nucleus, and it is likely that fibers originating from nuclei straddling the midline course in both third nerves (Bender and Weinstein, 1943). Fibers from proprioceptor end-organs in the extraocular muscles (muscle spindles) course centrally not only in the third nerve, but also in the fourth and in the sixth. Many of the fibers leave these nerves to enter the ophthalamic division of the fifth nerve, either at the level of the cavernous sinus or at more peripheral or even more central levels; however, the majority apparently pursue their entire course centrally in the third, fourth, and sixth nerves (Whitteridge, 1960). Fibers running in the third nerve have been described as skirting the lateral aspect of the third nucleus and as sending collaterals to this nucleus. The cell bodies of all these proprioceptor fibers are situated in the mesencephalic nucleus of the fifth nerve (Crosby, Humphrey, and Lauer, 1962; Warwick, 1964). The functional significance of these fibers is yet to be determined. No substantial evidence exists that they provide information, at the level of consciousness, concerning position of the eyes relative to the head (Merton, 1964). On the efferent side, gamma discharges appear to reach intrafusal fibers, altering sensitivity of the spindles and thus signaling small ocular movements when a target is being fixated (Whitteridge, 1960).

Subdivisions of the oculomotor nucleus. The oculomotor nucleus is divisible into three components: the lateral (or principal) nuclear group, the Edinger-Westphal

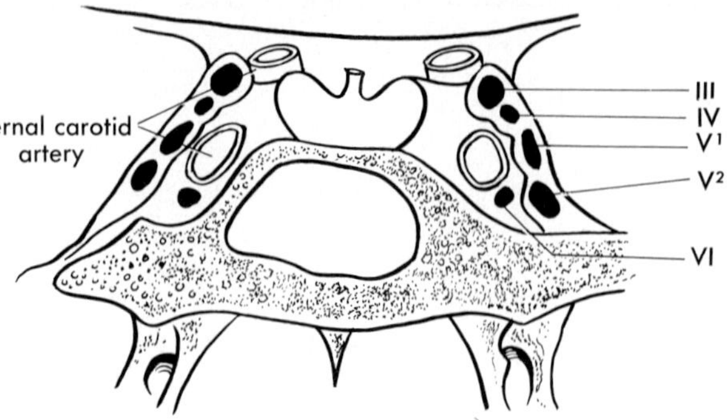

Fig. 16-1. Location of nerves III, IV, and VI, and of the ophthalmic *(V^1)* and maxillary *(V^2)* divisions of the trigeminus, in the lateral wall of the cavernous sinus. (The region of the cavernous sinus is left blank.) Shown here is the midlevel of the cavernous sinus. Somewhat farther forward the maxillary division leaves the region of the sinus. Beneath the pituitary is the sphenoid bone and sphenoid sinus.

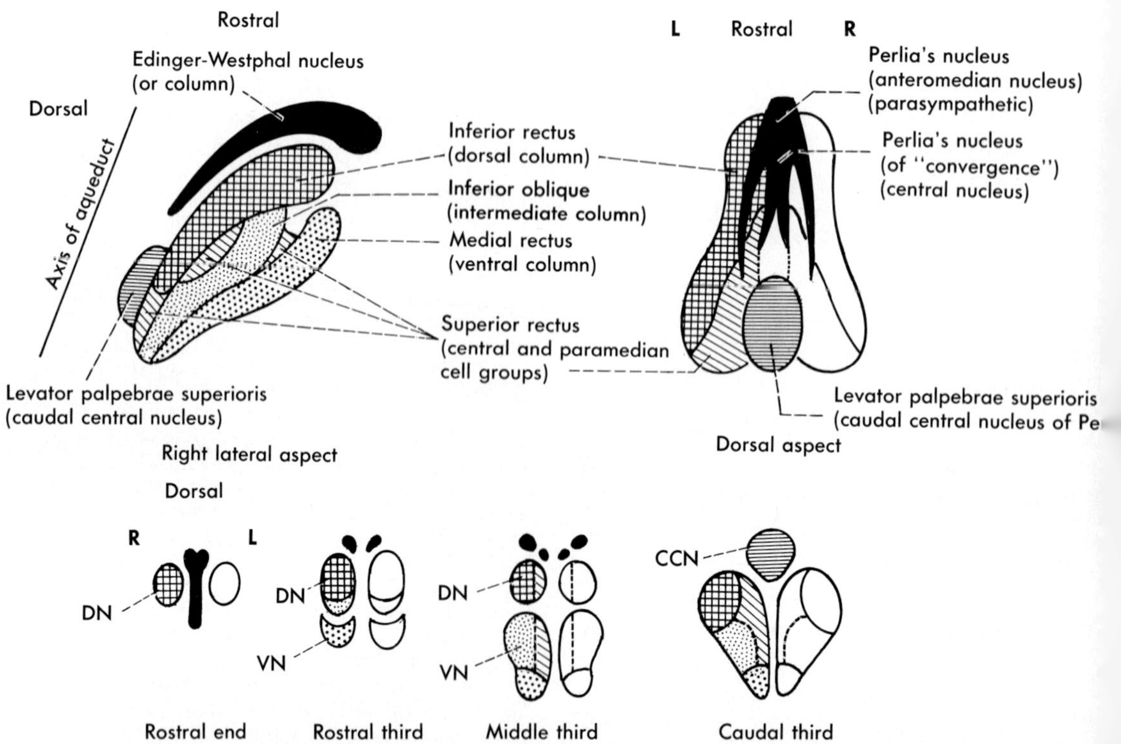

Fig. 16-2. The oculomotor-nucleus complex. *CCN*, caudal central nucleus (of Perlia); *DN*, dorsal nucleus or column; *VN*, ventral nucleus or column. (Redrawn from Warwick, 1964.)

nucleus, and the nuclei of Perlia (Fig. 16-2).

The *lateral nuclear* group is the largest of the three. Nuclear representation in terms of muscles, according to Warwick (1953, 1964), is indicated in Fig. 16-2. The nuclei are arranged in columns oriented dorsoventrally. Corresponding muscle representation is as follows: *inferior rectus* muscle, most dorsally; *inferior oblique,* in intermediate position; *medial rectus,* most ventrally. The *superior rectus*

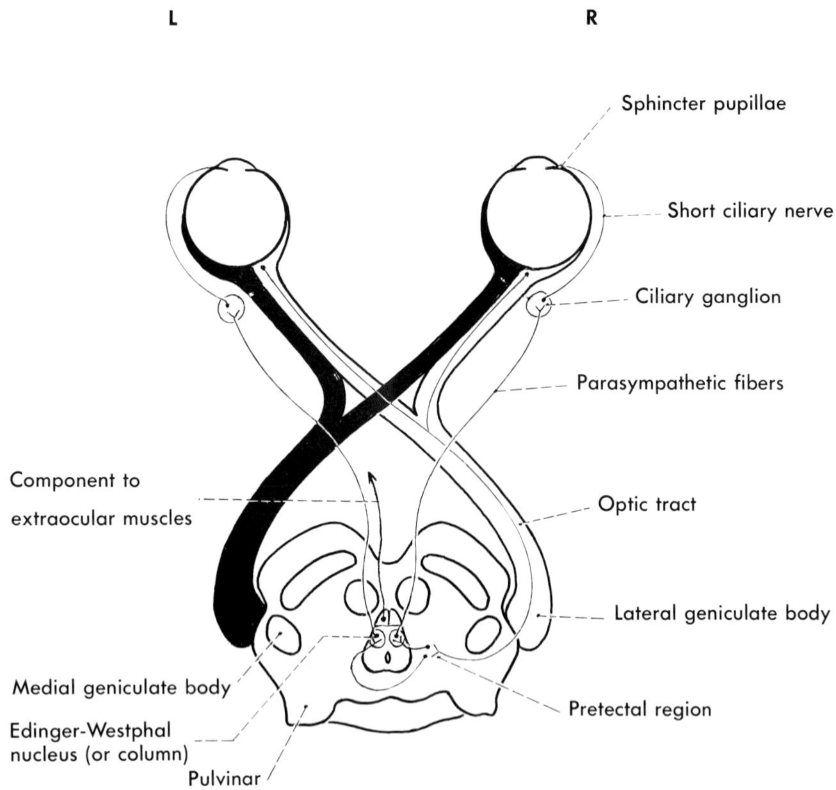

Fig. 16-3. The pupillary arc responsive to light.

receives its innervation from central and paramedian cell groups.

The *Edinger-Westphal nucleus,* a parasympathetic nucleus, consists of two columns of cells, one on either side of the midline. These cell columns lie dorsomedial to the rostral half of the lateral nuclear group.

The *nuclei of Perlia* consist conventionally of three cell aggregates. (1) The anteromedian nucleus is situated most rostrally and bridges the gap between the Edinger-Westphal cell columns of the two sides. Functionally, it is a parasympathetic nucleus. (2) The central nucleus, erroneously called the "nucleus of convergence," is poorly developed and can be identified in only 15 percent of brains (in monkeys). (3) The *caudal central nucleus,* straddling the midline inferiorly, provides the nerve supply for the levator palpebrae superioris.

Parasympathetic ocular innervation, pupillary responses, accommodation, convergence. Preganglionic fibers originating in the Edinger-Westphal–Perlia (anteromedian nucleus) complex course in the third nerve, gain the branch passing to the inferior rectus and inferior oblique muscles, then leave the branch as the so-called parasympathetic root to terminate in the ciliary ganglion; here arise postganglionic fibers that pursue their course in the short ciliary nerves, penetrate the back of the eyeball, run forward, and supply the constrictor muscle of the iris (sphincter pupillae) (Figs. 14-1 and 16-3). The fibers are concerned in pupillary constriction (miosis).

Other parasympathetic fibers running in the third nerve are concerned in accommodation of the eye for near vision. These fibers also originate in the Edinger-Westphal–Perlia nucleus complex. The preganglionic and postganglionic fibers take the same route as just indicated, but on reaching the anterior part of the globe the fibers turn off and supply the ciliary muscle. Some 90 percent of parasympathetic fibers bound for the eye terminate in this muscle. To put this in another way, the ciliary muscle is supplied by 30 times more neurons than the iris musculature (Warwick, 1964).

Under conditions in which the eyes are in their primary position, and when the optical system is so arranged that distant, or parallel, light rays from a fixated distant object come to a focus on the retinae at the maculae, the eyes are said to be accommodated for far vision. Under these conditions the lens is in a flattened state owing to the pull of the fibers of the suspensory ligament—the zonule of Zinn—which attaches the capsule of the lens to the ciliary body. During accommodation for far vision the circular fibers of the ciliary muscles (supplied by parasympathetic fibers) relax, and the radial fibers (supplied by the sympathetic) contract; this increases the tension on the fibers of the suspensory ligament and so aids in further flattening of the lens. Concomitantly the radial muscle of the iris (innervated by sympathetic fibers), undergoes contraction. As a result of the contraction the pupil enlarges; also, during accommodation from near to far vision the eyes diverge.

During accommodation of the eye for near vision the circular fibers of the ciliary muscle contract through the mediation of parasympathetic fibers. Contraction of these fibers pulls the ciliary processes forward and loosens the tension of the fibers of the suspensory ligament of the lens capsule, permitting the lens to bulge and to assume a more convex shape; accommodation for near vision is thus achieved. During this adjustment the circular muscle of the iris (the sphincter pupillae), innervated by parasympathetic fibers, undergoes contraction; decrease in pupillary size occurs. Moreover, during accommodation for near vision the eyes converge. (Morgan, Olmsted, and Watrous, 1940.)

Sighting of an object appears to be the stimulus for accommodation, with convergence or divergence and pupillary constriction or dilatation occurring simultaneously. Afferent fibers subserving accommodation pass by way of the optic pathway to the striate (calcarine) cortex, with a relay to the peristriate cortex (areas 19 and 22). From here, the fibers descend directly to the midbrain in a corticotegmental pathway. "Relay" sets of fibers reach the Edinger-Westphal–Perlia (anteromedian nucleus) complex. Electrical stimulation of the anteromedian nucleus (in the monkey) has resulted in prompt bulging of the lens—the result of contraction of circular fibers of the ciliary muscle—bringing about accommodation for near vision (Bender and Weinstein, 1943; Chin and others, 1968; Jampel and Mindel, 1967).

Warwick (1964) emphasizes that accommodation in man is under voluntary control—"Accurate regard without accurate focusing is of little value"—and he assumes that accommodation is, in some measure, under the control of the frontal eye field. Participation of cervical sympathetic fibers in the response is assumed from the frequency with which disturbances in the reaction of accommodation occur following cervical sympathectomy. Not only accommodation but also ocular convergence and pupillary constriction (the entire "near-response") has been obtained in the monkey by electrically stimulating cortical peristriate areas 19 and 22. A bilateral accommodation response was obtained by unilateral stimulation, and it was always accompanied by a bilateral convergence response. (Jampel, 1959.) Relevance of these observations to the anatomical situation in man still needs to be ascertained.

Trochlear, or fourth cranial, nerve

The nucleus of the fourth nerve is situated along the dorsal border of the medial longitudinal fasciculus at inferior colliculus levels (Fig. 10-14), overlapping slightly with the nucleus of the third nerve. Its fibers take a course dorsolaterally round the edge of the periaqueductal gray and reach the level of the caudal end of the inferior colliculus. Here all the fibers cross the midline (through the rostral part of the anterior medullary velum) and emerge on the dorsal aspect of the midbrain just below the lower border of the inferior colliculus (Figs. 10-2, 10-6, and 10-13). The nerve passes ventrally round the lateral aspect of the midbrain, courses between midbrain and temporal lobe, runs along the undersurface of the tentorium cerebelli (to which it is adhered through means of a membranous enclosure), passes across the free border of the tentorium cerebelli immediately lateral to the third nerve, and takes a position in the lateral wall of the cavernous sinus just below the third nerve, where it is enclosed by layers of dura (Fig. 16-1). From here it passes forward through the superior orbital fissure to gain the orbit and proceeds to the superior oblique muscle, which it innervates.

Abducens, or sixth cranial, nerve

The nucleus of the sixth nerve lies in the floor of the fourth ventricle near the midline, at a caudal pontile level (Figs. 10-3, 10-5, and 10-11). All its fibers pursue a strictly ipsilateral course. They extend ventrally and emerge from the brainstem near the midline at the junction of pons and medulla oblongata. The nerve then passes forward, then laterally, and enters Dorello's canal. This canal is in close relation to the posterior wall of the sphenoid sinus and is bounded by the posterior clinoid process, the apex of the petrous bone, and the petroclinoid ligament. Once through the canal the nerve penetrates the dura, then courses through the lateral wall of the cavernous sinus. Extending farther forward, it enters the superior orbital fissure and then traverses the orbit to terminate in the lateral rectus muscle.

FUNCTIONS OF THE EXTRAOCULAR MUSCLES

The extraocular muscles have the following functions:

1. The levator palpebrae elevates the upper eyelid.
2. The medial and lateral recti turn the eyeball around the vertical axis—toward the nose and temple, respectively.
3. The superior and inferior recti turn the eyeball around the transverse axis—upward and downward, respectively.
4. The superior and inferior oblique muscles turn the eyeball around the sagittal axis: the former rolls the upper part of the eyeball toward the nasal wall of the orbit, and the latter rolls the lower part of the eyeball toward the nasal wall of the orbit.

The medial and lateral rectus muscles perform simple movements, the medial rectus acting exclusively as an adductor and the lateral rectus exclusively as an abductor. The two are thus mutually antagonistic. The functions of the other extraocular muscles are more complex: the superior and inferior recti have the additional function of adducting, and the two oblique muscles the additional function of abducting, though some of the fibers of the inferior oblique have the additional function of adducting. The superior oblique has a depressing action, the inferior oblique an elevating action. The foregoing statements that the eyeball moves around the transverse and sagittal axes are therefore not absolute.

All the extraocular muscles are engaged when the eyes focus on an object. The combinations of muscles used vary in accordance with the movement undertaken. In ocular convergence the medial rectus acts in unison with the other medial rectus, and in conjugate lateral deviation the medial rectus acts with the opposite lateral rectus.

INFRANUCLEAR AND NUCLEAR PALSIES

Highly varied clinical disturbances result from lesions involving nuclei III, IV, or VI, or their nerves. Isolated paralysis of the lateral rectus or of the superior oblique muscle can readily occur because each is separately innervated—by the sixth and fourth nerves, respectively. By contrast, isolated paralysis of individual muscles supplied by the third nerve is uncommon because a nuclear lesion must be very circumscribed to produce such an effect.

Manifestations of infranuclear and nuclear palsies

Third nerve. Total interruption of the third nerve is manifested by marked drooping of the upper eyelid (ptosis) (due to the unopposed action of the orbicularis oculi, supplied by the seventh nerve) and by fixation of the eyeball in a position in which the pupil is directed downward and laterally (divergent strabismus) (a position due to the unopposed action of the lateral rectus and the superior oblique). The pupil is somewhat dilated, nonresponsive to light, but responsive in accommodation. Variations are, however, numerous; for instance, the lens may be adjusted permanently for distant vision, with absence of a convergence pupillary reaction. A person with complete third nerve palsy turns his head away from the paralyzed side in an effort to compensate for the abnormal position of the eye.

In internal ophthalmoplegia, when complete, the pupil is maximally dilated, it reacts neither to light or in convergence, and the accommodation reaction is totally absent. Again, variations occur; any one of these components may be missing. Lesions at various levels of the third nerve or its nucleus or the ciliary ganglion may be responsible, as brought out in the subsequent text.

Rapid paralysis of all the muscles supplied by the third nerve is almost certainly due to a lesion involving the nerve in its peripheral course. On the other hand, rapid paralysis of a single extraocular muscle supplied by the third nerve is most likely due to destruction of a part of the third nerve nucleus by an infarct. Progressive paralysis of extraocular muscles (without intraocular muscle palsy) may result from a peripheral third nerve lesion (for example, in involvement of the nerve by chromophobe adenoma [François and Neetens, 1968]), but it is usually due to a nuclear lesion (Mauthner's rule). In regard to intraocular muscle paralysis, it is usually due to a lesion in the peripheral part of the nerve, but not always; paralysis of intraocular muscles will occur if the superior part of the nerve (in which the parasympathetic fibers course [Goldstein and Cogan, 1960]), but not if the lesion interrupts solely the axial part of the nerve. Whether extraocular or intraocular muscle palsy is most likely to occur in a lesion of this or that part of oculomotor nerve complex depends on so many factors that generalizations have little value.

Fourth nerve. When the head of a patient with fourth nerve palsy is in the upright position, the pupil of the affected eye is lower than that of the other eye. On downward and lateral gaze the eye of the

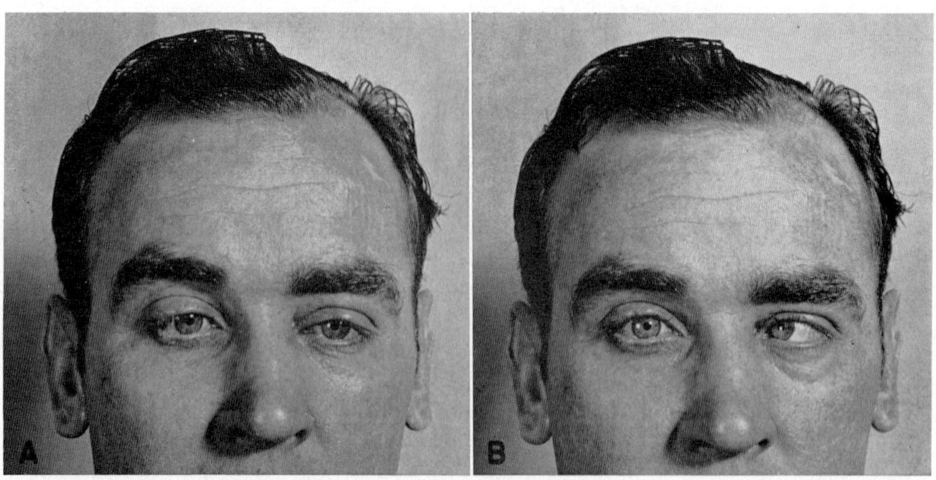

Fig. 16-4. Paralysis of the right lateral rectus due to head injury. In **A** the patient is looking straight ahead; in **B** he is attempting to look to the right. (From Bushnell General Hospital; Neg. 653.)

affected side undergoes rotation. Diplopia occurs when the patient turns his eyes in any direction except upward; this makes walking uncertain, particularly in descending stairs. To obviate this and to obtain binocular alignment, he tilts his head toward the opposite shoulder, suggesting torticollis. In palsy of the right superior oblique the false image is below and to the right of the true image (more peripheral than the true image); the greatest vertical separation of the images occurs when the eyes are turned downward and to the right.

Sixth nerve. In sixth nerve palsy the eyeball is rotated nasally (convergent strabismus) and is incapable of movement when the patient directs his gaze ipsilaterally (Fig. 16-4). Under such conditions the inferior oblique muscle may overact (Fig. 16-5). The diplopia may be obviated by turning the head toward the side of the lesion.

Third, fourth, and sixth nerves. When all three nerves are interrupted the eyeball is immobile and is directed straight ahead and the pupil is dilated and fixed (total ophthalmoplegia).

Oculomotor nuclear palsy is usually bilateral and is characterized by diplopia and strabismus. It is rarely total because the various components of the nucleus are spread over a relatively wide area of the midbrain. The involvement may be symmetrical or asymmetrical on the two sides. As may be gathered from the configuration of the third nucleus (Fig. 16-2), damage of its central inferior part first affects the levator palpebrae superioris, and damage of its central superior part affects the nuclei of Edinger-Westphal and Perlia. In an ascending lesion involving the third nu-

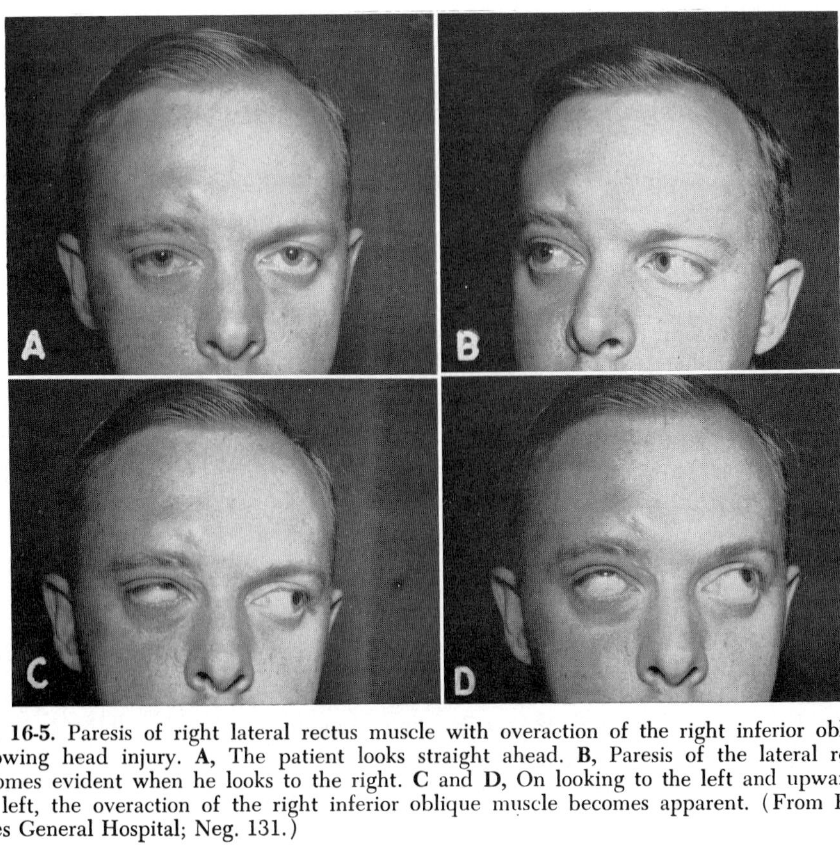

Fig. 16-5. Paresis of right lateral rectus muscle with overaction of the right inferior oblique following head injury. **A,** The patient looks straight ahead. **B,** Paresis of the lateral rectus becomes evident when he looks to the right. **C** and **D,** On looking to the left and upward to the left, the overaction of the right inferior oblique muscle becomes apparent. (From Percy Jones General Hospital; Neg. 131.)

cleus—for example, in expanding neoplasm—bilateral ptosis may be an initial sign. However, bilateral ptosis, when occurring abruptly, is usually the result of brainstem vascular disease. (Stevenson and Hoyt, 1963.) Generally speaking, the intraocular muscles tend to be spared in nuclear lesions. However, there are frequent exceptions.

Occasionally in lesions of the upper midbrain in the region of the posterior commissure, retraction of the eyelids rather than ptosis occurs. This may be an isolated phenomenon or it may occur in association with ophthalmoplegia. Commonly an eyelid is involved unilaterally. The retraction may give way to ptosis (Collier, 1927). Infarct in the region of the cerebral aqueduct may be responsible (Hatcher and Klintworth, 1966). The neural mechanism concerned is situated in the tegmentum at the level of the inferior colliculus; as shown in human patients, retraction of the eyelids occurs upon electrical stimulation in this region (6 mm. lateral to the aqueduct) (Nashold and Gills, 1967).

Since the orbicularis oculi muscles are innervated partly from the seventh nucleus and partly by fibers arising in the third nucleus—in a manner analogous to the partial innervation of the orbicularis oris by the twelfth nucleus (Fig. 14-5)—damage of the third nucleus of both sides may give rise to paresis of the orbiculares oculi (inability to close the eyes). The paresis is of localizing value because it is not produced by lesions of the third nerve trunk. Occasionally in midbrain lesions the pupils are small because of the involvement of descending sympathetic fibers. In bilateral sixth nerve palsy, the lesion usually involves the sixth nerve in a region either in or near the pons (Sachs, 1938).

Abnormal associated movements may occur following extraocular muscle palsy, usually after considerable time lapse. For example, although voluntary elevation of the eyelid of the affected side may be impossible, the eyelid rises when the patient looks downward or to the contralateral side (Bender and Alpert, 1937; Wartenberg, 1946). In cases in which no ptosis exists when the eye is in the primary position, the eyelid rises rather than falls when the patient looks downward. This may occur after basal skull fracture, basal meningitis, or brain tumor. It may also occur in internal carotid aneurysm, and may be noted in the latter before oculomotor nerve paralysis becomes evident. New growth of axons reaching the wrong muscles is doubtless responsible (Dailey and others, 1964).

Ocular nerve palsies in disease states

Infections, including syphilis. The granulomatous forms of meningitis, particularly tuberculous meningitis, are likely to affect nerves III, IV, and VI. Nerve VI may, however, be alone affected, sometimes unilaterally. Tuberculous meningitis is probably the most common cause.

Infection in various locations may result in cavernous sinus thrombosis, and in this manner lead to palsies of the third, fourth, and sixth nerves and of branches of the fifth nerve as well. Although usually the consequence of infection of the face and forehead, the thrombosis may be secondary to orbital abscess, peritonsillitis (Hara and Courville, 1942), tooth extraction (Haymaker, 1945), or otitis media.

Periostitis (with or without osteitis) in the region of the inferior orbital fissure may also give rise to oculomotor nerve palsy. The periosteal lesion may occur for no evident reason, or it may originate from a septic condition in the nose or the paranasal sinuses. Overexposure to cold can bring it on. The malady can occur at any age from puberty onward. Severe orbital pain marks the onset. Soon afterward proptosis of minor degree is evident, and tenderness is elicited on pressing on the eyeball. The nerve first affected is the sixth, and it may be the only nerve to suffer. Usually, however, there is subsequent involvement of the fourth nerve, the ophthalmic division of the fifth and then the maxillary division, and finally the third nerve, with total ophthalmoplegia and trigeminal anesthesia dolorosa resulting. Lasting and sometimes excruciating pain in the region of the orbit also characterizes this condition. (Collier, 1937.)

In chronic sphenoid sinusitis with spread of the infection to the base of the skull by contiguity, the third nerve is commonly involved, most frequently in the region in which it passes through the superior orbital fissure. The palsy is preceded by frontal aching pain on the corresponding side. The fourth nerve may also be affected as it enters the superior orbital fissure, as may the sixth nerve, chiefly in its course through Dorello's canal. The ophthalmic division of the fifth nerve may also suffer. When the infectious process is widespread, the clinical manifestations include headache, ipsilateral intraocular and extraocular palsy, deterioration of vision, proptosis, papilledema, and edema of the upper eyelid. Even "uncinate attacks" and hemiplegia may occur. (Dimsdale and Phillips, 1950; Feiling, 1924.)

Erosion of the tip of the petrous bone in subacute or chronic mastoiditis may, with spread to the infection locally to the arachnoid, lead to paralysis of the sixth nerve with or without involvement of the ophthalmic division of the fifth nerve; diplopia, pain behind the eye, and deep-seated headache are the main complaints *(Gradenigo's syndrome).*

Streptococcus pneumoniae infection is commonly the basis. Acute otitis media is an early complication, and aural discharge ensues. Aside from the sixth nerve palsy and the other disorders mentioned, the diagnosis rests on evidence of sepsis and lessened density of the petrous bone in x-ray films (Symonds, 1944; Yaskin and Kornblum, 1937). More common complications of chronic active petrositis are frank meningitis, extradural abscess, brain abscess (usually temporal lobe abscess), and labyrinthitis. Observed occasionally as complications are thrombosis of the petrosal and lateral venous sinuses, occlusion of the carotid artery, retropharyngeal abscess, and palsies from involvement, variously, of cranial nerves IX through XII. (Allam and Schuknecht, 1968.)

In syphilis involving the central nervous system, pupillary abnormalities occur relatively soon after the infection in about 25 percent of cases and ultimately in some 50 percent. In earlier stages of syphilis, isolated sixth nerve palsy is fairly frequent, and isolated third nerve palsy less so; pain in the periorbital region is commonly an early complaint, as are ptosis and diplopia (Green, Hackett, and Schlezinger, 1964; Shrader and Schlezinger, 1960). In basal syphilitic meningitis all three extraocular nerves may be affected, the third nerve most frequently.

In tabes dorsalis one extraocular muscle after another usually becomes involved. Transitory diplopia is common and is occasionally the initial ocular symptom. Ptosis is frequent, varies in degree, is slight, is usually more pronounced on one side than on the other, and is permanent. The ptosis is probably due to interruption of sympathetic fibers extending to the involuntary muscle of the upper lid. The patient counteracts the ptosis by elevating the eyebrows. Also frequent (in 70 percent of cases in early stages of the disease) is a reduced and ill-sustained pupillary reaction to light. Moreover, in tabes, miosis is the rule and mydriasis the exception. (Leimbach, 1895; Merritt and Moore, 1935.)

The *Argyll Robertson pupil* is observed in some 30 percent of cases of tabes dorsalis. Incidence in general paresis is lower. The pupillary disturbance tends to develop late in both conditions. The disturbance is usually bilateral; it has been found limited to one eye in as many as 26 percent of cases when eye examination was carried out with use of the slitlamp biomicroscope (Apter, 1954a). The pupil has the following characteristics: (1) it is small (miosis); (2) when miosis is moderate the pupil contracts slowly on exposure to light, and when pronounced (with pupillary diameter less than 2.5 mm.) it does not react at all to light (the same is true consensually); (3) the pupil contracts promptly in ocular convergence-accommodation and is supposedly hyperactive in this respect. The pupillary reactions to psychosensory stimuli are preserved. The two pupils are unequal in size. The iris is atrophic and the pupillary edge is irregular. The pupil dilates when mydriatics (belladonna, atropine, cocaine) are used, but the dilatation is slow and incomplete.

The lack of pupillary reaction to light has been attributed to interruption of fibers either in their course from the lateral geniculate body to the pretectal nuclei or in their passage from the pretectal nuclei to the Edinger-Westphal nuclei (Fig. 16-3); site of interruption is usually assumed to be prenuclear (Ingvar, 1928; Merritt and Moore, 1933). An experimentally induced lesion in this region does not, however, produce a small pupil. Sphincter spasm mediated by parasympathetic fibers and perpetuated by the continuous influence of transmitter substance (acetylcholine) in the region of the Edinger-Westphal nucleus has been postulated as the basis of the miosis (Lowenstein, 1956). Preservation of pupillary reaction to near vision presupposes a separate neural mechanism subserving this function. In the monkey, and presumably in man, a pathway subserving accommodation runs from peristriate areas 19 and 22 to the region of the tegmentum (the corticotegmental pathway), then to the Edinger-Westphal-Perlia complex (p. 267). This could be the neural mechanism spared, allowing a normal pupillary reaction to near vision. According to Lowenstein (1956), no clear evidence exists that the Argyll Robertson pupil results from a lesion involving the central sympathetic fibers for the iris musculature or the ciliary ganglion, the postsynaptic parasympathetic fibers, or the iris muscles themselves. An alternate hypothesis is that the Argyll Robertson pupil is due to a pathological process affecting the iris (Apter, 1954a, b). This is based partly on the finding of a colloidal gold curve in the aqueous humor identical with that found in the cerbrospinal fluid, and also on the presence of widespread involvement of nerves of the iris by an inflammatory exudate (Langworthy and Ortega, 1943).

The Argyll Robertson pupil in its classical form (as just described) is generally considered pathognomonic of syphilis. Some, but not all, of the features of the Argyll Robertson pupil are encountered in numerous cases of syphilis and in other conditions. For instance, large pupils nonreactive to light but responsive in convergence-accommodation may be observed in juvenile taboparesis and in midbrain damage—from tumor (particularly pineal tumor), encephalitis, multiple sclerosis, traumatic midbrain injury, third nerve injury, and herpes ophthalmicus. Typical Argyll Robertson pupils have, however, been observed in sarcoidosis involving the central nervous system (Suchenwirth, 1963).

Tonic pupil. The tonic pupil is the outcome of a benign, nonprogressive disorder, and is unilateral in 80 to 90 percent of cases. Women aged 20 to 40 years are most commonly affected. Both acute and chronic types of tonic pupil exist. The disorder may be heredofamilial, either as a dominant type of inheritance or as a double recessive with imperfect penetrance (Hedges, 1968).

The tonic pupil is characterized by an increase in size as compared with the other pupil. Other characteristics are: very slow reaction to light and to darkness, and, occasionally, impaired or delayed accommodation. The tonic pupil is never miotic. On ocular convergence the pupil contracts very slowly, though after a time the pupillary contraction may be greater than that on the sound side. Dazzle and photophobia on emerging into bright light are common complaints. In some cases a loss of accommodation occurs acutely and then slowly reverses. The pupil dilates to atropine and contracts briskly to methacholine chloride (2.5 percent) (the normal pupil and the Argyll Robertson pupil fail to react to the methacholine) (Scheie, 1940). Some 8 to 11 months may pass after onset of symptoms before the hypersensitivity to methacholine sets in (Hedges, 1968).

Tonic pupil is frequently found associated with loss of one or more deep reflexes (Holmes-Adie syndrome). The knee and ankle jerks are most commonly lost, though in about 50 percent of the cases tendon jerks in the upper limbs are also not elicitable. Total areflexia is occasionally noted, and in some instances the contraction phase of the reflex is normal, and the relaxation phase is slow and prolonged. Muscle tonus in the limbs appears in the normal range; deep sensibility may be slightly reduced, though it is usually unaltered; deformities in the spinal column are sometimes observed. Motor nerve conduction appears unaffected. (Lowenstein and Lowenfeld, 1965.)

The sudomotor system is impaired in some cases either in local or widespread areas (Hardin and Gay, 1965; Petajan and others, 1965).

Involvement of postsynaptic cholinergic fibers has been suggested as the basis of the pupillary disturbance (Petajan and others, 1965; Scheie, 1940); destruction of the ciliary ganglion was observed in one case (Ruttner, 1947). The refractoriness to methacholine occurring with the passage of time appears to be attributable to reinnervation of the iris musculature by regenerated postganglionic fibers, and it is supposed that a greater than normal population of regenerated fibers may account for the stronger near-reaction of the pupil (Hedges, 1968). The defect in deep reflexes has been considered due (1) to dysfunction of a central synaptic mechanism (Hardin and Gay, 1965; Levy, 1967), or (2) to loss of cells in spinal dorsal-root ganglia (Harriman and Garland, 1968).

Ectopia pupillae. This is a condition in which the pupil no longer occupies the center of the iris. Pupillary reflexes in this disorder are intact. The ectopia is occasionally noted in lesions of varied cause involving the midbrain (Wilson, 1906).

Defective pupillary response during accommodation. Selective loss of the pupillary reaction in accommodation occurs most commonly in diphtheria (p. 264). The disorder is also noted occasionally in other infectious states such as neurosyphilis, encephalitis lethargica, influenza, and measles. Faulty accommodation is frequently observed in patients receiving ganglionic blocking agents or belladonna in the treatment of parkinsonism, asthma, and hypertension. A blow on the eyeball is occasionally responsible. The same may be said for tumor of the midbrain (Cox, 1937). Precise location of the mechanism(s) involved appears unknown.

Trauma. Trauma may involve extraocular nerves in various ways: (1) contusion of extraocular muscles with consequent intramuscular hemorrhage (the levator palpebrae superioris is most vulnerable); (2) orbital fracture (the obliques suffer most commonly, but a number of other muscles may also be immobilized by intra-orbital hemorrhage); (3) fracture of the apex of the orbit in the region of the superior orbital fissure and optic foramen (immobility of the eye, with ptosis and with anesthesia in the realm of the ophthalmic division of the fifth nerve, and exophthalmos if hemorrhage has occurred into the orbit; also, loss of vision if the optic nerve is involved); (4) damage of the cavernous sinus by fracture (pulsating exophthalmos due to internal carotid–cavernous sinus fistula with extraocular palsy in which lateral rectus palsy may predominate); (5) fracture in the region of the clinoids or apex of the petrous bone (involving particularly the sixth nerve); and (6) compression of the third and/or the fourth nerve as a result of herniation of the hippocampal gyrus into the incisura tentorii. In basal skull fracture involving the petrous bone, the sixth is the extraocular nerve most frequently damaged. (Brain, 1942; Feiling, 1924; McKenzie, 1938; Terrien, 1922.) Internal ophthalmoplegia or faulty pupillary accommodation alone, as mentioned above, occasionally results from a blow to the eyeball; this disturbance may possibly be due to concussion involving the ciliary ganglion. Moreover, isolated third nerve paralysis may be of traumatic origin—for example, from a blow on the head with a baseball bat, fall in which the head hits the ground, or impact in an automobile accident. The superior rectus muscle is the most commonly and the most severely involved. (Green, Hackett, and

Schlezinger, 1964.) Isolated sixth nerve palsy also occurs under these conditions (Shrader and Schlezinger, 1960).

Epidural hemorrhage situated in the parietotemporal region, with expanding hematoma, displaces the temporal lobe medialward and downward, herniating it under the edge of the tentorium cerebelli. In about 50 percent of cases the third nerve of the ipsilateral side is severely compromised. Pupillary dilatation results, then fixation of the dilated pupil. Signs of pyramidal tract damage (occurring on the side contralateral to the lesion) are noted in a large percentage of cases. For reasons not clear, the contralateral pupil alone becomes dilated in 5 percent of cases and is considered to be related to shift of the hemisphere far across the midline. In such cases the pyramidal tract signs are ipsilateral to the site of the epidural hemorrhage. Other cranial nerves may also be affected. Commonly the patient, if conscious, points to the affected side of the head, indicating to the examiner the side on which the surgeon will find the hemorrhage.

In chronic subdural hematoma paresis of extraocular muscles occurs in about 12 percent of cases, the sixth nerve most frequently. Parasympathetic fibers of the third nerve are affected in some 18 percent of cases, as manifested by pupillary dilatation, usually ipsilaterally. The dilatation may be noted one day and not the next. Less frequently affected is the fifth nerve, then the fourth. (Jelsma, 1930.)

Neoplasms. Metastatic tumor of varied origin and carcinoma arising in the nasopharynx or sphenoid sinus, or parasellar meningioma, may compress the lateral wall of the cavernous sinus or encroach on the superior orbital fissure and involve one or more of the extraocular nerves. Sometimes all these nerves and the ophthalmic division of the fifth nerve as well are involved. Incidence of neoplasm in some series of oculomotor nerve palsy comes to about 10 percent (Goldstein and Cogan, 1960; Rucker, 1958). In tumor in the regions indicated, internal as well as external ophthalmoplegia commonly occurs. However, pupillary dilatation may in some cases be slight or absent when both the pericarotid sympathetic and the third nerve parasympathetic nerve fibers are affected (Terrien, 1922). Isolated third nerve or sixth nerve palsy is occasionally noted. In nasopharyngeal carcinoma, the ophthalmoplegia may be painless for a time, but when pain sets in it is often severe and intractable (Green, Hackett, and Schlezinger, 1964; Shrader and Schlezinger, 1960).

In neoplasms of the cerebellum and certain other neoplasms occupying the posterior cranial fossa, sixth nerve palsy is commonly encountered; but since it is related to the accompanying increase in intracranial pressure, the palsy has no localizing value. Third nerve palsy also occurs under these conditions, but it is rare.

Miscellaneous disorders involving the ocular nerves. *Diabetes mellitus* may involve the ocular nerves as the result of pathological changes in the nutrient vessels that course in the nerves. The main vessel is situated in the axial part of each of the nerves and, when occluded, infarction predominates in that part of the nerve (Goldstein and Cogan, 1960).

In diabetic ophthalmoplegia the third nerve is most commonly affected, then the sixth, then the fourth; only rarely is more than one of these nerves compromised. In third nerve involvement the intraocular muscles are affected in 10 to 40 percent of cases, but complete iridoplegia does not occur. Sparing of the intraocular muscles in most patients appears attributable to lack of involvement of the circumferential portion of the third nerve, in which the autonomic fibers run (Goldstein and Cogan, 1960). Diplopia frequently marks the onset. In some cases the diplopia occurs intermittently for a few days, then becomes constant. Associated with the diplopia is pain in the eye or ipsilateral frontotemporal headache. Third nerve palsy with headache and pain on that side occasionally occurs unilaterally, and the same is true for isolated sixth nerve palsy. (Friedman and others, 1967; Green, Hackett, and Schlezinger, 1964; Shrader and Schlezinger, 1960; Zorrilla and Kozak, 1967.)

The extraocular nerves may be affected in *nutritional deficiency*, particularly in thiamine deficiency. The sixth nerve suffers most frequently. In thiamine deficiency associated with chronic alcoholism the incidence of intraocular and extraocular nerve palsy is between 10 and 20 percent; horizontal nystagmus, usually poorly sustained, is the most common manifestation. In Wernicke's encephalopathy, palsy of the sixth nerve is common. The palsy is usually bilateral.

Myasthenia gravis is limited to the extraocular muscles in a small proportion of persons having this disease. Ptosis alone, either monocular or binocular, sometimes occurs, but much more commonly the ptosis is combined with weakness in ocular movement. Diplopia is a common initial symptom. Complete third nerve palsy never occurs. Occasionally the disorder is of congenital origin. (Schlezinger and Fairfax, 1959.)

Besides visual disturbances, ophthalmoplegia is a common manifestation in *migraine*. Recurrent attacks of typical migraine occur at first and are followed, in months or years, by more severe attacks in which periorbital pain and ocular palsy occur. The nerve most often affected is the third; in some 12 percent of cases, the sixth nerve suffers, and in rare instances the fourth nerve. In succeeding attacks the palsy usually involves the same eye. The palsy appears as the headache is subsiding. Internal ophthalmoplegia may accompany the external ocular palsy; the pupil may be dilated and reactive or dilated and fixed. The ophthalmoplegia may last several days to a month or more. In the initial attacks the ophthalmoplegia resolves completely, but subsequently (after a period of years) it may, in occasional instances, become permanent. Pressure exerted on the third nerve or other nerve as a consequence of dilatation and edema of the wall of the internal carotid artery at the level of the cavernous sinus is considered the basis of the ophthalmoplegia. (Friedman, Harter, and Merritt, 1961; Pearce, 1968.)

Dysglobulinemia is occasionally responsible for recurrent cranial nerve palsies. The third and seventh nerves tend to be affected the most often, and the fifth nerve and the optic nerve as well in some instances. Now and then the palsies occur in association with migrainous or other kind of headache. Those affected are usually between 30 and 40 years of age, the course of the disease is long; intervals between attacks are irregular, and the attacks brief. In some cases the protein disorder assumes the form of cryoglobulinemia. Varied hypotheses as to the basis of the palsies have been proposed. (Kreindler and Macovei-Patrichi, 1968.)

In *multiple sclerosis* the third nerve is affected in about 65 percent of cases, with pupillary changes more frequent than palsy of extraocular muscles. Sixth nerve palsy occurs in some 20 percent of cases. Ataxic movements of the eyes on lateral or vertical gaze are also fairly common (Carter, Sciarra, and Merritt, 1950). Diplopia is sometimes the initial symptom in multiple sclerosis; rapid loss of central vision is, however, more frequently the presenting symptom. Both together occur initially in 10 to 30 percent of cases (Leibowitz and Alter, 1968).

Aneurysm of the internal carotid and neighboring arteries commonly affects the extraocular nerves (Chapter 27), as does aneurysm of the basilar artery, though less frequently (Chapter 18). Ophthalmoplegia, external or internal, is also met with as a manifestation of vertebral-basilar arterial disease, but the incidence is extremely low. Thrombosis and intermittent insufficiency are the diagnoses usually made. The sixth nerve may be affected, usually unilaterally. Either diplopia is complained of or frank palsy is evident. In occasional instances diplopia is the presenting symptom. Even complete ophthalmoplegia, unilateral or bilateral, may occur. (Harel, Lavy, and Schwartz, 1967.)

Bilateral ptosis and slight third, fourth, and sixth nerve palsy together with other disturbances (generalized weakness, bilateral facial, palatal, lingual, and neck weakness) are characteristic signs of *botulism.* A hemoagglutination factor is involved. Thrombi are found in many vessels, systemically and in the brain, and nerve cells in some regions show minor loss of Nissl substance. (Tyler, 1968.)

Diphtheria, through its exotoxin, commonly involves nerves III, IV, and VI, in addition to other cranial nerves, particularly IX and X. Palsies appear in 2 to 4 weeks after the throat infection. Weakness or loss of visual accommodation (from involvement of the ciliary ganglion) is particularly frequent. There may also be palsy of extraocular muscles, most commonly the lateral rectus. Ptosis may also occur. (Cohen and Flora, 1962.)

In certain *infectious or presumably infectious states,* nerves III, IV, and VI are also apt to be involved. Acute internal and external ophthalmoplegia has been noted in cases of suspected viral origin, and severe ophthalmoplegia has also been encountered in *mumps infection* (Gibberd and Kelly, 1964). In generalized radiculoneuritis of unknown cause (the *Landry-Guillain-Barré syndrome),* lateral rectus palsy and ptosis are fairly common, and medial rectus palsy, total ophthalmoplegia, and paralysis of accommodation-convergence less common (Haymaker and Kernohan, 1949; Matsuyama and Haymaker, 1967). *Benign palsy of the sixth nerve* sometimes occurs in children. The disorder is painless, and develops in some 7 to 21 days after a nonspecific febrile or upper respiratory illness. The disorder may occur without warning. Improvement usually sets in within 3 to 6 weeks. The illness is without residua. Both otitis media and a viral systemic disease have been considered as instrumental. (Knox, Clark, and Schuster, 1967.)

PROGRESSIVE EXTERNAL OPHTHALMOPLEGIA

Progressive external ophthalmoplegia together with ptosis may represent an isolated phenomenon; or it may occur in conjunction with generalized myopathy or in association with disturbances in other systems. The ophthalmoplegia has its onset in persons of almost any age up to 60 years. Evolution of the disorder is slow. No sex preference is shown. Some cases are of a familial or heredofamilial nature, with signs of the disorder evident from the time of infancy; in such cases, congenital facial diplegia (Moebius' syndrome) is a frequent accompaniment (Hurwitz, Maguire, and Fannin, 1968).

Earliest recognized (by von Graefe in 1868) was the form limited to the extraocular muscles. Onset of this form, as recognized today, is in childhood or in early adult life. The disorder is characterized by ptosis, usually bilateral, followed gradually by paresis of extraocular muscles, until all muscles moving the eye may be paralyzed. The muscle involvement is usually symmetrical on the two sides. Strabismus therefore does not occur, or is not apparent; nor, with occasional exceptions, is double vision complained of. This is attributable not only to the symmetry of muscle involvement on the two sides but also to occlusion of one eye by a ptotic lid or suppression of the image on one side. The intraocular muscles are occasionally affected, sometimes totally.

Dystrophic changes in extraocular muscle were observed by Kiloh and Nevin (1951) (in biopsy from the medial rectus muscle in one case), and they concluded that the dystrophy was the basis of the disorder. They referred to the condition as "ocular myopathy." Subsequent autopsy or biopsy studies have led to the same conclusion (Hurwitz, Maguire, and Fannin, 1968; Rosenberg and others, 1968). In such cases neither eserine nor neostigmine is of benefit, which distinguishes the disorder from myasthenia gravis, in which there may also be complete external ophthalmoplegia. Progressive dystrophy of the extraocular muscles has, on the one hand, been considered a variant of the dystrophic process (Beckett and Netsky, 1953) and, on the other, a specific type of progressive muscular dystrophy (Magora and Zauberman, 1969).

Degenerative changes have been observed in cranial nerve nuclei III, IV, and VI and have been considered secondary to the muscular dystrophic process. However, the degree of severity of the change in these nuclei leaves this interpretation in doubt (Adams, Denny-Brown, and Pearson, 1962). The question of whether progressive external ophthalmoplegia must necessarily represent a muscular dystrophy was recently reopened by Daroff and co-workers (1966). In the case they reported the extraocular muscles showed "changes suggestive of or which could be interpreted as due to a myopathic process." Histologically, neuron degenerative atrophy and neuron loss occurred in nuclei III, IV, and VI; moreover, coarse vacuolation was noted in these nuclei and in the medial longitudinal fasciculi and elsewhere in this general region, including the paramedian reticular formation of the midbrain and pons. Retinal degeneration and heart block occurred in this case and, as an exception to the rule in progressive external ophthalmoplegia, the cerebrospinal fluid protein was increased, and there were EEG abnormalities. Rosenberg and associates (1968) have found lesions in the brainstem but did not consider them significant.

Ocular muscle biopsy in other cases has revealed regressive muscle change, but whether it represented myopathic or neuropathic atrophy could not be decided (Drachman, 1968). Uncertainty as to the basis of the palsy thus continues to prevail.

Varied ocular palsies occur when the ophthalmoplegia is a component of a neurological syndrome, suggesting, by inference, that the ocular disorder might also be neurogenic. Difficulty both in opening and closing the lids may be noted. Unilateral pupillary fixation may occur. Optic atrophy is common. Proptosis due to laxity of the extraocular muscles may develop and be severe. The many conditions in which ocular disturbances of these kinds may be observed are indicated in Table 16-1.

Table 16-1. Syndromes featuring progressive external ophthalmoplegia (from Drachman, 1968)

Progressive external ophthalmoplegia (progressive nuclear ophthalmoplegia; ocular myopathy)
Oculopharyngeal dystrophy
Chronic progressive external ophthalmoplegia and muscular dystrophy
Muscular dystrophy (features of ocular myopathy, distal myopathy, and myotonic dystrophy)
Ocular myopathy associated with retinitis pigmentosa
Retinitis pigmentosa, external ophthalmoplegia, heart block
Retinitis pigmentosa, ophthalmoplegia, spastic quadriplegia
Abiotrophic ophthalmoplegia externa
Retinitis pigmentosa, acanthocytosis, heredodegenerative neuromuscular disease (Bassen-Kornzweig syndrome; a-beta-lipoproteinemia; acanthocytosis)
Spongiform encephalopathy with chronic progressive external ophthalmoplegia
Generalized disorder of nervous system, skeletal muscle, and heart, resembling Refsum's disease and Hurler's syndrome
Refsum's syndrome
Hereditary ataxia of Sanger Brown
Familial ataxia, neural amyotrophy, associated with progressive external ophthalmoplegia

MARCUS GUNN AND RELATED SYNKINESES

The Marcus Gunn, or "jaw-winking," phenomenon represents a congenital disorder in persons having unilateral ptosis. The eyelid of that side cannot be raised voluntarily but becomes elevated automatically when the subject opens his mouth or moves his mandible to the opposite side. Upward gaze is restricted in some subjects, particularly on the side of the ptosis. Rarely is the Marcus Gunn phenomenon bilateral. The synkinetic movement may be abolished by sectioning the nerve to the external pterygoid muscle (Grant, 1936). In occasional instances, lid position when looking straight ahead is normal, but from time to time the lid droops slightly. In such a case the lid of one eye would fall during ipsilateral ocular adduction or elevation (synkinetic levator inhibition), and the upper lids would retract, together or alternately, during various jaw movements (synkinetic levator excitation); tonus in the ptotic lid could be restored by voluntary effort. Electromyographic and other evidence suggests that the disorder is mediated by the actions of inhibitory interneurons of the midbrain (Hepler, Hoyt, and Loeffler, 1968).

The inverted Marcus Gunn phenomenon (Maṛin-Amat syndrome) consists in closure of the eyelids when the mandible is moved maximally and forcibly. It is usually observed in later stages of peripheral facial palsy. The disorder is considered to be an intrafacial associated movement in which the closure of the eye is contingent on movement of the lower facial muscles and not the muscles of the mandible (Wartenberg, 1948).

Certain reflex changes relate to the mandible. Normally on closing one eye briskly, no alteration occurs in the position of the mandible. However, in lesions affecting corticotrigeminal pathways above the level of the pons, such closure (with all possible strength against resistance) evokes a quick movement of the mandible to the other side (winking-jaw phenomenon). The lesion responsible for the disturbances is situated on the side on which the eyelid is closed. The phenomenon is consistently elicitable in amyotrophic lateral sclerosis when corticotrigeminal fibers are affected. It may also be observed during the first few weeks after hemorrhage into the internal capsule. (Ornsteen, 1935; Wartenberg, 1948.)

CONJUGATE OCULAR MOVEMENTS

Anatomical and functional considerations

Practically all conjugate ocular movements represent combinations of the movements produced by four separate neurological control systems. Each can be excited independently. These are the saccadic, smooth pursuit, vestibular, and vergence systems, concerned, respectively, with acquiring targets, tracking them if they move in the environment, compensating for movements of the head in the environment, and tracking in depth. Through the mediation of the mesencephalic and pontile reticular formations, each of these systems converges on the motor nuclei that innervate the extraocular muscles. All the systems depend on visual information derived from the retina, except for the vestibular system, which receives information as to movement of the head in space from the vestibular labyrinth. (Robinson, 1968.)

The saccadic system. This system is specialized in moving both eyes from one position to another very rapidly in acquiring a target. Saccades (ocular flicks or jerks) are produced during ocular fixation so as to keep the image of the target on the retinal fovea—for example, during reading or during examination of an object when the object and the observer are stationary. On the afferent side are impulses of retinal origin that act either through cortical and subcortical mechanisms in controlling and maintaining fixation (Holmes, 1936). A possible factor in bringing about finer adjustments in ocular fixation is gamma efferent discharge on intrafusal fibers of the extraocular muscles (Whitteridge, 1960).

The saccadic system is under volitional control. In man, conjugate horizontal ocular deviation can be produced by electrically stimulating cortical area 8 (also areas 6 and 9), situated in the region indicated in Fig. 16-5 (Foerster, 1936; Penfield and Rasmussen, 1950). In the monkey, saccadic movements indistinguishable from those occurring spontaneously have been evoked by stimulation of area 8. Size and direction of the saccade depend not so much on how the cortex is stimulated (above threshold) as on where, in area 8, it is stimulated. Stimulation of different subdivisions of the frontal eye fields produces saccades ranging from 2 to 60 degrees in amplitude, depending only on stimulus location (Robinson, 1968). These observations support the contention of many observers, as brought out by Holmes (1936), that the frontal eye fields are the cortical outlet for the voluntary saccadic system. The pathway concerned descends through the genu of the internal capsule to the brainstem reticular formation, where much of the oculomotor signal processing takes place and where the pulse of activity associated with saccades is generated. To date, there is no evidence based on experimental degeneration studies following cortical ablations in monkeys that supranuclear fibers proceed directly to cranial nerve nuclei III, IV, and VI.

A much wider region of the cortex has, however, been found responsive to electrical stimulation in the monkey (Feldman and Bender, 1965; Wagman, 1964), indicating participation of subcortical nuclei in oculomotor function. Further, from cortical stimulation and ablation studies it has been concluded that ocular function is represented widely over the cortex, that although conjugate ocular movements in the lateral direction are most easily elicited electrically from area 8, it is unquestioned that numerous other corticofugal pathways are utilized, and that they converge toward the brainstem tegmentum (Pasik and Pasik, 1964). In mapping ocular responses of deeper regions of the cerebrum (in monkeys), Bender and Schanzer (1964) noted that conjugate contralateral ocular deviation could be elicited from the thalamus, pretectal region, and upper midbrain, and that on stimulation at sites caudal to the upper midbrain the conjugate ocular movements were to the ipsilateral side. Decussation of the supranuclear oculomotor pathway at the level of the third and fourth nuclei was thus demonstrated. The most electrically responsive area was in the paramedian zone of the mesencephalic tegmentum. On electrical stimulation of various deeper areas in the human brain, conjugate gaze to the opposite side could readily be produced by stimulation in the region extending from the level of field H of Forel down to the tegmentum of the rostral midbrain (Nashold and Gills, 1967).

The smooth pursuit system. Tracking a target so that the image remains on the retinal fovea requires the action of another system, the smooth pursuit system. Extrafoveal retinal stimuli bring the system into activity, whereupon it operates automatically. Target velocity rather than target position is the appropriate stimulus. Usually the smooth pursuit system tracks only one object at a time as it moves in a stationary environment. For correction, the saccadic system comes into play.

The smooth pursuit system utilizes information extracted from the visual system by cortical areas 19 and 18. The pathway mediating this information appears to be the internal corticotectal system. This pathway extends forward along the medial edge of the visual radiation; it then follows the radiation into the internal capsule (the postlenticular part of its posterior limb) (Fig. 19-11), courses caudally through the pulvinar (without synapsing), and takes a position along the dorsolateral edge of the midbrain; most of the fibers then move farther dorsally and terminate in the superior colliculus (Crosby and Henderson, 1948). It is not at all clear whether these corticotectal fibers are actually concerned in smooth ocular pursuit, nor have fibers been traced from the superior colliculus to the reticular core or to the oculomotor nuclei. Apparently, the fibers concerned in smooth pursuit movement leave the internal corticotectal system at a point short of the superior colliculus and terminate in the mesencephalic tegmentum, from which a relay reaches nuclei III and IV. Some of these postulated fibers may belong to the occipitotegmental system identified by Mettler (1935). Part of this system extends into the pons, making connections with nucleus VI (Jampel, 1959).

In the foregoing discussion, the saccadic system was identified with the frontal eye fields, and the smooth pursuit system with fields in the occipital lobe. Inasmuch as conjugate ocular deviation can be elicited (in the monkey) by electrical stimulation in the frontal lobes in the absence of the occipital lobes, and vice versa, it has been suggested that the oculomotor mechanisms in the two lobes can operate independently (Pasik and Pasik, 1964). Bundles of association fibers connecting the two are, however, available for integrated activity. These bundles run forward from the striate area to the middle frontal gyrus, passing en route beneath the supramarginal and angular gyri.

The vestibular system. This system has the function of stabilizing the target image on the fovea during tracking. Through it the eyes move in the head when the head is in motion, such that gaze is not deflected from the object in central vision. Influence of the system can be illustrated by the disturbances that occur under abnormal conditions. Thus, on destruction of the labyrinth, on severance of one vestibular nerve, or on isolated degeneration of the vestibular nuclei from cerebrospinal meningitis, the object looked at seems to oscillate or jerk whenever the head is moved, and vision becomes jumbled when the subject is transported over rough terrain (Ford and Walsh, 1936; Holmes, 1936; Whitteridge, 1960). Moreover, on section of the vestibular nerves bilaterally, ocular fixation during head movements may be lost (Ford and Walsh, 1936). Further, in unilateral loss of vestibular function ocular stabilization becomes defective at much lower head velocities than in normal subjects (Atkin and Bender, 1968). These disturbances are usually only temporary, indicating that the vestibular system is not essential to ocular fixation. Neural mechanisms involved are indicated in Chapter 13.

The vergence system. This system is concerned in tracking in depth. It functions comparatively slowly and maintains the correct degree of convergence of the visual axes necessary to the retention of the target image on each fovea. The appropriate stimulus determining whether the eyes are to converge or diverge appears to be the difference between the retinal errors perceived by each eye. Moreover, the system has the function of actively maintaining fusion of the two retinal images by controlling vertical and torsional muscle balance. (Robinson, 1968.) Ocular convergence together with accommodation and pupillary constriction has been produced (in the monkey) by electrically stimulating cortical areas 19 and 22 (peristriate cortex). A corticotegmental pathway connects, by relay, with appropriate components of the third nucleus bilaterally, but predominantly ipsilaterally. Since convergence could be elicited as an isolated phenomenon, it follows that a separate pathway is concerned. (Jampel, 1959.) Whether all this applies to man is yet to be ascertained.

Clinical disturbances

Disturbances in eye centering. Eye centering is considered a patterned excitatory process leading to integrated contraction of the extraocular muscles concerned, not a function solely of the tonus inherent in these muscles (Bender, 1955). As shown by electrical stimulation, the cortical areas from which ocular centering is mediated are in intimate spatial relation with those concerned in ocular deviation, and the pathways utilized appear to be identical in their course from the cerebrum to the brainstem; however, at the brainstem level (paramedian zone of the tegmentum), the evidence suggests two sets of fibers, the smaller portion mediating deviational and the larger, centering movements (Bender, 1955). Under abnormal conditions the eyes may become centered in response to an excitatory state, or there may be paralysis of eye centering. No evidence exists that either results from interruption of the afferent side of the neural fixation mechanism.

Staring straight ahead or fixating the eyes on an object without accompanying ocular convergence, such as occurs in petit mal or grand mal, constitute apt examples of excitation of the eye-centering mechanism(s). Another is a form of oculogyric crisis in which spasms of fixation in forward gaze occur. So firmly is the ocular gaze anchored to a visual target in this condition that turning of the eyes to some other target can be brought about only if the fixation is abolished by cutting off all retinal impulses—by blinking or by covering the eyes with the hand. In such cases, apparently the mechanism for ocular fixation is intact but cannot readily be inhibited so as to allow the gaze to be transferred to another target. (Bender, 1955, 1962.)

Disturbances in ocular fixation in con-

jugate gaze away from the center (primary) position. A condition exists in which the most striking feature is considerable difficulty or an inability to keep the eyes fixed on an object outside their center position, even though all ocular movements are intact.

The disturbance is most common on deviation of the eyes to one side, as the cerebral lesions to which it is due are usually unilateral. It has, however, been observed in attempts to fixate objects in any direction in space. On request to look at an object—for example, to the side—under conditions in which the lesion is ipsilateral, the patient moves his eyes promptly and accurately but he cannot keep them directed on the object. Almost immediately his eyes return toward their center position, then are brought back by a series of movements that are obviously volitional. The same disturbance occurs when the eyes attempt to follow a moving object, and when the head is moved passively during an attempt on the part of the patient to maintain ocular fixation. When the cerebral lesion is bilateral, as in pseudobulbar palsy following meningoencephalitis, the patient is unable to move his eyes on command. Although it is difficult for him to fix his gaze on an object in the peripheral visual field, once he does so he may be able to control his gaze and follow a slowly moving object; however, during the excursion his eyes frequently revert to their primary position. Reading of one entire line is achieved only if the eyes wander aimlessly until all the words in the line are recognized. Whether the responsible lesion is unilateral or bilateral, labyrinthine stimulation with cold or warm water usually reveals full ocular excursion. Such a reaction distinguishes the condition from conjugate ocular paralysis of peripheral or nuclear origin, in which labyrinthine stimulation fails to excite extraocular muscle contraction.

The disturbance, in Holmes' view (1936), is due to interruption of impulses in the pathway extending from the region of the calcarine cortex to the midbrain (component of the internal corticotectal system).

Disturbances in conjugate horizontal gaze. In the presence of an irritative lesion above the midbrain level that involves the supranuclear system concerned in conjugate horizontal gaze—for example, in hemorrhage into the internal capsule—the patient is unable to turn his eyes away from the side of the lesion, and his head and eyes may deviate toward the side of the lesion. By contrast, in a destructive lesion involving the frontal eye field unilaterally, little if any conjugate ocular deviation exists, and the same is true for destruction of the frontal eye fields bilaterally (Holmes, 1936). Under either condition, however, the patient may be unable to move his eyes when requested to do so, despite all attempts. If he looks at an object and the object is slowly moved in any direction, his eyes will follow the object (involuntary smooth pursuit movement), and the movement may be of the normal full range. With rapid movement of the object, the eyes follow it only for a short distance, then return to their original position. Furthermore, on passive turning of the head the eyes will remain directed on the object. (Foerster, 1936; Holmes, 1936, 1938.)

A center for lateral gaze has long been considered to be situated in the dorsal pontile tegmentum. Evidence is strong that the abducens nucleus itself contains a mechanism for conjugate lateral gaze. In human cases lesions more or less limited to this nucleus have resulted in paralysis of conjugate gaze to the side of the lesion (Bennet and Saville, 1889; Garel, 1882; Wernicke, 1877). Destruction of the ventral part of the abducens nucleus in the monkey has had the same effect (Carpenter, McMasters, and Hanna, 1963). Thus, among the motor cranial nerves, the sixth is unique in that lesions of the nucleus and lesions of the nerve produce different phenomena. Fibers from the sixth nucleus proceed to the medial longitudinal fasciculus, more passing up in the contralateral part of the fasciculus than in the ipsilateral part. However, these abducensfugal fibers are few as compared with the number of fibers derived from the vestibular nuclei that course in this fasciculus (Carpenter, McMasters, and Hanna, 1963). Normally, in conjugate lateral gaze—for example, to the right—the lateral rectus turns the right eye to the right through the mediation of the sixth nucleus, and the medial rectus turns the left eye to the right through the mediation of a specific group of cells in the third nucleus—a group established electrophysiologically (though not anatomically) by Bender and Weinstein (1943) and by Warwick (1953).

Excitation of the pontile mechanism under discussion—for example, by hemorrhage into the pons—causes the eyes to move conjugately toward the contralateral side. In destructive lesions the patient cannot voluntarily turn his eyes toward the side of the lesion, and because of the weakness his eyes may turn to the contralateral side. This disturbance in looking toward the side of the lesion is considered to be due both to damage inflicted on motor cells of the sixth nucleus and to interruption of secondary vestibulbar fibers as they traverse the sixth nucleus and areas near it to reach (and ascend in) the contralateral medial longitudinal fasciculus. That the vestibular system comes into play in this respect is supported by the observation (in the monkey) that paresis of contralateral ocular adduction results from lesions involving portions of the lateral vestibular and probably other vestibular nuclei. (Carpenter, McMasters, and Hanna, 1963.) Destruction limited to the superior colliculi (in monkeys) does not induce disturbances in conjugate lateral gaze (Pasik and Pasik, 1964; Pasik, Pasik, and Bender, 1966 a, b).

Conjugate vertical ocular paralysis. In man, lesions made unilaterally in the mesencephalic tegmentum at the level of the posterior commissure (for the treatment of pain) commonly produced paralysis of upward gaze. Paralysis of downward gaze resulted from damage inflicted in the region of field H of Forel. (Nashold and Gills, 1967.) In a human case both upward and downward ocular movements were paralyzed by a small lesion of vascular origin that destroyed the interstitial nucleus of Cajal and Darkschewitsch's nucleus bilaterally as well as adjacent structures (Angelergues, de Ajuriaguerra, and Hécaen, 1957). A unilateral lesion near the aqueduct can also produce conjugate vertical ocular paralysis (Hatcher and Klintworth, 1966). How such a lesion can lead to paralysis of vertical ocular movement bilaterally remains a problem. Környey (1966) postulates the presence of crossed and uncrossed supranuclear pathways reaching the nuclei of Cajal and Darkschwitsch, destruction of both by a unilateral lesion accounting for the paralysis. He assumes the presence of a ventral decussation in the vicinity of the interstitial nucleus of Cajal. Whether a dorsal decussation (in the posterior commissure) may carry such fibers is not settled, since destruction of the commissure has not led to paralysis of vertical gaze in man (Angelergues, de Ajuriaguerra and Hécaen, 1957; Molnár, 1959), though it has in the monkey (Bender, 1965; Pasik and Pasik, 1964).

Conjugate ocular paralysis in the vertical plane together with pupillary areflexia to light and loss of convergence *(Parinaud's syndrome)* is probably attributable to damage of the pretectal area that may also involve the interstitial nucleus of Cajal and Darkschewitsch's nucleus. Patients with Parinaud's syndrome may be unable to turn their eyes upward, downward, or in either direction. Paralysis of upward gaze is frequently accompanied by paralysis of pupillary reaction to light, and paralysis of downward gaze by loss of convergence and accommodation. Conjugate vertical ocular paralysis may occur in encephalitis of various kinds and can result from pressure exerted on the lamina quadrigemina by pineal or other tumor, also in intrinsic tumor growing in the periaqueductal region. This form of conjugate paralysis occasionally occurs in association with the thalamic syndrome as a consequence of a lesion extending into the region of the subthalamus. Older persons with advanced atheroma commonly exhibit minor degrees of vertical ocular paralysis. (Cogan, 1956; Globus and Silbert, 1931; Holmes, 1921; Laignel-Lavastine and Bernal, 1929.) No evidence exists that damage limited to the colliculi gives rise to Parinaud's syndrome (Dereux, 1926).

Conjugate convergence or divergence ocular paralysis. Voluntary convergence of the eyes is probably mediated from the caudal part of the middle frontal gyrus bilaterally, and from other cortical areas as well. The oculomotor nucleus itself appears not to contain any special cell group or center for convergence (Warwick, 1964). However, responsive areas exist not far from the third nucleus. In human patients, convergence (together with downward deviation) of the eyes was noted upon electrical stimulation of the posterior thalamic region 13 mm. lateral to midsagittal plane of the third ventricle, and also (together with ipsilateral tilting of the head) upon stimulation of the midbrain ventral and lateral to the aqueduct at the level of the inferior colliculus (Nashold and Gills, 1967). It would follow that paralysis of convergence could be due to a lesion in this general region. A convergence mechanism appears not to be present in the pons, as in a lesion in this region convergence has been found preserved in the presence of paralysis of lateral ocular movements (Reese and Yaskin, 1940). Paralysis of convergence is especially apt to occur in encephalitis; in such circumstances the medial rectus muscles often act normally in the execution of conjugate lateral gaze (Spiller, 1919).

In paralysis of ocular divergence, distant objects appear double. The diplopia, present when the eyes are in the medial horizontal plane, does not increase when the test object is moved to either side. Weakness of the lateral rectus muscles is not at issue, as there is no evident impairment in their function. In a case of paralysis of ocular divergence, a small cavernous hemangioma was found occupying the region of the periaqueductal gray at the level of the superior colliculus, just caudal to the level of the posterior commissure (Bender and Savitsky, 1940).

Compulsive eye opening. Inability to maintain the eyes closed, together with an inability to keep the mouth open or to keep the tongue protruded, constitutes a triad observed in diffuse brain damage, as from vascular thrombosis involving a cerebral hemisphere. Within 10 to 30 seconds after the eyes are closed, they again open, and the same applies to the other movements. Sometimes the eye on the paretic side opens before the other. Even when instructed to keep his eyes closed, a patient can do so for only the period of time indicated. The disorder decreases in severity in time. Berlin (1955) reasons that keeping the eyes open in the waking state is part of the basic vigilance attitude, which the intact person can overcome on command, but to which the patient with widespread brain damage compulsively reverts.

Conjugate spasmodic ocular deviation (oculogyric crises). Characteristically in this disorder the eyes turn spasmodically upward for a few seconds to a few hours, but in some instances they turn downward or in the horizontal or the oblique plane. These "oculogyric crises" may come on at frequent intervals—for example, daily—or appear a few weeks apart. During a crisis the pupils may be dilated and fixed. Additional features in some cases are compulsive running and the occurrence of hallucinations. Although of most frequent occurrence in late stages of postencephalitic parkinsonism, spasmodic ocular deviation may develop as an isolated phenomenon or a manifestation of brain tumor or tabes dorsalis. (Jelliffe, 1929.)

Convergence nystagmus and retraction nystagmus. Both convergence nystagmus and retraction nystagmus are rare events, but, when occurring, they have localizing significance. Convergence nystagmus consists in an intermittent, quick, jerky (saccadic) movement of convergence in which the eyeballs rhythmically move toward each other and then slowly return to the midposition; the next movement then begins. Similarly, retraction nystagmus consists in intermittent, quick retraction of both eyeballs (from contraction of the rectus muscles), followed by slow return of the eyes to the original position. Both may occur independently, in succession, or in combination; in rare instances, convergence nystagmus is noted in one eye and retraction nystagmus in the other. Either may occur spontaneously or only on gaze to one side (the side showing weakness in gaze). One or the other or both forms of nystagmus may be observed in lesions involving the region of the more rostral part of the aqueduct, the tegmentum of the midbrain, and/or the posterior wall of the third ventricle (Segarra and Ojeman, 1961). Retraction nystagmus may be observed under conditions in which the tectum is compressed, as by pineal tumor, or by a lesion situated in the region of the cerebral aqueduct (Hatcher and Klintworth, 1966). The disorder can be induced, and persists, following tissue destruction in the region of the cerebral aqueduct for the relief of pain (Nashold and Gills, 1967).

Sylvian-aqueduct syndrome. Making up the sylvian-aqueduct syndrome are combinations of ocular signs: impaired vertical gaze, vertical nystagmus, convergence nystagmus, convergence spasm, retraction nystagmus, extraocular palsy, and poor pupillary contraction to light and in adjustment to close vision. Neoplasm in the region of the aqueduct or vicinity (including the diencephalon) may be responsible, as may infarction involving the periaqueductal gray matter (Hatcher and Klintworth, 1966).

Disturbances produced by lesions made in the upper midbrain in the amelioration of painful conditions were as follows: paralysis of upward gaze, retraction nystagmus, convergence nystagmus, vertical nystagmus, pathological lid retraction, diplopia, and changes in pupillary responses. In general, lesions located in the more rostral tegmentum tended to produce phasic movements of the eyes, those in more caudal tegmentum, tonic movements. (Nashold and Gills, 1967.)

Internuclear ophthalmoplegia. The term *internuclear ophthalmoplegia* refers to the disturbances in conjugate ocular movements that result from lesions of the medial longitudinal fasciculus (MLF) situated rostral to the level of the sixth nucleus. Two types are usually distinguished in accordance with the nature of the disturbances produced: *superior* and *inferior*. Both may be unilateral or bilateral. The superior type is more frequently bilateral than the inferior type. Nystagmus can be induced by caloric stimulation of the labyrinth in both types.

Superior internuclear ophthalmoplegia is characterized (1) by weakness or paralysis of ocular adduction on attempted lateral gaze, with preservation of convergence, and (2) by horizontal nystagmus, occurring either exclusively in the abducting eye or predominantly so. *Inferior internuclear ophthalmoplegia* is characterized by weakness of ocular abduction; the lateral rectus fails to contract on attempted conjugate lateral ocular deviation toward one or both sides. Nystagmus is occasionally an added feature. Difficulty may be encountered in distinguishing this form from palsy of the sixth nerve(s).

Experimental studies in monkeys in which lesions were made at various levels of the MLF make it likely that the superior and inferior types of internuclear ophthalmoplegia represent variations of essentially the same syndrome. In the *superior type*, produced by a lesion of the medial part of the MLF bilaterally, paresis of ocular adduction bilaterally was found to be the most outstanding feature; moreover, there was monocular horizontal nystagmus in the abducted eye on each side. The responsible lesion was considered to be located in the MLF near the sixth nucleus, interrupting ascending vestibular fibers running to the sixth nucleus and interrupting also the vestibular fibers coursing to specific parts of the third nucleus bilaterally. Where the lesion in the MLF is unilateral, the disturbance in adduction is in the eye of the corresponding side. In the *inferior type,* the weakness of ocular abduction was greater than for the superior type, resulting in a limitation by ocular abduction. The level of the responsible lesion was presumed to be much the same as for the superior type. The disturbance appeared to be due to interruption either of MLF vestibular fibers passing to the sixth nucleus or interruption of collaterals that might interconnect the sixth nucleus of the two sides. Lesions involving relatively large parts of the MLF at the level of the two sixth nuclei produced bilateral paresis (or restriction) both of adducting and abducting ocular movements. (Carpenter and McMasters, 1963; see also Bender and Weinstein, 1950.)

Diplopia occurs as a feature of the MLF syndrome, but is uncommon; blurred vision from the oscillopia that sometimes accompanies the nystagmus is even more uncommon. These disturbances are noted on horizontal gaze toward the side on which adduction weakness and monocular nystagmus are elicited. (Gordon and Bender, 1966.)

The lesion most commonly encountered in unilateral internuclear palsy is infarct, and in bilateral internuclear palsy, multiple sclerosis. Unilateral or bilateral internuclear palsy may also be observed in pontile glioma, syphilis, encephalitis of varied kind, alcoholism, or traumatic injury. (Cogan, Kubik, and Smith, 1950; Collier, 1927; Savitsky and Rangell, 1950; Spiller, 1924.)

REFERENCES

Adams, R. D., Denny-Brown, D., and Pearson, C. M. 1962. Diseases of muscle; a study in pathology, ed. 2. New York, Harper & Row, Publishers, pp. 360, 366.

Allam, A. F., and Schuknecht, H. F. 1968. Pathology of petrositis. Laryngoscope **78**:1813-1832.

Angelergues, R., de Ajuriaguerra, J., and Hécaen, H. 1957. Paralysie de la verticalité du regard d'origine vasculaire. Rev. Neurol. **96**:301-319.

Apter, J. T. 1954a. The significance of the unilateral Argyll Robertson pupil: a report of 13 cases. Amer. J. Ophthal. **38**:34-43.

Apter, J. T. 1954b. The significance of the unilateral Argyll Robertson pupil: a critical review of the theories of its pathogenesis. Amer. J. Ophthal. **38**:209-222.

Atkin, A., and Bender, M. B. 1968. Ocular stabilization during oscillatory head movements: vestibular system dysfunction and the relation between head and eye velocities. Arch. Neurol. **19**:559-566.

Beckett, R. S., and Netsky, M. G. 1953. Familial ocular myopathy and external ophthalmoplegia. A.M.A. Arch. Neurol. Psychiat. **69**:64-72.

Bender, M. B. 1955. The eye-centering system: a theoretical consideration. A.M.A. Arch. Neurol. Psychiat. **73**:685-699.

Bender, M. B. 1962. Neuroophthalmology. In Baker, A. B., editor: Clinical neurology, ed. 2, vol. 1. New York, Harper & Row, Publishers, pp. 275-349.

Bender, M. B. 1965. Anatomic and physiologic basis for vertical eye movement. 23d Internat. Congr. Physiol. Sci., Tokyo, abstr. 986.

Bender, M. B., and Alpert, S. 1937. Abnormal ocular and pupillary movements following oculomotor paralysis; report of a case. Arch. Ophthal. **18**:411-414.

Bender, M. B., and Savitsky, N. 1940. Paralysis of convergence. Arch. Ophthal. **23**:1046-1051.

Bender, M. B., and Shanzer, S. 1964. Oculomotor pathways defined by electrical stimulation and lesions in the brainstem of monkey. In Bender, M. B., editor: The oculomotor system. New York, Harper & Row, Publishers, pp. 81-140.

Bender, M. B., and Weinstein, E. A. 1943. Functional representation in the oculomotor and trochlear nuclei. Arch. Neurol. Psychiat. **49**:98-106.

Bender, M. B., and Weinstein, E. A. 1950. The syndrome of the median longitudinal fasciculus. Res. Publ. Ass. Res. Nerv. Ment. Dis., Proc. **28**:414-420.

Bennet, A. H., and Savill, T. 1889. A case of permanent conjugate deviation of the eyes and the head, the result of a lesion limited to the sixth nucleus. Brain **12**:102-116.

Berlin, L. 1955. Compulsive eye opening and associated phenomena. A.M.A. Arch. Neurol. Psychiat. **73**:597-601.

Brain, W. R. 1942. Discussion on rehabilitation after injuries to the central nervous system. Proc. Roy. Soc. Med. **35**:295-308.

Carpenter, M. B., and McMasters, R. E. 1963. Disturbances of conjugate horizontal eye movements in the monkey: physiological effects and anatomical degeneration resulting from lesions of the medial longitudinal fasciculus. Arch. Neurol. **8**:347-368.

Carpenter, M. B., McMasters, R. E., and Hanna, G. R. 1963. Disturbances of conjugate horizontal eye movements in the monkey: physiological effects and anatomical degeneration resulting from lesions of the abducens nucleus and nerve. Arch. Neurol. **8**:231-247.

Carter, S., Sciarra, D., and Merritt, H. H. 1950. The course of multiple sclerosis as determined by autopsy proven cases. Res. Publ. Ass. Res. Nerv. Ment. Dis., Proc. **28**:471-511.

Chin, N. B., Ishikawa, S., Lappin, H., Davidowitz, J., and Breinin, G. M. 1968. Accommodation induced by midbrain stimulation. Invest. Ophthal. **7**:386-396.

Cogan, D. G. 1956. Neurology of the ocular muscles, ed. 2. Springfield, Illinois, Charles C Thomas, Publisher.

Cogan, D. G., Kubic, C. S., and Smith, W. L. 1950. Unilateral internuclear ophthalmoplegia: report on 8 clinical cases with 1 postmortem study. Arch. Ophthal. **44**:783-796.

Cohen, M. M., and Flora, G. C. 1962. Cerebral intoxication. In Baker, A. B., editor: Clinical neurology, ed. 2, vol. 2. New York, Harper & Row, Publishers, pp. 980-1053.

Collier, J. 1927. Nuclear ophthalmoplegia, with special reference to retraction of lids and ptosis, and to lesions of the posterior commissure. Brain **50**:488-498.

Collier, J. 1937. Affections of the cranial nerves. In Price, F. W., editor: A textbook of the practice of medicine, ed. 5. London, Oxford University Press, p. 1498.

Cox, L. B. 1937. Tumours of the base of the brain: their relation to pathological sleep and other changes in the conscious state. Med. J. Austr. **1**:742-752.

Crosby, E. C., and Henderson, J. W. 1948. The mammalian midbrain and isthmus regions: fiber connections of the superior colliculus: pathways concerned in automatic eye movements. J. Comp. Neurol. **88**:53-91.

Crosby, E. C., Humphrey, T., and Lauer, E. W. 1962. Correlative anatomy of the nervous system. New York, The Macmillan Company.

Dailey, E. J., Holloway, J. A., Murto, R. E., and Schlezinger, N. S. 1964. Evaluation of ocular signs and symptoms in cerebral aneurysms. Arch. Ophthal. **71**:463-474.

Daroff, R. B., Solitare, G. B., Pincus, J. H., and Gilbert, G. H. 1966. Spongiform encephalopathy with chronic progressive external ophthalmoplegia: central ophthalmoplegia mimicking ocular myopathy. Neurology **16**:161-169.

Dereux, J. 1926. Paralysie verticale du regard (syndrome de Parinaud): contribution à l'étude de la localisation de la lésion. Thèse, Paris.

Dimsdale, H., and Phillips, D. G. 1950. Ocular palsies with nasal sinusitis. J. Neurol. Neurosurg. Psychiat. **13**:225-236.

Drachman, D. A. 1968. Ophthalmoplegia plus: the neurodegenerative disorders associated with progressive external ophthalmoplegia. Arch. Neurol. **18**:654-674.

Feiling, A. 1924. Ocular palsies. Brit. Med. J. **1**:223-226.

Feldman, M., and Bender, M. B. 1965. Neuro-ophthalmology: the oculomotor system. Progr. Neurol. Psychiat. **20**:270-285.

Foerster, O. 1936. Symptomatologie der Erkrankungen des Rückenmarks und seiner Wurzeln. In Bumke, O., and Foerster, O., editors: Handbuch der Neurologie **5**:1-400.

Ford, F. R., and Walsh, F. B. 1936. Clinical observations upon the importance of the vestibular reflexes in ocular movements: the effects of section of one or both vestibular nerves. Bull. Johns Hopk. Hosp. **58**:80-88.

François, J., and Neetens, A. 1968. Oculomotor paralyses and tumors of the pituitary gland. Confin. Neurol. **30**:239-252.

Friedman, A. P., Harter, D. H., and Merritt, H. H. 1961. Ophthalmoplegic migraine. Trans. Amer. Neurol. Ass. **86**:169-172.

Friedman, S. A., Feinberg, R., Podolak, E., and Bedell, R. H. S. 1967. Pupillary abnormalities in diabetic neuropathy: a preliminary study. Ann. Int. Med. **67**:977-983.

Garel, J. 1882. Nouveau fait de paralysie de la sixième paire avec déviation conjugée dans un cas d'hémiplégie alterné. Rev. Méd. **2**:593-599.

Gibberd, F. B., and Kelly, R. E. 1964. Acute internal and external ophthalmoplegia with polyradiculitis of probable virus aetiology. Brain **87**:657-664.

Globus, J. H., and Silbert, S. 1931. Pinealomas. Arch. Neurol. Psychiat. **25**:937-985.

Goldstein, J. E., and Cogan, D. G. 1960. Diabetic ophthalmoplegia with special reference to the pupil. Arch. Ophthal. **64**:592-600.

Gordon, R. M., and Bender, M. B. 1966. Visual phenomena in lesions of the median longitudinal fasciculus. Arch. Neurol. **15**:238-240.

Grant, F. C. 1936. The Marcus Gunn phenomenon: report of a case with suggestions as to relief. Arch. Neurol. Psychiat. **35**:487-500.

Green, W. R., Hackett, E. R., and Schlezinger, N. S. 1964. Neuro-ophthalmic evaluation of oculomotor nerve paralysis. Arch. Ophthal. **72**:154-157.

Hara, H. J., and Courville, C. B. 1942. Intracranial complications of tonsillar origin: with special reference to their incidence and pathogenesis. Arch. Otolaryng. **35**:530-571.

Hardin, W. B., and Gay, A. J. 1965. The phenomenon of benign areflexia: review of the Holmes-Adie syndrome, with case reports and a study of the Achilles reflex. Neurology **15**:613-621.

Harel, D., Lavy, S., and Schwartz, A. 1967. Ophthalmoplegia as a manifestation of basilar artery disease. Amer. J. Ophthal. **63**:519-523.

Harriman, D. G. F., and Garland, H. 1968. The pathology of Adie's syndrome. Brain **91**:401-418.

Hatcher, M. A., and Klintworth, G. K. 1966. The sylvian aqueduct syndrome: a clinicopathologic study. Arch. Neurol. **15**:215-222.

Haymaker, W. 1945. Fatal infections of the central nervous system and meninges after tooth extraction: with an analysis of twenty-eight cases. Amer. J. Orthodont. (Oral Surg. Sect.) **31**:117-188.

Haymaker, W., and Kernohan, J. W. 1949. The Landry-Guillain-Barré syndrome: a clinicopathologic report of fifty fatal cases and a critique of the literature. Medicine **28**:59-141.

Hedges, T. R. 1968. The tonic pupil: familial

incidence, recognition, and progression. Arch. Ophthal. **80**:21-25.

Hepler, R. S., Hoyt, W. F., and Loeffler, J. D. 1968. Paradoxical synkinetic levator inhibition and excitation: an electromyographic study of unilateral oculopalpebral and bilateral mandibulopalpebral (Marcus Gunn) synkineses in a 74-year-old man. Arch. Neurol. **18**:416-424.

Holmes, G. 1921. Palsies of the conjugate ocular movements. Brit. J. Ophthal. **5**:241-271.

Holmes, G. 1936. Looking and seeing. (Movements and fixation of the eyes.) Irish J. Med. Sci., ser. 6, no. 129, pp. 565-576.

Holmes, G. 1938. The cerebral integration of the ocular movements. Brit. Med. J. **2**:107-112.

Hurwitz, L. J., Maguire, C. J. F., and Fannin, T. 1968. Congenital ophthalmoplegia: a myopathic aetiology in two siblings. J. Neurol. Neurosurg. Psychiat. **31**:372-378.

Ingvar, S. 1928. On the pathogenesis of the Argyll Robertson phenomenon. Bull. Johns Hopk. Hosp. **43**:363-396.

Jampel, R. S. 1959. Representation of the near-response on the cerebral cortex of the macaque. Amer. J. Ophthal. **48**:573-582.

Jampel, R. S., and Mindel, J. 1967. The nucleus for accommodation in the midbrain of the macaque. Invest. Ophthal. **6**:40-50.

Jelliffe, S. E. 1929. Oculogyric crises as compulsion phenomena in postencephalitis: their occurrence, phenomenology and meaning. J. Nerv. Ment. Dis. **69**:59-68.

Jelsma, F. 1930. Chronic subdural hematoma: summary and analysis of forty-two cases collected from the literature, with report of two additional cases. Arch. Surg. **21**:128-144.

Kiloh, L. G., and Nevin, S. 1951. Progressive dystrophy of the external ocular muscles (ocular myopathy). Brain **74**:115-143.

Knox, D. L., Clark, D. L., and Schuster, F. B. 1967. Benign VI nerve palsies in children. Pediatrics **40**:560-564.

Környey, S. 1966. Klinische Erfahrungen bei Hirnstammprozessen. Acta 25th Meeting on Neuropsychiatry and EEG, Budapest, pp. 41-51.

Kreindler, A., and Macovei-Patrichi, M. 1968. Recurrent cranial nerve palsies of dysglobulinaemic origin. J. Neurol. Sci. **6**:117-123.

Laignel-Lavastine, M., and Bernal, P. 1929. Encéphalite aiguë avec syndrome de Parinaud précoce compliqué et transitoire. Rev. Neurol. **1**:479-480.

Langworthy, O. R., and Ortega, L. 1943. The iris. Medicine **22**:287-361.

Leibowitz, U., and Alter, M. 1968. Optic nerve involvement and diplopia as initial manifestations of multiple sclerosis. Acta Neurol. Scand. **44**:70-80.

Leimbach, R. 1895. Statistisches zur Symptomatologie der Tabes dorsalis. Deutsch. Z. Nervenheilk. **7**:493-503.

Levy, R. 1967. The tendon reflexes in the Holmes-Adie syndrome. Neurology **17**:1213-1218.

Lowenstein, O. 1956. The Argyll Robertson pupillary syndrome: mechanism and localization. Amer. J. Ophthal. **42**:105-121.

Lowenstein, O., and Lowenfeld, I. E. 1965. Pupillotonic pseudotabes (syndrome of Markus-Weill and Reys-Holmes-Adie): a critical review of the literature. Survey Ophthal. **10**:129-185.

Magora, A., and Zauberman, H. 1969. Ocular myopathy. Arch. Neurol. **20**:1-8.

Matsuyama, H., and Haymaker, W. 1967. Distribution of lesions in the Landry-Guillain-Barré syndrome, with emphasis on involvement of the sympathetic system. Acta Neuropath. **8**:230-241.

McKenzie, K. G. 1938. Extradural haemorrhage. Brit. J. Surg. **26**:346-365.

Merritt, H. H., and Moore, M. 1933. The Argyll Robertson pupil: an anatomic-physiologic explanation of the phenomenon, with a survey of its occurrence in neurosyphilis. Arch. Neurol. Psychiat. **30**:357-373.

Merritt, H. H., and Moore, M. 1935. Acute syphilitic meningitis. Medicine **14**:119-183.

Merton, P. A. 1964. Absence of conscious position sense in the human eyes. In Bender, M. B., editor: The oculomotor system. New York, Harper & Row, Publishers, pp. 314-320.

Mettler, F. A. 1935. Corticofugal fiber connections of the cortex of *Macaca mulatta:* the occipital region. J. Comp. Neurol. **61**:221-256.

Molnár, L. 1959. Die lokaldiagnostische Bedeutung der vertikalen Blicklähmung; ein Beitrag zur mehrdimensionalen Diagnostik präseniler Psychosen. Arch. Psychiat. Nervenkr. **198**:523-534.

Morgan, M. W., Jr., Olmsted, J. M. D., and Watrous, W. G. 1940. Sympathetic action in accommodation for far vision. Amer. J. Physiol. **128**:588-591.

Nashold, B. S., and Gills, J. P., Jr. 1967. Ocular signs from brain stimulation and lesions. Arch. Ophthal. **77**:609-618.

Ornsteen, A. M. 1935. Palpebromandibular synkinesis in a patient with acute polyneuritis and facial diplegia. Arch. Neurol. Psychiat. **34**:625-630.

Pasik, P., and Pasik, T. 1964. Oculomotor functions in monkeys with lesions of the cerebrum and the superior colliculi. In Bender, M. B., editor: The oculomotor system. New York, Harper & Row, Publishers, pp. 40-80.

Pasik, P., Pasik, T., and Bender, M. B. 1966a. The pretectal syndrome in monkeys. Trans. Amer. Neurol. Ass. **91**:316-318.

Pasik, T., Pasik, P., and Bender, M. B. 1966b. The superior colliculi and eye movements: an experimental study in the monkey. Arch. Neurol. **15**:420-436.

Pearce, J. 1968. The ophthalmological complications of migraine. J. Neurol. Sci. **6**:73-81.

Penfield, W., and Rasmussen, T. 1950. The cerebral cortex of man: a clinical study of localization of function. New York, The Macmillan Company.

Petajan, J. H., Danforth, R. C., D'Allesio, D., and Lucas, G. J. 1965. Progressive sudomotor denervation and Adie's syndrome. Neurology **15**:172-176.

Reese, W. S., and Yaskin, J. C. 1940. Preservation of convergence with paralysis of all lateral movements in a case of intramedullary tumor of the pons. Trans. Amer. Ophthal. Soc. **76**:1-10.

Robinson, D. A. 1968. Eye movement control in primates. Science **161**:1219-1224.

Rosenberg, R. N., Schotland, D. L., Lovelace, R. E., and Rowland, L. P. 1968. Progressive ophthalmoplegia: report of cases. Arch. Neurol. **19**:362-376.

Rucker, C. W. 1958. Paralysis of third, fourth and sixth cranial nerves. Amer. J. Ophthal. **46**:787-794.

Ruttner, F. 1947. Die tonische Pupillenreaktion. Klinische und anatomische Untersuchungen. Mschr. Psychiat. Neurol. **114**:265-330.

Sachs, E. 1938. The importance of ocular signs in the diagnosis of brain tumor. Ann. Int. Med. **11**:1395-1400.

Savitsky, N., and Rangell, L. 1950. The ocular findings in multiple sclerosis. Res. Publ. Ass. Res. Nerv. Ment. Dis., Proc. **28**:403-413.

Scheie, H. G. 1940. Site of disturbance in Adie's syndrome. Arch. Ophthal. **24**:225-237.

Schlezinger, N. S., and Fairfax, W. A. 1959. Evaluation of ocular signs and symptoms in myasthenia gravis. A.M.A. Arch. Ophthal. **62**:985-990.

Segarra, J. M., and Ojeman, R. L. 1961. Convergence nystagmus. Neurology **11**:883-893.

Shrader, E. C., and Schlezinger, N. S. 1960. Neuro-ophthalmologic evaluation of abducens nerve paralysis. A.M.A. Arch. Ophthal. **63**:84-91.

Spiller, W. G. 1919. Contracture occurring in partial recovery from paralysis of the facial nerve and other nerves. Arch. Neurol. Psychiat. **1**:564-566.

Spiller, W. G. 1924. Ophthalmoplegia internuclearis anterior: a case with necropsy. (Paralysis of each rectus internus in lateral associated movement, with preservation of function of these muscles in convergence and of the function of each rectus externus.) Brain **47**:345-357.

Stevenson, G. G., and Hoyt, W. F. 1963. Metastasis to midbrain from mammary carcinoma: cause of bilateral ptosis and ophthalmoplegia. J.A.M.A. **186**:514-516.

Suchenwirth, R. 1963. Zur Klinik der Meningoencephalitis Besnier-Boeck-Schaumann. Arch. Psychiat. Z. Neurol. **204**:370-388.

Symonds, C. P. 1944. Venous thrombosis in the central nervous system. Proc. Roy. Soc. Med. **37**:386-388.

Terrien, F. 1922. Les ophtalmoplégies traumatiques. Presse Méd. **30**(1):267-270.

Tyler, H. R. 1968. Vascular thrombi and neuronal alterations in human botulism. Acta Neuropath. **10**:82-85.

von Graefe, A. 1868. Verhandlungen ärztlicher Gesellschaften. Berl. Klin. Wschr. **5**:125-127.

Wagman, I. H. 1964. Eye movements induced by electric stimulation of cerebrum in monkeys and their relationship to bodily movements. In Bender, M. B., editor: The oculomotor system. New York, Harper & Row, Publishers, pp. 18-39.

Wartenberg, R. 1946. Associated movements in the oculomotor and facial muscles. Arch. Neurol. Psychiat. **55**:439-488.

Wartenberg, R. 1948. "Inverted Marcus Gunn phenomenon" (so-called Marin Amat syndrome). Arch. Neurol. Psychiat. **60**:584-596.

Warwick, R. 1953. Representation of the extraocular muscles with oculomotor nuclei of the monkey. J. Comp. Neurol. **98**:449-504.

Warwick, R. 1964. Oculomotor organization. In Bender, M. B., editor: The oculomotor system. New York, Harper & Row, Publishers, pp. 173-204.

Wernicke, C. 1877. Ein Fall von Ponserkrankung. Arch. Psychiat. **7**:513-538.

Whitteridge, D. 1960. Central control of eye movements. In Handbook of physiology, sect. 1, vol. 2. Washington, D. C., Amer. Physiol. Soc., pp. 1089-1109.

Wilson, S. A. K. 1906. Ectopia pupillae in certain mesencephalic lesions. Brain **29**:524-536.

Yaskin, J. C., and Kornblum, K. 1937. Neurologic aspects of petrositis. Arch. Neurol. Psychiat. **37**:307-333.

Zorrilla, E., and Kozak, G. P. 1967. Ophthalmoplegia in diabetes mellitus. Ann. Int. Med. **67**:968-976.

Chapter 17

Disorders of cerebellar origin

ANATOMICAL AND FUNCTIONAL CONSIDERATIONS

The cerebellum, enclosed in the walls of the posterior cranial fossa and covered by the tentorium cerebelli, lies separated from the rest of the brain except where it is connected to the brainstem by means of three conspicuous pairs of fiber bundles: the inferior, middle, and superior cerebellar peduncles, also referred to respectively as restiform body, brachium pontis, and brachium conjunctivum (Fig. 17-1). Nerve fibers enter the cerebellum by passing through all three of these structures, and they leave chiefly by way of the superior cerebellar peduncle. The juxtarestiform body, which forms the medial part of the restiform body, carries mostly efferent cerebellar fibers.

The cerebellum consists of vermis, which straddles the midline, and hemispheres. All of the cerebellum is subdivided into lobules, each containing a number of folia. Midsagittal section of the cerebellum exposes the characteristic arbor vitae, with the gray matter lying superficial and the white matter central. The largest accumulation of gray matter within the cerebellum is the dentate nucleus, situated deep in the white matter of the hemisphere. Another mass of gray matter is the fastigial nucleus, which lies medially in the white matter, beneath the vermis. Situated between the fastigial and dentate nuclei are two small cell masses, the globose and emboliform nuclei. (Fastigial, globose, and emboliform nuclei are known collectively as the *roof nuclei,* though only the fastigial nucleus lies in the roof of the fourth ventricle.) Most of the fibers passing into the cerebellar peduncles terminate in the cerebellar cortex. The Purkinje cells constitute the link between the cerebellar cortex and the four nuclei just mentioned, their axons terminating in these nuclei. In turn, fibers originating in these cerebellar nuclei pass out of the cerebellum by way of the superior cerebellar peduncle and, in small measure, the juxtarestiform body.

For clinical purposes, it suffices to consider the cerebellum as made up of vermis and two hemispheres. Although many promising attempts have been made toward the localization of lesions in smaller units of the cerebellum, clinically one must be satisfied if he can ascertain whether a lesion is situated in the region of the inferior vermis, involving the flocculonodular lobe, or in one of the hemispheres. One reason is that the cerebellum is so hemmed in by bone and tentorium cerebelli (thus having little room for expansion) that in the presence of an expanding lesion it tends to suffer generalized compression injury. Another reason is that since the cerebellum has no direct motor function and is not concerned in the mediation of (conscious) sensibility, one cannot rely on disturbances in these realms in reaching a conclusion as to the site of a cerebellar lesion.

In earlier days the cerebellum was re-

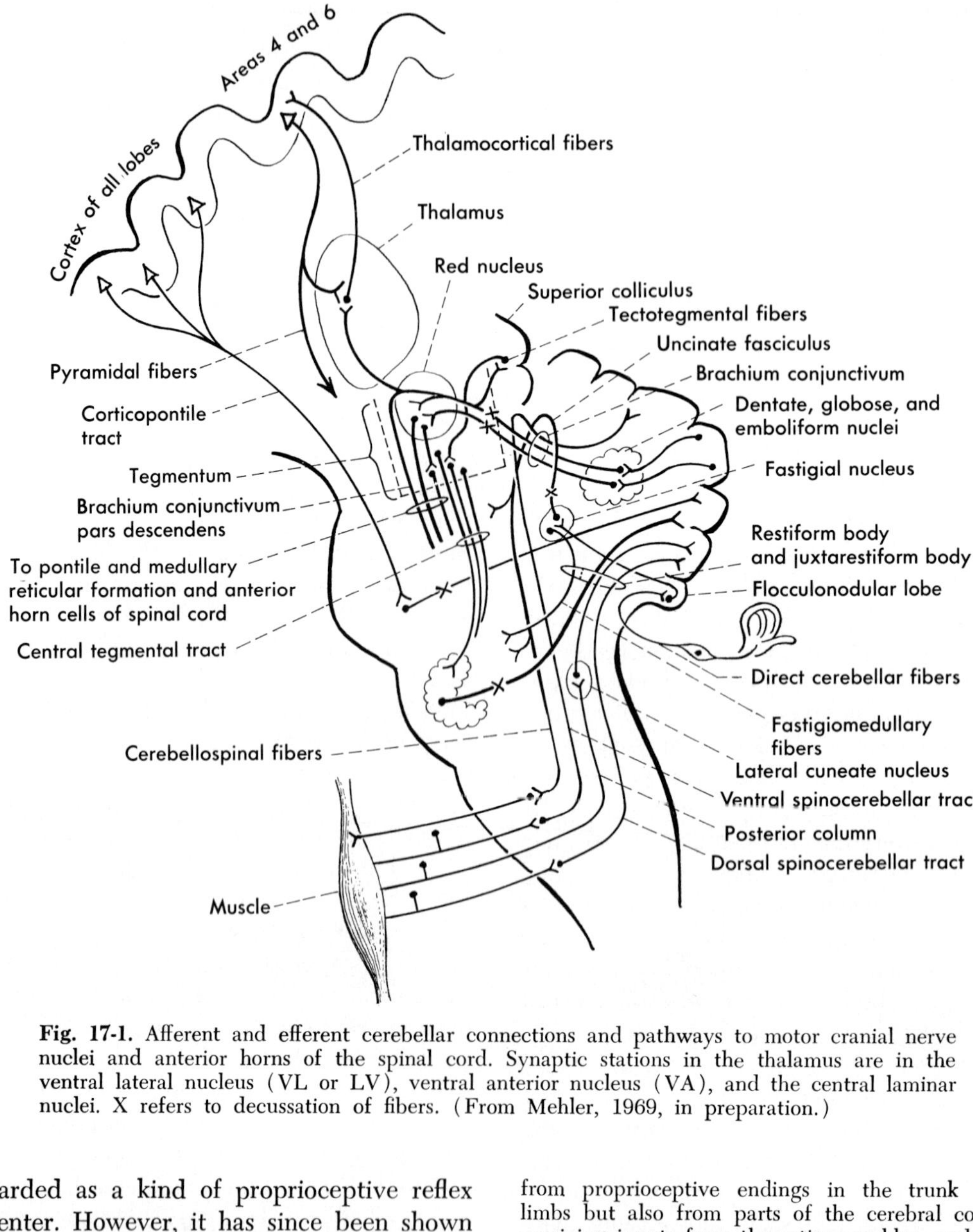

Fig. 17-1. Afferent and efferent cerebellar connections and pathways to motor cranial nerve nuclei and anterior horns of the spinal cord. Synaptic stations in the thalamus are in the ventral lateral nucleus (VL or LV), ventral anterior nucleus (VA), and the central laminar nuclei. X refers to decussation of fibers. (From Mehler, 1969, in preparation.)

garded as a kind of proprioceptive reflex center. However, it has since been shown that the cerebellum is a suprasegmental structure having inherent activity (as manifested by persistence of high-frequency potential waves after section of all cerebellar peduncles) and that its discharges are influenced by incoming impulses (Eccles, Ito, and Szentágothai, 1967).

On the *afferent side* the electrical recording of impulses reaching the cerebellar cortex following peripheral stimulation has indicated that afferent connections extend to the cerebellum not only from proprioceptive endings in the trunk and limbs but also from parts of the cerebral cortex receiving inputs from the retina, cochlea, and cutaneous tactile end-organs (Snider, 1967). Through fibers extending from the nuclei of the extraocular muscles to the superior and medial vestibular nuclei, the cerebellum also receives impressions as to the degree of contraction of the extraocular muscles, hence the position of the eyes (Szentágothai, 1964).

On the *efferent side* the cerebellum sends a massive contingent of fibers to the thalamus (to VL, VA, and the central laminar nuclei; Fig. 24-1, *E*) for the regulation of afferent impulses reaching the cortex in general; moreover, impulses received by the cerebellar cortex from the cerebral cortex are presumably relayed back to the parts of the cerebral cortex concerned in tactile, visual, and auditory perception. Further, the cerebellum sends fibers to the vestibular nuclei that project to the nuclei of the extraocular nerves (Carpenter and Strominger, 1964; Manni, Azzena, and Dow, 1965) (Chapter 13).

The cerebellum also exerts an influence on certain visceromotor neural mechanisms. Pupillary dilatation, for example, may be induced by stimulation over much of the cerebellar cortex, and pupillary constriction and bladder contraction by stimulation of certain circumscribed cerebellar cortical areas. Moreover, vasomotor responses have been found increased after cerebellar ablations. (Dow and Moruzzi, 1958; Snider, 1967.) Further, some fibers may reach the cerebellum from the gastrointestinal tract, judging from the observation that vomiting and other symptoms of motion sickness no longer occur after decerebellation or after ablation of the flocculonodular lobe (Tyler and Bard, 1949).

Feedbacks from the cerebral cortex reach nuclei to which the cerebellum projects. The stratum profundum of the superior colliculus is among them; it receives feedback connections from cortical areas 4 and 6. A cortical feedback is also received by the red nucleus (the *corticorubral tract*). Further, the same holds for the midbrain reticular nuclei receiving fibers from the red nucleus *(corticoreticular fibers)* (Holmes, 1939; Kuypers and Lawrence, 1967; Niemer and Magoun, 1947).

In various ways, then, the cerebellum has a much wider functional scope than is evident clinically.

Afferent pathways

Afferent impulses that activate this subtle regulating mechanism are transmitted to the cerebellum from various sources, most of which have already been indicated. From the clinical standpoint the chief of these are the spinocerebellar, vestibulocerebellar, olivocerebellar, and pontocerebellar pathways.

The *spinocerebellar tracts* (dorsal and ventral) transmit impulses arising in the muscles and joints of the vertebral column and the limbs, especially the lower limbs. Most of the spinocerebellar fibers are derived from cells of the lumbar and thoracic cord, which is understandable from the fact that in equilibration, whether in standing or in walking, the control of the legs and trunk is of primary importance. The general course of these tracts is shown in Fig. 1-5. Contributing also to the maintenance of equilibration are cervical dorsal root fibers that course up the posterior column, synapse in the lateral cuneate nucleus, and extend by way of the ipsilateral restiform body to the cerebellum. All these fiber systems terminate chiefly in the vermis.

The *vestibulocerebellar pathway* is described elsewhere (p. 192). Some nerve fibers from the vestibular apparatus that extend centrally in the vestibular nerve pass directly to the cortex of the flocculonodular lobe, from which Purkinje cell axons extend to the fastigial nucleus (Fig. 17-1). These fibers convey information to the cerebellum regarding position of the body, and particularly the head, in space.

The *olivocerebellar tract* originates in the principal and accessory inferior olivary nuclei, decussates in large part, proceeds up the restiform body, and ends diffusely in the cerebellar cortex of that side. The dorsal lamina of the principal inferior olivary nucleus projects to the superior part of the cerebellar hemisphere, and the ventral lamina to the inferior part of the hemisphere. On the other hand, the dorsal accessory nucleus projects to the superior part of the vermis. The flocculonodular lobe of the cerebellum receives fibers not only directly from the vestibular labyrinth—that is, from the cristae of the semicircular canals (Fig. 13-5)—but also from the rostral part of the medial accessory olivary nucleus. (Holmes and Stewart, 1908; Jansen and Brodal, 1954.)

The *corticopontocerebellar pathway* consists of two sets of neurons, the first of which originates from the cortex of the frontal, temporal, parietal, and occipital lobes and extends to the ipsilateral nuclei pontis. From here a second set, after decussating, courses in the brachium pontis, and terminates in the cortex of all parts of the cerebellum except that of the flocculonodular lobe. Like most other systems, these fibers do not decussate after entering the cerebellum.

Efferent pathways

Cerebellofugal impulses concerned in influencing muscular contraction reach their destinations (the motor cranial nerve nuclei and the anterior horn cells) largely through the mediation of the lateral vestibular nucleus and the red nucleus (Figs. 13-5 and 17-1). Other intermediate synaptic stations include the superior colliculus, the nucleus of Darkschewitsch, and the interstitial nucleus of the medial longitudinal fasciculus (of Cajal). The cerebellofugal pathways reaching these various structures emerge (1) via the juxtarestiform body, which carries some fibers from the fastigial nucleus, and (2) via the superior cerebellar peduncle, which carries other fibers from the fastigial nucleus and a large contingent of fibers from the dentate, globose, and emboliform nuclei.

The fibers originating in the fastigial nucleus and leaving via the juxtarestiform body are relatively few (Fig. 17-1). They terminate in medial reticular nuclei. Larger numbers of fibers emanating from the fastigial nucleus decussate (Fig. 13-5), extend upward to the brachium conjunctivum, arch round it, forming a hook (*uncinate fasciculus*, or *hook bundle of Russell*), then course downward in the descending component of the superior cerebellar peduncle; they proceed to the lateral vestibular nucleus and on into the medullary reticular formation. These fibers continue caudalward, giving off additional fiber groups to the lower brainstem, and some (as *cerebellospinal fibers*) enter and traverse the anterior column of the cord in the region next to the midline and terminate on anterior horns at cervical levels. (Eccles, Ito, and Szentágothai, 1967; Jansen, 1954; Pompeiano, 1967; Rand, 1954.) Functionally, these fibers may be concerned in bringing about changes in the position of the head.

The fiber pathway from the fastigial nucleus to the lateral and other vestibular nuclei is shown in Fig. 13-5. The lateral vestibular nucleus projects to the anterior horns at all levels of the spinal cord via the vestibulospinal tract (p. 5), and to cranial nerve nuclei III, IV, and VI via the medial longitudinal fasciculus (p. 193). The anterior horn cells of the upper cervical cord (for the supply of the neck musculature) receive additional connections via the medial longitudinal fasciculus and, as already indicated, via the uncinate fasciculus (Fig. 17-1). Thus the cerebellum, in addition to exercising control over trunk and limb movements, also has the function of maintaining synergy of head and ocular movements.

Other cerebellofugal fibers—by far the greatest number leaving the cerebellum—originate in the dentate, globose, and emboliform nuclei and pursue their course through the brachium conjunctivum. On reaching the midbrain tegmentum, practically all these fibers decussate. Many, after decussation, reach the *stratum profundum of the superior colliculus;* others terminate in the *nucleus of Darkschewitsch* and the *interstitial nucleus of Cajal.* Still others terminate in the red nucleus. Most, however, traverse the red nucleus and proceed to the thalamus. In degeneration studies (Nauta technique) following lesions made in various parts of the cerebellum in monkeys, no cerebellofugal fibers have been found terminating in the mesencephalic tegmentum (Mehler, personal communication).

More specifically, after passing through the red nucleus, the fibers bound for the thalamus traverse the (prerubral) field H of Forel and spread out in field H_1, in which they ascend to terminate in the ventral lateral (VL or LV) and ventral anterior (VA) thalamic nuclei; from these nuclei, thalamocortical relays proceed to areas 4 and 6 of the cortex. A significant portion of this thalamic limb of the brachium conjunctivum ascends via the internal medullary lamina and terminates in the central lateral intralaminar nucleus. Such a dual distribution, to principal and intralaminar thalamic nuclei, was suggested by earlier findings in man (Probst, 1901) and in the chimpanzee (Walker, 1938) in studies utilizing the Marchi method; more recently the sites of termination of these fibers have been confirmed in the monkey and other species by means of the Nauta method (Mehler, 1965; Mehler, Vernier, and Nauta, 1958).

From the stratum profundum of the superior colliculus an imposing contingent of fibers proceeds to the midbrain tegmentum, as has been observed in Nauta preparations. Morphological evidence suggests that cerebellar influence exerted by this cerebellotectotegmental route rivals that exerted by the cerebellorubrotegmental system.

From the red nucleus and/or midbrain tegmentum and cerebellum, three main fiber systems proceed caudally. (1) Fibers originating in the red nucleus and midbrain tegmentum, joined by the pars descendens of the brachium conjunctivum (Fig. 17-1), proceed to the reticular formation of the pons and medulla oblongata and to the anterior horns of the spinal cord *(rubrobulbar and rubrospinal tracts)*. (2) Fibers making up the *central tegmental tract* originate mainly in the midbrain tegmentum and terminate chiefly in the inferior olivary nucleus. (3) Other fibers in the central tegmental tract originate in the nucleus of Darkschewitsch and the interstitial nucleus of Cajal and proceed (as Ogawa's bundle) to the dorsal and medial accessory olivary nuclei, thence to the cerebellum.

Earlier claims that a *rubro-olivary projection* exists (Papez and Stotler, 1940; Walberg, 1954) has been challenged by Kuypers, Fleming, and Farinholt (1962). Lesions made in the red nucleus (by angular stereotaxis without involving the dorsal mesencephalic tegmentum), they found, did not provide any evidence of a rubro-olivary connection.

The primary function of the cerebellum is to provide *synergy* in the maintenance of postures. It acts by coordinating and modulating muscle contractions so that the body may be stabilized while in the standing position and may remain in equilibrium during locomotion. This means that during a motor act the cerebellum influences each participating muscle so that it may contract at the right time and to the proper degree, that is to say, chronometrically (Braitenberg, 1967).

CLINICAL MANIFESTATIONS OF CEREBELLAR LESIONS

The clinical manifestations of cerebellar lesions are a reflection of an asynergia of muscular activity. Although differences in the pattern of cerebellar deficit exist depending on the site of the lesion, the cerebellar deficit is expressed in terms of disturbances of equilibrium, posture, and voluntary movement.

Cerebellar ataxia

Disturbances in gait and static adaptation. Ataxia is the most important sign of damage of the cerebellum and is easily detectable. Cerebellar ataxia occurs only when movement is attempted. In contrast to *posterior column* or *posterior root ataxia*, in which all movements are carried out in an incoordinate fashion, cerebellar ataxia is restricted to the muscles participating in complex movements, for example, movement of a leg. Further, posterior column or posterior root ataxia is modified by the aid of vision, cerebellar ataxia is not. In cerebellar ataxia, simple movements such as flexion and extension at the ankle, knee, and hip can be well executed; however,

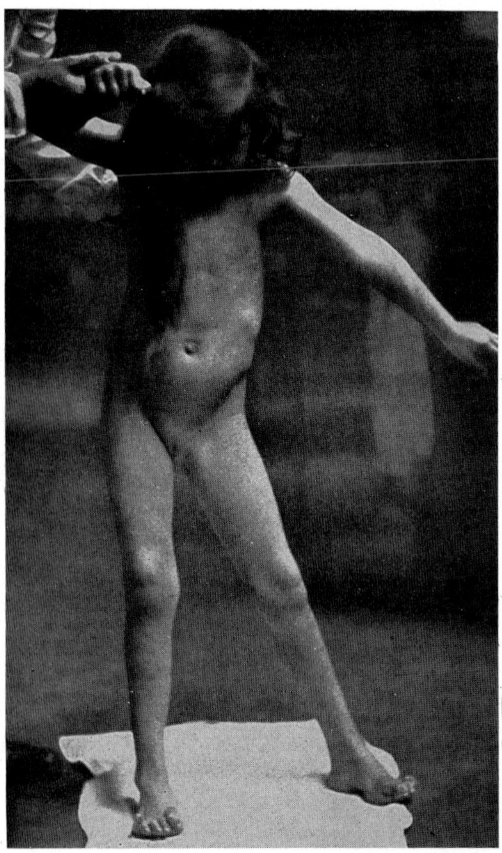

Fig. 17-2. Position resulting from cerebellar ataxia.

when they become part of a complex movement their dynamic and static unity is disrupted in such a manner that the gait is staggering and zigzag like that of a drunken man, and the erect posture characterized by more or less pronounced swaying (Fig. 17-2). Individual trunk and limb muscles are no longer capable of coordinating their contractions in the interest of immobilization and stabilization. In acute injury of the cerebellum all movements are ataxic.

The loss of static adaptation—due usually to damage inflicted on cerebellar nuclei—can be demonstrated in a patient with cerebellar ataxia by means of a simple test. The patient kneels on the examining table blindfolded with hands unsupported. When the table is tilted, his body fails to undergo the movements necessary to the maintenance of the center of gravity and he will therefore fall if not supported. Cerebellar asynergia may also be manifested when the patient walks; the head and trunk lag behind his limbs, endangering balance. When the patient attempts to rise from a prone position, his legs rise first instead of his trunk. Furthermore, when he leans over to pick up an object, the postural adjustments at the hip, knee, and ankle do not occur simultaneously, as in a normal person, but, instead, successively *(decomposition of movement)*.

A simple means of detecting incipient ataxia of the lower limbs is to ask the patient, lying prone with his legs flexed at the knees, to keep the legs vertical. With the slightest leg movement, oscillations of the leg will occur.

Disturbances in function of the upper limbs. The upper limbs are usually less affected than the lower limbs in cerebellar disorders because of the minor role they play in the maintenance of balance. In a lesion of the cerebellar hemispheres, disturbances of coordination of the upper limbs can, however, usually be induced by having the patient perform certain movements.

Ataxia of the upper limbs can easily be detected by means of the *finger-to-nose test.* With arms hanging loosely at his sides and eyes closed, the patient is asked to raise one arm slowly and touch his nose with the tip of his index finger. Normally this movement is carried out in a direct line. When cerebellar damage exists, the movement begins normally but soon becomes tremulous, with the tremor increasing in amplitude as the finger approaches the nose (*action*, or *intention, tremor*). Finally the finger comes to a halt somewhere near the nose. When the movement is normally performed and yet a cerebellar lesion is suspected, certain other tests may be carried out. Thus in the finger-to-nose test, ataxia and ataxic tremor may be induced by offering resistance to the movement of the limbs, for example, by means of a rubber band around the patient's wrist, held by the examiner, or merely by applying a finger or two to the volar aspect of the wrist while the movement is in progress.

Latent disturbances in the upper limbs may also be brought to light by having the patient perform rapidly alternating movements. Thus, with the arms bent at the elbow, the forearms upright, and the elbows a short distance in front of the body, the patient is requested to execute rapid pronation-supination movements. In the presence of a cerebellar lesion the movements of that side are slow and irregular, and the elbow undergoes wider excursions than normally. In short, there is a loss of the subtle cooperation normally existing between antagonistic muscles. This disturbance is called *adiadochokinesis* (*a*, absence of; *diadocho*, succeeding; *kinesis*, motion).

Slowing of speech *(bradylalia)* together with jerkiness and irregularity of articulation and phonation are characteristic of cerebellar damage; the speech is usually described as "staccato" or "scanning." These disturbances are expressions of adiadochokinesis.

Another manifestation of cerebellar ataxia is *dysmetria.* When, for example, a patient with a unilateral cerebellar lesion

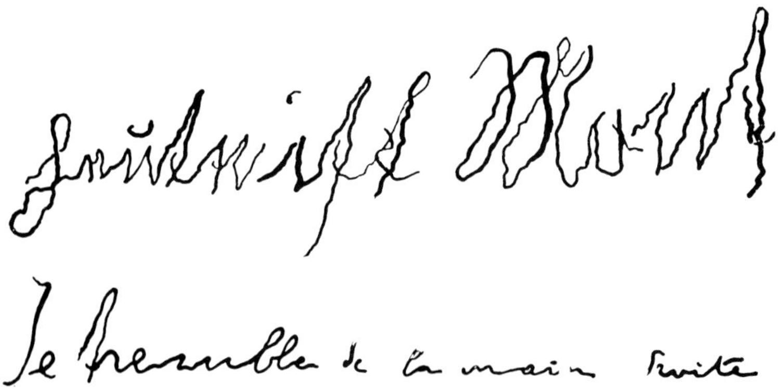

Fig. 17-3. Megalographia in cerebellar disease, and micrographia in the Parkinson syndrome.

attempts to grasp a glass of water with the hand of the affected side, he opens the hand in an exaggerated, superfluous manner before grasping it, and the same happens when he releases the glass. Asked to place the heel of the affected side on the opposite knee, the patient excessively flexes his leg so that the heel is placed on the thigh rather than on the knee. If he walks forward "on all fours," he raises the limbs of the affected side much higher from the floor than he does the limbs of the normal side. In contrast with the ataxia of posterior column origin, cerebellar ataxia is constant no matter whether the eyes are open or closed, and in the performance of simple movements no significant deviation from the normal occurs.

Cerebellar dysmetria, which consists in hypermetria, is also noticeable in the handwriting, which is larger than normal, particularly at the end of a word or sentence *(megalographia)*. By way of contrast, *hypometria and micrographia* prevail in Parkinson's disease and the other amyostatic states (Fig. 17-3).

Cerebellar hypotonia

The cerebellum is instrumental not only in the performance of harmonious movement but also in the maintenance of *statotonus*. Ataxia together with atonia results when the cerebellum or its afferent or efferent pathways are sufficiently damaged to induce an imbalance of the cerebellar impulses reaching rubroreticular systems

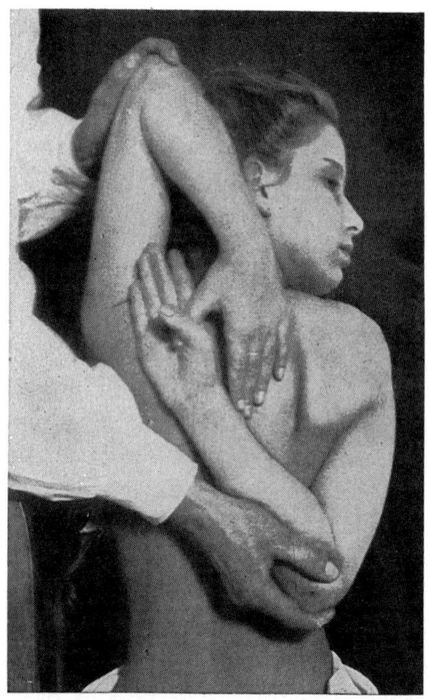

Fig. 17-4. Contortionist movement as the result of cerebellar hypotonia.

or the cerebral cortex (via the dentatorubrothalamic pathway) or both.

Cerebellar hypotonia is also manifested by flabbiness of muscles, by the ease with which the limbs may be placed in abnormal positions (Fig. 17-4), and by the decreased resistance offered by muscles to passive stretching. If the patient flexes his arm at the elbow and the examiner resists the movement by pulling on the forearm, then suddenly releases the forearm, the patient's hand flies up with considerable force and may strike him in the face. There is little if any of the forearm rebound that occurs under normal conditions. Both the exaggerated movement in flexion and the lack of extensor rebound are the expression of a defect in synergic balance and a general lack of inhibition. Hypotonia can also readily be demonstrated by grasping the patient's forearms and shaking them. The hand of the affected side exhibits far greater excursions, both in flexion and in extension, than that of the normal side. Moreover, if the two arms are outstretched, with the hands resting on a bar, and the bar is suddenly removed, the arm of the affected side falls farther than the other arm. This is all the more striking if the hands carry a weight. (Holmes, 1939.) A further manifestation of hypotonia is increased *pendulousness* of the lower limbs. A patient sits on the examining table with his legs dangling; each leg is then lifted passively and allowed to swing. The swinging time is longest for the limb on the side of the cerebellar lesion. The same may be brought out by tapping the patellar tendon. By contrast, owing to dyssynergia, pendulousness of the upper limbs in walking is diminished in cerebellar disease. (Wartenberg, 1954.)

While hypotonia resulting from posterior root lesions is associated with hyporeflexia or areflexia, in hypotonia of cerebellar origin the *deep reflexes* are unaffected. It is true that following extirpation of one-half of the cerebellum for cerebellar tumor the deep reflexes may be absent postoperatively, but they soon return and sometimes are exaggerated despite hypotonia. Enduring areflexia (particularly with respect to the knee and ankle jerks) in the presence of an expanding cerebellar lesion is attributed to the effects of increased cerebrospinal fluid pressure on the posterior root fibers at their site of penetration of the dura mater; even posterior column degeneration may develop secondarily, as may arachnoidal cysts (O'Connell, 1953).

Cerebellar hemihypotonia may occasionally be of sufficient degree to cause *hemiparesis,* or it may be reflected in retardation of muscular contraction. The hemiparesis is distinguishable from that of cerebral origin, which is spastic in nature, by the hypotonia. Moreover, in cerebellar hemiparesis the Babinski reflex is not elicitable.

Disorders occurring in association with ataxia and hypotonia

Laterality of disturbances. In unilateral lesions of the cerebellum, the ataxia and hypotonia that occur in the trunk and limbs are, as a rule, solely ipsilateral. This is understandable anatomically, for, with the exception of a part of the ventral spinocerebellar tract, the spinocerebellar tracts do not decussate in their course to the cerebellum. Most of the spinocerebellar fibers decussate in the vermis (Fig. 1-5), but they terminate so close to the midline that for clinical purposes they may be regarded as ending in the median plane.

Also from the efferent standpoint each half of the cerebellum exerts its influence almost entirely on the ipsilateral side of the cord, either through double-decussating pathways (such as the cerebellorubrospinal) or through non-decussating pathways (such as the cerebellovestibulospinal).

Assessment of the weight of an object. A patient with a unilateral cerebellar lesion and ipsilateral incoordination and atonia is often unable (with eyes shut) to assess the weight of an object placed in the hand of the affected side. As a rule the weight is underestimated. When this disturbance is not entirely evident, it can be unmasked by having the patient distinguish weights. No difference will be noticed, for instance, between a 50 or a 100 gram weight placed in the hand of the affected side, whereas on the normal side a 15 gram weight can readily by distinguished from a 20 gram weight. In some instances of unilateral cerebellar damage, even though the patient has an appreciation of position and movement and has intact stereognosis and cutaneous sensibility, he is unable to evaluate dimensions with the hand of the ipsilateral side and is unaware of the duration of a movement he has performed on that side.

Overestimation of weight may occasionally be noted in serous meningitis involving the posterior cranial fossa and in hemorrhage over the surface of the cerebellum. In such cases the cerebellar lesion appears to be irritative rather than destructive. The overestimation is now and then associated with muscular hypertonia, presumably of brainstem origin. (Bing, 1912.)

Pointing test. Disturbances of tonus and coordination can be demonstrated by the pointing test. If a normal individual is asked to touch the outstretched finger of the examiner with his own finger—first with eyes open, then closed—he can do so with ease. However, in unilateral cerebellar damage the finger deviates during the excursion, particularly when the eyes are closed.

Tendency to walk toward side of the lesion. Some authors contend that the gait disturbance occurring in the presence of cerebellar damage is such that the patient, when asked to walk straight ahead with eyes closed, always deviates toward the side of the lesion and tends to fall to that side. This is not altogether true; occasionally the patient has a tendency, while walking, to deviate or fall toward the side opposite the lesion. The tendency to walk in a circle *(compass gait)* is characteristic of a unilateral cerebellar lesion, but its diagnostic value is limited because this disturbance may also be observed in unilateral labyrinthine disorders. This type of gait may be tested by having the patient walk five steps forward and then five backward and continue in this exercise. Each time he walks forward his path is toward the side of the lesion, until after the fifth time or so he is walking in a direction 90 degrees off that he originally pursued *(starwise gait)*.

Abnormal positions of limbs and head. The spontaneous assumption of abnormal positions by the limbs may be a sign of a lesion of a cerebellar hemisphere. A glance at the foot of a patient lying in bed reveals that it is turned inward (in the sense of slight pes varus). In a patient standing, the arm on the side of the lesion lacks the slight flexion at the elbow and finger joints seen on the normal side. When the patient is asked to stretch out his arms in front of him, the arm on the side of the lesion will extend incompletely and at times remain at a lower level than the other arm. These are obvious expressions of cerebellar deficiency.

Asymmetry of position as a manifestation of vestibulocerebellar irritation occurs fairly frequently in cerebellopontile angle tumors: the head is tilted toward the sound side, the shoulder of that side is elevated, and the face is turned somewhat toward the side of the lesion *(vestibular tilt)*.

Arm and leg deviation. Certain postural reflexes tend to be exaggerated on the side of a cerebellar lesion. In a unilateral cerebellar lesion the outstretched arm of the affected side has a tendency to deviate laterally. Lateral deviation of the leg on the affected side may also occur when the patient, seated on a chair with eyes closed, is asked to lift both outstretched legs and hold them steady.

Ocular nystagmus. See Chapter 13.

Opsoclonus. "Opsoclonus" denotes conjugate, irregular jerking of the eyes occurring continually in all directions, but mostly in the horizontal plane. The movements are random, very rapid, and of unequal amplitude. The disturbance is thus altogether different from nystagmus and quite unlike the "lightning movements," the "flutter-like oscillations," and the "jelly-like" oscillations of the eyes observed in some cases of cerebellar disease. Myoclonus in the limbs or elsewhere may be an accompaniment of the opsoclonus.

A rare disturbance, opsoclonus is noted particularly in association with subacute cerebellar degeneration in persons having neoplasm (sometimes occult) at a distant site, for example, bronchogenic carcinoma or carcinoma of the breast or uterus. Generalized cerebellar atrophy and Purkinje cell loss are features of the cerebellar degeneration, as are also loss of nerve cells from the dentate nucleus and alterations in the neuropil in this nucleus. (Ellenberger, Campa, and Netsky, 1968; Ross and Zeman, 1967.) Opsoclonus can also occur in children and adults having a febrile illness. In some of these cases the opsoclonus is reversible. A chronic inflammatory state involving hypothalamus, midbrain, and pons was noted in one case. (Cogan, 1954.) In infants, not only may there be opsoclonus ("dancing eyes") but also spectacular somatic myoclonic ataxia and irritability, all developing suddenly and running a nonprogressive protracted course often marked by exacerbations and remissions. The condition ("infantile polymyoclonia") is considered a distinct clinical and immunopathological entity, that is, a disease, not merely a constellation of signs and symptoms. (Dyken and Kolář, 1968.)

Importance of ataxia as a sign of cerebellar disturbance

Ataxia is the cerebellar sign *par excellence.* From a practical standpoint, cerebellar hypotonia is not nearly so important. This is because the hypotonia may be blotted out or replaced by hypertonia as a result of brainstem (corticospinal tract) damage brought about by pressure from expanding cerebellar tumor, by an infiltrative process secondarily involving the brainstem, and so on. This is not true for cerebellar ataxia, for it persists even in the presence of pronounced spasticity, and it is always easily recognizable.

None of the other signs that aid in the localization of lesions to the cerebellum is necessarily to be regarded as an integral component of the cerebellar syndrome, for each may also be provoked by noncerebellar lesions. Where cerebellar ataxia is absent, one cannot be certain that a cerebellar lesion exists. Indeed, strictly speaking, not even the combination of ataxia and hypotonia is pathognomonic of a cerebellar lesion, for the two are demonstrable in lesions of cerebellofugal and cerebellopetal tracts outside of the cerebellum—whether in the midbrain, pons, medulla oblongata, or, as in Friedreich's ataxia, even in the spinal cord.

Ataxia may be the only cerebellar manifestation of tumor involving the *vermis,* of which medulloblastoma is the most notable example. Swaying while standing and staggering when walking are striking, and there may be some unsteadiness of the hands. The gait is peculiar in that the pelvis is tilted forward and the trunk projected slightly backward relative to the lower limb. Nystagmus is present in 40 to 70 percent of cases in early stages. If the tumor invades the cerebellar hemispheres later in the clinical course, nystagmus, dysdiadochokinesis, dysmetria, and other signs of cerebellar deficiency become evident. In compressing the medulla oblongata, the tumor may induce opisthotonos and extensor rigidity of the limbs. (Abbott and Kernohan, 1943; Bailey and Cushing, 1925; Walker and Botterell, 1937.) In damage of a cerebellar *hemisphere,* for example, by tumor, the signs just mentioned are elicitable. Weakness is encountered in the upper limb, not the lower (Holmes, 1922).

The most frequent *focal* pathological processes occurring in the cerebellum are neoplasm, infarction, hemorrhage, and abscess. Tuberculoma and gumma are rare. All these conditions usually induce unmistakable signs of cerebellar deficiency.

Hemorrhage into the cerebellum is fairly common, constituting about 10 percent of all brain hemorrhages occurring in hypertensive patients. The hemorrhage originates from the branches of superior cerebellar artery in the region of the dentate nucleus; it can be massive or can merely infiltrate the white matter, and blood can be found in the cerebrospinal fluid in most cases. Loss of consciousness succeeded by coma may occur, and in such patients there may be preliminary vertigo, sweating, vomiting, and occipital headache. In the presence of massive hemorrhage a bilateral or unilateral spastic syndrome may be encountered. Signs of cerebellar deficiency are detectable in patients whose condition is such that they can be examined. (Poór, 1967.)

In *cystic arachnoiditis* involving the posterior cranial fossa, seventh nerve palsy may occur and there may be vertigo; by contrast, cerebellar ataxia may be slight and cerebellar nystagmus absent (Bing, 1911).

Heredofamilial spinocerebellar degeneration, often combined with olivary and pontile atrophy (Fig. 17-5), is characterized by enduring signs of cerebellar deficiency (Greenfield, 1954).

Subacute diffuse cerebellar atrophy with florid signs of cerebellar deficiency (ataxia of gait and of individual movements of the lower and upper limbs, dysarthria, and, commonly, nystagmus) occurs now and then in carcinoma in various loca-

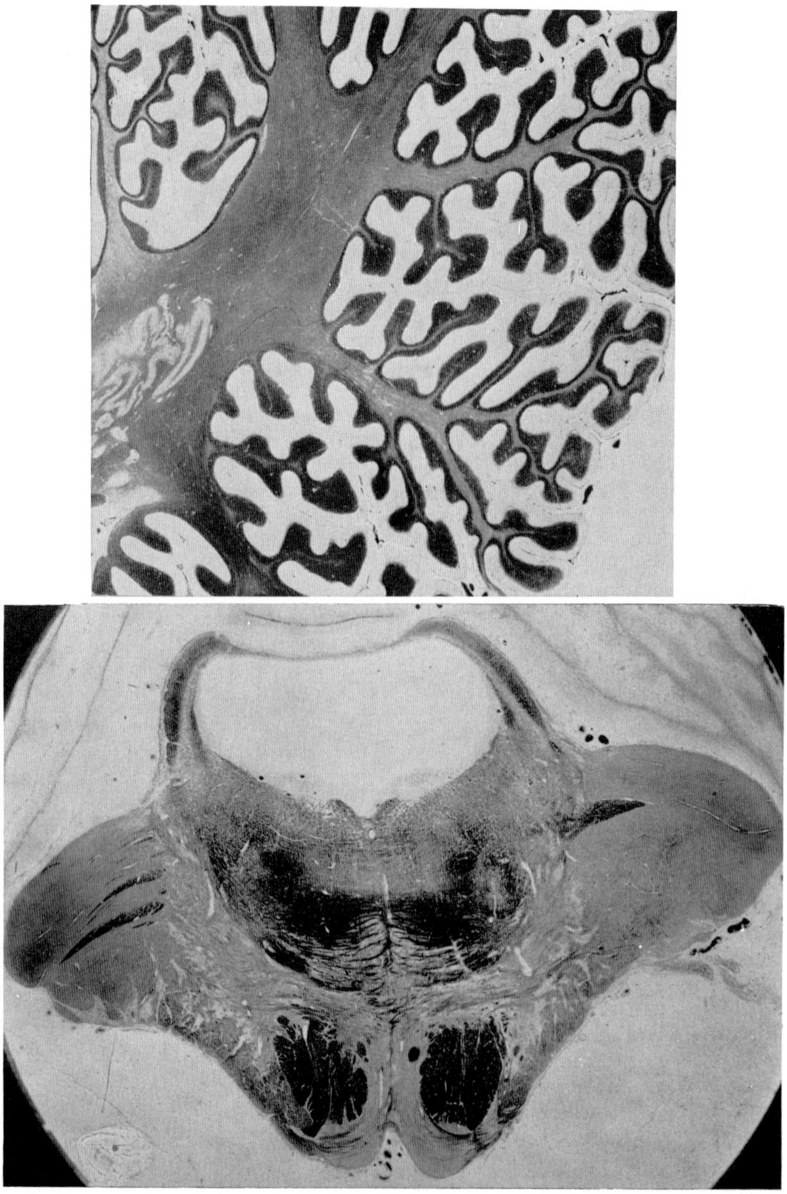

Fig. 17-5. Atrophy of pars basilaris pontis and cerebellum in case of hereditary ataxia. The medullary center of the cerebellum is demyelinated, the granular layer somewhat rarefied, and the molecular layer narrowed. The section from the pons shows severe demyelination of the pontocerebellar fibers and of the brachium pontis. (The myelin in these structures should normally stain as intensely as that in the tegmentum.) The brachium conjunctivum on the two sides is narrowed, and there is dilatation of the fourth ventricle. (From Schut and Haymaker, 1951.)

tions, such as the bronchi, breast, ovary, or uterus. Both cerebellar cortex and nuclei show evidence of rapid evolution of lesions, characterized histologically by prominent microglial activity, fat-laden macrophages, and (frequently) by perivascular and cerebellar meningeal accumulations of inflammatory cells (mostly lymphoid cells). Purkinje cell loss is conspicuous, and the granular layer of the nodulus may also suffer cell loss. Fastigial and dentate nuclei may share in the pathological process. The olivary nuclei in the medulla oblongata are usually affected, though, as a rule, slightly. (Brain, Daniel, and Greenfield, 1951; Victor, 1965.) In one case of bronchogenic carcinoma, postmortem study revealed not only the characteristic subacute degeneration and inflammation in the cerebellum but also a florid inflammatory reaction in numerous other structures (putamen, brainstem, and spinal roots and posterior root ganglia), suggesting to the authors (Vick, Schulman, and Dau, 1969) an associated infectious process. (See p. 88 for a description of other cases.)

The *cerebellar atrophy in malnutrition occurring in alcoholics* is slow in evolution (developing over a period of several weeks or months) and is manifested by ataxia of stance and gait and of individual movements of the lower limbs; the upper limbs are much less ataxic. Hypotonia is scarcely detectable. Spontaneous (static) tremor of the head and of distal parts is mild if it occurs at all. Nystagmus and dysarthria are usually lacking. Atrophy of the cerebellar cortex is limited to the anterior and superior lobules of the vermis and hemispheres, involving particularly the Purkinje cells. The dentate nucleus is not affected, the roof nuclei inconsistently; in contrast, the olivary nuclei are almost always heavily damaged. (Skillicorn, 1955; Victor, Adams, and Mancall, 1959.)

Another condition in which cerebellar atrophy occurs is *heat stroke*. The main clinical manifestations are ataxia of the limbs and dysarthria. These disturbances usually appear during the convalescence phase of the illness and may be temporary or permanent (Freeman and Dumoff, 1944). Cerebellar atrophy or cerebellitis may also occur in other conditions: *acute rheumatism* (Cruikshank, 1951), *ischemia and hypoxidosis* (Scholz, 1953), *atherosclerotic state, typhoid fever,* and *typhus* (Spielmeyer, 1922), *infectious mononucleosis* (Dowling and Van Slyck, 1966), *various intoxications or poisonings,* such as by lead, methyl mercury salts, manganese, and carbon monoxide (de Villaverde, 1927; Pentschew, 1958; Zülch, 1948), and sundry other pathological conditions (Victor, Adams, and Mancall, 1959).

Ataxia is a fairly common manifestation of *myxedema* and may be a presenting manifestation of the disease. It may occur suddenly or insidiously. The changes in the cerebellum are of a degenerative nature; moderate numbers of Purkinje cells disappear, especially from the vermis, and the granular layer becomes depleted of cells. Vessels are thickened. Rather numerous glycogen-containing "neural myxedema bodies" (resembling altered corpora amylacea) have been found in the cerebellar cortex and white matter and in other parts of the central nervous system (Price and Netsky, 1966). Broad-based ataxic gait is characteristic. Coordination tests of limbs frequently reveal ataxia. Dysarthria, nystagmus, and intention tremor carry a lower incidence, and in some series of cases are lacking. Peripheral neuropathy also occurs and includes involvement of the eighth nerve, as manifested by deafness; the neuropathy is attributed to mucinous deposits in the endoneurium and perineurium. Prompt and usually complete or nearly complete clearing of the ataxia is brought about with the use of thyroid hormone. In some instances the ataxia observed in hypothyroidism may be due not to the cerebellar disturbance under consideration but to some coexistent condition, such as familial spinocerebellar ataxia or diphenylhydantoin (Dilantin) toxicity. (Cremer and Paris, 1969; Jellinek and Kelly, 1960.)

One might assume that the most clear-cut clinical manifestations of cerebellar deficiency would be found in the total and partial aplasias and atrophies, since they do not produce irritative phenomena or signs of damage of adjacent extracerebellar structures. This is, however, usually not the case. Partial defects that render as much as half of the cerebellum functionless may remain clinically silent, while in extensive defects of both halves of the cerebellum the only disturbance may be ataxia.

Involvement of extracerebellar structures by cerebellar tumor, abscess, or hemorrhage

Manifestations of increased intracranial pressure. In cerebellar tumor, the intracranial pressure increases more frequently and more rapidly than in tumor in most other parts of the brain. The headache, caused by an increase in tension within the richly innervated tentorium cerebelli, is extraordinarily severe and deep-seated. Its site is in the region of the occiput and the back of the neck, and from here it usually radiates forward into the frontal region and downward into the trunk. The occipitonuchal headache is usually most intense on the same side as the lesion, while the frontal headache is diffuse. Stiffness of the neck is a fairly common accompaniment. Flexion of the head is more objectionable to the patient than extension. The occiput of the affected side is sometimes tender to pressure and to percussion. Pain may at times be elicited by applying pressure upward on the tip of the mastoid process of the affected side. The headache, which is intermittent in 90 percent of patients and continuous in the others, tends to be worst early in the morning and is aggravated by coughing, bodily effort, and a systemic infection. Throbbing as a feature of the headache is uncommon. (Wolff, 1948.)

Papilledema, usually bilateral, almost always occurs early and becomes marked.

In initial stages the blind spots enlarge, and later a concentric constriction of the fields occurs, and, ultimately, blindness (pp. 355 and 356).

Paralysis of the lateral rectus muscle, manifested by convergent squint, is fairly common and apparently results from pressure exerted upon the sixth nerve or from stretching of that nerve. The paralysis may be ipsilateral or contralateral to the lesion, or it may be bilateral. Thus the paralysis is of no lateralizing value.

Disturbances in conjugate ocular deviation. One of the more common "neighborhood" manifestations of an expanding cerebellar lesion (such as abscess) is weakness or paralysis of conjugate ocular gaze toward the side of the lesion. Persistent conjugate deviation of the eyes to the opposite side occasionally occurs. In early stages one may find, on the contrary, that conjugate deviation occurs toward the side of the lesion. This is a sign of irritation rather than of destruction (pp. 158 and 270).

Other cranial nerve disturbances. Anteriorly situated vermis tumors may cause fourth nerve palsy. Late in the clinical course, the seventh nerve may be implicated, giving rise to facial weakness. When occurring on one side the weakness is of lateralizing value. The eighth nerve may also be involved, but the reduction in hearing occurs late and is slight to moderate. The fifth nerve may also suffer, as manifested by hemihypalgesia of the face and loss of the corneal reflex ipsilaterally. The fifth nerve involvement is sometimes due to extension of the tumor to the pons by way of the brachium pontis. In rare instances, the bulbar cranial nerves are implicated later in the course, resulting in disturbances of phonation, respiration, deglutition, and articulation. Occasionally, either spasm or relaxation of the pylorus of the stomach is observed when the region of the dorsal nucleus of the tenth nerve is compressed by a cerebellar tumor. Sudden death is known to occur under such conditions.

Hemiplegia. Hemiplegia may develop either on the same side as the cerebellar tumor or on the opposite side, depending on whether a pyramid has been compressed above or below its decussation. Hemiplegia or quadriplegia may result from pressure exerted by expanding medulloblastoma.

Hypokinetic and hyperkinetic phenomena. Catatonic phenomena now and then are encountered in cerebellar abscess (p. 385). Acute cerebellar lesions, such as brought about by hemorrhage into the cerebellum or by rapidly expanding tumor, may occasionally be manifested by a turning of the trunk and head around their long axis or toward one side. Presumably the brachium conjunctivum or brachium pontis is implicated. There is no rule by which one can predict whether such movements will occur on the same side as the lesion or on the opposite side. Patients with cerebellar lesions may also exhibit unilateral choreoathetotic movements. These appear to be dependent upon associated or secondary alterations in the intramesencephalic part of brachium conjunctivum or in the mesencephalic tegmentum or both. Static tremor (tremor at rest) resulting from mesencephalic tegmental involvement may also occur in expanding cerebellar neoplasm or abscess.

Late in the clinical course in some cerebellar tumors, especially medulloblastoma, there may be *tonic seizures,* characterized by loss of consciousness, generalized muscular rigidity, retraction of the head, and opisthotonos. Such seizures, called "cerebellar fits," mimic the attitude of decerebration. Virtually every type of seizure has occasionally been noted in expanding cerebellar tumor. (Webster and Weinberger, 1940.)

"Frontal ataxia" and related disturbances

Ataxia and other "cerebellar" signs occur in a sizable proportion of cases in which the *frontal lobe* (or *lobes*) is damaged, whether the lesion be deep or superficial. Tumor is commonly responsible, not only frontal lobe tumor, but also temporal, parieto-occipital, occipital, suprasellar, thalamic, lenticular, or pineal tumor (Bing, 1925; Grant, 1928; Riese and Meredith, 1951). Meningioma in the region of the superior lateral surface of the frontal lobe rostral to the central sulcus has a strong tendency to induce "signs of ataxia," as noted by Frazier (1936) in 13 of 15 cases. The "ataxic disturbances" were bilateral in nine of the patients, contralateral to the meningioma in three, and ipsilateral in one. Further, in 49 percent of patients with frontal lobe tumor, he observed one or more of the following: staggering gait, Romberg sign, dyssynergia, difficulty in performing rapid alternating movements, dysmetria, and nystagmus.

In bilateral frontal lobe lesions the gait tends to be reeling and zigzag. In frontal lobe lesions occurring unilaterally, the patient, in walking forward, advances the contralateral foot awkwardly, usually setting it down too far laterally. Less frequently, he has the tendency during locomotion to place the contralateral foot in front of the normal foot. Occasionally a patient with "frontal ataxia" who is trying to stand still takes short, tripping steps backwards as though his center of gravity had been displaced in that direction. Practically all of these signs may also be noted in cerebellar lesions. There are, however, some points of distinction. In frontal lobe lesions, but not in cerebellar lesions, the Romberg sign is often elicitable. The dysmetria and dysdiadochokinesis so typical of cerebellar lesions are absent in about 40 percent of cases of frontal lobe lesions in which there is ataxia. Nystagmus is absent in frontal lobe lesions in about 65 percent of cases. Spontaneous tremor of the limbs commonly occurs in deep-seated frontal lobe lesions, which is another point of distinction. Past-pointing in frontal lobe lesions has also been described, especially in traumatic injuries, but in contrast to the past-pointing of cerebellar origin it is open to voluntary compensation. (Bruns, 1892.) The presence of a tonic plantar reflex, characteristic of frontal lobe lesions, is also helpful in differential diagnosis.

As to the basis of "frontal ataxia," most authors have considered it to be due to direct or indirect functional impairment of cerebellar structures brought about by way of the brachium pontis (frontopontocerebellar pathway), though without providing any histological backup or giving any clear reasons. In such cases Petrovici (1968) investigated the "postural set" in the initiation of gait by means of polymyographic recording ("postural set" referring to the postural change required for the initiation of a motor performance); he noted lack of initiative and motor spontaneity in almost all cases, also a delay in the appearance of muscular contraction and a dysharmonic distribution of the activity. Apraxia of gait and of trunk movements was postulated as the basis of "frontal ataxia."

Ataxia together with paresis of a lower limb, and occasionally of an upper limb as well, appearing acutely, constitutes a syndrome observed in *cerebral thrombosis* apparently occurring in the territory of supply of the lateral striate artery (or arteries) or of a branch of the anterior cerebral artery running to the corona radiata. Both the ataxia and the paresis occur on the side contralateral to the lesion. Striking dysmetria is noted both in the upper and the lower limb. The paresis in the lower limb is associated with an exaggerated knee jerk and the Babinski sign. These are the main changes observed on neurological examination. Transient "ischemic" attacks developing over a period of a few hours precede the stroke in some cases, while in others the stroke comes on without warning. Commonly noted at the onset are difficulty in walking and, on the same side, incoordination of the upper limb. Transient paresthesias, such as the feeling that the hand is swollen or the leg bandaged, also occur. The lower limb is weak, more so distally than proximally; in some cases only the toes and ankle are involved. Little or no weakness is encountered in the upper limb and none at all in the face. Sensibility is intact. The Romberg test is positive; the patient falls toward the affected side.

In a study of the brain in such a case, the responsible lesion was found in the upper part of the posterior limb of the internal capsule contralateral to the side of the stroke, the border zone between anterior and middle cerebral arteries being affected. The paracentral lobule was intact. The ataxia was thought to be attributable to direct involvement of corticopontile pathways. (Fisher and Cole, 1965.)

"Parietal ataxia"

Signs similar to those resulting from cerebellar lesions have also been noted occasionally in the presence of lesions involving the parietal lobe, namely, traumatic lesions (Claude and Lhermitte, 1916; Foix, Chavany, and Levy, 1927), abscess (Critchley, 1953; Thomas, 1918), tuberculoma (Foix and Thévenard, 1922), and infarct (Appenzeller and Hanson, 1966; Foix, Chavany, and Levy, 1927). The paracentral lobule was the main site of the lesion in some cases, the postcentral and adjacent parts of the parietal cortex in others, and the parietal lobe in general in still others. Signs of sensory impairment and corticospinal tract involvement were noted, except in Appenzeller and Hanson's case (1966) in which neither was observed. Incoordination of movement was the chief if not the only "cerebellar" sign in all these cases. The disturbance, easily brought out by testing, occurred in a contralateral limb or limbs. Severe apraxia on dressing was noted in one instance (for example, great difficulty in maneuvering a jacket with one sleeve turned inside out in order to get it on) (Appenzeller and Hanson, 1966), raising the question as to whether "parietal ataxia" could represent a form of apraxia.

REFERENCES

Abbott, K. H., and Kernohan, J. W. 1943. Medulloblastomas: concerning the problems of spinal metastasis and malignancy: a report of six cases and discussion of the problems involved. Bull. Los Angeles Neurol. Soc. **8**:1-10.

Appenzeller, O., and Hanson, J. C. 1966. Parietal ataxia. Arch. Neurol. **15**:264-274.

Bailey, P., and Cushing, H. 1925. Medulloblastoma cerebelli: a common type of midcerebellar glioma of childhood. Arch. Neurol. Psychiat. **14**:192-224.

Bing, R. 1911. Die Meningitis cystica serosa der hinteren Schädelgrube. Med. Klin. **1**:207-211.

Bing, R. 1912. Die Lokalisation der Kleinhirnerkrankungen, Deutsch. Med. Wschr. **38**:881-884.

Bing, R. 1925. Séminologie des affections cérébelleuses. Schweiz. Arch. Neurol. Psychiat. **16**:3-26.

Brain, W. R., Daniel, P. M., and Greenfield, J. G. 1951. Subacute cortical cerebellar degeneration and its relation to carcinoma. J. Neurol. Neurosurg. Psychiat. **14**:59-75.

Braitenberg, V. 1967. Is the cerebellar cortex a biological clock in the millisecond range? Progr. Brain Res. **25**:334-346.

Bruns, L. 1892. Ueber Störungen des Gleichgewichtes bei Stirnhirntumoren. Deutsch. Med. Wschr. **18**:138-140.

Carpenter, M. B., and Strominger, N. L. 1964. Cerebello-oculomotor fibers in the rhesus monkey. J. Comp. Neurol. **123**:211-229.

Claude, H., and Lhermitte, J. 1916. Les paraplégies cérébello-spasmodique et ataxo-cérébello-spasmodique consécutives aux lésions bilatérales des lobules paracentraux par projectiles de guerre. Bull. Soc. Méd. Hôp. Paris **40**:796-804.

Cogan, D. G. 1954. Ocular dysmetria; flutter-like oscillations of the eyes, and opsoclonus. Arch. Ophthal. **51**:318-335.

Cremer, G. M., Goldstein, N. P., and Paris, J. 1969. Myxedema and ataxia. Neurology **19**: 37-46.

Critchley, M. 1953. The parietal lobes. Baltimore, The Williams & Wilkins Company, p. 480.

Cruickshank, E. K. 1951. Hyperpyrexia with cerebellar damage in acute rheumatism. Lancet **1**: 1052-1053.

de Villaverde, J. M. 1927. Lesions du cervelet dans l'intoxication par le plomb. Tr. Lab. Invest. Biol. Univ. Madrid **25**:41-79.

Dow, R. S., and Moruzzi, G. 1958. The physiology and pathology of the cerebellum. Minneapolis, University of Minnesota Press.

Dowling, M. D., Jr., and Van Slyck, E. J. 1966. Cerebellar disease in infectious mononucleosis. Arch. Neurol. **15**:270-274.

Dyken, P., and Kolář, O. 1968. Dancing eyes, dancing feet: infantile polymyoclonia. Brain **91**: 305-320.

Eccles, J. C., Ito, M., and Szentágothai, J. 1967. The cerebellum as a neuronal machine. New York, Springer-Verlag.

Ellenberger, C., Jr., Campa, J. F., and Netsky, M. G. 1968. Opsoclonus and parenchymatous degeneration of the cerebellum: the cerebellar origin of abnormal movement. Neurology **18**: 1041-1046.

Fisher, C. M., and Cole, M. 1965. Homolateral ataxia and crural paresis: a vascular syndrome. J. Neurol. Neurosurg. Psychiat. **28**:48-55.

Foix, C., Chavany, J. A., and Levy, M. 1927. Syndrome pseudothalamique d'origine pariétale. Rev. Neurol. **1**:68-76.

Foix and Thévenard. 1922. Symptômes pseudocérébelleux d'origine cérébrale, tubercle de la région paracentrale postérieure. Rev. Neurol. **29**:1502-1504.

Frazier, C. 1936. Tumor involving the frontal lobe alone. Arch. Neurol. Psychiat. **35**:525-571.

Freeman, W., and Dumoff, E. 1944. Cerebellar syndrome following heat stroke. Arch. Neurol. Psychiat. **51**:67-72.

Grant, F. C. 1928. Cerebellar symptoms produced by supratentorial tumors: a further report. Arch. Neurol. Psychiat. **20**:292-308.

Greenfield, J. G. 1954. The spino-cerebellar degenerations. Oxford, Blackwell Scientific Publications Ltd., p. 5.

Holmes, G. 1922. Clinical symptoms of cerebellar disease and their interpretation. Lancet **1**:1172-1182; **2**:111-115.

Holmes, G. 1939. The cerebellum of man. Brain **62**:1-30.

Holmes, G., and Stewart, F. G. 1908. On the connections of the inferior olives with the cerebellum in man. Brain **31**:125-137.

Jansen, J. 1954. Efferent cerebellar connections. In Jansen, J., and Brodal, A., editors: Aspects of cerebellar anatomy. Oslo, Johan Grundt Tanum, pp. 189-248.

Jansen, J., and Brodal, A. 1954. Aspects of cerebellar anatomy. Oslo, Johan Grundt Tanum.

Jellinek, E. H., and Kelly, R. E. 1960. Cerebellar syndrome in myxoedema. Lancet **2**:225-227.

Kuypers, H. G. J. M., Fleming, W. R., and Farinholt, J. W. 1962. Subcorticospinal projection in the Rhesus monkey. J. Comp. Neurol. **118**:107-137.

Kuypers, H. G. J. M., and Lawrence, D. G. 1967. Cortical projections to the red nucleus and the brain stem in the Rhesus monkey. Brain Res. **4**:151-188.

Manni, E., Azzena, G. B., and Dow, R. S. 1965. Cerebellar influence on the unitary discharge of oculomotor nuclei and adjacent structures. Exp. Neurol. **13**:252-263.

Mehler, W. R. 1965. A comparison of cerebellar projections to vestibular, reticular and diencephalic nuclei in the monkey, cat, and rat. Proc. 8th Int. Congr. Anat. Stuttgart, Georg Thieme Verlag, p. 63.

Mehler, W. R., Vernier, V. G., and Nauta, W. J. H. 1958. Efferent projections from dentate and interpositus nuclei in primates. Anat. Rec. **130**:430-431.

Niemer, W. T., and Magoun, H. W. 1947. Reticulospinal tracts influencing motor activity. J. Comp. Neurol. **87**:367-379.

O'Connell, J. E. A. 1953. The cerebrospinal fluid pressure as an aetological factor in the development of lesions affecting the central nervous system. Brain **76**:279-298.

Papez, J. W., and Stotler, W. A. 1940. Connections of the red nucleus. Arch. Neurol. Psychiat. **44**:776-791.

Pentschew, A. 1958. Intoxikationen. In Lubarsch, O., Henke, F., and Rössle, R., editors: Handbuch der Speziellen Pathologischen Anatomie und Histologie, vol. 13 (edited by Scholz, W.), pt. 1B. Berlin, Springer-Verlag, pp. 1907-2502.

Petrovici, I. 1968. Apraxia of gait and of trunk movements. J. Neurol. Sci. **7**:229-244.

Pompeiano, O. 1967. Functional organization of the cerebellar projections to the spinal cord. Progr. Brain Res. **25**:282-321.

Poór, G. 1967. Über hypertonische Kleinhirnblutungen. Acta Med. Acad. Sci. Hung. **24**:81-88.

Price, T. R., and Netsky, M. G. 1966. Myxedema and ataxia: cerebellar alterations and "neural myxedema bodies." Neurology **16**:957-962.

Probst, M. 1901. Zur Kenntnis des Bindearmes, der Haubenstrahlung und der Regio subthalamica. Mschr. Psychiat. Neurol. **10**:288-309.

Rand, R. W. 1954. An anatomical and experimental study of the cerebellar nuclei and their efferent pathways in the monkey. J. Comp. Neurol. **101**:167-223.

Riese, W., and Meredith, J. M. 1951. Clinically unsuspected carcinoma of the lung with multiple metastatic lesion in the brain; neurologic findings not readily explained by location of metastases in the brain. J. Neuropath. Clin. Neurol. **1**:278-284.

Ross, A. T., and Zeman, W. 1967. Opsoclonus, occult carcinoma, and chemical pathology in dentate nuclei. Arch. Neurol. **17**:546-551.

Scholz, W. 1953. Selective neuronal necrosis and its topistic patterns in hypoxemia and oligemia. J. Neuropath. Exp. Neurol. **12**:249-261.

Schut, J. W., and Haymaker, W. 1951. Hereditary ataxia: a pathologic study of five cases of common ancestry. J. Neuropath. Clin. Neurol. **1**:183-213.

Skillicorn, S. A. 1955. Presenile cerebellar ataxia in chronic alcoholics. Neurology **5**:527-534.

Snider, R. S. 1967. Functional alterations of cerebral sensory areas by the cerebellum. Progr. Brain Res. **25**:322-333.

Spielmeyer, W. 1922. Histopathologie des Nervensystems. Berlin, Springer-Verlag, pp. 382-389.

Szentágothai, J. 1964. Pathways and synaptic articulation patterns connecting vestibular receptors and oculomotor nuclei. In Bender, M. B., editor: The oculomotor system. New York, Harper & Row, Publishers, pp. 205-223.

Thomas, A. 1918. Etude sur les blessures du cervelette. Paris, Vigot Frères.

Tyler, D. B., and Bard, P. 1949. Motion sickness. Physiol. Rev. **29**:311-369.

Vick, N., Schulman, S., and Dau, P. 1969. Carcinomatous cerebellar degeneration, encephalomyelitis, and sensory neuropathy (radiculitis). Neurology **19**:425-441.

Victor, M. 1965. The effects of nutritional deficiency on the nervous system: a comparison with the effects of carcinoma. In Brain, W. R., and Norris, F. H., Jr., editors: The remote effects of cancer of the nervous system. New York, Grune & Stratton, Inc.

Victor, M., Adams, R. D., and Mancall, E. L. 1959. A restricted form of cerebellar cortical degeneration occurring in alcoholic patients. Arch. Neurol. **1**:579-688.

Walberg, F. 1954. Descending connections to the inferior olive. In Jansen, J., and Brodal, A.,

editors: Aspects of cerebellar anatomy. Oslo, Johan Grundt Tanum, pp. 249-263.
Walker, A. E. 1938. The thalamus of the chimpanzee. Confin. Neurol. **1**:99-127.
Walker, A. E., and Botterell, E. H. 1937. The syndrome of the superior cerebellar peduncle in the monkey. Brain **60**:329-353.
Wartenberg, R. 1954. Cerebellar signs. J.A.M.A. **156**:102-105.
Webster, J. E., and Weinberger, L. M. 1940. Convulsions associated with tumors of the cerebellum: clinical and pathophysiologic features. Arch. Neurol. Psychiat. **43**:1163-1184.
Wolff, H. G. 1948. Headache and other head pain. New York, Oxford University Press, Inc., p. 587.
Zülch, K. J. 1948. Über die anatomische Stellung der Kleinhirnrindenatrophie und ihre Beziehung zur Nonne-Marieschen Krankheit. Deutsch. Z. Nervenheilk. **159**:501-513.

Chapter 18

Syndromes of arterial occlusion, circulatory insufficiency, and aneurysms in the region of the brainstem and cerebellum

The brainstem (medulla oblongata, pons, and midbrain) and the cerebellum receive their blood supply chiefly from the two vertebral arteries, the basilar artery, and the two posterior cerebral arteries (Fig. 18-1). A subsidiary blood supply reaches the upper midbrain by way of the anterior choroidal and posterior communicating arteries.

Syndromes resulting from occlusion of any one of these arteries tend to differ in nature because of variations in arterial origin and distribution, degree of anastomosis between arterial beds, and extent of arterial occlusion. Because of these factors, some of the syndromes will be considered in terms of regions of the brainstem involved rather than in terms of specific vessels occluded.

Syndromes of arterial *occlusion* are presented in the following pages. The term "occlusion" is used for ease in description. The tissue infarction giving rise to these syndromes may be caused not only by arterial occlusion resulting from the formation of a thrombus or the lodgement of an embolus but also by arterial stenosis; the infarction may also be due to circulatory insufficiency unrelated to occlusion or stenosis. This is brought out in connection with cerebral arterial syndromes (Chapter 27), and what is said there applies also to some of the syndromes described in the present chapter.

VERTEBRAL ARTERIES

The vertebral arteries normally arise from the subclavian artery. In its extracranial course the vertebral artery gives off vessels that supply upper segments of the spinal cord (Fig. 1-9). In its course from the atlas to the foramen magnum (during which it traverses the dura), the artery is S-shaped. While in the foramen magnum, it gives off branches for the supply of the dura of the posterior cranial fossa, including the tentorium cerebelli.

The two vertebrals run along the ventral surface of the medulla oblongata, between the rootlets of the twelfth nerve and the anterior roots of spinal segment C1. They terminate at the lower border of the pons by uniting to form the basilar artery. The main branches of the vertebral artery are the anterior spinal, the posterior spinal, and the posterior inferior cerebellar arteries (Figs. 1-9 and 18-1).

The arteries irrigating the medulla oblongata may be subdivided into two main groups, the paramedian bulbar and the lateral bulbar. A third group is the posterior bulbar, given off by the posterior inferior cerebellar artery and supplying the inferior cerebellar peduncle and the adjoining posterolateral part of the medulla oblongata.

Paramedian bulbar syndromes

The paramedian part of the medulla oblongata receives its blood supply from slender arteries branching from the anterior spinal, the vertebral, and the basilar arteries (Figs. 18-1 and 18-2). Occlusion of paramedian branches of the vertebrals or of branches of the anterior spinal (or of the anterior spinal artery itself) is characterized by paralysis of the tongue of the ipsilateral side and hemiplegia involving the contralateral side *(hemiplegia alternans infima),* with predominant involvement of the upper limb. Quadriplegia sometimes occurs. In some cases there is transitory contralateral hypesthesia (involving tactile and deep sensibility). Occlusion of twigs from the anterior spinal artery may give rise to *hemiplegia cruciata* (p. 150). Some of the paramedian branches supply the medial lemniscus. If they are occluded, there will be ataxia and a reduction of deep sensibility either unilaterally or bilaterally. Now and then, horizontal or, rarely, vertical nystagmus occurs. (Davison, 1944; Davison, Goodhart, and Savitsky, 1935; Hiller, 1952; O'Brien and Bender, 1945.)

Lateral bulbar syndrome

The lateral part of the medulla oblongata is supplied superiorly by branches from the lower part of the basilar artery, and inferiorly by the posterior inferior cerebellar artery. When the latter artery is absent (as it is in 10 to 25 percent of cases), all the lateral part of the medulla oblongata is supplied by small branches (short circumferential arteries) coming from the basilar and vertebral arteries and occasionally from the

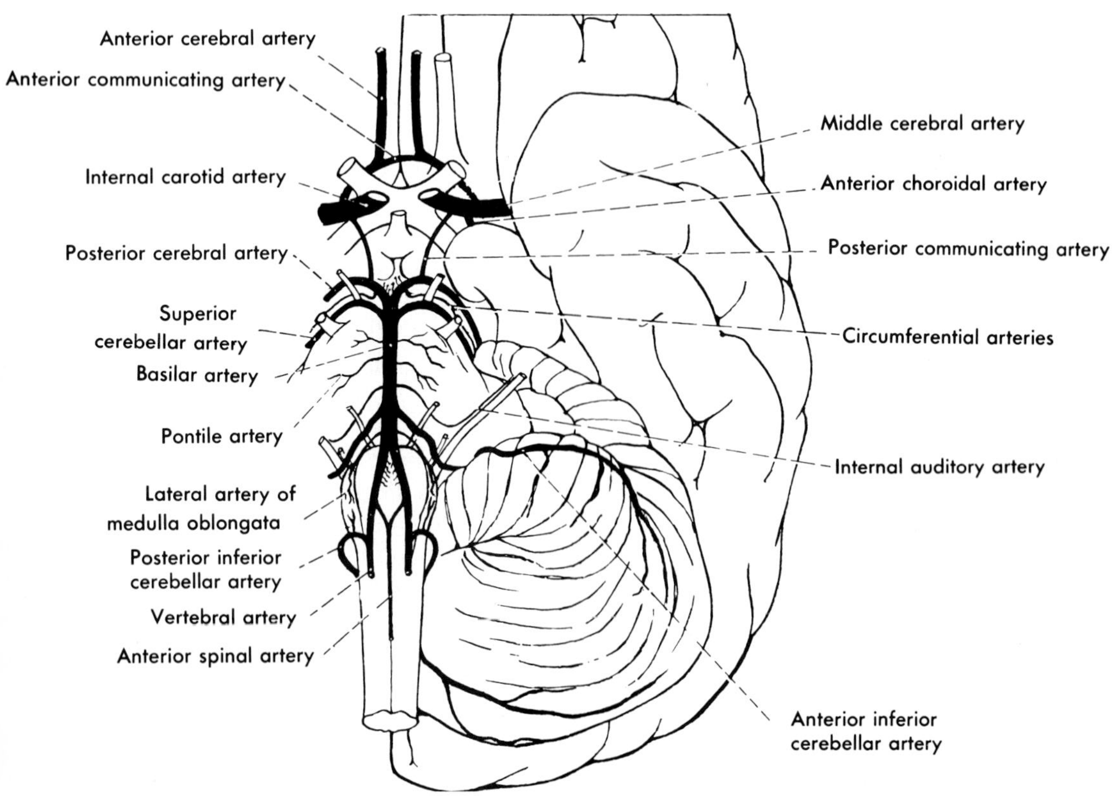

Fig. 18-1. Arteries at the base of the brain and brainstem, including the arterial circle of Willis.

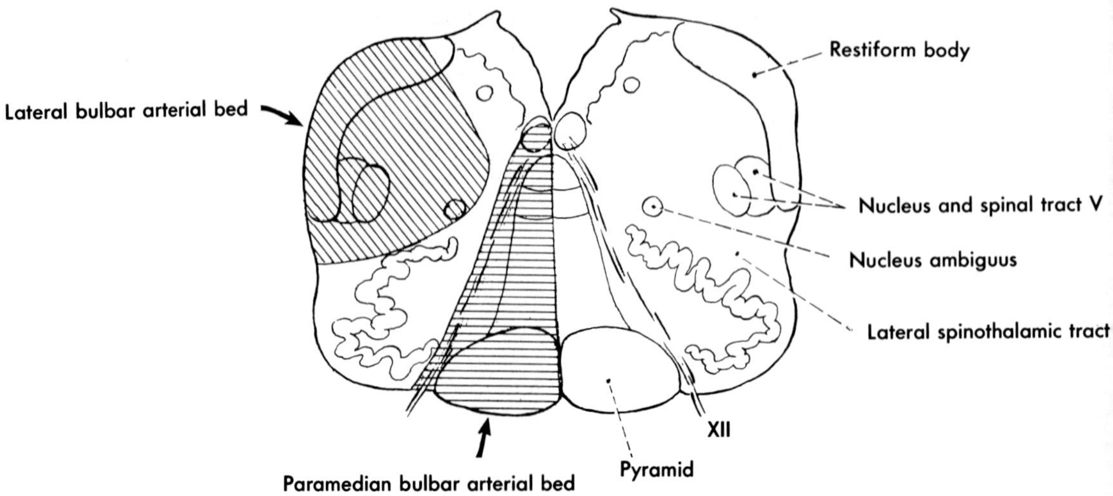

Fig. 18-2. The lateral bulbar and paramedian bulbar arterial beds.

anterior inferior cerebellar artery. The posterior inferior cerebellar artery usually arises fom the vertebral, about 1.5 cm. caudal to the level where the two vertebrals unite to form the basilar artery (Fig. 18-1), but it sometimes originates from the lower part of the basilar. After curving laterally just caudal to the twelfth nerve, it passes dorsalward, giving off branches to the lateral side of the medulla oblongata, and then extends to the cerebellum, where it divides into branches that ramify in the inferior vermis and the inferior part of the hemisphere. Other branches reach the emboliform and globose nuclei (Lazorthes, 1961) and possibly the fastigial nucleus as well. The posterior inferior cerebellar artery also gives off a branch to the choroid plexus of the fourth ventricle. (Baker, 1961; Hiller, 1952.)

Since the arterial branches reaching the lateral part of the medulla oblongata are numerous and their sources varied, infarcted areas within the irrigated field will vary in distribution and size. The retro-olivary area extending laterally to the surface of the medulla oblongata is most frequently infarcted, and then more commonly in its caudal than in its rostral part. To be held accountable in most cases is thrombosis of the vertebral artery or arteriosclerosis of the vertebral artery involving the site of origin of the posterior inferior cerebellar artery or of smaller vertebral or basilar arterial branches.

Vascular occlusion involving much of the lateral bulbar area is usually characterized by sudden onset, with dizziness or vertigo the chief symptoms. Headache also occurs, the pain being situated in the eye, nose, and/or cheek; aching occurs in the suboccipital region (Fisher, 1968). Often the person falls to the ground. Consciousness is seldom disturbed. Vomiting usually occurs and is nonprojectile. Dysesthesias occur in the upper part of the face ipsilaterally; pains occur less frequently. Difficulty in swallowing is characteristic and may be one of the initial complaints. Power of phonation is greatly reduced to the extent that the patient may speak only in a whisper. Diplopia is a common complaint. Rotary or horizontal nystagmus almost invariably occurs and is most pronounced when the eyes are turned toward the side of the lesion; the rapid movement is also toward that side. Hiccup is fairly common. Hypotonia and ataxia of the ipsilateral limbs, especially the upper, are also characteristic. Lateropulsion may be noted from the beginning, the patient falling to the side when he attempts to sit up (Bjerver and Silfverskiöld, 1968).

Examination in the period within a week after the infarction usually discloses paralysis of the ipsilateral soft palate, pharynx, and vocal cord. Slight weakness commonly occurs in the limbs, usually ipsilateral to the lesion but occasionally contralaterally; the Babinski sign is elicitable in as many as 40 percent of cases. Facial weakness ipsilaterally also occurs. Dissociated anesthesia of the ipsilateral side of the face (analgesia and thermoanesthesia with preserved tactile sensibility) is evident in most cases. Occasionally the contralateral side of the face is similarly affected (from involvement of the crossed quintothalamic tract). Tactile sensibility is affected slightly, if at all. (Alexander and Suh, 1937; Foix, Hillemand, and Schalit, 1925; Lewis, Littman, and Foley, 1952; Merritt and Finland, 1930; Stopford, 1916; Wallenberg, 1895, 1901.)

Dissociated anesthesia (pain and temperature appreciation lost but tactile sensibility preserved) involves not only the ipsilateral side of the face but also the contralateral side of the body and limbs. The sensory defect is of irregular distribution, not of segmental type, and can be such that two lesions—one involving the medulla oblongata and the other the spinal cord—may be suspected. For example, there may be: (1) initial loss of pain and temperature sensibility over half of the body, then resolution, with the upper level of the sensory defect retreating to the upper trunk, and the lower level retreating half way down the thigh; (2) the same, with only a band-like sensory defect remaining in the upper trunk; (3) sensory loss in the limbs, not in the trunk; (4) a larger area of thermal loss than of pain loss. (Currier, Giles, and DeJong, 1961; Soffin, Feldman, and Bender, 1968.)

Facial pain ipsilateral to the lesion occurs in a considerable proportion of patients in early stages after the infarction, while pain in the contralateral trunk and limbs occurs less commonly. The pain in the face is burning or stinging and is also described as "unbearable" or as "soreness." Occasionally it is referred to as "thalamic" pain.

Ipsilateral Horner's syndrome occurs in most cases; miosis is most frequent, ptosis uncommon, and "enophthalmos" rare (Currier, Giles, and DeJong, 1961; Sheehan and Smyth, 1937). There may also be vasodilatation and lack of sweating in the region of the face and body ipsilaterally and an increase in sweating on the opposite side. Although the pulse may be normal or slowed, it is usually accelerated. Glycosuria, with as much as 2 percent sugar in the urine, has been observed shortly after onset of the occlusion, with albuminuria an additional feature (Müller, 1906).

For a discussion of partial syndromes, see Currier, Giles, and DeJong (1961).

Disturbances having the greatest tendency to persist over weeks or longer are: lateropulsion together with staggering on walking (Bjerver and Silfverskiöld, 1968), pain in the face on the side of the infarction, loss of pain and temperature sensibility in the ipsilateral side of the face and contralateral side of the body and limbs, nystagmus (slight), diplopia, difficulty in phonation, Horner's syndrome, and loss of sweating on the ipsilateral side of the face and body (Currier, Giles, and DeJong, 1961).

Syndromes of occlusion of branches of the vertebral artery

Each of the vertebral arteries sends a few twigs to the paramedian region of the medulla oblongata, irrigating the area between the inferior olivary nucleus and pyramid (Fig. 18-2). The syndrome of occlusion of these twigs is discussed on pages 153 and 295.

In the event of thrombosis, the clinical features of occlusion of the vertebral artery itself will vary depending on whether the thrombus has propagated into the posterior inferior cerebellar artery or the basilar artery. Steady increase in the severity of the signs indicates enlargement of the initial field of infarction. Occlusion of the vertebral artery may, in acute stages, be accompanied by conjugate deviation of the eyes toward the side of the lesion together with nystagmus, which may be horizontal on one side and rotatory on the other (Thompson, 1929).

Syndrome of total occlusion of the vertebral artery

Onset of total occlusion is sudden and characterized by vertigo so severe that the patient falls to the ground. Vomiting is common. Spontaneous coarse nystagmus, usually toward the side of the lesion, almost invariably occurs, and there is ataxia and hypotonia of the ipsilateral limbs, especially the upper, which renders them useless. These initial disorders indicate involvement of the region of vestibular nuclei and of the dorsal nucleus of the tenth nerve, and of the restiform body and cerebellum. Consciousness is usually preserved. Characteristic are pain and dysesthesias in the face, most often of the upper part, indicating involvement of the spinal nucleus and tract of the fifth nerve. Moreover, there is dissociated anesthesia, with postural and tactile sensibility preserved on both sides (the medial lemniscus is spared) and appreciation of pain and temperature stimuli decreased or lost on the contralateral side of the body (through involvement of the lateral spinothalamic tract). The neck and upper thorax are frequently spared because of the medial position of their fibers in the lateral spinothalamic tract (Fig. 11-3). In the face, dissociated anesthesia ipsilaterally is usually found, with the ophthalmic division and/or the maxillary division most affected. In addition, there are paralysis of the ipsilateral vocal cord, dysarthria, and dysphagia, all resulting from involvement of the nucleus ambiguus. The diminished pharyngeal sensibility is attributed to involvement of the nucleus and tractus solitarius by the lesion. Ipsilateral miosis is frequent because of interruption of sympathetic fibers descending in the reticular formation. Ptosis is, however, uncommon. Vasodilatation involving the ipsilateral side of the face and body often occurs, and it may be followed in later stages by vasoconstriction and loss of sweating. (Böhne, 1927; Foix and Hillemand, 1925; Goodhart and Davison, 1936; Hiller, 1952.)

Occlusion of one vertebral artery through ligation performed for the control of vertebral artery aneurysm has frequently been accomplished without ill effects. *Occlusion of both vertebrals* is, however, rapidly fatal, at least when the occlusion is sudden. Such a case was reported by Dandy (1944). One vertebral artery had been successfully ligated in an effort to control tortuous arteriosclerotic aneurysms of the vertebral and basilar arteries. Subsequently an attempt was made to ligate the other vertebral artery. "Before the vessel was ligated it was compressed with the forceps for perhaps two seconds and then released. Death was immediate. Pulse and respiration ceased, and despite release of the compression and artificial respiration there was no return of pulse or breathing. There could be no more speedy death."

Syndrome associated with disease of cervical vertebrae

In its passage through the foramina in the transverse processes of the cervical vertebrae, the vertebral artery normally runs a straight course. However, the vessel may be considerably distorted in the presence of vertebral disease in this region, particularly spondylosis, in which osteoarthritic protuberances may displace the vertebral artery by more than 1 cm. Greater displacement occurs when the head is moved (Yates and Hutchinson, 1961). This is the background on which occipital headache, nystagmus, slight dysarthria, and (transient) abnormal plantar response may occur on extension or rotation of the head, in subjects with cerebral arteriosclerosis (Biemond, 1951).

Effects of aneurysm of the vertebral artery

In aneurysm of the vertebral artery, varied syndromes may result from pressure exerted on the medulla oblongata and/or by circulatory insufficiency brought about by altered hemodynamics. The disturbances are chiefly bulbar. There may be violent episodes of vertigo, unilateral tinnitus, and deafness, and diminished corneal reflex, ataxia, dysarthria, dysphagia, and unilateral anesthesia. The pulse may become irregular, and respiratory embarrassment may prove fatal. (Bassoe, 1939; Dial and Maurer, 1937.)

BASILAR ARTERY

The basilar artery, formed by the union of the two vertebral arteries, arises at the lower border of the pons, extends upward in the median groove of the pons, and terminates at the upper edge of the pons by dividing into the two posterior cerebral arteries. Phylogenetically, the basilar artery is derived from two independent arteries which have fused (Critchley, 1930), but in about 10 percent of brains the doubling persists.

The basilar artery gives off a number of branches, as follows.

Anterior inferior cerebellar artery

Constant (present in 96 percent of brains), but highly variable in its origin, the anterior inferior cerebellar artery may branch from the vertebral or from the basilar jointly with the posterior inferior cerebellar artery, but it usually arises as an independent vessel from the proximal third of the basilar artery (Fig. 18-1).

When originating from the basilar or the vertebral artery, the anterior inferior cerebellar artery extends lateralward across the pons, and in the cerebellopontile angle it passes just rostral to the root of the eighth nerve. In the region of the porus acusticus it lies in close relation both to the eighth and the seventh nerve. Here, the vessel (in 39 percent of brains according to Sunderland, 1945, and in a much smaller percentage according to Rhoton, Kobayashi, and Hollinshead, 1968) descends for a short distance into the internal auditory meatus, gives off the internal auditory artery, then turns on itself and emerges from the canal. Again in the cerebellopontile angle, the artery divides into two branches, a medial and a lateral (though variations exist; Lazorthes, 1961). The *medial* branch courses caudal to the flocculus, then along the medial border of the hemisphere, while the *lateral* branch (not shown in Fig. 18-1) passes along the rostral edge of the flocculus, then on to the brachium pontis, then the surface of the adjoining part of the hemisphere. The artery supplies the anterior and adjoining inferior aspects of the cerebellar hemispheres, including the flocculus. Vessels are given off to the restiform body, the caudal third of the lateral pontile tegmentum, the dorsolateral part of the rostralmost medulla oblongata, and the caudal part of the brachium pontis (Fig. 18-3). Included in the region of irrigation are the lateral spinothalamic tract, lateral lemniscus, vestibular nuclei, cochlear nuclei, nucleus of the spinal tract of the fifth nerve, and the intramedullary fibers of the seventh nerve.

Since in some brains the lateral pontile arteries share the supply of lateral pontile tegmentum with the anterior inferior cerebellar artery, the richness of the anastomosis between the two beds may be such that the manifestations of anterior inferior cerebellar artery occlusion are few. The posterior inferior cerebellar artery also comes into consideration, for when its capillary bed is small the area of infarction following anterior inferior cerebellar artery occlusion can be correspondingly large.

In a fairly large proportion of cases of occlusion of the anterior inferior cerebellar artery, the onset of symptoms is fulminant and marked by nausea and vomiting, vertigo, nystagmus, and ipsilateral tinnitus. Consciousness is seldom disturbed. Blood pressure is usually raised. When complete, the syndrome includes *contralateral* hypalgesia and thermohypesthesia of the trunk and limbs, and *ipsilateral* loss of pain and ther-

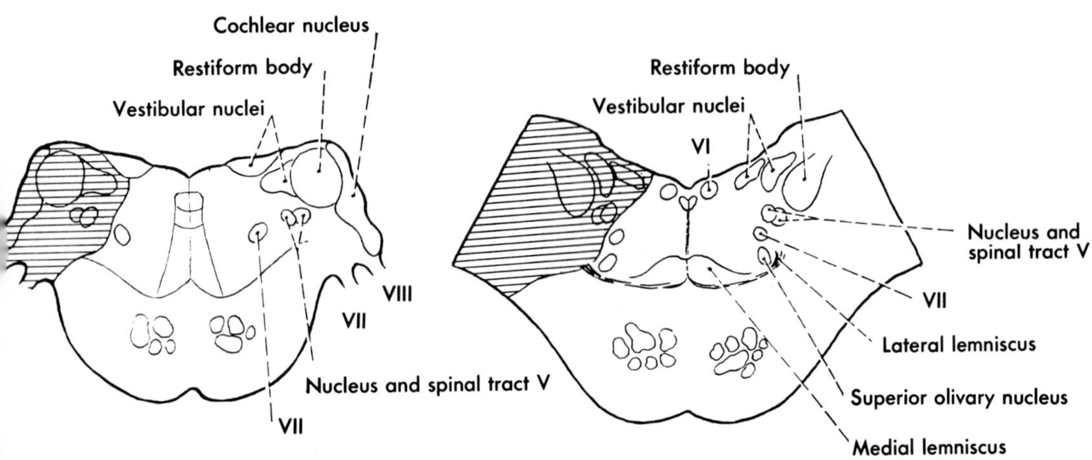

Fig. 18-3. Area of supply of the anterior inferior cerebellar artery.

mal sensibility of trigeminal distribution, facial paralysis, deafness, Horner's syndrome, ataxia, and other signs of cerebellar deficiency. (Adams, 1943; Atkinson, 1949; Hitselberger and House, 1966; Sunderland, 1945.)

A middle inferior cerebellar artery is frequently present. It arises from the middle third of the basilar artery. It is conspicuous in brains in which the anterior inferior cerebellar artery is absent. In its course lateralward, this vessel usually comes to lie near the root of the fifth nerve, but may pass between the roots of the seventh and eighth nerves. It supplies the flocculus and a variable portion of the tonsil and cerebellar hemisphere. (Hiller, 1936; Lazorthes, Poulhès, and Espagno, 1950a, b; Lindenberg, 1955.)

Internal auditory artery

This vessel, also called the *labyrinthine artery,* springs directly from the basilar artery in most brains (Fig. 18-1) and from the anterior inferior cerebellar artery in the remainder. Hypacusis is a common manifestation of occlusion of the internal auditory artery (Stopford, 1916; Sunderland, 1945).

Pontile arteries

Smaller branches of the basilar artery reaching the pons may be subdivided as follows (Figs. 18-4 and 18-5):

Paramedian branches. At all pontile levels these branches irrigate the more medial part of the pars basilaris (pontile nuclei, corticobulbar and corticospinal tracts, and, depending on the level, corticopontile fibers) and, in the upper third of the pons, the tegmentum as well.

Lateral branches. These supply the brachium pontis and the ventral half of the intermediate area of the tegmentum. Occasionally they supply the motor and the main sensory nucleus of the fifth nerve. Both the paramedian and the lateral branches supply rather minor parts of the medial lemniscus.

Paramedian pons syndrome. In the field of supply of the paramedian arteries, focal lesions due to vascular disease are common and are often limited to the more dorsal part of the pars basilaris pontis (Stern, 1935). Rarely, a lesion thus induced is more or less limited to pyramidal bundles (in the form of a large lacuna), giving rise contralaterally to paresis, then spasticity, of the limbs and paresis of the tongue (Brown and Fang, 1961; Fisher and Curry, 1965).

Larger lesions also give rise to contra-

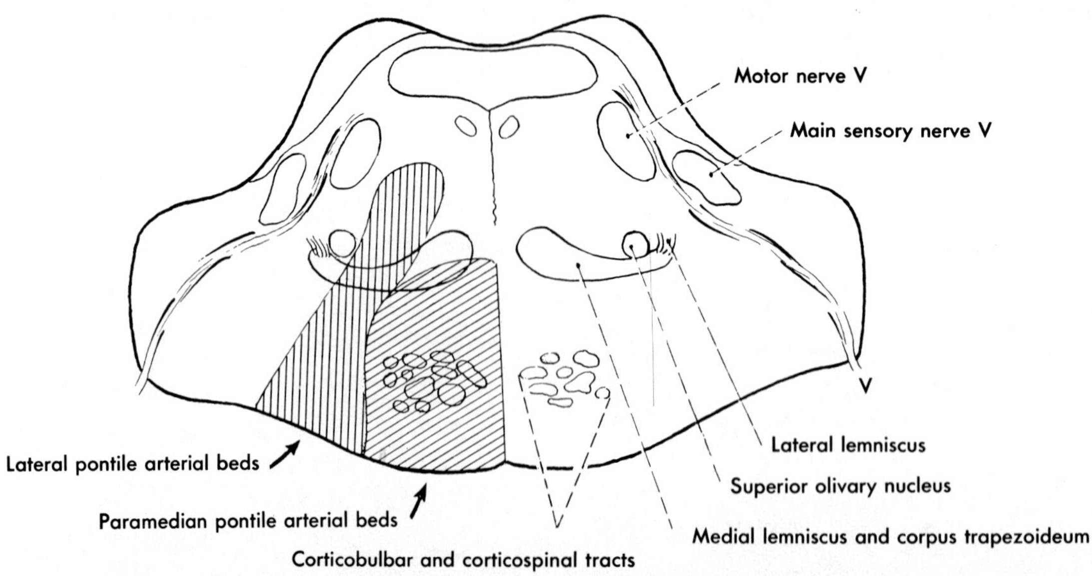

Fig. 18-4. Areas of supply of the paramedian pontile and lateral pontile branches of the basilar artery.

lateral hemiparesis, at first flaccid and later spastic. Not uncommonly the paresis is limited to a lower limb. Contralateral hemianesthesia occurs only in initial stages. A characteristic feature is that even when hemiplegia is sudden and severe, consciousness is preserved. Now and then the pontile lesions are bilateral, in which case paraplegia occurs. Manifestations of pyramidal tract involvement may disappear and then recur. Observed occasionally in tegmental lesions is conjugate ocular deviation to the contralateral side.

Lateral pons syndrome. In its pure form, this uncommon syndrome is characterized chiefly by ipsilateral cerebellar disturbances owing to involvement of pontocerebellar fibers. To be noted on the involved side is generalized hypotonia, a tendency to fall to that side when stand-

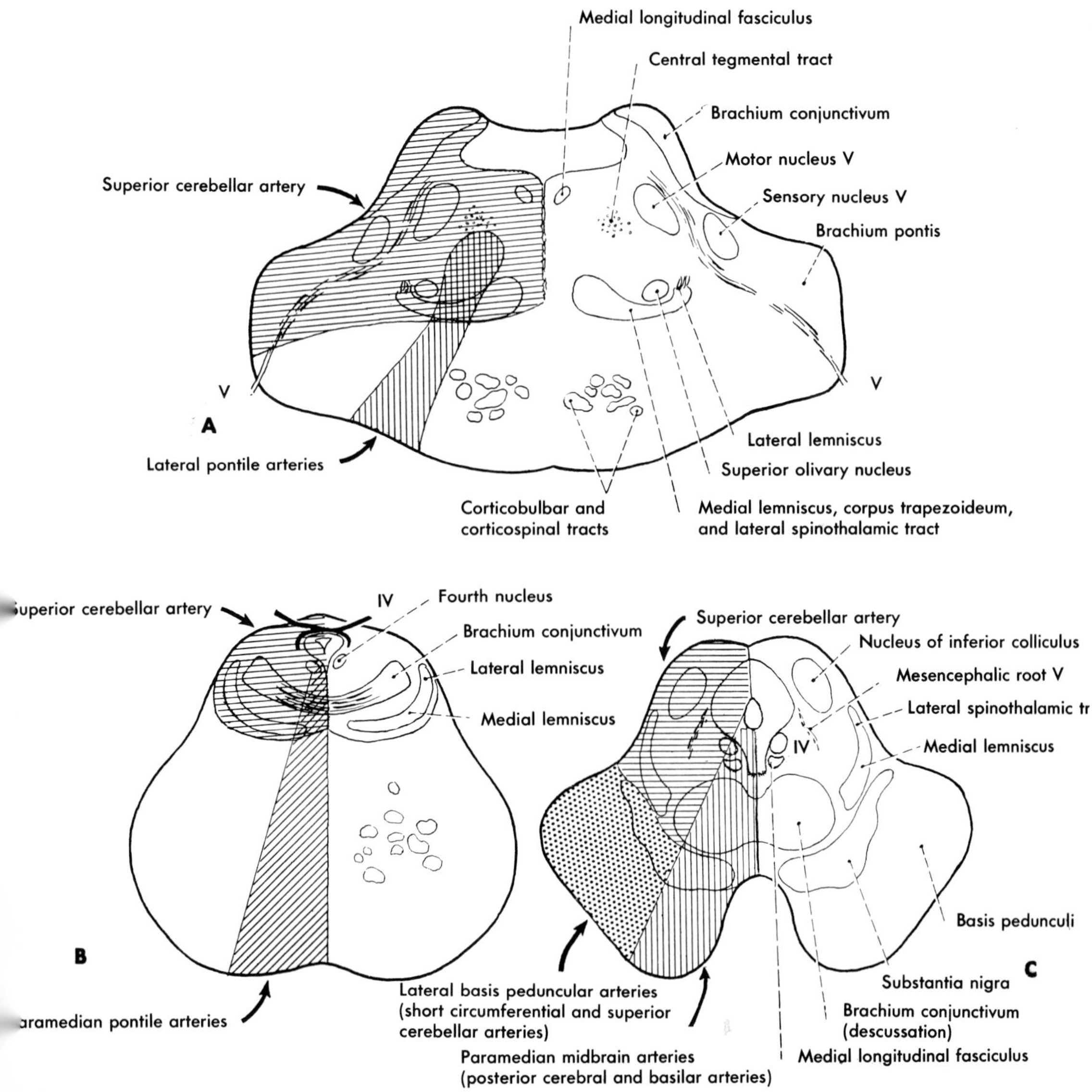

Fig. 18-5. The area of supply of the lateral pontile branches of the basilar artery is shown in **A**, and of the paramedian pontile branches in **B**. The regions of superior cerebellar artery supply are indicated in **A, B,** and **C**. In **C**, the regions of supply of the paramedian midbrain and lateral basis peduncular arteries are indicated.

ing, and increased pendulousness of the lower limb. Coarse tremor may occur in the arm and leg when the patient attempts to hold them in a semiflexed position, and, in rare instances, involuntary rolling movements of the body occur when the brachium pontis is implicated. Ocular nystagmus is characteristically absent. In addition to the cerebellar disorder there may be contralateral hemianesthesia and, occasionally, sensory deficit of the ipsilateral side of the face. Occipital headache and dizziness or vertigo are common. In the initial stages of vascular occlusion, as well as subsequently, consciousness is preserved.

Additional disturbances have been described as components of the lateral pons syndrome, but these are caused by wider involvement of the pontile tegmentum than ordinarily occurs. Thus there may be a Millard-Gubler (p. 153) or Foville syndrome (p. 153), or contralateral analgesia and thermoanesthesia. An occasional patient has Horner's syndrome *ipsilaterally* and hyperhidrosis, pallor, coldness, and thermohypesthesia *contralaterally,* alterations explicable on the basis that some descending sympathetic fibers decussate, while others pursue an ipsilateral course. Where lesions are bilateral and predominantly ventral and involve both the paramedian region and the lateral pars basilaris, supranuclear bulbar palsy is likely to occur.

Pontile syndromes in general. Basilar pontile syndromes may be subdivided into four forms: hemiplegia, paraplegia, cerebellar, and supranuclear bulbar. The latter two are frequently combined. Where the *tegmentum* is involved, facial paresis and anesthesia of the limbs, either unilaterally or bilaterally, may occur. Headache following the stroke varies as to its site. Most commonly it is situated in the occipital region; sometimes the patient complains of a constrictive or hat band-like sensation round the head. (Fisher, 1968.) *Complete occlusion of the basilar artery* is usually rapidly fatal. The most obvious neurological signs are flaccid quadriplegia with bulbar paralysis (Foix and Hillemand, 1926; Hiller, 1952; Lhermitte and Trelles, 1934). Some patients struck down with *thrombosis of the vertebral-basilar system* survive for a time. Such a case, in which the survival period was about 3 months, was described by Messimy and his associates (1966).

Prodromal disturbances in this case included occipital headache and homonymous hemianopia. Clouding of consciousness, nausea, and vomiting then set in. In the following days the torpor persisted. Deep reflexes on one side became hyperactive; dysmetria occurred unilaterally; dysarthria also developed. A week after onset sudden clouding of consciousness occurred, and with it, hemiplegia with a Babinski reflex. Within 3 or 4 minutes these disturbances had resolved. During the ensuing days, there were disturbances in consciousness (but no hypersomnia), hypertonia of the decerebration type (predominantly unilateral, and a rarity in basilar artery thrombosis), modifications of deep and superficial reflexes, and vertical nystagmus (from pontile involvement). *Akinetic mutism* was conspicuous during most of the time; the eyes were continually kept open during the day and often at night. Much of the tegmentum of the pons was found softened bilaterally, as were other structures such as the brachium conjunctivum unilaterally and the cerebellar hemispheres. Partial destruction of the reticular formation was favored as responsible for the akinetic mutism, which is in agreement with the view of others (pp. 390 and 391).

Primary pontile hemorrhage involving the pars basilaris pontis or the tegmentum, or both, and occurring either unilaterally or bilaterally (the latter most commonly), has points of similarity and dissimilarity when comparison is made with pontile infarction. Hemorrhage into the pons represents about 10 percent of all hemorrhages occurring in the central nervous system; its highest incidence is in persons between 40 and 50 years of age (and, in infarction, between 50 and 80 years). In 75 percent of cases the clinical course is characterized by sudden onset with or without prodromal symptoms followed by quadriplegia, bloody spinal fluid, and often a stormy course ending fatally within 24 hours. (In infarction the course tends to be less stormy, the coma less deep, and death not as rapid.) Incomplete paralysis, a combination of flaccid and spastic paralyses, and the absence of a history of transient ischemic episodes, all favor hemorrhage. In the other 25 percent the survival period ranges from 2 to 10 days. In these cases the location of the hemorrhage is sometimes suggested by the clinical findings, for example, dysphagia and dysarthria, palsies of cranial nerves III, V, and VII, and the occurrence of alternate syndromes. Miosis is more prevalent in hemorrhage, and dilated, fixed pupils in infarction. Convulsive seizures seem more common in hemorrhage than in infarction. In hemorrhage, a rapid loss of consciousness favors the central tegmentum as the location of the hemorrhage, while clouded consciousness suggests hemorrhage in the lateral tegmentum. Hyperthermia (which occurs in 40 percent of cases of hemorrhage) is apparently more common in hemorrhage than in infarction. (Silverstein, 1967.)

Patients lying unconscious following pontile hemorrhage or basilar artery thrombosis occasionally exhibit rapid upward and downward movements of the eyes *(ocular bobbing)*. The assumption is that conjugate lateral gaze is in abeyance, making roving movements of the eyes impossible,

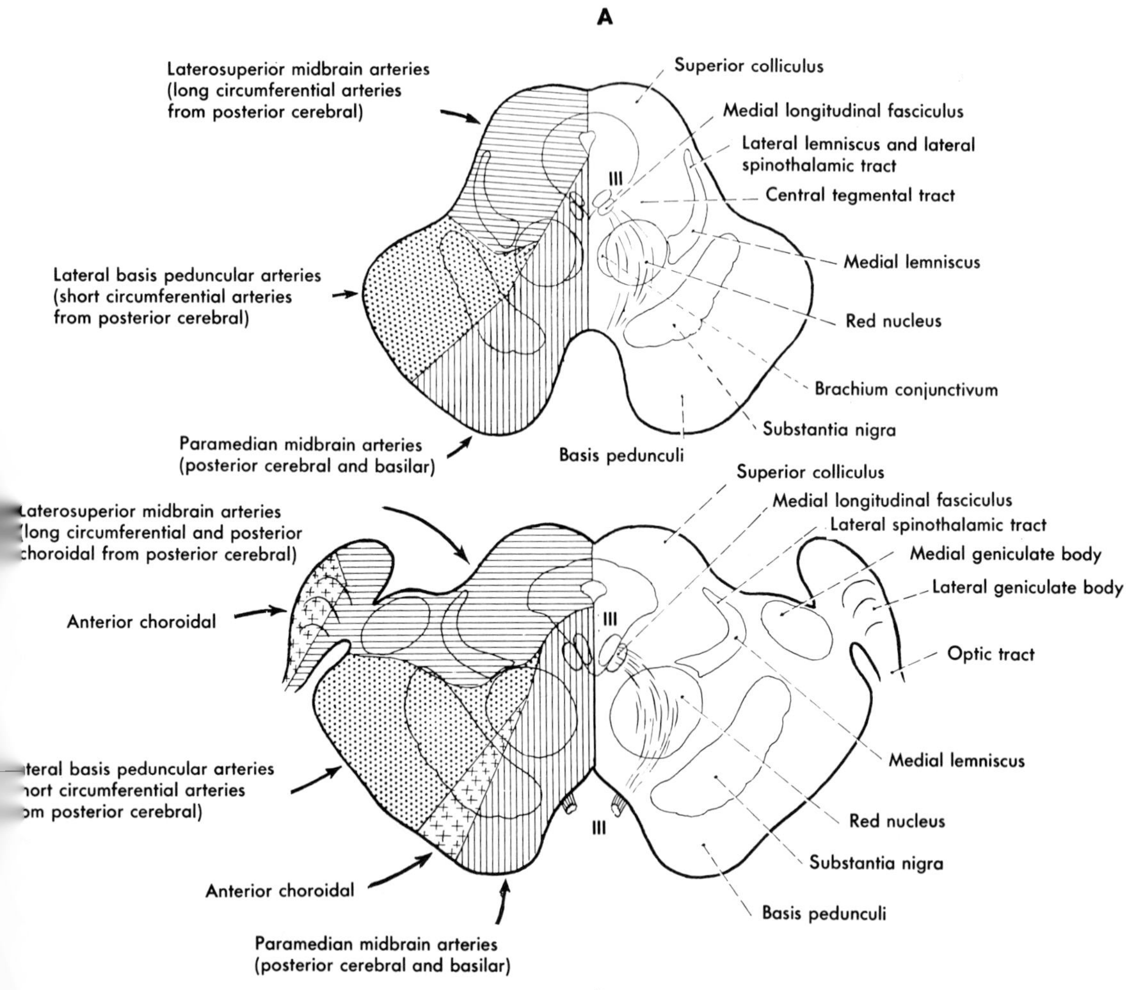

Fig. 18-6. Arterial supply of the upper midbrain. The fields of supply of the paramedian midbrain, lateral basis peduncular, and laterosuperior midbrain arteries are indicated, as are also the fields of supply of the anterior choroidal artery.

and that ocular movements take on a bobbing form owing to persisting activity meditated from mesencephalic mechanisms (Fisher, 1964).

Superior cerebellar artery

Arising from the basilar artery at the uppermost pontile level and rounding the caudal aspect of cerebral peduncle (Fig. 18-1), the superior cerebellar artery, which is subject to extraordinarily little variation, reaches and supplies the superior surface of the cerebellum and arborizes in the dentate nucleus (Lazorthes, 1961; Lazorthes, Poulhès, and Espagno, 1950a, b). (The globose and emboliform [and possibly the fastigial nucleus] are supplied by the posterior inferior cerebellar artery.) En route the superior cerebellar artery sends slender twigs to the lateral part of the basis pedunculi and much of the tegmentum of the upper pons and lower midbrain, and provides a *quadrigeminal artery* for the supply not only of the more caudal part of lamina quadrigemina but also the brachium conjunctivum and other dorsal structures at caudal levels of the midbrain. Along the surface of the lamina quadrigemina the quadrigeminal artery anastomoses with the quadrigeminal branches of the long circumferential artery derived from the posterior cerebral artery (Figs. 18-6 and 18-7).

All branches considered, in caudal parts of the midbrain the superior cerebral artery irrigates the lamina quadrigemina, brachium conjunctivum, and lateral tegmentum, and in the rostral pons much of the tegmentum and brachium pontis. Among the structures supplied are the medial lemniscus and lateral spinothalamic tract (Figs. 18-5 and 18-6).

Dorsolateral midbrain syndrome. Due predominantly to occlusion of the quadrigeminal artery, the dorsolateral midbrain syndrome is characterized by *ipsilateral* signs of cerebellar deficiency and Horner's syndrome, and *contralateral* sensory deficit (chiefly analgesia and thermoanesthesia) and hypacusis. Nystagmus is rare and signs of third and fourth nerve involvement absent, though there may be a rudimentary Nothnagel's syndrome (p. 154).

Midbrain tegmentum syndrome. This

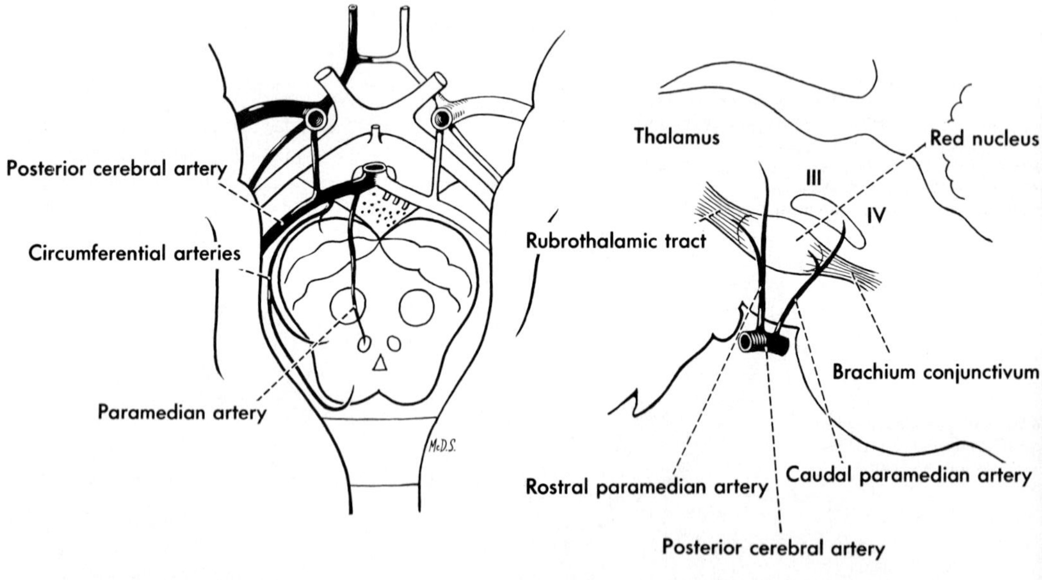

Fig. 18-7. Arterial supply of the midbrain. To the *left* the paramedian and short and long circumferential arteries are illustrated; and to the *right*, the rostral and caudal paramedian arteries. *Left:* The long circumferential artery is called the "quadrigeminal artery." It anastomoses with the quadrigeminal artery springing from the superior cerebellar artery. *Right:* Occlusion of the rostral paramedian artery gives rise to the "superior red nucleus syndrome," and of the caudal paramedian artery, the "inferior red nucleus syndrome." *III* and *IV*, Nuclei of the oculomotor and trochlear nerves. (Modified from Foix and Masson, 1923.)

syndrome results from occlusion of branches penetrating the lateral part of the tegmentum at caudal midbrain levels. Characteristic clinical features are tremor, ataxia, dyssynergia, adiadochokinesis, muscular hypotonia, astasia-abasia, and choreiform movements. The third and fourth nerves and the medial lemniscus are spared.

Pontile tegmentum syndrome. Occlusion of the branches of the superior cerebellar artery that penetrate the lateral surface of the midbrain and extend into the rostral pontile tegmentum is responsible for this syndrome. Certain features distinguish it from the midbrain tegmentum syndrome. For instance, the manifestations of cerebellar deficiency are considerably less pronounced and hyperkinesis less frequent. Myoclonus is, however, fairly common when the central tegmental tract is involved. Another feature of vascular occlusion of the rostral pontile tegmentum, when the lesion lies medially and well caudal to the decussation of the brachium conjunctivum, is the syndrome of Raymond-Cestan (p. 154). Disturbances in space perception (p. 158) may also be encountered in the presence of lesions in this general area. (Critchley and Schuster, 1933; Davison, Goodhart, and Savitsky, 1935; Freeman and Jaffe, 1941; Tscherny-scheff and Grigorowsky, 1930.)

Midbrain branches of the posterior cerebral, basilar, and anterior choroidal arteries

The branches to the midbrain from these sources may be divided into three groups: paramedian, basis pedunculi, and latero-superior.

Paramedian midbrain syndromes. The vessels concerned here are predominantly the branches from the proximal part of posterior cerebral artery that reach the paramedian part of the midbrain by penetrating the posterior perforated substance. A few of the vessels come from the most rostral part of the basilar artery (Figs. 18-1, *C*, 18-6, and 18-7). At upper midbrain levels an adjoining wedge of the basis pedunculi receives a branch from the anterior choroidal artery (Fig. 18-6, *B*). Among the structures supplied by the paramedian vessels are the more medial part of the basis pedunculi (including corticobulbar and corticospinal fibers), the medial part of the substantia nigra and red nucleus, the brachium conjunctivum both before and after decussation, the third and fourth nuclei, and the medial longitudinal fasciculus (Figs. 18-5 and 18-6).

Syndromes of vascular occlusion vary depending on the vessel or vessels involved and on the extent of the occlusion. One of the most common consists in paralysis of the third and fourth nerves ipsilaterally and hemianesthesia contralaterally. Two other paramedian syndromes are recognized: the inferior red nucleus or rubro-oculomotor syndrome (of Claude, 1912) and the superior red nucleus or rubro-thalamic syndrome (of Marie and Guillain, 1903) (Fig. 18-7).

The *inferior red nucleus syndrome* is characterized by Weber's syndrome (third nerve paralysis ipsilaterally and hemiplegia contralaterally) together with signs of ipsilateral cerebellar deficiency. (Isolated Weber's syndrome is rarely of vascular origin.) Occasionally the medial lemniscus is implicated, resulting in contralateral reduction in deep and superficial sensibility. The fourth nerve may also be affected. If the lesion is confined to the paramedian area, sparing the medial lemniscus but involving the crossed part of brachium conjunctivum and the medial longitudinal fasciculus, there will be *contralateral* ataxia together with tremor and choreo-athetotic movements and *ipsilateral* paralysis of conjugate lateral ocular movement. With involvement of the decussation of the brachium conjunctivum there may be bilateral choreo-athetotic movements.

The *superior red nucleus syndrome,* due to involvement of the red nucleus, rubrothalamic tract, and inferior caudal thalamus, is characterized by ipsilateral hemiasynergia and intention tremor without extraocular palsy or sensory deficit. The third nerve may also be affected, in which case oculomotor palsy occurs.

In general, lesions of the tegmentum and red nucleus give rise to tremor, athetotic and choreiform movements, ataxia, and disturbances of equilibrium. The tremor, usually coarse and either spontaneous or intentional, occurs in the limbs contralateral to the lesion. The athetotic movements are usually ipsilateral to the lesion and are also either spontaneous or intentional. The intentional variety (that is, characterized by athetotic movements when a voluntary act is attempted) has been noted in association with lesions of the medial lemniscus: this condition is called *athetoid static ataxia* (Gagel, 1949). Milder disturbances of equilibrium include the tendency to fall backward and away from the side of the lesion, particularly when the rubrotegmental area is involved unilaterally. Astasia-abasia may also occur.

Embolic occlusion of the rostral paramedian artery (or arteries) may, however, not result in involuntary movements, but, instead, in prolonged lethargy in association with oculomotor paralysis (Fig. 18-8).

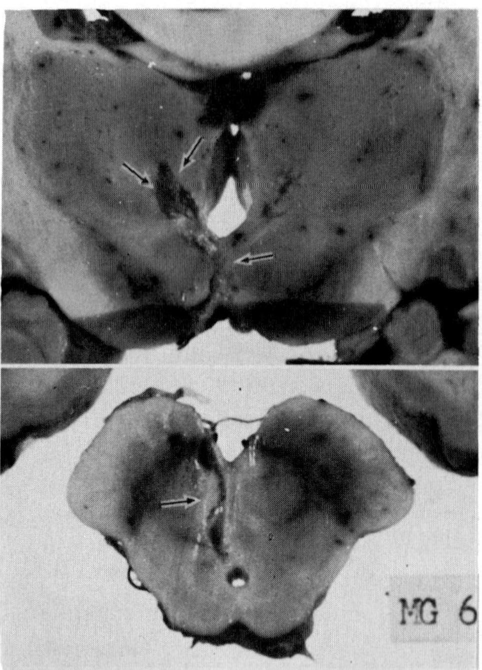

Fig. 18-8. Small areas of tissue cavitation (arrows) in region of distribution of the rostral paramedian midbrain artery. This is the end-stage probably of embolic infarction. The damaged area skirts the medial side of the red nucleus at both levels, lies in the path of the third nerve and nucleus, and extends up into the medial dorsal (MD) thalamic nucleus. The patient, 74 years of age, suddenly became unconscious while eating, and he remained severely lethargic during the 2 months prior to death. Oculomotor paralysis occurred ipsilaterally; the pupil remained dilated and never reacted to light. (Courtesy Dr. Richard Lindenberg, Baltimore.)

Basis pedunculi syndrome. The lateral half or more of the basis pedunculi is supplied by branches of the circumferential arteries (Fig. 18-6), which arise from the posterior cerebral artery. At lower midbrain levels, the superior cerebellar artery sends twigs to this area (Fig. 18-5, *C*). The field of irrigation includes the corticospinal tract. The most common effect of occlusion is the occurrence of Weber's syndrome, the third nerve being involved in its intramedullary course. The eye of that side is turned temporalward because of the unopposed action of the lateral rectus. Occlusion of these arteries bilaterally in association with lesions in the cerebrum may give rise to pseudobulbar palsy.

Laterosuperior midbrain syndrome. The vessels chiefly supplying the tectum and the lateral part of the tegmentum at superior collicular levels are the long and short circumferential arteries arising from the posterior cerebral artery (Figs. 18-6 and 18-7). The long circumferential arteries are also called *quadrigeminal arteries;* over the surface of the lamina quadrigemina they form an anastomosis with the quadrigeminal branch of the superior cerebellar artery. The syndrome of occlusion consists chiefly in contralateral hemihypesthesia and hemihypalgesia and sometimes in contralateral hypacusis.

Combined paramedian and laterosuperior midbrain syndrome. Occlusion of the several vessels referred to may give rise to combined paramedian and lateral midbrain syndromes. The same may occur when the more distal part of the *basilar artery* or the more proximal part of the *posterior cerebral* is occluded. If in the latter instance the calcarine cortex is spared, it is likely that the posterior cerebral artery is receiving a larger supply of blood from the posterior communicating artery than usual.

Manifestations of insufficiency of the vertebral-basilar arterial system; effects of aneurysm

Circulation provided by any of the local branches of this arterial system may become insufficient and induce neurological disturbances (Fig. 18-9). Fragments of material originating from the wall of such vessels can be carried centrally and lodge, for example, in the cerebellum or the calcarine cortex and produce "distant" symptoms. The problem is much the same with respect to aneurysm of the basilar artery. The usual basilar artery aneurysm is large, fusiform, and tortuous (McDonald and Korb, 1939). Only a few are syphilitic in origin (Bassoe, 1939).

Clinical syndromes vary. Frequently met with are transient recurrent attacks of binocular blurring of vision, which may be forerunners of a stroke. The blurring may last less than a minute, or as long as five minutes, and arouse so little concern that the person does not mention the episode unless specifically questioned. Embolization of the calcarine cortex by fibrin-platelet fragments originating from an atherosclerotic plaque and propelled into the calcarine branch of the posterior cerebral artery is considered to be the basis of such episodes (Hoyt, 1963). Where an attack of this kind lasts an hour or more, an *homonymous* visual field defect, resulting from occlusion of arteries which supply the calcarine cortex, usually results.

Recurrent attacks originating from a stenotic vertebral-basilar arterial system may be more severe than just indicated and may masquerade as "cerebral vasospasm." Included are dizziness, vertigo, dysarthria, dysphagia, facial numbness, weakness of the limbs, confusion, and somnolence. Diagnosis is suggested by involvement of one side of the body in one attack and of the other side in another, and is usually borne out, in any one attack, by disturbances referable to the pons, midbrain, and/or the visual cortex. (Denny-Brown and Foley, 1952; Kubik and Adams, 1946; Millikan and Siekert, 1955.)

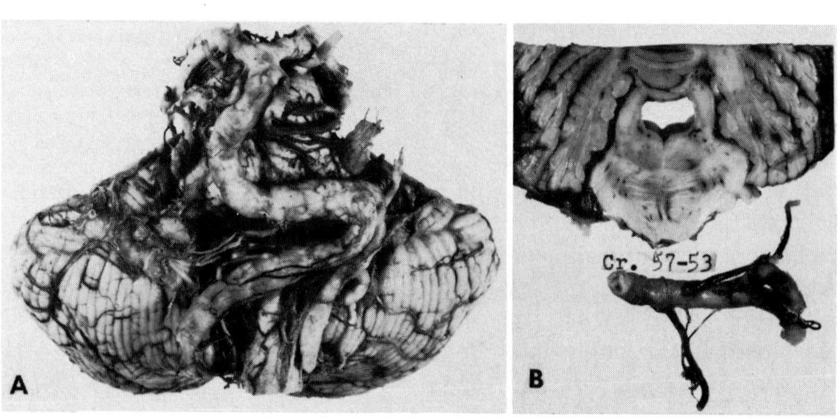

Fig. 18-9. A, Severe atherosclerosis involving the vertebral-basilar-posterior cerebral system. Nerves XII, VIII, VII, VI, III, and, to some extent, nerve V, are compressed. **B,** Severe atherosclerosis of the basilar with atrophy of the pons. The patient had no overt paralysis but, instead, a kind of ataxia, slight dysarthria and dysphagia, and psychosis. (Courtesy Dr. Richard Lindenberg, Baltimore.)

Of the disturbances just mentioned, *dizziness* and *vertigo* are among the most revealing. According to Thiébaut and colleagues (1968), dizziness (nonsystematized vertiginous sensations) signifies transitory vertebral artery insufficiency, brought about by ischemia involving the lateral vestibular nucleus. Further manifestations are spontaneous unidirectional or multidirectional nystagmus, reduced ocular responses to rotation and to douching of the ear with warm water, and nystagmus of cervical origin. By contrast, permanent basilar artery insufficiency, considered due to involvement of vestibular receptors, vestibular nerve, or vestibular nuclei, is marked by vertigo, which, later on, is succeeded by dizziness upon change in body or head position. Findings are much the same as those just mentioned, except that nystagmus of cervical origin is not elicitable. Thiébaut and colleagues noted that neither dizziness nor vertigo occurred in about a fourth of their cases of vertebral-basilar arterial insufficiency.

Vertigo as an isolated symptom of vertebral-basilar arterial insufficiency is rare. In one series (Bergen and others, 1967), vertigo was noted in association with visual disturbances in 32 percent of cases, dysarthria in 27 percent, and disorders of equilibrium in 18 percent. Without treatment, brainstem infarction eventually occurs in 50 to 75 percent of patients (Loeb and Meyer, 1965).

Another manifestation of vertebral-basilar arterial disease is *ophthalmoplegia*, which is, however, a rarity. It is a sign of arterial insufficiency or occlusion. Ophthalmoplegia, partial or complete, external or internal, unilateral but sometimes bilateral, may be a presenting sign. Diplopia is frequent, internuclear ophthalmoplegia rare. Stretching or displacement of nerves III, IV, and/or VI through pressure from the basilar artery or its branches is considered the basis in some cases, infarction within the brainstem in others. Angiography may be necessary to determine whether the ophthalmoplegia is of vertebral-basilar or internal carotid artery origin. (Harel, Lavy, and Schwartz, 1967; Kubik and Adams, 1946.)

Basilar artery aneurysm is manifested by attacks of sudden onset, fluctuating course, and highly variable symptoms and signs. During an attack there may be severe dizziness, ataxia, weakness of both legs, weakness of one side of the face, twitching of facial muscles, dysarthria, vomiting, nystagmus, sudden unilateral or bilateral deafness, abdominodiaphragmatic myoclonus, mental confusion, and disorientation. Bilateral hemiparesis is common; both sides of the body may be affected simultaneously, but, more frequently, one side is affected after the other. Trigeminal neuralgia may occur and rarely there is a slow jacksonian-like sensory march from one side of the face into the other. Ocular palsy with or without diplopia sometimes occurs; the palsy is usually bilateral. Pseudobulbar palsy has also been observed. (Denny-Brown, 1953; Denny-Brown and Foley, 1952; Duvoisin and Yahr, 1965; Harel, Lavy, and Schwartz, 1967; Höök, Norlén, and Gúzman, 1963.)

REFERENCES

Adams, R. D. 1943. Occlusion of the anterior inferior cerebellar artery. Arch. Neurol. Psychiat. **49**:765-770.

Alexander, L., and Suh, T. H. 1937. Arterial supply of the lateral parolivary area of the medulla oblongata. Arch. Neurol. Psychiat. **38**:1243-1260.

Atkinson, W. J. 1949. The anterior inferior cerebellar artery: its variations, pontine distribution, and significance in the surgery of cerebello-pontine angle tumours. J. Neurol. Neurosurg. Psychiat. **12**:137-151.

Baker, A. B. 1961. Cerebrovascular disease: the medullary blood supply and the lateral medullary syndrome. Neurology **11**:852-861.

Bassoe, P. 1939. Aneurysms of the vertebral artery. Arch. Neurol. Psychiat. **42**:127-133.

Bergen, J. J., Levy, J. S., Trippel, O. H., and Jurayji, M. 1967. Vascular implications of vertigo. Arch. Otolaryng. **85**:292-297.

Biemond, A. 1951. Thrombosis of the basilar artery and the vascularization of the brain stem. Brain **74**:300-317.

Bjerver, K., and Silfverskiöld, B. P. 1968. Lateropulsion and imbalance in Wallenberg's syndrome. Acta Neurol. Scand. **44**:91-100.

Böhne, S. 1927. Über die arterielle Versorgung des Gehirns; über die arterielle Blutversorgung der Medulla oblongata. Z. Ges. Neurol. Psychiat. **84**:670-776.

Brown, W. J., and Fang, H. C. H. 1961. Spastic

hemiplegia in man: lack of flaccidity in lesion of pyramidal tract. Neurology **11**:829-835.

Claude, H. 1912. Syndrome pédonculaire de la région du noyau rouge. Rev. Neurol. **23**:311-313.

Critchley, M. 1930. The anterior cerebral artery and its syndromes. Brain **53**:120-165.

Critchley, M., and Schuster, P. 1933. Beiträge zur Anatomie und Pathologie der Arteria cerebelli superior. Z. Ges. Neurol. Psychiat. **144**: 681-741.

Currier, R. D., Giles, C. L., and DeJong, R. N. 1961. Some comments on Wallenberg's lateral medullary syndrome. Neurology **11**:778-791.

Dandy, W. E. 1944. Intracranial arterial aneurysms. Ithaca, New York, Comstock Publishing Associates, pp. 1-22, 67-90.

Davison, C. 1944. Syndrome of the anterior spinal artery of the medulla oblongata. Arch. Neurol. Psychiat. **37**:91-107.

Davison, C., Goodhart, S. P., and Savitsky, N. 1935. The syndrome of the superior cerebellar artery and its branches. Arch. Neurol. Psychiat. **33**:1143-1172.

Denny-Brown, D. 1953. Basilar artery syndromes. Bull. New Eng. Med. Center **15**:53-60.

Denny-Brown, D., and Foley, J. M. 1952. The syndrome of basilar aneurysm. Trans. Amer. Neurol. Ass. **77**:30-34.

Dial, D. L., and Maurer, G. B. 1937. Intracranial aneurysms: report of 13 cases. Amer. J. Surg. **35**:2-21.

Duvoisin, R. C., and Yahr, M. D. 1965. Posterior fossa aneurysms. Neurology **15**:231-241.

Fisher, C. M. 1964. Ocular bobbing. Arch. Neurol. **11**:543-546.

Fisher, C. M. 1968. Headache in cerebrovascular disease. In Vinken, P. J., and Bruyn, G. W., editors: Handbook of clinical neurology, vol. 5. Amsterdam, North-Holland Publishing Company, pp. 124-156.

Fisher, C. M., and Curry, H. B. 1965. Pure motor hemiplegia of vascular origin. Arch. Neurol. **13**: 30-44.

Foix, C., and Hillemand, P. 1925. Les artères de l'axe encéphalique jusqu'au diéncephale inclusivement. Rev. Neurol. **2**:705-739.

Foix, C., and Hillemand, P. 1926. Contribution à l'étude des ramollissements protuberantiels. Rev. Méd. **43**:286-305.

Foix, C., Hillemand, P., and Schalit, I. 1925. Sur le syndrome latéral du bulbe et l'irrigation du bulb supérieur: l'artère de la fossette latérale du bulbe: le syndrome dit de la cérébelleuse inférieure: territoire de ses artères. Rev. Neurol. **1**:160-179.

Foix, C., and Masson, A. 1923. Le syndrome de l'artère cérébrale postérieure. Presse Méd. **31**: 361-365.

Freeman, W., and Jaffe, D. 1941. Occlusion of the superior cerebellar artery: report of a case with necropsy. Arch. Neurol. Psychiat. **46**:115-126.

Gagel, O. 1949. Einführung in die Neurologie. Berlin, Springer-Verlag.

Goodhart, S. P., and Davison, C. 1936. Posterior inferior and anterior inferior cerebellar arteries. Arch. Neurol. Psychiat. **35**:501-524.

Harel, D., Lavy, S., and Schwartz, A. 1967. Ophthalmoplegia as a manifestation of basilar artery disease. Amer. J. Ophthal. **63**:519-523.

Hiller, F. 1936. Die Zirkulationsstörungen des Rückenmarks und Gehirns. In Bumke, O., and Foerster, O., editors: Handbuch der Neurologie, vol. 11. Berlin, Springer-Verlag, pp. 178-465.

Hiller, F. 1952. The vascular syndromes of the basilar and vertebral arteries and their branches. J. Nerv. Ment. Dis. **116**:988-1016.

Hitselberger, W. E., and House, W. F. 1966. Acoustic tumor surgery: the significance of vital sign changes. Arch. Otolaryng. **84**:245-291.

Höök, O., Norlén, G., and Gúzman, J. 1963. Saccular aneurysms of the vertebral-basilar arterial system: a report of 28 cases. Acta Neurol. Scand. **39**:271-304.

Hoyt, W. F. 1963. Transient bilateral blurring of vision: considerations of episodic ischemic symptom of vertebral-basilar insufficiency. Arch. Ophthal. **70**:746-751.

Kubik, C. S., and Adams, R. D. 1946. Occlusion of the basilar artery: a clinical and pathological study. Brain **69**:73-121.

Lazorthes, G. 1961. Vascularisation et circulation cérébrales. Paris, Masson & Cie.

Lazorthes, G., Poulhès, J., and Espagno, J. 1950a. Les artères du cervelet. C. R. Assoc. Anat. **37**: 279-288.

Lazorthes, G., Poulhès, J., and Espagno, J. 1950b. Les territoires vasculaires du cortex cerebelleux. C. R. Assoc. Anat. **37**:289-209.

Lewis, G. N., Littman, A., and Foley, E. F. 1952. The syndrome of thrombosis of the posterior inferior cerebellar artery: a report of 28 cases. Ann. Intern. Med. **36**:592-602.

Lhermitte, J., and Trelles, J. O. 1934. L'artériosclèrose du tronc basilaire et ses consequences anatomo-cliniques. J. Psychiat. Neurol. **51**:91-107.

Lindenberg, R. 1955. Die Gefässversorgung und ihre Bedeutung für Art and Ort von kreislaufbedingten Gewebsschäden und Gefässprozessen. In Lubarsch, O., Henke, F., and Rössle, R., editors: Handbuch der speziellen pathologischen Anatomie und Histologie, vol. 3 (edited by Scholz, W.), pt. 1B. München, Springer-Verlag, pp. 1071-1164.

Loeb, C., and Meyer, J. S. 1965. Strokes due to vertebrobasilar disease. Springfield, Illinois, Charles C Thomas, Publisher, p. 138.

Marie, P., and Guillain, G. 1903. Lésion ancienne du noyau rouge; dégénérations secondaires. Nouv. Icong. Salpêtrière **16**:80-83.

McDonald, C. A., and Korb, M. 1939. Intracranial aneurysms. Arch. Neurol. Psychiat. **42**:298-328.

Merritt, H. H., and Finland, M. 1930. Vascular lesions of the hind-brain (lateral medullary syndrome). Brain **53**:290-305.

Messimy, R., Da Lage, C., David, M., and Harispe, L. 1966. Mutisme akinétique avec rigidité décérébrée par thrombose vertébro-basilaire: confrontation clinique et anatomo-pathologique. Rev. Neurol. **115**:1015-1028.

Millikan, C. H., and Siekert, R. G. 1955. Studies in cerebrovascular disease: the syndrome of intermittent insufficiency of the basilar arterial system. Proc. Staff Meet., Mayo Clin. **30**:61-68.

Müller, E. 1906. Ueber ein eigenartiges, scheinbar typisches Symptomenbild bei apoplektiformer Bulbärlähmung (nebst Bermerkungen über perverse Temperaturempfindungen und bulbäre Sympathicusparesen). Deutsch. Z. Nervenheilk. **31**:452-471.

O'Brien, F. H., and Bender, M. B. 1945. Localizing value of vertical nystagmus. Arch. Neurol. Psychiat. **54**:378-380.

Rhoton, A. L., Jr., Kobayashi, S., and Hollinshead, W. H. 1968. Nervus intermedius. J. Neurosurg. **29**:609-618.

Sheehan, D., and Smyth, G. E. 1937. A study of the anatomy of vertebral thrombosis, with reports on two cases. Lancet **2**:614-618.

Silverstein, A. 1967. Primary pontile hemorrhage: a review of 50 cases. Confin. Neurol. **29**:33-46.

Soffin, G., Feldman, M., and Bender, M. B. 1968. Alterations of sensory levels in vascular lesions of lateral medulla. Arch. Neurol. **18**:178-190.

Stern, K. 1935. Über gefässabhängige Störungen im Brücken-Mittelhirngebiet und ihre Entstehungsweisen. Z. Ges. Neurol. Psychiat. **152**: 497-518.

Stopford, J. S. B. 1916. The arteries of the pons and medulla oblongata. J. Anat. **50**:131-164.

Sunderland, S. 1945. The arterial relations of the internal auditory meatus. Brain **68**:23-27.

Thiébaut, F., Collard, M., Conraux, C., and Thiébaut, M. S. 1968. Les atteintes vestibularies au cours des syndromes vasculaires du tronc cérébral. Rev. Otoneuroophtal. **40**:77-87.

Thompson, R. H. 1929. Occlusion of the posterior inferior cerebellar artery. Arch. Neurol. Psychiat. **22**:530-546.

Tschernyscheff, A., and Grigorowsky, I. 1930. Über die arterielle Versorgung des Kleinhirns. Arch. Psychiat. **89**:482-569; **92**:8-85.

Wallenberg, A. 1895. Akute Bulbäraffection (Embolie der art. cerebellar. post. inf. sinistr.?). Arch. Psychiat. **23**:504-540.

Wallenberg, A. 1901. Anatomischer Befund in einem als "acute Bulbäraffection (Embolie der Art. cerebellar. post. inf. sinistr.?)" beschriebenen Falle. Arch. Psychiat. **34**:923-959.

Yates, P. O., and Hutchinson, E. C. 1961. Cerebral infarction: the role of stenosis of the extracranial cerebral arteries. Med. Res. Council Rep. No. 300. London, Her Majesty's Stationery Office.

Chapter 19

Cerebral landmarks; organization of the cerebral cortex and descending and ascending pathways

Webb Haymaker
Francis Schiller

GROSS LANDMARKS

Craniocerebral topography is illustrated in Figs. 19-1 and 19-2. The central sulcus (of Rolando) and the lateral cerebral fissure (of Sylvius) are two of the most important landmarks, for they serve as base lines from which the position of other sulci and fissures can be determined.

The positions of the two vertical lines indicated in Fig. 19-2, known as the *anterior* and *posterior ear lines,* are plotted as follows. The anterior ear line extends from the anterior rim of the external auditory canal to the midsagittal line of the skull, meeting the latter at a right angle. The posterior ear line runs parallel with the anterior ear line and has as its lowermost extremity the posterior rim of the mastoid process. The *black dots* shown in Fig. 19-2 divide the anterior ear line into three equal parts; the *black diamond mark* halves the line. Trephine between the diamond mark and the lower black dot uncovers the lower end of the central sulcus, which, in adults, is approximately 7 cm. above the external auditory meatus. In many persons the lower end of the central sulcus is to be found directly under the anterior ear line. In short heads the relations are those depicted in Fig. 19-2; in long heads, the lower end of the central sulcus is somewhat posterior to the anterior ear line. The posterior ear line passes through the upper end of the central sulcus.

The *lateral cerebral fissure* lies from 1.0 to 1.5 cm. below the lower end of central sulcus. In its further course, this fissure extends for a distance parallel to the temporal suture. The posterior end of the lateral cerebral fissure (the region of its termination in the supramarginal gyrus) usually lies beneath the tuberosity of the parietal bone.

The *middle meningeal artery,* a branch of the internal maxillary artery, enters the cranial cavity through the foramen spinosum and then divides into two branches, the anterior and the posterior (Fig. 19-3). After entering the foramen spinosum the artery may, in some instances, run a part of its course embedded in bone. In surgical intervention for hemorrhage from the middle meningeal artery, it is necessary to trephine the skull just above the zygomatic process in order to tie off the artery proximal to its site of branching (Fig. 19-3). The anterior branch of the artery can be reached at a point two fingerbreadths above the middle of the zygomatic arch. The posterior branch is accessible at the same distance above the zygomatic process.

The surface projection of the *transverse venous sinus* is also shown in Fig. 19-3.

Further cerebral landmarks are the gyri, sulci, and fissures. These are shown in Figs. 19-4 and 19-5.

GENERAL ORGANIZATION OF THE CEREBRAL CORTEX

Considered cytoarchitecturally, the cerebral cortex is composed of more or less clearly distinguishable areas, as exemplified in the maps of Brodmann (1908) (Fig. 19-6) and Bailey and von Bonin (1951). From forty to two hundred or more areas have been identified, depending on the

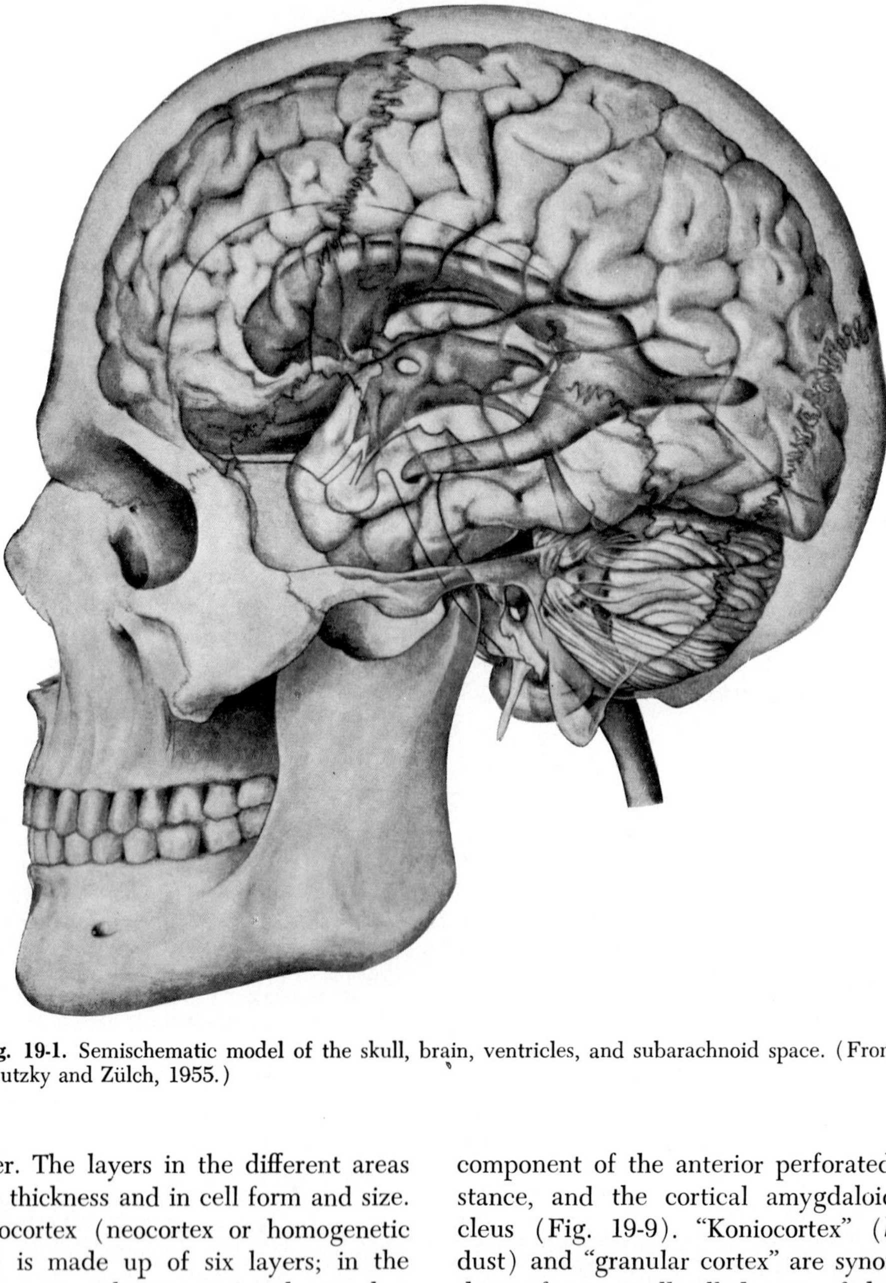

Fig. 19-1. Semischematic model of the skull, brain, ventricles, and subarachnoid space. (From Kautzky and Zülch, 1955.)

observer. The layers in the different areas vary in thickness and in cell form and size. The isocortex (neocortex or homogenetic cortex) is made up of six layers; in the calcarine cortex there appear to be ten, but those in excess merely represent subdivisions of layers IV, V, and VI. On the other hand, the allocortex (archicortex or heterogenetic cortex) contains less than six layers, usually three. The superficial layer of the allocortex is composed, here and there, not of a continuous row of cells, but of cell islands (islands of Calleja). Allocortex includes the piriform cortex, the cortical component of the anterior perforated substance, and the cortical amygdaloid nucleus (Fig. 19-9). "Koniocortex" (*konio,* dust) and "granular cortex" are synonyms; they refer to small-celled parts of the neocortex essentially comprising the primary receptive (sensory) areas. "Agranular" cortex refers to parts of the cortex containing large cells mixed with small cells, as in area 4 (of Brodmann). Ecto-, meso-, and entocortex are other terms that have been employed (Chapter 25).

A fundamental difference between the neocortex and the allocortex (if the choos-

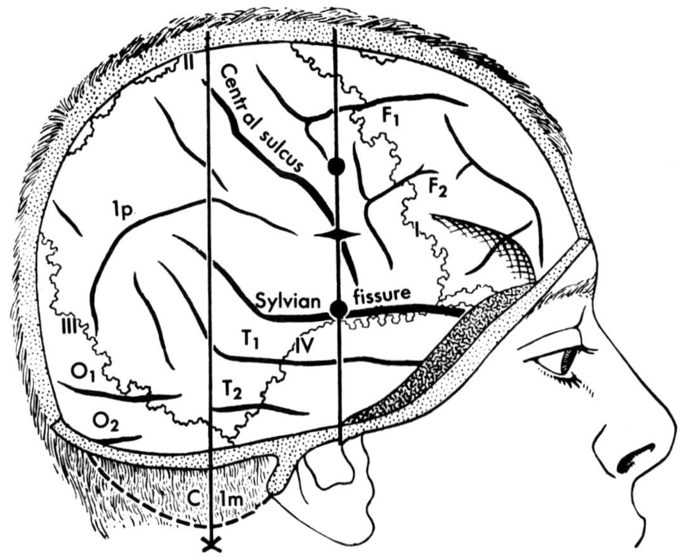

Fig. 19-2. Projection of the cerebral hemispheres and sulci on to the surface of the skull. *I,* Coronal suture; *II,* sagittal suture; *III,* lambdoid suture; *IV,* temporal suture; F_1 and F_2, superior and middle frontal sulci; *Ip,* interparietal sulcus; O_1 and O_2, superior and middle occipital sulci; T_1 and T_2, superior and middle temporal sulci; *Clm,* cerebellum; *X,* posterior border of the mastoid process.

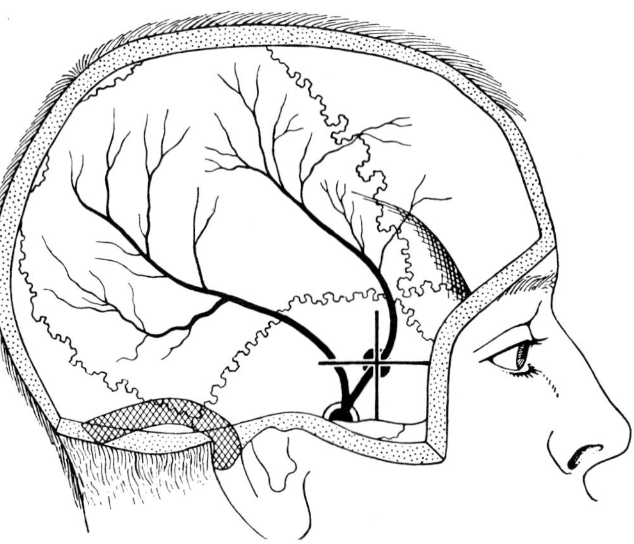

Fig. 19-3. Projection of the middle meningeal artery and the transverse venous sinus on to the surface of the skull.

ing of terms from two different classifications is in order) is in the course of incoming fibers. In the allocortex practically all of the incoming fibers first run along the cortical surface (in its molecular, or superficial plexiform, layer) and then descend into the other layers, while in the neocortex the incoming fibers first traverse the white matter and then ascend in the cortex.

Every part of the cerebral cortex is the terminus of an afferent path and the be-

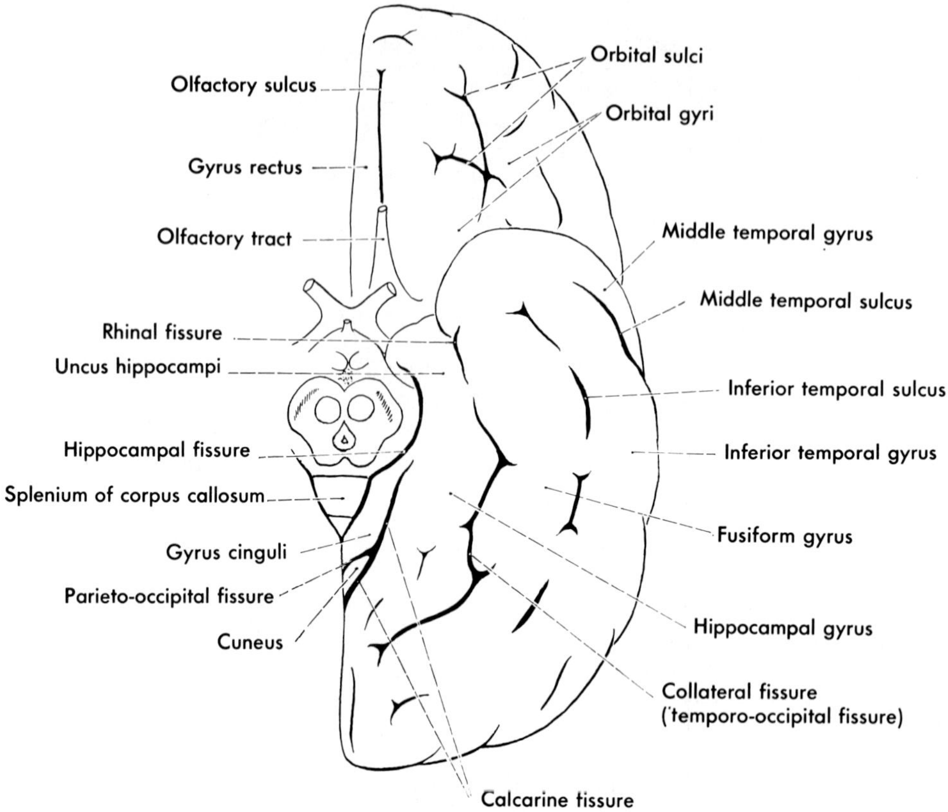

Fig. 19-4. The gyri and sulci of the inferior surface of the brain.

ginning of an efferent path. In the neocortex, layer IV is one of the main receptor layers; it receives most of the *specific* thalamic afferents (p. 450). On the other hand—according to Lorente de Nó (1938) —*nonspecific* thalamic efferents (those coming to the cortex from intralaminar thalamic nuclei) begin to give off horizontal collateral branches before reaching the cortex. These branches turn upward and ascend through the cortex to the outermost layer (the molecular layer), where, after running horizontally, they give off terminal branches. Layers V and VI are largely efferent; axons originating from some cell bodies in these layers enter the pyramidal tract or the corpus callosum, while the axons from other cell bodies form bundles of efferent association fibers that serve to interconnect parts of the cortex. Betz cells together with other large pyramidal* cells are situated in layer V (of area 4). Some incoming axons terminate directly (monosynaptically) on the bodies and dendrites of these and other motor cells. In other instances, internuncial neurons are interposed between afferent neurons and the dendrites and cell bodies of efferent neurons. Cortical neuron chains thus exist that, in principle, are no different from chains of internuncial neurons in any other part of the nervous system, such as the spinal cord.

FUNCTIONAL SUBDIVISIONS OF THE CORTEX

The cerebral cortex may be subdivided functionally.

*By a mere linguistic accident, the tract passing through the medullary pyramids, and hence named after *them,* originates partly from cells that happen to be shaped like pyramids also.

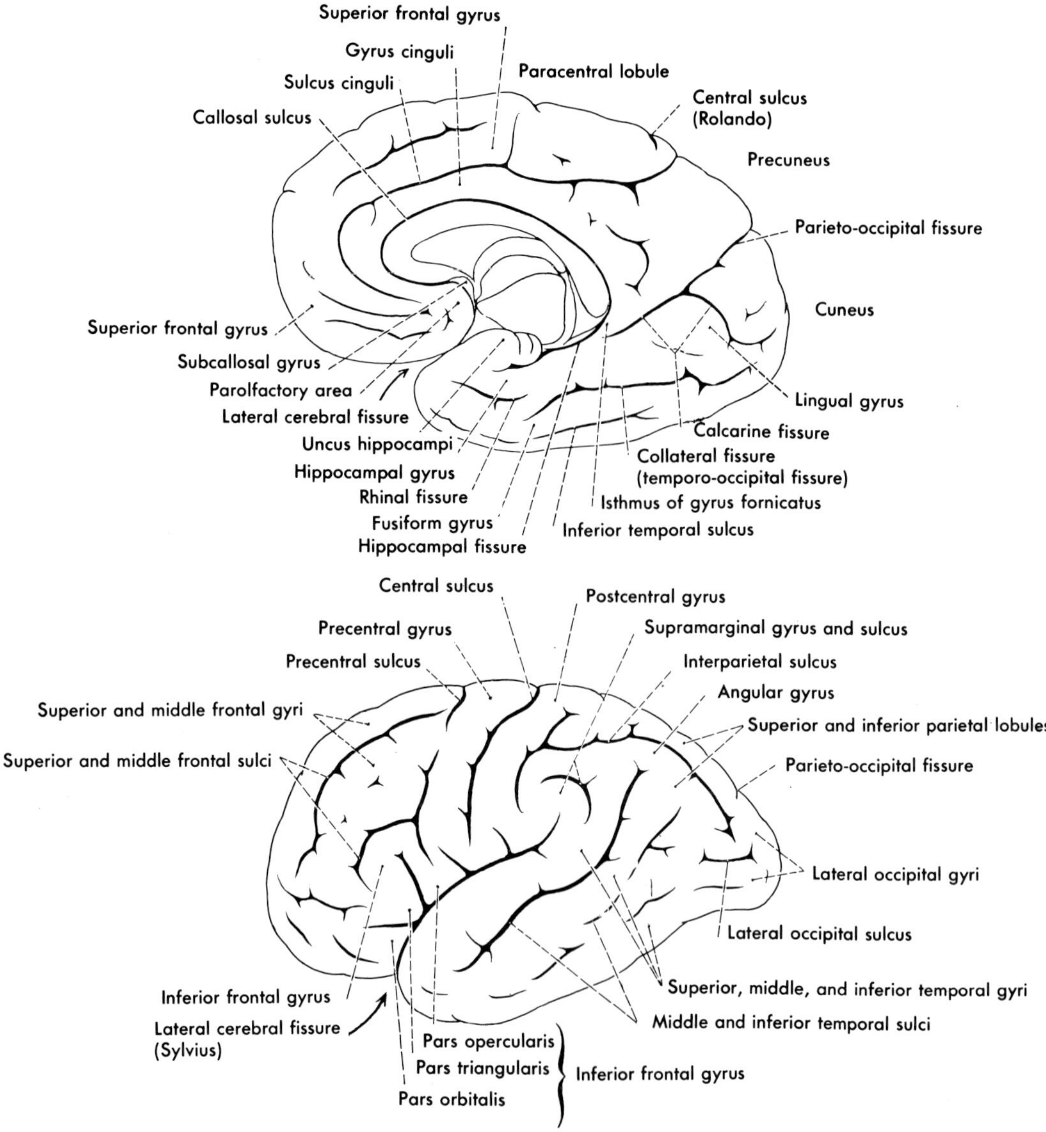

Fig. 19-5. The gyri and sulci of the brain.

Areas subserving voluntary motor functions. Nerve cell aggregates in numerous cortical areas contribute to the performance of voluntary movement via the corticospinal tract and other pathways. Fibers of the corticospinal tract concerned in the carrying out of skilled movement of a discrete nature originate widely. According to one count (made at the level of the pyramids) carried out in *Macaca rhesus,* 29 percent of the fibers of this tract originate in area 6, 31 percent in area 4, and 40 percent behind the central sulcus (areas 3, 1, 2, 5, 7) (Russell and DeMyer, 1961). The greatest concentration of the fibers is in the region of the central sulcus. Corticobulbar fibers projecting *directly* to cranial nerve nuclei V, VII, and XII are assumed to have a similar origin. Fibers passing to nuclei III, IV, and VI belong in a special category; they originate mainly in area 8 and find their way to these nuclei *indirectly* by way of the reticular substance. Similarly, *indirect* connections exist

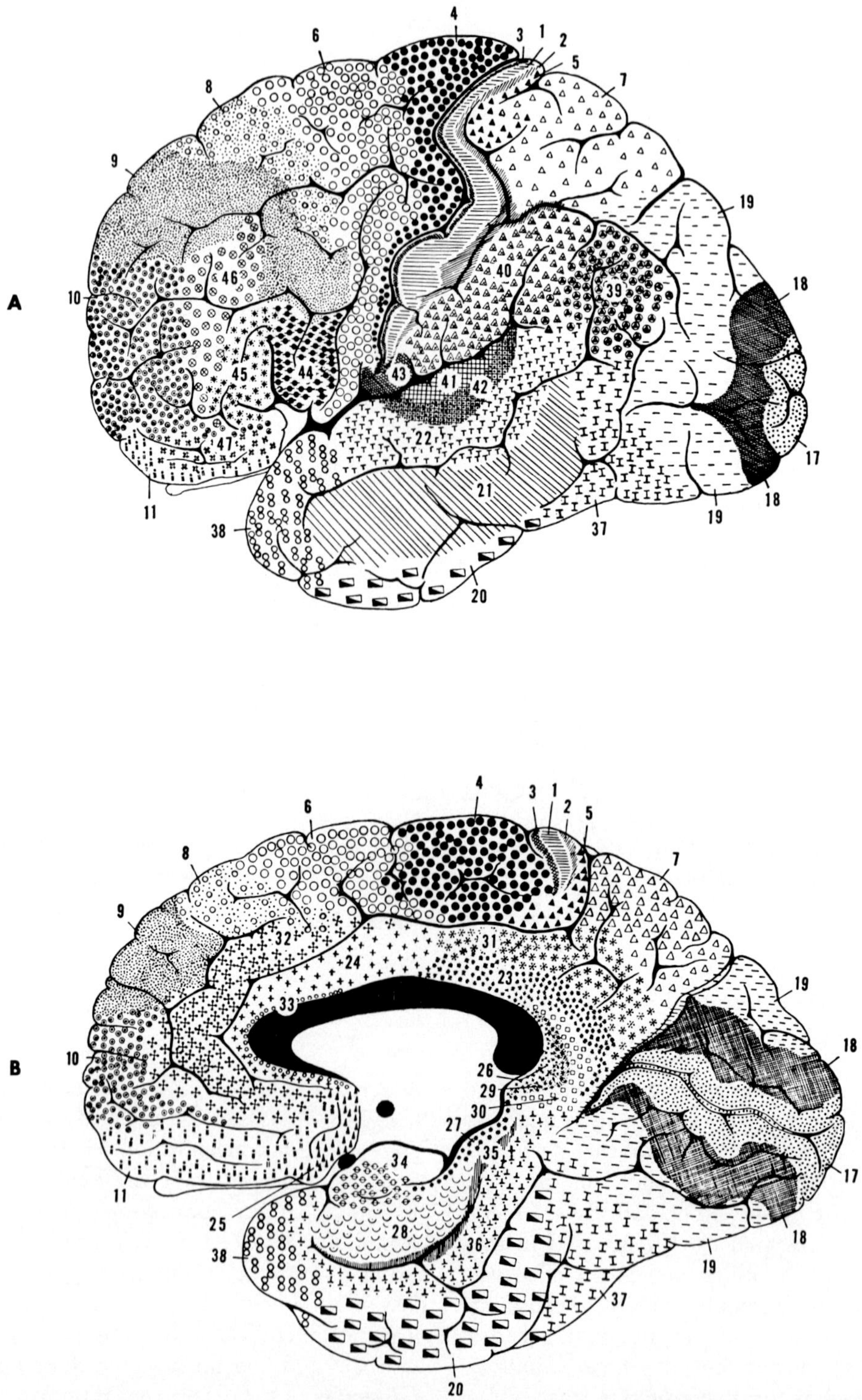

Fig. 19-6. The cytoarchitectural map of the cerebral cortex. (From Brodmann, 1908.)

with motor nuclei IX and X and with nucleus XI.

Each descending corticospinal fiber ultimately connects functionally through transsynaptic means with a muscle group. Thus, in this sense, *muscles* are represented in the cerebral cortex. However, in the aggregate, the cortex is more concerned in the performance of *movements*, each represented as indicated in Fig. 19-7. *Discrete* movements are being referred to; the cortex "thinks in terms of these movements." Each movement is brought about through the mediation of intracortical internuncial neurons having connections with Betz and other motor cells. (Lorente de Nó, 1938; Patton and Amassian, 1960; Penfield, 1954; Ruch and others, 1965.)

Area 4 in the precentral gyrus is considered the *primary motor sector* of the cortex. Areas 4 and 6 together with area 44 make up the *precentral motor cortex*. Only about 2.5 percent of the corticospinal fibers originating in area 4 and coursing down into the pyramids, arise from Betz cells, which are situated in layer V. Smaller cells of layers III through VI of area 4 contribute a greater proportion. (Lassek, 1942; Lassek and Evans, 1945, 1946; Mettler, 1944.)

Other motor areas, supplemental motor areas, areas concerned in adversive movements. Movements can be induced by electrical stimulation of numerous areas other than the primary motor sector. Many of these movements are brought about through fibers known collectively as the *cortically originating extrapyramidal sys-*

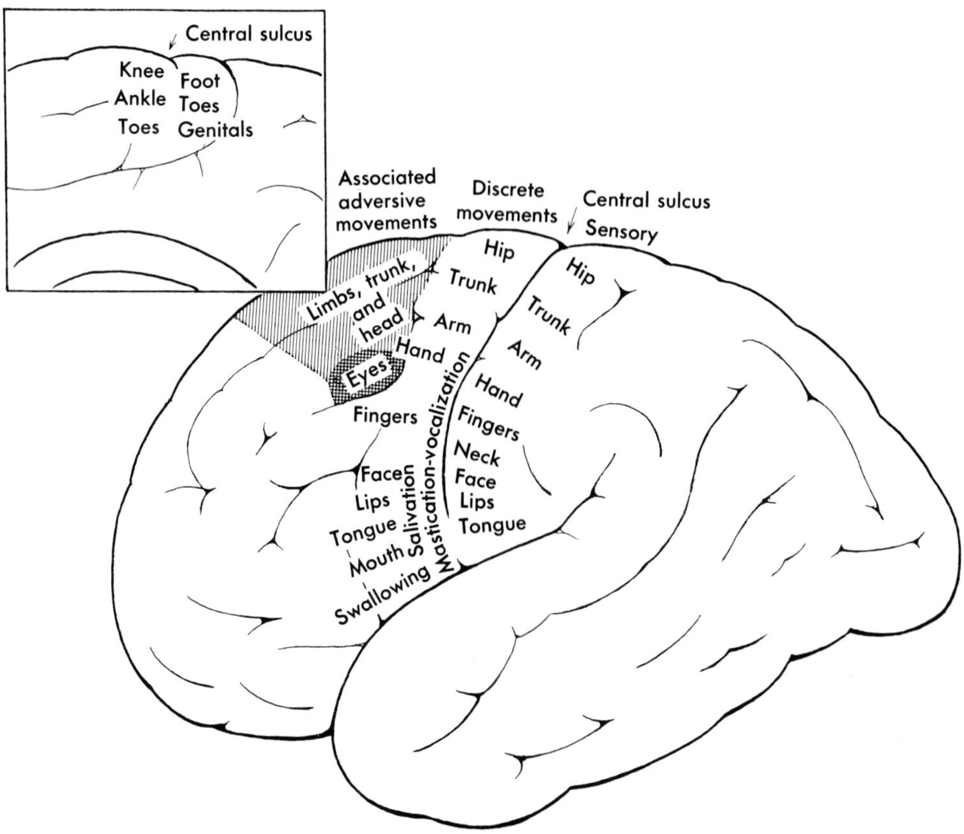

Fig. 19-7. Functional representation in the cerebral cortex. The inset illustrates the representation in the right paracentral lobule. (Mostly from Penfield, 1954, and Penfield and Rasmussen, 1950.)

tem (COEPS). COEPS originates both in front of the central sulcus (in areas 8, 6, and 4, in that order of decreasing number of cells) and behind this sulcus (in areas 3, 1, 2, 5, and 7) and in temporal cortical areas. Thus the cells of origin of COEPS and the corticospinal (and corticobulbar) tract overlap. COEPS terminates on basal ganglia and brainstem nuclei. A feedback to the cortex occurs from most of these structures. Through the cortex–basal ganglion system as well as through relays from basal ganglia to the brainstem and spinal cord, COEPS sends impulses that can *effect* and *affect* movement. (Ruch and others, 1965.)

Thus COEPS differs from the corticospinal (and corticobulbar) system in that it is composed of chains of neurons, with synaptic interruption at various levels of the neuraxis, and in that most of its fibers do not traverse the pyramids (Amassian, 1953; Hines, 1943; Rossi and Brodal, 1956; Tower, 1949). It is agreed, however, that both systems are heavily concerned in the performance of voluntary movement, an idea that seems to have been proposed first by Sir Victor Horsley (1909). In support of this view is the observation that, in man, a remarkable degree of recovery of motor skills occurs following pedunculotomy, in which all corticospinal fibers are supposedly interrupted (Bucy, 1957; Jane and others, 1968).

A further point about COEPS is that fibers issuing from the cortex of one hemisphere and terminating in the striatum (caudate nucleus and putamen) are supplemented by fibers originating in the sensorimotor cortex of the opposite hemisphere (in rat, rabbit, and cat); the fibers in point decussate via the corpus callosum (Carman and others, 1965). This observation provides an anatomical basis for the long-held view that striatal activity is governed by the cortex of both sides.

A *second motor area* is present in the portion of the precentral gyrus extending into the island of Reil—that portion tucked away in the upper lip of the Sylvian fissure. Electrical stimulation of this area reveals its order of representation as the *reverse* of that in the main part of the precentral gyrus (Sugar, Chusid, and French, 1948). The movements evoked by unilateral stimulation occur on both sides of the face (Crosby, Humphrey, and Showers, 1959; Furstenberg, 1958; Woolsey and others, 1952).

Supplementary motor areas, also identified under conditions in which the animal (or man) is unanesthetized or lightly anesthetized, coincide, in large part at least, with COEPS.

The supplementary motor area initially described (Hughes and Mazurowski, 1962; Woolsey, 1947, 1958; Woolsey and others, 1942, 1952) is situated in the *mesial* aspect of the cortex, in front of area 4, in a region corresponding roughly to area 6. In electrically stimulating this supplementary motor area in man, Penfield and Welch (1951) (also Penfield, 1950) observed the following: (1) vocalization—a vowel cry that may be sustained or rhythmically interrupted; (2) assumption of a posture in which the musculature of both sides of the body is employed (for example, the contralateral hand is raised and the head and eyes turn as though regarding it), or the appearance of a stepping rhythm; (3) arrest or slowing of voluntary action; (4) pupillary dilatation, less often acceleration of heart rate; and (5) a "feeling" in the epigastrium or head. Excision of this supplementary area was found without recognized effect. An important point is that after ablation of the rolandic motor and sensory gyri, stimulation of this supplementary area continued to induce the typical responses. This was taken to mean that the supplementary area "moves the opposite limbs which are paralyzed on voluntary effort" (Penfield, 1950).

Some cells in the anterior part of this supplementary area send their fibers to the prefrontal and precentral cortex; however, most of the fiber projections from these cells, as well as from cells of the posterior part of the supplementary motor area, extend into area 4 (the primary motor area). All these efferent fibers are components of COEPS (DeVito and Smith, 1959). At the cortical level the supplementary motor areas are interconnected with adjoining cortical areas by short association fibers (Showers, 1959), and with more distant portions of the same lobe or with adjoining lobes by long association fibers (Crosby, Humphrey, and Showers, 1959).

From ablations of the mesial cortical region in the monkey it has been concluded that each supplementary motor system acts bilaterally. The defects on a given side after simultaneous bilateral ablations are more pronounced than they are after unilateral ablations. Resistance to passive movements appears when lesions are made bilaterally, and after 2 to 4 weeks, contractures develop. The hypertonus even affects the flexor muscles, yet there is no paresis. (Travis, 1955a, b.)

Numerous other areas are "supplementary," for various kinds of movements have been induced by electrical excitation elsewhere in the cortex (Lilly, 1958)—for example, in the posterior parietal area and the temporal cortex. Crosby, Humphrey, and Showers (1959) assessed the situation as follows:

> Supplementary motor areas augment, broaden, in some respects, and may, to some degree (but not completely), substitute for the activities of the primary motor areas. They provide the cortical associated movements which enrich the motor responses. They are an important link in a chain of neurons by which emotions are translated into overt behavior. Through their relations with cerebellar discharges at cortical, basal ganglion, and midbrain levels, they regulate body tonus to fit it to the needs of voluntary and automatic movements. They play a significant part in the adjustment mechanism represented in the complex interplay of hypothalamic, tectal, cortical, cerebellar, and ascending multisynaptic reticular systems in the midbrain. Yet with it all, their basic function is to provide efferent discharge paths for sensory and associative areas of the cerebral cortex. (Original in German.)

Adversive movements, or the sustained conjugate turning of the eyes, with simultaneous turning of head and upper trunk to the same side, receive their innervation mostly from the contralateral area 8. Such movements are particularly evident in an epileptic seizure. Adversive movement of the upper trunk and sometimes of the head as well have been elicited from electrical stimulation farther forward in the mesial cerebral cortex, also from area 22 in the superior temporal gyrus. (Foerster, 1931; Penfield and Jasper, 1954; Woolsey and others, 1952.)

Areas subserving sensibility. Projecting on to the *postcentral gyrus* (areas 3, 1, 2) (Figs. 19-6 and 19-7) are fibers arising from the ventral posterior nuclei (VPM and VPL in Fig. 25-1) of the thalamus, which relay impulses conveyed by the spinothalamic tract, medial lemniscus, and trigeminal lemniscus. The pattern of distribution of the fibers reaching the postcentral gyrus from cutaneous sources is dermatomal, not regional (Dejerine, 1914; Woolsey, Marshall, and Bard, 1942). The sequence of representation is (inferior to superior): face, cervicothoracic segments, more caudal segments, the sequence being the same as in VPM and VPL, in which face, cervicothoracic segments, more caudal segments are represented medial to lateral. Although much of the sensory zone overlaps with the motor zone (hence the term "sensorimotor cortex"), some parts of the sensory may be independent. Impulses to the postcentral gyrus come only from the opposite side of the body, with the probable exception of the face area, which, according to Woolsey and Fairman (1946), receives fibers from both sides.

Another projection system is that reaching areas 5 and 7, in the posterior parietal cortex, from the lateral posterior (LP) and lateral dorsal (LD) thalamic nuclei and the pulvinar (Figs. 25-1 and 25-2), that is, from "association" thalamic nuclei as contrasted with "relay" thalamic nuclei. The distinction is that while relay nuclei receive afferent fibers from brainstem and spinal sources, association nuclei receive their fibers from other thalamic nuclei. It has been postulated that impulses carried in the anterolateral and posterior columns of the spinal cord and from bulbar nuclei reach areas 5 and 7 through the mediation of transthalamic fibers originating in VPL, via a bypass system (Ruch and others, 1965).

A *sensory area II* ("somatic sensory area II," as contrasted with "somatic sensory area I" in the postcentral gyrus) is present in the island of Reil, from the foot of the postcentral gyrus to the bottom of the sylvian fissure. Here the sensory representation is the reverse of that in the postcentral gyrus, that is (dorsal to ventral): face, upper limb, and, most distant from the postcentral gyrus, lower limb. An important point is that sensory area II receives fibers from both sides of the body.

The area has been identified in man (Penfield and Jasper, 1954; Penfield and Rasmussen, 1950), monkey, and other animals (Woolsey, 1958; Woolsey, Marshall, and Bard, 1942). A *sensory area III* has been mapped on the mesial surface of the cortex in the same frontal plane as the postcentral gyrus (Woolsey and others, 1952). Campbell (1965) suggests that these recently discovered sensory areas are, phylogenetically speaking, the primary ones, and that with increasing specialization and advancing skills, special "secondary" areas evolved, now designated as "sensory area I" simply because they were discovered first. The same may apply to the other supplementary areas.

It appears that the phylogenetically older sensory area II receives tactile impressions from large cutaneous areas, such as a hand or a whole limb, while sensory area I receives tactile impressions from small sensory fields, particularly from the periphery of the limbs (Denny-Brown, 1965).

Areas subserving the special senses. The cortical areas concerned in *vision* are described in Chapter 21. In subprimate forms (cat, rabbit, dog) a *visual area II* apparently corresponds to areas 17 and 18. Its pattern is a mirror image of the primary visual area (area 17). Corticopulvinar fibers may represent its discharge path (Crosby, Humphrey, and Lauer, 1962).

Hearing is represented in the superior aspect of the temporal lobe (Flechsig, 1908), that is, in *auditory area I*, or the primary auditory area. This part of the cortex (area 41) is buried beneath the convex cerebral surface and forms the lower lip of the lateral cerebral fissure; here, one to three transverse gyri (Heschl, 1878) are located (Fig. 19-8). An *auditory area II* has been discovered in monkey, chimpanzee, cat, and dog. This area lies ventral to auditory area I. A tonotopic pattern appears to exist in the auditory area I, and the evidence suggests a reversal of the pattern for the reception of tones in area II (Campbell, 1965; Crosby, Humphrey, and Lauer, 1962).

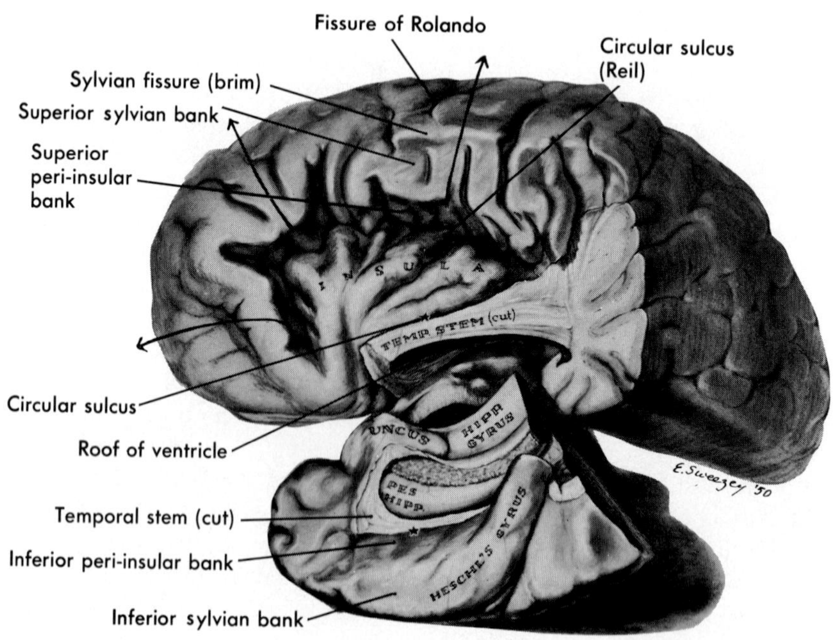

Fig. 19-8. The temporal lobe has been cut off and turned down. The orbital frontal and parietal opercula are pulled away from the insula to show the cortex down into the circular sulcus, which runs round the insula. Projecting from the inferior sylvian bank is a transverse gyrus, the gyrus of Heschl. (From Penfield and Jasper, 1954.)

Taste is generally considered to be represented either in the most inferior part of the postcentral and precentral gyri or in the contiguous part of the insular cortex, in the region of the circular sulcus bordering the island of Reil (Fig. 19-8) (Börnstein, 1940a, b; Penfield and Jasper, 1954).

Smell is probably represented in the more rostral part of the piriform cortex, which borders the outer side of the lateral olfactory stria. Smell might also be represented in the anterior perforated substance *(APS)* and its *olfactory tubercle (OLT)* and the cortex overlying the mesial aspect of the amygdala (Fig. 19-9, *C*) (Allison, 1954).

Situated behind the piriform cortex is the cortex of the hippocampal gyrus, which corresponds in large measure to the entorhinal cortex, or entorhinal area (Fig. 19-9). Deep to the hippocampal gyrus and continuous with it is the hippocampal formation. The hippocampus (cornu ammonis), a part of this formation, is divisible into a number of fields (Fig. 19-10). Projections going from these different hippocampal fields through the fimbria and fornix terminate differently.

Clinically speaking, the hippocampal formation is not considered of importance to olfaction; Penfield and Erickson (1941) could not induce any sensation of smell by electrically stimulating the hippocampal

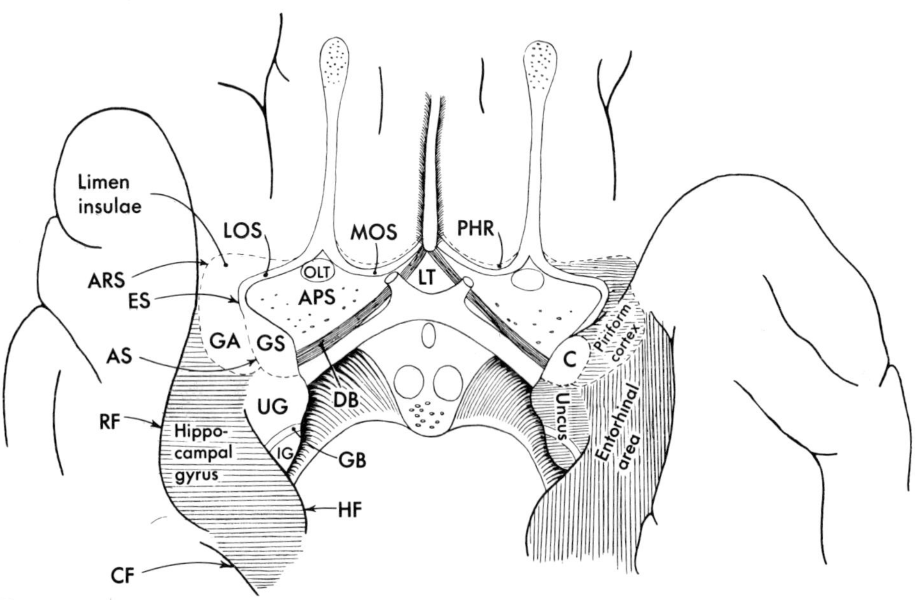

Fig. 19-9. Structures at the base of the brain. On the left the temporal lobe has been displaced laterally so as to expose underlying structures. The lateral olfactory stria *(LOS)* borders the anterior perforated substance *(APS)*, and extends caudally to reach the gyrus semilunaris *(GS)*, the pallium of which (see right side) constitutes the cortical amygdaloid nucleus *(C)*. On the left side, bordering the lateral olfactory stria and situated lateral to the gyrus semilunaris *(GS)* is the gyrus ambiens *(GA)*, the pallium of which (see right side) is piriform cortex. (The region labeled "Piriform cortex" is usually called "postpiriform cortex," and the horizontally lined area in front of it, "prepiriform cortex.") The gyrus ambiens coincides with the limen insulae. Caudal to the gyrus ambiens is the hippocampal gyrus, the cortex of which corresponds in general (see right side) with the entorhinal cortex. Medially the hippocampal gyrus is bounded by the hippocampal fissure *(HF)*, and laterally by the rhinal fissure *(RF)* and the collateral fissure *(CF)*. Caudal to the gyrus semilunaris is the uncus gyrus hippocampi: it is divided into three parts, the uncinate gyrus *(UG)*, Giacomini's band *(GS)* (which is the ventral continuation of the dentate gyrus), and the intralimbic gyrus *(IG)*.

ARS, anterior rhinal sulcus; *AS*, amygdalar, or semiannular, sulcus; *ES*, entorhinal sulcus; *MOS*, medial olfactory stria; *PHR*, prehippocampal rudiment. Not illustrated is the intermediate olfactory stria, passing to the olfactory tubercle *(OLT)*. (From Kuhlenbeck, 1927, with minor modifications.)

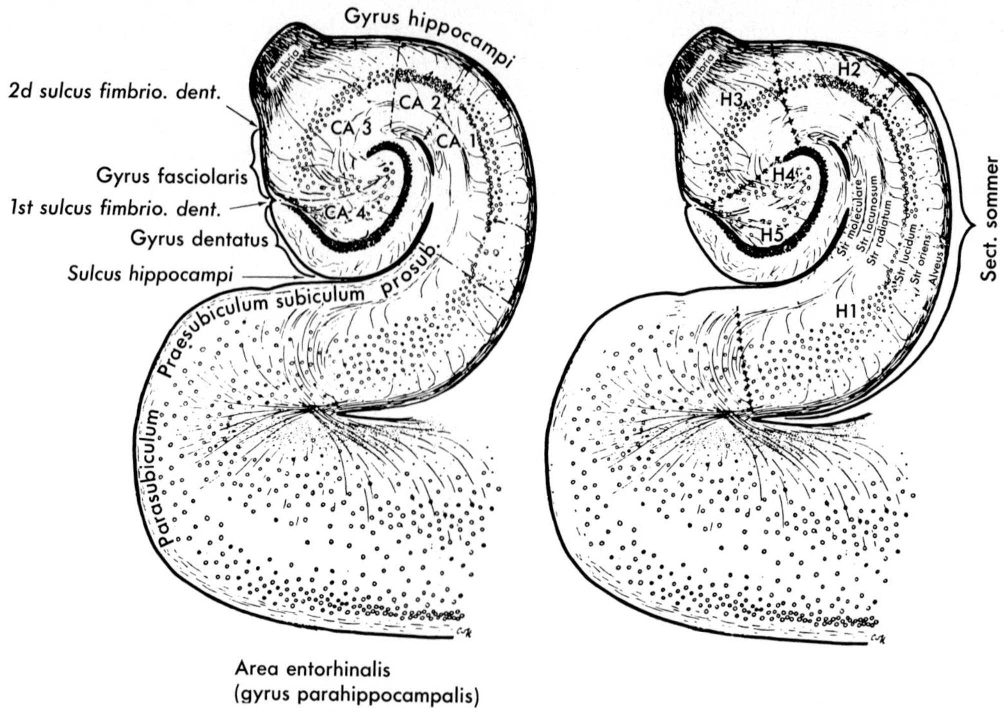

Fig. 19-10. Hippocampal formation, subiculum, and entorhinal area, according to Gastaut and Lammers (1961). "Gyrus parahippocampalis" is referred to by most authors as the *gyrus hippocampi.* The hippocampal fields of Lorente de Nó are indicated to the left *(CA 1-CA 4)*, and the fields of Rose to the right *(H 1-H 5)*. The strata (indicated to the right) are the following: stratum moleculare, stratum lacunosum, stratum radiatum, stratum lucidum, stratum oriens.

gyrus. Evidence, however, exists that the hippocampus does receive olfactory impulses by way of a perforant pathway from the hippocampal gyrus whose fibers terminate in the dendrites of hippocampal pyramidal cells; the olfactory stimuli reaching the hippocampus are considered analogous to conditioning stimuli (Yokota, Reeves, and MacLean, 1967).

Areas subserving vestibular function. Pathways conducting vestibular impulses to the cortex are described on page 194, and clinical aspects of the problem are presented on pages 381 and 382. Current views are that vestibular function is represented in the opercular cortex of the temporal lobe and the adjacent cortex of the superior temporal gyrus (lateral brain surface) at a level rostral to the auditory area (Schneider, Calhoun, and Crosby, 1968) and/or in preoccipital areas (Spiegel and others, 1965).

"Association" areas. The concept of cortical "association" areas is based on the premise that certain fiber systems convey directive stimuli from one part of the cortex to another without the intervention of fibers reaching the cortex from the thalamus or the geniculate bodies. Since somesthetic areas 5 and 7, previously considered to be association areas, receive projections from the thalamus (p. 319), and since other alleged association areas have been shown to receive projections from the thalamus, the concept of association areas has, in some circles, been abandoned. This is with the exception of the prefrontal cortex (p. 446). According to Campbell (1965), it is useful to look upon association areas "as places where more than one type of information (say, auditory together with visual) meet and are integrated to produce an appropriate response (say, head and eye movements toward or away from something heard or seen)."

Areas 18 and 19 are particularly rich in visual association fibers. Apparently in like manner, limbic structures are linked with the temporal neocortex (basal and lateral and temporal pole). For example, fibers from the inferior temporal gyrus interconnect with the hippocampal gyrus (which projects strongly to the hippocampus) and with the amygdala (which has important direct connections with the hypothalamus and the medial dorsal nucleus (MD) of the thalamus, and secondary connections with the hippocampus). The temporal cortex also projects to the posterior part of the cingulate region. (Akert and others, 1961; Bucy and Klüver, 1955; Geschwind, 1965.)

Association between the temporal cortex and the frontal cortex is brought about by the *uncinate fasciculus,* a bundle that connects frontal granular areas with temporal neocortex. Fibers of orbitocortical origin running alongside this bundle terminate in the rostral part of the superior, middle, and inferior temporal gyri, and it is possible that fibers from the amygdala pass by the same route to the orbitofrontal cortex (Klingler and Gloor, 1960; Nauta, 1962, 1964).

Limbic lobe. This part of the cerebrum is enclosed in two rings of cortex, an inner and an outer, the latter bordering the rest of the cerebrum (*limbus,* border or threshold) (Figs. 25-4 and 25-5). The *inner* ring, phylogenetically the older, includes the hippocampal formation, the septal and parolfactory areas, the anterior perforated substance with its olfactory tubercle (these two terms are often used synonymously), and the piriform cortex and the adjacent part of the amygdala (cortical and medial amygdaloid nuclei) (Fig. 19-9); and thus it is not entirely a ring. The *outer* ring includes the orbitoinsulotemporal cortex rostrolaterally, the cingulate cortex superiorly, and the entorhinal cortex and subiculum (Fig. 19-10) inferiorly. The olfactory bulb projects its fibers into various components of this system. Broca (1878, 1879), in his description of the "great limbic lobe"—so-called because he conceived of it as a threshold between pallium and brainstem, and belonging to the palii of the conventional lobes yet a phylogenetic entity—included both the inner and the outer ring, embracing in their confines certain basal structures (such as the anterior perforated substance), the parolfactory area ("carrefour de l'hémisphère"), cingulate and hippocampal gyrus, and the hippocampal complex. MacLean (1952) added certain noncortical structures to what he called the *limbic system:* the amygdaloid complex and the fornix.

Included in the limbic system are a number of fiber aggregates besides the fornix. Among them are the medial forebrain bundle (conveying fibers from the anterior perforated substance and elsewhere), the ventral amygdalofugal pathway, and the stria terminalis (the latter also from the amygdala). These are the most massive afferents reaching the hypothalamus from in front. Nuclei of the paramedian part of the midbrain ("limbic midbrain area," Nauta, 1958) unite with many of the rostrally lying structures in providing reciprocal connections with the hypothalamus. Another link between limbic cortex and hypothalamus is by way of the medial component of the medial dorsal thalamic nucleus and possibly the thalamic midline nuclei (MD, mc, and M, respectively, in Figs. 25-1 and 25-2). Direct neocortical projections to the limbic cortex (which, in its cingular part, is neocortical) are remarkably restricted as to origin, the major proportion coming from the inferior parietal lobule (Nauta and Haymaker, 1969).

Constituting a major part of the cerebrum, the limbic lobe has diverse functions. The fact that the olfactory bulb projects abundant fibers into this system (hence, the term, "rhinencephalon," for a sizable part of it) led in earlier days to an overemphasis of its role in olfactory function. Functionally the limbic lobe appears to be related mainly to mechanisms concerned in the execution of complex, yet primitive, semiautomatic sequences of action (Pribram, 1960), mechanisms in the cognitive sphere (Meissner, 1967), and mechanisms in the whole realm of affect, sexual function, and their somatic and autonomic accompaniments (MacLean, 1969).

Input from visceral structures. MacLean (1949) originally called the limbic system the "visceral brain." Besides abundant output, it receives an input from all viscera having autonomic innervation: heart, blood vessels, gastrointestinal tract, and so on (Kaada and Jasper, 1952; Kaada, Pribram, and Epstein, 1949).

The postcentral gyrus also receives an input from the viscera. Foerster (1936) noted girdle pains as well as abdominal and "cardiac" pains (in man) on stimulating the postcentral gyrus in the trunk area, and Woolsey, Marshall, and Bard (1942), utilizing the method of evoked potentials (in monkeys), noted that impulses from the splanchnic nerve reach the trunk area of the cortex at the exact site to which corresponding spinal segments project. The sensorimotor cortex is thus a "somato-viscerosensory" area. Autonomic function is represented in various parts of the neocortex. Generally speaking, *area 6* and, to a less degree, *areas 8* and *4* influence the circulation, pilomotor system, gastrointestinal tract, pupillary muscles, and the urinary bladder. The *orbitofrontal cortex* influences blood pressure, respiration, and gastric motility. The cingulate cortex, entorhinal, and insular parts of the cortex share in some of these functions (Kaada and Jasper, 1952). The hypothalamus provides the major autonomic outflow, and it seems that the cortex plays a controlling or regulating role in the carrying out of finer autonomic adjustments (Kennard, 1949).

Prefrontal and orbitofrontal areas and psychic function. Clinicopathological observations suggest that the more rostral part of the frontal lobe (the prefrontal area) is concerned in the formation of concepts and their synthesis in planning, forecasting and initiative, while the orbitofrontal cortex (basal neocortex) is correlated with temperament and character, the latter emphasized particularly by Spatz (1966). Although the cortex cannot be parcellated into regions, each subserving this or that psychic function (which are themselves ill defined), nonetheless differing constellations of psychic and behavioral disturbances are known to occur with lesions in different locations (Chapter 22).

CORTICOFUGAL AND CORTICOPETAL PATHWAYS

Corticofugal fiber systems

Corticonuclear tracts. These tracts originate from the primary motor cortex, which is centered about area 4, or in adjacent parts of the cortex, and extend downward to motor nuclei of the brainstem and the anterior horns of the spinal cord.

Corticosubcortical fibers. These fibers belong to COEPS. Issuing as relays from basal ganglia and brainstem nuclei are fibers which, through further relay, pass to motor cranial nerve nuclei of the brainstem or to anterior horn cells.

Corticopetal fiber systems

The cells of origin lie in subcortical structures. The most conspicuous subcortical station is the thalamus. It receives impulses concerned with sensibility by way of the spinal and cranial nerves and projects them to the cortex. Other clinically significant subcortical sensory structures are the medial geniculate body, which transmits impulses concerned in hearing to the superior aspect of the temporal lobe, and the lateral geniculate body, which transmits visual impulses to the calcarine cortex.

Components of the corona radiata and internal capsule

Corticofugal fibers converge as they pass in the corona radiata to reach the internal capsule, and corticopetal fibers diverge as they pass through the internal capsule and the corona radiata to end in the cortex.

The internal capsule is a half shell (the other half is in the external capsule) around the lentiform ("lens-shaped") nucleus. It consists of corticofugal and corticopetal fibers bounded laterally by the lentiform nucleus and medially by the caudate nucleus and thalamus. It surrounds the basal ganglia on their medial, anterior, posterior, and postero-inferior surfaces and connects the neopallium with nearly all subcortical structures. In lateral and horizontal sections of the hemisphere it is composed of five parts: anterior limb, genu, posterior limb, retrolenticular limb, and sublenticular limb (Fig. 27-10).

As viewed in the horizontal plane (Fig. 19-11), the *anterior limb* contains corticofugal fibers extending from the frontal cortex to the nuclei pontis and then, by way of a second neuron, to the contralateral hemisphere of the cerebellum (the frontopontocerebellar tract). The *genu* contains fibers destined to terminate in relation to the extraocular and facial nuclei. As to the *posterior limb,* the corticospinal tract is generally said to traverse its anterior two-thirds. Evidence from varied sources suggests, however, that the cortico-

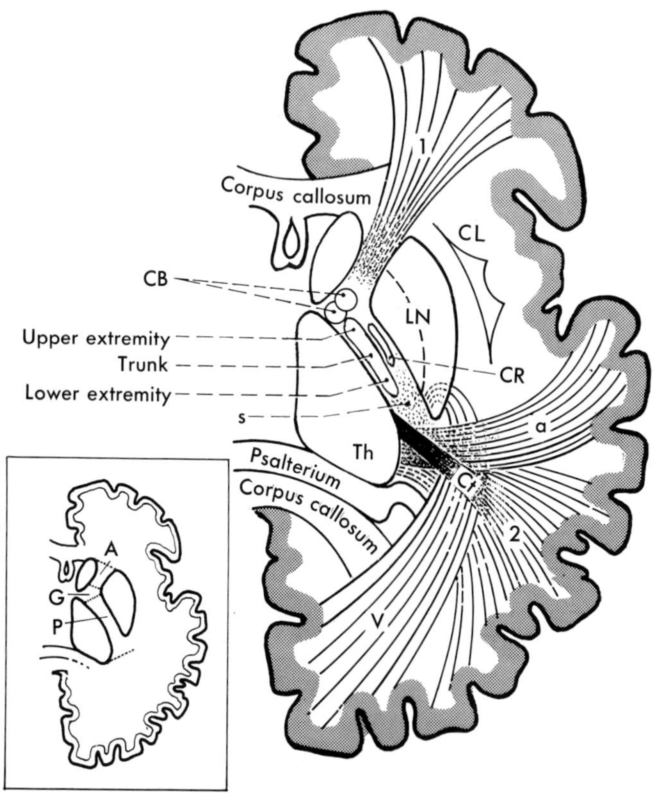

Fig. 19-11. Components of the internal capsule and corona radiata. In the inset, the positions of the anterior limb *(A)*, genu *(G)*, and posterior limb *(P)* of the internal capsule are indicated. The genu of the internal capsule contains corticobulbar pathways *(CB)*, and the anterior two-thirds of the posterior limb, the corticospinal tract for the supply of the upper extremity, trunk, and lower extremity. *CR* refers to the corticorubral tract together with the corticotegmental tract. The posterior third of the internal capsule contains sensory fibers (thalamocortical projection) *(s)* proceeding to the postcentral gyrus. The fiber radiatons comprise: *1*, the frontopontile tract and projections to and from the thalamus; *2*, pathways from the temporal, parietal, and occipital cortex to the pons; *a*, auditory radiation to the transverse gyri (of Heschl); *v*, visual radiation to the calcarine cortex. *CL*, claustrum; *Ct*, corticotectal and corticotegmental tracts; *LN*, lenticular nucleus; *Th*, thalamus.

spinal fibers pursue their course through the middle third or even more posteriorly, that is, through the third quarter of posterior limb (Brion and Guiot, 1964; Smith, 1960). The more rostral part of the internal capsule contains the corticorubral and corticotegmental pathways (from areas 4 and 6). The *posterior third of the posterior limb* contains the sensory radiation—fibers extending from the thalamus to the parietal cortex. Also traversing this part of the posterior limb are fibers extending from the temporal, parietal, and occipital cortex to the nuclei pontis, and thence via a second neuron to the cerebellum. Through these pathways, as well as through the frontopontocerebellar tract, cerebellar activity is brought under the control of varied areas of the cerebral cortex. The posterior limb also interconnects thalamus and striatum. A more or less horizontal course is taken by the retrolenticular and sublenticular parts of the internal capsule. Situated here are the visual and auditory fiber groups, which pass from the respective geniculate ganglia to the calcarine and superior temporal areas (Fig. 27-10).

Fiber pathways bringing the two hemispheres into communication. These include chiefly the corpus callosum and the anterior, posterior, and hippocampal commissures. The corpus callosum interconnects much of the cortex of the two sides. However, the visual cortex (area 17) receives no fibers from the corpus callosum, nor does any other primary sensory area, nor apparently does the prefrontal cortex (Geschwind, 1965). The anterior commissure interconnects the temporal poles; the temporal cortex in this region is referred to as *noncallosal cortex.*

REFERENCES

Akert, K., Gruesen, R. A., Woolsey, C. N., and Meyer, D. R. 1961. Klüver-Bucy syndrome in monkeys with neocortical ablations of temporal lobe. Brain **84**:480-498.

Allison, A. C. 1954. The secondary olfactory areas in the human brain. J. Anat. **88**:481-488.

Amassian, V. E. 1953. Evoked single cortical unit activity in the somatic sensory areas. EEG Clin. Neurophysiol. **5**:415-438.

Bailey, P., and von Bonin, G. 1951. The isocortex of man. Urbana, University of Illinois Press.

Börnstein, W. S. 1940a. Cortical representation of taste in man and monkey: functional and anatomical relations of taste, olfaction, and somatic sensibility. Yale J. Biol. Med. **12**:719-736.

Börnstein, W. S. 1940b. Cortical representation of taste in man and monkey: the localization of the cortical taste area in man and a method for measuring impairment of taste in man. Yale J. Biol. Med. **13**:133-156.

Brion, S., and Guiot, G. 1964. Topographie des faisceaux de projection du cortex dans la capsule interne et dans le pédoncule cérébral. Rev. Neurol. **110**:123-144.

Broca, P. 1878. Le grand lobe limbique (etc.) Rev. Anthropol., ser. 2, **1**:385-498.

Broca, P. 1879. Recherches sur les centres olfactifs. Rev. Anthropol., ser. 2, **2**:385-455.

Brodmann, K. 1908. Beiträge zur histologischen Lokalisation der Grosshirnrinde. VI. Mitteilung. Die Cortexgliederung des Menschen. J. Psychol. Neurol. **10**:231-246.

Bucy, P. C. 1957. Is there a pyramidal tract? Brain **80**:376-392.

Bucy, P. C., and Klüver, H. 1955. An anatomical investigation of the temporal lobe in the monkey (Macaca mulatta). J. Comp. Neurol. **103**: 151-251.

Campbell, H. J. 1965. Correlative physiology of the nervous system. New York, Academic Press, Inc.

Carman, J. B., Cowan, W. M., Powell, T. P. S., and Webster, K. E. 1965. A bilateral corticostriate projection. J. Neurol. Neurosurg. Psychiat. **28**:71-77.

Crosby, E. C., Humphrey, T., and Lauer, E. W. 1962. Correlative anatomy of the nervous system. New York, The Macmillan Company.

Crosby, E. C., Humphrey, T., and Showers, M. J. 1959. Einige Anordnungen, Verbindungen und Funktionen der supplementären motorischen Rinden. In Bauer, K. F., editor: Medizinische Grundlagenforschung, vol. 2. Stuttgart, Georg Thieme Verlag, pp. 101-124.

Dejerine, J. 1914. Sémiologie des affections du système nerveux. Paris, Masson et Cie.

Denny-Brown, D. 1965. The release of deep pain by nerve injury. Brain **88**:725-738.

DeVito, J. L., and Smith, O. A., Jr. 1959. Projections from the mesial frontal cortex (supplementary motor area) to the cerebral hemispheres and brain stem of the Macaca mulatta. J. Comp. Neurol. **111**:261-277.

Flechsig, P. 1908. Bemerkungen über die Hörsphäre des menschlichen Gehirns. Neurol. Zbl. **27**:2-7; 50-57.

Foerster, O. 1931. The cerebral cortex in man. Lancet **2**:309-312.

Foerster, O. 1936. Sensible corticale Felder. In Bumke, O., and Foerster, O., editors: Handbuch der Neurologie, vol. 6. Berlin, Springer-Verlag, pp. 358-448.

Furstenburg, A. C. 1958. Evidence of laryngeal participation in emotional expression: its relation to hysterical aphonia. Ann. Otol. **67**:516-527.

Gastaut, H., and Lammers, H. J. 1961. Anatomie

du rhinencéphale, vol. 1, p. 49, In Alajouanine, T., editor: Les grandes activités du rhinencéphale. Paris, Masson et Cie.

Geschwind, N. 1965. Disconnexion syndromes in animals and man. Brain **88**:237-294, 585-644.

Heschl, R. L. 1878. Ueber die vordere quere Schläfenwindung des menschlichen Grosshirns. Wien, Wilhelm Braumüller.

Hines, M. 1943. Control of movements by the cerebral cortex in primates. Biol. Rev. **18**:1-31.

Horsley, V. 1909. The Linacre Lecture on the function of the so-called motor area of the brain. Brit. Med. J. **2**:125-132.

Hughes, J. R., and Mazurowski, J. A. 1962. Studies on the supracallosal mesial cortex of unanesthetized, conscious mammals. II. Monkey. A. Movements elicited by electrical stimulation. EEG Clin. Neurophysiol. **14**:477-485.

Jane, J. A., Yashon, D., Becker, D. P., Beatty, R., and Sugar, O. 1968. The effect of destruction in the human cerebral peduncle upon motor function and involuntary movements: report of 11 cases. J. Neurosurg. **29**:581-585.

Kaada, B. R., and Jasper, H. 1952. Respiratory responses to stimulation of temporal pole, insula, and hippocampal and limbic gyri in man. A.M.A. Arch. Neurol. Psychiat. **68**:609-619.

Kaada, B. R., Pribram, K. H., and Epstein, J. A. 1949. Respiratory and vascular responses in monkeys from temporal pole, insula, orbital surface and cingulate gyrus: a preliminary report. J. Neurophysiol. **12**:347-356.

Kautzky, R., and Zülch, K. J. 1955. Neurologisch-Neurochirurgische Röntgendiagnostik und andere Methoden zur Erkennung intrakranialer Erkrankungen. Berlin, Springer-Verlag, pp. 5, 8-9.

Kennard, M. 1949. Autonomic function. In Bucy, P. C., editor: The precentral motor cortex, ed. 2. Urbana, University of Illinois Press, pp. 293-306.

Klingler, J., and Gloor, P. 1960. The connections of the amygdala and of the anterior cortex in the human brain. J. Comp. Neurol. **115**:333-369.

Kuhlenbeck, H. 1927. Vorlesungen über das Zentralnervensystem der Wirbelthiere. Jena, Gustav Fischer Verlag, pp. 52, 354.

Lassek, A. M. 1942. The human pyramidal tract: a study of the mature myelinated fibers of the pyramid. J. Comp. Neurol. **76**:217-225.

Lassek, A. M., and Evans, J. P. 1945. The human pyramidal tract: the effect of hemispherectomies on the fiber components of the pyramids. J. Comp. Neurol. **83**:113-119.

Lassek, A. M., and Evans, J. P. 1946. The human pyramidal tract: a study of the representation of the cortico-spinal tracts in the spinal cord. J. Comp. Neurol. **84**:11-16.

Lilly, J. C. 1958. Correlations between neurophysiological activity in the cortex and short-term behavior in the monkey. In Harlow, H. F., and Woolsey, C. N., editors: Biological and biochemical bases of behavior. Madison, University of Wisconsin Press, pp. 83-100.

Lorente de Nó, L. 1938. The cerebral cortex: architecture, intracortical connections and motor projections. In Fulton, J. F.: Physiology of the nervous system. London, Oxford University Press, pp. 291-346.

MacLean, P. B. 1949. Psychosomatic disease and the "visceral brain": recent developments bearing on the Papez theory of emotion. Psychosom. Med. **11**:338-353.

MacLean, P. D. 1952. Some psychiatric implications of physiological studies on frontotemporal portion of limbic system (visceral brain). EEG Clin. Neurophysiol. **4**:407-418.

Maclean, P. D. 1969. The hypothalamus and emotional behavior. In Haymaker, W., Anderson, E., and Nauta, W. J. H., editors: The hypothalamus. Springfield, Illinois, Charles C Thomas, Publisher, pp. 659-678.

Meissner, W. W. 1967. Memory function in the Korsakoff syndrome. J. Nerv. Ment. Dis. **145**:106-122.

Mettler, F. A. 1944. On origin of fibers in pyramid of primate brain. Proc. Soc. Exp. Biol. Med. **57**:111-113.

Nauta, W. J. H. 1958. Hippocampal projections and related neural pathways to the mid-brain in the cat. Brain **81**:319-341.

Nauta, W. J. H. 1962. Neural associations of the amygdaloid complex in the monkey. Brain **85**:505-520.

Nauta, W. J. H. 1964. Some afferent connections of the prefrontal cortex in the monkey. In Warren, J. M., and Akert, K., editors: The frontal granular cortex and behavior. New York, McGraw-Hill Book Company, pp. 397-409.

Nauta, W. J. H., and Haymaker, W. 1969. Hypothalamic nuclei and fiber connections. In Haymaker, W., Anderson, E., and Nauta, W. J. H., editors: The hypothalamus. Springfield, Illinois, Charles C Thomas, Publisher, pp. 136-209.

Patton, H. D., and Amassian, V. E. 1960. The pyramidal tract: its excitation and functions. In Field, J., Magoun, H. W., and Hall, V. E., editors: Handbook of physiology, sect. 1, vol. 2. Washington, D. C., American Physiological Society, pp. 837-861.

Penfield, W. 1950. The supplementary motor area in the cerebral cortex of man. Arch. Psychiat. Z. Neurol. **185**:670-674.

Penfield, W. 1954. Mechanisms of voluntary movement. Brain **77**:1-17.

Penfield, W. 1957. Vestibular sensation and the cerebral cortex. Ann. Otol. **66**:691-699.

Penfield, W., and Erickson, T. C. 1941. Epilepsy and cerebral localization. Springfield, Illinois, Charles C Thomas, Publisher, p. 12.

Penfield, W., and Jasper, H. 1954. Epilepsy and the functional anatomy of the human brain. Boston, Little, Brown and Company.

Penfield, W., and Rasmussen, T. 1950. The cerebral cortex of man: a clinical study of localization of function. New York, The Macmillan Company.

Penfield, W., and Welch, K. 1951. The supplementary motor area of the cerebral cortex: a clinical and experimental study. A.M.A. Arch. Neurol. Psychiat. **66**:289-317.

Pribram, K. H. 1960. A review of theory in physiological psychology. Ann. Rev. Psychol. **11**:1-40.

Rossi, G. F., and Brodal, A. 1956. Corticofugal fibres to the brain-stem reticular formation; an experimental study in the cat. J. Anat. **90**:42-62.

Ruch, T. C., Patton, H. D., Woodbury, J. W., and Towe, A. L. 1965. Neurophysiology, ed. 2. Philadelphia, W. B. Saunders Company.

Russell, J. R., and DeMyer, W. 1961. The quantitative cortical origin of pyramidal axons of Macaca rhesus: with some remarks on the slow rate of axolysis. Neurology **11**:96-108.

Schneider, R. C., Calhoun, H. D., and Crosby, E. C. 1968. Vertigo and rotational movement in cortical and subcortical lesions. J. Neurol. Sci. **6**:493-516.

Showers, M. J. C. 1959. The cingulate gyrus: additional motor area and cortical autonomic regulation. J. Comp. Neurol. **112**:231-302.

Smith, M. C. 1960. Nerve fiber degeneration in the brain in amyotrophic lateral sclerosis. J. Neurol. Neurosurg. Psychiat. **23**:269-282.

Spatz, H. 1966. Gehirnentwicklung (Introversion-Promination) und Endocranialausguss. In Hassler, R., and Stephan, H., editors: Evolution of the forebrain: phylogenesis and ontogenesis of the forebrain. Stuttgart, Georg Thieme Verlag, pp. 136-152.

Spiegel, E. A., Szekely, E. G., Moffet, R., Gildenberg, P., Lehman, R., and Robbins, A. 1965. Cortical projections of the labyrinth. In Kirikae, I., editor: Internat. symposium on vestibular and oculomotor problems. University of Tokyo, Japanese Society for Vestibular Research, pp. 9-14.

Sugar, O., Chusid, J. G., and French, J. D. 1948. A second motor cortex in the monkey (Macaca mulatta). J. Neuropath. Exp. Neurol. **7**:182-189.

Tower, S. S. 1949. The pyramidal tract. In Bucy, P. C., editor: The precentral motor cortex, ed. 2. Urbana, University of Illinois Press, pp. 149-179.

Travis, A. M. 1955a. Neurological deficiencies after ablation of the precentral motor area in Macaca mulatta. Brain **78**:155-173.

Travis, A. M. 1955b. Neurological deficiencies following supplementary motor area lesions in Macaca mulatta. Brain **78**:174-198.

Woolsey, C. N. 1947. Patterns of sensory representation in the cerebral cortex. Fed. Proc. **6**: 437-441.

Woolsey, C. N. 1958. Organization of somatic sensory and motor areas of the cerebral cortex. In Harlow, H. F., and Woolsey, C. N., editors: Biological and biochemical bases of behavior. Madison, University of Wisconsin Press, pp. 63-81.

Woolsey, C. N., and Fairman, D. 1946. Contralateral, ipsilateral, and bilateral representation of cutaneous receptors in somatic areas I and II of the cerebral cortex of pig, sheep, and other mammals. Surgery **19**:684-702.

Woolsey, C. N., Marshall, W. H., and Bard, P. 1942. Representation of cutaneous tactile sensibility in the cerebral cortex of the monkey as indicated by evoked potentials. Bull. Johns Hopk. Hosp. **70**:399-441.

Woolsey, C. N., Settlage, P. H., Meyer, D. R., Spencer, W., Hamuy, T. P., and Travis, A. M. 1952. Patterns of localization in precentral and "supplementary" motor areas and their relation to the concept of a premotor area. Res. Publ. Ass. Res. Nerv. Ment. Dis., Proc. **30**:238-264.

Yokota, T., Reeves, A. G., and MacLean, P. D. 1967. Intracellular olfactory response of hippocampal neurons in awake, sitting squirrel monkeys. Science **157**:1072-1077.

Chapter 20

Motor, sensory, reflex, and related disturbances of cerebral cortical and subcortical origin

The patterns of functional disturbance evoked by lesions involving motor and sensory structures of the cerebrum vary greatly, depending upon the site of the lesion—whether in the cerebral cortex, corona radiata, or internal capsule. The disturbances may represent either a functional deficit or an irritative (excitatory) phenomenon. Larger lesions involving the frontal lobe give rise to release and allied phenomena. These will be considered first.

FRONTAL RELEASE AND ALLIED PHENOMENA

Traction response, grasping, groping, perseveration. In the course of the development of normal infants, three forms of automatic grasping response occur (Twitchell, 1961).

In the neonate, a proprioceptive reaction in the form of a *traction response* is dominant. The stimulus consists in stretching the shoulder adductors and flexors by pulling at the forearm. In response, all fingers flex. When the infant is about 2 weeks of age this traction response can be facilitated by applying a distally moving, strong contact stimulus along the radial aspect of the palm in a distal direction. Flexion of the fingers is now accompanied by flexion at the wrist, elbow, and shoulder. As the infant matures, the traction response from the shoulder diminishes, that by contact stimulation at the palms increases.

At 4 weeks, the initial stage of the grasp reflex appears: a contact stimulus moving out between the thumb and index finger causes adduction of these two digits, immediately followed by synergistic flexion at all joints of the upper limb. Several days later the two digits will also flex in response to the same stimulus. The receptive field for the grasp reflex widens to include the entire radial aspect of the palm and volar surface of the proximal phalanges. The grasp reflex is fully developed at 3 to 4 months.

Another reaction, the *instinctive grasp reaction,* then appears. Initially, slight supination of the hand results from contact stimulation of the radial side of the hand. Some weeks later, pronation of the hand occurs upon stimulation along its ulnar border. In another 2 to 3 weeks slight palpating or *groping* movements of the hand are added to these orienting movements. Several weeks after the onset of the groping, the hand will pursue a retreating contact stimulus (applied to any part of the hand), orient to it, palpate it, and finally grasp it. The response is fully formed in infants 4 to 10 months of age. The adequate stimulus for the responses (orienting, groping, grasping) is light stationary or moving contact with any part of the hand.

Automatic traction, grasping, and groping responses, physiologically identical to those noted for the infant, may be obtained in the adult with acquired brain disease. The latter responses have been referred to as *forced grasping and groping* (Adie and Critchley, 1927), *grasp reflex* (Seyffarth and Denny-Brown, 1948), and *Zwangsgreifen und Nachgreifen* (Schuster, 1923, 1927). The strongest component of the grasp reflex is flexion with adduction of the thumb and index finger, elicited by contact stimulation in the area between these two digits. The *grasp reflex* and the *instinctive grasp responses* (including *groping*) are elicitable chiefly when lesions are located in the superior frontal gyrus in the region of area 4, but perhaps only when the mesial cortex in this region is also damaged. The two responses may occur independently of each other or together.

Unilateral grasping and groping strongly indicate the presence of tumor, infarction, or some other pathological process in the frontal lobe. Bilateral responses, as in internal hydrocephalus and Wernicke's encephalopathy, have less localizing importance. In patients in whom grasping and groping are elicited, psychic function is invariably impaired and consciousness may be clouded. The frontal lobe may be affected indirectly by a primary lesion elsewhere in the brain. In deep stupor and during sleep, grasping and groping are not elicitable.

In the *more tonic forms of the grasp reflex* the reaction outlasts the stimulus, and it may be difficult for the patient to relax his grasp. The responsible lesion is usually in the thalamus or striatum, but it is localizable only if the grasp reflex is unilateral. After shaking hands, *perseveratory grasping and groping* makes the patient grasp the examiner's hand again or catch hold of his coat. This is typical of diffuse cerebral cortical affections; here, the reaction occurs bilaterally. Perseveration can also take the form of constant buttoning and unbuttoning of the shirt, arranging and rearranging the bedclothes, pulling them a little higher, or turning them down a few inches, as has been observed in a patient with frontal lobe abscess (Williamson, 1896).

In patients with marked upper limb spasticity, a *traction response* can usually be obtained under these circumstances. Grasping and groping movements may, however, vanish when severe hemiplegia develops. In the recovery stage of hemiplegia all three forms of grasping automatism may occasionally be elicited. (Allison, 1966; Denny-Brown, Twitchell, and Saenz-Arroyo, 1949; Herman, 1952; Twitchell, 1965.)

The *grasp reflex of the foot* undergoes much the same evolution as the grasp reflex of the hand.

In a normal child 1 to 2 years old, the grasp reflex of the foot can be induced by exerting gentle pressure either on the sole, on the plantar surface of the toes, or in the grooves between the toes, though the most receptive area is the ball of the great toe. The reflex is characterized by a tonic flexion-adduction movement of all the toes that enables them to hold an object thrust between them for a period of 15 to 30 seconds. In infants there may also be a *Babinski reflex,* but its significance is doubtful in infants less than 3 years of age because the reflex is normally elicitable up to that time. In adults the grasp reflex of the foot is always pathological. (Brain and Curren, 1932.)

Analogous to the grasping reflex, and sometimes accompanying it, is the *bulldog reflex,* which consists in involuntary biting of an object placed between the teeth.

Other reflexes. *Bending reflexes* are affected in frontal lobe lesions. If the fingers of a normal person are passively folded into the hollow of his hand and his wrist then sharply flexed, the forearm undergoes simultaneous flexion at the elbow. In interruption of the pyramidal tract this reflex is abolished (forearm sign of Léri). However, in lesions of the frontal lobe, especially those situated parasagittally near the precentral gyrus, this reflex is greatly enhanced, as are bending reflexes elicited elsewhere in the limbs. The exaggerated reflex may be obtained most readily by deviating the hand either dorsally or radially at the wrist. Likewise, contraction of the arm adductors may occur following maximal passive abduction at the shoulder joint. The development of the bending and grasp reflexes is inversely related to the degree of increase of deep reflexes and other pyramidal signs. (Seyffarth, 1953.)

The *tonic plantar reflex* can frequently be elicited in frontal lobe lesions, especially in tumors and less commonly in hemorrhage or cerebral softening. It has little in common with the grasp reflex and is often present when the latter is absent.

The reflex is one of the earliest signs of a frontal lobe lesion; it appears before the Babinski and other pyramidal signs develop. Its presence is strongly suggestive of a lesion in or near the more anterior part of area 6. Not infrequently the lesion occupies the medial aspect of the hemisphere, to which it may have extended from an adjacent part of the cerebrum. The reflex is obtained only in cases in which voluntary movement of the toes is well preserved, and thus integrity of the precentral cortex is essential. The *tonic extensor reflex* of the toes and foot, by contrast, is obtainable only in lesions interrupting the cerebrospinal pathway. It may be elicited, for example, in cortical and subcortical lesions (such as bleeding into the internal capsule) that produce only slight paresis. The reflex may also be found in severe hemiplegia, for example, following occlusion of the internal carotid or the middle cerebral artery. Some long-lasting central excitatory state appears to be involved. (Grimby, 1965.)

To test for the tonic plantar reflex, the sole should be stimulated either with a moving blunt object or pressure upon the sole. Increase in pressure accentuates the response (Goldstein, 1938). The tonic plantar response is characterized by a slow, tonic flexion of the toes and distal part of the foot; the alteration in position persists a few seconds or longer, whereupon, with the same deliberate movement, the toes resume their previous position (Fig. 20-1). By contrast, in normal voluntary movement of the toes to a position of plantar flexion, the excursion of the toes is usually much more rapid and pronounced, with the toes reextending with equal rapidity.

The tonic plantar reflex may be interpreted as due to interruption of fronto-extrapyramidal con-

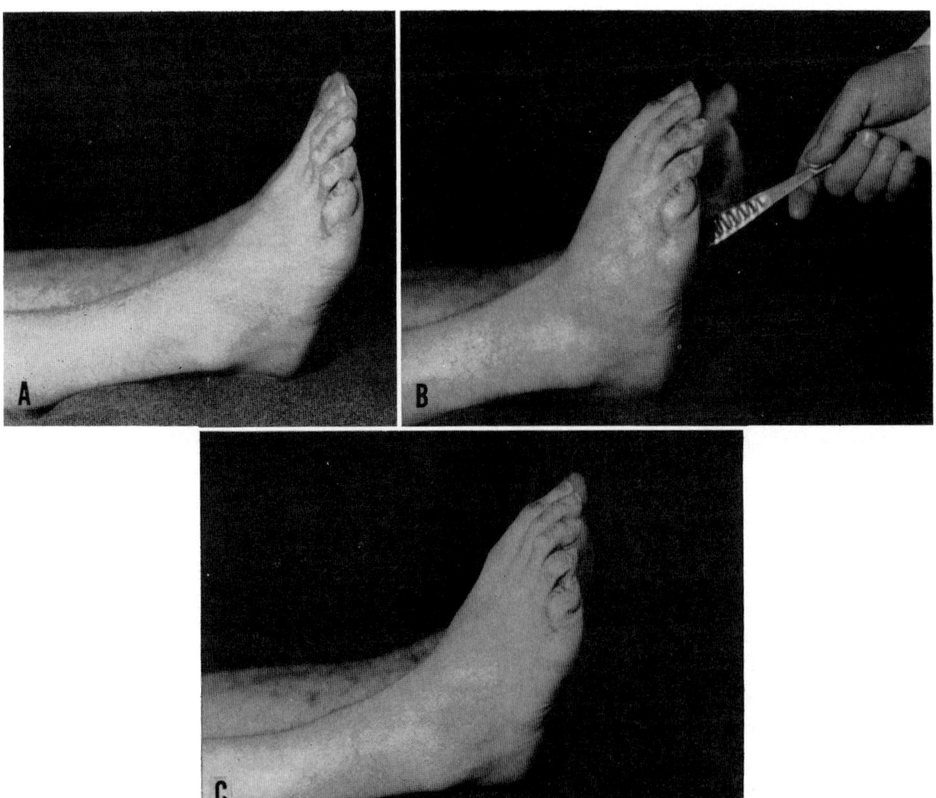

Fig. 20-1. Tonic plantar reflex. **A,** Normal position of the right foot before stimulation. **B,** Tonic plantar reflex on stimulation. **C,** Persistence of the reflex after stimulation. (Courtesy Prof. E. Herman, Lodz, Poland.)

nections. Since the extrapyramidal system functions both ipsilaterally and contralaterally, it is understandable that the tonic plantar reflex should in some cases be obtained ipsilateral to the lesion, in others contralateral, and in still others bilateral. The reflex is not to be regarded as an exaggerated physiological response but rather as evidence of disordered function of the extrapyramidal system. (Herman, 1952.)

In frontal lobe lesions a *crossed flexion reflex* is frequently elicitable in the lower limb; when one of the limbs is passively flexed at all joints, the other limb involuntarily assumes a similar position. The same applies to *diagonal reflexes:* for instance, when the examiner sharply flexes the patient's left hand at the wrist and at the same time rolls the patient's thumb over the palm of the hand, the right lower limb undergoes a similar flexion-reflex movement.

Tonic spasms of the fingers and toes. Such spasms are occasionally observed in frontal lobe lesions. They may be manifested simply by an inability of the muscles to relax after contraction. The spasms usually occur on the same side as the lesion, or, if bilateral, they are most pronounced ipsilaterally.

Diagonal rigidity. Occasionally in frontal lobe lesions there is rigidity of the arm contralateral to the lesion and of the leg on the same side as the lesion.

Gait disorders. When a patient with a frontal lobe lesion is asked to walk on his hands and knees, his gait is sometimes primitive; he moves forward by advancing simultaneously the arm of one side and the leg of the other, as would a baby or a four-legged animal (Engerth and Hoff, 1930). When the normal adult walks in this manner, the extremities of one side move forward first, then those of the other side. Furthermore, the normal adult uses the arms only for support and moves them forward before the legs undergo locomotion.

Automatisms. Automatisms resulting from lesions of the frontal lobe consist in repetitious movements performed by certain muscle groups—for instance, continual vigorous opening and closing of the eyes. The effect is often bizarre. The automatisms may be bilateral or confined to the side contralateral to the lesion.

Persistence of induced movements. When the examiner produces antagonistic movements in the patient's limb for a time—for example, flexion and extension or supination and pronation—and then suddenly ceases moving the part, active movement of the same kind will continue for awhile. This persistence of movement *(Kral's phenomenon)* is a frontal lobe sign.

MOTOR DISTURBANCES OF CORTICAL ORIGIN

Motor deficit caused by cortical lesions

Lesions situated in cerebral cortex can hardly fail to involve the subcortical white matter as well. Reference is made particularly to lesions resulting from neoplasms or vascular disorders. Even a meningioma that indents the cortex usually leaves its mark on the underlying white matter. In hypoxidosis of varied cause the cortex is a site of predilection of involvement, and so is the thalamus. The functional relationship between cortex and subcortical structures is such that the consideration of cortical injury in isolation seems artificial. Nonetheless, for ease in description, the expression "cortical" will be used in the following.

Monoplegia. Lesions involving the motor cortex are noted for the circumscribed pareses to which they give rise. Monoplegia, flaccid or spastic, is the essential criterion of a lesion in this location.

With the aid of Fig. 16-5, there should be no difficulty in localizing the lesion responsible for monoplegia. In facial monoplegia, only the muscles of the lower half of the face are prominently affected (Fig. 20-2). Isolated paralysis of the thumb may result from a circumscribed lesion in area 4, and mimic ulnar palsy (Foerster, 1931). A circumscribed lesion involving the more rostral part of the paracentral lobule leads to paresis of the contralateral

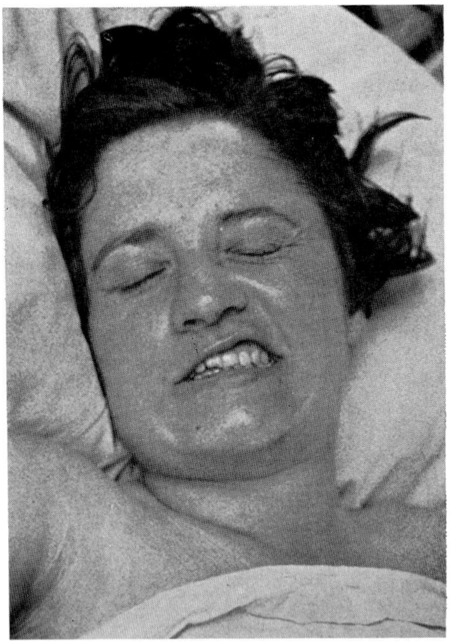

Fig. 20-2. Right facial palsy due to tumor of the left frontal lobe. On the attempt to smile, the right side of the face remains immobile. The eyelids close normally. (Courtesy Dr. A. Ornsteen, Philadelphia.)

foot, which at first glance may resemble common peroneal nerve palsy, but which on closer examination will be found to differ from it in scope of muscle involvement and by the lack of reaction of degeneration.

Monoplegia is frequently due to tumor involving the precentral gyrus, and under such conditions the paresis is slowly progressive. Paresis developing gradually in one lower limb suggests parasagittal meningioma, though other neoplasms and non-neoplastic lesions may have the same effect. By contrast, a small hemorrhage occurring in the corticosubcortical region may initially produce a hemiplegia that then fades into monoplegia. Following an epileptic seizure there may be transitory monoparesis or hemiparesis for a few hours or a day or two *(Todd's paralysis)*. Even shorter lived are the paretic phenomena in transient ischemic attacks. Only permanent monoplegia denotes destruction of the cortex. The spasticity of cortical origin is usually less pronounced than that of internal capsular origin and is rarely complicated by contractures.

Voluntary movement, muscle tonus, reflexes. Lesions involving area 4 are characterized clinically by loss of the capacity to carry out discrete, skilled movements contralaterally. In frontal or parietal corticosubcortical lesions, such movements can be performed as long as the precentral gyrus remains intact (Penfield, 1954). With removal of the hand area "the hand becomes completely paralyzed for any skilled movement whatever" (Penfield and Erickson, 1941). However, other movements can be performed: a boy from whom the uppermost part of the precentral and paracentral gyri was removed was subsequently (a year or less later) able to skate, hike, and dance (Bucy, 1949). In acute injuries or rapidly expanding lesions involving the motor areas (areas 4, 6, and 44), flaccid paresis occurs. There is a generalized depression of reflexes; and subsequently, spasticity develops. In slowly developing lesions involving these areas spasticity appears more quickly. Area 6 is mainly concerned; as in spastic hemiplegia of cortical origin, this area has been found consistently damaged. Flaccidity develops, however, in lesions involving area 6 if the postcentral cortex is also heavily damaged, or if deeper structures such as the thalamus share in the damage. Moreover, there may be flaccid hemiplegia in deep-seated cerebral lesions sparing the cortex. (Davison, 1949; Yakovlev, 1954.) Hypotonia is also enduring in lesions more or less limited to the postcentral gyrus (Head, 1918; Head and Holmes, 1911). In lesions involving areas 8 and 9, awkwardness, spasticity, and hyperreflexia appear early and are *followed* by motor weakness.

When lesions are confined to area 6, difficulty may be encountered in turning the head and the trunk to the opposite side and in stopping that movement. There may also be slowness in movement of the contralateral limbs and difficulty in carrying out complex movements (rapid or alternating) though simple movements can be adequately performed. (Foerster, 1936a.)

Appearance of the Babinski sign indicates damage of area 4, the Hoffmann sign, damage of areas 4 and 6, and the Rossolimo and Mendel-Bechterew signs, damage of more rostral areas as well (Davison, 1949).

Muscle atrophy and related disorders. Atrophy of muscles of the contralateral limbs is most frequent in severe damage of the sensorimotor cortex or parietal lobe in general (Hines, 1949). Lesions of vascular or traumatic origin may be responsible, as may neoplasm. The atrophy may be evident even within a few days after the onset of acute parietal lobe damage; its degree often runs parallel with the degree of hypotonus and sensory change (Guthrie, 1918). Hemiatrophy occasionally occurs in younger persons with a parietal lobe lesion, particularly porencephalic cyst. Under such conditions the shoulder and hand muscles may be most affected Arthropathy and bony rarefaction may also occur. Decrease in the size and length of the bones is common if parietal lobe injury occurs before the third year of life. (Garcin, Deparis, and Dimo, 1936; Gordon, 1927; Penfield and Robertson, 1943; Silverstein, 1955.)

In severe sensorimotor cortical damage, atrophy occurs in anterior horn cells and degeneration in anterior spinal roots and peripheral nerves, indicating a transsynaptic degenerative process. Degeneration has also been noted in the spinocerebellar tracts and the lateral spinothalamic tract, the outcome, apparently, of interruption of corticofugal fibers proceeding to the nuclei of origin of these tracts. In such cases the muscle atrophy has been considered due in part to "feedback degeneration": (1) short feedback to the cerebral cortex (via the spinal pathways mentioned) and (2) long feedback (via muscle spindles, then ascending pathways). (Botez and Carp, 1966.)

Monospasms, seizures, jacksonian epilepsy

Lesions of the sensorimotor cortex may give rise to signs and symptoms indicating motor cortical excitation, either alone or in combination with monoplegic paretic phenomena.

Preeminent among the manifestations of excitation of the motor cortex are *monospasms,* which consist in tonic-clonic muscular contractions. They may implicate either a normal or a paretic muscular region, for example, the face, the arm, or the hand. When they occur in an already paretic region, the paresis becomes much more pronounced.

Either *generalized or focal seizures* may occur in the presence of intracranial lesions, much more commonly in cerebral than in brainstem lesions. Seizures occur in some 35 percent of patients with intracranial tumor, with the focal form somewhat more common than the generalized form. The closer the tumor to the precentral gyrus, the greater the incidence of focal seizures; this applies also to lesions other than those caused by tumor. Where tumor is involved, focal seizures do not necessarily originate from tumor situated in the region of the sensorimotor cortex. They can be due to tumor elsewhere and constitute a false localizing sign. Such seizures have, for example, been noted in meningioma originating from the sphenoid wing. In such a case the meningioma forced the ipsilateral leg area of the cortex against the falx, resulting in subfalcal herniation of the gyri cinguli and the creation of an "irritable focus" (Beatty, 1965).

The type of tumor is of importance in the incidence of seizures. Seizures occur more commonly in slowly growing tumors (such as astrocytoma and oligodendroglioma) than in rapidly growing ones (such as glioblastoma multiforme), but once seizures begin in the more rapidly growing their frequency is greater than for the slower growing tumors. An average percentage incidence of all seizure types in astrocytoma, meningioma, and glioblastoma multiforme is 58:51:38. Percentage of seizure occurrence as the initial sign in these tumors comes to 68:60:51. In brain abscess, seizures occur in approximately 50 percent of cases, and in subdural hematoma in 5 to 25 percent of cases. (Hoefer, Schlesinger, and Pennes, 1947; Penfield and Erickson, 1941.) Further details on the occurrence of seizures in intracranial tumors are given in Chapter 28.

A manifestation of cortical excitation of a complex order is *epilepsy of the jacksonian type,* spoken of as "focal epilepsy" from the standpoint of its origin in the cerebral cortex and as "local epilepsy" from the circumscription of the bodily area initially affected. The muscular spasms are at first clonic, but if the discharges become more intense, both the agonists and the antagonists contract, leading to tetanic spasm. If the discharges reaching the muscles of a limb are sufficiently strong, movement will occur; the attitude assumed by the part will be determined by the comparative strength of the muscle groups affected.

Jacksonian seizures may begin in any part of the body, but most frequently in a part that has a relatively large cortical representation such as the face, hand, or foot. If it begins in the muscles at the corner of the mouth, for instance, the "jacksonian march" is not restricted to the lower part of the face, as in cortical monospasm, but spreads to the ipsilateral arm and, in turn, to the corresponding leg. The attack may begin in the lower limb and be propagated to the upper limb and then to the face. When the attack begins in the left side of the face, there may be an associated conjugate deviation of the eyes and the head to the left (Fig. 20-3) owing to excitation of the frontal cortical "adversive" field. In particularly severe cases the wave of excitation may pass to the other side of the brain by way of the corpus callosum, causing the attack to be propagated on the side opposite to where it began. In such cases consciousness may be temporarily lost and mental functioning held in abeyance for a time.

There may be many attacks per day, actually hundreds *(serial jacksonian seizures)*, and they may occur so rapidly one after the other than unconsciousness persists *(jacksonian status epilepticus)*. Sometimes an attack is limited to the general region where it began, and when occurring without cessation is referred to as *epilepsia partialis continua* (Juul-Jensen and Denny-Brown, 1966).

To be distinguished from jacksonian seizures is a rarity known as *diagonal epilepsy*, so named because of the order of involvement of the limbs in the course of the convulsive seizure—left arm → right leg → left leg → right arm. The responsible lesion is situated on the side contralateral to the site initially affected, in this case the right side.

To determine precisely in which muscles the very first spasm (the "motor aura") occurs is to give information about the exact site of the responsible cortical lesion. If, for instance, a jacksonian attack begins in the fingers of the right hand, the causative lesion must be located in the finger area of the left precentral gyrus (indicated in Fig. 19-7). The responsible lesion—which may be a scar, a small abscess, circumscribed meningitis, and so on, or be due to neoplasm or a foreign body—brings about a state of excitation, presumably in neighboring pyramidal cells, and then, like a wave initiated by a pebble falling on still water, the excitation spreads slowly over adjacent parts of the cortex, involving muscle groups concerned in movements in the order of their cortical representation.

If jacksonian seizures occur in the initial

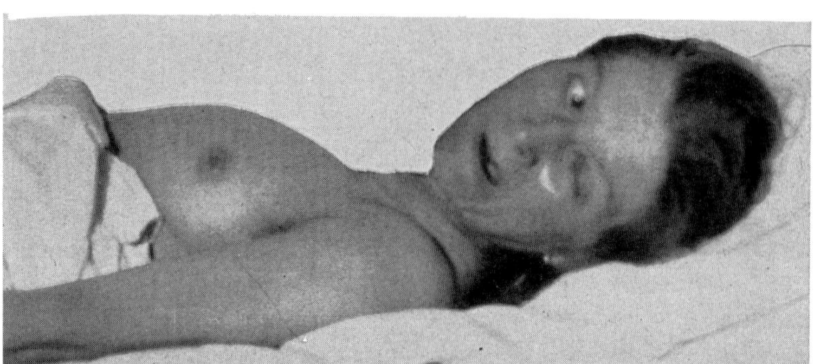

Fig. 20-3. Conjugate deviation of the head and eyes together with spasm of the left side of the face at the onset of a jacksonian attack. The patient has a tumor of the right side of the brain.

stage of a cerebral affection or as the initial sign, the responsible lesion is in all probability located at the surface of the brain. An expanding lesion as the cause of jacksonian epilepsy may in some instances be confirmed by manifestations of increased intracranial pressure. When no such evidence exists, other cortical conditions such as cysts, posttraumatic scars, and encephalitis should be considered. Tumors originating in the subcortical region may give rise secondarily to cortical excitatory phenomena, chiefly monospasms and hemispasms, but only after paresis and other signs of functional deficit have become established. Such seizures are much less stereotyped than jacksonian seizures. Regardless of the cause, jacksonian seizures are followed for a few minutes, hours, or even days by paresis of the muscles that had undergone spasm *(Todd's paralysis).*

SENSORY AND RELATED DISTURBANCES IN PARIETAL LOBE LESIONS

Sensory irritative phenomena

Lesions situated anywhere in the sensorimotor cortical region may give rise to sensory irritative phenomena, the most common of which are *dysesthesias,* often described by the patient as "tingling sensations." Sometimes the sensory phenomena are integral parts of a jacksonian seizure since they occur in the region involved by the initial spasms, for example, the face.

In *focal sensory epilepsy* the sensations may consist not only in dysesthesias but also in numbness, heaviness, or even lightning-like pain. The patient may have the sensation that a part of a limb is moving when actually it is lying motionless. Sometimes during a sensory seizure the limb does move, even violently.

In focal sensory seizures, the sensations are noted in the side contralateral to the lesion. As a rule, they remain confined to a functional unit, for example, an arm. However, as in jacksonian epilepsy, they may proceed from part to part, though the march is usually less consecutive than in jacksonian epilepsy. Sometimes several parts are simultaneously affected, for example, lips, tongue, and fingers. For some hours after termination of a seizure (in itself only a matter of seconds or a few minutes) a reduction of sensibility of the cortical type is noted in the parts in which the seizure occurred, the disturbances being in the realm of stereognosis, appreciation of passive movement, and twopoint discrimination. Appreciation of painful stimuli may be reduced, but only slightly.

Sensory deficit in parietal lobe lesions

Both the postcentral gyrus (areas 3, 1, and 2) and the posterior parietal cortex (areas 5 and 7) receive projections from the thalamic nuclei that are the recipients of exteroceptive and proprioceptive impulses from the body, limbs, and face. In addition, the precentral gyrus (area 4) receives an input from the dentatorubrothalamic system via relay thalamic nucleus LV (lateral ventral nucleus). Another system to be reckoned with is the tectothalamic pathway (originating in the superior colliculi), which, in the cat, terminates in the nuclei (lateral posterior [LP] and the pulvinar) that project to areas 5 and 7 (Altman and Carpenter, 1961); in the monkey a tectothalamic projection exists but terminations need yet to be ascertained. A strong association fiber system interconnects area 4 with areas 3, 1, and 2. These, then, are the major afferent systems that influence the activity of area 4, areas 3, 1, and 2, and areas 5 and 7.

Evidence is strong that no areal localization of sensory modalities as such exists in the sensorimotor cortex or posterior parietal cortex, for example, for touch, cold, warmth, pain, or kinesthesis. However, according to Head (1920), certain attributes of sensibility such as extensity, intensity, and quality (similarities and differences), have at least partially separate representations. From an analysis of many cases of hemianesthesia of cerebral origin, Dejerine (1914) went further in contending that the postcentral gyrus, like the precentral gyrus, is topographically organized in relation to spinal radicular fields, a conclusion confirmed by Woolsey, Marshall, and Bard (1942), who, in recording action potentials evoked in the postcentral gyrus by electrical stimulation of the skin (in the monkey), noted a detailed dermatomal pattern of representation in this part of the cortex. In the experience of Foerster (1936b), the same may be said for visceral representation in the cortex. With respect to tactile sensibility, electrical recordings from sensory units in the cerebral cortex (in the monkey) have revealed two distinct types, one type from small sensory fields (periphery of the limbs), the other from large fields (the entire hand or foot, a whole limb) (Mountcastle and Powell, 1959). Input from small fields reaches predominantly the postcentral cortex (sensory area I), and input from large fields the second sensory cortex (sensory area II) (Andersson, 1962). A map displaying sites of representation of various sensory functions in the sensorimotor cortex as based on clinical observations is shown in Fig. 20-4.

According to Head (1920) (also Head and Holmes, 1920), appreciation of spatial relationships is impaired mainly by lesions of the precentral gyrus. The recognition of similarities and dissimilarities between objects is most altered by lesions of the postcentral gyrus; response to graduated intensities suffers most from injury of the posterior parietal cortex. In this connection, Semmes and co-workers (1960), like others, found that a defect on any given test (such as point localization) might occur without concomitant impairment on any other given test. "The dissociations of defects . . . observed in individual subjects suggest that each test measures in part something that is specific to it."

Inherent differences in the cerebral organization for somesthesis in the two hemispheres were reported by Semmes and co-workers (1960), as based on an analysis in 232 war casualties with head injury. Testing was limited to the hands. Cortical representation for the right hand was found to be focally concentrated here and there within the somatosensory region of the left hemisphere, while representation of the left hand was more diffusely distributed within the right hemisphere and, occasionally, also in the left hemisphere. In contrast, Fennell, Satz, and Wise (1967), in studying pressure sensitivity thresholds for normal dextrals and sinistrals, could find no significant differences in mean thresholds for the right and left hands.

The nature and degree of sensory deficit depend on several factors other than the

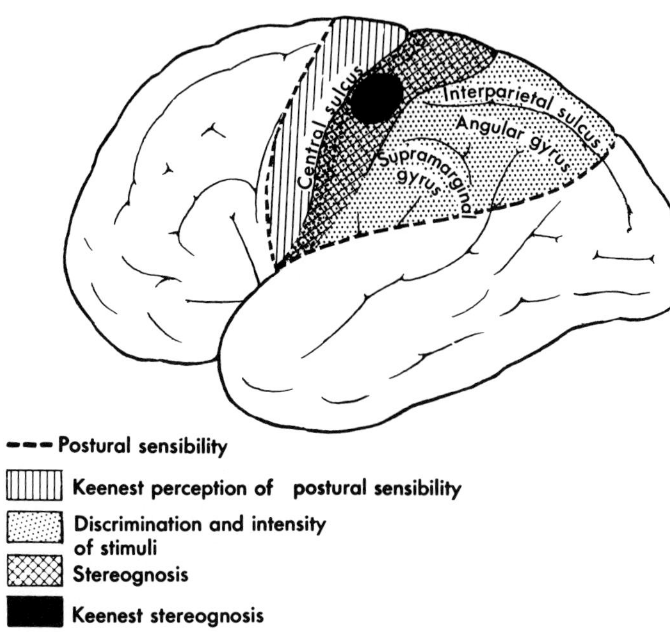

Fig. 20-4. Areas of the sensorimotor cortex concerned in different forms of perception, as based on clinical disturbances resulting from cortical-subcortical lesions, and partly on stimulation of the human cortex. The landmarks indicated are the central and interparietal sulci and the angular and supramarginal gyri.

site of the lesion, among them its kind, extent, mode of onset, and course (acute or chronic).

In *high-velocity missile wounds,* after a momentary stimulatory effect, immediate extinction of all local cerebral activity usually occurs, with total loss of sensibility in the affected contralateral limbs. After a few days or weeks, the area of total anesthesia shrinks; appreciation of pain returns, then appreciation of pressure, of vibratory stimuli, of warmth and cold. The remaining deficit, in a radicular or peripheral pattern, is in the tactile, proprioceptive, and stereognostic realms. Occasionally, little sensation returns, or none, particularly in cases where the damage is close to the central sulcus and where it involves deeper structures. (Head, 1920; Holmes, 1927; Russell, 1945; Walshe, 1942.)

In *acute lesions* of nontraumatic origin similar changes are encountered. In *slowly developing lesions,* such as those due to neoplasm, as a rule only the threshold for eliciting sensations is raised.

Lesions involving the parietal cortex interfere with certain isolated aspects of perception (Fig. 20-4):

1. *Pallesthesia* ("vibration sense") is *not* impaired in superficial lesions, but if the lesion lies deep and damages the thalamus, pallanesthesia usually is evident.

2. *Graphesthesia* (appreciation of numbers written on the skin) often suffers, but owing to the many factors involved in the test (degree of pressure exerted, speed of tracing, size of symbols traced), the results may be difficult to interpret.

3. *Appreciation of the position of the fingers or the hand (or of the toes and foot)* in space (proprioception) is interfered with when any part of the cortical area included within the heavy broken line indicated in Fig. 20-4 is seriously injured. The more rostral the lesion the greater the loss. Further, posture of all or only part of a limb thus affected may be altered. When only two or three fingers are affected, these fingers will droop when the arm is outstretched. Ataxia may accompany the postural deficit. Peculiar, uncomfortable postures may be assumed by an affected limb.

4. *Appreciation of passive movement* may likewise be affected. The highest incidence of defects in passive movement has been observed in lesions involving the posterior parietal region on the left side (determined by testing passive movement in the right hand) and in the lesions involving the postcentral gyrus on the right side (noted from carrying out passive motion in the left hand) (Semmes and others, 1960).

5. *Astereognosis* is encountered in lesions involving the postcentral gyrus, particularly its middle third (Bing and Schwartz, 1919) (Fig. 20-4), and may occur in lesions in deeper regions such as the subcortical parietal region and the thalamus (David and Askenasy, 1937; Rubenstein, 1938). In early stages of impaired stereognosis the patient may underestimate the size of objects *(micro-astereognosis);* upon recovery from total astereognosis he may overestimate them *(macro-astereognosis)* (Halpern, 1952).

6. *Disturbances in the perception of differences in weights* are encountered in lesions situated anywhere in the parietal area, but particularly in the region posterior to the postcentral gyrus. When objects of equal weight are placed in the two hands of a patient with a parietal lobe lesion, that in the affected hand seems the lighter. Moreover, the capacity to detect weight differences of objects placed in the hand, one after another, is less in the affected than in the other (normal) hand. (Bender, Teuber, and Battersby, 1950.)

7. *Faulty discrimination of tactile stimuli,* brought out with use of the compass test (two point discrimination), is seen in lesions involving any part of a rather wide area of the parietal cortex (Fig. 20-4). It is frequently the most conspicuous alteration in parietal cortical lesions (Holmes, 1927). In such lesions not only is the threshold of duality raised, but there may

also be tactile illusions. For example, a single stimulus may be interpreted as a duplex or a repetitive stimulus. The disturbances are valid only in the absence of gross cutaneous hypesthesia.

8. *Disturbances in the localization of stimuli* run a wide gamut and include tactile illusions and hallucinations. The simplest form consists in an inability to indicate precisely where touch has been applied; the error *(atopognosis)* is usually not more than an inch or two off the mark.

Tactile inattention, perseveration, allochiria, disturbances of body image

Tactile inattention (also called "sensory extinction") is a term used to denote a patient's failure to detect simultaneous stimuli. If two symmetrical parts are stimulated together (say, the hands), the patient will detect the stimulus clearly only on the sound side. When each side is tested singly, he appreciates fully every stimulus on the affected side. The same may occur when two similar objects are simultaneously placed in the hands, out of the patient's sight. The parts stimulated need not be symmetrical, for identical responses may be obtained on stimulating the hand on one side and the foot of the other. Tactile inattention is a sign of a parietal lobe lesion. The phenomenon can sometimes be accounted for by a lesion involving the thalamus or internal capsule. (Bender, 1945; Critchley, 1949.)

In occasional instances, a series of individual tactile stimuli may, after cessation of stimulus, evoke the hallucination of continuing touch; the patient, in a perseveratory manner, feels contacts where there are none *(tactile perseveration)*. Or the sensation of an object may persist after it has been removed from the hand. A tactile stimulus applied to one hand may be projected to a corresponding spot on the opposite hand *(tactile allochiria)*. Or, on having his hand stimulated, he may have the illusion that a distant part of the body (say, the ipsilateral cheek) has been stimulated. He may localize an initial touch correctly, but feel it again elsewhere after a few seconds. In other words, the stimulus is felt not on the affected side but is projected to the normal half of the body.

A rare variant or reversal of allochiria is the sensation that an object is being held in the affected hand when actually it is in the normal hand, and this faulty sensation may be delayed several minutes after the object has been released from the normal hand. Where causalgia coexists, pain in that limb may be precipitated or aggravated when a stimulus is applied to the sound side. Conversely, pain may be perceived in the normal limb when the opposite causalgic limb is stimulated *(synesthesialgia)*. (Bender, 1945; Critchley, 1953; Head and Holmes, 1911.)

Lesions involving the parietal lobe may give rise to a host of *disturbances of body-image* aside from allochiria. They are usually referred to as *anosognosia* (*a*, absence; *nosos*, disease; *gnosis*, knowledge—or unawareness of an affected part). Acute local lesions (hemorrhage, tumor, infarction) in the parietal lobe are much more likely to give rise to the disorder than diffuse cerebral lesions. Right preponderance of the denial has been noted in some series of cases but not in others. (Cole, Saexinger, and Hard, 1968.)

Critchley (1953) has subdivided the various modifications, which may merge one into another or appear in combinations, as follows: (1) unilateral neglect in the sensory motor or visual realm (for example, poverty of movement of a limb, failure to utilize a limb, application of cosmetics only to one side of the face or lips), which is one of the earliest and most characteristic manifestations of an expanding lesion in the parietal lobe; (2) lack of concern over the existence of hemiparesis; (3) unawareness of hemiparesis, occurring only in lesions in the right hemisphere in the right-handed; (4) defective appreciation of the existence of hemiparesis, with rationalization; (5) denial of hemiparesis; (6) denial of hemiparesis, with confabulation; (7) loss of awareness of one body-half; (8) undue heaviness, deadness, or lifelessness of one body-half; and (9) phantom third limb. For example, the patient may complain that his limb is in an entirely different position than is actually the case. If hemianopia co-exists, he "may be startled to see a hand appearing before his face, out of the blind sector, a hand which he does not recognize as his own, for it is devoid of proprioceptive cues."

Gerstmann's syndrome

Inability to recognize and use fingers, to perceive right and left, to write, and to calculate, most commonly resulting from lesions involving the angular and supramarginal gyri and the contiguous part of the occipital lobe, is known as Gerstmann's syndrome. Finger agnosia, the most important element of the syndrome, is bilateral and consists variously in an inability to recognize one's own fingers, to name them, or to point to an individual finger upon request *(autotopagnosia)*. The second, third, and fourth fingers offer the greatest source of confusion. There is no decrease in skill or strength of the fingers, either voluntary or involuntary. In advanced cases the disorder involves other parts of the limbs as well. The disorientation in right-left affects the entire body, not only the patient's, but also that of others. *Agraphia,* a kind of apraxia, may consist in an inability to write single letters or entire words. Letters and words are, however, copied correctly, and there appears to be a proper understanding of what is read. There is no disorder of verbalization, nor is there a disturbance in the comprehension of verbal symbols. *Dyscalculia* refers to the mistakes the patient makes in simple arithmetic, either "in his head" or on paper. Yet he may be able to enumerate even or odd numbers or to count backward. Various disorders may be associated with Gerstmann's syndrome, depending on the site of the lesion, for example, disturbances in drawing, alexia, ideokinetic apraxia, homonymous hemianopia, loss of optokinetic nystagmus, and pain asymbolia. (Critchley, 1953; Nielsen, 1938; Singer and Low, 1933.) Fragments of the syndrome may be encountered in lesions involving the parieto-occipital region, for example, dyscalculia (Spalding and Zangwill, 1950).

Metamorphopias

Distortions in the shape, size, and so on, of objects as they appear to the patient are not uncommon in lesions of the parietal lobe and environs. Examples are: "All the mats were crooked" (thrombosis of the right middle cerebral artery); "The furniture seemed to be turned around" (left parieto-occipital glioma); "The furniture sometimes appeared wider and fuller, and at other times smaller than normal" (right parieto-occipital lesion of vascular origin); "People's faces would frequently change; their eyes would swell and contract" (biparietal softening) (Critchley, 1953).

Chronotaraxis

Peculiar feelings regarding the passage of time, confusion with respect to time of the day or the date, and underestimation or overestimation of time intervals may occur in parietal lobe lesions (Critchley, 1953; Pötzl, 1928). The disorder can be induced by lesions made stereotactically in the medial dorsal nucleus of the thalamus (MD) or in the anterior thalamic nuclei bilaterally. Encroachment of the lesion on the intralaminar nuclei may play a role in the development of this disturbance (Spiegel and Wycis, 1967).

DISTURBANCES IN MOTILITY AND SENSIBILITY IN CORTICAL AND SUBCORTICAL LESIONS

This section deals with the disturbances in motility and/or sensibility resulting from assorted lesions involving, alone or in combination, the cerebral cortex, striatum, thalamus, region of the corona radiata and internal capsule, and the pars basilaris pontis. Differing combinations of spasticity versus rigidity and involuntary movements occur, depending on the site(s) of the lesion. Predominantly extrapyramidal disturbances are described elsewhere (Chapter 24).

Spastic diplegia and hemiplegia occurring in infancy

"Spastic diplegia" is a term signifying spasticity of like parts on both sides, due usually to damage involving, among other structures, the "motor area" of the cerebral cortex bilaterally. *Little's disease,* occurring congenitally, falls into this class. Causation is multiple. Hypoxemia and brain trauma occurring at the time of birth are the most frequent causes (Courville, 1953). Stiff, awkward movements of the lower limbs and their extended, adducted posture may be noted from the time of birth or not until the time the child tries first to walk (which is usually late), when the legs do not move properly. Later, on walking, the knees tend to cross, slight flexion is noted at the knees and hips, heels come off the ground and are everted, and toes and feet are turned inward. Pseudobulbar disturbances occur in some cases, and mobile spasms then athetosis in others, signifying coinvolvement of pyramidal tract and basal ganglia (Wilson, 1940). Where double athetosis prevails, bilateral pareses and spasticity occur in about 50 percent of cases; in such cases the lower limbs are, as a rule, predominantly involved. Added features commonly encountered are deficient speech development, dysarthria, and mental retardation (Carpenter, 1950). Occurring on the same basis as spastic diplegia is *hemiplegia* or *hemiparesis.* Though present from birth the disorder may go unrecognized until the age of 3 to 5 months.

Acute onset is the feature that distinguishes acquired hemiplegia from the congenital variety. Depending on the cause—of which there are many—the hemiparesis may either quickly disappear, slowly regress over a period of 3 to 4 months, or persist indefinitely. If lasting beyond 2 weeks, spasticity supervenes, to be followed in 1 to 3 months by contractures. During this time or later, hyperkinesias commonly develop. Complete recovery is unlikely when the hemiplegia occurs in infancy and when little or no improvement sets in during the subsequent week. The upper limb, particularly the hand, is most affected. (Carter and Gold, 1967.)

Striatal hemiplegia

Striatal hemiplegia is a disorder in which the lesion is limited to the striatum (caudate nucleus and putamen) of one side, leaving the adjoining internal capsule intact. In such a case an infarct in the region of distribution of the lateral striate group of arteries destroyed much of the striatum of one side (right side).

The patient, a woman aged 66 when death occurred, had had her disability since the age of 8 years, when the left leg and foot became stiff very shortly after an attack of unconsciousness. Besides the stiffness, both limbs were beset by recurring painless spasms, appearing either spontaneously or following mechanical stimuli or an emotional upset; during such episodes the upper arm would become flexed or extended at the shoulder, the forearm extended at the elbow, the wrist dorsiflexed, and the fingers flexed so as to form a fist. Increased resistance to passive movement at all joints was noted on that side. (Oppenheimer, 1967.)

Manifestations of lesions of the centrum semiovale

The motor disturbances produced by a lesion of the centrum semiovale vary with the size of the damaged area. Sometimes only monoplegia results. More commonly the motor disturbances are of wider distribution, though their scope is less than in hemiplegia. The nature of the motor disturbances is, however, basically the same under these conditions. Since lesions of the centrum semiovale also frequently interrupt commissural fibers of the corpus callosum, the motor deficit may be associated with apraxic disturbances. As to sensory changes, their scope and intensity correspond to the depth of the lesion when the latter involves fibers extending to the parietal cortex: the more superficial the lesion, the more profound the sensory changes in the discriminatory and orientation realms. The sensory deficit usually predominates in the hands and feet, either from the time of inception of the lesion or not until later when the sensory deficit elsewhere is receding.

Manifestations of acute lesions of the internal capsule

Acute lesions of the internal capsule usually give rise to more widespread disability than is encountered in lesions of the cortex or centrum semiovale, the reason being that the fibers affected in this region proceed to a wider area of the neuraxis than fibers damaged by a lesion of the same size at higher levels. Because of their compact grouping, there is little chance that the fibers innervating, for instance, the tongue or the upper limb, will be selectively damaged. Monoplegia from an internal capsular lesion is thus rare.

If the lesion also interrupts sensory fibers in the posterior third of the posterior limb, hemianesthesia (or hemihypesthesia) may occur, but this is uncommon. The reason for the infrequency of sensory deficit is not evident. Possibly the sensory fibers in this region are more diffuse than generally thought. By contrast, a destructive lesion in this location that extends backward and downward into the retrolenticular and sublenticular parts of the internal capsule, and interrupts the auditory and visual radiations (Fig. 19-11), more commonly gives rise to deficits which, when fully developed, are characterized by the triad: hemianesthesia, hemihypacusis, and hemianopia—all occurring contralaterally.

Motor irritative phenomena occur only in the early course of acute internal capsular injury. In apoplexy of internal capsular origin, especially in embolic occlusion of a vessel in the internal capsule, fasciculations may occur in muscles that soon thereafter become paretic. The fasciculations have little localizing value, for they may occur as the result of irritation of motor fibers of the cortex, cerebral peduncle, pons, medulla oblongata, or white or gray matter of the spinal cord.

Muscle power, muscle tonus, and reflexes are mainly affected. Immediately after an apoplectic attack the muscles of the hemiplegic side may be flaccid. Often some motor power is retained—more so proximally than distally, and more so in the lower than in the upper limb. At first, the deep reflexes and even the corneal reflex are usually unelicitable. Unilateral absence of these reflexes serves as a basis for determining which half of the body is paralyzed when the patient lies unconscious and totally flaccid shortly after apoplexy. Hypertonus develops and the deep reflexes become exaggerated in about 48 hours, and, if appearing earlier, probably denote escape of blood into the ventricular system. With the return of muscle tonus, voluntary movement sets in; capacity to flex at the shoulder and hip returns first, then at the elbow, wrist, and fingers, then at the knee and ankle.

In some cases of hemiplegia due to cerebral arterial thrombosis motility is completely restored within a few days. Such return of function can mean that an ischemic-edematous process has involved but not interrupted fibers of the pyramidal tract. Or a hemorrhage may have taken place solely in the putamen and induced hemiplegia through a complicating edematous process involving the internal capsule. But perhaps the lesion most commonly giving rise to transient hemiplegia is focal destruction of the internal capsule resulting in a lacuna or a small infarct. The hemiplegia which is to become persistent may develop in any one of various ways—by gradual onset over a period of a few hours up to several days, with the stroke reaching its peak in an average of 12 to 72 hours, or by abrupt onset when the subject is awake or is emerging from sleep, with the peak reached in 3 to 6 hours. Premonitory transient ischemic attacks and intermittent stepwise course almost always signify enduring hemiplegia. Slurring of speech, disturbances of conjugate gaze, and nystagmus are much less common and less pronounced than in pontile hemiplegia. (Fisher and Curry, 1965.)

Disturbances from chronic internal capsular lesions

Hemorrhage into the internal capsule is characterized by maximal initial defect. Slowly progressive hemiplegia may develop from involvement of the internal capsule or adjacent centrum semiovale by an expanding tumor or by occlusion of more and more arteriolar terminals as a result of propagation of a thrombus.

In the recovery phase following a "vascular accident," the paretic limb takes on certain abnormal attitudes caused by the

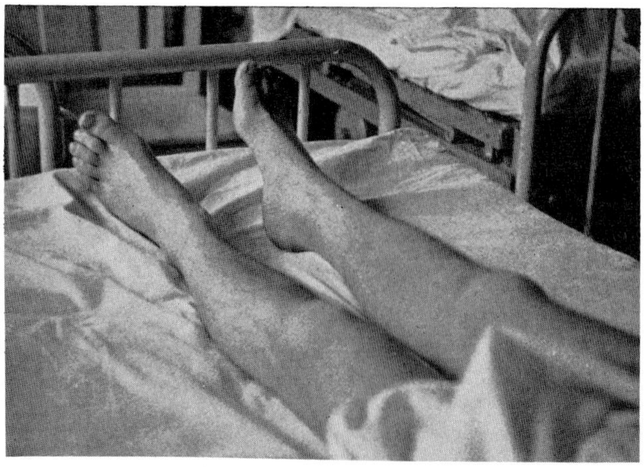

Fig. 20-5. Outward rotation of the paretic left leg in hemiplegia of internal capsular origin. (Courtesy Dr. A. Ornsteen, Philadelphia.)

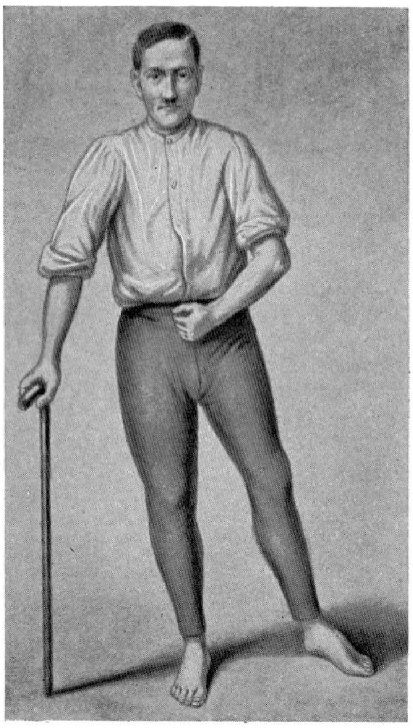

Fig. 20-6. Hemiplegia of the left side following hemorrhage involving the right internal capsule. The upper limb is in flexion-contracture, and the lower limb, in extension-contracture. In walking, the patient circumducts his leg.

unopposed action of the muscles that have undergone functional restitution (Fig. 20-5). Later the attitudes become fixed by muscular contraction. Long after the typical capsular stroke the patient has a typical appearance: an upper limb shortened by fixed flexion at the elbow and fingers, also in adduction and pronation, and a lower limb lengthened by fixed extension at the knee and by plantar flexion, also inversion of the foot, resulting in circumduction at the hip when the patient walks ("fauchage" or "scythe motion"), as well as the typical thumping sound as the healthy foot comes down (Fig. 20-6).

Sparing of movements having bilateral cortical innervation. The movements spared include those concerned in mastication and deglutition, and those of the larynx, eyes, and trunk. The lower part of the face is invariably affected, and the upper part of the face also but less strikingly so. Weakness of the frontalis is manifested by slight lowering of the eyebrow, and weakness of the orbicularis oculi is evident from the patient's inability to keep the affected eyelid closed for as long a period as on the normal side. In many patients these disorders are transitory.

Dissociated loss of facial movements. Weakness of the lower part of the face may be manifested only when voluntary movements are executed—for example, when the patient shows his teeth on command or when he talks. By contrast, emotional facial movements are performed normally, all traces of the facial hemiparesis disappearing when the patient cries or laughs. But minor movements, such as a smile, or in fact the face at complete rest, often reveal the defect better than intended innervation. In some instances, emotional facial movements of the hemiplegic side are exaggerated.

Limb muscles affected. While eventual return of function is the rule in many affected muscles, certain muscles fail to recover. These include the peroneal muscles, the knee and hip flexors, the elbow extensors, the hand and finger extensors, the external rotators of the upper arm, and the supinators of the forearm. The arm is usually affected much more than the leg. Paresis involving the arm is illustrated in Fig. 20-7.

Minor defects become manifest when the patient's affected limb is forced to maintain certain postures under the stress of gravity: the elevated arm or leg will droop before its healthy fellow does.

In rare instances, hypertonus predominates in certain extensor muscles of the upper limb, the arm being extended at the elbow, with minor flexion occurring at the wrist, hand, and finger joints. Moreover, the lower limb occasionally assumes the attitude of flexion-contracture rather than the customary extension-contracture (Yakovlev, 1954). Under such conditions extrapyramidal structures as well as the internal capsule are likely to have been damaged.

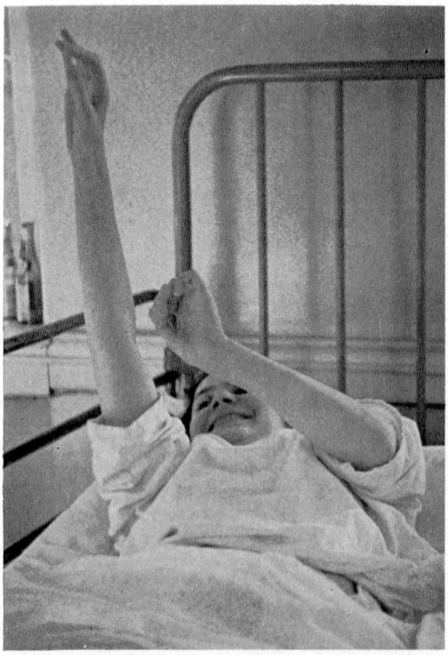

Fig. 20-7. Paresis of the left arm due to tumor of the right frontal lobe. On request to raise both arms only the right can be fully raised. (Courtesy Dr. A. Ornsteen, Philadelphia.)

Reflexes. Exaggeration of deep reflexes occurs in association with muscular hypertonia. These reflexes are, however, unelicitable if the spinal reflex arc is interrupted, for instance as a result of an increase in cerebrospinal fluid pressure (O'Connell, 1953), or rarely also with associated parietal lobe lesions. Further, numerous pathological reflexes (including the Babinski reflex) and muscle clonus (ankle, patellar) may be elicited. Latent reflexes such as the Rossolimo reflex are commonly activated. The superficial reflexes, for example, the abdominal, are usually permanently suppressed.

Associated movements. In the presence of an internal capsular lesion certain associated movements are lost. Among them is the *finger-thumb reflex* (of Mayer), which, in normal persons, consists in vigorous opposition of the thumb and extension at its terminal joint when the extended third or fourth finger is passively flexed; in lesions of the precentral gyrus the reflex may, however, be exaggerated. Also lost is the *forearm flexor response* (sign of Léri). If the fingers of a normal person are passively folded into the hollow of his hand, and the hand is then sharply flexed, the forearm flexes simultaneously at the elbow. In cerebral hemiplegia this movement is decreased or abolished, but it is retained in hysterical paralysis.

Symmetrical synkinesias (mirror movements). These are highly characteristic of cerebral hemiplegia. Examples: When the patient makes a tight fist with his normal hand, involuntary flexion movements of the fingers occur simultaneously on the affected side. When the patient energetically flexes his lower leg on the sound side, the paretic leg mimics the movement to some degree.

Sensory changes. In chronic hemiplegia

resulting from hemorrhage involving the internal capsule, sensory deficit occurs in at least 50 to 75 percent of cases. Pain sensibility and two point discrimination are commonly affected, and pallesthesia as well, the latter, according to one account (Zankel, 1969), being involved in practically all patients with prolonged stroke. The high incidence of sensory change is consistent with the fact that a common site of origin of spontaneous cerebral hemorrhage is in a region near the cortex, namely in the rostral part of the base of the external capsule. From here the hemorrhage spreads into the corona radiata and, in turn, into the internal capsule. (Critchley, 1953; Van Buskirk and Webster, 1955.) In arterial thrombosis involving the internal capsule, sensory deficit is less frequent.

Lacunar strokes

Autopsies show that outnumbering all cerebrovascular lesions described in the foregoing are those resulting from the development of lacunae or related lesions in the brain and brainstem.

In this context three terms need to be defined: *status cribratus (état criblé)* (Durand-Fardel), *status praecribratus (C. Vogt)*, and *status lacunaris (état lacunaire)* (Pierre Marie). All three are frequently found in association with cerebral arteriosclerosis, particularly when arterial hypertension coexists.

Status cribratus refers to a "sieve-like" state most commonly observed in the lenticular nucleus and fairly often in the corona radiata and internal capsule. Adventitia of arterial vessels is irregularly thickened or thinned, the sheath is distended or ballooned, and perivascular tissue is loculated or entirely destroyed. Emphasizing the change in the vascular sheath, Pierre Marie referred to the condition as *vaginalite destructive.* For the incipient stage, Cécile Vogt introduced the term *status praecribratus,* characterized by destruction of nerve cells, myelin, and glia perivascularly, but without distention of the vascular sheath. *Lacunae* are small, fluid-filled cavities in the tissue, usually no larger than a lentil or a small pea. They contain filmy strands of connective tissue and commonly are spanned by a thickened but patent vessel, frequently identifiable as an artery or arteriole. When numerous cavities exist the condition is called *status lacunaris* (or *état lacunaire*).

Differing opinions have been expressed regarding the pathogenesis of lacunae. Fig. 11-20 illustrates cavities in advanced *status cribratus* that merit the term "lacunae." Obviously the cavities are situated perivascularly. They are considered to represent, by and large, the end-stage of tissue destruction brought about by a disturbance in interchange between vascular and tissue compartments (Haymaker, 1951; Vogt and Vogt, 1951). According to Vogt and Vogt (1920), small softenings around vessels in the striatum and pallidum are to be called "lacunae." Fisher (1965a) regards lacunae (perhaps including the cavitations already mentioned) as ischemic infarcts brought about by occlusion of arteries or their branches, *presumably* due to an "unusual thrombotic process." Blackwood (1963) states that the term *status cribratus* applies to cavities in the centrum semiovale and other richly myelinated regions, and that *status lacunaris* is the term to be used for similar cavities in the basal gray nuclei; to him a lacuna differs from a "small softening in respect to its site of election, state of associated blood vessel and cell content within the cavity." The differing usages stem in part from the type of brain disease under consideration—whether "run-of-the-mill" arteriosclerosis or extrapyramidal disease.

Lacunae are found most frequently in the striatum and pars basilaris pontis, but are also noted in the pallidum, thalamus, and the region of the corona radiata and internal capsule. They are occasionally found in the corpus callosum and rarely in the cerebellum.

Neurological deficit occurred only in about 20 percent of cases in which lacunae were found (Fisher, 1965a). In such cases the type of clinical disorder varies in accordance with the site(s) of the lacunae.

Lacunar hemiplegia and *lacunar monoplegia,* purely motor, are the forms most commonly encountered. Onset is usually abrupt, the ictus mild and characterized, for example, by clumsiness of a limb and/or dysarthria together with temporary clouding or loss of consciousness. All functions may be rapidly restored, or paresis may persist and in rare instances be followed by contractures. Superficial reflexes are seldom disturbed. Prolonged illness may occasionally ensue and be characterized by "lacunar gait" *(démarche à petits pas),* impaired fine movements, the Babinski sign, and dysarthria, combined or not with manifestations of pseudobulbar palsy. In such patients there may be sensory disturbances in the limbs characterized by tingling, sensations of cold, slight hypesthesia, and pain. (Bing and Haymaker, 1939; Fisher, 1965a, b; Fisher and Curry, 1965; Foix and Hillemand, 1926; Foix and Levy, 1927.)

Lacunar stroke is in some instances characterized by *sensory disturbances.* In practically all cases the stroke is "benign" so far as subsequent vascular "accidents" are concerned. More or less complete hemianesthesia from involvement of the corona radiata is sometimes encountered. Numbness and paresthesias followed by transient or persistent sensory loss occur in the face, arm, and leg. One limb is first affected, then, in the course of minutes or hours, the other limb, then the face. Or only one side of the face, or the cheek and lips, may be affected. Headache does not occur. Motor power is preserved. Vertigo, dysarthria, diplopia, and nystagmus are lacking. In one case of sensory stroke, a "lacune" 7 mm. in diameter was found in the ventral posterior nucleus of the thalamus (Fisher, 1965b).

Lacunar stroke may also be characterized by a *dysarthria–clumsy hand syndrome* (Fisher, 1967). Like the others, this kind of stroke poses no threat of subsequent "vascular disaster." The clinical features are stereotyped and consist in dysarthria together with clumsiness of one hand. Some cases are also characterized by temporary facial weakness, deviation of the protruded tongue, slurred speech, and veering to one side while walking. The clumsiness is evident in the patient's inability to perform rapid alternating movements. Moreover, tapping of the index finger on the thumb is slow and dysmetric. In one such case a giant "lacune" 8 mm. in greatest diameter was found in the pars basilaris pontis.

REFERENCES

Adie, W. J., and Critchley, M. 1927. Forced grasping and groping. Brain **50:**142-170.

Allison, R. S. 1966. Perseveration as a sign of diffuse and focal brain damage—II. Brit. Med. J. **2:**1095-1101.

Altman, J., and Carpenter, M. D. 1961. Fiber projections of the superior colliculus in the cat. J. Comp. Neurol. **116:**157-178.

Andersson, S. A. 1962. Projection of different spinal pathways of the second somatic sensory area in cat. Acta Physiol. Scand. **56**(suppl. 194):1-74.

Beatty, R. A. 1965. The focal motor seizure as a false localizing sign. Neurology **15:**752-755.

Bender, M. B. 1945. Extinction and precipitation of cutaneous sensations. Arch. Neurol. Psychiat. **54:**1-9.

Bender, M. B., Teuber, H. L., and Battersby, W. S. 1950. Discrimination of weights by man with penetrating lesions of parietal lobes. Trans. Amer. Neurol. Ass. **75:**252-255.

Bing, R., and Haymaker, W. 1939. Textbook of nervous diseases. St. Louis, The C. V. Mosby Co.

Bing, R., and Schwartz, L. 1919. Contribution à la localization de la stéréoagnosie. Schweiz. Arch. Neurol. Psychiat. **4:**187-198.

Blackwood, W. 1963. Vascular disease of the central nervous system. In Greenfield's neuropathology, ed. 2. Baltimore, The Williams & Wilkins Co., pp. 71-137.

Botez, M. I., and Carp, N. 1966. Is there a feedback degeneration in the nervous system? Acta Neurol. Psychiat. Hellenica **5:**79-96.

Brain, W. R., and Curren, R. 1932. The grasp reflex of the foot. Brain **55:**347-356.

Bucy, P. C. 1949. Effects of extirpation in man. In Bucy, P. C., editor: The precentral motor cortex, ed. 2. Urbana, University of Illinois Press, pp. 353-394.

Carter, S., and Gold, A. P. 1967. Acute infantile hemiplegia. Pediat. Clin. N. Amer. **14:**851-864.

Carpenter, M. B. 1950. Athetosis and the basal ganglia: review of the literature and study of forty-two cases. Arch. Neurol. Psychiat. **63:** 875-901.

Cole, M., Saexinger, H. G., and Hard, A. 1968. Anosognosia—studies using regional intravenous anesthesia. Neuropsychol. **6:**365-371.

Courville, C. B. 1953. Contributions to the study of cerebral anoxia. Los Angeles, San Lucas Press.

Critchley, M. 1949. Phenomenon of tactile inattention with special reference to parietal lesions. Brain **72:**538-561.

Critchley, M. 1953. The parietal lobes. London, Edward Arnold (Publishers) Ltd.

David, M., and Askenasy, H. 1937. Ataxia and astereognosis of bulbar origin. Brain **60:**354-360.

Davison, C. 1949. Pathology. In Bucy, P. C., editor: The precentral motor cortex, ed. 2. Urbana, University of Illinois Press, pp. 425-457.

Dejerine, J. 1914. Semiologie des affections du système nerveux. Paris, Masson & Cie.

Denny-Brown, D., Twitchell, T. E., and Saenz-Arroyo, L. 1949. The nature of spasticity resulting from cerebral lesions. Trans. Amer. Neurol. Ass. **74:**108-113.

Engerth, G., and Hoff, H. 1930. Ein weiterer Beitrag zur Lehre von der Stirnhirnfunktion. Z. Ges. Neurol. Psychiat. **129:**332-341.

Fennell, E., Satz, P., and Wise, R. 1967. Laterality differences in the perception of pressure. J. Neurol. Neurosurg. Psychiat. **30**:337-340.

Fisher, C. M. 1965a. Lacunes: small, deep cerebral infarcts. Neurology **15**:774-784.

Fisher, C. M. 1965b. Pure sensory stroke involving face, arm and leg. Neurology **15**:76-80.

Fisher, C. M. 1967. A lacunar stroke: the dysarthria-clumsy hand syndrome. Neurology **17**: 614-617.

Fisher, C. M., and Curry, H. B. 1965. Pure motor hemiplegia of vascular origin. Arch. Neurol. **13**:30-44.

Foerster, O. 1931. The cerebral cortex in man. Lancet **2**:309-312.

Foerster, O. 1936a. Motorische Felder und Bahnen. In Bumke, O., and Foerster, O., editors: Handbuch der Neurologie, vol. 6. Berlin, Springer-Verlag, pp. 1-357.

Foerster, O. 1936b. Sensible corticale Felder. In Bumke, O., and Foerster, O., editors: Handbuch der Neurologie, vol. 6. Berlin, Springer-Verlag, pp. 358-448.

Foix, C., and Hillemand, P. 1926. Contribution à l'étude des ramollissements protubérantiels. Rev. Méd. **43**:287-305.

Foix, C., and Levy, M. 1927. Les ramollissements sylviens: syndromes des lésions en foyer du territoire de l'artère sylvienne et des ses branches. Rev. Neurol. **2**:1-51.

Garcin, R., Deparis, M., and Dimo, H. 1936. Hémiplégie spasmodique de l'adulte avec atrophie musculaire tardive considérable: contribution à l'étude pathogénique des atrophies musculaires de l'hémiplégie cérébrale de l'adulte. Rev. Neurol. **65**:158-167.

Goldstein, K. 1938. The tonic foot response to stimulation of the sole: its physiological significance and diagnostic value. Brain **61**:269-283.

Gordon, A. 1927. Segmental trophic edema of cerebral origin. J. Nerv. Ment. Dis. **66**:381-389.

Grimby, L. 1965. Pathological plantar response. Part I. Flexor and extensor components in early and late reflex parts. Part II. Loss of significance of stimulation site. J. Neurol. Neurosurg. Psychiat. **28**:469-481.

Guthrie, L. 1918. Muscular atrophy and other changes in nutrition associated with lesions of the sensory cortex of the brain, with especial reference to the possible existence of trophic representation in the postcentral area. Proc. Roy. Soc. Med. **11**:21-26.

Halpern, L. 1952. Secondary disturbances of perception. J. Nerv. Ment. Dis. **116**:783-788.

Haymaker, W. 1951. Cécile and Oskar Vogt: on the occasion of her 75th and his 80th birthday. Neurology **1**:179-204.

Head, H. 1918. Sensation and the cerebral cortex. Brain **41**:57-253.

Head, H. 1920. Studies in neurology. London, Oxford University Press.

Head, H., and Holmes, G. 1911. Sensory disturbances from cerebral lesions. Brain **34**:102-254.

Head, H., and Holmes, G. 1920. Sensory disturbances from cerebral lesions. In Head, H., editor: Studies in neurology, vol. 2. London, Oxford University Press, pp. 533-638.

Herman, E. 1952. The tonic plantar reflex and its localizing significance. J. Nerv. Ment. Dis. **116**:933-956.

Hines, M. 1949. Significance of the precentral motor cortex. In Bucy, P. C., editor: The precentral motor cortex, ed. 2. Urbana, University of Illinois Press, pp. 459-499.

Hoefer, P. F. A., Schlesinger, E. B., and Pennes, H. H. 1947. Seizures in patients with brain tumors. Res. Publ. Ass. Res. Nerv. Ment. Dis., Proc. **26**:50-58.

Holmes, G. 1927. Disorders of sensation produced by cortical lesions. Brain **50**:413-427.

Juul-Jensen, P., and Denny-Brown, D. 1966. Epilepsia partialis continua: a clinical, electroencephalographic, and neuropathological study of nine cases. Arch. Neurol. **15**:563-578.

Mountcastle, V. B., and Powell, T. P. S. 1959. Neural mechanisms subserving cutaneous sensibility, with special reference to the role of afferent inhibition in sensory perception and discrimination. Bull. Johns Hopk. Hosp. **105**:201-232.

Nielsen, J. M. 1938. Gerstmann syndrome: finger agnosia, agraphia, confusion of right and left and acalculia: comparison of this syndrome with disturbance of body scheme resulting from lesions of the right side of the brain. Arch. Neurol. Psychiat. **39**:536-560.

O'Connell, J. E. A. 1953. The cerebrospinal fluid pressure as an aetiological factor in the development of lesions affecting the central nervous system. Brain **76**:279-298.

Oppenheimer, D. R. 1967. A case of striatal hemiplegia. J. Neurol. Neurosurg. Psychiat. **30**:134-139.

Penfield, W. 1954. Mechanisms of voluntary movement. Brain **77**:1-17.

Penfield, W., and Erickson, T. C. 1941. Epilepsy and cerebral localization. Springfield, Illinois, Charles C Thomas, Publisher.

Penfield, W., and Robertson, J. S. M. 1943. Growth asymmetry due to lesions of the postcentral cerebral cortex. Arch. Neurol. Psychiat. **50**:405-430.

Pötzl, O. 1928. Optisch-agnostische Störungen. Vienna, Verlag Franz Deuticke.

Rubenstein, J. E. 1938. Astereognosis associated with tumors in the region of the foramen magnum. Arch. Neurol. Psychiat. **39**:1016-2032.

Russell, W. R. 1945. Transient disturbances following gunshot wounds of head. Brain **68**:79-97.

Schuster, P. 1923. Zwangsgreifen und Nachgreifen, zwei posthemiplegische Bewegungsstörungen. Z. Ges. Neurol. Psychiat. **83**:586-609.

Schuster, P. 1927. Autoptische Befunde bei Zwangsgreifen und Nachgreifen. Z. Ges. Neurol. Psychiat. **108**:715-733.

Semmes, J., Weinstein, S., Ghent, L., and Teuber, H.-L. 1960. Somatosensory changes after penetrating brain wounds in man. Cambridge, Massachusetts, Harvard University Press.

Seyffarth, H. 1953. The reaction to passive straining of joints (bending reflex) in patients with frontal lobe lesions. Brain **76**:457-472.

Seyffarth, H., and Denny-Brown, D. 1948. The grasp reflex and the instinctive grasp reaction. Brain **71**:109-183.

Silverstein, A. 1955. Diagnostic localizing value of muscle atrophy in parietal lobe lesions. Neurology **5**:30-55.

Singer, H. H., and Low, A. A. 1933. Acalculia (Henschen): a clinical study. Arch. Neurol. Psychiat. **29**:467-498.

Spalding, J. M. K., and Zangwill, O. L. 1950. Disturbance of number-form in a case of brain injury. J. Neurol. Neurosurg. Psychiat. **13**:24-29.

Spiegel, E. A., and Wycis, H. T. 1967. Multiple representation of various functions in the human subcortex. Confin. Neurol. **29**:163-167.

Twitchell, T. E. 1965. The automatic grasping responses of infants. Neuropsychologia **3**:247-259.

Van Buskirk, C., and Webster, D. 1955. Prognostic value of sensory defect in rehabilitation of hemiplegics. Neurology **5**:407-411.

Vogt, C., and Vogt, O. 1920. Zur Lehre der Erkrankungen des striären Systems. J. Psychol. Neurol., Erg. Heft 3, **25**:627-846.

Vogt, C., and Vogt, O. 1951. Importance of neuroanatomy in the field of neuropathology. Neurology **1**:205-218.

Walshe, F. M. R. 1942. Anatomy and physiology of cutaneous sensibility; critical review. Brain **65**:48-112.

Williamson, R. T. 1896. On the symptomatology of gross lesions (tumours and abscesses) involving the pre-frontal region of the brain. Brain **19**:346-365.

Wilson, S. A. K. 1940. Neurology, vol. 2. Baltimore, The Williams & Wilkins Co., pp. 755-769.

Woolsey, C. W., Marshall, W. H., and Bard, P. 1942. Representation of cutaneous tactile sensibility in the cerebral cortex of the monkey as indicated by evoked potentials. Bull. Johns Hopk. Hosp. **70**:399-441.

Yakovlev, P. I. 1954. Paraplegia in flexion of cerebral origin. J. Neuropath. Exp. Neurol. **13**:267-296.

Zankel, H. T. 1969. Pallesthesia studies in stroke patients. Southern Med. J. **62**:8-11.

Chapter 21

Localization of visual and associated reflex disturbances

ANATOMICAL CONSIDERATIONS

An overall view of the visual system is illustrated in Fig. 21-1. The visual system consists of the retinae, optic nerves, optic chiasm, optic tracts, geniculocalcarine tracts, and the calcarine cortex. The optic nerve is approximately 50 mm. in length and is divisible into four components: intraocular (0.7 mm. in length), orbital (33 mm.), intracanalicular (6 mm.), and intracranial (10 mm.). Like the brain, the optic nerve is surrounded by pia mater, arachnoid, and dura mater. The vaginal space surrounding the nerve is continuous with the subarachnoid space of the brain; the same does not apply to the subdural space. Rostrally, near the globe, the vaginal space ends blindly, there being no communication with any real or potential ocular or periocular space. A Virchow-Robin space surrounds vessels in the optic nerve and retina. The optic chiasm and optic tracts are bordered by a glial matting and are surrounded by pia and arachnoid. (Wolff, 1940.)

Visual and reflex systems

Visual pathways. Rods and cones, which lie deep in the retina, are the receptors of photic stimuli. These cells synapse with more superficial cells—bipolar cells—and these in turn synapse with cells of the most superficial cellular layer—the ganglion (large multipolar) cells. The axons of the ganglion cells constitute the most superficial layer of the retina. They assemble to form the intraocular part of the optic nerve, which leaves the bulb by passing through the lamina cribrosa of the sclera. The two optic nerves extend caudally to the optic chiasm.

The fibers arising from the half of each retina temporal to the fovea continue on caudally to enter the ipsilateral optic tract and proceed to the lateral geniculate body. On the other hand, the fibers arising in the half of each retina lying nasal to the fovea undergo decussation in the chiasm. Thus, the right optic tract is formed by the fibers both from the temporal half of the right retina and the nasal half of the left retina (Fig. 21-1). The fibers decussating in the chiasm do not pursue a direct course to reach the other side; instead, they swing into the optic chiasm in such a manner that the fibers from the superior nasal (extramacular) part of the retina traverse the more caudal ipsilateral part of the chiasm before crossing over, while those from the inferior (extramacular) retina pass through the anterior inferior part of the chiasm and the base of the opposite optic nerve (Fig. 21-2). The optic tracts diverge as they extend caudally to terminate in the lateral geniculate bodies.

The fibers arising in the lateral geniculate body extend to the calcarine cortex *(geniculocalcarine tract).* In leaving the

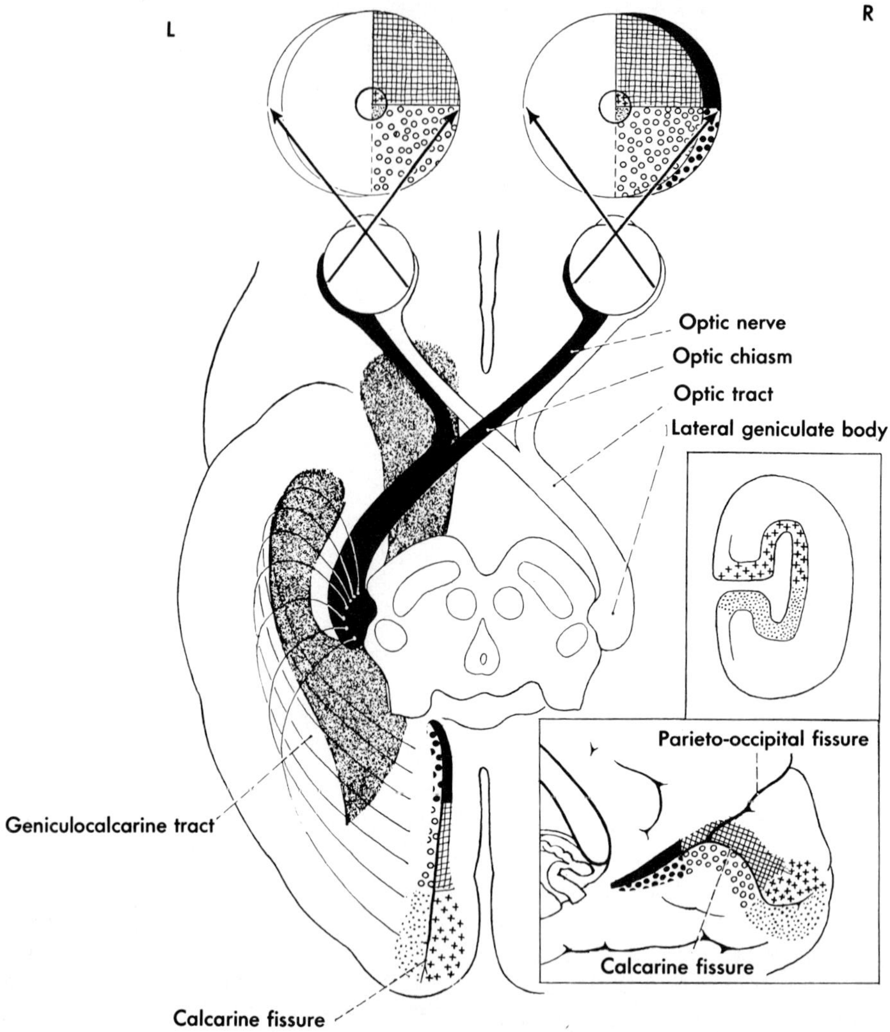

Fig. 21-1. The visual pathways. The visual cortex (area 17 of Brodmann) is illustrated as though it were on the medial surface of the cuneate and lingual lobules, whereas actually it is buried inside the calcarine fissure (upper inset, which illustrates a level in the caudal third of the visual cortex). The calcarine fissure is deepest (most opercularized) posteriorly and, hence, if the visual cortex were spread in one plane, it would have roughly the shape of a pyramid rounded at the bottom. The extension of the calcarine cortex rostral to the region of intersection by the parieto-occipital fissure is in accord with the descriptions given by Brodmann (1908) and von Economo and Koskinas (1925). (Diagram prepared in collaboration with Dr. Paul I. Yakovlev, Boston.)

lateral geniculate body, the fibers pass laterally through the sublenticular part of the internal capsule, then fan out (as the visual radiation). Beyond this level there are three contingents of visual fibers—dorsal, lateral, and ventral (Cushing, 1921). The dorsal and lateral are relatively direct in their passage to the calcarine cortex: they extend laterally over the posterior horn of the lateral ventricle, then backward along the edge of the ventricle; they then traverse the parietal lobe, then the occipital, to end in the upper half of the visual cortex (*calcarine cortex* or *area striata*). The ventral contingent sweeps forward and somewhat downward to the level of the uncus hippocampi, where it is situated 1 or 2 cm. or more short of the tip of the

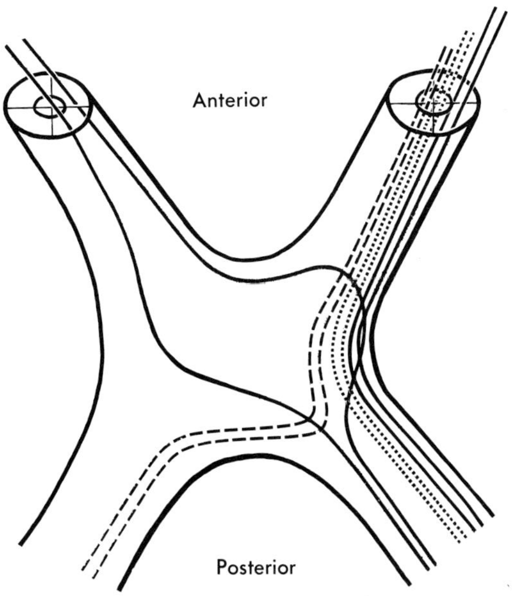

Fig. 21-2. Course of visual fibers through the optic chiasm. The macular fibers are represented by broken or dotted lines, the fibers from the peripheral part of the retina by solid lines. (After Hoyt, 1964.)

temporal horn (Marino and Rasmussen, 1968). It then passes lateralward over the inferior horn of the lateral ventricle (forming the *temporal loop*), then backward through the temporal and occipital lobes to terminate in the lower half of the visual cortex (Fig. 21-1). The latter group is called the *temporal loop*. At parietal, temporal, and occipital levels the caudally coursing geniculocalcarine tract runs lateral to the ventricle in the external sagittal stratum of fibers, separated from the ventricular cavity by the internal sagittal stratum, which is made up of a sheaf of fibers of the corpus callosum (tapetum) and the internal corticotectal tract.

The *external sagittal stratum* is a prominent, rather dense aggregate of fibers running medial to the posterior horn of the lateral ventricle. In addition to carrying the geniculocalcarine tract, it contains the inferior longitudinal fasciculus, which connects occipital cortex (lingula, cuneus, and lateral surface) with the cortex of the superior, middle, and inferior temporal gyri and the fusiform gyrus (Crosby, Humphrey, and Lauer, 1962).

Visual fields. Impressions gained in half of the binocular visual field are projected through the lens as a reversed image upon the opposite halves of the retinae. Therefore, the *right* optic tract transmits visual impressions from the *left* half of the binocular visual field, and vice versa. In Fig. 21-1 it will be noted that the fibers decussating in the chiasm originate in the *nasal* half of each retina and that they bring visual impressions from the *temporal* half of each monocular visual field. In the chiasm and beyond, there is a pairing of most of the fibers coming from corresponding receptor areas in the two homonymous fields, an exception being the most peripheral part of each temporal field (temporal "crescent" or "half moon"), which has an unpaired representation in the optic pathways and visual cortex. The fibers represented in the temporal "crescent" pass backward in the medial part of the optic nerve, form a ventral bundle in the chiasm and the optic tract, and terminate ventrally in the lateral geniculate body; continuing ventromedially in the geniculocalcarine tract they terminate in the most rostral part of the calcarine cortex. (Bender and Strauss, 1937; Walsh and Hoyt, 1969.)

Central and peripheral field representation. The part of the retina concerned in central vision is the macula (lutea), situated a little to the temporal side of the posterior pole of the eye. The macula is the region concerned in sharpest vision. The perception of shapes and contours depends largely on macular receptors, while the perception of motion depends on macular and peripheral retinal receptors. The macula being concerned in sharpest vision, ocular fixation is so regulated that the center of the image of any object looked at is brought on to the center of the macula. The fibers arising in the macula, constituting about a third of all the fibers originating in the retina, extend into the temporal aspect of the optic disk, or papilla, and shortly after leaving the disk they course in the central part of the optic nerve (as the papillomacular bundle).

The rest of the retinal fibers are disposed peripherally in the optic nerve.

At the chiasmal level the macular fibers derived from the nasal halves of the retinae undergo decussation, while those arising from the temporal halves course directly into the ipsilateral optic tract (Fig. 21-2). Thus, in these respects there are no differences between macular and other retinal fibers. The decussating macular fibers are most concentrated in the posterior superior part of the chiasm. (Jefferson, 1955; Naffziger, 1952; Walsh and Hoyt, 1969.)

Extending backward in the optic tract, the macular fibers occupy the central dorsal part of the tract and the peripheral retinal fibers the remainder of the tract. In the lateral geniculate body the macular fibers terminate superiorly, the fibers from the upper peripheral field inferolaterally, and the fibers from the lower peripheral field inferomedially (Chacko, 1948; Clark and Penman, 1934). The horizontal meridian of the visual field is represented approximately vertically (Spalding, 1952a).

In the visual radiation in its *anterior* part the macular fibers are spread out over the lateral aspect of the radiation (and tend to congregate toward the intermediate part of the radiation), while the fibers subserving peripheral vision are situated along the medial aspect of the radiation (and tend to congregate at the upper and lower margins of the radiation). The horizontal meridian of the visual field with respect to both the macular and the peripheral field is represented approximately horizontally. (Spalding, 1952a; Teuber, Battersby, and Bender, 1960.) In the *posterior* part of the visual radiation most of the fibers subserving peripheral vision leave the intermediate part of the radiation and congregate in the upper and the lower margins of the radiation. Thus, at posterior levels peripheral vision comes to be represented in the upper and the lower limbs of the "horseshoe," and central vision in between the two. (Brouwer, 1934; Polyak, 1942; Putnam, 1926.)

The *visual cortex (area striata, calcarine cortex)* includes all the cortex in the wall and floor of the calcarine fissure and also the adjoining parts of the cuneus and the lingual gyrus (Fig. 21-1). The area striata received its name from the prominent striation, or lamination, imparted to it by the white stripes of Gennari and Baillarger. In the Caucasian and Negro races the area striata, in relation to the sulcus lunatus, extends on to the lateral surface of the occipital pole in approximately 60 percent of brains (Connolly, 1950).

Central vision is represented most posteriorly in the calcarine cortex, with serial concentric zones of the visual field from the fixation point to the periphery represented in that order from behind forward. Peripheral vision is represented anterior to this area. The lower half of the field is represented in the upper half of the visual cortex, and vice versa. Central ("macular") vision is represented unilaterally (Spalding, 1952b). The horizontal meridian is represented in the floor of the calcarine fissure (Holmes, 1918, 1931; Spalding, 1952b).

Fibers subserving reflex responses. Fibers concerned in the pupillary light reflex leave the optic tract just rostral to the lateral geniculate body and pass to the pretectal region at the level of the posterior commissure (Fig. 21-3). From pretectal nuclei of each side, fibers course to the Edinger-Westphal nucleus of both sides. Fibers leaving this nucleus course in the oculomotor nerve to the ciliary ganglion, and from here a new set of fibers extends to the pupillary sphincter in the iris. The pupillary (light) reflex pathway consists of at least six neurons: rod and cone layer of the retina, bipolar cell layer of the retina, ganglion cell layer of the retina (the axons of which pass by way of optic nerve, chiasm, and tract to the pretectal region), axons extending from the pretectal region to the Edinger-Westphal nucleus, a relay from the Edinger-Westphal nucleus to the ciliary ganglia, and another relay from the ciliary ganglion to the sphincter pupillae. Because of the

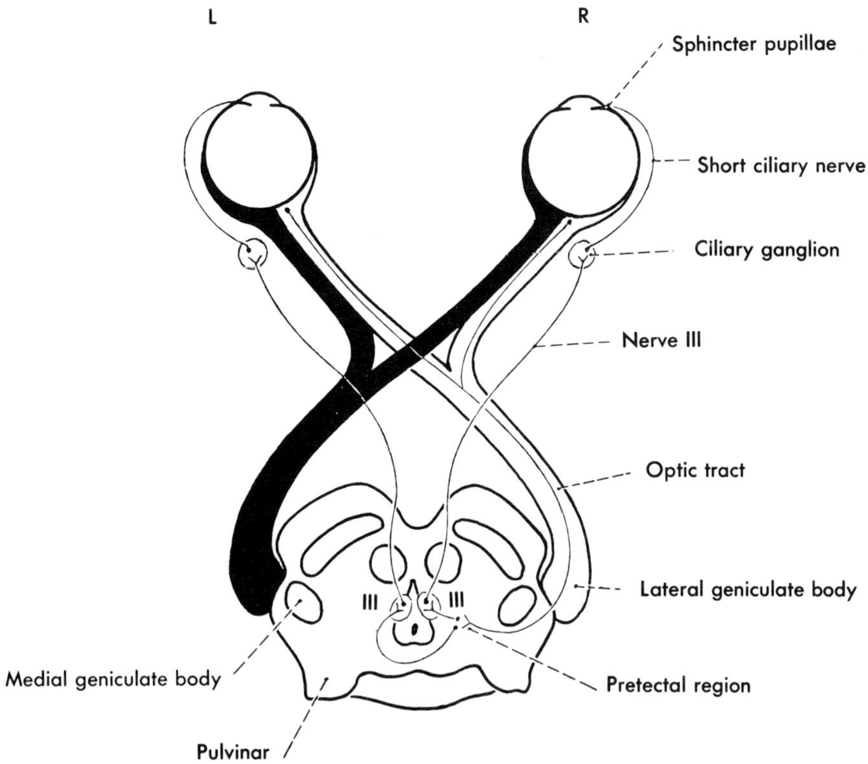

Fig. 21-3. The course of optic fibers concerned in pupillary constriction. *III*, Oculomotor nucleus.

presence of a connector pathway from the pretectal region of one side to the Edinger-Westphal nucleus of both sides, exposure of one eye to light results in constriction not only of the corresponding pupil *(direct reaction)* but also of the other pupil as well *(consensual reaction)* (Magoun and others, 1939).

Blood supply

Both the central artery of the retina and the vein (which are branches of the corresponding ophthalmic vessels) enter the optic nerve in its lower inner aspect, 10 to 20 mm. behind the posterior pole of the globe (François and Neetens, 1954). In reaching the optic nerve they run for a distance in the subarachnoid space.

The central artery and vein extend forward in the center of the optic nerve. In some brains the artery, in its forward course, gives off prominent branches that form the bulk of the capillary bed in the core of the nerve (in the region of the papillomacular bundle) (Steele and Blunt, 1956; Wybar, 1956). In other brains the core of the nerve receives only inconstant branches, which are of variable size (Fig. 21-4). In still other brains the central artery is strictly terminal (in the retina), providing blood only to the bulb. In such brains an anterior branch of the central artery, or a branch coming directly from the ophthalmic artery, gives off a short axial system of capillaries that supplies the core of the nerve (François and Neetens, 1954; François, Neetens, and Collette, 1955). Quite apart from this system are vessels in the leptomeninges that supply the periphery of the nerve; these vessels are fed mainly by the ophthalmic artery. Most rostrally the optic nerve also receives blood from the arterial circle of Zinn-Haller, which surrounds the nerve head. This arterial circle, present in the sclera, is fed through anastomotic channels by

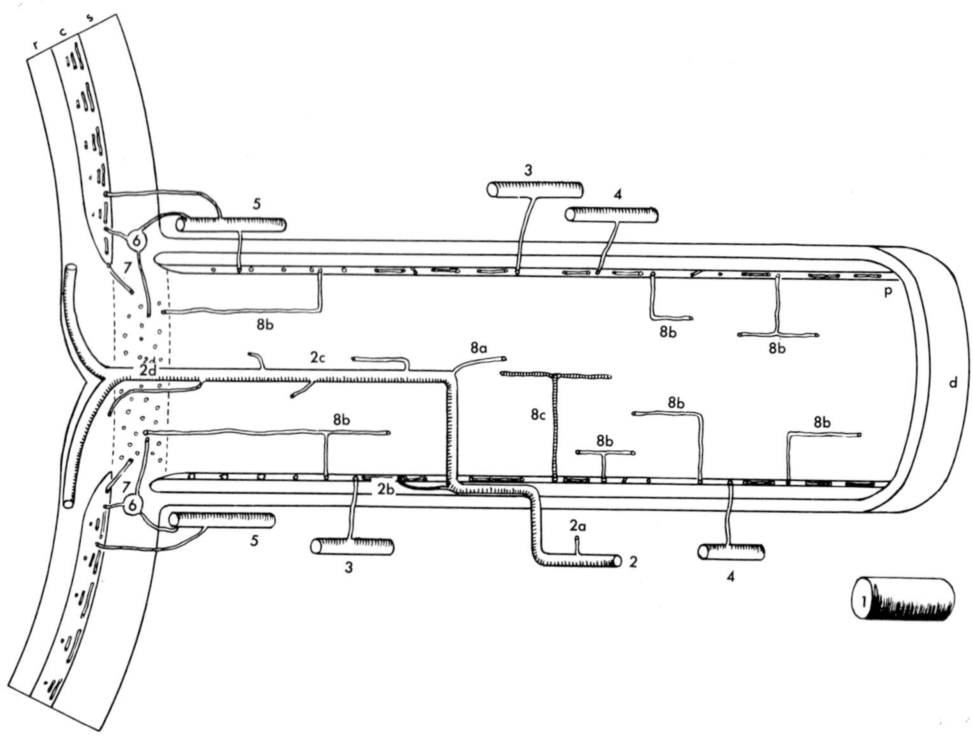

Fig. 21-4. Blood supply of the optic nerve and retina. (Courtesy Prof. J. François, Ghent, Belgium.)
r, retina; *c*, choroid; *s*, sclera; *p*, leptomeningeal arterial plexus: peripheral nerve supply; *d*, dural sheath.

1. Ophthalmic artery: main source of all arterial branches
2. Central retinal artery
   - 2a. Extraneural branch
   - 2b. Arachnoidal branch to leptomeningeal plexus
   - 2c. Intraneural branches: inconstant, variable in size, and few in number; precocious retinal branches
   - 2d. Absence of branches at the level of the lamina cribrosa
3. Ciliary arteries: branches to the leptomeningeal plexus and nerve
4. Muscular arteries: branches to the leptomeningeal plexus and nerve
5. Posterior short ciliary arteries: branches to the leptomeningeal plexus, the choroid, and origin of the arterial circle of Zinn-Haller
6. Arterial circle of Zinn-Haller
7. Recurrent arterial twigs to the lamina cribrosa
8. Peripheral and central optic nerve supply
   - 8a. Occasional central branch from central retinal artery
   - 8b. Peripheral supply with an anterior or posterior branch, or both, throughout the length of the nerve
   - 8c. One of these may reach the center of the nerve and, if of sufficient size, may constitute a central optic nerve artery

Variations of 2c, 8a, 8c are frequent.

the posterior short ciliary arteries (Fig. 21-4).

The central artery and vein enter the eye through the middle of the optic disk. The retina has a double blood supply. (1) The central artery supplies the retina down to the outer plexiform layer by means of a dense capillary network (Toussaint, Kuwabara, and Cogan, 1961), while the rod and cone layer is nourished by the choreocapillaris by diffusion through the pigment epithelium and Bruch's membrane. (2) Cilioretinal arterioles from the circle of Zinn-Haller contribute to the blood supply of the central part of the retina (François and Neetens, 1954). Owing to the latter source of supply, the central part of the retina may continue to function for a time after occlusion of the central retinal artery.

The part of the optic nerve situated behind the entrance of the central retinal artery and in front of the optic foramen is supplied mainly by recurrent branches of the central retinal artery together with vessels coming via the leptomeninges (Fig. 21-4) from the ophthalmic artery and other sources (Dawson, 1958; François and Neetens, 1954). The intracranial part of the optic nerve and the chiasm receive no significant contribution from the ophthalmic artery. From the chiasmal anastomotic arterial plexuses, a prechiasmal artery, derived either from the chiasmal anastomotic vessels (Dawson, 1958) or from the circuminfundibular plexus (Steele and Blunt, 1956), runs forward on the upper surface of the optic nerve. Hughes (1958), in summing up the situation, remarks that the major supply of the undersurface of the chiasm and presumably the undersurface of the intracranial part of the optic nerve is by way of the *anterior superior hypophysial artery*, the inferolateral aspect of the chiasm by *a branch from the internal carotid*, and the superior aspect of the chiasm by *branches from the anterior cerebral and anterior communicating arteries.*

LESIONS INVOLVING THE OPTIC SYSTEM, AND CLINICAL DISTURBANCES

Optic nerve and retina

Papilledema, optic atrophy, optic neuritis

Papilledema occurs in a variety of disease states. A common form is that caused by an increase in the normal pressure gradient existing between the intracranial contents and the interior of the eyeball. This increase is transmitted by way of the cerebrospinal fluid in the subarachnoid space surrounding the optic nerve; apparently the major factor concerned is obstruction of venous flow in the optic nerve resulting from compression of the central vein in its course across the subarachnoid space, the accompanying artery being spared because of its higher intraluminal pressure.

The disk can readily swell owing to its loose network of specialized glial cells ("spider" cells) situated just inside the lamina cribrosa and forming a wicker basket-like structure (Wolter, 1957). The structure of the retina surrounding the disk is different. Here, radial fibers (of Müller) form a rigid framework that does not yield readily to swelling. As a consequence, an edematous process in this region can lead to extensive irreversible damage in retinal components.

In an early stage, papilledema resulting from an increase in intracranial pressure is characterized by engorgement of the retinal veins, pinkness of the optic disk, and blurring of the disk margins. The blurring usually begins in the upper part of the disk and later extends to involve the nasal, then the temporal, side of the disk. Soon afterward the swelling obliterates the physiological cup, then causes an elevation of the disk as a whole. As the disk swells, it bulges laterally, displacing the peripapillary retina. As a consequence, swelling of axons occurs in the region next to the lamina cribrosa. If the papilledema persists, axonal interruption occurs in this region (Wolter, 1957).

In severe papilledema the edematous process may, in earlier stages, spread corona-like into the peripapillary retina (Fig. 21-5) and include the macula, in which case the intervening retina is thrown into folds that extend from disk to macula, the so-called "macular fan." Retinal veins are dilated and hemorrhages may occur in the peripapillary retina or even in the disk.

As papilledema develops, the blind spot in the binocular visual field increases in size, and if the more distal part of the papillary retina undergoes buckling, the blind spot enlargement will persist after the papilledema has subsided. Concentric peripheral constriction of the visual field also occurs in chronic severe papilledema, but it is seldom as pronounced as might be expected from the appearance of the papilledema. Commonly occurring in later stages are defects in the nasal visual field. Under conditions in which increase in intracranial pressure persists, the papilledema will give way to optic atrophy. This is characterized in later stages by pallor of the disk and constriction of the retinal arteries, and ultimately by a disk that is

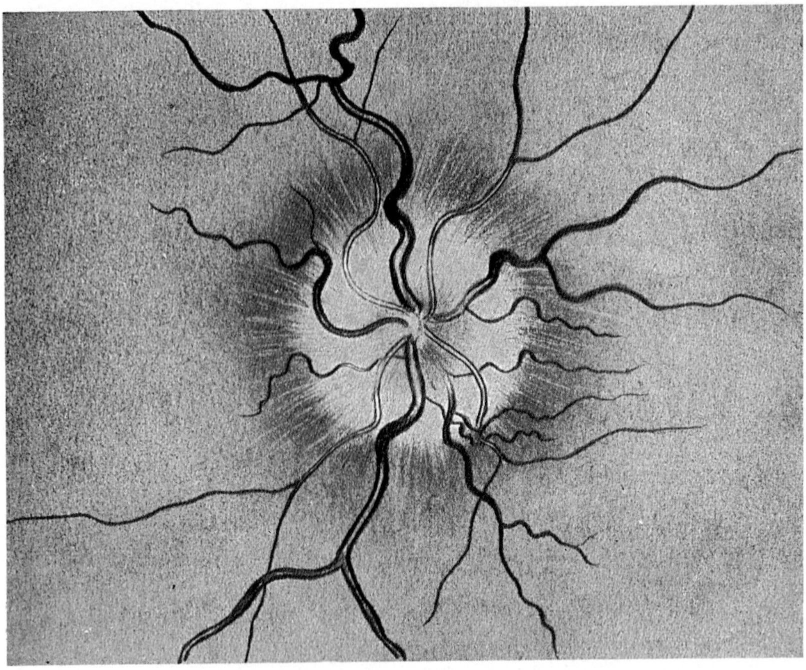

Fig. 21-5. Papilledema due to increased intracranial pressure brought about by cerebellar neoplasm.

flat, with indistinct edges, and with a physiological cup filled with glial tissue that obscures the lamina cribrosa. In due course, total blindness occurs. When this happens, the pupil enlarges and no longer reacts to light.

It is generally agreed that the visual field defects occurring in increased intracranial pressure are a direct expression of pathological changes in the optic nerve and optic nerve head bilaterally. The pathological process appears to commence in the sheath of the nerve head on the temporal side. A fibrosing process then gradually spreads around the nerves, constricting them, and resulting in concentric narrowing of the visual field. The periphery of the lower nasal field is first affected, and the involvement, if continued, can spread upward, resulting in nasal hemianopia. (Hughes, 1954.)

When a disk is irregularly elevated, lacks a physiological cup, but is not congested and has normal-appearing retinal vessels (Fig. 21-6), *pseudopapilledema* is probably the diagnosis; discrete, yellow, shining concretious or hyaline bodies (drusen) buried in the disk may be responsible for the altered appearance (Hoyt and Pont, 1962; Lyle, 1964). (The term "drusen" is probably derived from the Czechoslovakian word "drusa," meaning a hollow cavity in a rock, filled with crystals.

In *intraocular optic neuritis* (papillitis), in contrast to papilledema, the earliest visual field defect observed is centrally situated. The occurrence of central scotoma accounts for poor vision so often, but not always, complained of in this condition.

Intraocular optic neuritis and papilledema may, in earlier stages of development, be difficult to distinguish. The criterion that visual acuity suffers in intraocular optic neuritis but not in papilledema cannot always be relied on, because in as many as 21 percent of cases of optic neuritis visual acuity is preserved (Chamblin, 1953). Nor is pain on motion of the eye dependable as a criterion of intraocular optic neuritis, as it occurs in only 20 percent of cases (Henderson, 1956). Diagnosis of intraocular optic neuritis can be established by quantitative perimetry and confirmed by the presence of cells in the vitreous or by means of the Marcus Gunn pupillary sign, or both. The Marcus Gunn sign signifies a conduction defect in the prechiasmal afferent pupillary pathway (Thompson, 1966).

Perimetry reveals a field defect in intraocular optic neuritis, which distinguishes the disorder from papilledema. Scotoma in some of these cases

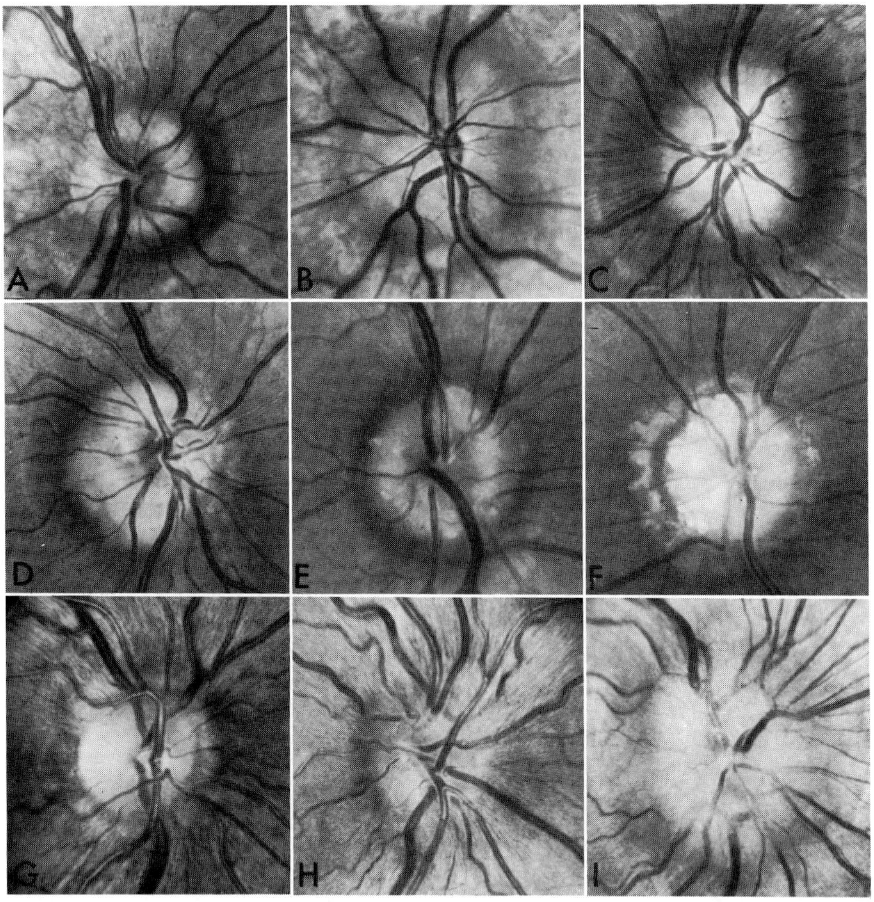

Fig. 21-6. Pseudopapilledema (anomalous elevation of the optic disk). These photographs were obtained from patients originally thought to harbor a brain tumor. **A** through **D** are examples from children with congenital disk elevation from intrapapillary drusen. Note normal, noncongested, and unobscured vessels and also the absence of the optic cup. The buried drusen are partially exposed in **E** (the disk of a young adult) and completely exposed in **F** (the disk of a 45-year-old man). None of these disks exhibit the capillary congestion, venous dilation, nerve fiber layer hemorrhages, or exudates, that accompany real papilledema. Disks **G** through **I** are examples of anomalies causing diagnostic confusion because of blurring of the disk margins; all are characterized by absence of the optic cup, anomalous branching of the vessels, and, in **I**, a congenital excess of glial tissue. (From Hoyt and Pont, 1962.)

spares fixation so that visual acuity remains normal. With severe optic nerve involvement, the classical "amaurotic pupil" is observed. A pupil of this kind does not react to direct light but responds consensually in a normal manner.

It is with incomplete optic nerve lesions in which routine clinical testing may not uncover a pupillary defect that the *Marcus Gunn sign* is of value. This test is based upon the fact that the direct light reaction in the involved (bad) eye is not as strong as its consensual reaction. The test is best performed in a dimly lighted room with the patient fixating in the distance. A light (from an ordinary flashlight) is presented to each eye for about 5 seconds and is moved alternately from one eye to the other. As the light is shifted from the good to the bad eye, the latter will be seen to dilate, apparently paradoxically. This direct light stimulus in the bad eye is no longer sufficient to maintain the previously evoked degree of consensual pupillary constriction, hence the dilatation. This may be striking even when both pupils, if tested separately, react well to light. For example, in optic neuritis involving the left eye, when the light is moved quickly to the left eye, the left pupil slowly dilates from the position it had attained due to the consensual response when the same light had been directed on the right eye. (Daroff and Smith, 1965.)

Retrobulbar optic neuritis, intraocular optic neuritis, and *neuroretinitis* are clinical terms denoting sites of involvement by a pathological process, not necessarily inflammatory. Although an inflammatory state may exist in nerve or disk (for example, in association with orbital cellulitis or meningitis), actually the basic process often consists in demyelination (as in multiple sclerosis) or nerve fiber destruction over a wide area (as in neuromyelitis optica). Generally speaking, if a destructive lesion is situated in front of the site at which the central artery and vein (of the retina) penetrate the optic nerve, papilledema, then atrophy of the papilla, will result; if behind this site, atrophy alone will occur. In *retrobulbar neuritis* (optic neuritis situated anywhere behind the globe) the atrophy may be slight. Thus, a patient with retrobulbar neuritis due presumably to demyelination of the optic nerve initially complains of unilateral blurred vision, most often a central scotoma; pain is usually experienced on movement of the eye; pupillary and color vision abnormalities occur; and in most cases the vision returns to normal or near normal within a few months. Often, but not invariably, only temporal pallor is left. (Rose, 1968.) In other cases complete loss of vision occurs (Bradley and Whitty, 1967). In such cases the optic disk becomes decidedly atrophic; the disk is characterized by a dead whiteness, flattening with exposure of the lamina cribrosa, sharpness of outline, retention of the physiological cup, and normal appearing vessels. On the other hand, following *intraocular optic neuritis* the disk outlines are irregular and fuzzy, the lamina cribrosa is obscured, and the physiological cup is filled in. In short, the disk is scarred.

Optic atrophy develops in a wide variety of other disorders involving eye, optic nerve, chiasm, or optic tracts. In *primary* optic atrophy—as occurs, for example, in multiple sclerosis or in traumatic involvement of the nerve—there is degeneration or gradual destruction of axons with little gliosis or mesodermal scarring and striking shrinkage of the entire nerve. The optic disk is characterized by sharply defined pallor and normal blood vessels. By contrast, in *secondary* optic nerve atrophy—resulting, for example, from inflammatory states—there is extensive gliosis and mesodermal scarring, less optic nerve shrinkage, and narrowed retinal arterioles.

The time required for atrophy of the disk to occur as a result of lesions in the optic nerve depends on the distance of the lesion from the retina and on other factors such as the degree of damage inflicted on the visual fibers. After compression of the optic nerve in its orbital course, a week or two is necessary for optic atrophy to become apparent in the disk, and in about 3 weeks after the nerve is interrupted in its intracanalicular course. This much time is required because the degenerative changes in the nerve fibers are retrograde.

Clinical manifestations of lesions involving the optic nerve vary in accordance with degree and site of interruption. Total interruption of an optic nerve causes complete blindness *(amaurosis)* in that eye. The pupillary reflex is not elicitable when the blind eye is exposed to light, but can be obtained in the blind eye when the unaffected eye is exposed to light. Pupillary constriction during accommodation-convergence is, however, retained in the blind eye. Some pathological processes involving the optic nerve (multiple sclerosis and intoxications by agents such as methyl alcohol) affect predominantly the papillomacular bundle, thus giving rise to a central scotoma (blind spot) that may or may not be associated with visual disturbances in the adjacent peripheral field. In most situations in which compression of the optic nerve takes place, a central scotoma also develops (Hughes, 1958); why the peripheral part of the nerve should be spared under these conditions remains an enigma. Other pathological processes (such as involvement of the nerve secondarily from spread of chronic syphilic meningitis) involve mostly the peripheral (periaxial) fibers in the nerve, in which case macular vision is preserved.

A parasellar tumor located in this region, particularly olfactory groove meningioma, frequently compresses the optic nerve in such degree (acutely or chronically) that optic atrophy occurs before papilledema can develop. Rarely in the growth of such a tumor, when intracranial pressure has increased, optic atrophy occurs on the compressed side and papilledema on the other side (Kennedy's syndrome, 1911, 1916; also syndrome of Gowers, 1909, and syndrome of Paton, 1909). Unilateral papilledema may also result from circumferential compression of the optic nerve by an intraorbital mass.

Lesions involving the optic nerve and retina

Vascular disease and circulatory disturbances. *Thrombosis* occurring locally in a retinal arteriole is most commonly a complication of arterial hypertension or diabetes mellitus. Visual field defects under these conditions vary in distribution. Thrombosis or other comparable interference with blood flow in the distal part of the internal carotid artery—for example, in its course near the pituitary—may lead to ischemia of the optic nerve and retina with visual disturbance and, in some cases, permanent residual blindness (Johnson and Walker, 1951). However, sudden and permanent blindness results only if the thrombus is propagated sufficiently far into the ophthalmic artery. This is because the ophthalmic artery (a branch of the internal carotid) possesses a rich anastomosis with vessels derived from the external carotid artery (anastomotic) branches between the ophthalmic artery and the external maxillary and the middle meningeal arteries, respectively (Gillilan, 1961; Vaernet, 1954; Yates and Hutchinson, 1961). Thrombotic occlusion of the more proximal part of the internal carotid artery can lead to much the same visual disturbances as just mentioned in connection with the distal part of the internal carotid. The same is true for sudden occlusion of the common carotid artery. The retinopathy (dilated retinal veins, hemorrhages, exudates, microaneurysms), resulting in loss of vision, is attributed to venous stasis in the retina occurring in association with reduced blood flow (Kearns and Hollenhorst, 1963).

Emboli originating from thrombotic material released from the wall of the left heart may lodge in the central artery of the retina, or material from ulcerated atheromatous plaques situated along the arch of the aorta or in the region of the bifurcation of the common carotid may lodge in this artery. More commonly, however, the emboli arrive in the retina itself. Perhaps the most common precipitating factor in retinal embolization is manipulation, either surgical or arteriographic, of a diseased carotid artery (Shillito and Rockett, 1963). Cholesterol crystals coming to a halt in fundal arterioles account for the glittering orange-yellow plaques not uncommonly found in the fundus (Ball, 1966). White or copper-colored plaques, previously regarded as local arteriosclerotic manifestations, may also owe their origin to emboli of this kind (Dark and Rizk, 1967; Hollenhorst, 1961).

Emboli from any source, if sufficiently small, may cause only a fleeting monocular blindness *(amaurosis fugax).* This is true, for instance, for cholesterol-crystal embolization. Patients thus affected also have recurrent transient ischemic episodes involving the brain; either kind of episode, ocular or cerebral, can herald catastrophic hemiplegia from acute carotid artery occlusion (Ehrenfeld, Hoyt, and Wylie, 1966). Infarct from lodgement of an embolus in a retinal arteriole sometimes gives rise to an *arcuate scotoma,* from involvement of a concentrically distributed bundle of nerve fibers issuing from one or more sectors of the retina; the same kind of field defect may result with a segmental optic nerve infarct and rarely from tumor involving the chiasm (Hoyt, 1962).

Occlusion of the central artery of the retina (or of an arterial branch supplying the papillomacular bundle) of whatever cause leads to ischemic infarction of the nerve, culminating in profound optic atrophy. In earlier stages the disk is pale and swollen, its arterioles are narrowed, and the peripapillary retina contains sparse, fluffy, white opacities *(cotton-wool spots).*

Among the disorders in which thrombotic occlusion of the ophthalmic artery or any of its branches may occur is *giant cell (temporal) arteritis.* Long stretches of an artery may be thrombosed, or the thrombosis may be segmental. Disturbances range from diplopia to complete blindness involving one or both eyes. There may be benign complications, such as diplopia, transient ptosis, pain in the eyeballs, and photophobia. As a result of thrombosis of the central artery of the retina, there may be profound visual disturbances in association with an edematous or pale papilla and other manifestations of ischemic optic neuritis. Prodromal symptoms may appear many months prior to acute onset. (Davidson, Schlezinger, and Mullen, 1959; Simmons and Cogan, 1962.)

In long-standing arterial hypertension associated with hyperplastic arteriosclerotic change, hemorrhages and edema may occur in the retina, and the retina may contain cotton-wool spots or patches. An additional feature of hypertensive retinopathy is a *star figure* in the area surrounding degenerative foci in the region of the fovea.

In *classical migraine* ("complicated migraine" in the European literature) visual scotoma or other visual aberrations usually precede the headache, as do other prodromes (hemianesthesia [involving usually the hands, fingers, and lips], mono- or hemiparesis, vertigo, inability to concentrate, disturbances of speech, aphasia). Occasionally, however, the visual disturbances are not followed by headache. Scotoma (for example, "holes in the vision") usually lasts 10 to 30 minutes. The defects usually have a homonymous hemianopic or quadrantanopic distribution, but may be central, peripheral, or altitudinal. The scotoma may, for example, commence in the macular region, then spread to the temporal field, then drift across the field so that its central margin withdraws from the macula. Not only scotomas but also photopia (sparks and flashes) and teichopia (bright spots or zigzags, commonly scintillating or vibrating) may also occur.

Defects in visual fields may persist after a migraine attack has ceased. Permanent hemianopia occasionally occurs. Observed now and then in association with permanent scotomas is evidence of retinal infarction, the result of occlusion of the central retinal artery or of a peripheral retinal arteriole.

During attacks the headache is usually contralateral to the scotoma, may be ipsilateral, and not uncommonly is bilateral. It tends to reach its peak of steady or throbbing pain in a half hour or an hour and usually lasts only a few hours, not more than 12 hours. Persons in their late teens or early twenties are most subject to migraine; only about 15 percent are beyond 20 years of age. (Bruyn, 1968; Graham, 1968; Klee and Willanger, 1966.)

Paroxysmal and nonprogressive course, lack of focal signs, lack of altered consciousness, and lack of epileptic attacks usually signify a vasomotor disturbance as the basis of the migraine, not some parenchymal lesion in association with angioma or neoplasm. (The latter have occasionally been found responsible; Pearce, 1968.) Dysfunction of the vertebral-basilar arterial system is doubtless responsible for some of the disorders—for example, hemianopia and teichopia (Klee and Willanger, 1966). Now and then "ophthalmic migraine," characterized by scotoma, turns out to be chronic glaucoma (Hobbs, 1964).

On the *venous* side, occlusion of the central retinal vein results in profound vascular engorgement, superficial hemorrhages, and focal necrosis of the inner layers of the retina, with subsequent cyst formation in the retina. Fibrovascular proliferation in the region of the macula is a late manifestation (Wise, 1957). Clinically, this is manifested by punctate microaneurysms, opacities in the wall of veins, and new vessel formation.

Syphilis. Involvement of the optic nerve by a syphilitic process (optic neuritis, juxtapapillary chorioretinitis, gumma) is in most instances secondary to chronic leptomeningitis affecting the periaxial part of the nerve intracranially or in the orbit. The end stage is marked either by primary or secondary optic atrophy or both. In late stages of syphilis (as in tabes dorsalis or general paresis), damage of the optic nerve and papilla may be severe and may be due to such factors as constriction of the nerve by arachnoidal scarring, arterial occlusion, and chorioretinitis.

Trauma. Contre-coup injuries sometimes affect the retina directly, rupturing particularly the internal limiting membrane. The macular region usually bears the brunt of the retinal damage. "Contusion necrosis" occurs and is followed by the development of cysts or crater-like defects in the macula; or a break in the cornea or rupture of the trabeculum at the scleral spur occurs. The optic nerve may be contused, lacerated, or otherwise damaged in its intracanalicular portion by frontal blows on the head, some of which cause fracture in the region of the optic foramen. Pallor of the disk develops in 3 weeks or less. (Hogan and Zimmerman, 1962; Wolter, 1963.)

Intracranial tumors and other masses. When papilledema is accompanied by headache, dizziness, projectile vomiting, bradycardia, and clouded consciousness, an expanding lesion within the intracranial cavity is to be suspected. When the increased intracranial pressure responsible for papilledema is the product of two factors, an increase in the volume of the intracranial contents and an obstruction in the flow of cerebrospinal fluid, there will be early and intense papilledema. As a general rule, the more rapid the growth of a tumor, the greater the tendency for papilledema to develop. After middle age, however, papilledema seldom occurs in earlier stages of tumor development, as diminished brain volume makes the disproportion between the cranium and its contents less critical.

No tumor gives rise more rapidly to intense papilledema than a colloid cyst in the third ventricle when impacted. Next in line are tumors of the cerebellum. Then come tumors of the medial part of the temporal lobe, cerebellopontile angle, pineal body, corpora quadrigemina, wall of the fourth ventricle, and after these, tumors of the parietal, occipital, and frontal lobes and pons. Papilledema occurs less readily in the presence of tumors of the lateral part of the temporal lobe, basal ganglia, and centrum semiovale, and is frequently minimal in tumors of the corpus callosum, wall of the third or lateral ventricle, cerebral peduncle, or medulla oblongata. Papilledema seldom results from tumors involving the base of the brain, the infundibulum, or the pituitary. An exception is craniopharyngioma developing in childhood. When there is severe *unilateral papilledema* or a conspicuous difference in the degree of papilledema on the right and left, the tumor is usually situated on the side on which the papilledema is most severe.

Papilledema can occur in the presence of tumors (or other masses) not giving rise to localizing signs. For instance, in 238 cases thus characterized clinically, Berg and his associates (1955) found lateral masses (glioma, meningioma, subdural hematoma) in 49 percent, midline masses (glioma, colloid cyst) in 26 percent, and in 11 percent the diagnosis made was "serous meningitis." Plain skull films were of diagnostic help in 30 percent.

Varied other causes of papilledema. A syndrome that includes manifestations of an intracranial expanding lesion—for example, papilledema, headache, vomiting, failing vision, diplopia, and dizziness—but that lacks signs of a focal lesion is sometimes referred to as the *syndrome of pseudotumor cerebri.* The term was coined to include those cases in which manifestations of intracranial tumor were evident during life but in which no lesions were found postmortem. As Kalbag and Woolf (1967) mention, it is historically incorrect to use the term in any other way. Higier (1926) made the plea that the term be used sparingly lest diagnosis be turned into pseudodiagnosis.

Causes of papilledema are dealt with in the following.

Venous sinus obstruction and serous meningitis. Papilledema occurring as a result of intracranial hypertension can result from obstruction in venous outflow from any major channel, such as the sagittal sinus, the torcular Herophili, and the lateral and sigmoid sinuses combined. For example, sagittal sinus thrombosis complicating closed head trauma may cause papilledema (Beller, 1964; Foley, 1955; Martin, 1955). Cavernous sinus thrombosis and arteriovenous fistula are further causes of papilledema. Infection originating in the middle ear or mastoid may also be responsible (Foley, 1955; Greer, 1962; Klestadt, 1924; Russell, 1949). Spread of the infective process to the lateral sinus, with thrombosis resulting, leads to serous meningitis (or acute meningeal hydrops), and if the lateral sinus thrombus extends in retrograde manner (by way of the veins on the convexity of the hemisphere) to the superior sagittal sinus, acute hydrocephalus develops. Changes resulting from infection rather than dural sinus obstruction per se appear to be the basis of the hydrocephalus in some cases. Symonds

(1931, 1937, 1940), in reaching these conclusions, coined the term "otitic hydrocephalus" for this condition. There was no alteration of the cerebrospinal fluid in his cases. Serous meningitis of cause other than otitis media can also lead to the development of papilledema and can be unaccompanied by ventricular enlargement or dural sinus thrombosis (Davidoff and Dyke, 1937); "toxic hydrocephalus" was proposed as a term to designate some of these cases (McAlpine, 1937). The hydrocephalus occurring in these states is generally conceded to be of the *external* type.

In many patients with papilledema thus caused, no abnormality in the visual fields can be found. When present, the defect usually consists in enlargement of the blind spots. In some instances of "toxic" or "otitic" hydrocephalus homonymous quadrant defects, central scotomas, and constricted fields have been noted (Foley, 1955). Quite commonly, inferior nasal quadrantanopia occurring unilaterally is observed (Dersh and Schlezinger, 1959; Dunn, Baker, and Wagener, 1955).

Hematological disorders. Pronounced papilledema is sometimes encountered in acute iron-deficiency anemia (Greer, 1967), in leukemia, and in acute blood loss. Under some of these conditions, not only may there be papilledema but also hemorrhages into the retina and, eventually, optic atrophy (Ashton, Pears, and Pickering, 1961). Similar changes, with variations, are observed in sickle cell anemia (Lieb, Geeraets, and Guerry, 1959) and in macroglobulinanemia of Waldenström (Carr and Henkind, 1963), the latter characterized also by polyneuritis and, in some cases, by hemiparesis or mono-

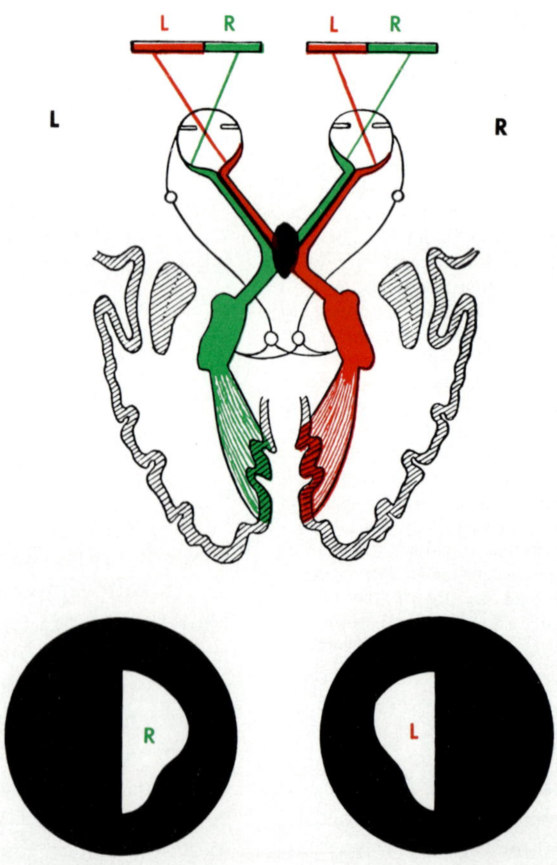

Fig. 21-7. Bitemporal heteronymous hemianopia resulting from interruption of the medial part of the chiasm.

paresis, and rarely by myelopathy or an extrapyramidal syndrome (Monteverde and others, 1966). Polycythemia vera is another disorder that falls into this group. Blurring of the optic disk is frequent, papilledema not uncommon. Hemorrhages are seen occasionally and thrombosis of the central retinal vein may occur. Still other disturbances are noted in polycythemia vera, such as headache, vertigo, paresthesias, hemiplegia, and extrapyramidal syndromes. (Johnson and Chalgren, 1951.)

Obstruction in cephalic blood flow of systemic origin. Examples in which papilledema can occur are right heart failure, respiratory insufficiency, severe pulmonary emphysema, and mediastinal tumor.

Diminished capacity of the cranium. Craniosynostosis (oxycephaly, plagiocephaly) due to premature fusion of the cranial vault, can give rise to increased intracranial pressure, with papilledema ensuing, then blindness (Andersson and Gomes, 1968).

Other states. Among other pathological states in which papilledema may occur are arterial hypertension, eclampsia, and premenstrual edema (Dunn, Baker, and Wagener, 1955), the Landry-Guillain-Barré syndrome or other polyneuritic state (Feldman, Landau, and Halpern, 1955; Janeway and Kelly, 1966; Joynt, 1958), vitamin A deficiency or excess (Cornfield and Cooke, 1952; Gerber, Raab, and Sobel, 1954), tetracycline administration (Fields, 1961), and certain endocrine disorders, such as hypothyroidism (Greer, 1967).

Involvement of the optic chiasm

Destruction of the central part of the chiasm interrupts decussating optic fibers that have originated in the nasal halves of the retinae. Bitemporal (heteronymous) hemianopia thus occurs (Fig. 21-7). Pressure exerted on the chiasm from below in-

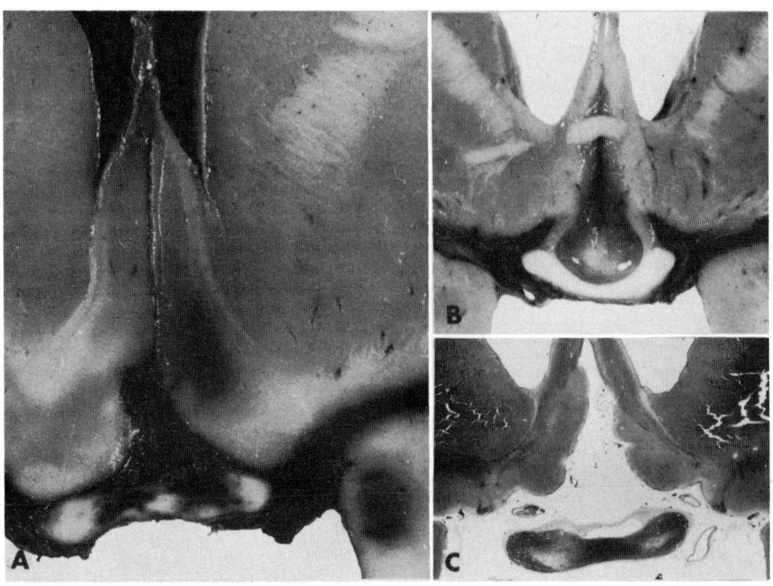

Fig. 21-8. A, Recent contusion with hemorrhages predominantly in the center of the chiasm resulting from a fall on the convexity of the forehead. Small contused areas are also present in the neighboring brain tissue. **B** and **C**, Bilateral focal loss of myelinated fibers in the chiasm occurring in association with a much enlarged preoptic recess. The demyelination is probably due to a circulatory disorder resulting from compression of vessels. The patient had internal hypertensive hydrocephalus caused by obstruction of the foramen of Magendie by cerebellar glioma. (Courtesy Dr. Richard Lindenberg, Baltimore.)

volves initially the fibers from the lower nasal quadrants of the retinae, and thus the earliest field defect is in the upper temporal quadrants. When pressure is applied from above, the reverse occurs. Usually the decussating fibers are compressed on one side before those on the other side, giving rise initially to a unilateral upper temporal quadrantic field defect, which may or may not be associated with a paracentral scotoma. Under such conditions the defect may extend into the lower temporal quadrant before a similar series of changes develop in the other visual field.

Bitemporal field defects involving the upper temporal quadrants may result, for example, from compression by chromophobe hypophysial adenoma or craniopharyngioma, but in these tumors atypical defects are the rule (see Chapter 26). Field defects in the lower temporal quadrants are less common. They may be seen, for example, in enlargement of the preoptic recess resulting from an increase in intraventricular pressure (Dott, 1936). Bitemporal field defects are also observed in traumatic laceration of the optic chiasm (Lindenberg and Walsh, 1964; Traquair, Dott, and Russell, 1935), of which an example is illustrated in Fig. 21-8, *A*. Stretching of the chiasm as a consequence of distortion of the skull (with or without fracture), separating the optic canals, appears to be the basis (Logan and Gordon, 1967). Purely local damage of the central part of the chiasm results, in time, in the classical chiasmal syndrome: optic atrophy and bitemporal defects without alteration in the sella turcica. Sclerotic anterior cerebral arteries may give rise to the syndrome. In

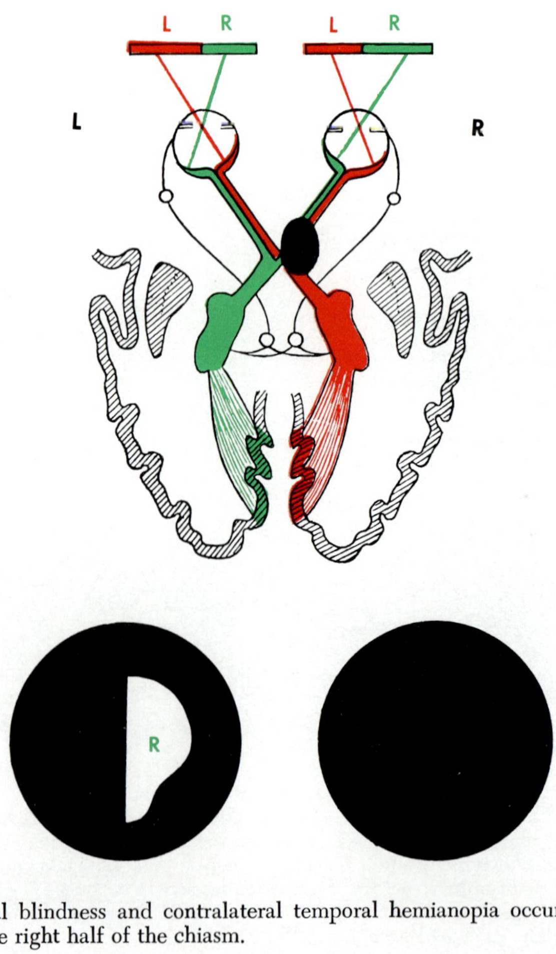

Fig. 21-9. Ipsilateral blindness and contralateral temporal hemianopia occurring as the result of interruption of the right half of the chiasm.

such cases the superior bitemporal field defects that occur may develop either abruptly or gradually. The disorder is probably due to impaired circulation in prechiasmal anastomotic vessels, brought about by traction upon or sclerotic obliteration of the small vessels that contribute to the anastomosis, including vessels derived from the anterior cerebral arteries. Where conditions in which inexplicable irregularities are present in the visual field pattern, a local ischemic process of varied cause involving chiasm or optic nerves may be largely at fault. (Dawson, 1958; Hilton and Hoyt, 1966; Hughes, 1958; Walsh and Gass, 1960.)

Pressure exerted on the *lateral* aspect of the chiasm produces a variety of visual field changes. In long-standing severe compression, blindness occurs in the ipsilateral eye and temporal hemianopia on the other side (Fig. 21-9). Compression of less scope is characterized by homonymous hemianopic defects with the predominant defect on the ipsilateral side, as occurs from pressure induced by a dilated internal carotid (Mitts and McQueen, 1965), or in suprasellar meningioma (p. 536). Monocular defects are not uncommon, and may occasionally be limited to the temporal "crescent." (Shenkin and Leopold, 1945; Walsh and Hoyt, 1969.)

Damage of the *lateral aspect of the chiasm bilaterally*, by interrupting fibers from the temporal halves of the retinae, results in binasal hemianopia (Fig. 21-10). The latter, which is uncommon, may be caused by pressure exerted by bilateral carotid aneurysms or by greatly dilated atherosclerotic carotids, by lateral outpocketings of

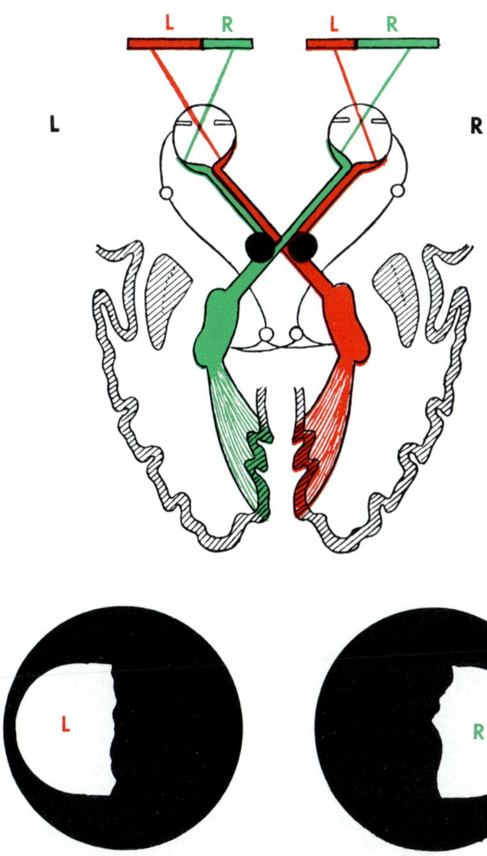

Fig. 21-10. Nasal heteronymous hemianopia due to interruption of the lateral parts of the chiasm.

pituitary cyst or by chromophobe adenoma. An enlarged and prolapsed preoptic recess (Fig. 21-8, *B* and *C*) due to increased intracranial pressure may also be responsible for binasal hemianopia; such a recess causes the anterior angles of the chiasm to be displaced laterally such that the lateral sides of the optic nerves are pressed against the carotid arteries (Traquair, 1949). Distention of sclerosed carotid arteries in their *supraclinoid* portion may lead not only to binasal field defects but also to arcuate or upper field defects (Hughes, 1958).

Damage of the *caudal aspect of the optic nerve* in the region in which the nerve merges with the chiasm may interrupt the loop of fibers coming from the opposite optic nerve (Fig. 21-2) and thus cause a defect in the temporal field of that eye.

Following compression of the optic chiasm sufficient to interrupt fibers, atrophy becomes evident in the optic disk in a month or so.

Involvement of the optic tract

Characteristic of optic tract damage is a contralateral homonymous hemianopic defect, "homonymous" meaning in the same position with respect to the two visual fields (Fig. 21-11). In compressive or inflammatory lesions in earlier stages of development there may be a contralateral homonymous quadrantanopia. Frequently the defect enlarges to the extent that homonymous hemianopia is complete (Fig. 21-12). Incomplete optic tract field defects are not entirely symmetrical, or congruous (they are not identical in size, shape, or density in the two hemianopic

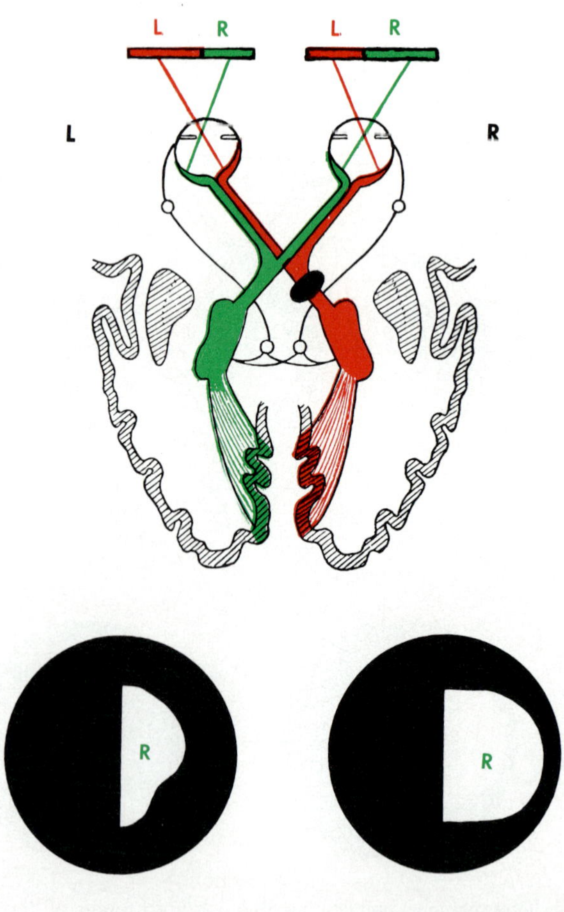

Fig. 21-11. Homonymous hemianopia to the left due to interruption of the right optic tract.

fields); instead, they are usually slightly larger on the side of the lesion (Fig. 21-13). With severe compression of the optic tract resulting in fiber interruption, pallor becomes evident in the optic disks, particularly in the disk contralateral to the lesion, after the lapse of 3 or 4 months. To be included with the conditions under which the optic tract can be seriously damaged is compression through lodgement of the tract against the free edge of the tentorium, the anterior part of which the tract crosses. This has been noted, for example, in displacement of the hemisphere medialward in subdural hematoma (Lindenberg and Walsh, 1964).

A hemianopic response of the pupils to light can be elicited with the aid of a slit lamp. With destruction of an optic tract, the pupillary light response is diminished or absent when the light beam is directed toward the temporal half of the retina of the ipsilateral eye or the nasal half of the retina of the contralateral eye, but the reflex *is* obtainable when the opposite sides of the retinae are exposed to the light. This is known as the "hemianopic pupillary reaction" *(Wernicke's hemianopic phenomenon).* On the other hand, if a lesion lies behind the lateral geniculate body (in the visual radiation or visual cortex), a light projected on the blind half of the retina will cause pupillary constriction.

Hemianopia caused by involvement of the caudal part of the optic tract by an expanding or inflammatory lesion may be associated with *contralateral paresis of the tongue and limbs.* This association may be explained by the proximity of the optic tract to the basis pedunculi and by the fact that the supranuclear pyramidal fibers

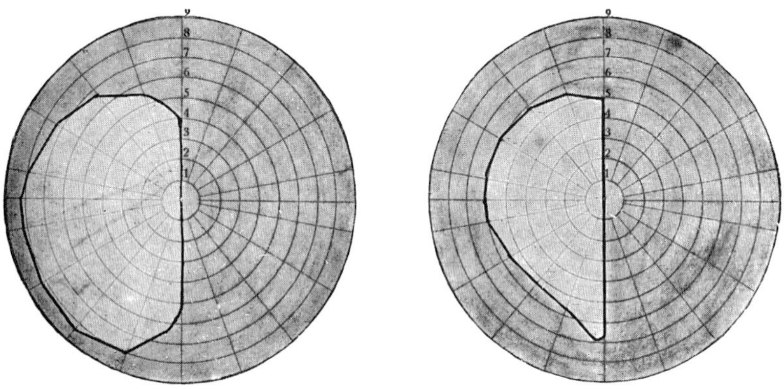

Fig. 21-12. Right-sided complete homonymous hemianopia due to severe damage of the left optic tract in basal skull fracture.

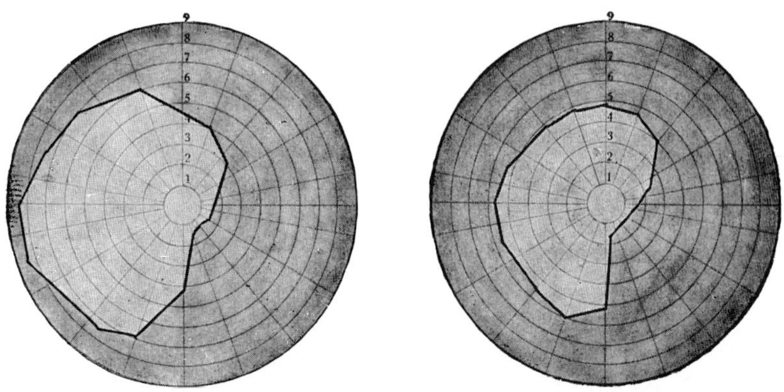

Fig. 21-13. Right-sided hemianopia due to destruction of the subcortical region of the left occipital lobe in traumatic porencephaly. The patient was unaware of his visual defect.

passing to the twelfth nucleus course superficially in the basis pedunculi and thus are exposed to lesions in this region.

Involvement of the visual radiation

As observed in a study of gunshot wounds of the brain, lesions involving the upper or the lower aspect of the *anterior part of the visual radiation* (in the region of Meyer's loop in the temporal lobe) cause partial quadrantanopia in which the field defect projects toward the fixation point in the vertical meridian. A lesion interrupting the upper aspect of the visual radiation at this level gives rise to partial quadrantanopia involving a lower quadrant, and the reverse holds for a lesion interrupting the lower aspect of the radiation. In contrast, a lesion involving the fibers situated in the *intermediate part of the radiation* produces a narrow, sector-shaped defect in the horizontal meridian, reaching the fixation point. (Spalding, 1952a.) It had been thought previously that field defects of this kind could occur only in lesions of the calcarine cortex, and indeed they are more prevalent in lesions at this site (Holmes, 1931). Marino and Rasmussen (1968), on the basis of their experience with temporal lobectomy, conclude that damage of the *anterior part of the temporal loop* results in superior quadrantic defects which are often somewhat incongruous, and that with extension of the lesion caudalward the incongruity gradually decreases as the defect enlarges toward the horizontal meridian and invades the inferior quadrant. Paracentral scotoma resulting from interruption of anterior part of the visual radiation is rare.

In tumors of the *temporal pole,* partial quadrantic field defects may be found (Cushing, 1921, 1922), as may also hemianopic defects (Horrax and Putnam, 1932; Sanford and Bair, 1939). Lesions of varied kind occupying the occipital lobe are more apt to damage a greater number of fibers of the visual radiation and thus give rise to hemianopic defects. Under such conditions, macular vision is usually spared (Fig. 21-12). This seems to be due to the comparatively large numbers of macular fibers in the visual radiation (Putnam, 1926). As the calcarine cortex is approached closer and closer by lesions, quadrantic or hemianopic defects tend to become more and more symmetrical (or congruous) in the two monocular fields (Fig. 21-14). However, in gunshot wounds involving the visual radiation in general, lack of congruence of homonymous field defects has been found the rule (Teuber, Battersby, and Bender, 1960). Regardless of the location of a lesion in the visual radiation, the homonymous hemianopias usually begin in the periphery of the field and advance toward the center. Rarely the initial disturbance is a unilateral (con-

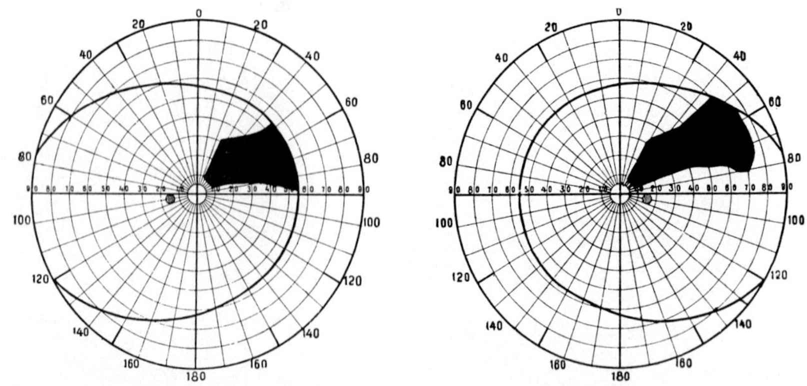

Fig. 21-14. Homonymous partial quadrantanopia due to involvement of part of the left geniculocalcarine tract.

tralateral) crescentic field defect (Shenkin and Leopold, 1945; Walsh and Hoyt, 1969).

The visual radiation and the visual cortex offer the most favorable terrain for the development of *horizontal* hemianopias. Central vision may either be spared or reduced in hemianopias of this kind. Horizontal hemianopia involving the *upper half* of the visual field, which is rare, has been attributed to occlusion of the posterior cerebral artery bilaterally. (This artery supplies the lower half of the radiation and the lower lip of the calcarine cortex, while the middle cerebral artery supplies the upper half of the radiation and the upper lip of the calcarine cortex.) In gunshot wounds occurring in the transverse plane of the occipital lobes, the *lower half* of the visual field is the more commonly involved because wounds in this region (in contrast with wounds involving the lower lip of the calcarine fissure) are compatible with life. (Schäublin, 1967.)

Involvement of the visual cortex

Destruction of the entire area striata of one side will give rise to homonymous hemianopia on the contralateral side. Lesions damaging the upper half of the area striata of one side will produce lower homonymous quadrantic defects, and the reverse holds for lesions of the lower half of the area striata of one side. Furthermore, in lesions of the upper part of the visual cortex bilaterally a defect occurs in both lower visual fields (horizontal inferior hemianopia). In lesions of the lower part of the visual cortex of the two sides the reverse holds (horizontal superior hemianopia). These statements should, however, be taken *cum grano salis,* because a lesion on one side of the calcarine fissure may encroach on the other side. For example, a scotoma resulting from damage to the cuneus may extend into the corresponding part of the upper quadrantic fields.

In lesions of the occipital lobe, central ("macular") vision is usually spared. This is true, for example, for posterior cerebral artery occlusion, an observation generally accounted for on the basis of a rich collateral blood supply received by the more caudal part of the area striata from the middle cerebral artery (Hiller, 1936, 1952). In bilateral occlusion of the calcarine arteries a sparing of central vision has also been noted (McDonald, 1943). Under such conditions there may be sparing of a contiguous area downward along the vertical meridian, a sparing explicable on the basis that in some brains the middle cerebral artery anastomoses more freely in the region of the cuneus than in the lingual gyrus (Shellshear, 1927). Complete homonymous hemianopia may, however, occur from posterior cerebral artery occlusion.

It is common experience that sudden hemorrhage or embolism involving the area striata of one side produces *bilateral complete blindness,* which later resolves into homonymous hemianopia. Such blindness has not been known to precede the hemianopia due to optic tract lesions.

Central vision is also usually spared in tumor of the occipital lobe. Hemianopia with splitting of the macula as been noted only in 12.5 to 32.5 percent of such cases (Allen, 1930; Horrax and Putnam, 1932).

Usually in small lesions involving one occipital pole the scotoma extends to the fixation point, as shown in Fig. 21-15. Further, Spalding (1952b) has noted in very slight unilateral occipital pole injury that a dense paracentral scotoma was present and that it extended to the fixation point. The evidence thus indicates that central vision is represented unilaterally.

Sparing of central vision may be more apparent than real. As a consequence of blindness of the entire half of his visual field, the patient automatically shifts the fixation of his eyes so that the blind area is brought into the field of intact vision. In other words, a patient with hemianopia, who, upon fixing his gaze, sees only half the field, unconsciously shifts his gaze to see as much as possible, like a sailor who wishes to see faint lights at night. It has been claimed that under such circumstances a functional rearrangement occurs, giving rise to a "pseudofovea." What has been said applies to vision at a distance; in fixation of the eyes on an object close at hand, the original fovea is used and central blindness becomes evident. (Critchley, 1953; Klüver, 1942; Spalding, 1952b.)

In superficial and circumscribed lesions

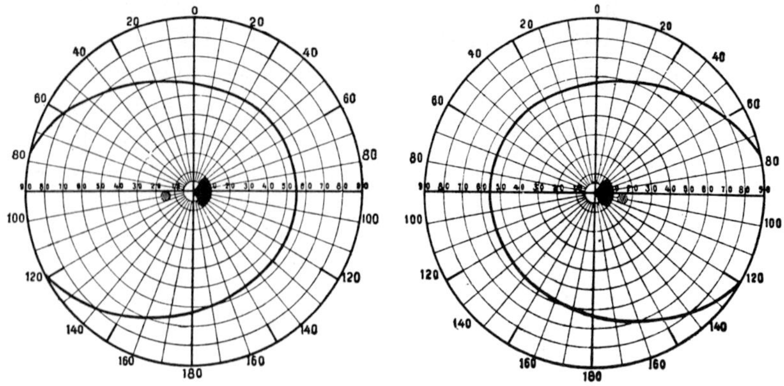

Fig. 21-15. Homonymous central scotoma to the right as the result of injury of the posterior part of the left calcarine cortex by a splinter of bone.

of the area striata of one occipital lobe, awareness of color in the homonymous field may be lost *(hemiachromatopia)*, while the perception of form is preserved; in such cases the color blindness is usually for red and green. In most cases, however, the degree of homonymous color blindness corresponds to the decrease in visual acuity. Of localizing and lateralizing importance is the *Riddoch phenomenon* (1917): the patient can detect moving objects but not stationary objects in the involved field. This is an occipital sign.

Following amaurosis due to striate cortex injury and during the time of resolution of vision to the stage in which bilateral large central scotomas are occurring, retinal functions return in a certain sequence, as shown by Bender and Furlow (1945). Light could be perceived at 2 days after injury, and then best with low illumination. Then movement of large objects was recognized. Subsequently the perception of form returned, first while objects were in motion, and later when they were stationary. Following this, appreciation of color returned—at first for red, and later for blue and green.

Awareness of scotomas

In lesions of the visual system the patient may be aware of a black spot in his visual field *(positive scotoma)* or not *(negative scotoma)*. Negative scotoma is more common in lesions behind than in front of the lateral geniculate body. A patient with a negative scotoma does not volunteer that he has visual trouble, and if asked usually denies it, but may admit that his vision is dim. Whether a scotoma is positive or negative depends on factors other than location of the lesion. Thus, in a slowly forming lesion, such as occurs with infiltrating neoplasm, the patient is less likely to notice visual loss than in acute damage to the visual pathway. Also the greater the integrity of central vision the less the patient will be aware of a blind area in his vision. Degree of intelligence is also an important factor. (Critchley, 1949; Hiller, 1952; Martin, 1952.)

In lesions of the visual radiation or cortex in which hemianopia is revealed only by perimetric examination, the visual defect may be suspected when the patient turns his head instinctively to the side of the defective half of the visual field so as to receive as much of the image as possible on the sensitive halves of his retinae. With the head thus turned, the patient sometimes thinks that he is "cross-eyed" on the side of the field defect. If one places before such a patient a piece of white paper on which a horizontal line is drawn, and asks him to draw a vertical line through the center of the horizontal one, he will draw the line to the right or the left of the center (in the center of the intact part of his visual field). An equally simple method of determining whether homonymous hemianopia exists is suddenly to thrust one's finger to within a short distance of the lateral side of each of the patient's eyes. The patient fails to wink when the blind half of the visual field is approached.

Optokinetic nystagmus

Optokinetic nystagmus (following movements of the eyes) is a normal phenomenon. Horizontal optokinetic nystagmus occurs, for example, when a person on a moving train looks at object after object in the passing terrain. It may also be elicited in a person placed inside a rotating cylinder when he watches parallel lines on a cylinder wall moving away from him, also when he watches a hand-operated drum that is rotated on a vertical axis. In the slow phase of the nystagmus the eyes follow an object in the direction in which it is moving, while in the quick phase the eyes move counterwise to fixate each succeeding object. Similarly, vertical nystagmus can be induced when the eyes follow a drum rotating on a horizontal axis. These tests unmask simulated blindness.

It has been postulated that the pathway concerned in optokinetic nystagmus runs from the homonymous sides of the retina to the lateral geniculate body, to the visual cortex (area 17), to the lateral surface of the occipital lobe (area 18), to the angular and supramarginal gyri, where the "supranuclear optokinetic center" is located, and that fibers from this cortical center course along the inferior medial aspect of the geniculocalcarine tract to reach the tectum, where an "optokinetic center" governing the oculomotor complex is located. Another view is that optokinetic nystagmus is governed by area 18, with pathways of one side coursing subcortically near the caudal part of the geniculocalcarine tract, to reach mainly the opposite side of the midbrain. However, clinical observations supported by autopsy study suggest a more complex reflex arc than thus far postulated.

Abnormal horizontal optokinetic nystagmus is interpretable only when the disturbances are clearcut, reproducible, and asymmetrical on the two sides. Abnormalities in the nystagmus may be observed in extensive lesions involving the central hemispheric white matter, deep areas of the forebrain (the diencephalon, particularly the thalamus), or tectal or other brainstem structures. The disturbance has lateralizing value: the fault in the nystagmus is on the side *contralateral* to the lesion. Abnormal horizontal optokinetic nystagmus may, however, fail to occur in the presence of extensive neoplastic lesions involving the parietal lobe, hypothalamus, pretectile region, tectum (and its superior colliculi), or ventral or lateral parts of the brainstem (Davidoff and others, 1966). In general, so far as the cerebral hemispheres are concerned, abnormality in the nystagmus is usually indicative of a lesion behind the central sulcus and probably in the parietal lobe. Lesions confined to the occipital lobe are said to be noneffective.

Between visual input and an oculomotor output lie numerous pathways that may carry the relevant impulses. Visual input can be implicated, as illustrated by the observation that in lesions involving the geniculocalcarine tract in its rostral part, horizontal optokinetic nystagmus may be abnormal before pronounced homonymous defects develop in the visual field. An abnormality in the optokinetic nystagmus is often associated with a homonymous field defect, but it is not dependent on the field defect.

Integrity of the nystagmus appears most dependent on an intact efferent oculomotor system. Interruption of varied cerebral pathways leading to this system is probably the main basis for faulty horizontal optokinetic nystagmus. That the oculomotor complex is heavily concerned is supported by the observation that practically all patients with a defect in gaze also have a disturbance in optokinetic nystagmus. When optokinetic nystagmus is disturbed, yet no alteration can be detected in ocular movements, it can be assumed that the test has uncovered a hidden deficit in oculomotor function. *Abnormalities in vertical optokinetic nystagmus* are commonly observed in lesions involving both hemispheres—in parkinsonism and multiple sclerosis, also in brainstem disease involving, among other structures, the pretectal region and the tectum. The close correspondence between deficits in vertical and horizontal optokinetic nystagmus suggests that the oculomotor pathways utilized may lie close to each other. (Carmichael, Dix, and Hallpike, 1954; Jung and Kornhuber, 1964; Norton, 1964; Smith, 1963; Smith and Cogan, 1960.)

Visual inattention and extinction

In the presence of a partial homonymous hemianopic field defect, an object that is correctly identified when placed in the defective side of the visual field may no longer be recognized when another object is placed in the opposite (normal) field of vision; or if two objects are shown such a patient, one on either side of the fixation point, the image on the normal side is perceived, while that on the defective side may appear indistinct, then fade completely. When, however, the object on the normal side is removed, the object remaining in the defective field is easily recognized. This phenomenon has been considered by some authors to be due to *visual inattention*. Others have contended that it is the result of *visual extinction*, on the premise that a strong stimulus extinguishes or suppresses a weaker one. The phenomenon is most often encountered in occipital lobe lesions. (Allen, 1948; Bender and Furlow, 1945; Head and Holmes, 1911.) Its parallel in the field of touch is described on page 339.

Metamorphopias

By "metamorphopias" are meant distortions of the images of objects, whether in their size, shape, color, orientation, or distance from the viewer. In addition to arising as the result of focal brain disease, metamorphopias (or hallucinations) may occur as an epileptic aura and as a symptom of psychosis and psychoneurosis; they may also appear in certain drug intoxications (for example, cannabis indica), in hemorrhage and thrombosis, and in delirium of febrile origin. The occurrence of colored, zigzag, glittering scotomas *(teichopsias)* in the course of an attack of ophthalmic migraine is a different phenomenon arising from the primary visual cortex. In general, in focal lesions the simpler metamorphopias denote a lesion of the occipital lobe, the more complex ones denote a lesion of the temporal lobe, and those intermediate between the two denote a lesion of the parietal lobe.

The classification of metamorphopias that follows is mainly from Critchley (1949, 1953).

Comparatively straightforward: (1) alterations in the size of objects, namely, *macropia* and *micropia*; (2) alteration in the size of objects in one dimension only, the objects appearing squeezed or compressed sideways; (3) tilting of objects; (4) waviness or fragmentation of linear components; (5) lack of color *(achromatopia)* or a bathing of everything in an illusory monochrome hue *(erythropia)*; and (6) apparent movement of stationary objects. Belonging in this category are *photopias* (spots of light or color in the visual field), and *photomas* (soaring clouds, moving waves, drifting fog, and shadowy figures).

More complex: (1) *teleopia,* in which objects seem not only small but also far away *(lilliputian hallucinations)*; (2) loss of stereoscopic vision, with objects appearing two-dimensional; (3) visual perseveration, both in time and place, characterized on the one hand by an illusory recurrence of visual perceptions after the stimulus-object has been removed and on the other by an illusory extension or expansion of an object; (4) inaccurate orientation of objects in space, which includes not only a confusion of spatial relations within a sagittal plane, but also in the up-down and right-left dimensions; and (5) disturbances in background, as in a landscape.

Still more complex: (1) objects, or the environment in general, appear unduly strange or mysterious or foreign; (2) they look ugly or sinister *(kakopia)* or beautiful and friendly *(kalopia)*; (3) they seem endowed with intense personal significance or meaning; (4) human faces appear distorted in a complicated way; and (5) *déjà vu.*

Of particular interest are the hallucinations (or metamorphopias) occurring in circumscribed lesions of the visual cortex. Hemianopic hallucinations may be limited to the intact half of the visual field, but in typical cases they are noted in the blind half though they usually tend to extend into the field of intact vision. Hallucinations of remembered scenes appearing in the form of epileptic attacks have been experienced in the blind half of the visual field in traumatic lesions involving the occipital lobe—flat, uncolored miniature pictures of past events appearing in a flash with different scenes, each a still picture, following one another quickly (Robinson and Watt, 1947).

Epileptogenic lesions of the occipital lobes usually give rise only to gross sensations of light or to sensations of darkness or color. The temporal lobe is the favored site of their initiation (Penfield and Kristiansen, 1951; Penfield and Rasmussen, 1950). Finding expression in the occipital lobe, such hallucinations may represent an even more "distant" symptom. Hemianopic visual hallucinations of occipital lobe origin may sometimes be associated with hallucinations not only of vision but also of taste and smell, indicating the relatively long distances across the cerebrum that discharges may travel.

Alexia, visual agnosia

Recognition of the significance of what is seen, whether the written word or an object, is dependent on pathways emerging from the area striata (area 17). From this area, association fibers extend through the subcortical white matter only to the peristriate areas of the occipital lobe (areas 18 and 19). The area striata neither sends nor receives fibers via the corpus callosum. On the other hand, area 18 and, in part, area 19, have wide two-way connections with various cortical regions through the long association bundles of the hemisphere. Through these bundles, relays go to the prefrontal, motor, sensory, and auditory cortical areas, and to the cortex of the island of Reil. The angular gyrus is the recipient of many of these fibers. Special mention should be made of fibers passing from the area striata to the basal temporal cortex, as they appear to be a link in a neuron chain extending from the area striata to the hippocampus. Fibers from most of these regions also run in the reverse direction and reach area 18. Areas 18 and 19 apparently also receive fibers from the cortex of the hippocampal gyrus (Geschwind, 1965). In addition, area 18 receives fibers from contralateral area 18 by way of the splenium of the corpus callosum. (Bailey, von Bonin, and McCulloch, 1950; Geschwind, 1965; von Bonin and Bailey, 1947.)

Alexia (better, dyslexia) is observed in lesions in various locations, such as splenium of the corpus callosum and splenium plus occipital lobe. Following surgical section of the corpus callosum in the course of removal of a colloid cyst from the third ventricle, alexia involving the left visual field was noted. By contrast, lesions limited to the occipital lobe do not cause alexia, nor does occipital lobectomy, except temporarily. (Foix and Hillemand, 1925; Gazzaniga, Bogen, and Sperry, 1962; Geschwind, 1962; Geschwind and Kaplan, 1962; Hécaen, de Ajuriaguerra, and David, 1952.)

The angular gyrus of the dominant hemisphere comes chiefly into consideration as responsible for alexia, as this gyrus is generally thought to contain a "visual memory center" for words. In "pure" alexia the angular gyrus of the dominant hemisphere is functionally active and in communication with the somesthetic area, as manifested, for example, by the patient's ability to "read" tactilely. In all likelihood, alexia represents a "disconnection" disturbance. It is proposed that alexia (in the right-handed) results from disconnection of fiber relays running from the right occipital lobe (area 17) to the right angular gyrus (due to a parietal lobe lesion), then to the left angular gyrus, or directly to the left angular gyrus by way of the splenium (with the site of disconnection in the splenium). Where alexia is combined with agraphia and with an inability to spell, a lesion has been found involving the angular gyrus and extending medialward to the occipital horn of the lateral ventricle—in some cases obviously affecting the splenium of the corpus callosum as well. For this combination of disturbances a lesion of a "memory center" in the parietotemporal region has been considered responsible. (Geschwind, 1965.)

Usually, however, the lesions in alexic patients are of wide scope, involving not only the angular gyrus but also the supramarginal gyrus and even more remote structures. Disturbances in addition to alexia are thus usually to be noted. These include loss of discriminative sensibility, Gerstmann's syndrome, and, occasionally, a disturbance of conjugate horizontal gaze. Difficulty in spelling and writing in alexic patients can frequently be traced to an associated disturbance in vision, such as blurring or oscillation of words or letters. (Adler, 1944; Critchley, 1953; Holmes, 1950.) A clinical picture characterized by alexia together with a right-sided homonymous hemianopic defect and Wernicke's syndrome (pp. 339-340) can be taken as evidence of a lesion involving the region of the angular gyrus and the subjacent geniculocalcarine tract.

In *visual agnosia* ("seeing without recognition," "mindblindness"), the patient is able to see a flat or three-dimensional object, but he fails to recognize its nature. If an object is shown him, be it a pencil, key, hat, or glove, he can state what form the object has, often also its color, and he is easily able to pick out like objects from an assorted collection, but he has lost the understanding of the significance of the object.

Partial "visual agnosias" have been described. Thus, in occipital lobe lesions there may be *simultanagnosia* (Wolpert, 1935): the patient recognizes and can name individual objects but fails totally to note the presence of other visual stimuli in the vicinity. Another form is *prosopagnosia* (Bodamer, 1947), in which the patient fails to recognize an acquaintance or friend by vision. Yet another is *defective Gestalt formation* (Bay, 1953): individual features of an object can be recognized, but the patient cannot synthesize them into a concept. Or, *Gestalt dissolution* (Bay, 1953): an object of relatively large size is at first seen in its entirety, but on further inspection becomes scattered into single components.

Lissauer (1889) distinguished two kinds of mindblindness (visual agnosia): *apperceptive,* described as a defect in identification produced by a distortion of visual perception, and *associative,* an inability to identify visual stimuli despite intactness of visual perception. There has been a question whether the apperceptive form exists, that is, whether any form of visual agnosia could alone be dependent on faulty visual discrimination. Or, in other words, can the mere occurrence of a visual defect in cases of visual agnosia be used as evidence that the failure of recognition is due to that defect? Bender and Feldman (1966) noted that whenever there was inability to recognize objects, defects were also found in vision, sensory function, and mentation. By appropriate testing the apperceptive form has, however, been established in a fair proportion of cases. In such a case, Benson and Greenberg (1969) noted that although the patient had normal visual acuity, he could not read, recognize faces, or name and match visual symbols of objects on confrontation; moreover, he had a keen ability to distinguish light intensity, object size, color, and direction, but he could not differentiate simple forms (circle versus square). The apperceptive form, according to Benson and Greenberg, "necessitates bilateral impairment of the primary visual analyzers," that is, the striate cortex. Lesions produced by prolonged bilateral circulatory insufficiency, or lesions resulting from hypoxidosis (for example, from carbon monoxide poisoning), have been found in such cases.

The patient with the associative type of visual agnosia (unlike the patient with the apperceptive form of visual agnosia) can easily describe or draw an outline of a visually presented object which he is unable to name. This may also be performed with letters, numbers, or drawings. (Benson and Greenberg, 1969.) Lesions responsible are often unilateral and focal. Usually the dominant visual cortex and the portion of the corpus callosum that carries fibers from the nondominant visual cortex to the dominant hemisphere are heavily damaged. Infarction of the left occipital cortex and callosal splenium due to occlusion of the left posterior cerebral artery was found postmortem (Hahn, 1895) in a case described clinically by Lissauer (1889). To Geschwind (1965), the associative type of visual agnosia represents a disconnection syndrome.

REFERENCES

Adler, A. 1944. Disintegration and restoration of optic recognition in visual agnosia. Arch. Neurol. Psychiat. **51**:243-259.

Allen, I. M. 1930. Clinical study of tumours involving occipital lobe. Brain **53**:194-243.

Allen, I. M. 1948. Unilateral visual inattention. New Zeal. Med. J. **47**:605-617.

Andersson, H., and Gomes, S. P. 1968. Craniosynostosis: review of the literature and indications for surgery. Acta Paediat. Scand. **57**: 47-54.

Ashton, N., Pears, M. A., and Pickering, G. W. 1961. Neuroretinopathy following hemorrhage, with discussion on the nature of cytoid bodies. Brit. J. Ophthal. **45**:385-394.

Bailey, P., von Bonin, G., and McCulloch, W. S. 1950. The isocortex of the chimpanzee. Urbana, University of Illinois Press.

Ball, C. J. 1966. Atheromatous embolism to the brain, retina, and choroid. Arch. Ophthal. **76**: 690-695.

Bay, E. 1953. Disturbances of visual perception and their examination. Brain **76**:515-550.

Beller, A. J. 1964. Benign post-traumatic intracranial hypertension. J. Neurol. Neurosurg. Psychiat. **27**:149-152.

Bender, M. B., and Feldman, M. 1966. The so-called "visual agnosias." Proc. 8th Internat. Congr. Neurology **3**:153-156.

Bender, M. B., and Furlow, L. T. 1945. Phenomenon of visual extinction in homonymous fields and psychologic principles involved. Arch. Neurol. Psychiat. **53**:29-33.

Bender, M. B., and Strauss, I. 1937. Defects in visual field of one eye only in patients with a lesion of one optic radiation. Arch. Ophthal. **17**:765-787.

Benson, D. F., and Greenberg, J. P. 1969. Visual form agnosia: a specific defect in visual discrimination. Arch. Neurol. **20**:82-89.

Berg, L., Rosomoff, H. L., Aronson, N., Silbermann, M., and Pool, J. L. 1955. The syndrome of increased intracranial pressure without localizing signs. Arch. Neurol. Psychiat. **74**:498-505.

Bodamer, J. 1947. Die Prosop-Agnosie. (Die Agnosie des Physiognomieerkennens.) Arch. Psychiat. **179**:6-53.

Bradley, W. G., and Whitty, C. W. M. 1967. Acute optic neuritis: its clinical features and their relation to prognosis for recovery of vision. J. Neurol. Neurosurg. Psychiat. **30**:531-538.

Brodmann, K. 1908. Beiträge zur histologischen Lokalisation der Grosshirnrinde. VI. Mitteilung. Die Cortexgliederung des Menschen. J. Psychol. Neurol. **10**:231-246.

Brouwer, B. 1934. Projection of the retina on the cortex in man. Res. Publ. Ass. Res. Nerv. Ment. Dis., Proc. **13**:529-534.

Bruyn, G. W. 1968. Complicated migraine. In Vinken, P. J., and Bruyn, G. W., editors: Handbook of clinical neurology, vol. 5. Amsterdam, North-Holland Publishing Company, pp. 59-95.

Carmichael, E. A., Dix, M. R., and Hallpike, C. S. 1954. Lesions of the cerebral hemispheres and their effects upon opticokinetic and caloric nystagmus. Brain **77**:345-372.

Carr, R. E., and Henkind, P. 1963. Retinal findings associated with serum hyperviscosity. Amer. J. Ophthal. **56**:23-31.

Chacko, L. W. 1948. Laminar pattern of lateral geniculate body in primates. J. Neurol. Neurosurg. Psychiat. **11**:211-224.

Chamblin, M. 1953. Visual field changes in optic neuritis. Arch. Ophthal. **50**:699-713.

Clark, W. E. Le G., and Penman, G. G. 1934. The projection of the retina in the lateral geniculate body. Proc. Roy Soc., B **114**:291-313.

Connolly, C. J. 1950. External morphology of the primate brain. Springfield, Illinois, Charles C Thomas, Publisher, pp. 252-253.

Cornfield, D., and Cooke, R. E. 1952. Vitamin A deficiency: case report; unusual manifestations in 5½ month baby. Pediatrics **10**:33-38.

Critchley, M. 1949. Phenomenon of tactile inattention with special reference to parietal lesions. Brain **72**:538-561.

Critchley, M. 1953. The parietal lobes. London, Edward Arnold (Publishers) Ltd.

Crosby, E. C., Humphrey, T., and Lauer, E. W. 1962. Correlative anatomy of the nervous system. New York, The Macmillan Company.

Cushing, H. 1921. The field defects produced by temporal lobe tumors. Brain **44**:341-396.

Cushing, H. 1922. Distortions of the visual fields in cases of brain tumor: the field defects produced by temporal lobe lesions. Brain **44**:341-396.

Dark, A. J., and Rizk, S. N. 1967. Progressive focal sclerosis of retinal arteries: a sequel to impaction of cholesterol emboli. Brit. Med. J. **1**: 270-273.

Daroff, R. B., and Smith, J. L. 1965. Intraocular optic neuritis with normal visual acuity. Neurology **15**:409-412.

Davidoff, L. M., and Dyke, C. G. 1937. Hypertensive meningeal hydrops: a syndrome frequently following infection in the middle ear or elsewhere in the body. Amer. J. Ophthal. **20**:908-927.

Davidoff, R. A., Atkin, A., Anderson, P. J., and Bender, M. B. 1966. Optokinetic nystagmus and cerebral disease: clinical and pathological study. Arch. Neurol. **14**:73-81.

Davidson, P., Schlezinger, N. S., and Mullen, C. R. 1959. Temporal arteritis: report of a case treated with cortisone. Penn. Med. J. **62**:1835-1838.

Dawson, B. H. 1958. The blood vessels of the human optic chiasma and their relation to those of the hypophysis and hypothalamus. Brain **81**: 207-217.

Dersh, J., and Schlezinger, N. S. 1959. Inferior nasal quadrantanopsia in pseudotumor cerebri. A.M.A. Arch. Neurol. **1**:695-699.

Dott, N. M. 1936. Bitemporal hemianopia in relation to hydrocephalic distention of the third ventricle. Brit. Med. J. **2**:296.

Dunn, J., Jr., Baker, G. S., and Wagener, H. P. 1955. Pseudotumor cerebri: a review and report of four cases. Proc. Staff Meet. Mayo Clin. **30**: 505-517.

Ehrenfeld, W. K., Hoyt, W. F., and Wylie, E. J. 1966. Embolization and transient blindness from carotid atheroma: surgical considerations. Arch. Surg. **93**:787-794.

Feldman, S., Landau, J., and Halpern, L. 1955. Papilledema in the Guillain-Barré syndrome. Arch. Neurol. Psychiat. **73**:678-684.

Fields, J. P. 1961. Bulging fontanel; a complication of tetracycline therapy in infants. J. Pediat. **58**:74-76.

Foix, C., and Hillemand, P. 1925. Rôle vraisemblable du splénium dans la pathogénie de l'alexie pure par lésion de la cérébrale postérieure. Bull. Mém. Soc. Méd. Hôp. Paris **49**:393-395.

Foley, J. 1955. Benign forms of intracranial hypertension—"toxic" and "otitic" hydrocephalus. Brain **78**:1-41.

François, J., and Neetens, A. 1954. Vascularization of the optic pathway. I. Lamina cribrosa and optic nerve. Brit. J. Ophthal. **38**:472-487.

François, J., Neetens, A., and Collette, J. M. 1955. Vascular supply of the optic pathway. II. Further studies by micro-arteriography of the optic nerve. Brit. J. Ophthal. **39**:220-232.

Gazzaniga, M. S., Bogen, J. E., and Sperry, R. W. 1962. Some functional effects of sectioning the cerebral commissures in man. Proc. Nat. Acad. Sci. **38**:1765-1769.

Gerber, A., Raab, A. P., and Sobel, A. E. 1954. Vitamin A poisoning in adults; with description of a case. Amer. J. Med. **16**:729-745.

Geschwind, N. 1962. The anatomy of acquired disorders of reading. In Money, J., editor: Reading disability: progress and research needs in dyslexia. Baltimore, The Johns Hopkins Press, pp. 115-129.

Geschwind, N. 1965. Disconnexion syndromes in animals and man. Brain **88**:237-294, 585-644.

Geschwind, N., and Kaplan, E. 1962. A human cerebral deconnection syndrome: a preliminary report. Neurology **12**:675-685.

Gillilan, L. A. 1961. The collateral circulation of the human orbit. A.M.A. Arch. Ophthal. **65**: 684-694.

Gowers, W. 1909. A case of unilateral optic neuritis from intracranial tumour. Lancet **2**: 65-68.

Graham, J. R. 1968. Migraine: clinical aspects. In Vinken, P. J., and Bruyn, G. N., editors: Handbook of clinical neurology, vol. 5. Amsterdam, North-Holland Publishing Company, pp. 45-58.

Greer, M. 1962. Benign intracranial hypertension: mastoiditis and lateral sinus obstruction. Neurology **12**:472-476.

Greer, M. 1967. Benign intracranial hypertension (pseudotumor cerebri). Pediat. Clin. N. Amer. **14**:819-830.

Hahn, E. 1895. Pathologisch-anatomische Untersuchung des Lissauer'schen Falles von Seelenblindheit. Psychiat. Klin. Breslau **21**:109-119.

Head, H., and Holmes, G. 1911. Sensory disturbances from cerebral lesions. Brain **34**:102-254.

Hécaen, H., de Ajuriaguerra, J., and David, M. 1952. Les déficits fonctionnels après lobectomie occipitale. Mschr. Psychiat. Neurol. **123**:239-290.

Henderson, J. W. 1956. Diseases of the optic nerve: anatomy and physiology; signs and symptoms. Trans. Amer. Acad. Ophthal. Otolaryng. **60**:8-13.

Higier, H. 1926. Zur Klinik der residierenden Formen der Polyneuritis, Myelitis und Meningencephalitis (Meningitis serosa, Pseudotumor cerebri). Z. Ges. Neurol. Psychiat. **104**:453-465.

Hiller, F. 1936. Die Zirkulationsstörungen des Rückenmarks und Gehirns. In Bumke, O., and Foerster, O., editors: Handbuch der Neurologie **11**:178-465.

Hiller, F. 1952. The vascular syndromes of the basilar and vertebral arteries and their branches. J. Nerv. Ment. Dis. **116**:988-1016.

Hilton, G. F., and Hoyt, W. F. 1966. An arteriosclerotic chiasmal syndrome: bitemporal hemianopia associated with fusiform dilatation of the anterior cerebral arteries. J.A.M.A. **196**: 1018-1020.

Hobbs, H. E. 1964. Headache. Trans. Ophthal. Soc. **84**:637-662.

Hogan, M. J., and Zimmerman, L. E., editors. 1962. Ophthalmic pathology: an atlas and textbook, ed. 2. Philadelphia, W. B. Saunders Co.

Hollenhorst, R. W. 1961. Significance of bright plaques in the retinal arterioles. J.A.M.A. **178**: 23-29.

Holmes, G. 1918. Disturbances of vision by cerebral lesions. Brit. J. Ophthal. **2**:353-384.

Holmes, G. 1931. A contribution to the cortical representation of vision. Brain **54**:470-479.

Holmes, G. 1950. Pure word blindness. Folia Psychiat., Neerl. **53**:279-288.

Horrax, G., and Putnam, T. J. 1932. Distortion of the visual fields in cases of brain tumor: the field defects and hallucinations produced by tumors of the occipital lobe. Brain **55**:499-523.

Hoyt, W. F. 1962. Anatomic considerations of arcuate scotomas associated with lesions of the optic nerve and chiasm: a Nauta axon degeneration study in the monkey. Bull. Johns Hopk. Hosp. **111**:57-71.

Hoyt, W. F. 1964. The human chiasm: a neuroanatomical review of current concepts, recent investigations, and unsolved problems. In Smith, J. L., editor: The University of Miami Neuro-Ophthalmology Symposium, Springfield, Illinois, Charles C Thomas, Publisher, pp. 64-111.

Hoyt, W. F., and Pont, M. E. 1962. Pseudopapilledema: anomalous elevation of optic disk; pitfalls in diagnosis and management. J.A.M.A. **181**:191-196.

Hughes, B. 1954. The visual fields: a study of

the applications of quantitative perimetry to the anatomy and pathology of the visual pathways, Springfield, Illinois, Charles C Thomas, Publisher.

Hughes, B. 1958. Blood supply of the optic nerves and chiasma and its clinical significance. Brit. J. Ophthal. **42**:106-125.

Janeway, R., and Kelly, D. L., Jr. 1966. Papilledema and hydrocephalus associated with recurrent polyneuritis: Guillain-Barré type. Arch. Neurol. **15**:507-514.

Jefferson, G. 1955. Further concerning compression of the optic pathways by intracranial aneurysms. In Clinical neurosurgery, Proc. Congr. Neurological Surgeons, vol. 1. Baltimore, The Williams & Wilkins Co., pp. 55-103.

Johnson, D. R., and Chalgren, W. S. 1951. Polycythemia vera and the nervous system. Neurology **1**:53-67.

Johnson, H. C., and Walker, A. E. 1951. The angiographic diagnosis of spontaneous thrombosis of the internal and common carotid arteries. J. Neurosurg. **8**:631-659.

Joynt, R. J. 1958. Mechanism of production of papilledema in the Guillain-Barré syndrome. Neurology **8**:8-12.

Jung, R., and Kornhuber, H. H. 1964. Results of electronystagmography in man: the value of optokinetic, vestibular, and spontaneous nystagmus for neurologic diagnosis and research. In Bender, M. B., editor: The oculomotor system. New York, Harper & Row, Publishers, pp. 428-482.

Kalbag, R. M., and Woolf, A. L. 1967. Cerebral venous thrombosis: with special reference to primary aseptic thrombosis. London, Oxford University Press.

Kearns, T. P., and Hollenhorst, R. W. 1963. Venous-stasis retinopathy of occlusive disease of the carotid artery. Mayo Clin. Proc. **38**: 304-312.

Kennedy, F. 1911. Retrobulbar neuritis as an exact diagnostic sign of certain tumors and abscesses of the frontal lobes. Amer. J. Med. Sci. **142**:355-368.

Kennedy, F. 1916. A further note on the diagnostic value of retrobulbar neuritis in expanding lesion of the frontal lobes: with a report on this syndrome in a case of aneurysm of the right internal carotid artery. J.A.M.A. **67**:1361-1363.

Klee, A., and Willanger, R. 1966. Disturbances of visual perception in migraine: review of the literature and a report of eight cases. Acta Neurol. Scand. **42**:400-414.

Klestadt, W. 1924. Zerebrale Symptomenkomplexe bei ontogener Sinusphlebitis. Z. Laryng. Rhin. **13**:83-105.

Klüver, H. 1942. Visual mechanisms. In Biological symposia, vol. 7. Lancaster, Cattell.

Lieb, W. A., Geeraets, W. J., and Guerry, D., III. 1959. Sickle cell retinopathy: ocular and systemic manifestations of sickle cell disease. Acta Ophthal., suppl. **58**:1-45.

Lindenberg, R., and Walsh, F. B. 1964. Vascular compressions involving intracranial visual pathways. Trans. Amer. Acad. Ophthal. Otolaryng. **68**:677-694.

Lissauer, H. 1889. Ein Fall von Seelenblindheit nebst einem Beitrag zur Theorie derselben. Arch. Psychiat. Nervenkr. **21**:222-270.

Logan, W. C., and Gordon, D. S. 1967. Traumatic lesions of the optic chiasma. Brit. J. Ophthal. **51**:258-260.

Lyle, T. K. 1964. Optic disc oedema: the differential diagnosis of its causes. J. Neurol. Sci. **1**:309-324.

Magoun, H. W., Atlas, D., Hare, W. K., and Ranson, S. W. 1939. The afferent path of the pupillary light reflex in the monkey. Brain **59**: 234-249.

Marino, R., Jr., and Rasmussen, T. 1968. Visual field changes after temporal lobectomy in man. Neurology **18**:825-835.

Martin, I. H. 1952. Cortical neurology: visual disturbances and the optic part of the body image. Med. J. Aust. **1**:211-220.

Martin, J. P. 1955. Signs of obstruction of the superior longitudinal sinus following closed head injuries (traumatic hydrocephalus). Brit. Med. J. **2**:467-470.

McAlpine, D. 1937. Toxic hydrocephalus. Brain **60**:180-203.

McDonald, P. R. 1943. Bilateral thombosis of posterior calcarine arteries with sparing of macular vision. Arch. Ophthal. **29**:92-97.

Mitts, M. G., and McQueen, J. D. 1965. Visual loss associated with fusiform enlargement of the intracranial portion of the internal carotid artery. J. Neurosurg. **23**:33-37.

Monteverde, D. A., Morgenfeld, M. C., Somoza, M. J., Bomchil, G., and Cabrini, R. L. 1966. Manifestations neurologiques de la macroglobulinémia de Waldenström. Rev. Neurol. **115**: 1029-1049.

Naffziger, H. C. 1952. Remarks on the treatment of pituitary tumors: indications and results. J. Nerv. Ment. Dis. **116**:760-765.

Norton, E. W. D. 1964. Nystagmus. In Smith, J. L., editor: University of Miami neuro-ophthalmology symposium. Springfield, Illinois, Charles C Thomas, Publisher, pp. 288-305.

Paton, L. 1909. A clinical study of optic neuritis in its relationship to intracranial tumours. Brain **32**:65-91.

Pearce, J. 1968. The ophthalmological complications of migraine. J. Neurol. Sci. **6**:73-81.

Penfield, W., and Kristiansen, K. 1951. Epileptic seizure patterns. Springfield, Illinois, Charles C Thomas, Publisher.

Penfield, W., and Rasmussen, T. 1950. The cerebral cortex of man: a clinical study of localization of function. New York, The Macmillan Company.

Polyak, S. L. 1942. Representation of central foveal and of horizontal meridians in visual radiation (radiatio optica) of human brain. J. Mt. Sinai Hosp. **9**:689-707.

Putnam, T. J. 1926. Studies on the central visual system: IV. The details of the organization of the geniculostriate system in man. Arch. Neurol. Psychiat. **16**:683-707.

Riddoch, G. 1917. Dissociation of visual perceptions due to occipital injuries, with especial reference to appreciation of movements. Brain **40**:15-57.

Robinson, P. K., and Watt, A. C. 1947. Hallucinations of remembered scenes as epileptic aura. Brain **70**:440-448.

Rose, F. C. 1968. Recent advances in neuro-ophthalmology. [Summary.] Proc. Roy. Soc. Med. **61**:122-123.

Russell, D. 1949. Observations on the pathology of hydrocephalus. London, Her Majesty's Stationery Office.

Sanford, H. S., and Bair, H. L. 1939. Visual disturbances with tumors of the temporal lobe. Arch. Neurol. Psychiat. **42**:21-43.

Schäublin, A. F. 1967. Horizontal hemianopias: a review prompted by a case of bilateral horizontal hemianopia affecting the upper half of the visual field. Confin. Neurol. **29**:327-350.

Shellshear, J. L. 1927. A contribution to our knowledge of the arterial supply of the cerebral cortex in man. Brain **50**:236-253.

Shenkin, H. A., and Leopold, I. H. 1945. Localizing value of temporal crescent defects in the visual fields. Arch. Neurol. Psychiat. **54**:97-101.

Shillito, J., and Rockett, F. X. 1963. Retinal artery embolism: a complication of carotid endarterectomy. J. Neurosurg. **20**:718-720.

Simmons, R. J., and Cogan, D. G. 1962. Occult temporal arteritis. Arch. Ophthal. **68**:8-18.

Smith, J. L. 1963. Optokinetic nystagmus: its use in topical neuro-ophthalmologic diagnosis. Springfield, Illinois, Charles C Thomas, Publisher.

Smith, J. L., and Cogan, D. G. 1960. Optokinetic nystagmus in cerebral disease: a report of 14 autopsied cases. Neurology **10**:127-137.

Spalding, J. M. K. 1952a. Wounds of the visual pathway. Part I: The visual radiation. J. Neurol. Neurosurg. Psychiat. **15**:99-109.

Spalding, J. M. K. 1952b. Wounds of the visual pathway. Part II: The striate cortex. J. Neurol. Neurosurg. Psychiat. **15**:169-183.

Steele, E. J., and Blunt, M. J. 1956. Blood supply of optic nerve and chiasma in man. J. Anat. **90**:486-493.

Symonds, C. P. 1931. Otitic hydrocephalus. Brain **54**:55-71.

Symonds, C. P. 1937. Hydrocephalic and focal cerebral symptoms in relation to thrombophlebitis of dural sinuses and cerebral veins. Brain **60**:531-550.

Symonds, C. P. 1940. Cerebral thrombophlebitis. Brit. Med. J. **2**:348-352.

Teuber, H.-L., Battersby, W. S., and Bender, M. B. 1960. Visual field defects after penetrating missile wounds of the brain. Cambridge, Harvard University Press.

Thompson, H. S. 1966. Afferent pupillary defects: pupillary findings associated with defects of the afferent arm of the pupillary light reflex arc. Amer. J. Ophthal. **62**:860-873.

Toussaint, D., Kuwabara, T., and Cogan, D. G. 1961. Retinal vascular patterns: human retinal vessels studied in three dimensions. A.M.A. Arch. Ophthal. **65**:575-581.

Traquair, H. M. 1949. An introduction to clinical perimetry, ed. 6. St. Louis, The C. V. Mosby Co.

Traquair, H. M., Dott, N. M., and Russell, W. R. 1935. Traumatic lesions of the optic chiasma. Brain **58**:398-411.

Vaernet, K. 1954. Collateral ophthalmic artery circulation in thrombotic occlusion. Neurology **4**:605-611.

von Bonin, G., and Bailey, P. 1947. The neocortex of Macaca mulatta. Urbana, University of Illinois Press.

von Economo, C., and Koskinas, G. N. 1925. Die Cytoarchitektonik der Hirnrinde des erwachsenen Menschen. Wien, Springer-Verlag, p. 63.

Walsh, F. B., and Gass, J. D. 1960. Concerning the optic chiasm: selected pathologic involvement and clinical problems. Amer. J. Ophthal. **50**:1031-1047.

Walsh, F. B., and Hoyt, W. F. 1969. Clinical neuro-ophthalmology, ed. 3. Baltimore, The Williams & Wilkins Co.

Wise, G. N. 1957. Macular changes after venous obstruction. A.M.A. Arch. Ophthal. **58**:544-557.

Wolff, E. 1933 and 1940. The anatomy of the eye and orbit; including the central connections, development, and comparative anatomy of the visual apparatus. London, Lewis; ed. 2, New York, McGraw-Hill Book Company.

Wolpert, I. 1935. Die Simultanagnosie (Störungen der Gesamtauffasung). Z. Ges. Neurol. Psychiat. **34**:1055-1064.

Wolter, J. R. 1957. The human optic papilla: a demonstration of new anatomic and pathologic findings. Amer. J. Ophthal. **44**:48-65.

Wolter, J. R. 1963. Coup-contrecoup mechanism of ocular injuries. Amer. J. Ophthal. **56**:785-796.

Wybar, K. C. 1956. Anastomoses between retinal and ciliary arterial circulation. Brit. J. Ophthal. **40**:65-81.

Yates, P. O., and Hutchinson, E. C. 1961. Cerebral infarction: the role of stenosis of the extracranial cerebral arteries. Med. Res. Council Rep. No. 300, London, Her Majesty's Stationery Office.

Chapter 22

Disturbances of behavior, memory, awareness, smell, taste, and hearing

Francis Schiller and Webb Haymaker

ANATOMICAL DEFINITIONS

Many disturbances of behavior, memory, awareness, smell, taste, and hearing, heterogeneous though they may seem, involve one large anatomical structure—the temporal lobe. On the superior surface of the temporal lobe are Heschl's one, two, or three transverse gyri: the receptor area of hearing (Fig. 19-8), connected by associative fibers to other cortical areas. The inferomesial surface has the hippocampal gyrus with its uncus (Figs. 19-8 and 19-9). The hippocampal formation is continuous ventrally with the hippocampal gyrus; it projects into the inferior horn of the lateral ventricle, and consists of hippocampus (cornu ammonis) and dentate gyrus, to which the alveus and fimbria may be added (Fig. 19-10). The rostral continuation of the hippocampal formation extends into the uncus and on its mesial surface the dentate gyrus becomes superficial as Giacomini's band (Fig. 19-9). Immediately anterior to the hippocampal formation and bulging into the tip of the inferior horn of the lateral ventricle is the amygdala. A great stretch of neocortex completes what is called the temporal lobe. There is thus something unique about the temporal lobe as compared with the other lobes. Its uniqueness lies in the fact that it contains systems concerned in all three spheres of motility—visceration, expression, and effectuation—derived, respectively, from ento-, meso-, and ectopallium (the hippocampus and the olfactory system leading into it, in the first instance; the hippocampal gyrus and the rest of gyrus fornicatus leading into it, in the second; and neocortex in the third instance) (Yakovlev, 1948) (see Chapter 25). Hence, the temporal lobe is that part of the cerebrum most intimately involved in the ultimate experiential and behavioral consequences of sensations and emotions which in turn dominate all the internal milieu, that is, visceral activity.

Another part of the brain with which this chapter is concerned is the *island of Reil,* especially the region of the circular sulcus (Fig. 19-8). Here, lesions may affect the sense of taste.

The *piriform cortex* (Fig. 19-9) is another landmark. It is a part of the entopallium of Yakovlev, or, in another sense, a component of the limbic system. This part of the cortex is concerned in the sense of smell.

Also to be mentioned is the *septum telencephali,* the septum verum of which corresponds to the septum of lower forms. Except for one of its nuclei (the triangular nucleus) this part of the septum has progressively increased in size during primate development. It is a component of the limbic system, and in primates is not connected with the olfactory apparatus (via the medial olfactory stria). (Andy and Stephan, 1968; Nauta and Haymaker, 1969.)

In considering abnormal states of consciousness the *reticular formation* necessarily comes into consideration; its site is illustrated in part in Fig. 26-2. The reticular formation is a nonspecific system made up of small neurons of the isodendritic type (with long, rectilinear, and sparsely branching dendrites), the dendrites of which overlap with other dendritic fields and mingle freely with the fascicles of transit axons. The reticular formation occupies much of the inner core of the brainstem. It extends up to the thalamus and the subthalamic and subpallidal region. Input consists of collaterals from ascending pathways and axons descending from higher centers, all arranged in an orderly and precise manner. Output is directed both upward and downward. The reticular formation is also included in the hypothalamus and reaches forward into the septal region, as was proposed by Dejerine (1895). Also included are the nonspecific thalamic cell groups. The portion in the upper brainstem contains the *reticular activating substance* (or *system*), many fibers of which extend into the thalamus. Quite apart from this reticular activating system there is another—the *midbrain-hypothalamic pituitary activating system.* It originates mainly from the dorsal and ventral tegmental nuclei of Gudden and extends into much of the hypothalamus, including the medial tuberal region (Nauta, 1963). There is also an area which Penfield (1952, 1967) called the *centrencephalic integrating system;* he postulated that it serves in the organization of the two hemispheres and makes possible those changing patterns of cerebral activity that constitute the indispensable accompaniment of consciousness. This system surmounts the cephalic end of the brainstem reticular formation and includes the thalamus.

It may seem unorthodox to present the hypothalamus as a part of the "reticular formation," as its neuron pattern differs in some ways from that in the brainstem. Here, "excitation can spread from a given focus in any direction and can establish an infinite number of closed self-re-exciting chains" (Szentágothai and others, 1968). But that term also implies a heterogeneity of afferent connections, and the hypothalamus *does* receive heterogenous fiber systems. Moreover, both the hypothalamus and the brainstem reticular formation contain certain highly specific neural mechanisms; the latter has the bulbar mechanism governing respiration, and the hypothalamus contains highly specific mechanisms concerned in visceral spheres. (Nauta and Haymaker, 1969; Ramon-Moliner and Nauta, 1966.)

SITES INVOLVED IN DISTURBANCES IN FUNCTION OF SPECIAL SENSES AND THE VESTIBULAR APPARATUS

Hearing is represented in the transverse gyri of Heschl (Fig. 19-8). Lesions of these gyri unilaterally, or lesions of pathways reaching them from the medial geniculate body, occasionally cause transitory contralateral or bilateral impairment of hearing. Removal of a temporal lobe tumor may be followed by transient deafness, and by inability to localize or evaluate sounds coming from a distance. The observation that any such hearing deficit is transitory permits the assumption that the cochlear nuclei of each side send relays of fibers to the auditory cortex of each temporal lobe, but that the connection with the contralateral side predominates. Permanent deafness, in the absence of aphasia, may result from severe damage of the auditory area bilaterally (Bramwell, 1927; Clark and Russell, 1938). A patient with such a lesion may, however, be able to hear sounds and recognize differences in the pitch of tones, suggesting representation of these qualities in subcortical structures, including the medial geniculate body (Crosby, Humphrey, and Lauer, 1962).

Taste is represented in the most inferior part of the postcentral and precentral gyri and the contiguous part of the insular cortex, in the region of the circular sulcus (Fig. 19-8) (Patton, Ruch, and Walker, 1944; Penfield and Jasper, 1954). Sour-bitter taste is sometimes experienced as an aura of an epileptic attack originating in this region. In such a case, in which a hemangioma was found near the circular sulcus (on the *right* side), examination of the patient in intervals between attacks revealed loss of the sensation of sweetness over the contralateral *(left)* half of the tongue (Shenkin and Lewey, 1943). Much more commonly observed in lesions in this region is a syndrome characterized by weakness of the contralateral masticatory muscles, increased salivation, impairment of sensory and motor functions of the tongue, mouth, lips, and thumb, and motor aphasia. The thalamus also comes into consideration regarding abnormalities in taste. It is the ventral posteromedial (arcuate) nucleus of the thalamus that projects taste impulses to the region of the circular sulcus. Loss of the appreciation of taste (except for slight recognition of bitter) was noted in the contralateral half of the tongue in a patient who was subsequently found to have a tuberculoma involving this nucleus (Adler, 1933).

Olfactory acuity may be decreased following destructive lesions involving the more rostral piriform cortex—including the region of the gyrus ambiens (see Fig. 19-9 for the location of this gyrus) (Frazier and Rowe, 1934). Far more commonly, a reduction in the appreciation of odors results from lesions of the olfactory bulb or stalk, for example, in contre-coup injury involving this region in head trauma (Sumner, 1964). Olfactory groove meningioma is another frequent cause. In rare instances unilateral anosmia is due to congenital absence of the olfactory bulb and tract (Uyematsu, 1921).

While the frequencies and wave lengths produced by some stimuli are limited in number, those produced by odoriferous stimuli number in the thousands. This is true because most odors are blends of primary sensations, the latter being relatively few. Capacity to discriminate odors may be dependent on cell arrangement in the olfactory bulb, where the central processes of as many as one hundred olfactory neurons (in the olfactory membrane) come into contact with a single second neuron, the mitral cell, and where converging and diverging pathways apparently form reverberating circuits. Perception, identification, and associations of odors, based on past experience, appear to be functions dependent on the piriform cortex. (Schneider, 1967.)

The units employed to express threshold of olfactory sensitivity are arbitrary and include volume (Elsberg and Levy, 1935), percentage concentration of odors, molality, and even absolute number of molecules. However, the problem is very involved; nearly all odors are "impure" and sometimes it is not known whether smell or taste is being tested. Olfactory adaptation (accommodation, refractory state)—cessation of awareness of continuous olfactory stimulation—is a significant attribute of smell; it varies with many factors.

Olfactory responses vary in a given age group. Disgust for malodorous substances appears only after infancy. About 25 percent of persons lose some discrimination of olfactory test substances as they grow old (Gorman, 1964; Tucker and Biedler, 1956).

Olfactory stimulation resulting in pleasure (as from perfume, savor of food) or displeasure (exhaust fumes, rancid fats) initiates reflexes and excitatory states affecting gastric function, sexual interest, breathing, the state of awareness, and so on. Abnormal olfactory excitatory reactions involving recollections, behavior, and emotional state are consequences of lesions in various locations; this condition is discussed later in the text.

Vestibular function is represented in the cerebral cortex, but little of a precise nature is known of the areas concerned. On the basis of "labyrinthine sensations" ("dizziness") elicited by electrical stimulation of the cortex in human subjects, Penfield (1957) considered that vestibular function may be represented in the superior temporal gyrus just lateral to the area subserving hearing (the transverse gyri of Heschl). Stimulation at points in the parietal lobe occasionally resulted in a sensation of rotation or bodily displacement, and stimulation of an area of the occipital cortex responsive to conjugate eye turning evoked what seemed to be nystagmus. Extirpation of any of these areas led to no observed defect in vestibular function.

Vestibular symptoms of one kind or another, accompanied or not by convulsive phenomena, were noted in 20 of 200 patients with temporal lobe lesions; the lesions in 107 of the patients were due to tumor (Paillas, Piganiol, and Bonnet, 1956; Strobos, 1953). *Tinnitus* occurs in occasional cases of temporal lobe tumor and is usually experienced on the contralateral side. *Vertigo* is now and then noted in tumor occupying the region of the lateral cerebral fissure; during an attack there may be a tendency to fall to that side. *Disturbances of equilibrium,* with the tendency to fall to the side opposite the lesion, have been encountered in tumors involving the convex portion of the temporal lobe in its caudal part (Spector, 1967; Spiegel and Alexander, 1936). Furthermore, vertigo or rotational movements ("spinning sensations") were noted in seven patients with brain tumor; six of the tumors were in the frontotemporal region and one was in the parietal region. In one patient a shift occurred from vertiginous symptoms to a motor vestibular response, such as torsional circling movement of the head; in another patient, a shift occurred from vertigo to auditory hallucinations to a tingling sensation on the right side of the face and finally to memory impairment and mental confusion. Representation of vestibular function was considered to be in the opercular portion of the temporal lobe and the adjacent lateral surface of the superior temporal gyrus, rostral to the auditory area. A lesion in this region may be manifested by a motor sequence in which the subject gets up, walks around an object (such as a table), then, as a climax, turns somersaults. (Schneider, Calhoun, and Crosby, 1968.)

LOCALIZATION OF DISORDERS OF BEHAVIOR, MEMORY, AND CONSCIOUSNESS

Notwithstanding the merits of the argument against "localizing" a phenomenon like disturbed behavior in some particular area (Gooddy, 1956; Lashley, 1938; Riese, 1967), it is imperative to list the evidence in favor of the historic working hypothesis that the "highest" functions must be regarded no less bound to structure than the "lowest." Some of this evidence is admittedly conflicting and confusing; other aspects are convincing and practical,

Psychomotor seizures

Paroxysmal disturbances of behavior and/or feeling are usually called "psychomotor" and are usually associated with lesions of the temporal lobe. They have been noted in as high as 94 percent of cases of temporal lobe tumor (Keschner, Bender, and Strauss, 1936), but glial scars resulting from trauma are probably the most common source of seizures (Freytag and Lindenberg, 1964). Psychic disturbances in temporal lobe lesions may occur as the sole component of a seizure or may precede a generalized convulsion as an aura (Ostow, 1952). They are frequently ushered in by peculiar sensations either in the abdomen (especially the epigastrium), the thorax, or the throat. Dysesthesias may spread from the face or epigastrium down toward the limbs; hallucinations of hearing various sounds and sequence of sounds also occur (Moore, 1952; Penfield and Jasper, 1954; Schneider, Calhoun, and Crosby, 1968).

The seizures often take a form called *uncinate epilepsy* (Jackson, 1890, 1931). Among its several components the most telltale are hallucinations of smell and taste. Their content is familiar or not, but usually unpleasant and sometimes "horrible." Fear may be experienced, either alone or in combination with the other sensations mentioned. These "recollective hallucinations" may accompany the frequently seen involuntary movements of sniffing, tasting, or chewing. Other accompaniments are stereotyped, purposeless, rarely violent movements, and phrases, likewise repetitive, sometimes unintelligible and often expressing bewilderment or fear. Such automatisms also occur without hallucinations; usually they are covered by amnesia.

Dazed, dreamy states with memory disturbances are frequently encountered in expanding temporal lobe lesions. During a seizure, events that occurred in the past loom up vividly into consciousness and are relived as though they were occurring in the present, or an uncanny familiarity attaches to a new event or scene. This is referred to as the *déjà vu phenomenon.* (Although frequently observed in temporal lobe lesions, by itself this is so common a phenomenon, especially in hospitalized psychiatric patients, that in such a population, and without other manifestations of epilepsy, it has questionable localizing value [Richardson and Winokur, 1967].) Memory disturbances may also be reflected in the patient's feeling of unfamiliarity in accustomed surroundings or he may recognize a familiar milieu that nevertheless seems far away *(microteleopia);* perception of the size of objects may also be faulty—*micropia* and *macropia.* These three disorders—microteleopia, micropia, and macropia—are less closely related to uncinate attacks. They may be due to pathological changes in the retina (for example, detachment complicated by rarefaction of retinal elements), to tumor involving the optic chiasm, or to "vascular accident" in the parieto-occipital region. (Bender and Savitsky, 1943; Halpern, 1952.) Williams (1968) suggests that these elaborate, highly organized visual experiences may dominate the temporal lobe epilepsies presumably because man is primarily a "visual animal," and so visualization pervades his activities in connation as well as in cognition.

Temporal lobe epilepsy of the "uncinate" form is usually due to lesions, apparently of an irritative nature, situated in the close vicinity of the uncus hippocampi or amygdala. Gliosis of the uncus and adjoining hippocampal gyrus brought about presumably by reduction in blood flow in the posterior cerebral and anterior choroidal arteries due to compression during the birth process ("incisural sclerosis") has been cited as a common cause (Earle, Baldwin, and Penfield, 1953). Ammon's horn sclerosis is thought to be the inciting cause of the seizures or, on the other hand, the product of seizures if limited to Sommer's sector (Meyer, 1957; Sano and Malamud, 1953).

In a large series of medicolegal autopsies—trauma 25 percent, tumors 7 percent, malformation 7 percent, cerebrovascular disease 10 percent—incisural sclerosis was the sole lesion in 4 percent of epileptics, and the sclerosis was combined with other lesions in 10 percent (Freytag and Lindenberg, 1964).

Lesions outside the temporal lobe, or lesions involving more of the brain than the temporal lobe, may also give rise to "temporal lobe" epilepsy.

Thus, lesions involving the orbitofrontal cortex (from abscess, olfactory groove meningioma, aneurysm of the anterior communicating artery) can trigger the disorder (including *déjà vu* phenomena and olfactory and auditory hallucinations) through the mediation of the uncinate, inferior fronto-occipital, and related fasciculi (Schneider and others, 1961). Cerebral trauma and glioma are further precipitating factors (Frazier and Rowe, 1934; Freytag and Lindenberg, 1964). Kernicterus and posticteric encephalopathy, which invariably involve the hippocampus, carry a low incidence of seizures (5 to 10 percent). By contrast, in herpes simplex and acute inclusion encephalitis, which often severely involve the temporal lobe, the incidence of seizures is high (65 percent) (Haymaker, 1949; Haymaker and others, 1958).

In patients with temporal lobe epilepsy the sex drive is usually much decreased and is restored after temporal lobectomy (Blumer and Walker, 1967; Gastaut and Collomb, 1954). Coexisting chronic personality disorders are widely recognized but are disputed by some authors (Guerrant and others, 1962). *Erotomania (nymphomania)* has been found in one instance to be an expression of epileptic discharge brought about by a small neoplasm (hemangioendothelioma) involving the cortex of the right paracentral lobule. The disorder disappeared after removal of the tumor (Erickson, 1945).

Disturbances in space perception are encountered now and then in patients with lesions in the temporo-occipital region, and less commonly in patients with lesions involving the tegmentum pontis near the floor of the fourth ventricle. The patient may complain that he sees people in his room step through the walls into an adjacent room and still be visible as they walk about. The walls of a room may seem bent or otherwise distorted or they may seem to be collapsing. Such visual illusions (unaccompanied by diplopia or nystagmus), when occurring in the presence of pontile lesions, may be due to interference with the blending of ophthalmostatic and vestibular impulses (Bender and Jung, 1948).

Paroxysmal attacks surcharged with pseudoaffective phenomena may be traceable to various structures, including the temporal lobe together with its hippocampal formation and amygdala, and the more caudal part of the orbitofrontal cortex. The patterning is effected largely by hypothalamic and mesencephalic neural mechanisms.

Some of the paroxysms have the features of rage. For instance, a patient with scarred temporal cortex complicating an ear infection had attacks beginning with a growling cry, followed shortly by violent rage; he walked the streets screaming and assaulted anyone he met. After scar resection the attacks ceased (Sjöqvist, 1941). Scarred temporal pole in association with hemangioma in a man subject to epilepsy and spells of irritability and abusiveness who eventually killed his wife while in a state of "epileptic furor" is shown in Fig. 22-1 (Walker, 1961). Similar phenomena occur with lesions outside the temporal lobe. With a developing abscess in orbitofrontal gyri, following traumatic laceration in this region, a previously cheerful child became morose, aggressive, and, at times, savage. Recovery ensued as the abscess healed. (Dott, 1938.) A patient with chiasmal glioma extending into the third ventricle acted, for a time, like a wild animal (Cushing, 1932). A woman recovering somewhat from carbon monoxide poisoning would grind her teeth and emit hissing sounds, and during attacks generalized sweating and piloerection were noted over her entire body (Wortis and Maurer, 1942). Colloid cyst in the third ventricle may give rise to "diencephalic epilepsy" (Penfield, 1929) or to less dramatic episodic phenomena (Nelson and Haymaker, 1957; Yenermen, Bowerman, and Haymaker, 1958). Attacks of rage and the like may also occur in lesions situated more caudally in the hypothalamus or in the subthalamus or midbrain (Alpers, 1940; Cox, 1937).

Disorders of posture, affect, social attitudes

Extirpation of anterior temporal cortex bilaterally for psychomotor seizures has resulted in reduction in the incidence of seizures and improvement in the psychic state (Bailey and others, 1953). But bilateral removal of most of the hippocampal formation and uncus is followed by profound and permanent disturbances. These include (1) loss of recognition, even of close relatives, and other serious disturbances of memory (Scoville and Milner, 1957), (2) changes in emotional behavior, such as abolition of fear, (3) psychomotor slowness, (4) increase in sexual

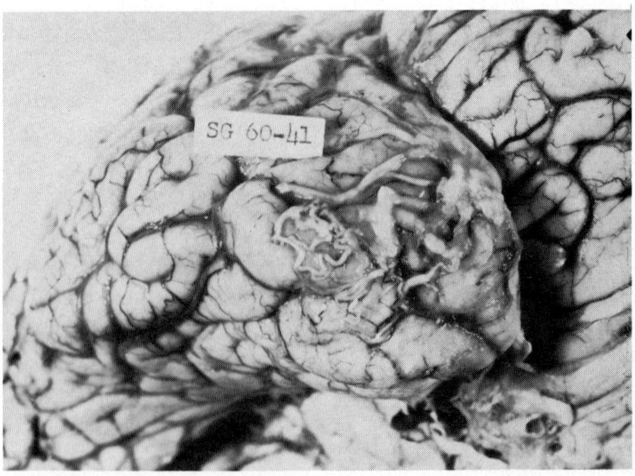

Fig. 22-1. Hemangioma in region of right temporal pole. The patient had had epilepsy over the previous 16 years. In the 3 years before death he exhibited increasing irritability. During cloudy states he became very aggressive. During one episode he repeatedly stabbed his wife while in an "epileptic furor," but he never could believe that he had murdered her. (From Walker, 1961.)

activity in some cases, and (5) hyperphagia (Terzian and Ore, 1955). Under other conditions—those leading to atrophy of the mediobasal part of the temporal lobe bilaterally (Pick's disease, Alzheimer's disease, hypoglycemic cerebral damage)—an added feature is a peculiar oral behavior that takes the form of grasping any object and placing it in the mouth (Pilleri, 1966).

This syndrome (Klüver and Bucy, 1939) has been considered traceable to interference with one or more of three routes: (1) hippocampus, to mamillary bodies, thence to the anterior thalamic nuclei, the cingular gyrus, and back by way of the retrosplenial cingular cortex to the hippocampal gyrus, then to the hippocampus (Papez, 1937); (2) in the reverse direction, from the septal region by way of the fornix to the hippocampus, to much of the rostral part of the temporal cortex, and from here by various pathways to the brainstem (Adey, Merrillees, and Sunderland, 1956; Votaw, 1960); and (3) from the visual association cortex (areas 18 and 19) to the lateral and basal parts of the temporal lobe, thence to the hippocampus (Geschwind, 1965). The sexual phase of the syndrome is thought to be related to lesions in the amygdala or vicinity (Pilleri, 1966). However, stereotaxic amygdalotomy—unilateral or bilateral—in man has not evoked hypersexuality (except temporarily in one instance), nor has it precipitated the Klüver-Bucy syndrome; what the operation accomplished was reduction of emotional excitability and normalization of social behavior and adaptation (Narabayashi and others, 1963).

An aspect of the hippocampal formation is that it may be concerned in the *perception of pain*, severe intractable pain having yielded to bilateral hippocampectomy. (Gol and Faibish, 1967.)

Catatonia may be encountered with cerebral lesions and resemble akinetic mutism, but the patients appear fully conscious. They assume and maintain the immobility of a wax figure without showing signs of fatigue. For instance, a catatonic patient may lie for hours on his back with legs separated and his hips and knees flexed, a posture no normal person would be able to maintain for long.

In *catalepsy* (waxy flexibility) the limbs placed in any position by the examiner are actively maintained by the patient. When the examiner moves the forearm at the elbow, the resistance offered by the muscles is inconstant. In extrapyramidal rigidity, by contrast, the resistance is either constant or cogwheel-like. Catatonia (and catalepsy) resemble the parkinsonian state in no other way, aside from facial immobility.

Catalepsy is frequently a manifestation of hysteria, and *catatonia* a sign or a form of schizophrenia. However, catatonia may be due to lesions in various locations, even the cerebellum, where an abscess has been found (Bing, 1925). The disorder is more commonly seen in frontal lobe lesions (tumor, abscess, acute or subacute encephalitis, infarct, or a degenerative disease). Catatonic schizophrenia has occasionally occurred as a prelude to the postencephalitic parkinsonian state. Catatonia has been produced in the monkey by damaging cortical area 6 (Crosby, Humphrey, and Showers, 1959), and in the cat through damage either of the rostral neocortex bilaterally or the retromamillary region (Barris, 1937; de Jong, 1945; Ingram, Barris, and Ranson, 1936). It may be considered as a kind of decerebrate rigidity or akin to "cerebellar fits" (p. 289).

Autonomic disturbances prevail in a kaleidoscopic disorder known as *familial dysautonomia*, or Riley-Day syndrome, which commences in infancy (Riley and others, 1949; Riley and Moore, 1966). In rare instances a similar disorder is observed in adulthood (Shy and Drager, 1960).

Onset of the familial variety is usually in early infancy. Characteristic features are defective lacrimation, blotching of the skin with eating and/or excitement, excessive sweating, drooling, abnormal esophageal motility, and absence of fungiform papillae on the tongue with decrease in taste perception. Also of frequent occurrence are bouts of hyperthermia and postural hypotension with intermittent hypertension. Abnormal swallowing reflexes and cyclic vomiting, characteristic of the disorder, make feeding difficult. Among other disorders are relative indifference to pain, emotional lability, mental retardation, motor incoordination, kyphoreflexia, and convulsions. Charcot joints and kyphoscoliosis may develop as the child grows older. Clinical testing reveals absence of an erythematous flare in response to histamine given intradermally, exaggerated response to intravenous infusion of methacholine (hydrochloride) or norepinephrine, and potentiated miosis following instillation of methacholine (2.5 percent) or physostigmine into the conjunctival sac and mydriasis from instillation of phenylephrine. It thus appears that familial dysautonomia represents an autonomic denervation syndrome. The tetrad consisting in absence of lacrimation, corneal hypesthesia or anesthesia, and pupillary constriction following the local application of methacholine is distinctive and virtually diagnostic of the disorder. (Goldberg, Payne, and Brunt, 1968; Shinebourne, Sneddon, and Turner, 1967; Smith and Dancis, 1964; Smith, Dancis, and Breinin, 1965.)

Postmortem study in one case revealed a thalamic lesion of vascular origin (Aring and Engel, 1945). Demyelinative lesions in the anterior commissure and fornix were found in another case, and multiple tiny hamartomas of the base of the hypothalamus and widespread calcification of the surface of the brain in still another (Stevens, unpublished). These findings may be incidental. In another case gastrointestinal ganglion cells and the myenteric plexuses were found normal (Linde and Westover, 1962). Great dilatation of the vestibular aqueduct bilaterally was observed in another case (Keleman, 1968).

In the adult the syndrome is characterized by orthostatic hypotension, anhidrosis, impotence, loss of sphincter control, and other disorders—for example, external ophthalmoparesis, iris atrophy, incoordination (cerebellar), tremor, rigidity, loss of associated movements, and neuropathic muscle wasting. Nerve cell damage or loss has been noted in autonomic ganglia and in many locations in the central nervous system (Schwarz, 1967; Shy and Drager, 1960).

Episodic phenomena, not as yet traceable to any particular series of neural mechanisms or to a trigger site, characterize the *Kleine-Levin syndrome.* (Kleine, 1925; Levin, 1936.)

This disorder is occasionally met with in adolescent males. Periodic sleepiness or somnolence and megaphagia (compulsive eating), often in association with motor unrest or apathy and abnormal behavior, characterize the syndrome. The episodes last a few days to 2 weeks or so, and they end abruptly or gradually. They usually recur every few days or months but may make their appearance only every year or so. During an episode the subject may be apathetic, fatuous, distracted, childishly querulous, feel persecuted, berate his relatives as though he were drunk, and have outbursts of laughter, peculiar singing, or shouting. Afterward he may be gay and excited, often sexually. Delusions and visual hallucinations may also occur, headache is occasionally complained of, and retrospective recollection is usually vague. The disorder usually ceases spontaneously. (Critchley, 1962; Critchley and Hoffman, 1962; Ronald, 1946.)

There has been a question whether the syndrome just described is too restrictive. In the experience of some, adolescent females may also be affected. Hypersomnia may be replaced by insomnia. The syndrome may alternate with episodes of narcolepsy; polydipsia and hyperhidrosis may be additional features. Psychological manifestations occurring during an attack or afterward range from clouding of sensorium or amnesia to classical depressive syndromes, none of which is of psychogenic origin. "Periodic quantitative dysregulation of food intake and sleep with periodic mental aberrations" has been suggested as a definition of the Kleine-Levin syndrome (Gallinek, 1967).

In occasional instances the syndrome has been noted following (or in association with) febrile illness of uncertain case, influenza, head injury, or hypothalamic tumor. There has been a tendency to attribute the syndrome to dysfunction of the hypothalamus and possibly of the midbrain reticular substance as well. Occasionally the patient presents a "pseudo-tumor" syndrome. (Andermann, 1967; Gallinek, 1967; Gilbert, 1964.)

Lack of social inhibition and appropriate affect are particularly apt to occur in lesions of the orbitofrontal cortex (or basal neocortex) bilaterally. This is the cortical region last to appear in simian evolution, and it reaches its greatest degree of development in the human brain (Spatz, 1966). Despite these considerations intelligence suffers relatively little (Kleist, 1934; Spatz, 1966).

The main *afferent* fibers received by the orbitofrontal cortex are from the medial, magnocellular part of the medial dorsal thalamic nucleus; a feedback from cortex to nucleus also occurs (Locke, 1967; Nauta, 1962, 1964). On the *efferent* side, the orbitofrontal cortex also projects to various nuclei of the more rostral part of the hypothalamus (Clark and Meyer, 1950, Nauta, 1962, 1964; Wall, Glees, and Fulton, 1951).

Pathologically inappropriate and uninhibited *affect*—indifference or euphoria—is seen in extensive lesions of the more rostral part of the frontal cortex and others situated deep in the white matter. Examples are presenile and senile atrophy, trauma (including psychosurgical), and lesions resulting from tumor (Frazier, 1936). The pathways concerned are frontal-thalamic; presumably they also involve basal ganglia (forced laughing and crying may occur, for example, when extrapyramidal pathways are involved) and the limbic system, considering the latter's role as a link between neopallium and brainstem by way of the diencephalon, between the intellectual and the visceral representations (Malamud, 1967).

Memory

Disturbances in memory characterize many of the disorders referred to previously. The mechanism of storage and recall of information is unknown. Memory, like intelligence, is best regarded as multifactorial. The loss of a function, experience, or skill (loss of the appropriate response to any given stimulus) is related to the specific area of its representation, its "cortical analyser." Diffuse bilateral and extensive lesions affecting the cortex-subcortex of the frontal, temporal, and parietal lobes are often to blame for this loss. But some evidence points to a general factor of memory, such as recognition, and the matching of past and recent experiences. The limbic circuit, which partakes of all three lobes, and its temporal portion in particular, seems to play a special role in the disorders of remembering.

Small unilateral lesions in the hippocampal formation in man have no noticeable effect, but where bilateral small lesions exist, or where partial temporal lobe resection is carried out sufficiently caudal to previously damaged parts of the anterior hippocampal formation and adjoining gyrus, a loss of memory for recent events has been noted (Milner and Penfield, 1955; Penfield, 1955; Penfield and Milner, 1958; Scoville and Milner, 1957). DeJong, Itabashi, and Olson (1969) record a case of severe memory impairment in association with infarction of the entire hippocampal formation bilaterally together with damage of the cortex in the region of the collateral fissure on one side and parts of the paracalcarine cortex bilaterally (from occlusion of branches of the posterior cerebral artery); the most pronounced memory loss was for "emotionally charged" events. The view was advanced that the hippocampus is not the primary center for the "storage" of memories, but rather a region for integration and sorting of information, for storage elsewhere. Loss of memory for recent events may also occur following section of the anterior column of the fornix bilaterally (Sweet, Talland, and Erwin, 1959), and following removal of the temporal lobe unilaterally (Dimsdale, Logue, and Pierey, 1964). Moreover, varied recollections (auras) can be elicited in epileptic patients on electrically stimulating the temporal cortex, exclusive of the hippocampal gyrus and amygdala. From this "storehouse of remembered experience," stimulation in patients with seizures arouses not only recent and past events but also the thought and emotion bound to the events (Penfield, 1950, 1952).

The *Korsakoff syndrome* (lack of recognition of recently acquired information, retention of older material, and confabulation) is encountered in association with transient or permanent lesions (traumatic, toxic, metabolic, neoplastic, or infectious) that affect the limbic system mainly from the region of the mamillary bodies rostrally. Most constant is damage of the medial parts of the medial dorsal and anterior nuclei of the thalamus and the mamillary body; less frequently affected are the periaqueductal region and nuclei of the floor of the fourth ventricle (Collins, Victor, and Adams, 1961; Delay, Brion, and Elissalde, 1958; Malamud and Skillicorn, 1956). The pars tecta fornicis was heavily affected (demyelination was the chief finding) in a case of Korsakoff's syndrome occurring as a manifestation of suprasellar craniopharyngioma (Orthner and Rettinger, 1965). Other parts of the limbic system may also be implicated in the development of Korsakoff's syndrome, judging from the marked frequency with which this syndrome follows operation for ruptured aneurysm of the anterior communicating artery (Lindqvist and Norlén, 1966; Talland, Sweet, and Ballantine, 1967). The marked alterations in behavior observed in aneurysm of this artery have been regarded as due to damage inflicted secondarily on the parolfactory and septal areas (Taren, 1965).

It has long been contended that the primary defect is in memory, the patient tending to compensate for his forgetfulness and confusion by confabulating (Barbizet, 1963).

As viewed by Meissner (1967), the initial registration and short-term storage of sensory input is intact in the patient with Korsakoff's syndrome and enables him to function at relatively normal levels on simple learning tasks and at the initial stages of more complex tasks. Primary memory is thus unaffected. Secondary memory—that is, longer-term storage—requires sequential organization of material transferred from primary memory. Impairment of some functions on which secondary memory depends seems to be at fault. As memory for events long past (childhood) is also relatively intact, the view is put forward that the peculiar malfunctioning in the Korsakoff patient is not a defect in memory at all. In accord is in the view of Orthner and Rettinger (1965) that the defect in the Korsakoff syndrome is in the *power of registration (Merkfähigkeit, mémoire de fixation)*, not in the capacity for recent memory.

The lesions encountered in the central nervous system in the Korsakoff syndrome are of much the same nature as in the disorder now to be described.

Wernicke's encephalopathy, a disorder due mostly to thiamine deficiency occurring in starvation and alcoholism, and also in hyperemesis gravidarum, occlusion of the stomach (for example, by carcinoma), and rarely as a complication of chronic uremia (Lopez and Collins, 1968). The structures most affected are the mamillary bodies, periaqueductal region, and lamina quadrigemina, in that order of decreasing frequency; characteristically, the lesions extend all along the periventricular system and are most prevalent in the floor of the fourth ventricle and the wall of the third. Affected areas tend to have a lacunar appearance, occasional nerve cells are lost, astroglial cells are hypertrophic and their nuclei assume varied shapes, endothelial cells of vessels are enlarged and aggregates of lipid-filled cells are found perivascularly, and hemorrhages frequently occur terminally. In occasional instances invasive tumor (for example, ependymal tumor) occupying most of the structures mentioned in the foregoing, and extending far downward in the periventricular region, has been found the basis of Wernicke's syndrome (Környey, 1967).

Moreover, as observed by Lopez and Collins (1968), there may be *central pontile myelinolysis*, an obscure demyelinative disorder first described by Adams, Victor, and Mancall (1959) and subsequently observed by others. The lesion develops under numerous conditions: alcoholism, malnutrition, following continual vomiting, subacute and chronic bronchopulmonary infections,

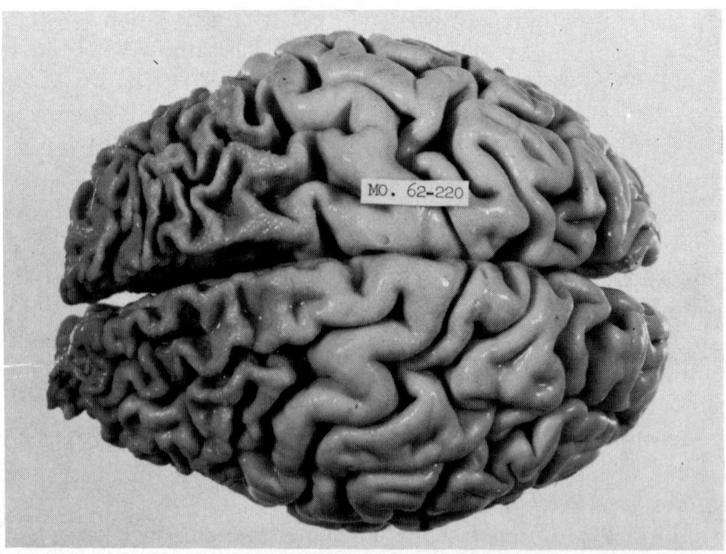

Fig. 22-2. Pick's disease, showing profound atrophy of the frontal lobe. (Courtesy Dr. Richard Lindenberg, Baltimore.)

hepatic cirrhosis, ketosis in diabetes mellitus, water-electrolyte depletion following operation for brain tumor, subdural abscess, and Wilson's disease (Castan, 1967; Shiraki, 1968). The demyelination occurs symmetrically in the tegmentum of the pons and commonly includes the pars basilaris of the pons. Oligodendroglial cells in these lesions undergo hypertrophy such that they take on the appearance of macrophages.

Wernicke's encephalopathy is characterized by acute onset of ocular muscle pareses, nystagmus, ataxia, and mental disturbances. Apathy and severe confusion mark this acute phase. Commonly observed soon afterward are confabulation, disorientation, and hallucinations (Korsakoff's syndrome), culminating in amnestic dementia. Optic neuritis with papilledema, occasionally associated with retinal hemorrhages, may also occur; in later stages the deep reflexes are lost. (Frantzen, 1966; Victor and Adams, 1953; Victor and Yakovlev, 1955; de Wardener and Lennox, 1947; Willanger, 1966.)

In some cases of Wernicke's encephalopathy, somnolence is the leading symptom, and it may persist for weeks; in such cases typical lesions have been found in a number of locations (mamillary bodies, nuclei tuberis laterales, tuberomamillary and supraoptic nuclei), or in the mamillary bodies alone (Gagel, 1936).

Among the diffuse and extensive pathological processes that lead to memory loss, *Alzheimer's disease* is to be included. In this disorder the pathological process usually commences in the parietal region.

Patients with Alzheimer's disease are forgetful from the beginning and complain that their memory is falling apart. According to Lindenberg (personal communication): "One of my patients complaining of total forgetfulness was previously an excellent typist. Now sitting in front of a typewriter, she did not recognize the typewriter as such, and putting her hands on the machine did not help. She was totally unaware of what is done with this kind of object." Later stages of the disease are characterized by spatial disorientation and further defects in cognitive function, such as disturbed speech and thinking.

In *Pick's disease,* memory may be retained over extraordinarily long periods of time whether the atrophy begins in the frontal convex cortex, orbitofrontal cortex, or temporal cortex.

If the disease process starts in the frontal convex cortex, the patient initially exhibits the akinetic frontal lobe syndrome of Kleist (1934): severe inhibition of all motor activity and initiative without confusion or loss of memory (unaccompanied by lower limb or sphincter disturbances) similar to that occurring in other types of lesions that destroy frontal convolutions. Appearance of the cortex at the end-stage of Pick's disease involving the frontal lobe is illustrated in Fig. 22-2. If the disease begins in the temporal cortex the patient will show the expected signs of aphasia. If the orbitofrontal cortex suffers first the patient may initially show a loss of social inhibitions and a euphoria similar to that observed in general paresis or in hebephrenia. (Lindenberg, personal communication.)

Consciousness

An even wider area is involved in disturbances of drive and consciousness. This becomes clear if we take "consciousness" in its most general connotation, which includes all mental functioning. The clinical "levels" of consciousness (coma, stupor, confusion, somnolence) may, however, be equated with anatomical levels. The fundamental level appears to be the *brainstem reticular formation;* as we move from there by way of the thalamus to the cortex, conscious operations become more specialized. Thus, coma results from gross interference with the reticular formation. Lesser degrees—from stupor (in which the subject is capable of crude awakening and sleeping) to confusion—are due either to minor interference of the brainstem or to extensive cortical malfunction. Confusion may therefore represent a primary diffuse cortical condition (as in toxic delirium) or it may occur as a consequence of brainstem injury. (Eccles, 1966; Plum and Posner, 1966.)

In closed head injury, the amnesia elicited after recovery coextends with the period of confusion (von Wowern, 1966) and remains the most reliable measure of the severity of the injury (Symonds, 1962). The structure of consciousness by anatomical levels may also be inferred from the presumable sites of pharmacological action: brainstem and cortex for barbiturates, the limbic system for phenothiazines (Himwich, 1958). Case reports bear out these generalizations.

Coma lasting 4½ months followed massive and extensive infarction of tegmentum and base of the pons, tegmentum of the midbrain, and unilaterally in the thalamus (including the pulvinar), from occlusion of the basilar artery. During this time the eyeballs were fixed in forward gaze. The patient responded to noxious stimuli by generalized flexion of the limbs at all joints. At no time did the EEG assume the quality of sleep. (Neumann and Cohn, 1965.) Damage of the cephalic part of the tegmentum predominated in three cases in which coma or stupor lasted 6 to 9 months. All showed hypokinesis, spasticity, altered pupillary and ocular muscle activity, pathological reflexes, apparent insensitivity to sensory stimuli, mutism, loss of deglutition, impaired sphincter control, and amentia. One patient had a stroke (from infarction in the midbrain) and the other two sustained severe head injury. (French, 1952.)

While alerting activity is attributed to the reticular activating substance (or system), the *reticular formation of the brainstem* in general has a far wider functional connotation. This is inferred from observations in three cases of a particularly complex form of heredoataxia in which the pallidum and subthalamic region were atrophic and in which the reticular formation from the subthalamic nuclei and thalamus down to the spinal cord was selectively atrophic. The study suggested that the part of the reticular formation related to the subpallidal-subthalamic region was far more abundant than the part extending to the nonspecific nuclei of the thalamus. Besides a cerebello-pyramido-extrapyramidal syndrome, the clinical disturbances in these patients included severe defects in attention, character, and behavior. From its influence in the spheres of hormonal activity and in the milieu intérieur, its role in conditioned reflexes, discrimination perception, stress, and muscle tonus, and its participation in diverse hyperkinesias, hallucinations, and epilepsy, the reticular formation was considered an apparatus concerned in the regulation of the "equilibrium" of the neuraxis—an equilibrium (or homeostasis), of which behavior, attention, vigilance, variations in muscle tonus, and the physiognomy of movements are the major expressions. Pathologically the disorder in the three patients was referred to as *reticulocerebellar atrophy,* and clinically as the *dyshomeostasis syndrome of the neuraxis.* (Varela, 1967.)

Akinetic mutism occurs with lesions in a number of locations. The disorder is considered to be a fragment of the dyshomeostasis syndrome just mentioned. Patients with akinetic mutism are motionless and speechless; their eyes usually remain open for long periods, moving in all directions, apparently at random ("coma vigil"). Reflex-type movements are usually maintained; for example, painful stimuli may induce a withdrawal reaction. The patient usually swallows fluids monitored into his mouth. Sphincter control is lost. In many cases what has been called akinetic mutism is, however, not that stereotyped. Since the patient lies immobile his state of consciousness may be difficult to judge; hence, instead of *coma vigil,* he may be said to be unconscious, stuporous, lethargic, or somnolent ("somnolent coma"); deep coma may precede any of these states. There may be associated extraocular muscle palsy or, on the other hand, an ability of the eyes to follow an object moved in his visual field (hence such a patient is not akinetic in this respect). Preservation of intellectual faculties is sometimes noted (the patient may be able to add or multiply, as indicated by gestures; Lhermitte and others, 1963) or he may lack these faculties (Cravioto, Silberman, and Feigin, 1960). The patient may even be able to speak occasionally in monosyllables or whispered voice. Static tremor and/or increased muscle tone are noted in some patients

In cases of this kind, there may be infarcts (for example, from thrombosis of the basilar artery) or other lesions in the brainstem involving the tegmentum and its reticular formation, particularly the tegmentum of the rostral part of the midbrain. Pars basilaris pontis and the periaqueductal region may also be affected. (Cravioto, Silberman, and Feigin, 1960; French, 1952; Lhermitte and others, 1963; Neuman and Cohn, 1965; Williams and Parsons-Smith, 1951.) Brainstem tumor has been encountered in occasional patients (Messert, Henke, and Langheim, 1966). Central myelinolysis has also been noted (Adams, Victor, and Mancall, 1959; Kepes, Reece, and Oxley, 1965). Cerebellar tumor can also give rise to the disorder, as can cerebellar abscess (Bing, 1925). Skultety (1968) concludes that a syndrome of hypokinesis or decreased vocal output, or both, can arise (1) from loss of a critical amount of *afferent* input into the cerebrum as a consequence of destruction of the lemniscal or the reticular activating system, (2) from lesions that destroy a critical amount of the rostral reticular system, resulting in a failure of activation of appropriate integrating mechanisms, and (3) from lesions that destroy a critical amount of certain *efferent* systems. Retention of sensory functions, retained awareness, and retention of the ability to move and speak if inhibition of motor function is overcome led Klee (1961), on the other hand, to conclude that long sensory and motor tracts can be relatively intact.

Akinetic mutism may also occur in the presence of obstructive hydrocephalus (Moore, 1969; see also next section, on dementia). Epidermoid cyst of the third ventricle was observed by Cairns and coworkers (1941) in a case for which they coined the term "akinetic mutism." Craniopharyngioma and other tumors in the region of the third ventricle may also be responsible (Kepes, Reece, and Oxley, 1965; Klee, 1961). According to Messert, Henke, and Langheim (1966), both obstructive hydrocephalus and variations in the gradients of intracranial pressure seem to be major underlying factors in the production of akinetic mutism. Return of voice and facial expression together with the occurrence of spontaneous movement of the limbs followed ventricular, cisternal, or even lumbar tap. All features of the akinetic mutism syndrome may, in fact, disappear after elimination of aqueductal block. For reasons not altogether clear, atrophy of the periventricular fiber system was held responsible for the akinetic mutism in these cases, not akinetic mutism per se, but, instead, increased sensitivity of the atrophied system to sudden pressure change. To them, akinetic mutism represents a global apraxia. Ataxia of gait, then apraxia of gait, occurred in earlier stages in some of their patients (with brainstem tumor) and was followed by akinetic mutism—or, according to them, by "global apraxia."

Lesions in certain other locations may also give rise to akinetic mutism. Diencephalic-mesencephalic involvement from pineal tumor may bring it about (Cairns, 1952). The disorder has been observed in carbon monoxide poisoning, in which lesions occurred mainly in the frontal cortex and the globus pallidus (Cravioto, Silberman, and Feigin, 1960). Unilateral or bilateral subdural hematoma may also be responsible. The akinetic frontal syndrome of Kleist (p. 389) appears to be a fragment of the akinetic mutism syndrome. The limbic system has been found to be affected in some instances. Barris and Schuman (1953) found severe lesions in the cingulate gyrus bilaterally in one case, and Ogata, Fukiyama, and Iwata (1966) noted softening of the septal nuclei, rostral part of the cingulate gyri, fornices, and mamillary bodies (due partly at least to anterior cerebral artery insufficiency) in another. In two cases of ruptured aneurysm of the anterior communicating artery characterized by akinetic mutism, Faris (1969) found softening of much of the limbic system (cingulate, hippocampal, and basal frontal gyri, gyri recti, amygdala, and septal region). Damage of the limbic system may fit into the schema of a disconnection syndrome by virtue of interruption of pathways from certain structures—for example, the hippocampus—that project to the temporal cortex, or from interruption of pathways from parolfactory and certain septal nuclei that project to the cingulate cortex or hypothalamus, thence to the reticular formation.

Severe head trauma, with or without skull fracture, which at first—over weeks or months—is characterized by loss of consciousness in association with muscle rigidity, quadriparesis, hyperpnea, and autonomic disturbances (hyperhidrosis, salivation) may, with the passage of time, be manifested by akinetic mutism. The clearing of consciousness characteristic of this syndrome usually occurs spontaneously, not through the stages from coma, stupor, confusion, and somnolence; nor is there a delirium-amentia intermediate stage. The EEG may be dominated by intermediate and delta waves over both hemispheres and a lack of alpha waves. Pathologically, the main findings may include widespread degenerative atrophy of the cerebral white matter, "contusion foci" in the cortex in some cases but not in others, hydrocephalus, and degeneration of fiber pathways, including pathways to the brainstem. (Ule, Döhner, and Bues, 1961.) Or, in akinetic mutism following trauma the chief lesions may, as mentioned earlier, be situated in the upper midbrain tegmentum (French, 1952).

For those cases of head trauma heavily involving the cerebrum, Yakovlev postulates deafferentiation of the thalamus from the striatum and epistriatal cortex as the basis (p. 462). Elimination of afferent input into the neocortex through cerebral white matter destruction, hence lack of pallial (or cortical) function was considered by Ule, Döhner, and Bues (1961) as the basis of akinetic mutism of traumatic origin, and thus they called the condition the *apallic syndrome* (absence of pallial, or cortical, function).

In summary, the akinetic mutism syndrome represents a spectrum of altered states of consciousness. For numerous cases there is much to commend the view that disconnection of the reticular activating substance from the nonspecific (intralaminar) thalamic nuclei—hence from the cerebral neocortex—is responsible. For other cases disconnection of the neocortex owing to white matter destruction may be the explanation (see also page 462). The basis of limbic cortex destruction as a cause needs yet a convincing working hypothesis. Atrophy of periventricular fiber pathways as responsible remains nebulous. Interruption of the cerebellorubrothalamic pathway can scarcely be invoked as a cause, as there is no incoordination of movement in akinetic mutism. Interruption of long descending pathways seems of importance in the development of the syndrome.

Kemper and Romanul's (1967) patient did not move and could not speak, but could retract her eyelids and move her eyes conjugately. Infarction of the pons that spared the tegmentum, lemnisci, and cranial nerve nuclei led them to consider the condition (in her case) not as akinetic mutism but as a state of paralysis secondary to interruption of corticopontile, corticobulbar, and corticospinal pathways. However, it would be difficult to rule out the possibility that the reticular substance was deactivated by lack of impulses ordinarily received from downgoing pathways.

Dementia

In organic dementia, large sectors of judgment and memory are defective. The disorder is seen in the senile and presenile dementias such as Alzheimer's disease, in cerebrovascular disease, in post-ictal states, in brain tumor, and in inclusion body encephalitis. Damage of the brain is often widespread and irreversible.

However, dementia may be symptomatic and reversible. This has been noted in *hydrocephalus* either of the communicating or the obstructive type in association with "normal" cerebrospinal fluid (C.S.F.) pressure.

In early stages the patient has slight impairment of memory, paucity of thought and action, slight horizontal nystagmus, unsteadiness of gait, and urinary incontinence. Neither papilledema nor headache occur. There may be episodes of weakness, giddiness, and pallor. Progressive dementia follows, and in advanced stages there may be akinetic mutism and signs of severe pyramidal tract and extrapyramidal system involvement. C.S.F. pressure remains below 180 to 200 mm. H_2O. Diagnosis, established by pneumoencephalography, reveals great dilatation of all or part of the ventricular system, depending on the site and nature of the obstruction. Rapid restitution of health occurs following lowering of the C.S.F. pressure through surgical shunting. (Adams and others, 1965.)

Another pathological state that may lead to reversible dementia is *chronic subdural hematoma.* Little of clinical significance may be noted shortly after the hemorrhage, aside from transient pupillary dilatation ipsilaterally. Months or years later there may be headache, hemiparesis, and epileptic seizures. Mental deterioration amounting to dementia, or to fluctuating psychosis, may ensue, and disappear after surgical intervention. The degree to which brain atrophy may occur as a consequence of subdural hematoma occurring bilaterally is illustrated in Fig. 28-7.

Other pathological states associated with "normal-pressure hydrocephalus" may also be manifested by akinetic mutism succeeded by dementia. To be cited is cerebellar hemangioblastoma with manifold brainstem disturbances resulting from brainstem compression. Removal of the tumor in a case of this kind increased the severity of the patient's mental state. However, great improvement followed ventriculoatrial shunting. (Moore, 1969.)

REFERENCES

Adams, R. D., Fisher, C. M., Hakim, S., Ojemann, R. G., and Sweet, W. H. 1965. Symptomatic occult hydrocephalus with "normal" cerebrospinal-fluid pressure: a treatable syndrome. New Eng. J. Med. **273**:117-126.

Adams, R. D., Victor, M., and Mancall, E. L. 1959. Central pontine myelinolysis: a hitherto undescribed disease occurring in alcoholic and malnourished patients. Arch. Neurol. Psychiat. **81**:154-172.

Adey, W. R., Merrillees, N. R. C., and Sunderland, S. 1956. The entorhinal area; behavioral, evoked potential, and histological studies of its interrelationships with brain stem regions. Brain **79**:414-439.

Adler, A. 1933. Zur Topik des Verlaufes der Gesmacks sinnsfasern und anderer afferenter Bahnen im Thalamus. Z. Ges. Neurol. Psychiat. **149**:208-220.

Alpers, B. J. 1940. Personality and emotional disorders associated with hypothalamic lesions. Res. Publ. Ass. Res. Nerv. Ment. Dis., Proc. **20**:725-752.

Andermann, F. 1968. Observaciones sobre el síndrome de Kleine-Levin. Proc. 2d Panam. Congr. Neurology, San Juan, Puerto Rico.

Andy, O. J., and Stephan, H. 1968. The septum in the human brain. J. Comp. Neurol. **133**:383-392.

Aring, C. D., and Engel, G. L. 1945. Hypothalamic attacks with thalamic lesion: anatomic considerations. Arch. Neurol. Psychiat. **54**:44-50.

Bailey, P., Green, J. R., Amador, L., and Gibbs, F. A. 1953. Treatment of psychomotor states by anterior temporal lobectomy: a report of progress. Res. Publ. Ass. Res. Nerv. Ment. Dis., Proc. **31**:341-346.

Barbizet, J. 1963. Defect of memorizing of hippocampal-mammillary origin: a review. J. Neurol. Neurosurg. Psychiat. **26**:127-135.

Barris, R. W. 1937. Cataleptic symptoms following bilateral cortical lesions in cats. Amer. J. Physiol. **119**:213-220.

Barris, R. W., and Schuman, H. R. 1953. Bilateral anterior cingulate gyrus lesions: syndrome of the anterior cingulate gyri. Neurology **3**:44-52.

Bender, M. B., and Jung, R. 1948. Abweichungen der subjectiven optischen Vertikalen und Horizontalen bei Gesunden und Hirnverletzten. Arch. Psychiat. **181**:193-212.

Bender, M. B., and Savitsky, N. 1943. Micropsia and teleopsia limited to the temporal fields of vision. Arch. Ophthal. **29**:904-908.

Bing, R. 1925. Sémiologie des affections cérébelleuses. Schweiz. Arch. Neurol. Psychiat. **16**: 3-26.

Blumer, O., and Walker, E. A. 1967. Sexual behavior in temporal lobe epilepsy. Arch. Neurol. **16**:37-43.

Bramwell, E. 1927. A case of cortical deafness. Brain **50**:579-580.

Cairns, H. 1952. Disturbances of consciousness with lesions of the brainstem and diencephalon. Brain **75**:109-146.

Cairns, H., Oldfield, R., Pennybacker, J., and Whitteridge, D. 1941. Akinetic mutism with epidermoid cyst of third vestricle. (With a report of the associated disturbances of brain potentials.) Brain **64**:273-290.

Castan, P. 1967. La myélinolyse centrale dans la dégénérescence hépatolenticulaire: essai sur la signification. Rev. Neurol. **117**:391-409.

Clark, W. E. Le G., and Meyer, M. 1950. Anatomical relationships between the cerebral cortex and the hypothalamus. Brit. Med. Bull. **6**:341-345.

Clark, W. E. Le G., and Russell, W. R. 1938. Cortical deafness without aphasia. Brain **61**: 375-383.

Collins, G. H., Victor, M., and Adams, R. D. 1961. A neuropathological study of Wernicke's disease and Korsakoff's psychosis. J. Neuropath. Exp. Neurol. **20**:289-291.

Cox, L. B. 1937. Tumours of the base of the brain: their relation to pathological sleep and other changes in the conscious state. Med. J. Aust. **1**:742-752.

Cravioto, H., Silberman, J., and Feigin, I. 1960. A clinical and pathologic study of akinetic mutism. Neurology **10**:10-21.

Critchley, M. 1962. Periodic hypersomnia and megaphagia in adolescent males. Brain **85**:627-656.

Critchley, M., and Hoffman, H. L. 1942. Syndrome of periodic somnolence and morbid hunger (Kleine-Levin syndrome). Brit. Med. J. **1**:137-139.

Crosby, E. C., Humphrey, T., and Lauer, E. W. 1962. Correlative anatomy of the nervous system. New York, The Macmillan Company.

Crosby, E. C., Humphrey, T., and Showers, M. J. 1959. Einige Anordnungen, Verbindungen und Funktionen der supplementären motorischen Rinden. In Bauer, K. F., editor: Medizinische Grundlagenforschung, vol. 2. Stuttgart, Georg Thieme Verlag, pp. 101-124.

Cushing, H. 1932. Intracranial tumors: notes upon a series of two thousand verified cases. Springfield, Illinois, Charles C Thomas, Publisher.

Dejerine, J. 1895. Anatomie des centres nerveux, vol. 2. Paris, Rueff.

de Jong, H. H. 1945. Experimental catatonia: a general reaction-form of the central nervous system and its implications for human pathology. Baltimore, The Williams & Wilkins Co.

DeJong, R. N., Itabashi, H. H., and Olson, J. R. 1969. Memory loss due to hippocampal lesions: report of a case. Arch. Neurol. **20**:339-348.

Delay, J., Brion, S., and Elissalde, B. 1958. Corps mamillares et syndrome de Korsakoff: étude anatomique de huit cas de syndrome de Korsakoff d'origin alcoolique sans altération significative du cortex cérébral. Presse Méd. **66**: 1849-1852, 1965-1968.

de Wardener, H. E., and Lennox, B. 1947. Cerebral beriberi (Wernicke's encephalopathy): review of 52 cases in a Singapore prisoner-of-war hospital. Lancet **1**:11-17.

Dimsdale, H., Logue, V., and Pierey, M. 1964. A case of persisting impairment of recent memory following right temporal lobectomy. Neuropsychologia **1**:287-298.

Dott, N. M. 1938. Surgical aspects of the hypothalamus. In Clark, W. E. Le G., and others: The hypothalamus. Edinburgh, Oliver & Boyd Ltd., pp. 131-185.

Earle, K. M., Baldwin, M., and Penfield, W. 1953. Incisural sclerosis and temporal lobe seizures produced by hippocampal herniation at birth. Arch. Neurol. Psychiat. **69**:27-42.

Eccles, J. C. 1966. Conscious experience and memory. In Eccles, J. C., editor: Brain and conscious experience. New York, Springer Publishing Co., Inc., pp. 314-344.

Elsberg, C. A., and Levy, I. 1935. Sense of smell: new and simple method of quantitative olfactometry. Bull. Neurol. Inst. New York **4**:5-19.

Erickson, T. C. 1945. Erotomania (nymphomania) as an expression of cortical epileptiform discharge. Arch. Neurol. Psychiat. **53**:226-231.

Faris, A. A. 1969. Limbic system infarction: a report of two cases. Neurology **19**:91-96.

Frantzen, E. 1966. Wernicke's encephalopathy: 3 cases occurring in connection with severe malnutrition. Acta Neurol. Scand. **42**:426-441.

Frazier, C. H. 1936. Tumor involving the frontal lobe alone: a symptomatic survey of one hundred and five verified cases. Arch. Neurol. Psychiat. **35**:525-571.

Frazier, C. H., and Rowe, S. N. 1934. Certain observations upon localization in fifty-one verified tumors of the temporal lobe. Res. Publ. Ass. Res. Nerv. Ment. Dis., Proc. **13**:251-258.

French, J. D. 1952. Brain lesions associated with prolonged unconsciousness. Arch. Neurol. Psychiat. **68**:727-740.

Freytag, E., and Lindenberg, R. 1964. 294 medicolegal autopsies on epileptics: cerebral findings. Arch. Path. **78**:274-286.

Gagel, O. 1936. Symptomatologie der Erkrankungen des Hypothalamus. In Bumke, O., and Foerster, O., editors: Handbuch der Neurologie **5**:482-522.

Gallinek, A. 1967. The Kleine-Levin syndrome. Dis. Nerv. System **28**:448-451.

Gastaut, H., and Collomb, H. 1954. Étude du comportement sexuel chez les épileptiques psychomoteurs. Ann. Médicopsychol. **112**:657-696.

Geschwind, N. 1965. Disconnexion syndromes in animals and man. Brain **88**:237-294, 585-644.

Gilbert, G. J. 1964. Periodic hypersomnia and bulimia: the Kleine-Levin syndrome. Neurology **14**:844-850.

Gol, A., and Faibish, G. M. 1967. Effects of human hippocampal ablation. J. Neurosurg. **26**: 390-398.

Goldberg, M. F., Payne, J. W., and Brunt, P. W. 1968. Ophthalmologic studies of familial dysautonomia: the Riley-Day syndrome. Arch. Ophthal. **80**:732-743.

Gooddy, W. 1956. Cerebral representation. Brain **79**:167-187.

Gorman, W. 1964. The sense of smell: a clinical review. EENT Monthly **43**:54-58.

Guerrant, J., Anderson, W. W., Fischer, A., Weinstein, M. R., Jaros, R. M., and Deskins, A. 1962. Personality in epilepsy. Springfield, Illinois, Charles C Thomas, Publisher.

Halpern, L. 1952. Secondary disturbances of perception. J. Nerv. Ment. Dis. **116**:783-788.

Haymaker, W. 1949. Herpes simplex encephalitis in man. J. Neuropath. Exp. Neurol. **8**:132-154.

Haymaker, W., Pentschew, A., Margoles, C., and Bingham, W. G. 1958. Occurrence of lesions in the temporal lobe in the absence of convulsive seizures: with especial reference to the hippocampus, amygdala, and anterior perforated substance. In Baldwin, M., and Bailey, P., editors: Temporal lobe epilepsy. Springfield, Illinois, Charles C Thomas, Publisher, pp. 166-202.

Himwich, H. E. 1958. Psychopharmacologic drugs. Science **127**:59-72.

Ingram, W. R., Barris, R. W., and Ranson, S. W. 1936. Catalepsy: an experimental study. Arch. Neurol. Psychiat. **35**:1175-1197.

Jackson, J. H. 1890. Case of tumour of the right temporosphenoidal lobe bearing on the localization of the sense of smell and on the interpretation of a particular variety of epilepsy. Brain **12**:346-357.

Jackson, J. H. 1931. Selected writings, edited by J. Taylor, vol. 1. London, Hodder & Stoughton Ltd., pp. 385-473.

Kelemen, G. 1968. Familial dysautonomia (Riley-Day): aural histopathology. Pract. Oto-Rhino-Laryng. **30**:194-200.

Kemper, T. L., and Romanul, F. C. A. 1967. State resembling akinetic mutism in basilar artery occlusion. Neurology **17**:74-80.

Kepes, J. J., Reece, C. A., and Oxley, D. K. 1965. Central pontine myelinolysis in a 7-year-old boy. J. Neurol. Neurosurg. Psychiat. **28**:39-47.

Keschner, M., Bender, M. B., and Strauss, I. 1936. Mental symptoms in cases of tumor of the temporal lobe. Arch. Neurol. Psychiat. **35**: 572-596.

Klee, A. 1961. Akinetic mutism: review of the literature and report of a case. J. Nerv. Ment. Dis. **133**:536-553.

Kleine, W. 1925. Periodische Schlafsucht. Monatschr. Psychiat. **57**:285-320.

Kleist, K. 1934. Gehirnpathologie. Leipzig, Barth, pp. 1159 *et seq.*

Klüver, H., and Bucy, P. C. 1939. Preliminary analysis of functions of the temporal lobes in monkeys. Arch. Neurol. Psychiat. **42**:979-1000.

Környey, S. 1967. Geschwulst des Hirnstammes mit der Symptomatologie des Wernicke-Korsakow-Prozesses. In Zukunft der Neurologie. Stuttgart, Thieme, pp. 157-168.

Lashley, K. S. 1938. Factors limiting recovery after central nervous lesions. J. Nerv. Ment. Dis. **88**:733-755.

Levin, M. 1936. Periodic somnolence and morbid hunger: a new syndrome. Brain **59**:494-504.

Lhermitte, F., Gautier, J. C., Marteau, R., and Chain, F. 1963. Troubles de la conscience et mutisme akinétique: étude anatomo-clinique d'un ramollissement paramédian, bilatéral, du pédoncule cérébral et du thalamus. Rev. Neurol. **2**:115-131.

Linde, L. M., and Westover, J. L. 1962. Esophageal and gastric abnormalities in dysautonomia. Pediatrics **29**:303-306.

Lindqvist, G., and Norlén, G. 1966. Korsakoff's syndrome after operation on ruptured aneurysm of the anterior communicating artery. Acta Psychiat. Scand. **42**:24-34.

Locke, S. 1967. Thalamic connections to insular and opercular cortex of monkey. J. Comp. Neurol. **129**:219-240.

Lopez, R. I., and Collins, G. H. 1968. Wernicke's encephalopathy. Arch. Neurol. **18**:248-259.

Malamud, N. 1967. Psychiatric disorder with intracranial tumors of limbic system. Arch. Neurol. **17**:113-123.

Malamud, N., and Skillicorn, S. A. 1956. Relationship between the Wernicke and the Korsakoff syndrome. A.M.A. Arch. Neurol. Psychiat. **76**:585-596.

Meissner, W. W. 1967. Memory function in the Korsakoff syndrome. J. Nerv. Ment. Dis. **145**: 106-122.

Messer, B., Henke, T. K., and Langheim, W. 1966. Syndrome of akinetic mutism associated with obstructive hydrocephalus. Neurology **16**: 635-649.

Meyer, A. 1957. Hippocampal lesions in epilepsy. In Williams, D., editor: Modern trends in neurology. New York, Harper & Row, Publishers, ser. 2, pp. 301-316.

Milner, B., and Penfield, W. 1955. The effect of hippocampal lesion on recent memory. Trans. Amer. Neurol. Ass. **80**:42-48.

Moore, M. T. 1952. Within the realm of epilepsy. J. Nerv. Ment. Dis. **116**:841-861.

Moore, M. T. 1969. Progressive akinetic mutism in cerebellar hemangioblastoma with "normal-pressure hydrocephalus." Neurology **19**:32-36.

Narabayashi, H., Nagao, T., Saito, Y., Yoshida, M., and Nagahata, M. 1963. Stereotaxic amygdalotomy for behavior disorders. Arch. Neurol. **9**:1-16.

Nauta, W. J. H. 1962. Neural associations of the amygdaloid complex in the monkey. Brain **85**: 505-519.

Nauta, W. J. H. 1963. Central nervous organization and the endocrine motor system. In Nalbandov, A. V., editor: Advances in neuroendocrinology. Urbana, University of Illinois Press, pp. 5-28.

Nauta, W. J. H. 1964. Some afferent connections of the prefrontal cortex in the monkey. In Warren, J. M., and Akert, K., editors: The frontal granular cortex and behavior. New York, McGraw-Hill Book Company, pp. 397-409.

Nauta, W. J. H., and Haymaker, W. 1969. Hypothalamic nuclei and fiber connections. In Haymaker, W., Anderson, E., and Nauta, W. J. H., editors: The hypothalamus. Springfield, Illinois, Charles C Thomas, Publisher, pp. 136-209.

Nelson, E., and Haymaker, W. 1957. Colloid cyst of the third ventricle: report of three fatal cases. J. Aviation Med. **28**:356-363.

Neumann, M. A., and Cohn, R. 1965. The neurology of reticular formation apoplexy. Arch. Neurobiol. (Madrid) **28**:725-752.

Ogata, J., Fukiyama, K., and Iwata, Y. 1966. Akinetic mutism in extensive cerebral softenings: clinical and pathological observations. Clin. Neurol. (Tokyo) **6**:125-130.

Orthner, H., and Rettinger, E. 1965. Ein intraventrikuläres Kraniopharyngeom, zugleich ein Beitrag zum hypothalamisch auslösbaren Störüngen der Merkfähigkeit und des Trieblebens bei Mensch und Tier. Ftschr. Neurol. Psychiat. **33**:299-331.

Ostow, M. 1952. Psychodynamic disturbances in patients with temporal lobe disorders. Trans. Amer. Neurol. Ass. **77**:79-83.

Paillas, J. E., Piganiol, G., and Bonnet, J. 1956. Séméiologie cochléovestibulaire après lobectomie temporale (étude de 25 épileptiques opérés). Rev. Neurol. **94**:281-283.

Papez, J. W. 1937. A proposed mechanism of emotion. Arch. Neurol. Psychiat. **38**:725-743.

Patton, H. D., Ruch, T. C., and Walker, A. E. 1944. Experimental hypogeusia from Horsley-Clarke lesions of thalamus in Macaca mulatta. J. Neurophysiol. **7**:171-184.

Penfield, W. 1929. Diencephalic autonomic epilepsy. Arch. Neurol. Psychiat. **22**:358-374.

Penfield, W. 1950. Observations on anatomy of memory. Folia Psychiat. Neurol. Neurochir. Neerl. **53**:349-351.

Penfield, W. 1952. Symposium on brain and mind: memory mechanisms. A.M.A. Arch. Neurol. Psychiat. **67**:178-191.

Penfield, W. 1955. The role of the temporal cortex in certain psychical phenomena. J. Ment. Sci. **101**:451-456.

Penfield, W. 1957. Vestibular sensation and the cerebral cortex. Ann. Otol. **66**:691-699.

Penfield, W. 1967. Epilepsy, the great teacher: the progress of one pupil. Acta Neurol. Scand. **43**:1-10.

Penfield, W., and Jasper, H. 1954. Epilepsy and the functional anatomy of the human brain. Boston, Little, Brown and Company.

Penfield, W., and Milner, B. 1958. Memory deficit produced by bilateral lesions in the hippocampal zone. Arch. Neurol. Psychiat. **79**: 475-497.

Pilleri, G. 1966. The Klüver-Bucy syndrome in man: a clinico-anatomical contribution to the function of medial temporal lobe structures. Psychiat. Neurol. (Basel) **152**:65-103.

Plum, F., and Posner, J. B. 1966. Diagnosis of stupor and coma. Philadelphia, F. A. Davis Co.

Rámon-Moliner, E., and Nauta, W. J. H. 1966. The isodendritic core of the brain stem. J. Comp. Neurol. **126**:311-335.

Richardson, T. F., and Winokur, G. 1967. Déjà vu in psychiatric and neurosurgical patients. Arch. Gen. Psychiat. **17**:622-625.

Riese, W. 1967. Changing concepts of cerebral localization. Clio Med. **2**:189-230.

Riley, C. M., Day, R. L., Greeley, D. M., and Langford, W. S. 1949. Central autonomic dysfunction with defective lacrimation: report of 5 cases. Pediatrics **3**:468-478.

Riley, C. M., and Moore, R. H. 1966. Familial dysautonomia differentiated from related disorders. Pediatrics **37**:435-446.

Ronald, J. 1946. Hypersomnia associated with abnormal hunger: the Kleine-Levin syndrome. Brit. Med. J. **2**:326-327.

Sano, K., and Malamud, N. 1953. Clinical significance of sclerosis of the cornu Ammonis (ictal "psychic phenomena"). A.M.A. Arch. Neurol. Psychiat. **70**:40-53.

Schneider, R. A. 1967. The sense of smell in man—its physiological basis. New Eng. J. Med. **277**:293-303.

Schneider, R. C., Calhoun, H. D., and Crosby, E. C. 1968. Vertigo and rotational movement in cortical and subcortical lesions. J. Neurol. Sci. **6**:493-516.

Schneider, R. C., Crosby, E. C., Bagchi, B. K., and Calhoun, H. D. 1961. Temporal or occipital lobe hallucinations triggered from frontal lobe lesions. Neurology **11**:172-179.

Schwarz, G. A. 1967. The orthostatic hypotension syndrome of Shy-Drager: a clinicopathologic report. Arch. Neurol. **16**:123-139.

Scoville, W. B., and Milner, B. 1957. Loss of recent memory after bilateral hippocampal lesions. J. Neurol. Neurosurg. Psychiat. **20**:11-21.

Shenkin, H. A., and Lewey, F. H. 1943. Aura of taste preceding convulsions associated with a lesion of the parietal operculum: report of a case. Arch. Neurol. Psychiat. **50**:375-378.

Shinebourne, E., Sneddon, J. M., and Turner, P. 1967. Evidence for autonomic denervation in familial dysautonomia, the Riley-Day syndrome. Brit. Med. J. **4**:91-92.

Shiraki, H. 1968. Comparative neuropathologic study of Wilson's disease and other types of hepatocerebral disease. In Bergsma, D., editor: Wilson's disease. New York, National Foundation–March of Dimes, pp. 64-73.

Shy, G. M., and Drager, G. A. 1960. A neurological syndrome associated with orthostatic hypertension: a clinico-pathologic study. A.M.A. Arch. Path. **2**:520-527.

Sjöqvist, O. 1941. Hypothalamic discharge and its relation to epilepsy: with the report of a case of "sham rage" in man with surgical verification. Acta Chir. Scand. **85**:235-247.

Skultety, F. M. 1968. Clinical and experimental aspects of akinetic mutism: report of a case. Arch. Neurol. **19**:1-14.

Smith, A. A., and Dancis, J. 1964. Exaggerated response to infused norepinephrine in familial dysautonomia. New Eng. J. Med. **270**:704-707.

Smith, A. A., Dancis, J., and Breinin, G. 1965. Ocular responses to autonomic drugs in familial dysautonomia. Invest. Ophthal. **4**:358-361.

Spatz, H. 1966. Gehirnentwicklung (Introversion-Promination) und Endocranialausguss. In Hassler, R., and Stephan, H., editors: Evolution of the forebrain: phylogenesis and ontogenesis of the forebrain. Stuttgart, Georg Thieme Verlag, pp. 136-152.

Spector, M. 1967. Dizziness and vertigo. New York, Grune & Stratton, Inc.

Spiegel, E. A., and Alexander, A. 1936. Vertigo in brain tumors, with special reference to the results of labyrinth examination. Ann. Otol. **45**: 979-987.

Strobos, R. R. J. 1953. Tumors of the temporal lobe. Neurology **3**:752-760.

Sumner, D. 1964. Post-traumatic anosmia. Brain **87**:107-120.

Sweet, W. H., Talland, G. A., and Erwin, F. R. 1959. Loss of recent memory following section of fornix. Trans. Amer. Neurol. Ass. **84**: 76-82.

Symonds, C. 1962. Concussion and its sequelae. Lancet **1**:1-5.

Szentágothai, J., Flerkó, B., Mess, B., and Halász, B. 1968. Hypothalamic control of the anterior pituitary: an experimental-morphological study, ed. 3. Budapest, Akadémiai Kiadó, p. 56.

Talland, G. A., Sweet, W. H., and Ballantine, H. T. 1967. Amnesic syndrome with anterior communicating aneurysm. J. Nerv. Ment. Dis. **145**: 179-192.

Taren, J. A. 1965. Anatomical pathways related to the clinical findings in aneurysms of the anterior communicating artery. J. Neurol. Neurosurg. Psychiat. **28**:228-234.

Terzian, H., and Ore, G. D. 1955. Syndrome of Klüver and Bucy reproduced in man by bilateral removal of the temporal lobes. Neurology **5**:373-380.

Tucker, D., and Biedler, L. M. 1956. Autonomic nervous system influence on olfactory receptors. Amer. J. Physiol. **187**:637.

Ule, G., Döhner, W., and Bues, E. 1961. Ausgedehnte Hemisphärenmarkschädigung nach Hirntrauma mit apallischem Syndrom und partieller Späthabilitation. Arch. Psychiat. Nervenkr. **202**: 155-176.

Uyematsu, S. 1921. A study of the cortical olfactory center, based on two cases of unilateral involvement of the olfactory lobe. Arch. Neurol. Psychiat. **6**:146-156.

Varela, J. M. 1967. Atrophie systématisée globale de la formation réticulaire: syndrome de dyshoméostasie du névraxe. Rev. Neurol. **1**:437-440.

Victor, M., and Adams, R. D. 1953. The effect of alcohol on the nervous system. Res. Publ. Ass. Res. Nerv. Ment. Dis., Proc. **32**:526-573.

Victor, M., and Yakovlev, P. I. 1955. S. S. Korsakoff's psychic disorder in conjunction with peripheral neuritis: a translation of Korsakoff's original article with brief comments on the author and his contribution to clinical medicine. Neurology **5**:394-406.

von Wowern, F. 1966. Posttraumatic amnesia and confusion as an index of severity in head injury. Acta Neurol. Scand. **42**:373-378.

Votaw, C. L. 1960. Certain functional and anatomical relations of the cornu ammonis of the macaque monkey: anatomical relations. J. Comp. Neurol. **114**:283-293.

Walker, E. A. 1961. Murder or epilepsy? J. Nerv. Ment. Dis. **133**:430-437.

Wall, P. D., Glees, P., and Fulton, J. F. 1951. Corticofugal connections of posterior orbital surface in rhesus monkey. Brain **74**:66-71.

Willanger, R. 1966. The amnestic syndrome in the early phase of Wernicke's encephalopathy. Acta Neurol. Scand. **42**:442-454.

Williams, D. 1968. Man's temporal lobe. Brain **91**:639-654.

Williams, D., and Parsons-Smith, G. 1951. Thalamic activity in stupor. Brain **74**:377-398.

Wortis, H., and Maurer, W. S. 1942. "Sham-rage" in man. Amer. J. Psychiat. **98**:638-644.

Yakovlev, P. I. 1948. Motility, behavior and the brain: stereodynamic organization and neural co-ordinates of behavior. J. Nerv. Ment. Dis. **107**:313-335.

Yenermen, M. H., Bowerman, C. I., and Haymaker, W. 1958. Colloid cyst of the third ventricle: a clinical study of 54 cases in the light of previous publications. Acta Neuroveg. **17**: 211-277.

Chapter 23

Dysarthria, aphasia, and apraxia

Francis Schiller

Although first in the line of valid cortical localizations ever made (Broca, 1961), speech is not an elementary function. Speaking is an acquired social skill—the skill to handle an ethnically shared property called language. Everybody acquires it for himself in a gradual way from the second year of life on. Hence we are able to correlate speech to cerebral structure even less closely than simpler performances laid down at an earlier phylogenetic and ontogenetic stage (kinesthesis, sight, or even walking). Localization is further hampered by the immensely complex, multilevelled feedback that comes into play when we speak, both with a healthy and with a diseased sensorimotor system (Goldstein, 1948; Luria, 1966). Indeed, we do not localize language in a lobe, or grammar in a gyrus, or a noun in a neuron.

Disease, nevertheless, produces several notorious clinical signs that allow us to determine the approximate site at which the neuronal or muscular mechanism has broken down. The three most distinctive of these clinical features—clusters, rather, or breaks in a continuous chain of failure—are *dysarthria, aphasia,* and *dementia.*

DYSARTHRIA

Dysarthric speech is indistinct through lack of phonetic precision and because of slurring, "scanning," and poor "resolution" of speech sounds. The pronunciation of phonemes is at fault, not the vocabulary of morphemes and semantemes. Articulation suffers; so also do rhythm, phonetic stress, and variety of pitch or inflection. All this leads to monotony.

Tongue-twisters ("methodist episcopal"), or fast alternating movements of the tongue ("la-la-la-la"), the lips ("ba-ba-ba-ba"), and the jaw muscles ("ga-ga-ga-ga") reveal some of this inadequacy. Cerebellar, corticobulbar, and striatal (supranuclear and bilateral) pathways are disrupted; their disruption is usually corroborated by the associated clinical evidence. Inspecting the peripheral speech organs one finds the cause for the nasal and other abnormal speech sounds that match the lower motor neuron or the muscular lesions.

Dysarthric or anarthric disturbances of articulation may, however, result from cortical lesions. This poses a problem in localization and the diagnosis of aphasia.

APHASIA

The oldest, the most fundamental, and the least contested fact about aphasia is its association with the left hemisphere (Joynt and Benton, 1964). It has led to the concept of *hemispheric dominance,* or functional asymmetry of the human brain, the distinction between a "major" and a "minor" hemisphere. Asymmetry presents a biological exception in man. The sensorimotor framework of vertebrates is organized on strictly symmetrical bilaterally equivalent lines, where unity between right and left is achieved by an extensive commissural arrangement. (Sever optic chiasm and corpus callosum by a sagittal cut: each half of this animal's "split-brain" now learns new performances and uses old tracts independently and without the benefit of the other—Sperry, 1961.) In right-handed man it can be demonstrated that section of the cerebral commissures denies to the left hemisphere, when suitably tested, the information gathered by the left hand and the left visual field. In this experimental situation only, with stimuli reaching only the minor hemisphere, the subject has a nominal aphasia (see p. 399); but comprehension by the minor hemisphere is not found to be totally abolished (Gazzaniga and Sperry, 1967). Human speech favors the left hemisphere, handedness the right hand. Implicit in the term "sinistrality" is the popular tradition that what is not right must be gauche and most likely is also wrong. Some of this ancient prejudice is based on biological fact; eloquence is verbal dexterity in every respect. Exceptions to this rule are rather uncommon. For in the majority of left-handed people not the right but again the left hemisphere exerts dominance for speech, the right remaining the "minor" one that takes its cues from the left (Hécaen and Ajuriaguerria, 1964; Mountcastle, 1962; Penfield and Roberts, 1959; Zangwill, 1960). This is true for the adult trained brain of the left-handed or ambidextrous subject, but it is not true in the small child. If his left hemisphere is severely damaged before speech has been developed, right hemisphere dominance will result. A corollary is the relatively fast and complete recovery from aphasia acquired before the age of 10 years; here, too, the right hemisphere "takes over" (Guttmann, 1942). The problem of congenital reading disability—*developmental dyslexia*—is presumably tied to cerebral right-left ambivalence and failure to establish dominance. So far no pathoanatomical basis for it has been found. The ambidextrous or left-handed as a group are, of course, far from being poor readers (Critchley, 1964; Hermann, 1959; Orton, 1937).

Aside from clinicopathological proof and correlations made in surgical excisions (Penfield and Roberts, 1959), dominance may be tested in any individual case by injecting sodium amytal into each carotid artery in turn. The side on which transient aphasia results is so proved to be dominant (Wada, 1949).

Right as well as left hemisphere lesions may cause musical capabilities to suffer *(amusia)* (Brain, 1965). By and large, the influence of the right parietal lobe is confined to the opposite (left) intracorporeal and extracorporeal space, while the left plays a more general and bilateral role (Hécaen and Ajuriaguerria, 1964).

Types of aphasia and their localization

Speaking is a mode of expression; like gesture it is a motor act (to talk of "sensory speech," normal or disturbed, does not sound logical). But as speaking implies understanding, it is also a sensory process. For this reason—and others that are historical, anatomical, practical, and controversial—aphasic disorders have been divided into *expressive* or motor and *receptive* or sensory. Areas involved are indicated in Fig. 23-1.

Motor aphasia. Originally called *aphemia* by Broca (1861), motor aphasia combines, in various degrees, *dysarthria* (anarthria when severe*) with the reduced drive to communicate, and the unavailability of the desired words. When urged to speak, the patient cannot form his words *(verbal aphasia)* (Head, 1926). Worse, he cannot find them, and so they may be reduced to a minimum of phrases, syllables, expletives, or grunts. In the test situation, the aphasic's inability to name the objects shown has been variously

***Dys*phasia and *dys*lexia are terms correspondingly used to denote lesser degrees.

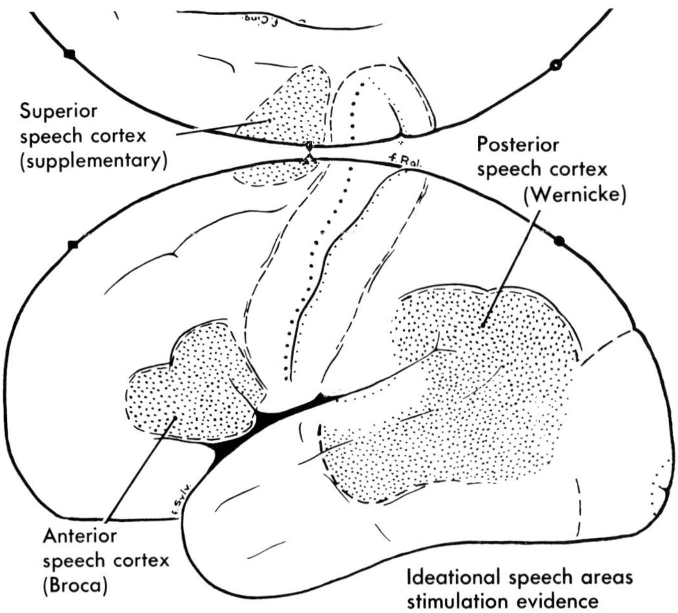

Fig. 23-1. Areas of cortex in the dominant hemisphere normally concerned in the ideational elaboration of speech, derived by electrical speech mapping. Almost identical maps were obtained from studies of the effects of cortical ablations. (From Penfield and Roberts, 1959.)

called *nominal (anomia), central,* and *amnesic.* All three terms were ostensibly coined to get at the core and essence of aphasia which, in simple terms, is a defective memory for words. Unfortunately for the schematist and localizer, expressive and receptive aphasia share this lack of appropriate recall (Schiller, 1947). "Central aphasia" is used in this way, and in others (Geschwind, 1965).

Anterior or Broca's area. The type of aphasia just described is associated with lesions of the hind end of the left third frontal convolution and the frontal operculum (Brodmann's area 44). Penfield's term "speech arrest," caused by galvanic stimulation of this area, includes all these shortcomings (Penfield and Roberts, 1959).

Precentral gyrus. A lesion or galvanic stimulation of the lower third of the left somatomotor area, lying just posterior to Broca's, produces anarthria. The same lesion on the right side may, in the ambidextrous or left-handed, have a similar result. There is a contralateral lower facial weakness, and rarely, weakness of tongue and palate.

Supplementary motor area. Speech arrest has been observed upon stimulation of area 6; other evidence for an aphasic center here is scanty (Penfield and Roberts, 1959; Petit-Dutaillis and others, 1954).

Sensory aphasia. There are two helpful negative aspects to this variety in distinguishing it at once from motor aphasia: the absence of dysarthria and the lack of reticence. What garbled words this kind of patient has are fluently pronounced. In some extreme instances there is even a vast stream of well-produced, well-inflected, and well-rhythmed utterances. But these—and here lies the positive aspect of sensory aphasia—tend to be imprecise, circumlocutory, metonymous, or even entirely devoid of the desired meaning. On this scale of disintegration we get either correct but misused items of the language (malapropisms) or neoformations of the patient's own making (jargon). Between these two poles of misuse lies the substitution of a word by another member of its phonetic or semantic class, a word replaced by one with a similar sound or meaning (Kussmaul, 1877; Lotmar, 1919-20; Weisenburg and McBride, 1935). This is *paraphasia;* in its most elementary manifestation ("pledger" for "pleasure") it is merely a high degree of dysarthria. Much of what is said to these patients falls on deaf ears; questions and requests of increasing complexity remain increasingly unrequited. Their lost ability for decoding auditory symbols may extend to the incomprehension of other meaningful noises; *word-deafness* may extend to *psychic deafness* or *auditory agnosia.* The loss of "memory" for what sounds—especially phonemes—really mean may well be at the root of the patient's inability to instill his own copious utterances with the appropriate meaning of words, or to monitor them while he speaks. (In like manner the motor aphasic may be said to have forgotten how to produce words.)

Posterior or Wernicke's area. The posterior end of the first temporal convolution (area 22) is the focal point for what goes by the name of "sensory aphasia" (Wernicke, 1874). The adjacent temporal, parietal, and occipital areas and the supramarginal and angular gyri tend to be involved functionally and anatomically. Agraphia and alexia are frequently associated with such lesions, as well as right-left confusion and finger-agnosia, in various combinations (Benton, 1959; Gerstmann, 1940).

Agraphia and alexia. For the literate, language also means written or printed communication. All western and some non-western script is a notation corresponding more or less fully to the phonetic pattern of spoken words. In our minds these auditory symbols very closely duplicate their visual counterparts. The translation from one into the other is likewise divided into a motor act: writing (involving the hand), and its sensory complement, reading (involving visual perception). Their respective disturbances are called *agraphia* and *alexia.* (The examiner of an aphasic disorder is always equipped with pencil and paper and a small printed text.)

Subcortical lesions of the dominant hemisphere

It is quite rare that a patient who is not otherwise dysphasic or mentally disturbed displays a rather isolated or "pure" defect. This may be *word-blindness,* or the inability to repeat words and phrases, or, on the contrary, the compulsion to repeat utterances made by himself or others (*palilalia* and *echolalia*). These and similarly isolated abnormalities have suggested to several authors, especially before the neuron theory was established, what is variously called a *conduction* aphasia or a *disconnection* syndrome. The idea here is that not cortical areas but their subcortical connections are damaged and that bits of functioning cortex have become isolated from the rest. (For a recent discussion, see Brain, 1965, and Geschwind, 1965.) It is questionable, however, whether lesions of cell bodies (gray matter) differ in their effect from lesions of axis cylinders (white matter) and whether there can be destruction anywhere without isolation of the neighboring areas.

Thalamocortical connections explain the arrest as well as the acceleration of speech; both of these have been observed in stereotaxic galvanic stimulation of the ventrolateral thalamus (Guiot and others, 1961), and after thalamotomy (Bell, 1968).

Size of the lesion is important. Small lesions produce minor disturbances. These take the character of the closest elementary projection area or "analyser," to use Pavlov's term (Luria, 1966). Motor defects will thus be found with lesions close to the motor area—sensory defects of the corresponding type with lesions close to where the tactile, auditory, and visual cortex meet (Freud, 1953). The areas in question are included in the territory of the middle cerebral artery: in short, around the Sylvian fissure, more particularly at its anterior superior end, and around its posterior termination. Considering this close mutual relationship it is therefore not surprising to find frequently together, in lesions of some magnitude, both defective speaking and understanding, the two components mixed in various degree *(global aphasia)* (Schiller, 1947). Rarely, however, does the severity of sensory aphasia equal that of the expressive kind; patients who can *say* nothing are common, those who can *understand* nothing are very rare. *Total aphasia*—the complete breakdown of communication—does occur in conscious patients; it is usually due to extensive destruction of brain substance. In such cases the overall intellectual deficit is as a rule considerable. The bulk of tissue destroyed is an important, if not the only, factor in assessing the extent of present and future disability.

Distinguishing features—aphasia and dementia

Intelligence and speech are not identical. Nor are they quite independent. The interchanges between thought and its formulation, even between the internal and external kind of formulation, are subtle and extensive (Vygotsky, 1962); any major disruption in one sphere will be noticeable in the other.

The minds of aphasic patients "limp" (Trousseau, 1865) to varying degrees. Foresight, decision making, judging the effect of one's action, and making efficient use of past experience are in abeyance. Another aspect the aphasic shares with the extensively brain-damaged person's behavior is *perseveration*. A patient perseverates by repeating the same task against the challenge of a new demand; inertly he gets stuck in a groove (Denny-Brown, 1958). This may be failure of inhibition, as is lewd behavior and loose talk, a general disregard for what is nice and appropriate and becoming—including *Witzelsucht (moria)*—or excessive euphoria, seen in frontal and sometimes in temporal lobe lesions. Parietal lobe lesions cause a more or less isolated unlearning of numerical operations: *acalculia*, a congener of sensory aphasia; alexia; and the failure to handle what is not obviously inherent in the present situation or context, "abstract," and without immediate application (Goldstein, 1948). But "concrete behavior" of this sort is not necessarily the outcome of damage of this or that cerebral lobe (Keschner, Bender, and Strauss, 1936). For the untrained observer (and sometimes for the trained) it may be hard to decide whether any given patient with gross behavioral breakdown has merely lost the means of verbal communication and perhaps some other special skill; or whether, in fact, he is a "case" of general dementia. In another instance a sensory aphasic may become agitated and so appear psychotic merely because he cannot grasp the reason why he cannot make himself understood. His motor counterpart is often a person who has no initiative, is withdrawn, and is depressed (Frazier, 1936). More important is the reverse observation where aphasic manifestations form part of a widespread organic dementia and large sectors of judgment and memory are defective (senile and presenile dementia, post-ictal states). Clinical judgment is guided by the relative preponderance of symptoms.

Finally, there are mental retardation and the nonorganic psychiatric disorders such as schizophrenia, depression, and that more doubtful entity, hysteria: all these may affect speech. Schizophrenia produces "word-salad" (associated with other elements of bizarre behavior); in any of the other conditions the withdrawal symptom of *mutism* may be exhibited. An organic form of mutism (total absence of speech without accompanying hemiplegia on the dominant side) also should be distinguished from total aphasia. The distinction is given by the patient's total inactivity *(akinetic mutism)* (Cairns and others, 1941); in some instances it results from midline lesions affecting the hypothalamus (craniopharyngioma), in others from lesions affecting the basal ganglia (in advanced parkinsonism). The subject is handled further in Chapter 22.

APRAXIA

Motor aphasia and agraphia have been called "apraxia"; their counterparts, sensory aphasia and alexia, have been called "agnosia" (Bing, 1910; Wilson, 1920). Apraxia in the narrower definition is the inability to perform skilled movements (other than speech), where no motor, sensory, ataxic, or extensive mental disturbance is detectable (Denny-Brown, 1958; Liepmann, 1900). There are degrees of this disability, possibly also gradations from motor to sensory, which imply differences in the site of the responsible lesion. Simple clumsiness is associated with the precentral and postcentral areas for the opposite hand and/or foot. The *grasp reflex,* normal from the third to sixth month of life onward ("grasping" is a mass reflex up to that time; see p. 329), is observed in deep-seated *frontal lobe* lesions, usually affecting the opposite hand, which compulsively closes down on any stimulus applied to the palm (Schuster and Pinéas, 1926). A similar pathological phenomenon, but also normal in the infant, may be observed in the foot (Brain and Curran, 1932); it may also be seen in the jaws that shut tight on any object placed between them ("bulldog phenomenon"). All these phenomena may be a form of perseveration due to frontal lobe damage; catatonic posturing and ataxia of gait under these circumstances may be similarly caused. All this may be summarily referred to as *kinetic apraxia* (Denny-Brown, 1958).

Lesions of either *parietal lobe* interfere with orientation, hence with performance in space and with the ability to put things together in a sequential, orderly, and meaningful way. Stepwise assembly may fail in producing words and other desired patterns with a pencil on paper, in building with toy blocks *(constructional apraxia),* or in putting on one's clothes. The latter, *apraxia for dressing,* may affect one side of the body only, the side (opposite the lesion) of which the patient has become unaware; it is usually the left (Brain, 1965; Critchley, 1953). The subtle role of the corpus callosum claimed for ideomotor apraxia is not supported by neurosurgical evidence (Akelaitis, 1944; Akelaitis and others, 1942).

Ideational apraxia, effected by left parietal lesions, is the patient's failure to initiate or imitate such performances as waving good-bye, threading a needle, or lighting a match, out of their natural context, and sometimes even within it. The relationship is obviously one to gyrus supramarginalis and angularis anatomically; and to writing, reading, arithmetic, or formulating concepts, functionally.

REFERENCES

Akelaitis, A. J. 1944. A study of gnosis, praxis and language following section of the corpus callosum and anterior commissure. J. Neurosurg. **1**:94-102.

Akelaitis, A. J., Risteen, W. A., Herren, R. Y., and Van Wagenen, W. P. 1942. Studies on the corpus callosum: a contribution to the study of dyspraxia and apraxia following partial and complete section of the corpus callosum. Arch. Neurol. Psychiat. **47**:971-1008.

Bell, D. S. 1968. Speech functions of the thalamus inferred from the effects of thalamotomy. Brain **91**:619-638.

Benton, A. L. 1959. Right-left discrimination and finger localization. New York, Harper & Row, Publishers.

Bing, R. 1910. Aphasie und Apraxie: Klinische Vorlesung. Würzburg, Abh. Gesamtgeb. Prakt. Med. **10**:239-261.

Brain, R. 1965. Speech disorders: aphasia, apraxia and agnosia, ed. 2. London, Butterworth & Co. (Publishers) Ltd.

Brain, W. R., and Curran, R. 1932. The grasp reflex of the foot. Brain **55**:347-356.

Broca, P. P. 1861. Remarques sur le siège de la faculté du language articulé, suivie d'une observation d'aphémie (perte de la parole). Bull. Soc. Anat. Paris **36**:330-357.

Cairns, H., Oldfield, R. C., Pennybacker, J. B., and Whitteridge, O. 1941. Akinetic mutism with an epidermoid cyst of the 3rd ventricle. Brain **64**:273-290.

Critchley, M. 1953. The parietal lobes. London, Arnold.

Critchley, M. 1964. Developmental dyslexia. London, William Heinemann Medical Books Ltd.

Denny-Brown, D. 1958. The nature of apraxia. J. Nerv. Ment. Dis. **126**:9-32.

Frazier, C. H. 1936. Tumor involving the frontal lobe alone: a symptomatic survey of one hundred and five verified cases. Arch. Neurol. Psychiat. **35**:525-571.

Freud, S. 1953. On aphasia. Translated by E. Stengel from 1891 edition. New York, International University Press.

Gazzaniga, M. S., and Sperry, R. W. 1967. Language after section of the cerebral commissures. Brain **90**:131-148.

Gerstmann, J. 1940. Syndrome of finger agnosia, disorientation for right or left, agraphia and acalculia: local diagnostic value. Arch. Neurol. Psychiat. **44**:389-408.

Geschwind, N. 1965. Disconnexion syndromes in animals and man. Brain **88**:237-294, 585-644.

Goldstein, K. 1948. Language and language disturbances. New York, Grune & Stratton, Inc.

Guiot, G., Hertzog, E., Rondot, P., and Molina, P. 1961. Arrest or acceleration of speech evoked by thalamic stimulation in the course of stereotaxic procedures for Parkinsonism. Brain **84**: 363-379.

Guttmann, E. 1942. Aphasia in children. Brain **65**:205-219.

Head, H. 1926. Aphasia and kindred disorders of speech, ed. 2. Cambridge, Cambridge University Press.

Hécaen, H. L., and Ajuriaguerria, J. 1964. Lefthandedness. New York, Grune & Stratton, Inc.

Hermann, K. 1959. Reading disability. Copenhagen, Munksgaard, International Booksellers and Publishers Ltd.

Joynt, R. J., and Benton, A. L. 1964. The memoir of Marc Dax on aphasia. Neurology **14**:851-854.

Keschner, M., Bender, M. B., and Strauss, I. 1936. Mental symptoms in cases of tumor of the temporal lobe. Arch. Neurol. Psychiat. **35**: 572-596.

Kussmaul, A. 1877. Die Störungen der Sprache: Versuch einer Pathologie der Sprache. Leipzig, Vogel.

Liepmann, H. 1900. Das Krankheitsbild der Apraxie (motorische Asmybolie). Mschr. Psychiat. Neurol. **8**:15-44, 102-132, 182-197.

Lotmar, F. 1919-20. Zur Kenntnis der erschwerten Wortfindung und ihres Bedeutung für das Denken des Aphasischen. Schweiz. Arch. Neurol. Psychiat. **5**:206-239; **6**:1-36.

Luria, A. R. 1966. Higher cortical functions in man. New York, Basic Books, Inc.

Mountcastle, V. B. 1962. Interhemispheric relations and cerebral dominance. Baltimore, Johns Hopkins University Press.

Orton, S. T. 1937. Reading, writing and speech problems in children. London, Chapman & Hall Ltd.

Penfield, W., and Roberts, L. 1959. Speech and brain-mechanisms. Princeton, Princeton University Press.

Petit-Dutaillis, O., Guiot, G., Messimy, R., and Bourdillon, C. 1954. A propos d'une aphémie par atteinte de la zone supplémentaire de Penfield, au cours de l'évolution d'un anévrisme arterio-veneux: guérison de l'aphémie par ablation de la lésion. Rev. Neurol. **90**:95-106.

Schiller, F. 1947. Aphasia studied in patients with missile wounds. J. Neurol. Neurosurg. Psychiat. **10**:183-197.

Schuster, P., and Pinéas, H. 1926. Weitere Beobachtungen über Zwangsgreifen und Nachgreifen und deren Beziehungen zu ähnlicher Bewegungsstörungen. Deutsch. Z. Nervenheilk. **91**:16-56.

Sperry, R. W. 1961. Cerebral organization and behavior. Science **133**:1949-1957.

Trousseau, A. 1865. De l'aphasie: Clinique Médicale de l'Hôtel-Dieu de Paris, ed. 2, vol. 2. Paris, Baillière.

Vygotsky, L. S. 1962. Thought and language. Translated by E. Hanfmann and G. Vakar from 1934 edition. Cambridge, M.I.T. Press.

Wada, J. 1949. A new method for the determination of the side of cerebral speech dominance . . . intracarotid injection of sodium amytal. Med. Biol. **14**:221-222.

Weisenburg, T., and McBride, K. E. 1935. Aphasia: a clinical and psychological study. New York, Commonwealth Fund.

Wernicke, C. 1874. Der aphasische Symptomenkomplex: eine psychologische Studie auf anatomischer Basis. Breslau, Cohn und Weigert.

Wilson, K. 1920. Discussion on aphasia. Brain **43**: 433-438.

Zangwill, O. L. 1960. Cerebral dominance and its relations to psychological function. Edinburgh, Oliver & Boyd Ltd.

Chapter 24

Extrapyramidal motor disorders

Since the turn of the century a large group of extrapyramidal motor disorders has gradually emerged from clinical and anatomical observations. The grouping is fostered by practical and didactic considerations, and it receives some support from animal experiment as well as from surgical intervention in patients. What the group has clinically in common is not one feature but, instead, single or multiple disabilities in the voluntary control of the limb, face, neck, trunk, diaphragm, and other structures, alone or in combination. The loss of control affects posture, on the one hand; on the other hand the patients are unable either to prevent unintended movement (*hyper-* and *dyskinesia*) or to overcome immobility (*hypo-* and *akinesia*). The increase in muscle tone—where it occurs—is called *rigidity*. Unlike spasticity, rigidity is not associated with increased reflexes, and the Babinski sign is flexor. The unintended movements may be essentially rhythmic or essentially arrhythmic. *Choreoathetosis* is easily distinguished from *tremor*. As a rule (there are exceptions) the muscles in extrapyramidal disorders are not paralyzed. Their coordination is interfered with in a manner distinguishable from the ataxia of cerebellar disease, though the latter distinction may be questioned on theoretical grounds.

What the group of extrapyramidal motor disorders has also in common is a certain unity of the anatomical structures involved. Again, this unity was in part derived from clinical considerations, just as anatomical considerations have helped in shaping the clinical group. Unity, finally, becomes all the more evident by exclusion: not considered responsible (yet sometimes involved) are the pyramidal system, the aggregates of lower motor neurons in brainstem and spinal cord, the hypothalamus and limbic system, and, in a certain sense, the cerebellum.

Anatomically, by and large, the structures involved in extrapyramidal disorders are the basal ganglia. Superimposed on some of these nuclear masses are systems of neurons arising in various areas of the cerebral cortex, known as the *centrally originating extrapyramidal system* (COEPS). (This system is described elsewhere; see pp. 317-318.) COEPS extends from the cortex to the striatum, pallidum, thalamus, red nucleus, reticular formation, pontile nuclei, and probably the substantia nigra.

Two features distinguish COEPS from the corticospinal tract: the system is multisynaptic, and its fibers do not pass through the pyramids. Instead, they discharge through reticulobulbar and reticulospinal pathways reaching, through these connections, certain cranial nerve nuclei and cell aggregates in the spinal gray matter. They are as concerned in voluntary, or volitional, motor activity as are the corticobulbar or pyramidal corticospinal neurons, perhaps even more so in some realms. In addition, certain basal ganglia discharge to thalamic cells that project back to the cerebral cortex, influencing the activity of the cells that give rise to the corticobulbar and corticospinal pathway and COEPS.

The *extrapyramidal nuclei* include (1) the striatum (or corpus striatum), by which is meant the caudate nucleus and putamen, (2) the pallidum (or globus pallidus), (3) the substantia nigra, and (4) the subthalamic nucleus (corpus Luysii). Putamen and globus pallidus form an anatomical unit called the *lenticular nucleus.* The term *extrapyramidal system* refers not only to these various masses of gray matter together with their emergent fibers but also to the reticular nuclei in the mesencephalic and pontile tegmentum and their emergent fibers. Used in its widest sense, the extrapyramidal system also includes the cerebellum. "Basal ganglia" is a term hard to define because it has been so variously used. In the present text the term refers to the extrapyramidal nuclei listed.

CONNECTIONS OF THE EXTRAPYRAMIDAL MOTOR SYSTEM

William R. Mehler

Connections of the extrapyramidal nuclei are indicated in Figs. 24-1 and 24-2, and those of the pyramidal system as well in Fig. 24-3.

Striatum. On the afferent side, both caudate nucleus and putamen receive an input from cortical areas 8, 6, and 4 (that is, from components of COEPS). The caudate receives them by way of the subcallosal fasciculus and as collaterals from fibers descending in the internal capsule (Glees, 1944; Papez, 1942). Connections also exist with the prefrontal area (De Vito and Smith, 1964) and the temporal cortex (Whitlock and Nauta, 1956). Another fiber system, coming from the thalamus, reaches the caudate and putamen from below. The caudate receives its input from the parafascicular thalamic nucleus, and the putamen from the nucleus centrum medianum (Mehler, 1966; Vogt and Vogt, 1941).

On the efferent side, the striatum projects to the pallidum and substantia nigra (Fig. 24-1, *A*). The major outflow is to the reticular portion of the substantia nigra (Ogawa, 1952; Papez, 1942; Szabo, 1963, 1967). Fibers from the substantia nigra reportedly extend back to the medial division of the pallidum (Ranson and Ranson, 1941) and to the thalamus (Fig. 24-1, *D*) (Carpenter and Strominger, 1967; Cole, Nauta, and Mehler, 1964). Fibers en route from striatum to substantia nigra give off collaterals both to the lateral and the medial division of the pallidum (Fig. 24-1, *A*) (Szabo, 1963, 1967).

Results of electrical stimulation of the caudate nucleus have suggested that the caudate functions in an integrative capacity. Controversive head and eye movements occur on weaker stimulation; running in a circle away from the side stimulated occurs on stronger stimulation (Laursen, 1961). Further, the striatum appears to be involved in the ordering of the component parts of complex movement (Wang and Akert, 1962). All this activity seems to be mediated from the cortex, since there is little proof that the striatum has any function independent of that of the cortex.

Pallidum. The pallidum is partly afferent and partly efferent in its orientation. On the afferent side, it receives fibers chiefly from the striatum. The pallidum is a component of a circuit: cortex → striatum → pallidum → thalamus → motor cortex. On the efferent side, it is an important discharging center.

Topologically organized fibers originating from the striatum and coursing through the pallidum en route to the substantia nigra issue collaterals both to the lateral and the medial segment of the globus pallidus (Fig. 24-1, *A*) (Szabo, 1963, 1967). Some fibers originating in the lateral segment of the pallidum (Fig. 24-1, *B*) proceed to the subthalamic nucleus, terminating in its lateral part (Beck and Bignami, 1968); in their course to the subthalamic nucleus, they appear to contribute collaterals to the medial segment of the globus pallidus (Nauta and Mehler, 1966). Reciprocal connections linking the subthalamic nucleus and substantia nigra with the pallidal segments have also been described (Carpenter and Strominger, 1967).

Fibers of the larger-celled medial division of the pallidum exit in one of two efferent groups: (1) in the *ansa lenticularis,* which loops around the undersurface of the most inferior part of the internal capsule (near the basis pedunculi) and takes an upward, then caudal, course; or (2) as a component of the *fasciculus lenticularis,* which penetrates, or "combs," through the posterior limb of the internal capsule, then proceeds medialward in the region between the subthalamic nucleus and zona incerta (the zona incerta is not labeled in Fig. 24-2).

These two groups of fibers join in field H_2 of Forel, situated in the subthalamic region (Fig. 24-2). Some of the pallidal fibers reaching field H_2 course downward from H_2 into the hypothalamus (as the so-called pallidohypothalamic fasciculus), then, without synapsing in any hypothalamic nucleus, they turn upward to rejoin field H_2 (Beck and Bignami, 1968; Nauta and Mehler, 1966); other pallidal fibers in field H_2 pass caudally and terminate in field H (that is, in the nucleus of the prerubral field, known also as the nucleus campus Foreli); still other pallidal fibers, forming a small but significant contingent (Fig. 24-2), continue caudally and reach the caudal mesencephalic reticular formation.

However, the majority of the fibers reaching field H_2 execute a recurrent trajectory in that field; then, as the *fasciculus thalamicus,* they pass

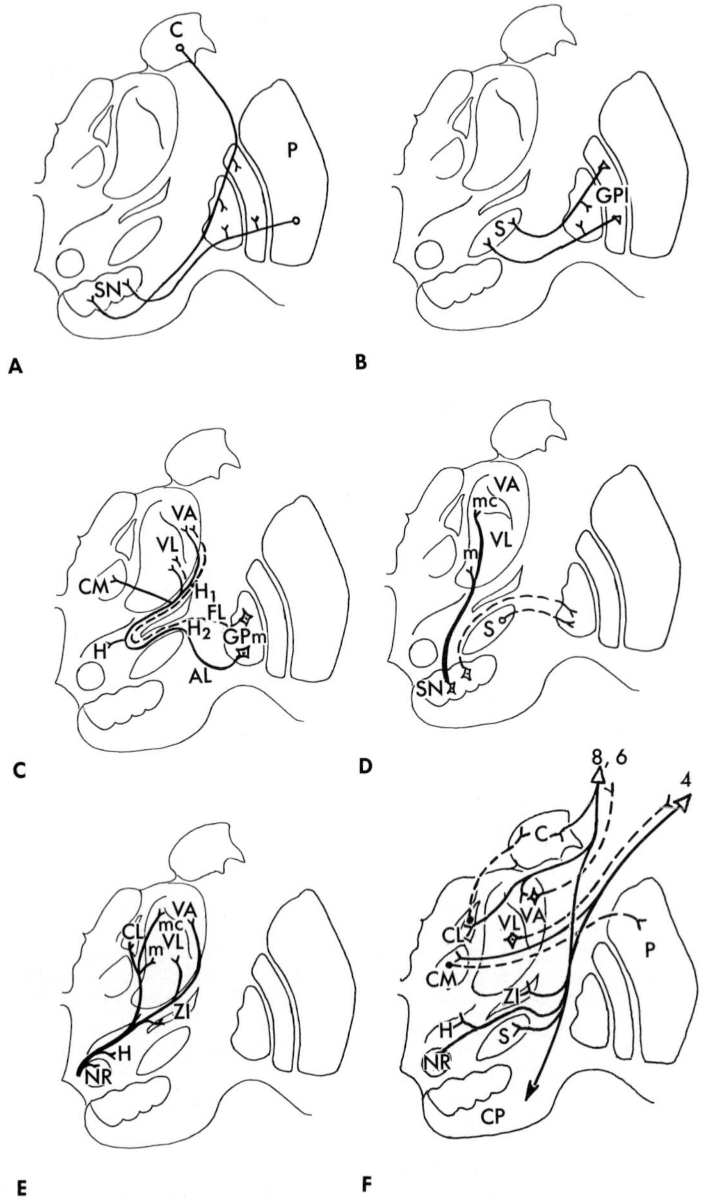

Fig. 24-1. A to **F**, Transverse sections depicting: **A**, striatonigral connections; **B**, connections of the lateral pallidum; **C**, connections of the medial pallidum; **D**, nigrothalamic and pallidal connections; **E**, brachium conjunctivum–diencephalic connections; **F**, thalamocortical, thalamostriatal, and corticodiencephalic connections.

KEY FOR ABBREVIATIONS USED IN FIGS. 24-1 AND 24-2

AL—ansa lenticularis
C—caudate nucleus
CL—central lateral intralaminar nucleus
FL—fasciculus lenticularis
CM—nucleus centrum medianum
CP—basis pedunculi
GPL—globus pallidus, lateral segment
GPM—globus pallidus, medial segment
H, H_1, H_2—H-fields of Forel
IC—internal capsule
NR—red nucleus
P—putamen
RF—reticular formation
S—subthalamic nucleus
SN—substantia nigra
VA—ventral anterior nucleus
(mc—magnocellar part)
VL—ventral lateral nucleus
(m—medial part)
ZI—zona incerta

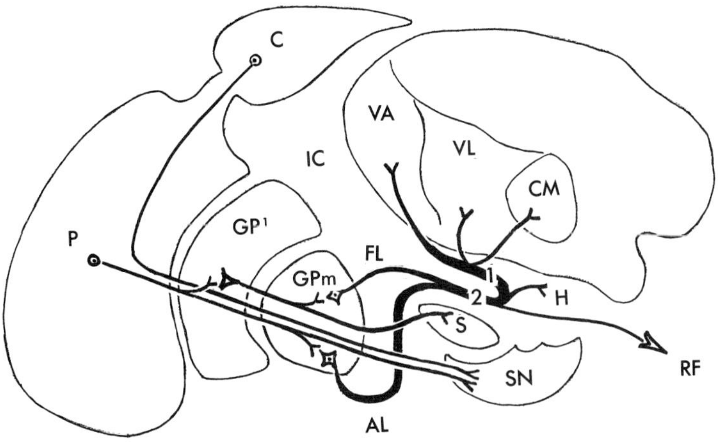

Fig. 24-2. Sagittal view of striatal and pallidal pathways illustrated in **A**, **B**, and **C** of Fig. 24-1. *1* refers to Forel's field H_1 (in which the fasciculus thalamicus runs), and *2* refers to Forel's field H_2. For key to abbreviations see Fig. 24-1.

above the zona incerta (in field H_1) and terminate in the ventral lateral (VL)* and ventral anterior (VA) nuclei of the thalamus (Fig. 24-1, *C*), which in turn project fibers to the precentral and the premotor cortex (Fig. 24-1, *F*). In addition to the aforementioned pallidothalamic connections, a strong projection from the medial pallidum proceeds to the nucleus centrum medianum (CM) (Figs. 24-1, *C* and 24-2) (Nauta and Mehler, 1966). CM also receives a major afferent fiber system from the precentral motor cortex (Petras, 1964). Thus, it appears that the motor cortex, the keystone of the "pyramidal system," projects on to two thalamic nuclei (VL and CM) that receive major "extrapyramidal" connections from the medial pallidum. However, of these two nuclei, only VL is dependent upon (projects to) area 4, for CM projects only to the striatum (Fig. 24-1, *F*) (Mehler, 1966; Vogt and Vogt, 1941).

These essentially dual closed circuits (cortex → striatum → pallidum → thalamus → cortex, or reciprocally from thalamus back to the striatum) suggest various combinations of reverberating mechanisms incorporated in current COEPS hypotheses. Viewed accordingly, except for the numerically small and topologically limited pallidal projections to the reticular formation, the combined anatomical and neurophysiological data appear to support the previously stated contention that the striatum has no function independent of that of the cerebral cortex.

Subthalamic nucleus. Both ascending and descending connections with the subthalamic nucleus have been described. Descending connections are nebulous. The major established pathway is to the medial pallidal segment (Fig. 24-1, *D*) (Carpenter and Strominger, 1967). Lateral pallidum → subthalamic nucleus → medial pallidum presents still another closed extrapyramidal circuit to be considered in the interpretation of neural mechanisms involved in extrapyramidal disorders. In manganese poisoning, for example, this unit is selectively destroyed (Pentschew, Ebner, and Kovatch, 1963). Moreover, COEPS projections from the precentral (motor) cortex proceed to the subthalamic nucleus and also to the zona incerta, field H, and the red nucleus. En route all these fibers course through field H_2.

Substantia nigra. The substantia nigra is divisible into two parts, the *pars reticularis* (red zone) and the *pars compacta* (black zone). On the afferent side, there is suggestive evidence of a corticonigral pathway issuing from areas 8, 6, and 4 (as a component of COEPS). Much more clear cut are striatonigral connections, the fibers reaching the pars reticularis of the substantia nigra both from the caudate and the putamen (Nauta and Mehler, 1966; Szabo, 1963, 1967). In addition, there appears to be a pallidal input into the substantia nigra; the fibers, which are relatively few, extend from the medial pallidum to the pars compacta of the nigra (Nauta and Mehler, 1966) (not shown in Fig. 24-1). The main efferent pathway from the substantia nigra (Fig. 24-1, *D*) is to the thalamus (pars medialis of the ventral lateral nucleus [m] and pars magnocellularis [mc] of the ventral anterior nucleus) (Fig. 24-1, *D*) (Cole, Nauta, and Mehler, 1964). Ascending nigral fibers may also terminate in the pallidum (Carpenter and Strominger, 1967). These are illustrated in Fig. 24-1, *D*. Whether some nigral fibers descend from nigra into the tegmentum and effect connections with reticulospinal fibers, as contended by Hassler, 1938, and by Jung and Hassler, 1960, is still not clear.

Red nucleus. The red nucleus of the human brain is composed of a large parvocellular portion (pc) and a small magnocellular portion (mc). Somatotopic arrangement exists in the cortical fibers extending to the red nucleus, area 4 projecting to pc and areas 8 and 6 to mc (Kuypers and Lawrence, 1967). The position of the corticorubral pathway in the internal capsule is illustrated in

*This nucleus corresponds to the lateral ventral nucleus (LVB and LVD) in Fig. 25-1.

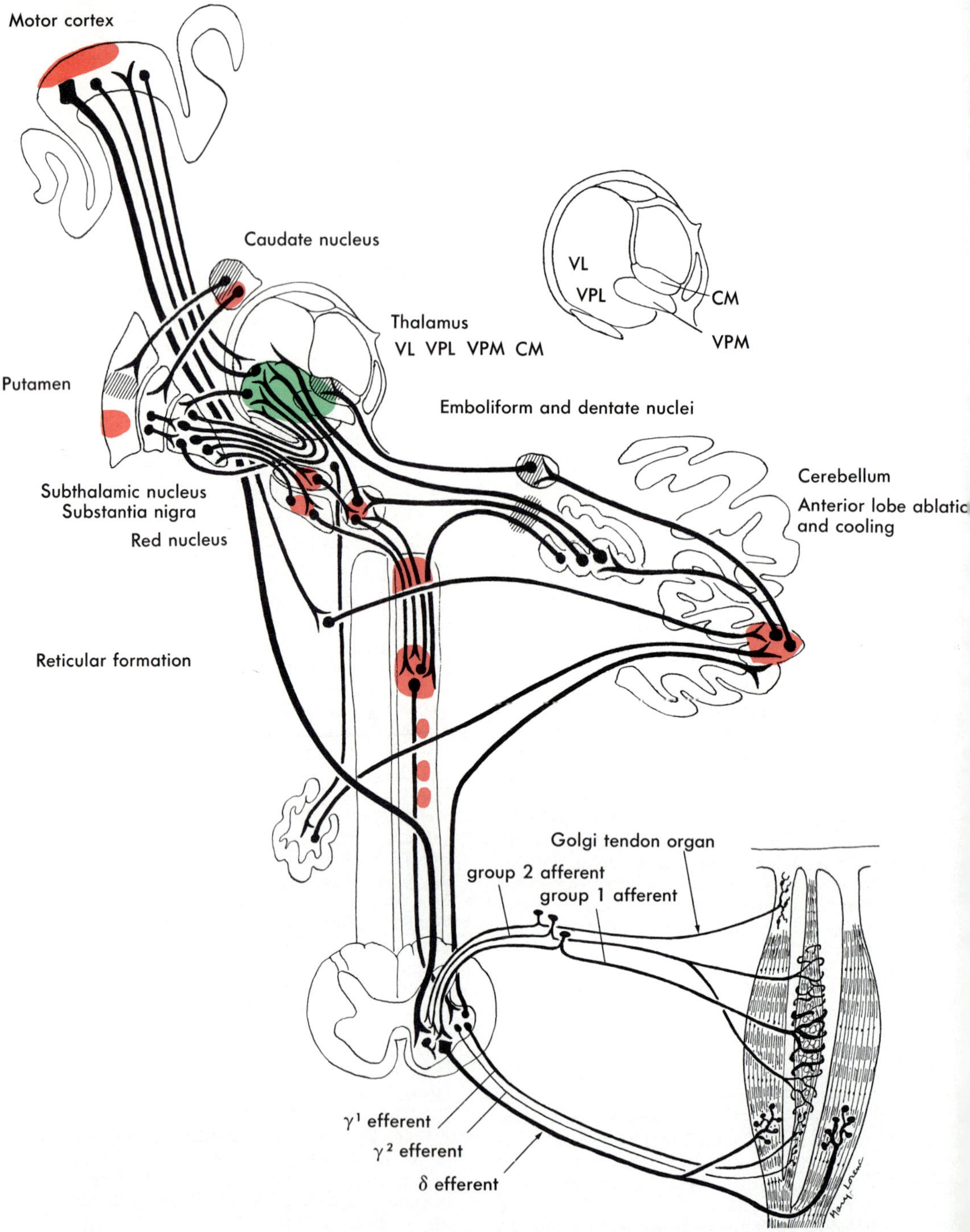

Fig. 24-3. Connections at various levels, with ultimate innervation of muscle. *Areas shaded by slanted lines:* the main sites at which lesions have been noted in cases of intention tremor, dystonia, and Wilson's disease. These involve the caudate nucleus, putamen, dentate nucleus, brachium conjunctivum, and nucleus centrum medianum, all of which subserve afferent communication and feedback, modulating the activity of the motor cortex. *Areas shaded in red:* loci that, when electrically stimulated, facilitate or inhibit the gamma fusiform motor system. *Area shaded in green:* sites of thalamic lesions that have proved most efficacious in abolishing intention tremor, manifestations of dystonia, and torticollis. *CM*, nucleus centrum medianum; *VL*, ventral lateral (or lateral ventral) nucleus; *VPL* and *VPM*, ventral posterolateral and ventral posteromedial (arcuate) nuclei. (From Cooper, 1965.)

Fig. 19-11; fibers traversing this region on one side appear to terminate in the red nucleus of both sides, judging from the results of fiber degeneration studies in cases of parkinsonism subjected to stereotactic lesions in this region (Beck and Bignami, 1968). Another afferent connection (to both parts of the red nucleus) is provided by collaterals from the dentate-thalamic pathway. As to efferent connections, the parvocellular part of the red nucleus projects chiefly to the lateral reticular formation, while its magnocellular part sends fibers down into the spinal cord as the rubrospinal tract (Kuypers, 1964; Massion, 1967; Poirier and Bouvier, 1966).

Connections with the reticular formation. In the previous sections it was indicated that the medial pallidum projects to the reticular formation as far caudally as the lowermost part of the midbrain, and that the red nucleus gives off rubroreticular fibers. Other reported sources are illustrated in Fig. 24-3. From area 4 of the precentral cortex, corticospinal fibers course downward, giving off collaterals to the reticular formation of the midbrain, pons, and medulla oblongata. Direct corticonuclear connections have also been found to originate from the same region in the precentral cortex in which corticoreticular projections take origin. These direct systems proceed to cranial nerve nuclei V, VII, and XII and to the anterior horns of the spinal cord. Nuclei III, IV, and VI receive connections by way of the reticular substance, as do also motor nuclei IX, X, and XI.

Other descending systems exist. The postcentral sensory cortex (particularly areas 3, 1, and 2) projects fibers to the reticular formation. Moreover, this part of the cortex provides feedback connections to sensory nuclei of the brainstem and various cell aggregates in the spinal cord. For example, from the face area of the postcentral cortex extensive connections project back specifically upon the spinal trigeminal nucleus and adjacent regions of the reticular formation. From the arm and leg regions of the postcentral cortex, strong projections feed back upon reticular-like basal cell groups of the spinal dorsal funicular nuclei and to cells situated in the posterior horn of the spinal cord (Kuypers, Fleming, and Farinholt, 1962; Kuypers and Lawrence, 1967). The full significance of these connections in regard to notions of the COEPS and extrapyramidal systems is yet to be ascertained. Magni and Willis (1964a, b), in finding that many reticulospinal neurons are driven by stimulation of widespread areas of cortex, suggested that the extrapyramidal system is invoked both in motor and sensory control. Efferent fibers from cells in the medullary and pontile reticular formation constitute reticulospinal tracts (Kuypers, 1958; Kuypers, Fleming, and Farinholt, 1962). These are described in Chapter 1.

Cerebellum. The dentate nucleus projects through the brachium conjunctivum to the thalamus—to its ventral lateral (VL), ventral anterior (VA), and central lateral laminar (CL) nuclei (shown in part in Fig. 24-3; see also Fig. 17-1). En route, after decussating, the pathway gives off collaterals to both portions of the red nucleus, to field H (the nucleus campus Foreli), and to the zona incerta (Fig. 24-1, *E*).

Thalamus. The secondary somesthetic pathways —the spinothalamic and the trigeminothalamic systems—project to the ventral posterolateral and ventral posteromedial thalamic nuclei, respectively (VPL and VPM in Fig. 24-3). In VPL the spinothalamic tract overlaps with incoming fibers of the lemniscal systems ascending from the spinal dorsal funicular nuclei, and in VPM the trigeminothalamic system overlaps with incoming fibers ascending from the principal nucleus of the trigeminus. Similarly, major constituents of the extrapyramidal system (pallidum, nigra, cerebellum) converge in varying degree upon subdivisions of the ventral lateral (VL) and ventral anterior (VA) nuclei.

The course and distribution of the pallidothalamic connections have been outlined in the foregoing. Nigrothalamic connections have also been indicated. Considered from the standpoint of density and areal distribution, the cerebellothalamic connections constitute numerically by far the most massive thalamic afferent input system. It distributes to practically all the VL and VA complex, completely overlapping the distribution of the pallidothalamic connections except for the latter's connection with the nucleus centrum medianum.

Although somatotopic arrangement has been established with respect to the afferent and efferent connections of the somesthetic thalamic nuclei, the existence of such an organization in the thalamic nuclei that receive proprioceptive fibers is less clear. Somatotopic cerebellar connections with VL and VA have not been established. Likewise, the nonconvergence of the pallidothalamic and nigrothalamic projections, respectively, to the lateral and medial subdivisions of VL and VA is not understood. At best, on the basis of the cortical connections of the various regions of VL and VA, respectively, with the precentral (area 4) and premotor (areas 6 and 8) parts of the cortex, a somatotopic motor homunculus might be envisaged. However, Walker (1959) has concluded that any functional analysis of lateral nuclear mass-thalamocortical mechanisms would vary according to the functional cortical map adopted by the author. With respect to those nuclei (VL, VA) related to the extrapyramidal basal ganglia, Walker indicates that infarcts occurring in them may result in tremor or choreo-athetoid movements or both. Intrinsic thalamic functional mechanisms cannot, however, be separated from the afferent fiber connections interrupted in such cases.

Thalamus to cortex. Completing some circuits are fibers from thalamus to cortex. The essentials are given in Chapter 25.

CLINICAL SYNDROMES, PATHOLOGY, MECHANISMS INVOLVED

Webb Haymaker and Francis Schiller

In order to identify the neural mechanisms involved in extrapyramidal disease, the following pathways must be considered: (1) those extending from the cerebral cortex to the cranial nerve nuclei and the anterior horns of the spinal cord (the alpha system), either directly or via synaptic stations; (2) pathways originating in the cortex (the COEPS system) which, through multisynaptic means, loop back to the cortex to influence the activities of the descending pathways; and (3) the basal ganglia and their efferent pathways, including the reticulospinal tracts (the latter, at least, belonging to the gamma system).

Recurrent or feedback systems from cortex back to cortex (mentioned in the second point above) are illustrated in Figs. 24-1 to 24-3. The main potential pathways are, first, cortex → striatum → pallidum → thalamus → motor cortex, and, second, cortex → pons → cerebellum → thalamus → cortex. A possible third recurrent system is: cortex → subthalamic nucleus → globus pallidus → thalamus → motor cortex. They all converge as thalamopetal fibers in the region between subthalamus and thalamus (colored green in Fig. 24-3). Remember that the largest contingent of incoming fibers is of cerebellar origin.

Not belonging to these recurrent or feedback systems are (1) the substantia nigra (since it apparently does not project to those thalamic nuclei that send fibers to the motor or premotor cortex), and (2) the red nucleus and other tegmental nuclei (whose fibers pursue only a downward course).

Consequently it appears that the basal ganglia modulate motor activity both indirectly through the cortex and directly through convergence at lower levels.

The grasp and classification of extrapyramidal disorders is made difficult by the tangle of permutations in which similar assortments of symptoms and signs (chorea, athetosis, ballism, dystonia, akinesia, rigidity, tremor, dementia, and occasionally muscle wasting and spasticity) are distributed throughout a series of metabolic, genetic, apparently degenerative and other etiologies, all these in turn being tied to the variety of cerebral sites (such as the basal ganglia) mentioned previously. Wherever possible, we have followed the tradition of making an impressive and coherent clinical syndrome the starting point for classifying disease. But the frontiers of research form untidy lines; advances made in pathology, both anatomical and biochemical, cannot be easily matched in the clinic, nor can the physiological interpretations be expected to keep step with observations made on the examining and the operating table.

Chorea, athetosis, ballism

Chorea and choreoathetosis

Sydenham's chorea. Sydenham's chorea, no longer a frequent disorder, is a symptom rather than a disease entity. It is also called *chorea minor* to distinguish it from *chorea major*—or Sancti Viti—the medieval mass hysteria, the dancing mania. It occurs most often in childhood and adolescence as a complication of rheumatic fever, with or without evidence of arthritis and endocarditis; a heart murmur is heard in 30 percent of cases (Aron, Freeman, and Carter, 1965). Among the etiological agents, a prior streptococcal infection has now and then been established; emotional stress and genetic predisposition have been postulated. The involuntary movements are ceaseless, often surprisingly well coordinated but grotesque, and affect limbs, face, tongue, and eyelids ("chorea" is the "act of dancing"). They are rapid, jerky, irregular, quasi-expressive and quasi-purposive ("There is some method in their madness"—Hughlings Jackson). They may be most pronounced unilaterally. Associated movements may be excessive: the impulse of grasping an object may spread from the limb to the face and trunk. Hypotonia is invariable, hyperextension of the fingers at the metacarpophalangeal joints and flexion at the wrist are characteristic. Hemiplegia, aphasia, convulsions, disorientation, even major functional psychoses may be associated. (Aron, Freeman, and

Carter, 1965; Brain, 1928; Lhermitte and Pagniez, 1930; Majewska and Szelożyńska, 1967; Winkelman and Eckel, 1932.) The condition runs a course averaging 5 months, with a maximum of about 2 years.

The *pathological changes* in Sydenham's chorea are nonspecific, the pathophysiology is obscure. Vasculitis, diffuse perivascular cell infiltrates, and neuronal degeneration or necrosis are commonly observed. These changes predominate at one site or another, such as the caudate nucleus, putamen, thalamus, substantia nigra, or subthalamic nucleus. The cerebellum and cerebral cortex may share in the pathological process. Hyalinization of vessel walls may occur, as may also infarction, though the latter is rare. In some instances nothing more than toxidegenerative changes in nerve cells could be found. (Colony and Malamud, 1956; Greenfield and Wolfsohn, 1922; Kernohan, Woltman, and Barnes, 1939; von Sántha, 1932.)

Chorea of other cause. Adults with this disorder are often primiparae in the earlier months of pregnancy *(chorea gravidarum).* The statement that an anxiety reaction ushered in the disorder is common. Chorea may develop following epidemic encephalitis or pertussis, and it has been noted in lupus erythematosus, cerebrovascular syphilis, or other infections, including diphtheria (Critchley, 1924). Other conditions giving rise to chorea are polycythemia vera (Gautier-Smith and Prankerd, 1967), embolization in the region of the basal ganglia, cerebral syphilis, a primary tumor (rare), carbon monoxide poisoning, and hypocalcemia. In all these conditions the disorder may be unilateral and confined to the face or to one limb, particularly in cerebral syphilis (Münzer, 1935). Chorea of a benign nature may be a familial disorder that first becomes manifest during the first two decades of life or in adulthood; in addition to choreic movements, these patients may have intention tremor (Pincus and Chutorian, 1967).

Progressive chorea may develop in other disorders involving the striatum. For example, it is said to complicate encephalitis and chronic edema (Vogt and Vogt, 1920, 1951). Senile chorea (which appears in persons in their forties or older) is characterized by choreoathetotic movements. The clinical course is benign, and mental deterioration is slight or absent. The only conspicuous pathological change consists in moderate atrophy of the striatum and pallidum. (Alcock, 1936.)

Choreoathetosis in hepatic and portosystemic encephalopathy. Chronic liver disease is associated with varied neurological syndromes. Choreoathetosis together with dysarthria, ataxia of gait, intention tremor, dementia, and less frequently, diffuse muscular rigidity, nystagmus, tremor in repose (static tremor), and grasp reflexes, characterized twenty-seven cases described by Victor, Adams, and Cole (1965). These disturbances persisted and were unrelated to hepatic coma. In acquired forms of liver disease, such as alcoholic cirrhosis, portal blood may be shunted into the inferior vena cava and thus bypass the liver and lead to encephalopathy. The ensemble of clinical disturbances may be formidable, as reported by Toghill, Johnston, and Smith (1967). The movements in these patients were both choreiform and athetotic: there was choreiform frowning, smiling, and pursing of lips, in rapid succession with slow protrusion and withdrawal of the tongue, and athetotic writhing of arms and legs. Sometimes postural distortions ("flexion dystonia") affect the proximal portions of the limbs in the wake of purposive movements; they simulate the distortions of Wilson's disease but are nonprogressive. Some cases are characterized by akinetic mutism. (Denny-Brown, 1964; Shiraki, 1968.) In impending hepatic coma a peculiar flapping motion and inability to maintain extension at the wrists and ankles, called *liver flap* or *asterixis,* may be observed (Adams and Foley, 1953; Victor, Adams, and Cole, 1965).

Pathologically the changes observed in the brain under these conditions resemble those of Wilson's disease or Westphal's pseudosclerosis. Commonly there are tiny cavities in the putamen and caudate nucleus, but they are less conspicuous than in Wilson's disease. Laminar or pseudolaminar necrosis reminiscent of hypoxic change is also frequently seen in deeper laminae of the cerebral cortex (Adams and Sidman, 1968). Classification of pathological changes reflecting differences in clinical disturbances has been proposed. Excluding changes in the basal ganglia, the types are: (1) laminar or pseudolaminar cortical necrosis, foci of destruction in the thalamus, and "ischemic" nerve cell changes in various locations (Inose type); (2) widespread, confluent necrosis, severe atrophy, and spongy necrosis involving the cerebral cortex, also the white matter (pseudo-ulegyric type); and (3) "ischemic" nerve cell changes in the cerebral cortex and occasional areas of cortical necrosis or pallor (ischemic type) (Shiraki, 1968). Glycogen deposition in astroglia was pronounced in these different types (Shiraki, 1968), but was not observed in any substantial degree in "Wilson-pseudosclerosis" (Inose, Ichikawa, and Nomura, 1960). The glycogen deposition probably represents nothing specific; it appears to be merely a reflection of a reduction in oxidative metabolism of brain tissue (Haymaker, 1969).

Huntington's disease. The cardinal criteria for the diagnosis of Huntington's disease are choreoathetoid hyperkinesis and hereditary disposition (monohybrid dominant without anticipation or sex-linked inheritance). Progressive mental deterioration occurs in a rather large proportion of cases. Although usually first appearing in adult life (late thirties), the disorder may, in some 15 percent of cases, first manifest itself before the age of 20, and develop even in childhood (Brothers, 1964). Hyperkinesias usually precede the mental disturbances. Continuous choreoathetotic movements involve the limbs and face and ultimately the entire body. Speed of progression of the disorder varies greatly. Parkinson-like rigidity may ultimately develop (Dunlap, 1927; Spillane and Phillips, 1937). In *juvenile Huntington's disease* two variants are recognized, one in which a hyperkinetic syndrome culminates in Parkinson-like rigidity, and the other in which progressive rigidity develops in the absence of involuntary movements. Only rarely does torsion dystonia or athetoid hyperkinesis occur. (Campbell and others, 1961; Hansotia, Cleeland, and Chun, 1968.)

The most conspicuous *pathological changes* (nerve cell necrobiosis with advanced astrogliosis) are in the striatum and cerebral cortex, particularly the frontal cortex (laminae III and IV). The caudate nucleus is, as a rule, most severely affected. The small nerve cells of both caudate and putamen are the most vulnerable; large nerve cells suffer less. Striatal vessels are commonly fibrosed. (Adams and Sidman, 1968.) The globus pallidus may also share in the pathological process, as illustrated in Fig. 24-4. Structures less altered are the subthalamic nucleus and certain brainstem nuclei. However, in a case marked by a disorder of rapid eye movements, the nucleus of the

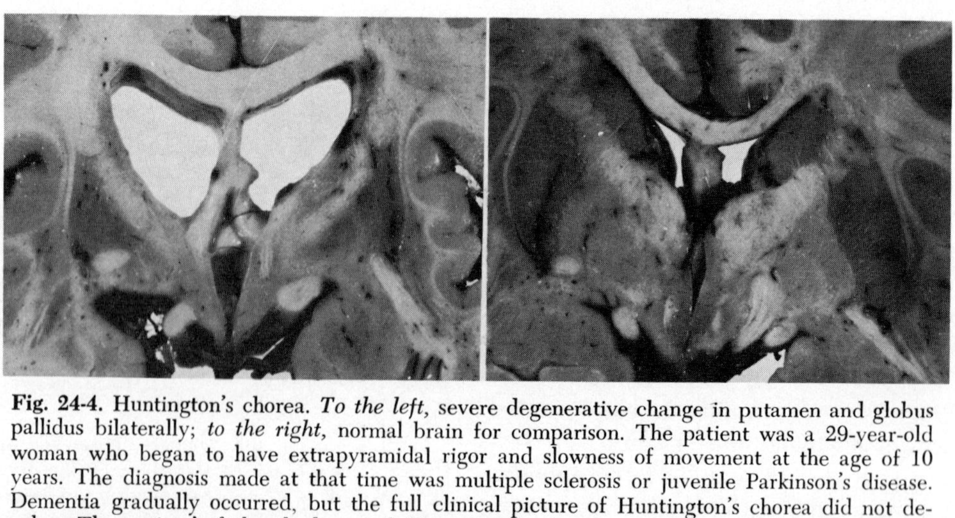

Fig. 24-4. Huntington's chorea. *To the left,* severe degenerative change in putamen and globus pallidus bilaterally; *to the right,* normal brain for comparison. The patient was a 29-year-old woman who began to have extrapyramidal rigor and slowness of movement at the age of 10 years. The diagnosis made at that time was multiple sclerosis or juvenile Parkinson's disease. Dementia gradually occurred, but the full clinical picture of Huntington's chorea did not develop. The patient's father had typical Huntington's chorea, starting at the age of 45 years. Changes in the brain were the same as shown here. (Courtesy Dr. Richard Lindenberg, Baltimore.)

third nerve was severely affected, as manifested by nerve cell loss, neurofibrillary tangles in remaining nerve cells, and gliosis (Starr, 1967). In the rigid form of juvenile Huntington's disease, atrophy of the cortex occurs mostly in the postcentral gyri and occipital lobes, the striatum shows loss mainly of small cells, and the globus pallidus is most damaged in its lateral segment (Campbell and others, 1961).

Pathophysiology. Choreiform movements presumably result from imbalance caused by interruption of those neuronal arcs that relate such systems as caudate and putamen, pallidum, and ventral nuclear group of thalamus to the motor pathways as they originate in the cerebral cortex. Transitory choreiform activity has been produced in monkeys by making lesions bilaterally in the brachium conjunctivum (Carrea and Mettler, 1954). In man choreiform movements have been provoked by unilateral lesions in the ventrolateral part of the thalamus and in the subthalamic nucleus. Release of inhibitory influences ordinarily exerted by the putamen on the pallidum has been considered the basis of the hyperkinesis (Dierssen, Gioino, and Cooper, 1961).

Considered from the standpoint of serotonin (5-HT) metabolism, it has been postulated that such release may be associated with a relative overresponsiveness to the activity of mesencephalic-pallidal 5-HT neurons, the latter of which are situated mainly in the raphe nuclei of the pons and midbrain, and which send their axons to the globus pallidus as well as to limbic structures. The therapeutic use of 5-HTP (the immediate precursor of 5-HT) in patients with Huntington's disease has been found to worsen their condition. Increase in 5-HT in cells that normally do not contain a significant level of 5-HT has been suggested as an alternative explanation of the worsening of the patients' condition following the giving of the drug. (Lee, Markham, and Clark, 1968.)

Disorders primarily characterized by athetosis

Double athetosis. Hypoxemia occurring in utero or during the birth process is frequently the basis of double athetosis. Prolonged spasm of the upper limbs (in flexion) and the lower limbs (in extension) in response to startle may be the initial sign in early infancy. A mobile type of spasm becomes more prominent when the child reaches for objects or tries to sit up. Tonus in antagonistic muscle groups increases and decreases in irregular sequence. The child's arms become rigid as it clasps a bar and is raised off the ground.

Athetotic movements (athetosis, "without fixed position") ultimately develop. They resemble coordinated voluntary move-

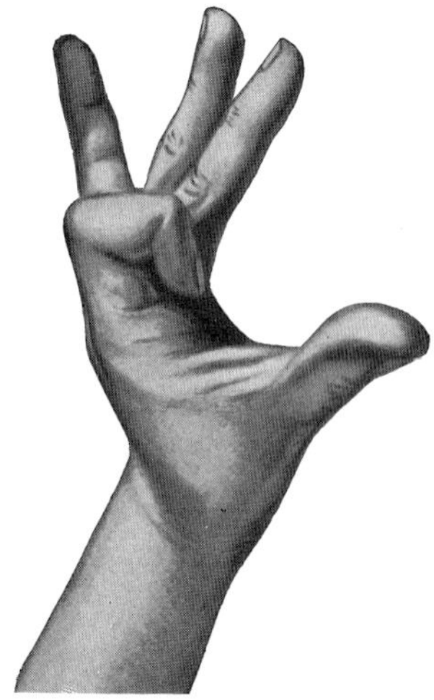

Fig. 24-5. Position of hand and fingers during athetotic movement.

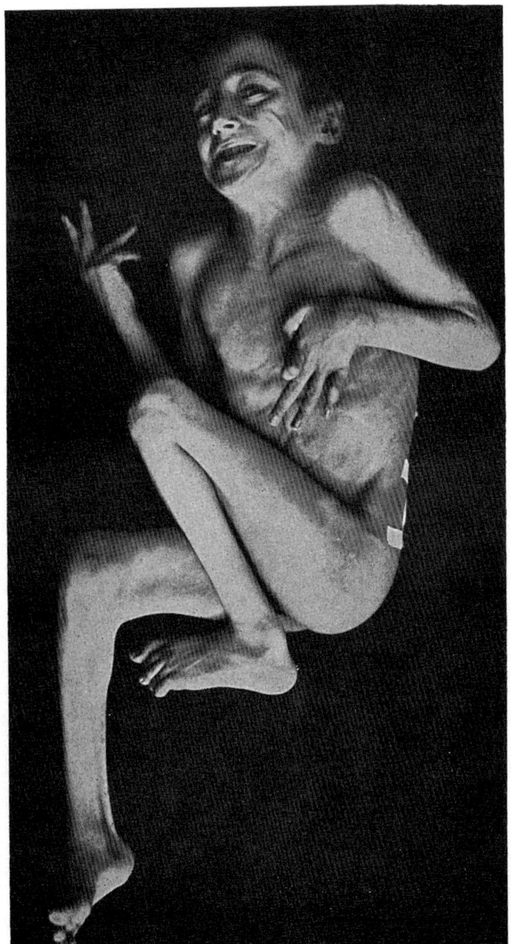

Fig. 24-6. Far-advanced choreoathetosis of congenital origin.

ments much less than the movements of chorea do. Athetotic movements are essentially confined to the limbs and predominate distally. Hands and feet, especially individual fingers and toes, undergo slow grotesque excursions that culminate momentarily in an attitude of hyperextension (Fig. 24-5). They simulate the motions of certain oriental dances, the hands of a piano player, or attempts at grasping. Their amplitude may be temporarily reduced with intended movements or increased by emotional excitement. They cease during sleep. Spasms of pharyngeal muscles causing dysphagia are rare. In a few patients, forceful, irregular athetoid movements also involve trunk, neck, and face, approaching the bizarre postures of dystonia musculorum deformans (Fig. 24-6). In later stages the movements usually become asymmetrical both in pattern and in amplitude. Since the limbs may become rigid, sooner or later the athetotic movements are reduced to mobile spasms.

Pathologically, the most constant change in congenital athetosis is bilateral atrophy, together with astrogliosis, of the putamen. The lesions appear inactive. In myelin preparations a marbled appearance of the putamen is commonly observed (*état marbré, status marmoratus*) (Fig. 24-7). This is due to new growth, here and there, of great numbers of myelinated axons. *Hypermyelination* is hardly the word for it, for no fiber has an excess of myelin. (The marbling found in Holzer preparations is a reflection of patchy gliosis associated with nerve cell fallout.) The caudate nucleus, and less commonly the thalamus, may be similarly affected. In the globus pallidus, myelin loss out of proportion to nerve cell loss sometimes occurs (*status dysmyelinisatus*); kernicterus, not hypoxemia occurring perinatally, is its chief basis. In one well-documented case of neonatal asphyxia, there was severe atrophy of the globus pallidus with fallout of at least 75 percent of cells from both pallidal segments, as well as degeneration of all pallidofugal pathways and the "corticonigral tract," while the rest of the brain was intact (Papez, Herzman, and Rundles, 1938).

Changes in the cerebral cortex, prominent in some cases, vary from patchy gliosis to microgyria, with the occasional finding of fibromyelin plaques containing newly grown nerve fibers. Almost any cerebral structure, including the brainstem, may be found damaged (Carpenter, 1950; Courville, 1953; Denny-Brown, 1962; Norman, 1947; Scholz, Wake, and Peters, 1938). Status marmoratus involving putamen and cortex (precentral, parietal, occipital) without concurrent athetosis has been observed by one author (Norman, 1938), who explained the discrepancy

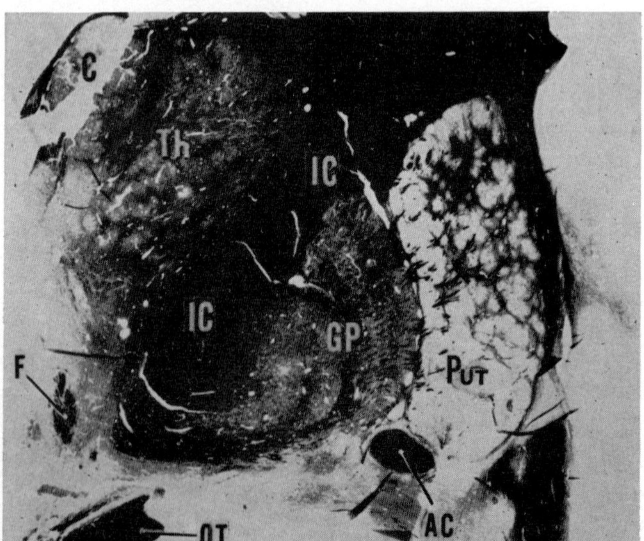

Fig. 24-7. Status marmoratus in a case of athetosis. The putamen *(Put)*, thalamus *(Th)*, and caudate nucleus *(C)* have a marbled appearance owing to myelination of regenerated nerve fibers. The globus pallidus *(GP)* shows perivascular myelin loss. *AC*, anterior commissure; *F*, fornix; *IC*, internal capsule; *OT*, optic tract. Myelin stain. (From the Deutsche Forschungsanstalt für Psychiatrie, Max-Planck-Institut, München.)

by pointing to the coincident damage of the precentral cortex (area 4).

Perinatal hypoxemia, however, has also given rise to hemichorea, double chorea, and associated pyramidal disorders. Belonging in this group is Little's disease, described on pp. 340 and 341.

Athetosis of other cause. Double athetosis develops not only from lack of oxygen at birth but also in morbus coeruleus and posticteric encephalopathy. In a small proportion of such cases, dystonic phenomena ensue. Once developed, conditions of this kind usually remain static.

Pathological changes in *posticteric encephalopathy* include myelin loss in the globus pallidus and subthalamic nucleus, as well as loss of nerve cells from these structures and from the hippocampus, the zona reticulata (red zone) of the substantia nigra, the interstitial nucleus of Cajal, the dentate nucleus, and the vestibular nuclei. Affected areas may show reactive astrogliosis. Putamen and thalamus now and then exhibit status marmoratus. The causative agent is bilirubin, which diffuses into the brain substance in the nonconjugated form after conjugation of bilirubin with serum albumin reaches the saturation point. This pigment is taken up by nerve cells and destroys them. (Haymaker and others, 1961; Malamud, 1963.)

Hemiathetosis may follow cerebral infarction, with hemiparesis preceding athetosis. Lesions are found in diverse and sometimes multiple structures: thalamus, striatum, globus pallidus, internal capsule, and cerebral peduncle (Carpenter, 1950). Athetosis in the adult is not infrequently a result of a lesion, vascular or neoplastic, in the subthalamic region (Bucy, 1942; Denny-Brown, 1962; Gowers, 1876; Papez, Hertzman, and Rundles, 1938; Spiller, 1920).

The putamen of both sides may be predominantly damaged when a *barbiturate* is taken in a dose large enough to cause cardiac arrest (Fig. 24-8). Or the lateral segment of the globus pallidus may bear the brunt and so give rise to bilateral athetoid hyperkinesias (Jervis and Joyce, 1948).

Athetosis occurs in a great variety of disorders, often only as one phase in the development of more inclusive extrapyramidal syndromes to be described later.

Athetosis has not been produced experimentally. Striatal ablations in the monkey result in motor hyperactivity but not athetosis; according to Mettler and Mettler (1942), the striatum becomes sensitized to proprioceptive stimuli. Bucy and Case (1937) have concluded that area 6 of

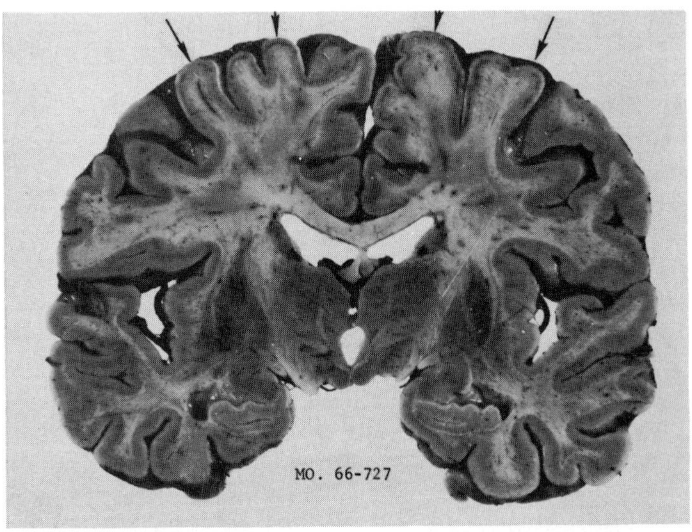

Fig. 24-8. Temporary cardiac arrest from an overdose of barbiturates, with survival period of about 7 weeks. Areas of the putamen are necrotic bilaterally. Cortex in the territory of supply of terminal branches of anterior and middle cerebral arteries is also necrotic (arrows). (Courtesy Dr. Richard Lindenberg, Baltimore.)

the cortex mediates the movements. In Bucy's view (1949, 1958), choreoathetosis is produced by a break in striatum, pallidum, or thalamus that disrupts the reverberating circuit: areas 8 and 4 → caudate nucleus → pallidum → VL of thalamus → area 6 and, in a lesser degree, area 4. An alternate view presupposes a fronto → thalamo → pallidal system; a state of pallidal overexcitability brought about by release from striatal inhibition would have an activating influence via this system and thus induce pathological hyperkinesis (Spiegel and Wycis, 1953).

In human cases the *nature* of the lesion is highly significant for the precipitation of hyperkinesis. While slowly progressive or subacute lesions in the striatum often result in athetosis, sudden widespread infarction results in hemiplegia, attended by only minor involuntary movements (p. 341).

Ballism. Ballism is an acute disorder of middle or late adult life, but has occurred in persons as young as 7 years of age. Usually unilateral *(hemiballism),* the hyperkinesis is a nonpatterned, violent hurling, flinging, or kicking (ballism—"throwing"). The left side is more commonly affected. The movements, contralateral to the lesion, are commonly of the same nature as in chorea; hence some authors stick to the term *hemichorea.* However, there is a difference in the muscles involved and in degree: proximal, and excessive, and mainly involving the upper limb in ballism. Torsion of the trunk is sometimes an integral part. When the face is implicated, speech, respiration, and swallowing suffer. The movements can be voluntarily checked, but not for more than a few moments at a time. They cease during sleep. Death from physical exhaustion may occur in a few weeks or months. Very rarely, ballism ceases spontaneously, for example, at the end of 7 weeks. (Carpenter, 1955; Christensen and Krabbe, 1945; Martin and Alcock, 1934; Vincent and van Bogaert, 1936.)

The most frequent pathological change consists in focal softening in and around the subthalamic nucleus, usually the outcome of vascular thrombosis, or, occasionally, embolism, rarely a small hemorrhage. Diabetes mellitus often underlies the thrombotic process. Other effective lesions include gumma, tuberculoma, and metastatic abscess, as well as lesions resulting from metastatic neoplasm. Cranial trauma may also be responsible. To be effective, the lesion can be so situated as to interrupt afferent pathways to the subthalamic nucleus or efferent pathways, for example, a lesion in the medial segment of the globus pallidus extending into the internal capsule. (Martin, 1957; Martin and Alcock, 1934; Meyers, Sweeney, and Schwidde, 1950.) While the lesion is usually contralateral to the movements, there are cases in which a suitable lesion produced both contralateral and ipsilateral hemiballism (or hemichorea), effects that have been duplicated in patients with parkinsonism subjected to chemopallidectomy or chemothalamotomy (Dierssen, Gioino, and Cooper, 1961). Hemiballism has occasionally been produced in monkeys by damaging the subthalamic nucleus (Carpenter, 1958); since severance of connections between the globus pallidus and subthalamic nucleus abolished the ballism, the ansa lenticularis may be necessary to produce the movements (Whittier and Mettler, 1949). Data from stereotaxic procedures in man indicate that hemiballism may result from lesions situated near the subthalamic nucleus, without direct injury to it, and even from lesions in pallidum, thalamus, or cerebral cortex (Cooper, Bergmann, and Caracalos, 1963; Fager, 1968; Hughes, 1965; Schwarz and Barrows, 1960). Conversely, a lesion made in the substantia nigra can abolish ballism (Wycis, 1958).

Neural mechanisms responsible for the disorder remain enigmatic. As already indicated, derangement of fiber systems coursing through or adjacent to the corpus Luysii can be effective. COEPS projections from precentral (motor) cortex to subthalamic nucleus, zona incerta, field H, and even the red nucleus, all course through field H_2 or contribute to the dorsal capsule of the subthalamic nucleus. Release of certain components of the corticospinal system from the influence of subcortical systems that ascend to the cortex represents a reasonable working hypothesis to explain how, for example, only an arm can be affected. In the monkey, the descending pathway mediating ballistic (or choreiform) movements produced by lesions of the subthalamic nucleus is situated in the dorsolateral quadrant of the spinal cord (Carpenter, Correll, and Hinman, 1960).

Dystonia

Dystonia musculorum deformans. Dystonic disturbances involving either posture or movement or both may be an expression of a number of extrapyramidal disorders, such as Wilson's disease and postencephalitic states. They may also be seen in such varied conditions as perinatal brain damage (Fig. 24-6) and senility associated with arteriosclerosis (Richter, 1923; Schmitt and Scholz, 1932; Wechsler and Brock, 1922). Dystonia may also occur paroxysmally, for example in familial cases of the disorder and in such diseases as multiple sclerosis (Weber, 1967). The lesions most apt to produce dystonic disturbances, according to Cooper (1965), are those situated in the caudate nucleus, putamen, brachium conjunctivum, or emboliform nucleus (Fig. 24-3).

However, most cases of dystonia musculorum deformans are unrelated to other clinical entities. They usually affect persons aged 5 to 12 years, less often those between 13 to 21 years (range in 148 cases: 1 to 33 years). In some cases the disorder seems to occur sporadically, but by and large, dystonia musculorum deformans is an heredofamilial disease transmitted through autosomal mendelian dominance with a penetrance rate between 0.5 and 0.7. (Zeman and Dyken, 1967.)

These are the diagnostic criteria for genetic dystonia musculorum deformans, as given by Zeman and Dyken (1967) in agreement with others: dystonic hyperkinesias and postures at rest or in action; dystonia (irregular alternation of hypotonus and hypertonus) elicited by passive movement; dystonic postures (most frequently manifested by scoliosis or kyphosis); writer's cramp; and restricted, sustained muscle spasms. In most cases the initial disturbance is in the lower limb; in the remainder the upper limb or axial musculature is affected first. Facial involvement is more frequent in older patients. In some cases the hyperkinetic feature is lacking. In some 30 percent of cases early crippling occurs. During sleep the movements cease and in some cases the fixed postures revert toward normal. The disorder is usually episodic in its evolution but may be steadily progressive. (Herz, 1944.)

Negative findings in earlier stages of dystonia musculorum deformans, and not uncommonly in later stages as well, are: no paresis; no atrophy; no sensory, perceptive, or sphincter disturbances; no cranial nerve paresis; no speech disturbances; no significant psychological abnormalities (Zeman and Dyken, 1967).

Formes frustes, characterized for example by writer's cramp or mild dystonia, are very common; diagnosis can sometimes be made only on the basis of a positive family history (Johnson, Schwartz, and Barbeau, 1962).

Strangely, in genetic dystonia musculorum deformans, no significant pathological change has thus far been encountered in the central nervous system (Zeman and Dyken, 1967).

Dystonia has not been reproduced experimentally. An effective lesion in nongenetic human cases, according to Hassler (1953), consists in loss of large cells in the putamen together with damage of the pallidum. In some cases the putamen exhibits status marmoratus (Davison and Goodhart, 1938). Lesions made in the region of the ventral lateral nucleus of the thalamus have ameliorated the dystonia, particularly that on the side contralateral to the lesion (Fig. 24-3).

Torticollis and retrocollis. Spasmodic torticollis and retrocollis, or sustained involuntary movement resulting in tonic deviation of the head and neck, are considered variants of dystonia musculorum deformans (Herz and Hoefer, 1949). The disorder may be familial (van Bogaert, 1941) but is more commonly sporadic. The spasmodic jerks that occur appear to be attempts to correct the forced abnormal attitude. Spasmodic lateral flexion of the head occurring in attacks from the time of childhood is illustrated in Fig. 24-9, *A*, and retrocollis associated with the Parkinson state in Fig. 24-9, *B*. Torticollis may be associated with action tremor in one or both upper limbs.

Torticollis and retrocollis have been experimentally produced in part by lesions injuring the brachium conjunctivum and mesencephalic tegmentum (Foltz, Knopp, and Ward, 1959), and by electrically stimulating the midline cerebellar nuclei (Koella, 1955). An abnormal cerebellar servo mechanism involving the cerebello → thalamo → cortical circuit is thought to contribute to the nuchal hyperkinesis characterizing the torticollis syndrome, the latter being brought about through modulation of somatic motor pathways maintaining the head in its normal position. (Cooper, 1964, 1965.)

Stationary, nonspasmodic torticollis is the result of local disorders. These include cervical vertebral defect, fibrosis of the sternocleidomastoid

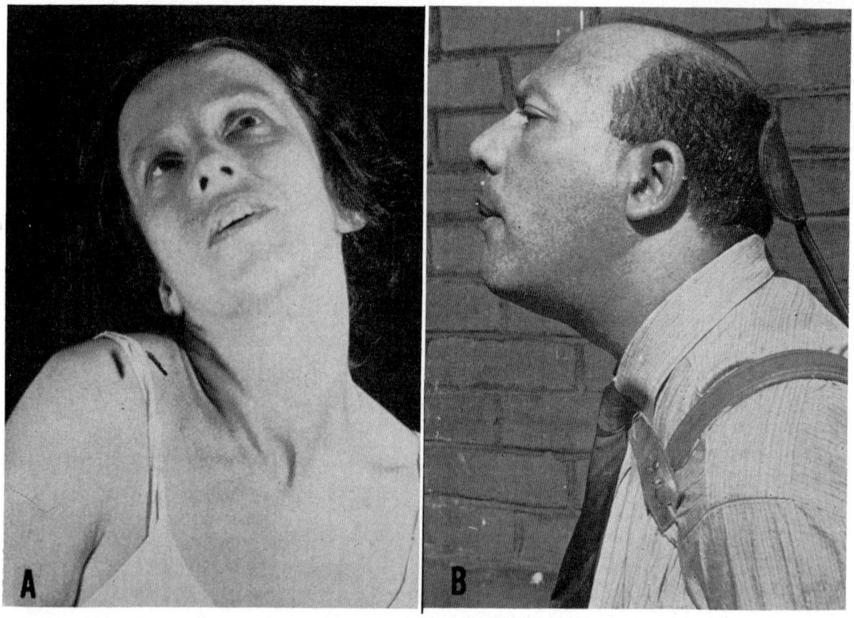

Fig. 24-9. A, Spasmodic torticollis occurring in attacks since childhood. **B,** Postencephalitic retrocollis. (Courtesy Dr. A. Ornsteen, Philadelphia.)

muscle following hemorrhage into the muscle, and cervical myositis (Cooper, 1965; Hassin, Schaub, and Voris, 1931; Herz and Glaser, 1949; Herz and Hoefer, 1949).

Hepatolenticular degeneration

Hepatolenticular degeneration is a disorder occurring in younger as well as older persons. It is characterized by the deposition of protein-bound copper (ceruloplasmin) in numerous structures, such as the brain (especially the putamen and thalamus), and in the peripheral zone of Descemet's membrane at the corneoscleral junction, giving rise to the "Kayser-Fleischer ring." Defective ceruloplasmin synthesis or the production of an abnormal tissue protein may be the basis of the disease. A disturbance of iron metabolism has also been noted (O'Reilly, Pollycove, and Bank, 1968). The disorder is also marked by aminoaciduria and peptiduria, apparently the results of a defect in renal tubular absorption (Adams and Sidman, 1968).

The disorder is referred to as *Wilson-pseudosclerosis,* particularly in German literature. The latter part of this term was coined by Westphal (in 1883) as a designation for a disorder (in an adult) in which intention tremor and spasticity suggested multiple sclerosis but in which no plaques were found (also no lenticular lesions) at autopsy. Hence the patient was said to have pseudosclerosis, not multiple sclerosis (no mention was made of liver cirrhosis). Wilson's description of a juvenile form in which he found liver cirrhosis and "progressive lenticular degeneration" appeared in 1912. Finding that the two clinical descriptions referred to the same disorder and to include the hepatic lesion, Hall (in 1921) chose the term *hepatolenticular degeneration* (see Eicke, 1957, and Wilson, 1912, 1940, for review of the history of the subject). The type of patient described by Westphal and Strümpell on one hand, and by Wilson on the other, may be said to form a spectrum: Wilson's disease occurs in younger persons and runs a slowly progressive course; pseudosclerosis appears at a later age and has an ingravescent or remittent course. On various grounds, mainly that of differing response to chelation therapy (reflecting a difference in "fundamental biochemical defect"), Denny-Brown (1964) considers Wilson's disease and pseudosclerosis as two "components" of hepatolenticular degeneration.

Wilson's disease (in younger persons) and Westphal's pseudosclerosis* (in older persons) are together a familial or heredofamilial disorder probably having auto-

*All terms containing "pseudo-" have always had a bad press, and rightly so. "Pseudosclerosis" expresses nothing characteristic of the disease and is only of historical interest, a fossil. The eponym "Westphal's disease," as a means of contrasting it with "Wilson's disease," has its merits.

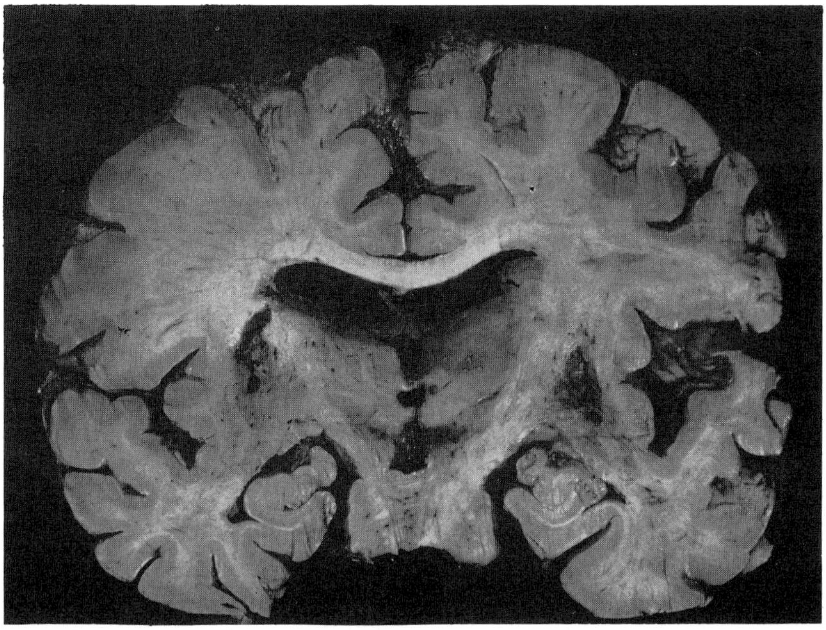

Fig. 24-10. Wilson's disease, showing degeneration of the lenticular nuclei with cavity formation. (AFIP Acc. 195199.)

somal recessive inheritance. The age at which the disease becomes manifest varies widely. Wilson's disease sets in most frequently in persons aged 7 to 15 years, the adult form *(pseudosclerosis)* at an age from 19 to 35, though symptoms and signs, including the Kayser-Fleischer ring, may not develop until the late forties. Duration of the disease varies from a few months to 40 years. (Denny-Brown, 1964; O'Reilly, 1967; Scheinberg, 1961; Sternlieb and Scheinberg, 1968.)

The patients display dystonic postures that are at first transient, a set expression of the face with open mouth and a spastic or vacuous smile (malocclusion of the teeth and high arched palate have been blamed), rhythmic action tremor of irregular amplitude at the wrists ("flapping") and the shoulders ("wingbeating") that increase with volitional movement, periodic athetoid overflexion of one arm or leg brought on by movement, ultimately a fixed dystonic posture, and finally, continuous overflexion, or "hemiplegic" dystonia. (Denny-Brown, 1962, 1964.) Speech is often slurred; spasmodic laughter and true emotional outbursts may develop. Attacks in which consciousness is altered can also occur, and they may dominate the clinical tableau. Moreover, personality changes occur and intelligence deteriorates in some cases to the point of outright dementia. "Schizophrenia" features in some cases. (Inose, 1968; Lichtenstein and Gore, 1955; Wilson, 1940.)

Outstanding in pseudosclerosis, according to Denny-Brown (1964), are tremor and dysarthria. As in the juvenile form of the disease, the tremor is at the wrists and shoulders. The dysarthria is slurring, with a tendency to scan. In contrast with Wilson's disease, dystonic fixity of posture is lacking. In the face, however, fixity of expression and infrequency of blinking are noted in some cases. As emphasized by Lichtenstein and Gore (1955), hemiparkinsonism may characterize the onset and "cerebellar" symptoms may suggest multiple sclerosis.

Of the cerebral structures involved in hepatolenticular degeneration, the most profound pathological changes are in the *putamen*. In the juvenile form, astrocytes in the putamen are enlarged and their cytoplasm contains numerous golden, copper-positive granules. These glial cells degenerate. Small cavities *(status spongiosus)* develop, and they commonly merge to form larger cavities (Fig. 24-10). Endothelial cells of capillaries bordering foci of early status spongiosus are enlarged or, in some cases, proliferated. Vessel walls show evidence of damage. The presence of vascular alterations has brought forward the suggestion that defective exchange between blood and tissue compartments may be a leading factor in the tissue disintegration. (Denny-Brown, 1964; Eicke, 1957; von Braunmühl, 1930.) However, nerve cells persist unaltered in affected areas, ruling out ischemia as the responsible process. Similar though less widespread changes take place in the cerebral cortex and convolutional white matter (mainly frontal), with spongy necrosis and cavitation sometimes occurring. Also affected, though in still less degree, are caudate nucleus, thalamus, and certain other structures such as globus pallidus, subthalamic region, red nucleus, zona compacta of the substantia nigra (Fig. 24-11, *B*), and the dentate and roof nuclei of the cerebellum. In the adult form of the disease the pathological change is the same except in the putamen, where no cavities develop and where the astrogliosis is possibly not as dense as in Wilson's disease. Also affected, as a rule, are the globus pallidus, red nucleus, and dentate nucleus of the cerebellum. (Denny-Brown, 1962, 1964; Eicke, 1957; Richter, 1948; Shiraki, 1968.) Multiple hemorrhages—an expression of the hepatic insufficiency—may be found in the brain (Lichtenstein and Gore, 1955).

Hallervorden-Spatz's disease

Hallervorden-Spatz's disease was established as an entity through the finding of abnormal iron deposits in the pallidum and the substantia nigra (its zona reticularis). Clinically the disorder includes not only extrapyramidal disturbances but also muscle wasting, spasms, and dementia. The diagnosis is to be suspected if, in persons 8 to 15 years old, walking becomes stiff-legged and pigeon-toed (equinovarus deformities). In the next few years all four limbs exhibit choreiform or athetoid movements, and mental disturbances may supervene. There may also be buccopharyngeal and laryngeal spasms. (Vincent and van Bogaert, 1936.) Some atypical cases are characterized by action tremor and slowness of speech suggesting multiple sclerosis; others have muscular hypotonia, fasciculations, atrophy of the interosseous muscles, and bulbar palsy. Parkinson-like tremor as well as dystonic postures may be observed during the evolution of the disorder. Also recognized is a rapidly evolving myoclonic form of the disease, again with dementia, but developing in adulthood (Eicke, 1940; Radermecker and Rizzuto, 1967; Rozdilsky, Cumings, and Huston, 1968). When running in families (siblings) the disorder usually becomes manifest earlier, at the age of 7 to 9 years. Onset soon after birth has even been re-

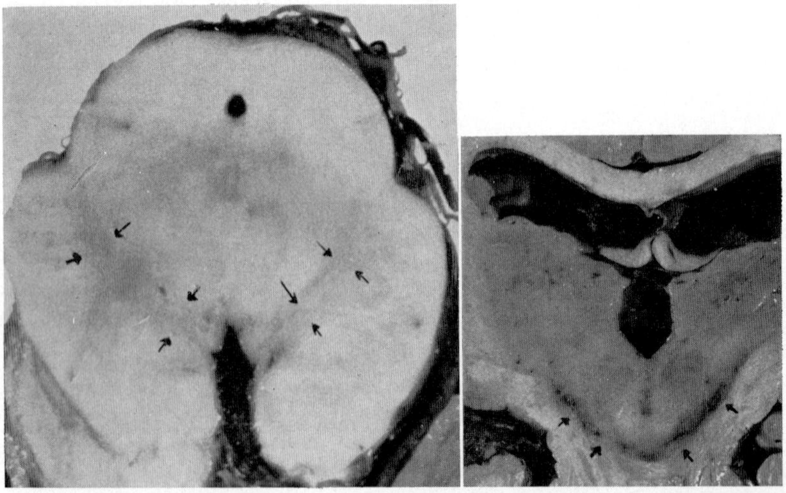

Fig. 24-11. *Left:* The midbrain in a case of postencephalitic Parkinson state, showing virtually complete depigmentation of the substantia nigra (arrows). (AFIP Acc. 266301.) *Right:* From a case of Wilson's disease, with preservation of most of the pigment (arrows). (AFIP Acc. 195199.)

ported. There may be seizures of various kinds. On the whole, speech disturbances are uncommon throughout much of the course of the disease (Sacks, Aguilar, and Brown, 1966). Optic atrophy and retinitis pigmentosa are occasionally seen.

Globus pallidus and substantia nigra (its nonpigmented zone, the zona reticularis) are predominantly affected. As viewed grossly, both of these structures have an intense rust brown hue; viewed microscopically, the affected cells (astrocytes) are a green blue. This is a reflection of the deposition of iron salts on these cells. Iron-containing material also accumulates in the tissue and in macrophages in regions of astrocytic disruption. Excessive amounts of physiological lipid are also found in glia and tissue. Areas of the globus pallidus may be converted to astroglial scars. Moreover, the globus pallidus may be characterized by status dysmyelinisatus. Occasionally, capillary vessels in the zona reticularis of the substantia nigra exhibit changes similar to those observed in Wernicke's encephalopathy. Striatum, thalamus, subthalamic nucleus, and cerebral cortex are additional sites of lesions. Severe atrophy of the cerebellum has also been noted. (DeJong and Scharenberg, 1952; Meyer, 1963; van Bogaert, 1940.) Rounded argyrophilic axonal swellings of varying diameter may be seen in substantia nigra, pallidum, putamen, and other structures such as the cerebral white matter, suggesting, according to Sacks, Aguilar, and Brown (1966), an almost volcanic activity in the dystrophic neurons. Lesions simulating those of Hallervorden-Spatz's disease have been noted in the amyotrophic lateral sclerosis occurring in Guam and Japan (Shiraki, 1966).

The following interpretations have been offered: (1) the pigmentation is the only specific change, hence it is the indispensable prerequisite to the diagnosis of the disease (Hallervorden and Spatz, 1922); (2) the main pathogenetic factor may be a primary disturbance in the metabolic function of glia (Bischoff and Regli, 1963); (3) the neuroaxonal dystrophy may be genetically determined and be the basic pathogenetic factor (Cowen and Olmstead, 1963; Seitelberger and Gross, 1957).

Creutzfeldt-Jakob's disease and subacute spongiform encephalopathy

Creutzfeldt-Jakob's disease is among the subacute dementias but has many extrapyramidal features. The disorder usually occurs spontaneously, but familial cases are recognized (May, 1968; May, Itabashi, and DeJong, 1968). Age at onset is usually between 35 and 55 years but may be in the sixties or seventies. There is no sex preference. Memory loss, disturbances in equilibrium, or slurring of speech may open the clinical tableau. Subsequent features include ataxia, intention tremor, dysarthria, spasticity, extrapyramidal disturbances (rigidity, tremor, athetosis, dystonic attitude), signs such as are found in amyotrophic lateral sclerosis (including bulbar palsy), myoclonus (in some cases), hallucinations, confusion, depression or euphoria, and ultimately dementia. The condition runs its course in a few months to 2 years. Variants of the disease are common (May, 1968).

Pathological features include widespread neuronal loss and degeneration together with prominent gliosis. In the cerebral cortex the alterations are maximal in the temporocentral region. Changes are also found in the cerebellum, thalamus, striatum, pallidum, and, in some cases, in motor cranial nerve nuclei and anterior horns of the spinal cord. Loculation, or honeycombing, of the tissue (status spongiosus), advancing to spongy necrosis, is common in the cerebral cortex but rarely if ever occurs in the basal ganglia. No pattern of damage common to all cases has emerged. (Bornstein and Jervis, 1955; Lafon and others, 1965; Nevin and others, 1960.)

Subacute spongiform encephalopathy may be familial, and become clinically evident in young persons (van Bogaert and Bertrand, 1949). However, it usually develops spontaneously and is manifested by subacute presenile dementia (most commonly in persons in their fifties). In adults, aside from general symptoms such as depression and malaise, the initial complaint in this ingravescent illness includes one or more of the following: impairment or distortion of vision, diplopia; stiffness, weakness, or loss of control of a limb, also involuntary movements, especially myoclonus; even epileptic seizures, dysphasia, blunting of memory; then dementia sets in. (Nevin and others, 1960.)

Pathological changes predominate in the cerebral cortex. The sponginess originates from ballooning of astroglial cells and the development of spaces within myelin sheaths from "splits" of the sheath at the interperiod line (Gambetti, Mellman, and Gonatos, 1969; van Bogaert and Bertrand, 1949). An edematous process is generally favored as the basis, though a primary change in astroglial cells has been contended (Foley and Denny-Brown, 1957), a view that may or may not be supported by the finding that astrocytic mitochondria are abnormal (Gambetti, Mellman, and Gonatos, 1969). In some cases nerve cell loss is rather minor, and no vascular change can be found. In others, neuron depletion does occur; loss of nerve cells is noted in all laminae in various regions of the cortex, particularly the occipital cortex. Astroglia and oligodendroglia vanish from softened areas, and there may be striking astrogliosis elsewhere in the cortex. Similar though less advanced lesions, including status spongiosus, have been noted on occasion in the striatum, thalamus, globus pallidus, and cerebellum. From these and other observations (such as lack of degenerative change in brainstem motor nuclei), it has been concluded that the condition is fundamentally different from Creutzfeldt-Jakob disease. (Nevin and others, 1960.)

According to May, Itabashi, and DeJong (1968), and in support of the majority view, the constellation of signs and symptoms, the occurrence of status spongiosus, and the occasional terminal myoclonic phenomena strongly suggest that the classical form of Creutzfeldt-Jakob's disease and subacute spongiform encephalopathy are one and the same disorder. In Crompton's (1968) view Creutzfeldt-Jakob's disease, subacute spongiform encephalopathy, and Alpers' disease (occurring in infants) have enough in common to suggest that they are manifestations of the same kind of reaction in the brain. Gaps, however, still exist: the pathological changes in the latter two are more restricted than in Creutzfeldt-Jakob's disease, while Alpers' disease, with some changes suggestive of malformation, has yet to be established as an entity. The controversial aspects of progressive cortical degeneration in infants are reviewed by Laurence and Cavanagh (1968).

As to cause, there is a growing impression that both Creutzfeldt-Jakob disease and subacute spongiform encephalopathy, when occurring spontaneously, may represent an infective process due to a "slow virus." Gibbs and his colleagues (1968) have observed a similar disorder in chimpanzees into which biopsy material from a human brain had been inoculated.

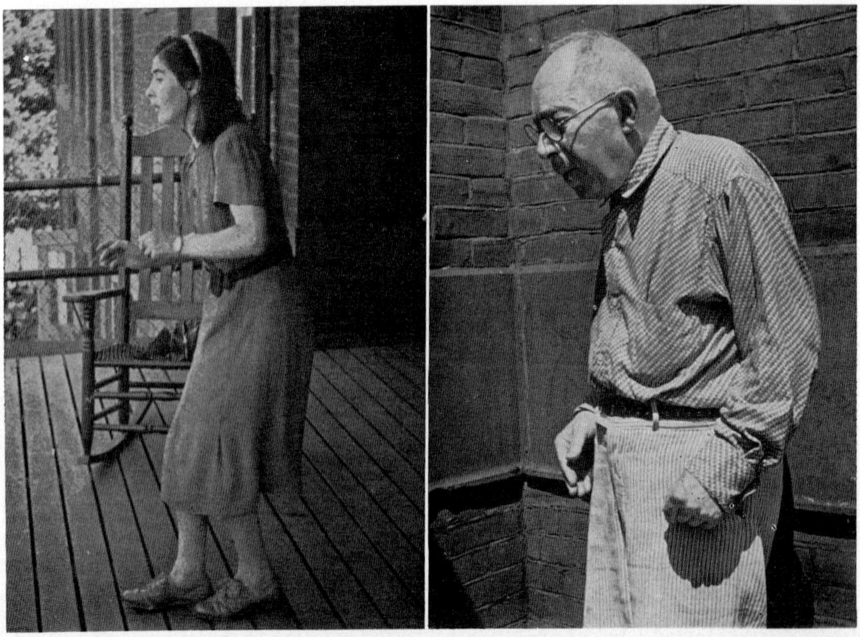

Fig. 24-12. Muscular rigidity in the Parkinson state. (Courtesy Dr. A. Ornsteen, Philadelphia.)

Parkinsonian states

Paralysis agitans and postencephalitic parkinsonism. The paralysis agitans, or shaking palsy, described by Parkinson usually becomes manifest in persons 50 to 60 years of age. Epidemic encephalitis occurring in the period from 1917 to 1924 ("von Economo's disease") affected persons of any age. In many of these patients parkinsonism developed either soon after termination of the acute stage or following a latency period up to 10 years and more. Both paralysis agitans and postencephalitic parkinsonism usually set in without indications of constitutional brain disease. (Bing and Haymaker, 1939; Siegfried, 1968.) Although the distinction between the two forms is thus somewhat arbitrary, it is usually made; the distinction is retained in the text that follows.

Both disorders are characterized by disturbances classed as *amyostatic,* which essentially is a synonym for *tremor.* The main features are: insidious onset and slow progress; a moderately rapid, rhythmic tremor, first fine, then coarse, pronounced during rest and virtually disappearing upon movement; generalized rigidity of the skeletal and mimetic muscles (Fig. 24-12); difficulty in initiating voluntary movement; poverty of movement in general; dissociation of movements; reduction in the scope of automatic movements; postural disturbances; autonomic disturbances, including seborrhea and alterations in sweat pattern and in skin temperature. The occasional urinary retention that occurs can be blamed on the disease as much as on the anticholinergic agents used in its treatment. Salivation is often quite troublesome; it results from infrequent swallowing rather than excess production of saliva (Yahr and Bering and others, 1966). Autonomic disturbances are usually more severe in the postencephalic form than in paralysis agitans. Symptoms of depression are frequent and directly correlated with vulnerability to stress.

The "resting" tremor in parkinsonism, due to reciprocal firing of antagonistic muscles, is especially notable in the thumb beating against the index finger. The tremor commonly begins here and in the wrist, then affects the lips and tongue; finally it may become almost generalized. It may be so violent as to make the entire body shake, especially in the postencephalitic form. Eyelids are also involved, with the tremor occurring at a faster rate than in the limbs (Loeffler, Slatt, and Hoyt, 1966). Severity of the tremor fluctuates during the day and the course of the disease.

The face freezes into a mask, there is no smile, no frown. As the years go by, the voice becomes monotonous, ill articulated, and low to the point of being inaudible as well as unintelligible. The walking stride gets smaller and smaller; the body's center of gravity being displaced forward, the patient endeavors to catch up with it; as the rate of stepping increases, festination and locomotor control is lost; he may fall. Finally, he ceases to be self-propelled.

As to the details of posture, there is that progressive lumbar stoop; the limbs, too, usually assume an attitude of flexion, the hand in hyperpronation, flexed at the metacarpophalangeal joints, but with fingers extended. The head may also be fixed in flexion. Minimal excursions of intercostal muscles and diaphragm lead to hypoventilation. The postural change, immobility, or akinesia can be quite independent of the rigidity and unrelated as to intensity (Denny-Brown, 1962). The end result is a totally bedridden patient who may develop bedsores, a silent, completely fixed, vibrating, horizontal, single mass, staring into space, with relatively well preserved mentation that distinguishes him from the catatonic schizophrenic. General health is usually excellent.

The rigidity is manifest both in extensor and flexor muscles but is most pronounced in the flexors. It is more "plastic" than the spasticity observed in a hemiplegic limb. To flex or extend at large joints feels like bending a "lead-pipe"; the rigid limb exhibits some resistance throughout the entire extent of the excursion. Interrupting the smooth flow of passive motion, however, is a series of "checks and gives" *(cogwheel phenomenon)* due to extensor contractions during flexion movements *(Westphal's paradoxical reaction, or tonic postural reflex).*

To bring out the *cogwheel phenomenon,* the examiner slowly moves the patient's forearm to produce, alternately, flexion and extension at the elbow. As the muscles yield to the stretching, they undergo rhythmic contractions, each of which momentarily impedes the movement. The phenomenon can also be elicited by pronation-supination at the elbow or by flexion-extension of the wrist (Ornsteen, 1929). Where rigidity is latent the phenomenon is reinforced through rapid tapping with the other hand, for example, by tapping the knee. The cogwheel effect, according to Denny-Brown (1962), is due to tremor, which, by virtue of its rhythmicity, allows steps of relaxation in the resistance to passive movement.

As to the *Westphal reaction,* if the plantar flexors of the foot or the palmar flexors at the wrist are suddenly stretched, the (shortened) extensors undergo brief contractions such that tautening of the extensor tendons is readily visible. Voluntary effort at extension induces rhythmic tremor in the same extensor muscles. The reaction is interpreted as "proprioceptive and related to the antagonistic autogenetic reflex excitatory state of the annulospiral endings versus the inhibitory secondary sensory flower-spray endings of the muscle spindles" (Denny-Brown, 1962).

Defects in posture, equilibrium, movements, and reflexes, may be brought out by various tests.

Pushing test. If a normal person standing upright is suddenly pushed backward or forward, an immediate contraction occurs in the muscles necessary to the maintenance of equilibrium. If the chest is pushed, there is a compensatory contraction of the abdominal muscles, quadriceps femoris, and tibialis anterior; if the back is pushed the contractions take place in the lumbosacral, hamstring, and calf muscles. However, in parkinsonism these muscular responses are retarded or absent, and as a result, retropulsion and propulsion occur—the patient is set in motion by a relatively feeble push. (The same factors are responsible for the hurried, festinating gait.) This disturbance, however, is likewise observed in focal lesions of the midbrain tegmentum in persons not having parkinsonism.

Arm swinging. Decrease in the range of arm swinging in walking is a noteworthy early sign of the Parkinson state, particularly when the involvement is unilateral. In addition the examiner can test arm swinging by jerkily moving the patient's shoulders to and fro to observe the relative excursions of the two arms.

Little toe reflex. Slow abduction of the little toe occurs when the outer edge of the foot is lightly stroked.

Flexion reflex of the toes. Percussion of the anterior surface of the lower leg produces flexion of the toes.

Pressure reflex. When certain bony prominences are firmly stroked, a slow muscular contraction ensues. Thus, when the ulna is stroked in a downward direction, the second, third, and fourth fingers flex. When the region of the radius is stroked, the thumb flexes.

Jendrassik maneuver. Normally, in this maneuver, hooking the flexed fingers together and pulling in opposite directions short of separating them facilitates the knee jerk and other stretch reflexes. This is due to muscle spindle activation resulting from increased muscle tension. This facilitation, generally useful in patients whose reflexes are hard to elicit, does not occur in parkinsonism: in patients with unilateral parkinsonism the response is absent only on the affected side. (Hassler, 1956; Ward, 1961.)

Certain phenomena may be classed among the riddles of parkinsonism. One is *paradoxical kinesis.* The rigidity in parkinsonism is not invariable, being influenced, for instance, by psychical stress: a Parkinson patient, though bedridden and unable to turn in bed, has been known to run out of a house that is on fire and lapse into frozen immobility on the front lawn. Ward (1961) suggests that massive driving of facilitatory circuits operating through the alpha motor system—circuits he believes ordinarily to be suppressed in such patients—may bring this about. Periodicity of motor activity is also recognized; fluctuations are linked with the sleep-waking mechanism. A patient unable to walk, hardly able to talk, confined to bed, and rigid during the day may be able to walk about the ward and be sociable at night (Abrahamson and Rabiner, 1924). Parkinsonian tremor is in abeyance during sleep.

The sequence in which various signs make their appearance in the parkinsonian state varies. According to Hoehn and Yahr (1967), tremor is the most frequent sign, then a gait disturbance, both in paralysis agitans and postencephalitic parkinsonism. In the postencephalitic form, Ornsteen (1936) has noted that generalized hypokinesis is commonly the first disturbance to appear. Degree and rapidity of progression may differ: in paralysis agitans, according to Denny-Brown (1962), tremor is gradually replaced by rigidity, then by dystonic attitudes, while in the postencephalitic form rigidity soon gives way to fixed attitudes of dystonia, leading to scoliosis, torticollis, and grotesque postures of the limbs. In contrast, according to Selby (1967a, b), in the form presumed to be postencephalitic, the signs of parkinsonism cease to progress after a few months of their onset. Dissociation of disturbances has been emphasized by the results of stereotaxic surgery but occurs naturally: some patients are rigid and beset by tremor, while others are free from rigidity and have little tremor, yet suffer from akinesia—mask-like facial expression, weak voice, shuffling gait, general lack of spontaneity (DeJong, 1965; Denny-Brown, 1962; Martin, 1965). Further, oculogyric crises (pp. 268 and 271) occur in postencephalitic patients and apparently not in paralysis agitans.

Parkinsonism and cerebellar disorders are, in principle, diametrical opposites in their manifestations. The rigidity of parkinsonism contrasts with the hypotonia and dysmetria of the cerebellar syndrome, where movements overrun their normal bounds. An example is in handwriting; micrographia occurs in the parkinsonian state and megalographia in cerebellar disorders (Fig. 17-3). The Parkinson patient overestimates the weight of an object placed in the affected hand; the cerebellar patient underestimates it. Tremor of the parkinsonian syndrome is usually reduced on movement; in the cerebellar syndrome it is provoked by movement.

Considered pathologically, pigmented cells suffer most. In *paralysis agitans* the substantia nigra is the structure most prominently affected. In some series it was found damaged in all cases (Adams and Sidman, 1968; Foix and Nicolesco, 1925; Hassler, 1938; Klaue, 1940). Pigmented cells in the pars compacta (black zone) undergo necrobiosis; the pigment spills over into the nervous tissue and is taken up by macrophages. Commonly the cell loss is more or less limited to certain cell groups of the nigra—the anterior medial group in the oral part of the nigra and the middle cell group in the caudal part (Forno, 1966; Greenfield and Bosanquet, 1953; Hassler, 1938; Klaue, 1940). Similar changes occur in pigmented cells of the *locus coeruleus,* as well as in cells of the *pigmented vagal nucleus.* The *globus pallidus* is much less frequently affected (Adams and Sidman, 1968). When affected, its lateral segment suffers the most. Here, according to Denny-Brown (1962), nerve cells are mainly lost focally. Patchy demyelination is seen in regions corresponding more or less to the areas of nerve cell loss. In advanced stages, all remaining pallidal nerve cells may be shrunken, and the myelin of striopallidal fibers is less stainable than the myelin of the efferent pallidal fibers in the ansa lenticularis. Greenfield (1963) and Hassler (1938) consider that most of the affected nerve cells in the globus pallidus show changes indistinguishable from those seen in the course of senility. Cell changes in the striatum are inconspicuous and late in appearance. Other cell aggregates that may be affected include substantia innominata of Reichert, subthalamic nucleus, zona incerta, superior and inferior olivary nuclei, and the dorsal nucleus of the vagus nerve. Vessels in certain affected structures may show hyaline change but usually appear unaltered. Considerable glial activation, mainly microglial, occurs in affected gray matter, and parallels the nerve cell loss. (Foix and Nicolesco, 1925; Hallervorden, 1957; Stadlan, Duvoisin, and Yahr, 1966; van Bogaert, 1930.)

In the *postencephalitic Parkinson syndrome* residual inflammatory cells may be found, particularly in the region of the midbrain, for as long as several years after the initial illness. Otherwise the pathological changes are qualitatively much the same as in paralysis agitans but frequently more widespread and, in the aggregate, more severe. For example, gliosis may occur in the hypothalamus, periaqueductal gray, subthalamic nucleus or thalamus, or in all these structures. (Foix and Nicolesco, 1925; Forno, 1966; Lewy, 1923.) Again, the *substantia nigra* (its pars compacta) is the structure most commonly and most seriously affected. Pigment disappears from the nigra (Fig. 24-11, A), not from certain cell groups (as in paralysis agitans) but from all cell groups. Accumulations of lipid (lipochrome) are found in persisting nerve cells. Where clinical disturbances are predominantly unilateral the greatest damage of the nigra is on the opposite side. The *locus coeruleus,* too, usually suffers heavily but is scarcely affected in some cases (Forno, 1966). The *globus pallidus* is variably affected. "Obvious nerve cell changes in the globus pallidus or striatum were seldom found" in one series (Denny-Brown, 1962). In others "degeneration of nerve cells throughout the pallidum [was of such degree] that it was doubtful whether any normal nerve cells remained in the outer segment, and few remained in the inner segment" (Martin, 1965). The lateral segment usually suffers most. Diffuse myelin pallor due partly to loss of striopallidal fibers is sometimes characteristic. In general, greater glial reaction occurs in affected structures than in paralysis agitans. (Earle, 1968; Stadlan, Duvoisin, and Yahr, 1966; von Braunmühl, 1949.) Foix and Nicolesco (1925) laid emphasis on the occurrence of status cribratus, lacuna development, small tissue softenings, "abiobiotrophic" degeneration, and neuroglial sclerosis in varied structures.

Whether and to what extent *brain atrophy* occurs in paralysis agitans and postencephalitic parkinsonism has received some attention. Adams, van Bogaert, and Vander Eecken (1964) commented that "slight brain atrophy, enlargement of the lateral and third ventricles and loss of cortical neurons with replacement gliosis is another feature of some cases of paralysis agitans which may prove more characteristic than has been realized in the past. We have observed these changes in a significant number of cases. . . ." Occasional cases of cerebral cortical lesions associated with atrophy are on record (Lhermitte and Cornil, 1921). Where such exist, they have been attributed to senility (Foix and Nicolesco, 1925). Hallervorden (1957) could find no macroscopic changes in the cortex and, from microscopic examination, concluded: "There are no changes in the cerebral cortex other than those attributable to aging." Nor could Forno (1966) find any alteration beyond "dropping out" of nerve cells, chronic nerve cell changes, and mild increase in astrocytic nuclei. Denny-Brown (1962) mentions myelin pallor of corticostriate fibers in postencephalitic parkinsonism and of "corticopallidal" fibers in paralysis agitans. Selby recently (1968) reopened the subject of cerebral atrophy in parkinsonism. In pneumoencephalograms in 250 cases, he noted evidence of cerebral cortical atrophy (as manifested by widening of the subarachnoidal and cisternal spaces) in 57.2 percent of the cases (26.8 percent in the control cases of varied neurological diseases) and ventricular enlargement in 30 percent. What this means in terms of the development of parkinsonism is not evident. If parkinsonism finds expression through the sensorimotor cortex, which is suggested by Selby as a possibility, observed pathological changes in the cortex as incitants carry so small an incidence as to be negligible.

Both in paralysis agitans and postencephalitic parkinsonism, *granular bodies* (composed of ill-defined eosinophilic granules) are occasionally found in the cytoplasm of nerve cells in both parts of the substantia nigra and less commonly in other grisea. They appear age-related, being most common in older persons. The same is true for *granulovacuolar cytoplasmic inclusions. Lewy bodies* (eosinophilic concentric hyalin cytoplasmic inclusions surrounded by an unstained halo) are almost always present in classical paralysis agitans but seldom in the postencephalitic brain. In paralysis agitans they are found almost exclusively in the age range between 45 and 75 years. The bodies are observed predominantly in the substantia nigra and locus coeruleus (Lewy, 1913). They are also seen in the brains of older persons not having had the stigmata of parkinsonism (Klaue, 1940). In the view of Stadlan, Duvoisin, and Yahr (1966), "Lewy bodies, in the absence of other evidence of nigral atrophy, do not appear to be related to parkinsonism." *Neurofibrillary tangles* are far more common in postencephalitic parkinsonism than in paralysis agitans. They are present mostly in the periaqueductal gray, putamen, hypothalamus, and thalamus. They are also found in inclusion encephalitis, senile and presenile dementia, and in the brains of at least 10 percent of older, "normal" persons. Lewy bodies and tangles are sometimes found in the same brain, although only after painstaking search. (Alvord, 1958, 1965; Beheim-Schwarzbach, 1952; Earle, 1968; Forno, 1966; Greenfield, 1963; Greenfield and Bosanquet, 1953; Hallervorden, 1935; Lipkin, 1959.) What the presence of the bodies and the tangles signify is not evident. Discussions on this point are available (Earle, 1968; Forno, 1966; von Braunmühl, 1949). Neither can be considered specific for parkinsonism.

Attempts have been to base different forms of parkinsonism (paralysis agitans versus postencephalitic group) on sites of major damage or on cytological changes.

Beheim-Schwarzbach (1952) distinguished nigral and supranigral forms of the disease. In paralysis agitans with changes in the nigra, Lewy inclusions were constantly found in cells of the locus coeruleus, but they were absent in the postencephalitic form of the disease and in "supranigral" parkinsonism. From a study of pigment-containing cells of the brainstem, Alvord (1958) distinguished nigral and extranigral forms, those with and those without significant loss of neurons and changes in the remaining neurons of the substantia nigra: "These two variations could mean that the basic change is somewhere else and that only some of the cases also have changes in the substantia nigra." Pakkenberg and Brody (1965) were, however, unable to make this distinction. Stadlan, Duvoisin, and Yahr (1966) expressed the view that parkinsonism could be subdivided into two types: one distinguished by the presence of Lewy bodies and manifested clinically by "classical" parkinsonism with tremor and rigidity, and the other, the akinetic form *(sine agitatione),* by neurofibrillary changes or symmetrical supranigral degeneration or both.

Some cases of paralysis agitans are hereditary (Hallervorden, 1957); familial incidence has been estimated as high as 16 percent (Denny-Brown, 1945). From a detailed survey of the literature, Siegfried (1968) noted that in a large percentage of such patients the disorder becomes evident before the age of 20 years.

For parkinsonism occurring without known heredofamilial background, various hypotheses concerning cause have been proposed.

It seems agreed that parkinsonism becomes manifest when a certain threshold of nerve cell dysfunction or loss in critical structures is exceeded. A decrease in melanin content in the substantia nigra in parkinsonism has long been recognized, as has a decrease in certain biogenic amines (dopamine, norepinephrine, serotonin), changes regarded as specific for the Parkinson brain (Hornykiewicz, 1963). Interrelation of these two defects was suggested by the fact that in melanocytes and sympathetic nerve cells, tyrosine is hydroxylated to dihydroxyphenylalanine (dopa), a precursor in the synthesis of both melanin and catecholamines (Poskanzer, 1969). Of especial current interest are observations that the prolonged administration of L-3,4-dihydroxyphenylalamine (L-dopa) in sufficient dosage can reverse the disease process. At latest count, twenty of twenty-eight patients on this regimen showed marked or dramatic improvement up to 2 years, and four others moderate improvement. The frequency of involuntary movements tended, however, to be increased by this therapy. (Cotzias and Papavasiliou, 1967; Cotzias, Papavasiliou, and Gellene, 1969; Cotzias, Van Woert, and Schiffer, 1967.) The basis of the deficiency still needs clarification. Possibly related to this problem is Gomirato and Hydén's (1963) observation that glial cells in the pallidum exhibit a marked alteration in the composition of RNA base with increased adenine and decreased guanine and uracil, findings suggesting to them an expression of a primary biochemical error of the glia. Disappearance of nerve cells due to an aging process has been postulated as the basis of acceleration in the pace of the disease. In utilizing the degree of mobility of joints as an index of the scope and the rate of development of brain damage in patients with parkinsonian disease, DeJong and Burns (1967) noted that the progress of the disease at age 65 was four times more rapid than for a patient aged 35. For postencephalitic parkinsonism an additional factor, infective changes in nerve cells so altering the cells that they are left less resistant to the ordinary involution of aging, has been proposed (Hallervorden, 1935, 1957; von Braunmühl, 1949). Asenjo (1968) has observed iron deposits in nerve cells and glial cells of the ventral lateral (VL) nucleus of the thalamus and in other central nuclei in biopsy material from Parkinson patients, and in the liver as well. Assessment is still needed.

Parkinsonism occurring under other conditions. Muscle rigidity, tremor, and akinesis are essentially of the same nature in all parkinsonian syndromes. However, the various disease states in which this triad is found are often clinically distinguishable in virtue of additional disturbances observed in one or another etiological variety and in virtue of the clinical course.

"Arteriosclerotic parkinsonism." Muscle rigidity, bent-forward attitude with the eyes looking toward the floor, slowness in turning around, fixed facial expression, and short-stepped gait *(démarche à petits pas)*, all developing insidiously or, occasionally, rapidly, are commonly called arteriosclerotic when the onset is in persons in their sixties or beyond. This rigidity is said to differ from that found in paralysis agitans in that the flexors at the elbow and the extensors at the knee are predominantly affected. The clinical course is described as more rapid than in paralysis agitans. The distinction seems justified when pyramidal tract signs are evident, when spastic contractures develop in bedridden patients, when pseudobulbar palsy occurs, or when aphasic and apraxic disturbances develop. Tremor may be absent in the "arteriosclerotic form" (Critchley, 1929).

Pathologically, nerve cells in the substantia nigra are shrunken, contain abundant lipids, and are poor in pigment. Free pigment is found in reactive glia and around vessels, indicating that some nerve cells have vanished. More striking changes occur in the striatum and pallidum. Here (as well as elsewhere) *status cribratus* and *status lacunaris* are common features; further, nerve cell loss is noted and glia are hypertrophic. According to von Braunmühl (1957), large cells in the striatum suffer most. The cerebral cortex also suffers severely, perhaps more so than any other structure. Laminar degeneration (layers 3 and 5) occurs, particularly in frontal and temporal areas, and neurofibrillary changes and lacunae are found not only in the cortex but also in the white matter. Sclerosis is noted in basal arteries, but it is no more pronounced than under conditions in which parkinsonism is lacking. Klaue (1940) has made the point that arteriosclerosis is less conspicuous in parkinsonism in general than in the brains of unaffected persons of comparable age.

There seems no way of attributing the cell changes and cell loss in the putamen, pallidum, and substantia nigra to arteriosclerosis per se, and thus the term "arteriosclerotic parkinsonism" has been regarded as a misnomer. "Arteriosclerosis in parkinsonism" (Eadie and Sunderland, 1964) is more in keeping with the facts.

Posttraumatic parkinsonism. The parkinsonism developing after head trauma is usually atypical and varied. *Formes frustes* are the rule. However, full-blown parkinsonism sometimes occurs. The disorder may take days, weeks, or even years to develop and is usually progressive. The incidence of parkinsonism was not increased among "shell-shocked" soldiers in wartime. Remarkable cases have been described, such as hemiparkinsonism in association with a grenade splinter in the contralateral substantia nigra (Lindenberg, 1964).

Parkinsonism may represent the only sequela of the trauma, but additional neurological disturbances are usually encountered, such as signs of pyramidal tract injury or, after an automobile accident, slowness of movement, decrease in associated movements, and amimic facial expression, coupled with intention tremor and diplopia (Pichard and Liber, 1934).

In one case an iron bar fell on a man's head, causing spastic paresis contralaterally. A few months later, athetotic restlessness appeared in the hand on the previously affected side. In another year, muscle tonus in the arm was increased, and the patient had a peculiar stare. In 5 years the athetotic movements had disappeared, but tonus in the lower limbs had increased and "rigor" was noted in the previously unaffected arm; moreover, all movements were slowed. At 7 years finger movements were stiff and tremor was noted in the fingers of both hands. Various changes in the brain were observed postmortem (for example, slight nerve cell loss together with gliosis in regions of the pallidum); the significant changes were found in the black zone of the substantia nigra bilaterally, multifocal loss of nerve cells, gliosis, and changes in arterial walls. (Lindenburg, 1964.)

"Punch-drunk" state. In boxers, besides signs of pyramidal tract and cerebellar damage and of a syndrome reminiscent of general paresis and another resembling multiple sclerosis, extrapyramidal disturbances may also occur (after an interval averaging some 16 years): masklike face, slurred monotonous speech, muscle rigidity, poverty of movement, and tremors of the head and arms. Both pallidum and striatum are among the structures damaged. Cortical atrophy with a profusion of senile plaques was noted in one such instance. (Critchley, 1957.)

Manganese poisoning. Numerous manifestations of the Parkinson syndrome may be observed in the end stage. Manganese poisoning also leads to deterioration of skilled coordination (at the beginning), peculiar gait disturbances, fixed athetotic posture of the hands, elevation of the upper lip, hypertrophy of neck muscles, torticollis, extensor plantar responses, symptoms of neuritis, and psychiatric disorders. Poor ocular convergence, weakness of facial muscles, raspy voice, and decreased hearing of high tones are also known to occur, as well as uncontrollable laughing and crying. (Mena and others, 1967; Pentschew, 1958; Whitlock, Amuso, and Bittenbender, 1966.) According to Turner (1955), manganese poisoning mimicks Wilson's disease more than it does parkinsonism.

The major pathological changes in one case of manganese poisoning with Parkinson syndrome consisted in multifocal glial scarring and atrophy equally involving caudate nucleus and putamen, globus pallidus, and thalamus (Canavan, Cobb, and Drinker, 1934). Globus pallidus and subthalamic nucleus were the structures most affected in manganese intoxication in monkeys, though the astroglial hypertrophy was widespread (Pentschew, Ebner, and Kovatch, 1963). Turnover studies of Mn^{54} given intravenously to Chilean miners have revealed that the rate of excretion of the radioactive nuclide is less in miners with parkinsonism and in non-miner controls than it is in "healthy" miners (Mena and others, 1967).

Carbon monoxide poisoning. In acute carbon monoxide poisoning, choreic or choreoathetoid movements may occur initially, but, as a rule, akinetic disturbances mark the early phase. Hemiplegia may be an early sign, but it is rare. Subsequently, in survivors, hyperkinesias may occur in some cases, but, again, parkinsonism is far more commonly encountered. However, the incidence of extrapyramidal disturbances is far outweighed by visual failure (of cortical origin), dysphasia, agnosia, apraxia, temporospatial disorientation, epileptic seizures, and mental changes ranging from retardation to frank psychosis.

Pathologically, damage of the cerebral cortex is probably the most constant finding. As to the basal ganglia, the pallidum suffers most frequently. Usually the damage is symmetrical on the two sides and occurs rostrally in the pallidum, involving the internal capsule. Only rarely do lesions extend into the putamen. Sometimes the lesions are situated in the caudal part of pallidum and extend backward into the red nucleus and substantia nigra. By contrast, in occasional cases the pallidum escapes damage. In children the striatum has, by some accounts, been found to be the most vulnerable subcortical structure. (Garland and Pearce, 1967; Pentschew, 1958.)

Phenothiazine effects. At least 40 percent of patients given sustained phenothiazine medication ultimately exhibit manifestations of intoxication. The disturbances appear, roughly, in the following order: vasomotor and other signs of autonomic dysfunction, acute dystonic reactions, akathisia and other signs of motor restlessness, parkinsonism, and persistent dystonias. Although these disturbances can be reversible, there is a growing clinical impression that the combined use of phenothiazine compounds and drugs to control rigidity and akathisia (for example, benzhexol and orphenadrine) may facilitate the development of an irreversible extrapyramidal syndrome. (Crane and Paulson, 1967; Haddenbrock, 1966.)

Since patients thus affected are usually well on in years and tend to acquire abnormalities in extrapyramidal nuclei, difficulties have been encountered in trying to establish the substrate of the neurological phenomena. Abnormal fibers (Marchi method) have been found in the globus pallidus, the pallidofugal system, the "capsule" of the subthalamic nucleus, and elsewhere, but mostly along the edge of the substantia nigra. The oligodendrogliamyelin unit thus seems implicated. (Hunter and others, 1968.)

Amyotrophic lateral sclerosis. Amyotrophic lateral sclerosis (ALS) with or without bulbar palsy occasionally develops in persons with postencephalitic parkinsonism (Greenfield and Matthews, 1954; Wimmer and Neel, 1928) and in some without known antecedent encephalitis (Siegfried, 1968), also in hereditary cases of parkinsonism in association with dementia (van Bogaert and Radermecker, 1954). Relatively large numbers of Chamorros on Guam and other Mariana Islands as well as natives of the Philippines (and occasionally elsewhere) have come down with ALS, parkinsonism with ALS, or both combined with dementia. A virus as a cause has been claimed but lacks substantiation. (Elizan and others, 1966; Hirano and others, 1966.)

Alzheimer's disease. Although the most prominent manifestation of Alzheimer's disease is dementia, there are heredofamilial cases (probably of autosomal dominant transmission) in which Parkinson's syndrome with pyramidal tract signs overshadows the dementia. Age at onset of the disturbances ranges from 22 to 52 years, with a mean of 37 years. The disease runs a progressive course, with mean duration about 3½ years. (Heston, Lowther, and Leventhal, 1966.)

Specific atrophies with Parkinson variants

Striatonigral degeneration. Striatonigral degeneration, sometimes referred to as the *rigid akinetic form of paralysis agitans* and hardly distinguishable clinically, is a rare disorder characterized by rigidity and slowness of movement spreading from one limb to the others and manifested as described in the foregoing text. Psychic disturbances such as instability of mood, disorientation, and confusion in the early stages are special features. There may also be recurring syncopal attacks.

Pathologically, the brain is usually atrophic. The putamen has a brown tint. Both substantia nigra and globus pallidus show advanced nerve cell loss, disappearance or thinning of myelinated fibers, and oligodendroglial loss. Astroglial cells in the affected areas are hypertrophic. Fibers of the ansa lenticularis are also thinned. Putamen, peripheral parts of the caudate nucleus, subthalamic nucleus, and locus coeruleus are similarly though less affected. Glial cells in some of these structures contain acid hematin, giving them a green-blue hue. (Adams, van Bogaert, and Vander-Eecken, 1961, 1964; Jellinger and Danielczyk, 1968.) In some cases a few neurofibrillary tangles and Lewy bodies are seen (Jellinger and Danielczyk, 1968; Stadlan, Duvoisin, and Yahr, 1966). The disorder is considered a possible variant of paralysis agitans or Huntington's chorea by some (Adams, van Bogaert, and Vander Eecken, 1964); others (Jellinger and Danielczyk, 1968) see it more closely related to Creutzfeldt-Jakob's disease. Choreoathetosis, even more than rigidity, might have been expected in these cases in view of the relatively severe lesion of the putamen. This may be masked by the nigral lesion affecting downcoming striatonigral fibers (see Fig. 24-1, A for the pathway) (Adams, van Bogaert, and Vander Eecken, 1964).

Pallidal and pallido-luysian degeneration. In this disorder autopsy has revealed atrophy limited to the globus pallidus or the subthalamus or both, before the degeneration had spread to other systems. The atrophy is bilateral and usually symmetrical.

In the *progressive atrophy of the pallidum* described by Hunt (1917), muscle rigidity was the main clinical disturbance in young persons, and was referred to as a sporadic, juvenile form of paralysis agitans. Similar instances were described by van Bogaert (1930, 1946), hence the disorder came to be known as the Hunt-van Bogaert syndrome. However, familial cases are also recognized.

In one of the two cases described by Jellinger (1968), where atrophy (with nerve cell loss) was again limited to the globus pallidus bilaterally, a progressive dystonic-dyskinetic syndrome developed, followed by double athetosis, with increasing muscle rigidity and terminal dystonic contractions in flexion. In the second patient involuntary movements of the face and tongue were followed by contractions of the neck muscles, disturbances in articulation, tremor of the hand, writer's cramp, rotational movements of the hand, and torticollis, terminating in double athetosis with hypotonia. Torsion dystonic disturbances and a ballistic component came last. There was no rigidity or akinesis. In addition to nerve cell loss in the pallidum, there was striking reduction in size of pallidal efferent pathways. In Case 1 the middle segment of the globus was the most profoundly affected (sometimes three divisions of the pallidum are discernible), with a secondary cell loss in the ventro-oral part of the thalamus. In Case 2 the oral part of the medial pallidal segment was most severely affected, with secondary cell loss in the thalamus and the dorsolateral part of the subthalamic nucleus together with loss of striopallidal fibers.

Neural mechanisms involved in parkinsonism. Despite uncertainties, some conclusions may be reached concerning the mechanisms involved in patients with extrapyramidal somatomotor disturbances. No matter which portion of the basal ganglia is damaged, the influences leading to the disorder must be mediated by fibers reaching the lower motor neurons in cranial nerve nuclei and anterior horns. Such fibers run in two systems: the pyramidal, or alpha, system, and the reticulospinal, or gamma, system. Accordingly, the problem is mainly one of circuitry. In other words, do the influences leading to these disorders pass from the basal ganglia, through the thalamus, and upward to the origin of the pyramidal system? Or do they pass downward to the brainstem reticular core and on through the reticulospinal system? Putting it this way, however, is an oversimplication, since the pyramidal system itself gives off collaterals to the reticular core (see p. 409). Finally, consideration must be given to the influence exerted on the reticular core by the exquisite sensing element of a proprioceptive servo system based on the muscle spindle.

Rigidity, akinesis, and postural disturbances. Considering the *mesencephalic reticular core* first, from the cytopathological standpoint, nothing seems to be known of its status in parkinsonism in man. However, monkeys with an electrolytic lesion in the region between the substantia nigra and red nucleus show a number of relevant disturbances. They include sluggishness of movements, rigidity, akinesia, a mask-like face, loss of mimicry, even tremor at rest (Carey and DeJong, 1954; Carrea and Mettler, 1954; Ward, 1958). In addition, lesions made in the rostral mesencephalic reticular formation have produced increased resistance to passive muscle stretch and also the cogwheel phenomenon (Schreiner, MacCarty, and Grindlay, 1958). These observations suggest the possibility that gamma system activity is an intrinsic property of the reticular core and that the disruption of this activity is instrumental in producing the disturbances.

Next, in parkinsonism the *substantia nigra* is probably more consistently damaged than any other structure; it may, in fact, be severely damaged in cases in which the globus pallidus is not perceptibly altered (Hassler, 1938, 1953). Yet experimentally it seems established that nigral lesions in monkeys do not result in rigidity or any other extrapyramidal disturbance (Carpenter and McMasters, 1964; Mettler,

1964). The pathway from nigra to pallidum is available, and disturbances originating in the nigra could be mediated through it (Fig. 24-1, *D*). Electrophysiological data indicate, moreover, that the nigra provides a potent source of inhibitory input to the gamma loop (Ward, 1961), hence a nigroreticular pathway is likely to exist. Whether such a nigroreticulospinal pathway is available anatomically needs yet to be settled (see p. 407). If there is such a pathway, and if nigral cell groups (Hassler, 1937) have a somatotopic arrangement, then certain manifestations in parkinsonism, such as akinesis beginning in the fingers (reflected in the handwriting), could be attributed directly to damage of the substantia nigra.

With regard to the *globus pallidus*, there are more data from which to draw. We know that pallidofugal pathways proceed, on the one hand, to the cortex (via the thalamus), on the other hand, to the reticular core (Fig. 24-2). The pallidum has two segments, each of which possesses distinctive functions. Integration of their activities is essential to the carrying out of normal motor function (Carpenter and Strominger, 1966; Hallervorden, 1957). In cases of *progressive pallidal atrophy* the clinical disturbances differ depending on whether the site of major damage is in the lateral or the medial segment. Damage of the *lateral segment*, together with the outer medullary pallidal lamella, is considered the basis of the hyperkinesias that occur. Damage of the *medial segment*, together with degeneration of its efferent systems, is considered the basis of the progressive rigidity that commonly supersedes the hyperkinesis. Concurrent lesions in the putamen seem to be irrelevant, because in progressive pallidal atrophy no correlation has been found between the hyperkinesis and the presence of lesions in the putamen. (Jellinger, 1968.) The relevance of the pallidum for rigidity is also evident from stereotactic interference either with the pallidum itself or with its outflow, the ansa lenticularis. Such interference immediately, and in fact paradoxically, abolishes rigidity in the contralateral limbs of patients with parkinsonism (Bravo and Cooper, 1959; Houspian and Pool, 1958; Spiegel and Wycis, 1954). Likewise, Martin (1965) has observed that in paralysis agitans, rigidity does not develop if the pallidum has suffered severe damage. The difficulty here is that damage, interference, and "lesions" caused by disease are far from identical with those made at operation. All these observations notwithstanding, parkinsonism may develop under conditions in which changes in the globus pallidus are minimal or absent.

The *ventrolateral (VL) nucleus of the thalamus* also comes into consideration inasmuch as stereotactically-produced lesions in it abolish (contralateral) tremor and rigidity (Cooper, Samra, and Bergmann, 1969). In such cases effective lesions commonly encroach on neighboring thalamic nuclei (ventral posterolateral and ventral posteromedial—VPL and VPM) (Cooper, Bergmann, and Caracalos, 1963). Pallidothalamic pathways, corticothalamic circuits, and intrathalamic connections are thus interrupted. Any attempt to ferret out from this array the mechanism(s) concerned in the abolition of the tremor and rigidity would seem fruitless.

Further, hypokinesis, but not rigidity, is a complication Spiegel and co-workers (1956) have found to develop in patients following surgical destruction of a small part of the pallidum together with ansa lenticularis. They postulated that some fibers given off by the pallidum that course into the ansa lenticularis conduct facilitating impulses down to lower tonus-maintaining reflex arcs. In monkeys it has further been noted that, following bilateral destruction of only about 10 percent of the pallidum, the animals had expressionless faces combined with reduced range of movement, poor associated movements, bizarre and forced postures, and righting disability (Carpenter and Whittier, 1952). Sometimes the head was bent over and rested on the floor ("somersault" posture) (Carpenter, Whittier, and Mettler, 1950). In man, too, progressive pallidal atrophy has led to postural deficiencies that were all the more pronounced the more severe the pallidal damage (Martin, 1965). Thus, the evidence suggests that mechanisms concerned in rigidity, in hypokinesis, and in postural change are separable and that any one of these disturbances can originate from pallidal damage either alone or in combination. It is possible that the disturbances result from disruption of influences fed into the reticular core through the pallidofugal system (illustrated in Fig. 24-2). Spiegel and Wycis (1967) ventured the hypothesis that damage of the hypothalamus may be responsible for hypokinesis, as others had observed in monkeys that lesions therein resulted in loss of initiative and slowing of movement. Detailed confirmatory studies are needed in support.

That increased activity of the gamma system is responsible for the production of rigidity has been contended by Jinnai and co-workers (1964a, b). In a patient with parkinsonism, the globus pallidus was electrically stimulated while electromyographic recordings were made from the contralateral soleus and anterior tibial muscles. During or immediately after stimulation, when the soleus muscle was passively stretched, the EMG showed increase in amplitude and spike frequency, prolongation of the after-discharge, as well as increase in the rigidity of the muscle on palpation. Apparently, then, stimulation of the pallidum per se can increase rigidity in the Parkinson patient. The stimulation did not alter the H-wave, hence the pyramidal tract was not activated (see Fig. 8-3, *B* for this wave). When, by contrast, the fibers at the border of the thalamus and internal capsule (presumably, pyramidal fibers) were stimulated, an increase in the amplitude of the H-wave resulted without change in the stretch reflex. Stimulation of the ventrolateral nucleus of the thalamus (VL or LV) produced no change in the EMG. These findings were thought to indicate an increase in impulses transmitted to gamma motoneurons. Since surgical lesions in the pallidum or in VL decrease the rigidity of the Parkinson patient, whereas stimulation does the reverse, it appeared to Jinnai and his associates that these structures constitute the upper end of the gamma system. That the gamma system is concerned in the production of rigidity is also in agreement with the views of others (Granit, 1950; Rushworth, 1960). Presumably the pathway extending from the pallidum to the mesencephalic tegmental region (*RF* in Fig. 24-2) conducts these impulses.

A different view is held by Hassler (1964), Jung and Hassler (1960), and Ward and Stern (Stern and Ward, 1962, 1963; Ward, 1958, 1961; Ward and Stern, 1963). Ward and Stern consider first the substrate of voluntary motor activity: (1) the alpha route, which is both direct and through relays to the alpha (or large anterior horn) cells; (2) the gamma route, composed of pathways reaching the gamma (or small anterior horn) cells. The excitation of gamma cells influences muscle spindles so that a barrage of afferent impulses is fed back to the cord over the dorsal roots; this barrage of impulses terminates monosynaptically on the alpha motoneuron, completing the "servo loop" (Fig. 2-1). Steady voluntary or postural muscle contraction is regarded as a result of the tonic innervation of the muscle spindle and consequent facilitation of the alpha motoneuron via this servo loop. Additional and much more complex feedback circuits might, according to the Ward-Stern view, exist at higher levels—within the brainstem, through the cerebellum, and at the cerebral cortical level.

On the basis of this proposed substrate, Ward and Stern suggested that any or all of the manifestations—akinesis and tremor as well—are the result of alterations of the balance between the alpha and gamma systems brought about at various levels. They expressed the view that if, in parkinsonism, the gamma loop is inhibited because the inhibitory activity generated in pallidum, thalamus, nigra, and reticular formation is unopposed, akinesia might well be the result. Facilitatory circuits may in this case be insufficient to permit a rapid initiation of voluntary phasic motor activity. Rigidity (as opposed to akinesia) they considered a consequence of increased alpha drive, and this possibly a result of reduced inhibitory inflow into the cord.

Tremor at rest. Tremor at rest (static tremor) can be induced by electrical stimulation at various sites, and again it can be abolished surgically by lesions made at some of those same sites.

In a Parkinson patient, tremor on one side was augmented by stimulating the contralateral *mesencephalic tegmentum* (reticular core) in a region just dorsal to the red nucleus. This tremor was then abolished by coagulating the stimulated area. In experimental animals this result could be obtained even after internal capsule degeneration (Spiegel and Wycis, 1958). Tremor simulating that of parkinsonism has been produced in monkeys, mostly in the contralateral limbs, by electrically stimulating the brainstem reticular core, and tremor of face, neck, and even the fingers on stimulation of the region just caudal to the red nucleus (Carey and DeJong, 1954; Jenkner and Ward, 1953). A pill-rolling rhythmic movement, also in monkeys, has been produced by stimulating the mesencephalic reticular core (Mettler,

1955). Thus it seems that the tremorogenic mechanisms of the reticular core are at least partly intrinsic.

In regard to the *putamen* and its role in tremor, Denny-Brown (1962) noticed that when tremor had been absent in patients with paralysis agitans, the putamen was more severely damaged than the pallidum. Tremor, according to Kaada (1963), also did not ensue with circumscribed lesions in any part of the striatum.

The *globus pallidus,* however, is clearly concerned in static tremor, for stimulation of this structure in awake Parkinson patients increases the amplitude or frequency or both of the tremor (Spiegel and Wycis, 1961).

So-called tremorogenic neurons are also situated in the *ventral lateral nucleus of the thalamus* (LV or VL). In Parkinson patients, cells in this nucleus fire in bursts that are precisely timed with the frequency of the tremor (Jasper and Bertrand, 1966). Tremor is abolished by lesions in VL that may also involve VPL and VPM (ventral posterolateral and ventral medial thalamic nuclei) (Bravo and Cooper, 1959; Cooper, 1965; Cooper, Bergmann, and Caracalos, 1963; Krayenbühl and Yasargil, 1961). "Tremorogenic neurons" are present even in the *cerebral cortex,* for tremor (in monkeys) has been diminished or abolished by lesions that interrupt the corticospinal pathway, both at its inception in the cortex and at the level of the basis pedunculi or pyramid. Yet this is not always the case, since tremor may persist despite degeneration of the fibers traversing the basis pedunculi (Mettler, Davidoff, and Grimes, 1947).

Cerebellar circuits appear nonessential to the development of static tremor. The tremor fails to occur (in monkeys) following damage inflicted on the brachium conjunctivum alone (Walker and Botterell, 1937; Ward, McCulloch, and Magoun, 1948). Cerebellar circuits do not appear essential to the elicitation of evoked tremor (in cats). Degeneration of the brachium conjunctivum does not prevent or alter the characteristics of the tremor induced by stimulating the mesencephalic reticular core (Wycis, Szekely, and Spiegel, 1957).

Jung (1941) has linked static tremor with the *reticular core.* Interruption of circuits sustaining this phylogenetically old motor system (it subserves, for instance, the swimming movements of fishes) would result in tremor. As to the *alpha system,* Ward (1961), like so many others, in finding that stimulation of pallidum or VL (thalamus) increased the tremor of Parkinson patients, postulated that pallidum and VL "drive" the reticular core and, over multisynaptic pathways, exert excitatory effects on the spinal alpha motoneurons. By contrast, little or no participation of the *gamma system* was suggested, as preexisting tremor in animals was unaffected by extensive unilateral dorsal root section.

In summary, no matter how comprehensive or how [judiciously] selective a reviewer tries to be, he must end up holding a certain number of pieces that do not fit his jigsaw puzzle, or missing those that have not yet been provided. He must be content with accepting such commonplaces as "disequilibrium" and such riddles as how to relate posture and movement, stimulus and lesion, facilitation and inhibition, simple and rhythmic innervation, voluntary and automatic control, and the "conflict of reflex factors" (Denny-Brown, 1962).

REFERENCES

Abrahamson, T., and Rabiner, A. N. 1924. Some phasic and permanent mutations in certain encephalitic syndromes. J. Nerv. Ment. Dis. **60**: 249-261.

Adams, R. D., and Foley, J. M. 1953. Disorders of movement in more common varieties of liver disease. EEG Clin. Neurophysiol. (suppl.) **3**: 51.

Adams, R. D., and Sidman, R. L. 1968. Introduction to neuropathology. New York, McGraw-Hill Book Company.

Adams, R. D., van Bogaert, L., and Vander Eecken, H. 1961. Dégénérescence nigrostriée et cerebello-nigro-striée. (Unicité clinique et variabilité pathologique des dégénérescences préséniles à forme de rigidité extrapyramidale.) Psychiat. Neurol. **142**:219-259.

Adams, R. D., van Bogaert, L., and Vander Eecken, H. 1964. Striato-nigral degeneration. J. Neuropath. Exp. Neurol. **23**:584-608.

Alcock, N. S. 1936. A note on the pathology of senile chorea (nonhereditary). Brain **59**:376-387.

Alvord, E. C., Jr. 1958. Pathology of parkinsonism. In Fields, W. S., editor: Pathogenesis and treatment of parkinsonism. Springfield, Illinois, Charles C Thomas, Publisher, pp. 161-183.

Alvord, E. C., Jr. 1965. The pathology of parkinsonism: etiologic, pathogenetic, and prognostic implications. Trans. Amer. Neurol. Ass. **90**:167-170.

Aron, A. M., Freeman, J. M., and Carter, S. 1965. The natural history of Sydenham's chorea: review of the literature and long-term evaluation with emphasis on cardiac sequelae. Amer. J. Med. **38**:83-95.

Asenjo, A. 1968. Cytosiderosis and iron deposits in ventrolateral nucleus of the thalamus in Parkinson's disease: clinical and experimental study. Johns Hopk. Med. J. **122**:284-294.

Beck, E., and Bignami, A. 1968. Some neuroanatomical observations in cases with stereotactic lesions for the relief of parkinsonism. Brain **91**:589-618.

Beheim-Schwarzbach, D. 1952. Über Zelleib-Veränderungen im Nucleus coeruleus bei Parkinson-Symptomen. J. Nerv. Ment. Dis. **116**: 619-653.

Bing, R., and Haymaker, W. 1939. Textbook of nervous diseases, ed. 5. St. Louis, The C. V. Mosby Co.

Bischoff, A., and Regli, F. 1963. Die Hallervorden-Spatzsche Krankheit: Diskussion der pathologisch-anatomischen Befunde anhand eines eigenen autoptisch bestätigten Falles. Arch. Psychiat. Nervenkr. **204**:589-602.

Bornstein, S., and Jervis, G. A. 1955. Presenile dementia of the Jacob type: corticostriospinal degeneration. Arch. Neurol. Psychiat. **74**:598-610.

Brain, W. R. 1928. Posture of the hand in chorea and other states of muscular hypotonia. Lancet **1**:439-441.

Bravo, G. J., and Cooper, I. S. 1959. A clinical and radiological correlation of the lesions produced by chemopallidectomy and thalamectomy. J. Neurol. Neurosurg. Psychiat. **22**:1-10.

Brothers, C. R. D. 1964. Huntington's chorea in Victoria and Tasmania. J. Neurol. Sci. **1**:405-420.

Bucy, P. C. 1942. The neural mechanisms of athetosis and tremor. J. Neuropath. Exp. Neurol. **1**:224-239.

Bucy, P. C. 1949. Relation to abnormal involuntary movements. In Bucy, C. P., editor: The precentral motor cortex, ed. 2. Urbana, University of Illinois Press, pp. 395-408.

Bucy, P. C. 1958. The cortico-spinal tract and tremor. In Fields, W. S., editor: Pathogenesis and treatment of parkinsonism. Springfield, Illinois, Charles C Thomas, Publisher, pp. 271-293.

Bucy, P. C., and Case, T. J. 1937. Athetosis. Surgical treatment of unilateral athetosis. Arch. Neurol. Psychiat. **37**:983-1020.

Campbell, A. M. G., Corner, B., Norman, R. M., and Urich, H. 1961. The rigid form of Huntington's disease. J. Neurol. Neurosurg. Psychiat. **24**:71-77.

Canavan, M. M., Cobb, S., and Drinker, C. K. 1934. Chronic manganese poisoning: report of a case, with autopsy. Arch. Neurol. Psychiat. **32**:501-512.

Carey, J. H., and DeJong, R. N. 1954. Preliminary studies on the production of Parkinson's syndrome. Trans. Amer. Neurol. Ass. **79**:28-35.

Carpenter, M. B. 1950. Athetosis and the basal ganglia: review of the literature and study of forty-two cases. Arch. Neurol. Psychiat. **63**:875-901.

Carpenter, M. B. 1955. Ballism associated with partial destruction of the subthalamic nucleus of Luys. Neurology **5**:479-489.

Carpenter, M. B. 1958. The neuroanatomical basis of dyskinesia. In Fields, W. S., editor: Pathogenesis and treatment of parkinsonism. Springfield, Illinois, Charles C Thomas, Publisher, pp. 50-85.

Carpenter, M. B., Correll, J. W., and Hinman, A. 1960. Spinal tracts mediating subthalamic hyperkinesia: physiological effects of selective partial cordotomies upon dyskinesia in Rhesus monkey. J. Neurophysiol. **23**:288-304.

Carpenter, M. B., and McMasters, R. E. 1964. Lesions of the substantia nigra in the rhesus monkey: efferent fiber degeneration and behavioral observations. Amer. J. Anat. **114**:293-312.

Carpenter, M., and Strominger, N. L. 1966. Corticostriate encephalitis and paraballism in the monkey. Arch. Neurol. **14**:241-253.

Carpenter, M. B., and Strominger, N. L. 1967. Efferent fibers of the subthalamic nucleus in the monkey: a comparison of the efferent projections of the subthalamic nucleus, substantia nigra and globus pallidus. Amer. J. Anat. **121**:41-72.

Carpenter, M. B., and Whittier, J. R. 1952. Study of methods for producing experimental lesions of the central nervous system with special reference to stereotaxic techniques. J. Comp. Neurol. **97**:73-132.

Carpenter, M. B., Whittier, J. R., and Mettler, F. A. 1950. Analysis of choreoid hyperkinesia in rhesus monkey. J. Comp. Neurol. **92**:293-332.

Carrea, R. M. E., and Mettler, F. A. 1954. The anatomy of the primate brachium conjunctivum and associated structures. J. Comp. Neurol. **101**:565-689.

Christensen, E., and Krabbe, K. H. 1945. Case of hemiballism with autopsy. Acta Psychiat. Neurol. **20**:149-157.

Cole, M., Nauta, W. J. H., and Mehler, W. R. 1964. The ascending efferent projections of the substantia nigra. Trans. Amer. Neurol. Ass. **89**:74-78.

Colony, H. S., and Malamud, N. 1956. Sydenham's chorea: a clinicopathologic study. Neurology **6**:672-676.

Cooper, I. S. 1964. Effect of thalamic lesions upon torticollis. New Eng. J. Med. **270**:967-972.

Cooper, I. S. 1965. Clinical and physiologic implications of thalamic surgery for disorders of sensory communication: intention tremor, dystonia, Wilson's disease and torticollis. J. Neurol. Sci. **2**:520-553.

Cooper, I. S., Bergmann, L. L., and Caracalos, A. 1963. Anatomic verification of the lesion which abolishes parkinsonian tremor and rigidity. Neurology **13**:779-787.

Cooper, I. S., Samra, K., and Bergmann, L. 1969. The thalamic lesion which abolishes tremor and rigidity of parkinsonism: a radiologico-clinico-anatomic correlative study. J. Neurol. Sci. **8**:69-84.

Cotzias, G. C., and Papavasiliou, P. S. 1967. Therapeutic studies of parkinsonian patients: long term effects of D L and L DOPA. Meeting, 2d Internat. Congr. Neuro-Genetics and Ophthalmology, Montreal, Sept. 19, 1967.

Cotzias, G. C., Papavasiliou, P. S., and Gellene, R. 1969. Modification of Parkinsonism—chronic treatment with L-dopa. New Eng. J. Med. **280**:337-345.

Cotzias, G. C., Van Woert, M. H., and Schiffer, L. M. 1967. Aromatic amino acids and modification of parkinsonism. New Eng. J. Med. **276**:374-379.

Courville, C. B. 1953. Contributions to the study of cerebral anoxia. Los Angeles, San Lucas Press.

Cowen, D., and Olmstead, E. M. 1963. Infantile neuroaxonal dystrophy. J. Neuropath. Exp. Neurol. **22**:175-236.

Crane, G. E., and Paulson, G. 1967. Involuntary movements in a sample of chronic mental patients and their relation to the treatment with neuroleptics. Internat. J. Neuropsychiat. **3**:286-291.

Critchley, M. 1924. Post-diphtheritic "chorea." Brit. J. Child. Dis. **21**:188-192.

Critchley, M. 1929. Arteriosclerotic parkinsonism. Brain **52**:23-83.

Critchley, M. 1957. Medical aspects of boxing, particularly from a neurological standpoint. Brit. Med. J. **1**:357-362.

Crompton, M. R. 1968. Alper's disease—a variant of Creutzfeldt-Jakob disease and subacute spongiform encephalopathy? Acta Neuropath. **10**:99-104.

Davison, C., and Goodhart, S. P. 1933 and 1938. Dystonia musculorum deformans: a clinicopathologic study. Arch. Neurol. Psychiat. **29**: 1108-1124; **39**:939-972.

DeJong, J. D. 1965. Some approaches to further investigation of Parkinson's disease. Monograph Biological Medicine, New York, Grune & Stratton, Inc., pp. 30-37.

DeJong, J. D., and Burns, B. D. 1967. Parkinson's disease—a random process. Canad. Med. Ass. J. **97**:49-56.

DeJong, R. N., and Scharenberg, K. 1952. The syndrome of Hallervorden and Spatz. Trans. Amer. Neurol. Ass. **77**:83-87.

Denny-Brown, D. 1945. Diseases of the basal ganglia and subthalamic nuclei. In Christian, H. A., editor: Oxford loose-leaf medicine, vol. 6. New York, Oxford University Press, pp. 261-302.

Denny-Brown, D. 1962. The basal ganglia and their relation to disorders of movement. London, Oxford University Press.

Denny-Brown, D. 1964. Hepatolenticular degeneration (Wilson's disease): two different components. New Eng. J. Med. **270**:1149-1156.

De Vito, J. L., and Smith, O. A., Jr. 1964. Subcortical projections of the prefrontal lobe of the monkey. J. Comp. Neurol. **123**:413-424.

Dierssen, G., Gioino, G. G., and Cooper, I. S. 1961. Participation of ipsilateral hemisphere lesions in the pathology of hemichorea and hemiballismus. Neurology **11**:894-898.

Dunlap, C. B. 1927. Pathologic changes in Huntington's chorea with special reference to the corpus striatum. Arch. Neurol. Psychiat. **18**: 867-943.

Eadie, M. J., and Sutherland, J. M. 1964. Arteriosclerosis in parkinsonism. J. Neurol. Neurosurg. Psychiat. **27**:237-240.

Earle, K. M. 1968. Studies of Parkinson's disease including x-ray fluorescent spectroscopy of formalin fixed brain tissue. J. Neuropath. Exp. Neurol. **27**:1-14.

Eicke, W.-J. 1940. Neue Beobachtungen über die Hallervorden-Spatzsche Krankheit. Arch. Psychiat. Nervenkr. **111**:514-546.

Eicke, W.-J. 1957. Wilsonsche Krankheit-Pseudosclerosis. In Lubarsch, O., Henke, F., and Rössle, R., editors: Handbuch der speziellen pathologischen Anatomie und Histologie, vol. 13 (edited by Scholz, W.), pt. 1A. Berlin, Springer-Verlag, pp. 851-899.

Elizan, T. S., Hirano, A., Abrams, B. M., Need, R. C., Vannius, C., and Kurland, L. T. 1966. Amyotrophic lateral sclerosis and parkinsonism —dementia complex of Guam: neurological evaluation. Arch. Neurol. **14**:356-368.

Fager, C. A. 1968. Evaluation of thalamic and subthalamic surgical lesions in the alleviation of Parkinson's disease. J. Neurosurg. **28**:145-149.

Foix, C., and Nicolesco, J. 1925. Les noyaux gris centraux et la région mésencephalo-sous-optique. Paris, Masson & Cie.

Foley, J. M., and Denny-Brown, D. 1957. Subacute progressive encephalopathy with bulbar myoclonus. J. Neuropath. Exp. Neurol. **26**:133.

Foltz, E. L., Knopp, L. M., and Ward, A. A., Jr. 1959. Experimental spasmodic torticollis. J. Neurosurg. **16**:55-67.

Forno, L. S. 1966. Pathology of parkinsonism: a preliminary report of 24 cases. J. Neurosurg. **24**:266-271.

Gambetti, P., Mellman, W. J., and Gonatos, N. K. 1969. Familial spongy degeneration of the central nervous system (van Bogaert-Bertrand disease): an ultrastructural study. Acta Neuropath. **12**:103-115.

Garland, H., and Pearce, J. 1967. Neurological complications of carbon monoxide poisoning. Quart. J. Med. **36**:445-455.

Gautier-Smith, P. C., and Prankerd, T. A. J. 1967. Polycythaemia vera and chorea. Acta Neurol. Scand. **43**:357-364.

Gibbs, C. J., Jr., Gajdusek, D. C., Asher, D. M., Alpers, M. P., Beck, E., Daniel, P. M., and Matthews, W. B. 1968. Creutzfeldt-Jakob disease (spongiform encephalopathy): transmission to the chimpanzee. Science **161**:388-389.

Glees, P. 1944. The anatomical basis of corticostriate connections. J. Anat. **78**:47-51.

Gomirato, G., and Hydén, H. 1963. A biochemical glia error in Parkinson disease. Brain **86**:773-780.

Gowers, W. 1876. On "athetosis" and post-hemiplegic disorders of movement. Med-Chir. Soc. Trans. **59**:271-327.

Granit, R. 1950. Receptors and sensory perception. New Haven, Yale University Press.

Greenfield, J. G. 1963. System degenerations of the cerebellum, brain stem and spinal cord. In Greenfield's neuropathology, ed. 2. Baltimore, The Williams & Wilkins Co., pp. 581-601.

Greenfield, J. G., and Bosanquet, F. D. 1953. The brain-stem lesions in parkinsonism. J. Neurol. Neurosurg. Psychiat. **16**:213-226.

Greenfield, J. G., and Wolfsohn, J. M. 1922. Sydenham's chorea. Lancet **2**:603-606.

Greenfield, J. G., and Matthews, W. B. 1954. Postencephalitic parkinsonism with amyotrophy. J. Neurol. Neurosurg. Psychiat. **17**:50-56.

Haddenbrock, S. 1966. Zur Wirkungsweise und zur Frage zentralorganischer Spätschäden der neuroleptischen Dauerbehandlung. Nervenarzt **37**:199-203.

Hallervorden, J. 1935. Anatomische Untersuchungen zur Pathogenese des post-encephalitischen

Parkinsonismus. Deutsch. Z. Nervenheilk. **136**: 68-77.

Hallervorden, J. 1957. Paralysis agitans. (Anhang: Essentieller Tremor.) In Lubarsch, O., Henke, F., and Rössle, R., editors: Handbuch der speziellen pathologische Anatomie und Histologie, vol. 13 (edited by Scholz, W.), pt. 1A. Berlin, Springer-Verlag, pp. 900-924.

Hallervorden, J., and Spatz, H. 1922. Eigenartige Erkrankung in extrapyramidalen System mit besonderer Beiteiligung des Globus pallidus und der Substantia nigra. Z. Ges. Neurol. Psychiat. **79**:254-302.

Hansotia, P., Cleeland, C. S., and Chun, R. W. M. 1968. Juvenile Huntington's chorea. Neurology **18**:217-224.

Hassin, G. B., Schaub, C. F., and Voris, H. C. 1931. Spasmodic torticollis. Arch. Neurol. Psychiat. **25**:1043-1052.

Hassler, R. 1937. Zur Normalanatomie der Substantia nigra. J. Psychol. Neurol. **48**:1-55.

Hassler, R. 1938. Zur Pathologie der Paralysis Agitans und des postenzephalitischen Parkinsonismus. J. Psychol. Neurol. **48**:387-476.

Hassler, R. 1953. Extrapyramidal-motorische Syndrome und Erkrankungen. In von Bergmann, G., Frey, W., and Schwiegk, H., editors: Handbuch der inneren Medizin, vol. 5, pt. 3. Berlin, Springer-Verlag, pp. 676-964.

Hassler, R. 1956. Die extrapyramidalen Rindensysteme und die zentrale Regelung der Motorik. Deutsch. Z. Nervenheilk. **175**:233-258.

Hassler, R. 1964. Spezifische und unspezifische Systeme des menschlichen Zwischenhirns. Progr. Brain Res. **5**:1-32.

Haymaker, W. 1969. Effects of ionizing radiation on nervous tissue. In Bourne, G. H., editor: The structure and function of the nervous system, vol. 3. New York, Academic Press, Inc., pp. 441-518.

Haymaker, W., Margoles, C., Pentschew, A., Jacob, H., Lindenberg, R., Sáenz Arroya, L., Stochdorph, O., and Stowens, D. 1961. Pathology of kernicterus and posticteric encephalopathy: presentation of 87 cases, with a consideration of pathogenesis. In Swinyard, C. A., editor: Kernicterus and its importance in cerebral palsy. Springfield, Illinois, Charles C Thomas, Publisher, pp. 221-228.

Herz, E. 1944. Dystonia: pathology and conclusions. Arch. Neurol. Psychiat. **52**:20-26.

Herz, E., and Glaser, G. H. 1949. Spasmodic torticollis: clinical evaluation. Arch. Neurol. Psychiat. **61**:227-239.

Herz, E., and Hoefer, P. F. A. 1949. Spasmodic torticollis: physiologic analysis of involuntary motor activity. Arch. Neurol. Psychiat. **61**:129-136.

Heston, L. L., Lowther, D. L. W., and Leventhal, C. M. 1966. Alzheimer's disease: a family study. Arch. Neurol. **15**:225-233.

Hirano, A., Malamud, N., Elizan, T. S., and Kurland, L. T. 1966. Amyotrophic lateral sclerosis and parkinsonism-dementia complex on Guam: further pathologic studies. Arch. Neurol. **15**:35-51.

Hoehn, M. M., and Yahr, M. D. 1967. Parkinsonism: onset, progression, and mortality. Neurology **17**:427-442.

Hornykiewicz, O. 1963. Die topische Lokalisation und das Verhalten von Noradrenalin und Dopamin (3-Hydroxytyramin) in der Substantia Nigra des normalen und Parkinson Kranken Menschen. Wien. Klin. Wschr. **75**:309-312.

Houspian, E. M., and Pool, J. L. 1958. An evaluation of pallido-ansal surgery: hypokinesis as a primary symptom of parkinsonism. In Fields. W. S., editor: Pathogenesis and treatment of parkinsonism. Springfield, Illinois, Charles C Thomas, Publisher, pp. 317-324.

Hughes, B. 1965. Involuntary movements following stereotactic operations for parkinsonism, with special reference to hemichorea (ballismus). J. Neurol. Neurosurg. Psychiat. **28**:291-303.

Hunt, J. R. 1917. Progressive atrophy of the globus pallidus (primary atrophy of the pallidal system): a system disease of the paralysis agitans type, characterized by atrophy of the motor cells of the corpus striatum: a contribution to the functions of the corpus striatum. Brain **40**:58-148.

Hunter, R., Blackwood, W., Smith, M. C., and Cumings, J. N. 1968. Neuropathological findings in three cases of persistent dyskinesia following phenothiazine medication. J. Neurol. Sci. **7**: 263-273.

Inose, T. 1968. Neuropsychiatric manifestations in Wilson's disease: attacks of disturbance in consciousness. In Bergsma, D., editor: Wilson's disease. New York, National Foundation–March of Dimes, pp. 74-84.

Inose, T., Ichikawa, Y., and Nomura, H. 1960. Eine histochemische Studie bei den hepatocerebralen Degeneration und bei Leberkrankheiten (Glycogenbefund). Arch. Psychiat. Z. Ges. Neurol. **200**:509-519.

Jasper, H. H., and Bertrand, G. 1966. Recording from microelectrodes in stereotactic surgery for Parkinson's disease. J. Neurosurg. **23**:219-221.

Jellinger, K. 1968. Progressive Pallidumatrophie. J. Neurol. Sci. **6**:19-44.

Jellinger, K., and Danielczyk, W. 1968. "Striatonigrale" degeneration. Acta Neuropath. **10**:242-257.

Jenkner, F. L., and Ward, A. A., Jr. 1953. Bulbar reticular formation and tremor. A.M.A. Arch. Neurol. Psychiat. **70**:489-502.

Jervis, G. A., and Joyce, F. T. 1948. Barbiturate-opiate intoxication with necrosis of the basal ganglions of the brain: report of case. Arch. Path. **45**:319-326.

Jinnai, D., Nishimoto, A., Numoto, M., and Adachi, I. 1964a. Electrophysiological studies in stereotaxic surgery for extrapyramidal disorders: electrophysiological study of globus pallidus, thalamus and their vicinity. Confin. Neurol. **24**: 281-288.

Jinnai, D., Nishimoto, A., Numoto, M., and Adachi, I. 1964b. Electrophysiological studies in stereotaxic surgery for extrapyramidal disorders: mechanisms of parkinsonism tremor. Confin. Neurol. **24**:289-300.

Johnson, W., Schwartz, G., and Barbeau, A. 1962. Studies on dystonia musculorum deformans. Arch. Neurol. **7**:301-313.

Jung, R. 1941. Physiologische Untersuchungen über den Parkinsontremor und andere Zitterformen beim Menschen. Z. Ges. Neurol. Psychiat. **173**:263-332.

Jung, R., and Hassler, R. 1960. The extrapyramidal motor system. In Field, J., Magoun, H. W., and Hall, V. E., editors: Handbook of physiology, sect. 1, vol. 2. Washington, D. C., American Physiological Society, pp. 863-927.

Kaada, B. R. 1963. The pathophysiology of Parkinsonian tremor, rigidity, and hypokinesia. Acta Neurol. Scand., suppl. 4, **39**:39-51.

Kernohan, J. W., Woltman, H. W., and Barnes, A. R. 1939. Involvement of the nervous system associated with endocarditis: neuropsychiatric and neuropathologic observations in forty-two cases of fatal outcome. Arch. Neurol. Psychiat. **42**:789-809.

Klaue, R. 1940. Parkinsonsche Krankheit (Paralysis agitans) und postencephalitischer Parkinsonismus: Versuch einer klinisch-anatomischen Differentialdiagnose. Arch. Psychiat. Nervenkr. **111**:251-321.

Koella, W. P. 1955. Motor effects from electrical stimulation of basal cerebellum in unrestrained cat. J. Neurophysiol. **18**:559-573.

Krahenbühl, H., and Yasargil, M. G. 1961. Ergebnisse der stereotaktischen Operationen beim Parkinsonismus, insbesondere der doppelseitigen Eingriffe. Deutsch. Z. Nervenheilk. **182**:530-541.

Kuypers, H. G. J. M. 1958. Corticobulbar connections to the pons and lower brain-stem in man. Brain **81**:364-388.

Kuypers, H. G. J. M. 1964. The descending pathways to the spinal cord, their anatomy and function. Progr. Brain Res. **11**:178-202.

Kuypers, H. G. J. M., Fleming, W. R., and Farinholt, J. W. 1962. Subcorticospinal projections in the Rhesus monkey. J. Comp. Neurol. **118**:107-137.

Kuypers, H. G. J. M., and Lawrence, D. G. 1967. Cortical projections to the red nucleus and the brain stem in the Rhesus monkey. Brain Res. **4**:151-188.

Lafon, R., Labauge, R., van Bogaert, L., and Castan, P. 1965. Sur l'unité histopathologiques des encéphalopathies subaigües (types Creutzfeldt, Jakob, Heidenhain et Nevin). Rev. Neurol. **1**:201-227.

Laurence, K. M., and Cavanagh, J. B. 1968. Progressive degeneration of the cerebral cortex in infancy. Brain **91**:261-280.

Laursen, A. M. 1961. Movements evoked from the region of the caudate nucleus in cats. Acta Physiol. Scand. **54**:175-184.

Lee, D. K., Markham, C. H., and Clark, W. G. 1968. Serotonin (5-HT) metabolism in Huntington's chorea. Life Sci. **7**:707-712.

Lewy, F. H. 1913. Zur pathologischen Anatomie der Paralysis agitans. Deutsch. Z. Nervenheilk. **50**:50-55.

Lewy, F. H. 1923. Tonus und Bewegung. Berlin, Springer-Verlag.

Lhermitte, J., and Cornil, L. 1921. Recherches anatomiques sur la maladie de Parkinson. Rev. Neurol. **37**:587-592.

Lhermitte, J., and Pagniez, P. 1930. Anatomie et physiologie pathologiques de la chorée de Sydenham. Encéphale **25**:24-47.

Lichtenstein, B. W., and Gore, I. 1955. Wilson's disease—chronic form: clinical-pathological observations in a brother and sister. Arch. Neurol. Psychiat. **73**:13-21.

Lindenberg, R. 1964. Die Schädigungsmechanismen der Substantia Nigra bei Hirntrauma und das Problem des posttraumatischen Parkinsonismus. Deutsch. Z. Nervenheilk. **185**:637-663.

Lipkin, L. E. 1959. Cytoplasmic inclusions in ganglion cells associated with parkinsonian states: a neurocellular change studied in 53 cases and 206 controls. Amer. J. Path. **35**:1117-1133.

Loeffler, J. D., Slatt, B., and Hoyt, W. F. 1966. Motor abnormalities of the eyelids in Parkinson's disease. Arch. Ophthal. **76**:178-185.

Magni, F., and Willis, W. D. 1964a. Cortical control of brain stem reticular neurons. Arch. Ital. Biol. **102**:418-433.

Magni, F., and Willis, W. D. 1964b. Subcortical and peripheral control of brain stem reticular neurons. Arch. Ital. Biol. **102**:434-448.

Majewska, Z., and Szelożyńska, K. 1967. Asymmetry of movements in cases of chorea minor. In Choróbski, J., editor: Neurological problems. London, Pergamon Press, pp. 165-169.

Malamud, N. 1963. Pattern of CNS vulnerability in neonatal hypoxaemia. In Schadé, J. P., and McMenemey, W. H., editors: Selective vulnerability of the brain in hypoxaemia. Oxford, Blackwell Scientific Publications, pp. 211-225.

Martin, J. P. 1957. Hemichorea (hemiballismus) without lesions in the corpus Luysii. Brain **80**:1-10.

Martin, J. P. 1965. The globus pallidus in postencephalitic parkinsonism. J. Neurol. Sci. **2**:344-375.

Martin, J. P., and Alcock, N. S. 1934. Hemichorea associated with a lesion of the corpus Luysii. Brain **57**:504-516.

Massion, J. 1967. The mammalian red nucleus. Physiol. Rev. **47**:383-436.

May, W. W. 1968. Creutzfeldt-Jakob disease. I. Survey of the literature and clinical diagnosis. Acta Neurol. Scand. **44**:1-32.

May, W. W., Itabashi, H. H., and DeJong, R. N. 1968. Creutzfeldt-Jakob disease: clinical, pathologic, and genetic study of a family. Neurology **19**:137-155.

Mehler, W. R. 1966. Further notes on the centre médian nucleus of Luys. In Purpura, D. P., and Yahr, M. D., editors: The thalamus. New York, Columbia University Press, pp. 109-127.

Mena, I., Marin, O., Fuenzalida, S., and Cotzias, G. C. 1967. Chronic manganese poisoning: clinical picture and manganese turnover. Neurology **17**:128-136.

Mettler, F. A. 1955. The experimental anatomophysiologic approach to the study of diseases of the basal ganglia. J. Neuropath. Exp. Neurol. **14**:115-141.

Mettler, F. A. 1964. Substantia nigra and parkinsonism. Arch. Neurol. **11**:529-542.

Mettler, F. A., Davidoff, L. M., and Grimes, R. 1947. Static tremor with hemiplegia. Arch. Neurol. Psychiat. **57**:423-429.

Mettler, F. A., and Mettler, C. C. 1942. The effects of striatal injury. Brain **65**:242-255.

Meyer, A. 1963. The Hallervorden-Spatz syndrome. In Greenfield's neuropathology, ed. 2. London, Edward Arnold (Publishers) Ltd., pp. 412-414.

Meyers, R., Sweeney, D. B., and Schwidde, J. T. 1950. Hemiballismus: aetiology and surgical treatment. J. Neurol. Neurosurg. Psychiat. **13**: 115-126.

Münzer, F. T. 1935. Choreatisches Syndrom der rechten oberen Extremität als Ausdruck einer monosymptomatischen Lues cerebri. Z. Ges. Neurol. Psychiat. **152**:12-18.

Nauta, W. J. H., and Mehler, W. R. 1966. Projections of the lentiform nucleus in the monkey. Brain Res. **1**:3-42.

Nevin, S., McMenemey, W. H., Behrman, S., and Jones, D. P. 1960. Subacute spongiform encephalopathy—a subacute form of encephalopathy attributable to vascular dysfunction (spongiform cerebral atrophy). Brain **85**:519-564.

Norman, R. M. 1938. An example of status marmoratus of the cerebral cortex. J. Neurol. Psychiat. **1**:7-12.

Norman, R. M. 1947. État marbré of the corpus striatum following birth injury. J. Neurosurg. Neurol. Psychiat. **10**:12-25.

Ogawa, T. 1952. Eine neue Auffassung über die Faserverbindung des Corpus striatum. J. Nerv. Ment. Dis. **116**:555-571.

O'Reilly, S. 1967. Problems in Wilson's disease. Neurology **17**:137-146.

O'Reilly, S., Pollycove, M., and Bank, W. J. 1968. Iron metabolism in Wilson's disease: kinetic studies with iron^{59}. Neurology **18**:634-644.

Ornsteen, A. M. 1929. Incipient parkinsonism: a diagnostic triad for its early recognition. Arch. Neurol. Psychiat. **22**:709-713.

Ornsteen, A. M. 1936. Incipient parkinsonism: diagnosis and treatment. Med. Clin. N. Amer., pp. 233-238.

Pakkenberg, H., and Brody, H. 1965. The number of nerve cells in the substantia nigra in paralysis agitans. Acta Neuropath. **5**:320-324.

Papez, J. W. 1942. A summary of fiber connections of the basal ganglia with each other and other portions of the brain. Res. Publ. Ass. Res. Nerv. Ment. Dis., Proc. **21**:21-68.

Papez, J. W., Hertzman, J., and Rundles, R. W. 1938. Athetosis and pallidal deficiency. Arch. Neurol. Psychiat. **40**:789-799.

Pentschew, A. 1958. Intoxikationen. In Lubarsch, O., Henke, F., and Rössle, R., editors: Handbuch der speziellen pathologische Anatomie und Histologie, vol. 13 (edited by Scholz, W.), pt. 2B. Heidelberg, Springer-Verlag, pp. 1907-2502.

Pentschew, A., Ebner, F. F., and Kovatch, R. M. 1963. Experimental manganese encephalopathy in monkeys: a preliminary report. J. Neuropath. Exp. Neurol. **22**:488-499.

Pichard, H., and Liber, A. F. 1934. Parkinsonisme fruste traumatique. Ann. Méd.-Psychol. **1**:1-6.

Pincus, J. H., and Chutorian, A. 1967. Familial benign chorea with intention tremor: a clinical entity. J. Pediat. **70**:724-729.

Poirier, L. J., and Bouvier, G. 1966. The red nucleus and its efferent nervous pathways in the monkey. J. Comp. Neurol. **128**:223-244.

Poskanzer, D. C. 1969. L-dopa in Parkinson's syndrome. New Eng. J. Med. **280**:382-383.

Radermecker, J., and Rizzuto, N. 1967. Forme myoclonique de la maladie de Hallervorden-Spatz. (Aspect clinique simulant une encéphalopathie spongieuse subaiguë.) Rev. Neurol. **1**: 184-188.

Ranson, S. W., and Ranson, S. W., Jr. 1941. Strio nigral or nigro striatal fibers. Trans. Amer. Neurol. Ass. **67**:168-171.

Richter, H. 1923. Beiträge zur Klinik und pathologischen Anatomie der extrapyramidalen Bewegungsstörungen. Arch. Psychiat. Nervenkr. **67**:226-294.

Richter, R. 1948. The pallial component in hepatolenticular degeneration. J. Neuropath. Exp. Neurol. **7**:1-18.

Rozdilsky, B., Cumings, J. N., and Huston, A. F. 1968. Hallervorden-Spatz disease—late infantile and adult types, report of two cases. Acta Neuropath. **10**:1-16.

Rushworth, G. 1960. Spasticity and rigidity: an experimental study and review. J. Neurol. Neurosurg. Psychiat. **23**:99-118.

Sacks, O. W., Aguilar, M. J., and Brown, W. J. 1966. Hallervorden Spatz disease: its pathogenesis and place among the axonal dystrophies. Acta Neuropath. **6**:164-174.

Scheinberg, I. H. 1961. Copper metabolism; a review. In Walshe, J. M., and Cumings, J. N., editors: Wilson's disease; some current concepts. Oxford, Blackwell Scientific Publications, pp. 14-17.

Schmitt, W., and Scholz, W. 1932. Klinischer und pathologisch-anatomischer Beitrag zur Torsionsdystonia. Deutsch. Z. Nervenheilk. **126**:53-79.

Scholz, W., Wake, J., and Peters, G. 1938. Der Status marmoratus, ein Beispiel systemähnlicher Hirnveränderungen auf der Grundlage von Kreislaufstörungen. Z. Ges. Neurol. Psychiat. **163**:193-232.

Schreiner, L., MacCarty, C. S., and Grindlay, J. H. 1958. Production and relief of tremor in the monkey. In Fields, W. S., editor: Pathogenesis and treatment of parkinsonism. Springfield, Illinois, Charles C Thomas, Publisher, pp. 118-137.

Schwarz, G. A., and Barrows, L. J. 1960. Hemiballism without involvement of Luy's body. Arch. Neurol. **2**:420-434.

Seitelberger, F., and Gross, H. 1957. Über eine spätinfantile Form der Hallervorden-Spatzchen Krankheit. Mitteilung: Histochemische Befunde, Erörterung der Nosologie. Deutsch. Z. Nervenheilk. **176**:104-125.

Selby, G. 1967a. Stereotactic surgery for the relief of Parkinson's disease: a critical review. J. Neurol. Sci. **5**:315-342.

Selby, G. 1967b. Stereotactic surgery for the relief of Parkinson's disease: an analysis of the results in a series of 303 patients (413 operations). J. Neurol. Sci. **5**:343-375.

Selby, G. 1968. Cerebral atrophy in parkinsonism. J. Neurol. Sci. **6**:517-559.

Shiraki, H. 1966. Some unusual neuropathologic features in Guam cases in comparison with those in the Japanese: with special reference to Hallervorden-Spatz disease-like lesions. Proc. 5th Internat. Congr. Neuropath., Amsterdam, Excerpta Medica Foundation, pp. 201-207.

Shiraki, H. 1968. Comparative neuropathologic study of Wilson's disease and other types of hepatocerebral disease. In Bergsma, D., editor: Wilson's disease. New York, National Foundation–March of Dimes, pp. 64-73.

Siegfried, J. 1968. Die Parkinsonsche Krankheit und ihre Behandlung. Wien, Springer-Verlag.

Spiegel, E. A., and Wycis, H. T. 1953. Role of pallidum in genesis of some choreic movements. Neurology **3**:261-266.

Spiegel, E. A., and Wycis, H. T. 1954. Ansotomy in paralysis agitans. Arch. Neurol. Psychiat. **71**:598-614.

Spiegel, E. A., and Wycis, H. T. 1958. Pallidoanatomy: anatomic-physiologic foundation and histopathologic control. In Fields, W. S., editor: Pathogenesis and treatment of parkinsonism. Springfield, Illinois, Charles C Thomas, Publisher, pp. 86-105.

Spiegel, E. A., and Wycis, H. T. 1961. Stimulation of the brain stem and basal ganglia in man. In Sheer, D. E., editor: Electrical stimulation of the brain. Austin, University of Texas Press, pp. 86-105.

Spiegel, E. A., and Wycis, H. T. 1967. The possible role of the hypothalamus in parkinsonian brady- and akinesia: a working hypothesis. Confin. Neurol. **29**:262-264.

Spiegel, E. A., Wycis, H. T., Baird, H. W., III, Rovner, D., and Thur, C. 1956. Pallidum and muscle tone. Neurology **6**:350-356.

Spillane, J., and Phillips, R. 1937. Huntington's chorea in South Wales. Quart. J. Med. **6**:403-423.

Spiller, W. G. 1920. Acquired double athetosis (dystonia lenticularis). Arch. Neurol. Psychiat. **4**:370-386.

Stadlan, E. M., Duvoisin, R., and Yahr, M. 1966. The pathology of parkinsonism. Proc. 5th Internat. Congr. Neuropath. Amsterdam, Excerpta Medica Foundation, pp. 569-571.

Starr, A. 1967. A disorder of rapid eye movements in Huntington's chorea. Brain **90**:545-564.

Stern, J., and Ward, A. A., Jr. 1962. Supraspinal and drug modulation of the alpha motor system: relation of supraspinal and drug modulation to parkinsonism. Arch. Neurol. **6**:404-413.

Stern, J., and Ward, A. A., Jr. 1963. The relationship of alpha and gamma motor systems to the efficacy of the surgical therapy of parkinsonism. J. Neurosurg. **20**:185-187.

Sternlieb, I., and Scheinberg, I. H. 1968. Prevention of Wilson's disease in asymptomatic patients. New Eng. J. Med. **278**:352-359.

Szabo, J. 1963. Topical distribution of the striatal efferents in the monkey. Exp. Neurol. **5**:21-36.

Szabo, J. 1967. The efferent projections of the putamen in the monkey. Exp. Neurol. **19**:463-476.

Toghill, P. J., Johnston, A. W., and Smith, J. F. 1967. Choreoathetosis in porto-systemic encephalopathy. J. Neurol. Neurosurg. Psychiat. **30**:358-363.

Turner, J. W. A. 1955. Metallic poisons and nervous system. Lancet **1**:661-663.

van Bogaert, L. 1930. Contribution clinique et anatomique à l'étude de la paralysie agitante, juvénile primitive (atrophic progressive du globe pâle de Ramsay-Hunt). Rev. Neurol. **2**:315-326.

van Bogaert, L. 1940. Associations anatomo-cliniques; dégénérescence pigmentaire pallido-nigrique (Hallervorden-Spatz) et encéphalite léthargique chronique. Rev. Neurol. **72**:448-456.

van Bogaert, L. 1941. Études anatomo-cliniques de syndrômes hypercinétiques complexes (Un torticollis héréditaire et familiale avec tremblement). Mschr. Psychiat. Neurol. **103**:312-342.

van Bogaert, L. 1946. Aspects cliniques et pathologiques des atrophies pallidales et pallido-luysiennes progressives. J. Neurol. Neurosurg. Psychiat. **9**:125-157.

van Bogaert, L., and Bertrand, I. 1949. Sur une idiotie familiale avec dégénerescence spongieuse du névraxe (note préliminaire). Acta Neurol. Belg. **49**:572-587.

van Bogaert, L., and Radermecker, M. A. 1954. Scléroses latérales amyotrophiques typiques et paralysies agitantes héréditaires dans une même famille, avec une forme de passage possible entre les deux affections. Mschr. Psychiat. Neurol. **127**:185-203.

Victor, M., Adams, R. D., and Cole, M. 1965. The acquired (non-Wilsonian) type of chronic hepatocerebral degeneration. Medicine **44**:345-396.

Vincent, C., and van Bogaert, L. 1936. Contribution à l'étude des syndromes du globe pâle: la dégénérescence progressive du globe pâle et de la portion réticulée de la substance noire. (Maladie d'Hallervorden-Spatz.) Rev. Neurol. **65**:921-959.

Vogt, C., and Vogt, O. 1920. Zur Lehre der Erkrankungen des striären Systems. J. Psychol. Neurol., Erg. Heft 3, **25**:627-846.

Vogt, C., and Vogt, O. 1941. Thalamusstudien I-III. J. Psychol. Neurol. **50**:32-154.

Vogt, C., and Vogt, O. 1951. Importance of neuroanatomy in the field of neuropathology. Neurology **1**:205-218.

von Braunmühl, A. 1930. Die Rinden-Markkomponente im anatomischen Bild der Wilson-Pseudosklerosegruppe nebst Bemerkungen zur Pathogenese des Leidens vornehmlich unter dem Gesichtspunkt einer vergleichenden Krankheitsforschung. Z. Ges. Neurol. Psychiat. **130**:1-65.

von Braunmühl, A. 1949. Encephalitis epidemica und Synäresislehre: Grundsätliches zur Anatomie und Pathogenese des postencephalitischen Parkinsonismus. Arch. Psychiat. Nervenkr. **181**:543-576.

von Braunmühl, A. 1957. Alterserkrankungen des Zentralnervensystems: Senile involution. Senile Demenz: Alzheimersche Krankheit. In Bumke, O., Henke, F., and Rössle, R., editors: Handbuch der speziellen pathologischen Anatomie und Histologie, vol. 13 (edited by Scholz, W.), pt. 1A. Berlin, Springer-Verlag, pp. 337-539.

von Sántha, K. 1932. Über Gefässveränderungen im Zentralnervensystem bei Chorea rheumatica. Virchows Arch. Path. Anat. **287**:405-420.

Walker, A. E. 1959. Normal and pathological physiology of the thalamus. In Schaltenbrand, G., and Bailey, P., editors: Introduction to stereotaxis, with an atlas of the human brain. Stuttgart, Georg Thieme Verlag.

Walker, A. E., and Botterell, E. H. 1937. The syndrome of the superior cerebellar peduncle in the monkey. Brain **60**:329-353.

Wang, G. H., and Akert, K. 1962. Behavior and reflexes of chronic striatal cats. Arch. Ital. Biol. **100**:48-85.

Ward, A. A., Jr. 1958. Physiological basis of involuntary movement. In Fields, W. S., editor: Pathogenesis and treatment of parkinsonism. Springfield, Illinois, Charles C Thomas, Publisher, pp. 106-117.

Ward, A. A., Jr. 1961. Physiological mechanism in parkinsonism. Rev. Canad. Biol. **20**:345-350.

Ward, A. A., Jr., McCulloch, W. S., and Magoun, H. W. 1948. Production of alternating tremor at rest in monkeys. J. Neurophysiol. **11**:317-330.

Ward, A. A., Jr., and Stern, J. 1963. Thalamic inhibition of the myotatic reflex in man. J. Neurosurg. **20**:1033-1039.

Weber, M. B. 1967. Familial paroxysmal dystonia. J. Nerv. Ment. Dis. **145**:221-226.

Wechsler, I. S., and Brock, S. 1922. Dystonia musculorum deformans with especial reference to a myostatic form and the occurrence of decerebrate rigidity phenomena: a study of six cases. Arch. Neurol. Psychiat. **8**:538-552.

Whitlock, C. M., Jr., Amuso, S. J., and Bittenbender, J. B. 1966. Chronic neurological disease in two manganese steel workers. Amer. Industr. Hyg. Ass. J. **27**:454-459.

Whitlock, D. G., and Nauta, W. J. H. 1956. Subcortical projections from the temporal neocortex in Macaca mulatta. J. Comp. Neurol. **106**:183-212.

Whittier, J. R., and Mettler, F. A. 1949. Studies on the subthalamus of the rhesus monkey: hyperkinesia and other physiologic effects of subthalamic lesions with special reference to the subthalamic nucleus of Luys. J. Comp. Neurol. **90**:319-372.

Wilson, S. A. K. 1912. Progressive lenticular degeneration: familial nervous disease associated with cirrhosis of the liver. Brain **34**:295-509.

Wilson, S. A. K. 1940. Neurology. Baltimore, The Williams & Wilkins Co.

Wimmer, A., and Neel, A. V. 1928. Les amyotrophies systématisées dans l'encéphalite épidémique chronique. Acta Psychiat. Scand. **3**:319-365.

Winkelman, N. W., and Eckel, J. L. 1932. The brain in acute rheumatic fever. Arch. Neurol. Psychiat. **28**:844-870.

Wycis, H. T. 1958. Discussion. In Fields, W. S., editor: Pathogenesis and treatment of parkinsonism. Springfield, Illinois, Charles C Thomas, Publisher, p. 137.

Wycis, H. T., Szekely, E. G., and Spiegel, E. A. 1957. Tremor on stimulation of the midbrain tegmentum after degeneration of the brachium conjunctivum. J. Neuropath. Exp. Neurol. **16**:79-84.

Yahr, M. D., Bering, E. A., Jr., and others. 1966. Parkinson's disease: present status and research trends. Public Health Service Publication Number 1491, U.S. Department of Health, Education and Welfare, Bethesda, National Institutes of Health.

Zeman, W., and Dyken, P. 1967. Dystonia musculorum deformans: clinical, genetic and pathoanatomical studies. Psychiat. Neurol. Neurochir. (Amst.) **70**:77-121.

Chapter 25

Localization of lesions of the thalamus

Paul I. Yakovlev

The general configuration of the two ovoid masses of gray matter called thalami conforms to the cerebral pallium covering them. Keeping in mind these respective configurations will help in visualizing the organization of thalamocortical connections in three planes of space.

Before the schema of these connections is provided, some of the terms to be used need to be defined.

ANATOMICAL DEFINITIONS

Subdivisions of the thalamus

The relative position and general configuration of most of the nuclei of the thalamus are shown diagrammatically in Figs. 25-1, 25-2, and 25-3, and the cortical zones of their projection in Figs. 25-4 and 25-5. The abbreviations used are presented in Table 25-1.

As shown in Figs. 25-1 to 25-3, the thalamus consists of aggregates of nerve cells surrounded by fibers called *lamina medullaris externa* (LME) and interwoven by a plexus of fibers called *lamina medullaris interna* (LMI) and accessory laminae. This plexus of fibers subdivides the thalamic mass into three zones.

(1) *Median zone* (black). This consists of a periventricular plate of generally small cells and thinly myelinated fibers joined with the periventricular plate of the opposite thalamus by the massa intermedia (mi), bridging the cavity of the third ventricle.

(2) *Paramedian zone.* This zone consists of discrete aggregates of cells, extremely heteromorphic in cell type, enmeshed in the septa of the lamina medullaris interna and accessory laminae and subdivided into a rostral group of nuclei (vertical lines in Figs. 25-1 to 25-3) overlying the hypothalamus and a caudal group (horizontal lines) overlying the subthalamus.

(3) *Dorsolateral and posterior zone* (areas left white). This consists of large and confluent aggregates, relatively homogenous in cell type, constituting approximately two-thirds of the thalamic mass and overriding posteriorly the paramedian zone as the pulvinar of the thalamus.

A shell-like plate of medium and small cells enmeshed in a plexus of fibers of the lamina medullaris externa (LME) is called the "reticular nucleus" (ReT). It surrounds the ventral and lateral walls of the thalamic mass and separates it from the posterior limb of the internal capsule. The habenular nuclei (Hb) are connected to the median thalamic zone by the fibers of the stria medullaris (taenia thalami) and the habenulo-interpeduncular tract (fasciculus retroflexus) (FR). The habenular nuclei (epithalamus) are generally regarded as formations distinct from the thalamus.

Subdivisions of the hemispheres

The thalamus and the cerebral hemispheres develop as a unit. On developmental grounds three zones are recognizable in the endbrain and correspond to three thalamic zones (Figs. 25-3 to 25-5).

(1) *Median zone.* This zone is made up of the rhinencephalon (solid black), which comprises the olfactory lobe (septal area [SpA], amygdala, and the anterior perforated substance and olfactory bulbs [OlB] and tracts) and the hippocampus (the hippocampal rudiment [HR] and Ammon's horn, or "hippocampus major" [H]).

(2) *Paramedian zone* (vertical lines). Forming this zone are the corpus striatum (caudatum and putamen) and the cortex of the inner border, or "limbus," of the hemisphere, which encircles the striatum and comprises the insula, the orbital border of the frontal lobe, the parolfactory lobule of Broca, the cingulate gyrus, and the parahippocampal gyrus with the uncus.

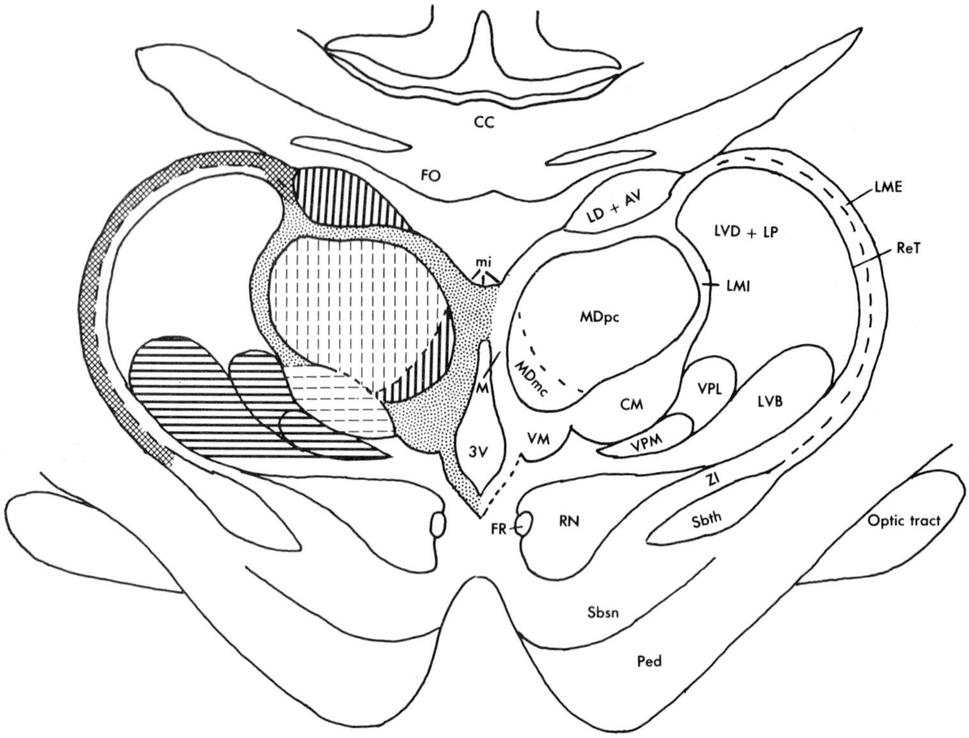

Fig. 25-1. Thalamic zones and nuclear groups projected in the transverse plane (the geniculate nuclei are omitted). *Fine dots:* median zone; nuclei of the midline and intralaminar nuclei. *Cross-hatch:* reticular nucleus. *Horizontal heavy lines:* lemniscal nuclei of the paramedian zone; specific nuclei. *Horizontal dash lines:* centrum medianum nucleus. *Vertical heavy lines:* limbic nuclei of the paramedian zone. *Vertical dash lines:* medial dorsal nucleus. *Area left white:* nuclei of the dorsolateral and posterior zone.

(3) *Dorsolateral and posterior zone* (horizontal lines and areas left white). This zone includes more than two-thirds of the mass of the hemisphere and comprises the frontal, parietal, temporal, and occipital lobes overlying the paramedian zone of the hemisphere.

On the grounds of comparative anatomy and of development during embryonal life, the paramedian and dorsolateral and posterior zones are regarded as characteristic of the brain of mammals. They are covered by a six-layered cortex called *isocortex* (O. Vogt, 1911) (synonym: "neocortex"; Edinger, 1904) and make up the hemispheres proper. The isocortex is laid down early in the third fetal month in the marginal layer of the lateral wall of the hemispheric evaginations and spreads gradually over the hemispheres as a mantle (hence the term *pallium*) separated from the striatum and lateral ventricle by a layer of white matter. Such a discrete mantle of stratified gray matter never develops in the part of the rhinencephalon situated between the hemispheres. The superficial gray matter of the rhinencephalon is covered by a layer of white matter (hence "white cortex"; Meynert, 1867) and is called *allocortex* (O. Vogt, 1911). In the olfactory lobe ("paleocortex") the gray matter is not stratified but is homogeneously reticular and blends with the deep gray matter of the striatum and hypothalamus. It may be regarded as the rostral extension of the reticular formation of the brainstem. The convoluted plate of gray matter of the hippocampus ("archicortex") develops in the mantle layer of the dorsal wall of the telencephalic vesicle between the hemispheric evaginations and is not comparable in development or structure to the isocortical plate. It is covered by a wide stratum zonale of afferent fibers entering the hippocampus from the limbus of the hemisphere, that is, from the surface of the brain.

The isocortex (pallium) of the hemispheres also exhibits wide differences in its structure and pattern of lamination. In the border or "limbus" of the hemisphere (vertical lines), the superficial layers are less developed than in the crown or "fundus" of the hemisphere, and the cortical plate departs from the standard six-layered pattern. This limbic cortex will be referred to as

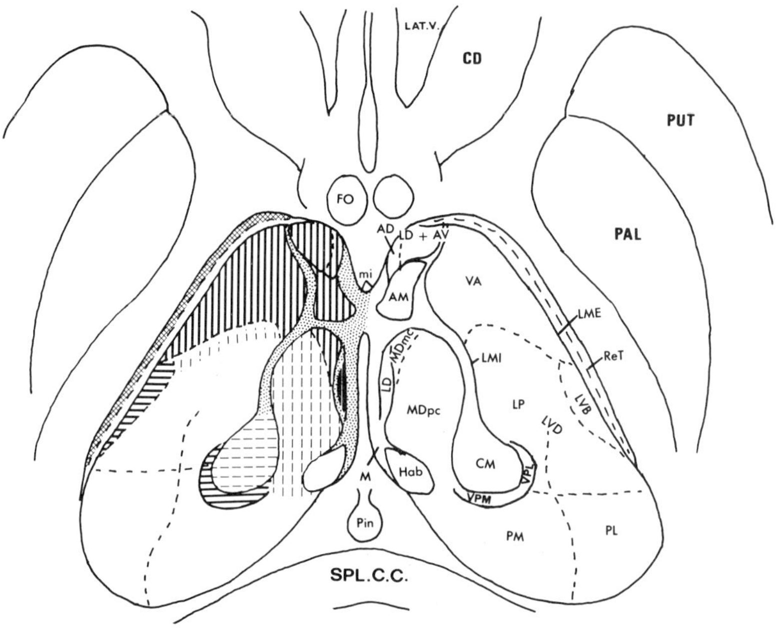

Fig. 25-2. Thalamic zones and nuclear groups in horizontal plane (geniculate nuclei are omitted). Schema of shadings is the same as in Fig. 25-1.

Table 25-1. Abbreviations used

For thalamic nuclei	
AD—anterior dorsal nucleus	M—midline nuclei
AL—anterior lateral nucleus	MD mc—medial dorsal nucleus, magnocellular part
AM—anterior medial nucleus	
AV—anterior ventral nucleus	MDpc—medial dorsal nucleus, parvocellular part
CM—nucleus centrum medianum	
Ant. Tub.—anterior tubercle of thalamus	MG—medial geniculate nucleus
FR—habenulo-interpeduncular tract	mi—massa intermedia
Hab—habenular nucleus (epithalamus)	PI—inferior pulvinar nucleus
IL—intralaminar nuclei	PL—lateral pulvinar nucleus
LD—lateral dorsal nucleus	PM—medial pulvinar nucleus
LG—lateral geniculate nucleus	Pulv—pulvinar
LME—external medullary lamina	ReT—reticular nucleus
LMI—internal medullary lamina	VA—ventral anterior nucleus
LP—lateral posterior nucleus	VM—ventral medial (submedial) nucleus
LVB—lateral ventral nucleus,* basal part	VPL—ventral posterolateral nucleus
LVD—lateral ventral nucleus,* dorsal part	VPM—ventral posteromedial (arcuate) nucleus
For other structures	
CC—corpus callosum	PUT—putamen
CD—caudate nucleus	RN—red nucleus
FO—fornix	SbsN—substantia nigra
FR—fasciculus retroflexus	Sbth—subthalamic nucleus
LAT.V.—lateral ventricle	SPL.C.C.—splenium of corpus callosum
PAL—pallidum	ZI—zona incerta
Ped—basis pedunculi	3V—third ventricle

*Also called ventral lateral nucleus.

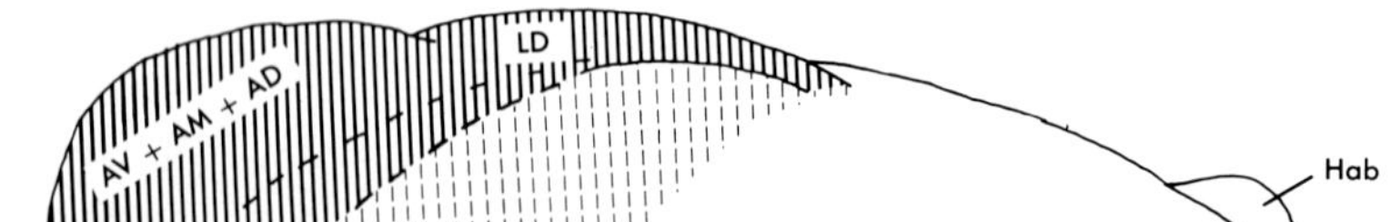

Fig. 25-3. Thalamic zones and nuclear groups projected in the parasagittal plane. The geniculate nuclei are also illustrated. Schema of shadings is the same as in Fig. 25-1.

Fig. 25-4. Telencephalic zones and cortical areas of thalamocortical projections as viewed on the lateral aspect of the cerebral hemisphere. *Solid black:* the median or rhinencephalic zone; allocortex or *entocortex.* Shown here is the olfactory lobe or "paleocortex" with the olfactory tract and bulb, which is the projection zone of the median thalamus. *Heavy vertical lines:* paramedian or limbic zone of the hemisphere; heterotypical isocortex, or mesocortex. Shown here is the insula, which is the projection zone of the limbic nuclei. *Vertical dash lines:* paralimbic or transitional ectocortex (isocortex). Included here is the insular operculum, which is the projection zone of the medial dorsal nucleus, at least anteriorly. *Heavy horizontal lines:* special heterotypical ectocortex (isocortex) of the sensory-motor analyser areas ("vector areas"). Included here are projection areas of the lemniscal nuclei. *Light horizontal dash lines:* heterotypical cortex surrounding analyses areas. *Areas left white:* homotypical ectocortex (isocortex). Shown here are epistriatal (frontal) and epihippocampal (temporoparietal) "association" ectocortical areas.

Fig. 25-5. Same shadings as in Fig. 25-4, the medial aspect of the cerebral hemisphere. Illustrated here is the entire median zone (solid black), including the olfactory lobe, e.g., olfactory bulb *(OB)* and tract *(Olf T),* septal area *(SA)* (paleocortex), subcallosal (area 25) and pericallosal *(SPL* and *HR)* hippocampal rudiments, hippocampus major *(H)* (archicortex), and uncus gyrus hippocampi *(U).* The paramedian zone (heavy vertical lines) includes the orbitomedial (parolfactory), cingular, and parahippocampal mesocortex of the medial limbus of the hemisphere. For the significance of the other shadings, see text and the legend to Fig. 25-4.

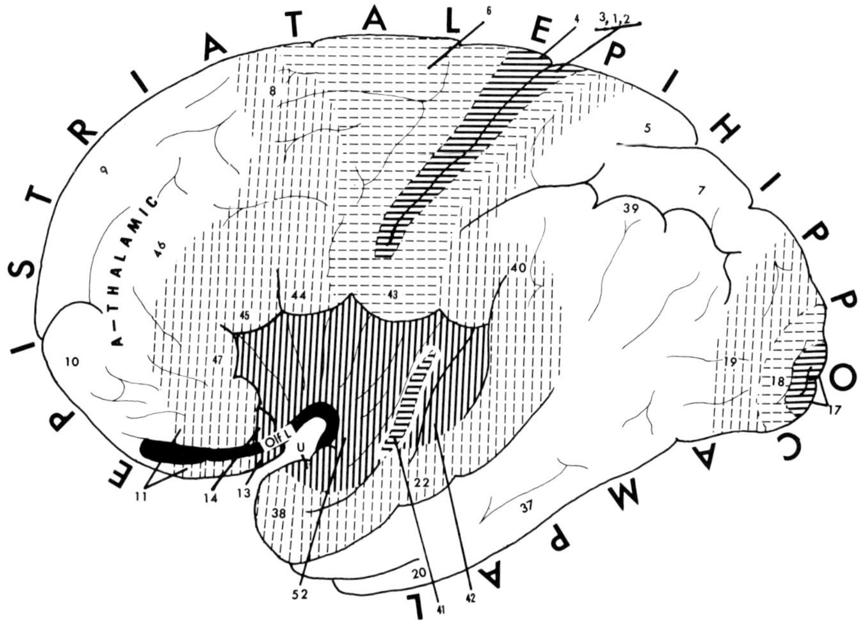

Fig. 25-4. For legend see opposite page.

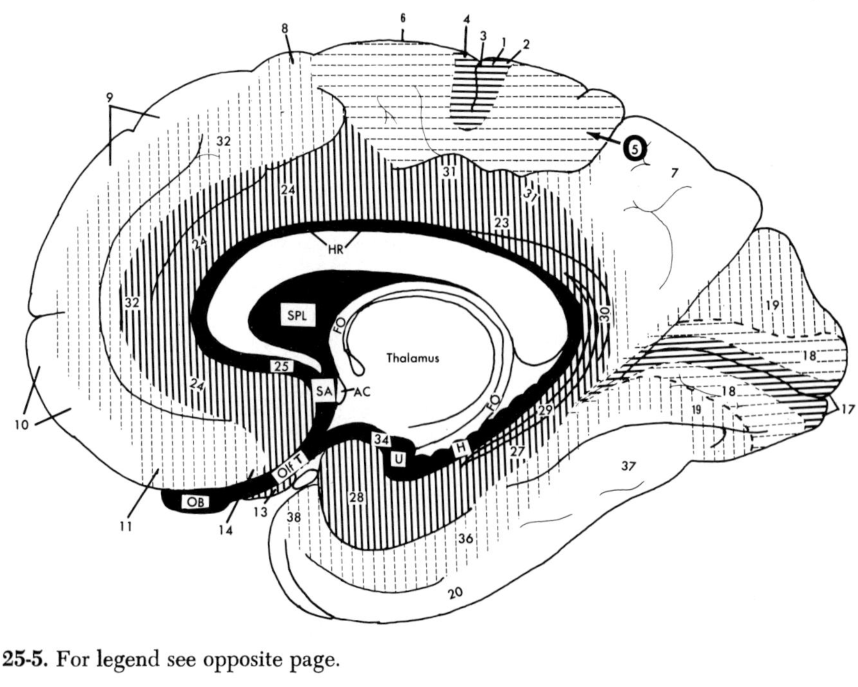

Fig. 25-5. For legend see opposite page.

heterotypical isocortex (von Economo and Koskinas, 1925). The cortex of the fundus of the hemisphere maintains the pattern of six-layered lamination (areas left white) and will be designated as *homotypical isocortex.* However, the areas of the cortex of the fundus that are most intimately thalamus-bound (areas shown by horizontal lines) exhibit the widest departures in pattern of lamination and structure from the areas of the homotypical cortex surrounding them and will be designated as areas of *special heterotypical isocortex* of the fundus of the hemisphere.

On these grounds, and to reduce the nomenclative palimpsest of overlapping designations to a manageable schema, the gray matter of the olfactory lobe and hippocampus (the median zone) will be designated as the *entocortex,* that is, the innermost gray matter nearest the third ventricle and median zone of the thalamus. The heterotypical cortex of the limbus of the hemispheres (the paramedian zone), bordering bilaterad on the entocortex and nearest the striatum and lateral ventricle, which it encircles and the configurations of which it duplicates, will be designated *mesocortex* or *limbic cortex;* the mesocortex is interposed between the rhinencephalon and the fundus of the hemisphere and corresponds in general position to that of the paramedian thalamic zone. The homotypical cortex of the fundus of the hemisphere overlying the insula, the cingulate gyrus, and the parahippocampal gyrus will be designated *ectocortex,* that is, the outermost cortex covering the dorsolateral and posterior free surface of the hemisphere and corresponding in relative position in the hemisphere to the position of the dorsolateral and posterior zone of the thalamus. Between the mesocortex of the limbus and the ectocortex of the fundus of the hemisphere is a gradient of structural transition. The areas of transition (shown by vertical dash lines) may be designated *paralimbic ectocortex.*

It is noteworthy that areas of the special heterotypical ectocortex (horizontal lines) are represented amidst wide areas of the homotypical ectocortex (in white) in three bands, all of which extend from the heterotypical mesocortex of the limbus of the hemisphere. These bands of special heterotypical isocortex represent the cortical ends of the afferent conduction paths, relayed through the thalamus to the hemisphere from the receptors of the *specific modalities of sensory experience,* such as sight (Figs. 25-4 and 25-5, area 17), sound (Fig. 25-4, area 41), touch (areas 3, 1, and 2), and muscle sense (areas 4 and 6). During the development of the isocortical plate these areas become recognizable early in the third fetal month by their distinctive structure and, in a sense, may be regarded as the "vector areas" of the growth and differentiation of the cortical plate about them. The largest and widest of the three bands of special heterotypical cortex extends across the fundus of the hemisphere from the insula to the cingular gyrus (Figs. 25-4 and 25-5) and is bisected in its long axis by the deep sulcus of Rolando into agranular macropyramidal areas 4 and 6, anterior to the sulcus and the highly granular areas 3 and 2 posterior to it. This transverse band divides the hemisphere into two parts—an anterior part or frontal lobe, overlying the striatum and developing upon the olfactory lobe of the rhinencephalon (median zone) as its pediment, and a posterior part developing upon the hippocampus as its pediment and overlying the thalamus in an arc (Fig. 25-5). The *epihippocampal* part is the recipient of most of the *afferent* fibers from the thalamus. The *epistriatal* part is the origin of most of the long *efferent* fibers descending from the hemisphere through the internal capsule to the striatum, thalamus, brainstem, and spinal cord. This part of the hemisphere receives afferent fibers from the thalamus only posteriorly in the heterotypical areas of the limbus (vertical lines) and in the transition paralimbic areas (dash lines) of the frontal lobe. The homotypical areas (white) covering the anterior convexity of the frontal lobe in the human brain receive few if any projection fibers from the thalamus and may be regarded as "a-thalamic" association areas of the frontal lobes emancipated in man from the direct influence of the thalamus on their activities (Yakovlev, 1954).

RETICULATE AND NUCLEATE COMPONENTS OF THE THALAMUS

In the cellular structure of the thalamus two components may be distinguished: (1) the *reticulate* component appearing early in the second embryonal month in the mantle layer of the dorsolateral wall of the diencephalic vesicle and (2) the *nucleated* component emerging gradually within the former during the third and fourth fetal months. The two patterns of neuronal assembly persist in the adult and are recognizable as differing degrees of prominence of one or the other component, in all three thalamic zones.

Reticulate component and the median thalamic zone

The reticulate component pervades the thalamus and consists of (1) stellate cells with *multiple* dendrites and a *short* axon ramifying close to the cell body in the thalamus ("intercalar" or "intercalated" neurons) and (2) cells with *few* dendrites and a *long* axon branching in the thalamus and in the extrathalamic gray masses (striatum, cortex) (Leontowich, 1959). Both types of cells are widespread in the thalamus and are found amidst cells in the discretely nucleated cell aggregates (nuclei) and in the fiber plexus between these nucleated formations. In the periventricular cell plate and massa intermedia they form a dense plexus of fine fibers that appears to correspond in position to the feltwork of fine fibers described by Herrick (1948) in the amphibian brain and designated by him as "deep" and "periventricular" neuropils. Basically, the reticulate component is not a bilateral formation but a median formation, continuous through the massa intermedia without any demarcation in the midplane. In the periventricular cell plate, massa intermedia, and the lamina medullaris, the cells of the reticulate component form loose, poorly delineated aggregates generally referred to as the "nuclei of midline" and "intralaminar nuclei."

It is probable that the cells of the reticulate component with long axons project widely and diffusely to all three zonal subdivisions of the endbrain, yet in an orderly topographical sequence.

1. The cells of the median thalamic zone ("nuclei of the midline") project to the entocortex of the olfactory lobe and septal area.

2. The cells of the paramedian zone ("intralaminar nuclei" and nucleus parafascicularis) project to the striatum and the mesocortex of the limbus of the hemisphere.

3. The cells of the reticular nucleus in the lamina medullaris externa project to the "ectocortex" of the fundus of the hemisphere.

Degree of density of the direct connections exchanged between the reticulate component of the thalamus and these formations of the endbrain is still conjectural. It is unlikely that there are many direct axonal fibers exchanged between the midline nuclei and the olfactory lobe and hippocampus. On developmental grounds—both phyletic and ontogenetic—it can be assumed that the continuum of neuronal reticulum (deep and periventricular neuropil of Herrick, 1948) mainly provides for the propagation of reciprocal activities between them.

Nucleate component of the thalamus

The nucleated component consists of more or less discrete aggregates of cells and fibers. The cells with *few* dendrites and *long* axons characteristic of the reticulate component are also present amidst cells of the nucleated aggregates, but are reduced in number as if crowded out by the prevalent cell type peculiar to each aggregate. In each aggregate the constituent cells are of a more or less similar type with regard to size, shape, and tinctorial properties of their cell bodies and with regard to the pattern of their dendritic and axonal branching and distribution of axonal terminals. The cells with *short* axons ramifying close to the cell body ("intercalar" cells) pervade the nucleated aggregates. The cells with *multiple*, profusely branching, *long* dendrites and a *long and thick* axon, which bifurcates in some cells close to the cell body and in other such cells only after coursing some distance from it and branching in extrathalamic structures (striatum, cortex), are the cell types that prevail in the nucleated aggregates (Leontowich, 1959, and personal communication, 1967).

The cell types, modes of branching, and zones of distribution of their axonal terminals are characteristic for each aggregate and "define" the "nucleus," but they vary widely in different aggregates.

During development of the thalamus the segregation of neuroblasts and the emergence of nucleated aggregates from the primordial reticulum of undifferentiated cells of the mantle layer is determined first (beginning already early in the *third* month) by the plexus of the ingrowing (afferent) and of the outgrowing (efferent) fibers. This is long before the neuroblasts differentiate (beginning in the *fourth* fetal month) into more or less mature neurons peculiar to each nucleus. These two processes of segregation by fibers and of ultimate differentiation of neuroblasts into definitive cell types follow an orderly sequence and correlate with the sequence of development of the cortical plate (pallium) of the corresponding zones of the cerebral hemispheres (Yakovlev, 1969). In the paramedian thalamic zone the segregation of nuclei by fibers is the earliest process to appear, beginning caudally already in the tenth fetal week; the differentiation of the neuroblasts into definitive cells is most rapid (exhibits the shortest "cycle" [Yakovlev, 1969]) and in a widest range of differentiation of cells into the most heteromorphic cell types in different nuclei. Accordingly, the nucleated aggregates of cells of this zone will be designated as the *heterotypical* nuclei of the thalamus (Figs. 25-1 to 25-3, horizontal and vertical lines). The early segregation and differentiation of nuclei of the paramedian zone correlates with the early appearance and short cycle of structural differentiation of the heterotypical mesocortex in the limbus and of the *special* heterotypical areas of the ectocortex in the fundus of the hemisphere (vertical and horizontal lines in Figs. 25-3 to 25-5).

In the dorsolateral and posterior thalamic zone (pulvinar), the segregation of the nuclei by fibers is the latest to appear (beginning in the fifth fetal month) and, in contrast to nuclei of the paramedian zone, is never sharp. The nuclei of the dorsolateral and posterior zone blend anteriorly and laterally in the thalamic mass with the rostral group of nuclei of the paramedian thalamic zone. The cytological differentiation of nuclei of the relatively homogeneous dorsolateral and posterior zone is, in contrast to those of the paramedian zone, characterized by a *long cycle* protracted beyond term with the nuclei exhibiting the least variation in their relatively homeomorphic cell types. Accordingly, the nuclei of the dorsolateral and posterior thalamic zone will be designated as the *homotypical nuclei* of the thalamus (Figs. 25-1 to 25-3, areas left white). These features of the dorsolateral and posterior thalamic zone correlate with the late development and protracted cycle of the areal differentiation of the homotypical ectocortex, particularly of the posterior (epihippocampal) part of the fundus of the hemisphere (areas left white in Figs. 25-4 and 25-5).

NUCLEI OF THE PARAMEDIAN ZONE (HETEROTYPICAL NUCLEI)

The heterotypical nuclei of the paramedian zone of the thalamus may be subdivided into two groups—*ventrocaudal* (horizontal lines) and *rostral group* (vertical lines) of nuclei—according to the order in which they emerge in the fetal thalamus, according to the sources of their afferent fibers, and according to the areas to which their efferent fibers project.

Ventrocaudal or lemniscal group of nuclei

The nuclei of this group (synonym: "relay" nuclei) are the earliest ones to emerge in the paramedian zone. They receive more or less compact ribbons of fibers ("lemnisci") from the receptors of the more or less "specific" modalities of sensory experience in the head region and body wall—the optic tract and the trigeminothalamic, the bulbothalamic (medial and lateral), the cerebellorubrothalamic, and the spinothalamic lemnisci. The fibers of the *spinal lemniscus* (lateral spinothalamic tract) carrying pain and the interoceptive (visceral) modalities of sensory experience over multiple relays via the reticular formation from the spinal cord and brainstem are diffuse fibers distributed widely in the nuclei of the lemniscal group and in the nuclei of the lemniscal group of the paramedian thalamic zone and in the intralaminar nuclei. The *medial* (somesthetic) and the *lateral* (auditory) lemnisci, the *brachium conjunctivum,* and the *optic tract,* carrying more discrete ("specific") modalities of sensory experience, are compact tracts of long fibers distributed each in the specific nucleus of the lemniscal group.

The nuclei of the lemniscal group, the first to emerge from the homogeneous reticulate component in the caudal part of the paramedian zone, exhibit the sharpest segregation into discretely nucleated formations and the widest range of heteromorphism in cell types of individual nuclei. According to these criteria, all these nuclei of termination of the lemniscal afferents to the thalamus will be referred to as the *special heterotypical nuclei* of the paramedian thalamic zone (horizontal lines in Figs. 25-1 to 25-3).

The nuclei of this group and some of their connections are described in the following paragraphs.

1. The *ventral posteromedial nucleus* (VPM) receives fibers of the trigeminal and glossopharyngeal lemniscus from the nuclei of termination of the respective sensory nerves. This nucleus is most medial in position in the crescent of lemniscal nuclei ventral to the nucleus centrum medianum (Fig. 25-1).

2. The *ventral posterolateral nucleus (VPL)* receives fibers of the anterior spinothalamic tract and the nuclei of the posterior columns of the spinal cord.

3. The *lateral ventral nucleus, basal part* (LVB),* receives fibers of the cerebellothalamic projection (the brachium conjunctivum) from the dentate and roof nuclei of the cerebellum; these fibers distribute throughout the nucleus. Regional connections from the substantia nigra and the medial segment of the globus pallidus have also been described. The ventral lateral nucleus is the largest and the most lateral in position in the thalamus (Fig. 25-1). It blends dorsad with the lateral part of the dorsolateral and posterior zone (LVD).

4. The *nucleus centrum medianum* (CM) of Luys represents the core of the special heterotypical nuclei of the lemniscal group. It is lodged in the capsule of the lamina medullaris interna, as if in a sling, and generally is included with the "intralaminar" nuclei (with the reticulate component of the thalamus as here defined). Posteriorly it is demarcated from the habenular complex and from the pretectal area of the dimesencephalic junction by the fiber bundles of the *fasciculus retroflexus.* The nucleus centrum medianum is a highly heterotypical nucleus of heteromorphic cells and consists of a small-celled, loosely cellular ventrolateral part and a larger-celled and denser dorsomedial part. The latter part blends with cells of

*The designation "lateral ventral" nucleus is not in conventional usage. Here it designates the part of the thalamic mass lateral to the lamina medullaris interna. This large part of the thalamic mass (lateral or "external" nucleus of early writers) is actually lateroventral to the medial part of the thalamic mass (the "internal" nucleus). The lateral ventral nucleus consists of two parts: the large-celled *basal* part and a smaller-celled *dorsal* part. The *basal* part (LVB) blends anteroventrally with the nucleus ventralis anterior (VA) of our "limbic group" and posteroventrally and medially with the nucleus ventralis posterolateralis of the lemniscal group (VPL). This basal part of the nucleus lateralis ventralis is assigned to the paramedian zone on developmental grounds and also because it receives the brachium conjunctivum. The medium- and small-celled *dorsal* part (LVD) is wedged between the ventral anterior nucleus (VA) and the lateral part of the medial dorsal nucleus (MD pc). Dorsad and posteriorly it blends with the lateral posterior nucleus (LP).

the *nucleus parafascicularis.* Ventrolaterally the nucleus centrum medianum is lodged in the arcuate crescent of the heterotypical nuclei 1 to 3 of the lemniscal group.

The nucleus centrum medianum is the first of the special heterotypical nuclei to emerge (early in the tenth week) in the caudal part of the paramedian thalamic zone. Its emergence is followed in rapid succession by the segregation of discrete, heteromorphic cell groups of the ventral posteromedial nucleus (VPM), ventral posterolateral nucleus (VPL), and by the segregation of the *basal part* of the lateral ventral thalamic mass (LVB) (Yakovlev, 1969). The nucleus centrum medianum has been called "the intrathalamic association nucleus" (Walker, 1938), and it deserves that name. It remains embedded more intimately, as it were, in the primordial reticulate component of the thalamus than the other thalamic nuclei. It reportedly receives fibers of the spinal lemniscus that carry the protopathic modalities of sensory experience such as pain. Ascending cerebellar, vestibular, and trigeminal fiber connections have also been described (Hassler, 1959). Walker (1938) and Mehler (1966), however, have questioned the notion of ascending fiber connections with the centrum medianum, and recent studies in primate species have revealed that the major afferent connections of the centrum medianum originate from the medial segment of the globus pallidus and the precentral "motor" cortex (Kuypers, 1966; Mehler, 1966; Nauta and Mehler, 1966). Nevertheless, this does not deny that "delegations" of collaterals enter the centrum medianum nucleus from the previously mentioned lemniscal systems of afferent fibers.

5. The *medial geniculate* (MG) and the *lateral geniculate* (LG) *nuclei* (or bodies) are the thalamic recipients, respectively, of the experience of sound and light. These nuclei occupy a special position in the group of lemniscal nuclei (Fig. 25-3). They arise from a common anlage of neuroblasts with other lemniscal nuclei in the caudal part of the paramedian zone and migrate (early in the third fetal month) ventrad and laterad from the nucleus centrum medianum. They eventually (in the seventh fetal month) become covered (opercularized) by the large and homotypical nuclei of the dorsolateral and posterior thalamic zone (pulvinar).

The *medial geniculate nucleus* (MG) is located immediately caudal to the ventral posterolateral nucleus (Fig. 25-3) and is covered by the fibers of the brachium of the superior colliculus and by the pulvinar. The medial geniculate nucleus is very large in mammals such as bats and cetacea, which depend in their modes of procurement for the needs of life more on sound "cues" than on sight; it receives its afferent fibers from the *lateral* (cochlear) *lemniscus* via relays in the intercalated nuclei and in the inferior colliculus.

The *lateral geniculate nucleus* (LG) migrates early in the tenth week and moves farthest laterad from the nucleus centrum medianum and the anlage of the lemniscal group. Up to about 15 weeks it is located on the free dorsolateral surface of the thalamus, outside the reticular nucleus and lamina medullaris externa. nucleus and lamina medullaris externa. By the twenty-fourth fetal week the lateral geniculate nucleus becomes displaced from the dorsolateral on to the ventral surface of the thalamus toward the medial geniculate nucleus, in consequence of the overgrowth and dorsolateral and posterior proplasia of the pulvinar. It receives afferent fibers from the retinae through the *optic nerves and tract.* This lemniscus of optic fibers forms a compact bundle of secondary sensory fibers, completely extruded from the brain and enclosed in its own meningeal sheaths. The lateral geniculate nucleus exhibits the most heterotypical structure of all the special heterotypical nuclei of the paramedian zone. The structure of the lateral geniculate is prominently stratilaminate and "corticoid" in appearance. It consists of six layers of cells, four of which are small celled and separated by plexuses of optic tract fibers, and the remaining two which are large-celled layers. All these cell layers receive terminal branches of optic tract fibers. However, not all the branches of optic tract fibers terminate in the lateral geniculate nucleus; some pass to the nuclei of the dorsolateral and posterior thalamic zone, others extend to the tectum of the midbrain (superior colliculus).

As to *projections* of these nuclei, the *nucleus centrum medianum* projects fibers to the *corpus striatum.* The cells of this nucleus are resistant to retrograde degeneration following destruction of the cortex of the cerebral hemispheres and are in this respect comparable to the cells of the reticulate component of the thalamus. Because of this and because of the dense capsule of fibers of the lamina medullaris interna, the nucleus centrum medianum is regarded by some authors as one of the intralaminar nuclei. This, however, is an unwarranted simplification. It is one of the phylogenetically oldest nucleated formations of the mammalian thalamus; it increases in prominence in primates and is the first nucleus to emerge in the human embryo and to become defined by its capsule of fibers and by fibers growing from it into the hemispheric stalk towards the striatum.

All other special heterotypical nuclei of the lemniscal group project fibers to the *special heterotypical areas* of the fundus of the hemisphere (Figs. 25-4 and 25-5). The *ventral posteromedial nucleus* (VPM) projects fibers to the banks of the inferior third of the sulcus of Rolando (the area of sensorimotor representation of the fifth, ninth, and seventh cranial nerves). The *ventral posterolateral nucleus* (VPL) projects to the banks of the upper two-thirds of the sulcus of Rolando in an orderly, topographical sequence; the cells of the rostral and medial part project to the middle third (the area of hand representation); the cells of the caudal and lateral part project to the upper third (the area of sensorimotor representation of the foot).

The *lateral ventral nucleus, basal part* (LVB), receiving afferent fibers from the cerebellar lemniscus, projects fibers more widely and more anteriorly to the entire transverse band of special heterotypical cortex (macropyramidal agranular areas 4 and 6).

The *medial geniculate nucleus* projects fibers to the highly granular area 41 on the banks of the transverse temporal sulcus and anterior transverse temporal gyrus (Heschl's gyrus). The *lateral geniculate nucleus* projects fibers to the band of the highly granular area 17 extending in the floor and banks of the calcarine sulcus from the parahippocampal limbus of the hemisphere to the occipital pole.

All of the projection fibers from the special heterotypical nuclei of the paramedian thalamic zone to the special heterotypical areas of the fundus of the hemisphere have this in common, that they branch in the thalamus and course through the internal capsule and corona radiata *without branching* until they come close to and enter the cortical plate in which they branch profusely in the internal granular (fourth) layer and in the supragranular layers. They all represent the thalamocortical "relay" fibers of the special modalities of sensory experience from the sensory receptors through the thalamus to these cortical "analyser" areas of the *stimuli-physical agents,* such as touch, pressure, force of gravity, sound, and light. The lemniscal nuclei degenerate more or less completely and rapidly, leaving few residual cells, following experimental ablations and lesions restricted to the special heterotypical areas of the cortex to which they project.

Rostral or limbic group of nuclei

The nuclei of the rostral or limbic group of the paramedian zone emerge from the homogenous reticulum of neuroblasts in the thalamic mantle layer during the fourth fetal month, that is, later than the special heterotypical nuclei of the lemniscal group. They become segregated into discrete nuclei by the accessory medullary laminae. In general, the nuclei of the rostral group exhibit a less pronounced heteromorphism of prevalent cell types as compared with the nuclei of the ventrocaudal (lemniscal) group. Yet they are nuclei prominently heteromorphic in cell type and heterotypical in architecture, as compared with the homeomorphic and homotypical nuclei of the dorsolateral and posterior zone. They are shown in Figs. 25-1 to 25-3 by vertical lining. It should be noted with regard to the general topography of these nuclei that they form an arc convex anterodorsad (Fig. 25-3), large anteriorly and attenuated posteriorly into a narrow tail, and in this configuration conform to the arcuate configuration of the corpus striatum and the epistriatal limbus of the hemisphere. The large and nearly spherical medial dorsal nucleus (MD pc) is lodged in the concavity of the arc and represents the core of the rostral group of nuclei of the paramedian zone. Because the nuclei of this group are disposed in the anteromedial border of the thalamic mass and project fibers to the mesocortex of the limbus of the hemisphere, they are called *limbic nuclei* (Angevine, Locke, and Yakovlev, 1964; Locke, Angevine, and Yakovlev, 1964; Yakovlev and Locke, 1960; Yakovlev and others, 1966).

The limbic group of nuclei of the paramedian zone consists of the following individual nuclei.

1. *The ventral anterior nucleus* (VA), the most lateral and largest limbic nucleus, is most heteromorphic in cell type and most heterotypical in architecture. It receives afferent fibers from the pallidum via the ansa lenticularis and fasciculus thalamicus (H_1 of Forel) and from the cerebellar lemniscus. The anterior and inferior thalamic radiations from these and from the other nuclei of the paramedian zone give the ventral anterior nucleus (VA) a characteristic fasciculate appearance.

2. *The magnocellular component of the medial dorsal nucleus* (MD mc) is located along the anterior medial border of the large, parvocellular component of the medial nucleus (MD pc). Mediad and ventrad from the latter nucleus the magnocellular part of medial dorsal nucleus blends with the periventricular cell plate of the median thalamic zone in the ventral medial (VM) (or submedial) nucleus situated ventral to the massa intermedia. The magnocellular medial dorsal nucleus receives afferents from the anterior hypothalamus and from the septohypothalamic junctional area. Afferent and efferent connections with the orbitofrontal cortex have been described in the monkey.

3. The *anterior ventral nucleus* (AV), the *anterior dorsal nucleus* (AD), and the *anterior medial nucleus* (AM) form the so-called anterior thalamic tubercle (Ant. Tub.) (Fig. 25-3). The latter is covered by the stratum zonale, while the three nuclei forming the tubercle are separated from one another by sheets of fibers of the accessory laminae medullares. These nuclei receive afferents from the hypothalamus through the hypothalamo-thalamic system and the mamillothalamic tract of Vicq d'Azyr. They blend mediad and ventrad with the periventricular cell plate of the median thalamic zone anterior and dorsal to the massa intermedia, and with the medial dorsal nucleus.

4. The *lateral dorsal nucleus* (LD)* represents a long posterior extension of the nuclei of the anterior thalamic tubercle (the nuclei included under 3, 4, and 5) over the medial dorsal nucleus, from which it is separated by a sheet of fibers of accessory lamina medullaris. This long and flat nucleus attenuates posteriorly in a tail-like extension and becomes broken over the pulvinar into small groups of cells ("nuclei disseminati"). The lateral dorsal nucleus receives afferents from the hypothalamus via the mamillothalamic tract.

5. The *medial dorsal nucleus* (MD pc) is the latest of the rostral group of nuclei of the paramedian zone to emerge from the reticulate component of this zone and to assume an anatomical identity as the so-called small-celled or *parvocellular* medial dorsal nucleus. In the group of the heterotypical nuclei of the paramedian zone it is the most homogenous in cell type. Its boundaries are defined only anterolaterally, by the lamina medullaris interna, which separates it anteriorly from the crescentic shell of heterotypical nuclei of the limbic group and laterally and ventrally from the lemniscal group. Dorsally and posteriorly the medial dorsal nucleus blends with the nuclei of the dorsolateral and posterior thalamic zone without cyto- and myeloarchitectonic boundaries (except arbitrary ones). Like the nuclei of the latter zone, it increases in size and prominence from carnivora to primates; in primates it appears to parallel in its evolution the pro-

*The lateral dorsal nucleus is, by position, "medial dorsal." The designation "lateral dorsal" is maintained to avoid confusion with the medial dorsal nucleus (MD pc) of traditional nomenclative usage.

gressive opercularization of the mesocortex of the lateral limbus (insula) of the hemisphere by the overgrowth of the paralimbic ectocortex (operculum). This comparative anatomical fact is important in connection with the cortical projections of the medial dorsal nucleus in the human thalamus and will be discussed below. The limbic group of nuclei receives a massive inflow of afferents from the basal forebrain, specifically, from the hypothalamus via the *mamillothalamic tract* of Vicq d'Azyr and from the striatum and pallidum via the *ansa lenticularis.*

Projections of the limbic nuclei of the paramedian zone. The discretely nucleated, heterotypical nuclei of the limbic group project to the heterotypical mesocortex of the limbus of the hemisphere, the limbic cortex (vertical lines in Figs. 25-4 and 25-5). The densest projections from the group of nuclei are distributed mainly anteriorly in the epistriatal limbus of the hemisphere—the insula, the orbitomedial border of the frontal lobe (areas 13 and 14), and the anterior part of the cingulate gyrus (area 24). The density of these projections appears to decrease posteriorly toward the parahippocampal limbus of the hemisphere (Fig. 25-5).

The projections from these nuclei form sheets of fibers that travel in broad arcs laterad and anteriorly through the stratum zonale of the thalamus and around the lateral wall of the anterior horn of the lateral ventricle. They perforate the callosal radiations to pass over the anterior horn mediad, then, with a strong posterior deflection, reach the cortex of the cingulate gyrus. The fibers that pass from the anterior and ventral nuclei of the limbic group to the orbital and insular limbus of the frontal lobe exit with the fibers of the *inferior* thalamic peduncle; those to the orbitomedial and cingular limbus exit with the *anterior* thalamic peduncle. The cells nearest the median thalamic zone in the arc of the limbic nuclei project fibers to the concentric cortical band in the arc of the limbic mesocortex nearest the olfactory lobe and hippocampal rudiment; those in the intermediate position project to the intermediate concentric bands, and those most lateral in the limbic nuclei project to the outermost bands of the mesocortex in the limbus of the hemisphere (Pribram and Fulton, 1954; Yakovlev and others, 1960).

The *ventral anterior nucleus* (VA) projects to the heterotypical cortex of the anterior insula (Angevine, Locke, and Yakovlev, 1964). The *magnocellular part of the medial dorsal nucleus* (MD mc) projects to the orbital limbus of the hemisphere (areas 13 and 14), the *anterior ventral nucleus* (AV) projects mainly to the parolfactory lobule of Broca and the subcallosal sector of the cingular gyrus (area 24). The *anterior medial* (AM) and *anterior dorsal* (AD) nuclei (the latter are small in man) project to the pregenual and to the supracallosal sector of the cingular gyrus. The *lateral dorsal nucleus* (LD) projects to the posterior part of this gyrus (areas 23 and 31), its longest projection fibers becoming scant and more diffuse behind the splenium of the corpus callosum.

The large *parvocellular part of medial dorsal nucleus* in the core of the limbic group projects, in cat, dog, and monkey, to the frontal lobe (areas 9, 10, 46) and degenerates in these animals when the frontal cortex is ablated. However, in the human brain the nucleus projects to the more posterior areas of the frontal lobe bordering on the limbic mesocortex in the opercula, and also to the orbital and medial walls of the frontal lobe (paralimbic areas shown in Figs. 25-4 and 25-5 by the vertical dash lines). The *posterior* frontal leukotomies which undercut the opercula, the orbital cortex, and the anterior cingulate gyrus result in severe degeneration of the anterior moiety of this nucleus. The *posteromedial* leukotomies limited to the orbitomedial quadrants of the frontal lobe produce degeneration of the *anteromedial* part of the nucleus, and the *posterolateral* leukotomies in which the orbital and frontal opercula are undercut (or destroyed by cortical infarcts) produce degeneration in the *anterolateral* part of the nucleus. The *anterior* frontal ("prefrontal") leukotomies (and infarcts) that undercut or destroy the cortex only in areas 9, 10, and 46 (situated on the frontal pole and anterior convexity of the frontal lobe) and that spare the paralimbic areas (areas shown by vertical dash lines in

Figs. 25-4 and 25-5) do not, *in man*, result in discernible degeneration of the medial dorsal nucleus (Angevine, Locke, and Yakovlev, 1964; Yakovlev, 1954).

In contrast to the nuclei of the lemniscal group, the nuclei of the limbic group do not degenerate completely, even after extensive ablation of the cortical areas to which they project. This feature may be accounted for in part by the diffuse and wide distribution of terminals in the overlapping areas of termination of projection fibers from the crescent of limbic nuclei to the long arc of the limbus of the hemisphere, and in part by the concentric disposition in this long arc of the narrow cortical bands of projection from the limbic nuclei. This pattern of distribution of terminals from each nucleus would make difficult a *selective* and complete destruction of all cortical terminals from any one of the nuclei, and would cause only partial degeneration of cells in several nuclei.

NUCLEI OF THE DORSOLATERAL AND POSTERIOR ZONE (HOMOTYPICAL NUCLEI)

Development

Up to the fifth fetal month of development, the dorsolateral thalamic zone represents not more than one-fourth of the whole thalamus. The dorsolateral zone consists of a small, homogenous area of neuroblasts between the habenular nuclei mediad and posteriorly and the anlage of the lateral geniculate nucleus laterad. At this stage, approximately three-fourths of the thalamus is represented by the anlage of the nuclei of the paramedian zone with the large nucleus centrum medianum in its core (Yakovlev, 1969). However, *pari passu* with the accelerated growth and dorsolateral and posterior expansion of the cerebral hemispheres, while the paramedian zone begins to lag in growth after the fifth month, there occurs a dramatic acceleration of the growth and an increasing proplasia of the homogenous dorsolateral and posterior thalamic zone, first laterad and then increasingly caudad (pulvinar), over the colliculi. It is a notable fact that this zone expands from the same homogenous anlage in which the medial dorsal nucleus develops in the core of the heterotypical nuclei of the limbic group, that is, from the rostral part of the thalamus. As a result of this dorsolateral and posterior proplasia of the thalamic mass, the lemniscal group in the caudal part of the paramedian zone and the lateral geniculate nucleus become crowded ventrad and mediad by the expanding pulvinar. The limbic group, anchored, as it were, to the striatum and the orbitoinsular and anterior cingular limbus of the frontal lobe by the anterior thalamic radiations, remains rostral and forms the rostral pole of the thalamus. Dorsad to the nucleus centrum medianum, however, the medial dorsal nucleus remains in continuity with the large and homogenous mass of homeomorphic cells of the dorsolateral and posterior zone. The confluent and homotypical nuclei of this zone are distinguished mainly by the greater density of the fibers that radiate from the dorsolateral border of this zone and pass through the lamina medullaris externa into the lenticulothalamic and the retrolenticular sectors of the posterior limb of the internal capsule.

The nuclei of this zone are discussed in the following paragraphs.

1. *The lateral ventral nucleus, dorsal part* (LVD)* is represented by the large and relatively homogenous cell mass in the rostral part of the dorsolateral and posterior zone. It lies dorsal and caudal to the ventral anterior nucleus (VA) and the basal part of the lateral ventral nucleus (LVB) and lateral to the lamina medullaris interna. The nucleus blends without clear demarcation with the basal part of the lateral ventral nucleus (LVB), from which it differs because of its smaller, more uniform, and evenly distributed cells.

2. The *lateral posterior nucleus* (LP) is a homogenous area of cells extending posteriorly from the dorsal part of the lateral ventral nucleus. It is wedged between the lateral ventral nucleus and the medial dorsal nucleus, from which it is not separated by the lamina medullaris interna. The lateral posterior nucleus blends caudad over the nucleus centrum medianum with

*See footnote, p. 448.

the lateral nucleus of the pulvinar (PL). It may be easily distinguished from the latter since it lacks the radial fibers that characterize the lateral nucleus of the pulvinar.

3. The *posterior lateral nucleus* (PL) or lateral pulvinar overlies the lateral geniculate nucleus (LG) and is heavily fasciculated by the comb of fiber bundles of the posterior thalamic radiations.

4. The *posterior medial nucleus* (PM) or medial pulvinar, the most homogenous of the nuclei of the dorsolateral zone in cellular and fiber structure, blends with the dorsal part of the medial dorsal nucleus (MD pc) and appears as a posteromedial extension of it. The posterior medial nucleus is wedged between the posterior lateral nucleus laterad and the habenular nucleus (epithalamus) mediad. It overlies the medial geniculate nucleus (LG) and projects posteriorly over the pretectal area and superior colliculus.

5. The *posterior inferior nucleus* (PI) or inferior pulvinar is situated ventrally between the medial (PM) and lateral (PL) pulvinar nuclei and is separated from the medial geniculate nuclei by the fibers of the brachium of the superior colliculus to the lateral geniculate nucleus. The posterior inferior nucleus consists of large and small cells and is the most heteromorphic in cell type among the homeomorphic nuclei of the pulvinar. With some reservations, it is included in the dorsolateral and posterior thalamic zone. The nucleus blends anteriorly with the caudal part of the ventral posterolateral nucleus (VPL) of the lemniscal group and is interwoven by the fibers of the brachium of the superior colliculus. It may possibly belong to the lemniscal group of the paramedian zone.

The nuclei of the dorsolateral and posterior thalamic zone receive collaterals of the brachia of the superior colliculus and of the other lemnisci of afferent fibers extending to the paramedian thalamic zone. This whole zone appears to be a massive elaboration of the limbic group of nuclei. The proplasia of these cell masses in the primate and human thalamus appears to have been conditioned in evolution by the same factors that led to the elaboration of the vast expanse of the homotypical ectocortex of the epihippocampal part of the hemisphere (temporal and occipital lobes) around the special heterotypical areas of projection of the nuclei of the lemniscal group, particularly the area of projection of the lateral geniculate nucleus (area 17).

The delayed and protracted cycle of architectural differentiation and massive growth of this zone (beginning late in the fourth fetal month) suggest that its main cell mass may arise by migration of neuroblasts from the median telencephalic zone (septal area), where the hippocampus arises. Some evidence in support of this has recently been procured by Sidman and Rakic (1968).

Cortical projections of the nuclei of the dorsolateral and posterior thalamic zone

The homotypical nuclei of the dorsolateral and posterior thalamic zone project to the homotypical ectocortex of the posterior parietal, temporal, and occipital lobes (Figs. 25-4 and 25-5, areas left white). In relation to the hemisphere and thalamus, these nuclei, or *dorsolateral* cell masses of the thalamus (the lateral ventral nucleus, dorsal part [LVD], the lateral posterior nucleus [LP], and the posterior lateral nucleus [PL]), project to the *dorsolateral* homotypical areas of the parietal and occipital lobe. The posterior medial nucleus (PM), *posteromedial* in position in the thalamus, projects to the *basomedial* areas of the temporal and occipital lobes. It has been proposed (Hassler, 1959) that the posterior inferior nucleus (PI) projects to area 18, surrounding area 17 in the medial wall of the occipital lobe as a narrow band. The projection fibers from these nuclei have this in common, that, in contrast to projection fibers from the lemniscal group, they give off branches already on their way through the white matter of the hemispheres. These projections are distributed widely in extensive areas and in all layers of the cortical plate. They represent a diffuse thalamic projection distributed in the homotypical cortex nevertheless in a gradient of density; the densest area is nearest the areas of special heterotypical cortex, with decreasing density "away" from these areas. The areas of homotypical cortex farthest removed from the special heterotypical areas are least supplied with the thalamocortical projections, and some of the areas in the posterior part of the hemisphere may be "a-thalamic," even as the frontal homotypical areas in the anterior part of the hemisphere are "a-thalamic."

Owing to the diffuse distribution and wide overlap of thalamocortical projection from the dorsolateral and posterior thalamic zone, the small ablations of the homotypical ectocortex in monkeys do not produce discernible retrograde degenerations in the nuclei of this zone. Extensive ablations are required. However, longstanding cortical infarcts in the human brain and circumscribed atrophy of the cerebral cortex, such as occurs in Alzheimer's disease and Pick's lobar sclerosis, result in selective and severe atrophies and retrograde degeneration of the nuclei of the dorsolateral and posterior zone.

FUNCTIONAL CONSIDERATIONS

The thalamus is generally regarded as a "relay station" in the afferent paths conducting different modalities of sensory experience ("feelings") from the receptor organs to the cerebral cortex. However, the development, structure, and organization of its main afferent and efferent connections clearly indicate that it is more than a switching station for the relay to the cortex of the stimuli aroused in the receptor organs. Its phyletic evolution and its development in mammals as a unit with the *posterior* part of the hemisphere overlying the hippocampus indicate that before the total input of sensory stimuli is sorted out in the "epihippocampal" cortex and becomes a *conscious* experience, the inchoate mass of incoming stimuli and of traces of past stimuli are integrated in the thalamus and become a "consciable" experience—the "stuff" of memory.

A distinction should be made between at least three main orders of sensory stimuli transmitted from the receptors to the effectors (muscle, glands) and elaborated in the thalamus and cortex into orderly behavioral responses, each *response* leaving a cumulative trace (change) in the material structure of the brain. These three orders of sensory stimuli are (1) stimuli-*physical agents,* (2) stimuli-*signals* of these agents, and (3) stimuli-*symbols* (signs) of the signals (Viaud, 1956).

(1) *Stimuli-physical agents* are physical forces such as heat and cold, mechanical and chemical agents, force of gravity, sound, light, and other radiations. All these agents besiege the organism with sovereign indifference, and the responses of the organism to these *random* stimuli are, at least at the level of single cells, also random.

(2) *Stimuli-signals* of the physical agents are nerve impulses circulating in the synaptic nerve net of the nervous system. This nerve net arises in the evolution of animal organisms as a *signaling* device (Poliakov, 1966) that permits the organism to respond to stimuli-physical agents *selectively* rather than randomly. Different stimuli-physical agents generate nerve impulses that are conducted as signals (messages) of changes in the environment forecasting the imminent changes in the internal states of the organism. The stimuli-signals *compel* pertinent responses adapted only to the meaning of the signals relevant to the well-being of the organism, lest the integrity of the organism be disrupted. The responses to stimuli signals are movements of posture, body attitude, mimicry, gestures, vocalizations, and articulate *speech* as a vocalized gesture (but not yet language) subsummed succinctly in the word "emotions" (Yakovlev, 1948). The "code" of the stimuli-signals and "repertory" of the "responses" to signals are *finite* and basically the same in all organisms endowed with a nervous system. All these movements have this in common, that their physiological *ends* (their functions) are the needs of the organism *itself.* The emotional movements consummate bodily energy but *produce no work* outside the body. They are movements of the body and of parts on the body and are generally referred to as "automatic," "involuntary," or "instinctive" movements. They answer adaptively the imminent changes in the internal state of the body and, in their turn, are signals of these changes. As signals, the emotional responses *communicate* the private (subjective) experiences to other organisms and the communication thus signalled is ever *candid.* However, the evolution of man from his ancestral animal stock has led to the development of responses that are wholly independent and free from the animal candor of the emotional responses to signals, but are responses to stimuli of an entirely different order.

(3) *Stimuli-symbols (signs) of the signals,* in man, are the elaboration of the stimuli-signals of the inexorable physical realities into stimuli-signs or symbols—abstract *models* of these realities (objects and events). This is *language.* The "models" of realities (words as ideas—*logos*) do not communicate; they *represent* the realities and are empirical generalizations upon innumerable past and present signals. They can be as compelling of a response as the most urgent stimuli-signals of an imminent catastrophe, or of an object of compelling need, yet they allow the widest range of *choice* in the "representation" of subjective reality from a candid "revelation" of an intimately personal truth to a deliberate deception or an artful disguise of a private sensory experience. (Thus a little tot who begins to articulate

speech and to "talk" at 1 year of age uses *language* when at 3 years he tells his mother his first "fib.") The responses that stimuli-symbols elicit are also movements (behavior). However, in contrast to the ever candid emotional responses to stimuli-signals and the body itself as their end, the ends (functions) of the responses to stimuli-symbols are physical forces as *goals* or targets of bodily action *outside* the body. They produce *work* and, in the case of man, as we are well aware, constantly transform the human environment into a new state of dynamic relationships between man and the random forces of the environment.

The function of the three zones of human thalamus will be considered in the framework of the above concept of evolutionary hierarchy of sensory stimuli and responses.

Reticulate component and median zone; visceral aging and states of consciousness

Different shadings in Figs. 25-1 through 25-5 are meant to convey the idea of the tectogenetic (developmental and connective) unity of the corresponding thalamic and telencephalic zones. The similarity in the pattern of neuronal assembly and structural continuity of both median divisions of the forebrain *(black)* with the hypothalamus and with the central gray and reticular formation of the brainstem and spinal cord implies a functional unity of this "centrencephalic integrating system"—to use the term proposed by Penfield (1952, 1967) for a postulated system of nerve fibers and gray matter situated in the "higher" brainstem (diencephalon, mesencephalon, and probably some of the metencephalon) and having the function of coordinating the activity of the two hemispheres.

This entire reticulate median zone of the forebrain ("centrencephalic system") represents an immense surface of synaptic interneuronal contact. This synaptic surface may be envisaged as being interposed between the olfactory and special and general visceral afferent neurons and the neurons of origin of the preganglionic fibers of the autonomic system. The afferent input propagates through this immense synaptic surface slowly, and is distributed widely in the forebrain, including the septal area and the olfactory lobes (entocortex).* The efferent output from the entocortex is, however, fed back to the reticulate median zone from the hippocampus, via the fornix, to the septal area, hypothalamus, and median thalamic zone, and thence to the reticular formation of the brainstem and spinal cord, and to the preganglionic neurons embedded in the reticular formation. The olfactory lobe may thus be regarded as the zone of telencephalic confluence of the olfactovisceral sensory input (Herrick, 1922, 1948), and the hippocampus as the origin of the common paths from the entocortex to the centrencephalic system and then to the effector organs of visceration (smooth musculature and glands). The disposition of the telencephalic origin of the efferent *visceral* path (fornix) from the hippocampus nearest the telencephalic end of the visceral afferent paths foreshadows the disposition of the origin of the *somatomotor* (pyramidal) path from the precentral cortex (area 4) nearest the end of the somatosensory path (muscle sense and touch) in the postcentral cortex of the hemispheres.

Summarizing the current consensus, the physiological role of the constituent neurons of the system (the median zone of the thalamus and its reticulate component) is to "condition" the activity of the rest of the thalamus and the cortical nerve nets. The function of the median reticulate component is of a conservative nature; it conditions states of quiescence and sleep (Hess, 1957). Contrariwise, the intralaminar and reticular nuclei of this reticulate component condition the "arousal" and "recruitment" of the cortical neurons to activity (Dempsey, Morison, and Morison, 1941; Jasper, 1949).

Any damage of the median zone of the forebrain by trauma, ventricular hemorrhage, neoplasm, or nutritional diseases such as Wernicke's and Korsakoff's encephalopathies (Adams, Collins, and Victor, 1962) are associated with states of profoundly altered consciousness, memory loss, severe metabolic disarray, trophic

*The "olfactory lobe" is the primordial part of the telencephalon and comprises the olfactory bulb and tract (peduncle), the lateral and medial olfactory gyri and striae (area paleocorticalis prepiriformis), olfactory tubercle (area paleocorticalis tubercularis), the diagonal band of Broca (area paleocorticalis diagonalis), and the "cortical nucleus of the amygdala" (area paleocorticalis periamygdalaris). The olfactory lobes are joined in the floor of the interhemispheric cleft by the septal area (area paleocorticalis septalis).

disturbances, cachexia, and, ultimately, dementia.

It is noteworthy that in the process of normal aging the median thalamic zone, including the massa intermedia, is the earliest (beginning at the sixth decade) to exhibit evidence of involutional atrophy, with resulting widening of the third ventricle and increasing frequency of resolution and absence of the massa intermedia, particularly in males (Morel, 1947; Yakovlev, 1962). This correlates, on one hand, with the greater longevity of females after the climacterium is reached without mishaps to general visceral health (Rabl, 1958) and, on the other hand, with the physiological changes of normal aging generally reflected first in the curtailment of activities of the visceral and endocrine apparatus, later in the performance of the somatic apparatus, and last, in the reduction of intellectual grasp and psychical vigor.

On these general empirical grounds the reticulate component of the median zone of the forebrain appears to represent the anatomical substrate whose integrity is essential to the maintenance of physiological functions in the spheres of visceration and conscious cerebration.

Paramedian zone; modalities of sensory experience and stimuli signals of physical agents

It is a notable fact of the anatomy of the lemniscal paths to the most sharply nucleated, special heterotypical nuclei of the paramedian thalamic zone that the degree of the anatomical discreteness of these afferent paths as "fiber tracts" correlates with the "specificity" of the subjective expression of each modality of sensory experience in language.

No words are usually "adequate" to express the subjective experience (feeling) of a "hurt," however eloquent may be the mimicry, gestures, and exclamations of a personal distress. The same is true of expressions of the feelings of hunger, satiety, and like experiences of the visceral needs. The more intense the distress of frustration, or the greater the pleasure of gratification, the less there are words to express them; they become "ineffable" experiences. In correlation with this stands the anatomical fact that the *spinal lemniscus,* which conducts the modalities of sensory experience the least "specifiable" in language, such as "pain" and the like—essentially ineffable sensory experiences—is a *diffusely* fibered "tract," consisting of multiple, overlapping, and mostly short relays, scattered also in the reticular formation throughout the breadth and length of the brainstem. In the thalamus, the terminal relays conducting pain and visceral sensations are distributed widely in the reticulate component of the thalamus, in the nucleus centrum medianum, and, probably, in all other nuclei of the thalamus, albeit they appear to be concentrated mainly in the median thalamic zone.

In contrast to pain and visceral sensations, the modalities of sensory experience such as touch, taste, pressure, muscular tension, and sound have a more explicit and precise vocabulary of symbolization in language. Impulses subserving these modalities reach the thalamus by discrete, relatively compact bundles (lemnisci) of long fibers, the latter sending off, on their way, abundant collaterals to the reticular formation and nuclei of the brainstem. The fibers are distributed in "specific" cell aggregates of the paramedian zone, the lemniscal nuclei, in accordance with the nature of the sensory impressions they convey. All these fibers course *within* the substance of the brainstem.

The most explicitly "specific" modality of sensory experience is that aroused by *light.* This modality has the richest vocabulary of expression. The impulses are conducted by the most discrete and most compact of all lemnisci—the optic tract, which runs *outside* the brain in a meningeal sheath. Similarly, the "specific" thalamic nucleus in which the fibers mainly terminate, the lateral geniculate nucleus, lies superficially.

In harmony with the foregoing, the visual thalamocortical radiations and the special heterotypical cortical area striata of the photo-analyser (area 17) exhibit the sharpest anatomical and histoarchitectonic boundaries. By contrast, the thalamocortical radiations and the boundaries of the cortical analyser areas of the acoustic (area 41), tactile (areas 3, 1, 2), and propriokinesthetic (areas 4 and 6) modalities of sensory experience are less discrete and blend gradually with the homotypical ectocortex and heterotypical mesocortex around them. There is no area of the cortex anatomically definable as an analyser area of pain experience nor, for that matter, of pleasure experience.

In this connection the results obtained by surgeons in the relief of otherwise unmanageable pain in patients suffering from inoperable cancer by cutting fiber tracts, undercutting or removing cortex (frontal leukotomies), or coagulating various parts of the thalamus (thalamotomies) has been instructive. Generally, the medial thalamotomies appear more effective than the lateral ones (Mark, Ervin, and Yakovlev, 1962). While in some patients the *complaint* of pain was resumed sooner or later after the operation with a greater or lesser clamor, in many other patients having undergone identical operations, the pain, "unbearable" before the operation, became "bearable," and in some patients the continued experience of pain was admitted casually and with complete detachment or was even stoutly denied. However, the common objective denominator of the beneficial results in all patients appears to be that the expression of the "catastrophic" experience loses, as it were, its "exclamation point" and no longer elicits a "catastrophic" response. The cancer is still there and the affected parts of the body must be assumed to send to the brain the signals of distress; the messages must reach the brain as before the operation, yet the neural and somatic apparatus of emotional response appears unavailable to the messages. All this is in sharp contrast to the effects of interruption of the discrete pathways subserving explicit modalities of sensory experience such as touch, position sense, and sense of sight. Ablation of visual cortex, a lesion of the lateral geniculate nucleus, or section of the optic tract produces unconditional blindness (hemianopia) for all visual signals from the part of the environment contralateral to the side of the lesion. The same applies to the anesthesias for touch, position sense, and parts of the acoustic scale following interruption of an appropriate lemniscal system, or resulting from damage of the special heterotypical ("specific") nucleus of the thalamus or of the cortical analyser area to which fibers from the nucleus project.

It follows that after thalamotomy or frontal leukotomy, the patients' subjective experience specifiable in language loses its "affective charge." Apparently the lesion dissociates the paramedian and dorsolateral thalamic zone (pulvinar) and the ectocortex from the median thalamic zone and from the entocortex, and so deprives the patients' subjective experience of bodily self of the affective charge.

The limbic group of nuclei of the paramedian thalamic zone, and the limbic mesocortex to which they project, appear to play an important role in the elaboration of the *stimuli-signals* of the imminent events within and outside the body into "automatic" or "instinctual" responses expressed in changes of respiration, heart beat, blood pressure, posture, mimicry, gestures, vocalizations, articulate speech, and like movements of the body *on the body itself* in the emotional expression of the internal states.

As an anatomical arrangement in keeping with such a role is the convergence upon the limbic group of nuclei of the extrathalamic afferents arising in the *hypothalamus* (mamillothalamic tract) and in the *striatum and pallidum* (ansa lenticularis), and the dense projections of these heterotypical nuclei to the *limbus* of the hemisphere and adjoining paralimbic areas.

The common efferent path from the limbus of the hemisphere is the *cingulum* bundle and its profuse collaterals distributed widely and bilaterally in the striatum of both hemispheres and in the hippocampus (Yakovlev and others, 1966). Thus, the activities of the limbic group of nuclei are exerted through the mesocortex of the limbic lobe and cingulum on the striatum and "extrapyramidal" motor system of the *somatic* emotional expression and, through the hippocampal fornix, upon the hypothalamus and autonomic nervous system of *visceral* expression of the emotional states.

Through these arrangements in the paramedian thalamic and telencephalic zones of the forebrain (the "intermediate neuropil" of Herrick, 1948) the stimuli-signals of the internal states are responded to by the automatic "instinctive" movements of the body wall and of the internal organs, fulfilling the *compelling* needs that tolerate no compromise, such as the needs of space to live in, of air to breathe, of nutrient to live by, and the need to reproduce in the act of procreation. The responses to signals of these compelling needs are ever *candid* and in their motor somatic and visceral expressions are "spoken out" louder and truer than any words of language or phrases of an abstract discourse.

Dorsolateral and posterior zone; stimuli-symbols and language

The extraordinary proplasia of the homotypical nuclei of the dorsolateral and posterior thalamic zone and of the homotypical ectocortex of the cerebral hemisphere to which these nuclei project is a characteristic feature of the human forebrain. Homologies notwithstanding, nothing comparable exists in the brain of a gorilla, macaque, dog, or swine.

It is significant that the nuclei of this thalamic zone develop late from a common anlage with the limbic group of nuclei and expand over the lemniscal group. The nuclei of the pulvinar may be regarded as a phyletic elaboration of the medial dorsal nucleus. They appear to play an important role in a *higher* elaboration of the sensory experiences mediated by the thalamus than that elaborated in the limbic nuclei. The nuclei of the dorsolateral and posterior thalamic zone and the homotypical cortex of the epihippocampal part of the hemisphere to which they project represent together the substrate of evolution of the uniquely human cerebral function which is a *language*.

Clinical experience implemented with anatomical control shows (Nielsen, 1946) that lesions of the *epihippocampal* cortex and thalamus are associated as a rule, with a more or less profound disarray (confusion) of senses and deprive the individual of *language* ("sensory" or "receptive" aphasias), without impairment of articulate speech. The latter tends, in fact, to increase in output in persons thus afflicted; patients with Wernicke's aphasia are loquacious. This is in contrast to the clinical effects of damage of the striatum and the *epistriatal* cortex of the frontal lobes, in which "apraxias of speech" ("motor" or "executive" aphasias) occur, depriving the person of the *means* of language; patients with Broca's aphasia appear mute.

The thalamocortical projections of the pulvinar radiate widely in the homotypical areas (white, in Figs. 25-4 and 25-5) of the epihippocampal cortex and overlap with the projections of the medial dorsal nucleus in the paralimbic areas (vertical dash lines in Figs. 25-4 and 25-5). These projections conjugate in the cerebral cortex with the corticocortical (association) fibers and with the corticopontile and other long, corticofugal fiber bundles that descend through the corona radiata and the internal capsule; collectively, these descending fibers may be regarded as the common path of the supralimbic division of the cerebral hemisphere.

The homogenous structure of the homotypical nuclei of the dorsolateral and posterior thalamic zone and of the areas of the homotypical epihippocampal cortex to which these nuclei project appear to be the least committed to any genetically fixed and specific function. Their late development and differentiation protracted long after birth indicate that the nuclei of this thalamic zone and the epihippocampal ectocortex of the supralimbic division of the hemisphere maintain their quasi embryonal structural plasticity and the potential for functional differentiation longer than any other part of the brain (Yakovlev, 1962). They appear to be the substrate of specifically human, *individual learning*—learning to think for the sheer fun of thinking in symbols of realities and for no other end. Of course, this also applies to the homotypical areas of the epistriatal cortex of the frontal lobes devoid of thalamic projections. The wide expanse of these epihippocampal and epistriatal homotypical areas in the human brain provides a stock of functionally labile gray matter relatively emancipated from the tutelage of thalamic activation and interposed between the thalamus-bound heterotypical mesocortex and the special heterotypical cortex of the sensory motor analyser areas.

Thus between the urgencies of the stimuli-signals and of candid motor responses to them, a barrier of large synaptic surface is interposed and permits thought and deliberation. The stimuli-symbols "appeal" to this substrate in the epihippocampal cortex and are responded to through the epistriatal cortex in the works of human endeavor as an end in itself.

VASCULARIZATION OF THE THALAMUS

The following account is based mainly on the studies of Foix and Hillemand (1925), which remain a classic in clarity of concept and exposition. The important details brought out by more recent observations of Abbie (1934), Lazorthes (1961), and Percheron (1966) are incorporated.

The thalamus receives blood from the internal carotid and the vertebral system of arteries. It is supplied mainly by the branches of the posterior cerebral artery. The anterior cerebral artery contributes no vessels to the thalamus. The proximal branches of the middle cerebral artery supply mostly the structures that surround the thalamic mass—the subthalamic region, the internal capsule, the pallidum, and the striatum. The thalamic branches of the middle cerebral artery converge on to the thalamus, supplying the lateral posterior (LP) and lateral dorsal (LD) nuclei. Since arterial vessels of the thalamus do not anastomose with one another except at the capillary level, occlusion of any one of them produces an area of softening which conforms to the territory supplied.

Each thalamic zone has its own scaffolding of blood vessels. The *median* thalamic zone as well as more rostral parts of the hypothalamus (Fig. 27-1) are supplied by numerous, thin, vertical twigs of the *posterior communicant* (or communicating) artery. The *paramedian* thalamic zone is supplied from three main sources (Fig. 25-6):

(1) The long, *lateral anterior branch* of the posterior communicant artery (Percheron, 1966)

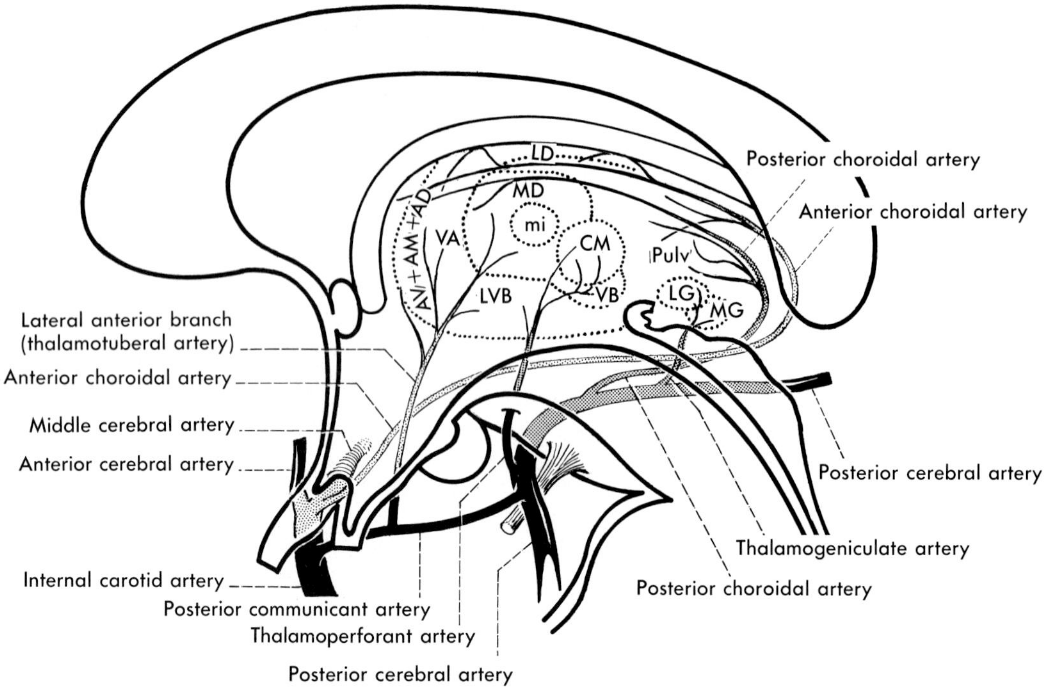

Fig. 25-6. Vascularization of the thalamus (redrawn and modified from Lazorthes, 1961, following in part the data of Percheron, 1966). For meaning of the abbreviations of the thalamic nuclei, see Table 25-1. Note that the rostral, the intermediate, and the caudal sectors of the paramedian thalamic zone are each supplied by its own "twig" of arterial scaffolding: the *lateral anterior* (or thalamotuberal) *branch* of the posterior communicant artery passes to the limbic nuclei and medial dorsal nucleus, the *thalamoperforant branch* of the basilar bifurcation to the lemniscal nuclei and nucleus centrum medianum, and the *thalamogeniculate branch* of the posterior cerebral artery to the geniculate nuclei of the lemniscal group. Note that the *posterior choroid branch* of the posterior cerebral artery supplies mainly the dorsolateral and posterior thalamic zone and supplements the arterial "twigs" to all three sectors. The *anterior choroid branch* of the internal carotid artery provides blood supply mostly for extrathalamic structures.

(also known as the thalamotuberal artery; Fig. 27-1) supplies the *limbic group* of nuclei and the medial dorsal nucleus, including the rostral part of the lateral zone.

(2) The *thalamoperforant* branches springing from the posterior cerebral artery near the basilar bifurcation supply the posterior hypothalamus and the adjoining parts of the *median* thalamic zone, the *nucleus centrum medianum* and the crescent of *lemniscal nuclei* about it, including the basal part of the lateral ventral nucleus *(LVB).*

(3) The *thalamogeniculate* branches of the posterior cerebral artery are generally said to supply the *lateral* and *medial geniculate nuclei* and the adjoining (caudal) parts of the dorsolateral and posterior thalamic zone (pulvinar). Variations must, however, exist. According to Percheron (personal communication, 1960), the "thalamogeniculate arteries" are a misnomer and do not exist as branches of the posterior cerebral artery. In his view the geniculate nuclei are supplied from branches of the posterior choroidal and from thalamoperforant arteries (but see Fig. 27-14.)

The *dorsolateral* and *posterior* thalamic zone in all its anteroposterior extent from the dorsal part of the lateral ventral nucleus *(LVD)* to the pulvinar is supplied by two long, circumferential arteries, designated as the *anterior choroidal* and the *posterior choroidal arteries,* arising, respectively, from the internal carotid (in about 75 per cent of cases; Carpenter, Noback, and Moss, 1954) and from the posterior cerebral artery. Both these arteries follow a nearly parallel course from their origins posteriorly, around the lateral geniculate nuclei and posterolateral border of the pulvinar, then dorsally and anteriorly toward the anterior tubercle and foramen of Monro. The contribution of the anterior choroidal artery to the blood supply of the anterolateral part of the thalamic mass appears to be small (Percheron, 1966). It supplies the choroid plexus, internal capsule, and pallidum. The posterior choroidal artery is often duplicated in the form of medial and lateral trunks. It is the main artery of the dorsolateral and posterior zone and supplements, along its circumferential course through its secondary branches, the thalamogeniculate, the thalamoperforant, and the lateral anterior branch (thalamotuberal artery) of the posterior communicant arteries supplying the nuclei of the paramedian zone.

It is noteworthy that the latter three arterial channels (lateral anterior, thalamogeniculate, and thalamoperforant) spring from the basal trunks of their origin and expand in their branching in the thalamus in planes at roughly a right angle to the choroidal arteries and supply the corresponding anterior, middle, and posterior sectors of the paramedian and dorsolateral zones (Fig. 25-6). The thalamoperforant twigs arising from the region of the bifurcation of the basilar artery commonly also undergo bifurcation and supply the posterior sector of the thalamus *bilaterad* from a common median stem.

THALAMIC SYNDROMES

Infarcts in the territory of the *thalamoperforant arteries* (derived from the posterior cerebral artery in the region of the basilar bifurcation) result in one or another of three syndromes or combinations thereof.

The *syndrome of Dejerine-Roussy* (1906) consists of mild and transient initial hemiparesis on the side contralateral to the thalamic lesion, persistent hemianesthesia involving tactile and proprioceptive (position sense) modalities of sensation, and thermoanalgesia with a complaint of ineffable pain referred to the parts affected, but usually not specifiable as to site or locus of distress. In addition, there is a more or less pronounced dislocation of posture in the affected extremities, usually most evident in the posture of the hand ("thalamic hand") at rest and during movements with a choreatic unrest in the wrist and fingers. The syndrome may be regarded as the result of deafferentation of the thalamus from the sensory periphery by softening in the lemniscal group of nuclei and nucleus centrum medianum but (in the classical form of the syndrome) sparing the geniculate nuclei. The stimuli-signals of the specific modalities of conscious experience become blocked or blurred and lose their meaning in the context of conscious sensory experience. They are perceived as an incoate "sensory noise" and expressed as ineffable distress (pain) or, occasionally, as a pleasurable experience, but then, as a rule, of an intense ("exquisite") pleasure (Head, 1920).

Thrombosis in the region of the basilar bifurcation produces softening in the territories supplied by thalamoperforant arteries that usually extend bilaterad from the posterior median zone through the nucleus centrum medianum and lemniscal nuclei to the internal capsule. The softening deafferents the thalamus from the reticular formation of the brainstem as well as from the lemniscal afferent input. Clinically the thrombosis is characterized by akinetic mutism and combinations of ophthalmoplegia and conjugate ocular palsy. Somatomotor paralysis occurs but is rather uncommon. The patients are hypersomnic and appear in a state of torpor. (Castaigne and others, 1962; Lhermitte and others, 1963.)

Finally, small infarcts in the territory of supply of the median branches of the basilar bifurcation may involve the rostral part of the red nucleus and the rubrothalamic lemniscus; the softening often implicates the pretectal area and supranuclear oculomotor fibers, producing the *suprarubral syndrome* of Chiray, Foix, and Nicolesco (1923). There is intention tremor without hemianesthesia or hemiparesis but usually with ophthalmoplegia and disturbances of conjugate eye movements.

Infarcts limited to the territory of the *thalamogeniculate* branches of the posterior cerebral artery (or, alternatively, of branches of the posterior choroidal arteries and of thalamoperforant arteries) are less common than infarcts from occlusion of the thalamoperforant arteries. The homonymous visual field defects that occur are frequently ushered in by an initial transitory hemiparesis, with or without hemianesthesia. The distortions in the perception of sounds and a distressful hyperacusis to normally indifferent sounds ("noises") may be associated with the visual field defects.

Infarcts involving the territory of supply of the *posterior communicant artery* usually also involve the areas of the cerebrum supplied by proximal branches of the middle cerebral and anterior choroidal arteries. In such instances, clinical survival is usually short. The resulting clinical syndromes may be subdivided into two groups in relation to extent rather than specific locus of infarcts in the general territory supplied by these branches of the internal carotid artery. These are the syndrome of akinetic mutism and the syndrome of frontal leukotomy.

The syndrome of *akinetic mutism* is discussed elsewhere (pp. 390-391). With infarction involving the territory of the posterior communicant artery, the akinetic mutism is often of the *coma vigil* type. Frequently there are clinical and EEG expressions of an *arousal* state, without hypersomnolence and in the absence of extraocular muscle palsy. The syndrome is frequently observed following head trauma in automobile accidents. The momentum of the forward impact of the head in motion disconnects the thalamus and striatum from the epistriatal cortex in the plane of cleavage between the centrum semiovale with the lateral ventricles in the core of the hemisphere, and the corona radiata with the cortical plate overlying it. The akinetic state (stupor) may be protracted, lasting for months and even years after the accident. The syndrome of coma vigil may be interpreted as a result of deafferentation of the thalamus from the striatum and epistriatal cortex through interruption of the striopallidal and hypothalamic "lemnisci" (ansa lenticularis and mamillothalamic tract) in their course to the limbic nuclei of the paramedian thalamic zone.

The effects of *leukotomies* in the region of the orbitomedial quadrants of the frontal lobes (Leyerly, Grantham operations) for the relief of states of compulsive-obsessive anguish and similar disorders of emotional expression of the internal states ("neuroses" and "psychoses") do not differ from the effects of *thalamotomies* in the region of the medial dorsal nucleus and of the anterior thalamic tubercle (Spiegel and Wycis, 1949). The resulting syndrome consists essentially of:

1. A rise in the threshold of responses particularly to stimuli-symbols of the "censorious" social exigencies ("ethics and morality"), with resulting flattening of the patients' emotional concern with "guilt" feelings (Freeman and Watts, 1950).
2. A rise in the threshold of responses to stimuli-signals of potentially "catastrophic" events, with resulting blunting of foresight.
3. Pronounced lowering of the threshold and an increase in compulsive (somatic and visceral) responses to distressful (unpleasant or "catastrophic") stimuli-physical agents, with resulting intolerance to pain, physical crowding, want of food, sexual deprivation, and like restraints on primordial bodily needs and instinctual drives.

The behavioral changes observed in patients thus operated may be expected also following the occurrence of infarcts of the rostral part of the thalamus and of its connections with the epistriatal limbus of the hemisphere.

Infarction in the territory of supply of the *anterior choroidal artery* results in softening in the internal capsule and pallidum. The infarcts impede the outflow of the corticofugal (motor) innervation to structures of the basal forebrain and so reduce the load of their cortical activation, essential to the functioning of these basal structures during the waking state. Moreover, the infarcts deafferent the pallidum and the thalamus from the striatum and epistriatal cortex. Except for passing initial confusion, such infarcts do not produce lasting changes in the state of consciousness, but, short of causing hemiplegia, they reduce the spontaneity and range of movements in the spheres of emotional expression (vigilant "coma") and of the performance of motor acts of occupation and of play. The wide range of individual variation in the distribution of the branches of the anterior choroidal artery (Carpenter, Noback, and Moss, 1954) may account for the variations in the *accessory* features of the above-mentioned "central" deficit in the clinical picture of the infarcts in this artery's main territory which is the pallidum and its capsule of *afferent* fibers.

Infarcts in the territory of the *posterior choroidal artery* and of its branches deafferent the *epihippocampal* part of the hemisphere from the thalamus and result in alterations of consciousness and language. These, however, do not essentially differ from those defects in the patient's conscious experience and language which result from infarcts limited to the area of supply of the *cortical* branches of the posterior cerebral artery. The infarcts in the territory of distribution of these long, circumferential (thalamic and cortical) branches of the posterior cerebral arteries all result in a confusion of "special senses" and of perceptions of stimuli-*signals* of physical agents (visual, tactile, acoustic, proprioceptive). Consequently, the ultimate elaboration of these stimuli-signals into symbols of physical realities in a relevant language is impaired. Such is, in my opinion, the essence of cerebral disorder in "sensory aphasias," "agnosias," "alexias," "right and left" confusion, "acalculia," disturbances of "body image," and like disorganizations in the symbolic context of private sensory experience, without impairment of speech and of the "executive" cerebral functions. These latter are the office of the anterior, *epistriatal* parts of the cerebral hemispheres.

REFERENCES

Abbie, A. A. 1934. The morphology of the forebrain arteries with especial reference to the evolution of the basal ganglia. J. Anat. **68**:433-470.

Adams, R. D., Collins, G. H., and Victor, M. 1962. Troubles de la mémoire et d'apprentissage chez l'homme: leurs relations avec des lésions des lobes temporaux et du diencéphale (Observations anatomo-cliniques). In Passouant, P., editor: Physiologie de l'hippocampe, Colloq. Internat. Centre Nat. Rech. Sci. No. 107. Paris, Publications du Centre National de la Recherche Scientifique, pp. 273-297.

Angevine, J. B., Jr., Locke, S., and Yakovlev, P. I. 1964. Limbic nuclei of thalamus and connections of limbic cortex: thalamocortical projections of the magnocellular medial dorsal nucleus in man. Arch. Neurol. **10**:165-180.

Carpenter, M. B., Noback, C. R., and Moss, M. L. 1954. The anterior choroidal artery: its origins, course, distribution, and variations. A.M.A. Arch. Neurol. Psychiat. **71**:714-722.

Castaigne, P., Buge, A., Escourolle, R., and Massou, M. 1962. Ramollissement pédonculaire médian, tegmento-thalamique avec ophthalmoplégie et hypersomnie. Rev. Neurol. **106**:357-367.

Chiray, P., Foix, C., and Nicolesco, I. 1923. Hémitremblement du type de la sclérose en plaques par lésion rubro-thalamo-sous-thalamique; syndrome de la région supéro-externe du noyau rouge avec atteinte silencieuse ou non du thalamus. Ann. Méd. **14**:173-191.

Dejerine, J., and Roussy, G. 1906. Le syndrome thalamique. Rev. Neurol. **14**:521-532.

Dempsey, E. W., Morison, R. S., and Morison, B. R. 1941. Some afferent diencephalic pathways related to cortical potentials in the cat. Amer. J. Physiol. **131**:718-731.

Edinger, L. 1904. Vorlesungen über den Bau der nervösen Centralorgane des Menschen und der Tiere, ed. 7. Leipzig, F. C. W. Vogel.

Foix, C., and Hillemand, P. 1925. Les artères de l'axe encéphaliques jusqu'au diencéphale inclusivement. Rev. Neurol. **2**:705-739.

Freeman, W., and Watts, J. W. 1950. Psychosurgery in the treatment of mental disorders and intractable pain, ed. 2. Springfield, Charles C Thomas, Publisher.

Hassler, R. 1959. Anatomy of thalamus. In Schaltenbrand, G., and Bailey, P., editors: Introduction to stereotaxis with an atlas of the human brain. New York, Grune & Stratton, Inc., pp. 230-290.

Head, H. 1920. Studies in neurology. London, Oxford University Press.

Herrick, C. J. 1922. An introduction to neurology, ed. 3. Philadelphia, W. B. Saunders Co.

Herrick, C. J. 1948. The brain of the tiger salamander. Chicago, University of Chicago Press.

Hess, W. R. 1957. The functional organization of the diencephalon. New York, Grune & Stratton, Inc.

Jasper, H. H. 1949. Diffuse projection systems: the integrative action of the thalamic reticular systems, EEG Clin. Neurophysiol. **1**:405-419.

Kuypers, H. G. J. M. 1966. Discussion. In Purpura, D. P., and Yahr, M. D., editors: The thalamus. New York, Columbia University Press, pp. 122-127.

Lazorthes, G. 1961. Vascularisation et circulation cérébrales. Paris, Masson & Cie.

Leontowich, T. A. 1959. Structure and function of the reticular formation and its role in the system of analyzers. Moscow, State Publications of Medical Literature (MEDGIZ), pp. 91-126. (In Russian.)

Lhermitte, F., Gautier, J. C., Marteau, R., and Chain, F. 1963. Troubles de la conscience et mutisme akinétique: étude anatomo-clinique d'un ramollissement paramédian, bilatéral du pédoncule cérébrale et du thalamus. Rev. Neurol. **109**:115-131.

Locke, S., Angevine, J. B., Jr., and Yakovlev, P. I. 1964. Limbic nuclei of thalamus and connections of limbic cortex: thalamocortical projections of lateral dorsal nucleus in cat and monkey. Arch. Neurol. **11**:1-12.

Mark, V. H., Ervin, F. R., and Yakovlev, P. I. 1962. Treatment of pain by stereotaxic methods. Confin. Neurol. **22**:238-245.

Mehler, W. R. 1966. Further notes on the centre médian nucleus of Luys. In Purpura, D. P., and Yahr, M. D., editors: The thalamus. New York, Columbia University Press, pp. 109-127.

Meynert, T. 1867. Quoted by von Economo, C., and Koskinas, G. N. 1925. Die Cytoarchitektonik der Hirnrinde des erwachsenen Menschen. Wien, Springer-Verlag, p. 9.

Morel, F. 1947. La massa intermedia ou commissure grise: contribution à l'étude statistique de cette formation inconstante chez l'homme. Acta Anat. **4**:203-207.

Nauta, W. J. H., and Mehler, W. R. 1966. Projections of the lentiform nucleus in the monkey. Brain Res. **1**:3-42.

Nielson, J. M. 1946. Agnosia, apraxia, aphasia: their value in cerebral localization. New York, Paul B. Hoeber, Inc.

Penfield, W. 1952. Epileptic automatism and the centrencephalic integrating system. Res. Publ. Ass. Nerv. Ment. Dis., Proc. **30**:513-528.

Penfield, W. 1967. Epilepsy, the great teacher: the progress of one pupil. Acta Neurol. Scand. **43**:1-10.

Percheron, G. M. J. 1966. Etude anatomique du thalamus de l'homme adulte et de sa vascularization artérielle (avec un atlas). Thesis No. 7989. J. Fac. Med. Univ. Paris.

Poliakov, G. I. 1966. The principles of the neuronal organisation of the brain. Moscow, Moscow University Press. (In Russian.)

Pribram, K. H., and Fulton, J. F. 1954. An experimental critique of the effects of the anterior cingulate to ablations in monkey. Brain **77**:34-44.

Rabl, R. 1958. Strukturstudien an der Massa intermedia des Thalamus opticus. J. Hirnforsch. **4**:78-112.

Sidman, R. L., and Rakic, P. 1968. Cerebral origin of pulvinar thalamic neurons in the human fetal brain. Anat. Rec. **160**:428-429.

Spiegel, E. A., and Wycis, H. T. 1949. Physiological and psychological results of thalamotomy. Proc. Roy. Soc. Med., suppl. **42**:84-92.

Viaud, G. 1956. Taxies et tropismes dans le comportment instinctif. In Autuori, M., and others, editors: L'instinct dans le comportment des animaux et de l'homme. Paris, Masson & Cie., pp. 4-49.

Vogt, O. 1911. Nouvelle contribution à l'étude de la myéloarchitecture de l'écorce cérébrale. Congr. 20e d. méd. alién. de France, 8 août 1910. Brussels, pp. 3-11.

von Economo, C., and Koskinas, G. N. 1925. Die Cytoarchitektonik der Hirnrinde des erwachsenen Menschen. Wien, Springer-Verlag.

Walker, A. E. 1938. The primate thalamus. Chicago, University of Chicago Press.

Yakovlev, P. I. 1948. Motility, behavior and the brain: stereodynamic organization and neural co-ordinates of behavior. J. Nerv. Ment. Dis. **107**:313-335.

Yakovlev, P. I. 1954. Anatomical studies on frontal leucotomies: cortical origin of the ponto-frontine tract and organization of thalamo-frontal projections in man. Trans. Amer. Neurol. Ass. **79**:53-56.

Yakovlev, P. I. 1962. Morphological criteria of the growth and maturation of the nervous system in man in mental retardation. Res. Publ. Ass. Res. Nerv. Ment. Dis., Proc. **39**:3-46.

Yakovlev, P. I. 1969. The development of the nuclei of the dorsal thalamus and of the cerebral cortex: morphogenetic and tectogenetic correlation. In Locke, S., editor: The modern neurology. Boston, Little, Brown and Company, pp. 15-54.

Yakovlev, P. I., and Locke, S. 1960. Limbic nuclei of thalamus and connections of limb cortex: corticocortical connections of the anterior cingulate gyrus, the cingulum, and the subcallosal bundle in monkey. Arch. Neurol. **5**:364-400.

Yakovlev, P. I., Locke, S., and Angevine, J. B., Jr. 1966. The limbus of the cerebral hemisphere, limbic nuclei of the thalamus, and the cingulum bundle. In Purpura, D. P., and Yahr, M. D., editors: The thalamus. New York, Columbia University Press, pp. 77-97.

Yakovlev, P. I., Locke, S., Koskoff, D. Y., and Patton, R. A. 1960. Limbic nuclei of thalamus and connections of limbic cortex: organization of the projections of the anterior group of nuclei and of the midline nuclei. Arch. Neurol. **3**:620-641.

Chapter 26

Hypothalamus, pituitary gland, midbrain, and related regions

A primitive part of the cerebrum occupying a strategic central position from the earliest stage of vertebrate evolution, the hypothalamus has come to have a controlling influence on all aspects of behavior. These include the whole realm of visceromotor and behavioral responses, especially those having homeostatic import. It is worth emphasis that the hypothalamus is also concerned in patterned somatomotor activity.

The base of the hypothalamus is illustrated in Fig. 26-1, and the approximate position of some of the hypothalamic nuclei in Fig. 26-2. Nuclei of the hypothalamus appear not to be organized in terms of specific functions, excepting those having connections with the pituitary gland—the supraoptic, paraventricular, and infundibular (arcuate) nuclei—and excepting the nucleus concerned in satiety, the ventromedial nucleus. Not any particular hypothalamic nucleus, but, instead, circumscribed regions contain specialized neuroreceptors and set-point regulators that maintain the constancy of the internal milieu by modifying bodily reactions. This occurs in part through local neurochemical systems. Five biogenic amines are known to be present in the brainstem—serotonin (5-HT), dopamine, norepinephrine, epinephrine, and histamine—and of these, the first three have been detected in individual cells in the hypothalamus, implying functional specificity of these cells (Myers, 1969b).

The hypothalamus can most logically be subdivided into three longitudinal zones: lateral, medial, and periventricular (Crosby and Woodburne, 1940). Nerve cells in the lateral zone form a continuous longitudinal column making up the lateral preoptic and lateral hypothalamic nuclei. The medial zone is more differentiated and contains a number of conspicuous cell aggregates, some of which are illustrated in Fig. 26-2. The periventricular zone is poor in nerve cells. All these cell groups are interconnected, though the greatest number of intrahypothalamic connections originate from the ventromedial nucleus.

Fiber systems conveying impulses to the hypothalamus come from numerous sources and terminate in varied hypothalamic nuclei.

The largest system, the medial forebrain bundle, runs caudally in the *lateral preoptic–hypothalamic area* (or zone); it is derived from parts of the limbic lobe: amygdala, piriform cortex, anterior perforated substance, septal nuclei, and, to some extent, the hippocampus. By virtue of its size, its compactness, and its many sources of origin, the medial forebrain bundle is to the limbic lobe what the internal capsule is to the neocortex of the cerebral convexity. The *medial zone of the hypothalamus* receives fibers mainly from (1) the amygdala (via the stria terminalis, the fibers ending in the more rostral part of the medial hypothalamus and the ventromedial nucleus), (2) the hippocampus (via the fornix, with the terminus in the medial mamillary nucleus), and (3) from some of the septal nuclei. The *periventricular region* is a route

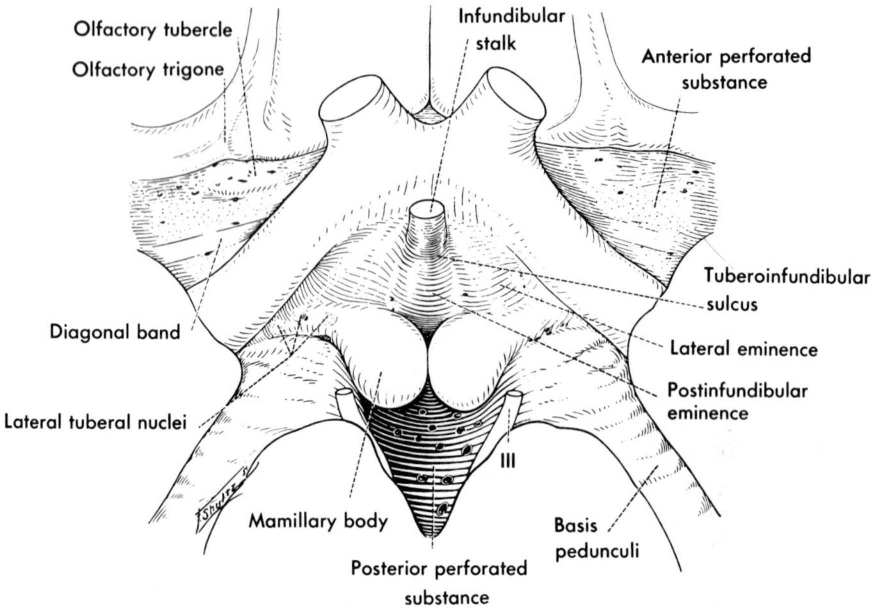

Fig. 26-1. Base of the brain, showing the hypothalamus and adjacent structures.

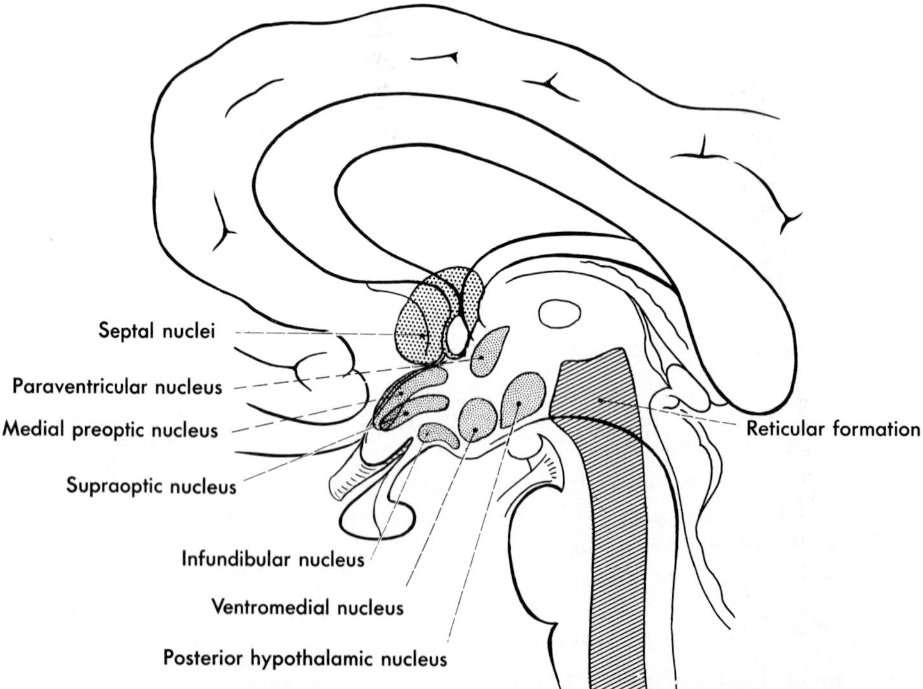

Fig. 26-2. Approximate sites of septal nuclei, medial hypothalamic nuclei, and reticular formation. The mamillary body, which belongs to the medial hypothalamus, is not labeled.

for the passage of fibers to the medial hypothalamus, the fibers coming from the thalamus (medial dorsal and midline thalamic nuclei) and the central gray midbrain substance (via the dorsal longitudinal fasciculus [of Schütz]).

The *lateral zone of the hypothalamus* also receives a heavy complement of fibers from the upper brainstem, mainly from the periaqueductal gray matter and some of the paramedian mesencephalic tegmental nuclei. Sensory impulses reach the hypothalamus through the medium of the midbrain tegmental nuclei in which sensory fibers of the classical lemnisci terminate. Through synaptic stations in these mesencephalic nuclei, as well as through related multisynaptic systems, signals related to states of pain and altered visceral function, including signals from the periphery of the body (Feldman, 1965), are transmitted to the hypothalamus via the dorsal longitudinal fasciculus, the mamillary peduncle, and the tractus solitarius.

Most of the fiber pathways mentioned are two-way systems through which reciprocal reactions between the hypothalamus and the respective parts of the cerebrum and brainstem are brought about. The main points to be mentioned are the following:

1. The hypothalamus receives a major input via the olfactory radiation (originating from the piriform cortex and anterior perforated substance).
2. The hypothalamus has very strong associations with these and other limbic forebrain structures, also with the paramedian region of the midbrain.
3. The lateral preoptic–hypothalamic area is the zone most immediately involved in the interaction of the hypothalamus with adjoining medial hypothalamic and with more or less remote central nervous structures.
4. The most abundant *intra*hypothalamic connections originate from the ventromedial nucleus.
5. Biogenic amines appear to provide functional specificity to hypothalamic nerve cells.
6. Hypothalamic *(efferent)* projections to known visceral motor nuclei are probably established only by the medium of the mesencephalic and bulbar reticular formation and related nuclei. (Nauta and Haymaker, 1969.)

Two efferent pathways from the hypothalamus extend to the neurohypophysis. They are separate and distinct anatomically and are presumed to be separate and distinct functionally. Both represent final common pathways; functionally, their neurons are under the influence of the many afferent systems (humoral, as well as neural) reaching the hypothalamus. One of the pathways is the *tuberohypophysial tract*, the fibers of which terminate on vascular loops in the upper neurohypophysis. There is evidence to suggest that hypophysiotrophic ("releasing") hormones produced in the hypothalamus are conveyed downward in this tract to capillary loops, enter the bloodstream circulating in these loops, and are then carried through the hypophysioportal system to the anterior pituitary. Here, hypothetically, they trigger the production and the release of various hormones of anterior pituitary cells; these pituitary hormones then enter the systemic bloodstream. (Anderson, 1966; Christ, 1966; Harris, Reed, and Fawcett, 1966; Reichlin, 1966; Szentágothai and others, 1968.) The other pathway to the pituitary is from the supraoptic and paraventricular nuclei; it is commonly called the *supraopticohypophysial tract.* Its fibers terminate in relation to capillaries situated in the infundibular process (neural lobe) and apparently in the infundibulum as well. This system is concerned in water balance (through vasopressin production and release) and in smooth muscle contraction (oxytocin production and release). Effects of damage of this system only on water balance are considered in the following.

DIABETES INSIPIDUS AND ADIPSIA

Diabetes insipidus is usually due to a deficiency of the antidiuretic hormone (ADH) brought about by degenerative change in the supraopticohypophysial system. In some instances, however, primary hyperdipsia results from hypothalamic injury. These are the forms that concern us most in the following. Other forms are known.

Diabetes insipidus may be heredofamilial in origin and is sometimes sex-linked. This form has been considered to result from a submicroscopic renal lesion, the defect consisting in a resistance of the renal tubules to the water-retaining effect of ADH (Darmady and others, 1964; Martin, 1959; Williams and Henry, 1947). However, in hereditary as well as in idiopathic types of diabetes insipidus, profound loss of cells from the supraoptic nucleus and of the large cells from the paraventricular nucleus has been observed, which would account for the diabetes insipidus (Green and others, 1967). Another form of diabetes insipidus, associated or not with active hepatitis, is the result of abnormal ADH inactivation. Various tissues in addition to liver tissue contain enzymes capable of inactivating ADH. Accelerated inactivation of the hormone appears to be responsible for the diabetes insipidus. (Hankiss, Keszthelyi, and Siro, 1961; Lee, 1966.)

ADH conserves body water by reabsorbing glomerular filtrate through the walls of distal-convoluted and collecting tubules of the kidney. The hormone is produced by cells of the *supraoptic and paraventricular nuclei* and is transported down into the neurohypophysis by way of the supraopticohypophysial tract. An important determinant of ADH secretion is osmolality of the blood perfusing these nuclei. Small increases in the osmolality cause a release of sufficient ADH to produce marked antidiuresis. Conversely, small *decreases* in osmolality prevent ADH release and lead to maximal water diuresis unless ADH release is maintained by some nonosmotic stimulus, such as decreased blood pressure in carotid baroreceptors (Kleeman and Fichman, 1967). Superimposed on the hypothalamic osmoreceptors —situated anteriorly in the hypothalamus (Jewell and Verney, 1957)—are volume receptors (Stricker and Wolf, 1967). These respond under conditions in which body-water depletion as well as hypo-osmolality occurs, such as following hemorrhage.

Destruction of more than 80 percent of the supraoptic nucleus or the supraopticohypophysial tract in experimental animals results in diabetes insipidus. The antidiuretic activity of the neurohypophysis is counterbalanced by the diuretic action of the anterior lobe of the pituitary—mainly through growth hormone, ACTH, and thyrotrophic hormone—so that if both the anterior pituitary and the neural lobe are removed, no significant change in water output occurs. Under these conditions, however, if the uppermost part of neurohypophysis (infundibulum, or median eminence) is also destroyed, or if the supraoptic nuclei are destroyed, diabetes insipidus will set in. In man much the same applies. The degree to which the supraopticohypophysial system is destroyed determines the severity of the diabetes insipidus: with low stalk section (carried out for therapeutic reasons) the diabetes is minimal or absent; it is severe only when the median eminence or adjoining hypothalamic region is damaged (Sharkey, Perry, and Ehni, 1961).

Primary polydipsia also occurs. It has been called *compulsive water drinking*. It may develop in the absence of any demonstrable renal, endocrine, or central nervous system abnormality (Barlow and De Wardener, 1959; Swanson and Iseri, 1958). The mechanism concerned is obscure; no postmortem studies are known to have been carried out. Apparently related to this category are cases in which drinking in excess sets in shortly after head trauma. Nothnagel's (1881) patient drank profusely within a half hour after being kicked in the head by a horse, but no urine was voided for 3 hours. Other cases in which intense thirst preceded polyuria are known (Futcher, 1904; Kennaway and Mottram, 1919; Weir, Larson, and Rowntree, 1922). Children with diseases that result in diabetes insipidus may subsequently have primary polydipsia, possibly related to psychogenic factors (Stevko, Balsley, and Segar, 1968). Conceivably, primary polydipsia may be attributable to blockage of a releasing mechanism necessary to the entrance of ADH into the neurohypophysial circulation (Orthner and Meyer, 1967).

In experimental diabetes insipidus, hyperdipsia is sometimes the initial phenomenon, preceding polyuria by a day or so (Bellows and Van Wagenen, 1939). A "thirst" center situated in the lateral part of the hypothalamus at about the level of the hypophysial stalk has been postulated (Anand and Dua, 1958; Andersson and McCann, 1956). The evidence suggests that while water intake is inhibited in a medial area by a "thirst satiety" center (whose destruction results in diabetes insipidus), it is stimulated by a mechanism in the lateral area (Smith and McCann, 1961; Teitelbaum and Epstein, 1962). While water intake appears to be controlled by these tiny centers, it is probable that the whole limbic system is involved in drinking, both in the motivation of drinking (Fitzsimons, 1966) and in transforming of a need for water ingestion into appropriate behavior (Kleeman and Fichman, 1967).

Normally, thirst sensation is satiated well before water intoxication has a chance to develop. However, thirst persists in the presence of hyponatremia. Sodium chloride depletion with resultant polydipsia is observed in normal infants given large amounts of very dilute feedings (Dugan and Holliday, 1967), also in a number of disease states, for example, in diarrhea, adrenocortical insufficiency, and diabetic acidosis. Polydipsia due to hyponatremia and progressing to a state of water intoxication may also be observed in the presence of intracranial infections (such as acute meningitis), tumor, or trauma (Gonzalez, Finberg, and Bluestein, 1964; Nyhan and Cooke, 1956). The old question of whether the hypothalamus is concerned primarily in electrolyte metabolism as well as in water exchange remains unresolved.

Lesions of the hypothalamus may alter thirst to the point where *adipsia* associated with severe hypertonic dehydration and hypernatremia occurs (Allen, 1953; Biemond, 1949). Hypodipsia together with hypernatremia has been produced experimentally through destruction of the lateral part of the ventromedial hypothalamic nucleus (Montemurro and Stevenson, 1956). Clinical cases of asymptomatic "neurogenic hypernatremia," sometimes associated with hypothalamic lesions, have been reported (Bauer, 1959; Kastin and others, 1965), but such cases are rare. Whether a faulty thirst mechanism is chiefly concerned, or whether a new set-point for plasma osmolality has been established, is unknown. Kleeman and Fichman (1967) emphasize that whenever negative water balance and hypernatremia develop in a conscious person without a desire to drink, a defect in the thirst-regulating mechanism exists.

HYPERPHAGIA AND APHAGIA

It is generally acknowledged that the quantity of food consumed is largely controlled by the hypothalamus. The suggestion has been made that in certain species (the rat) the neocortex is involved in qualitative modifications of food intake. The orbital neocortex is clearly concerned (in the monkey) in the quantitative consumption of food: a lesion made caudally in this part of the cortex will reduce food intake, although only slightly, while a lesion made in an adjacent cortical area will increase it (Anand, Dua, and Chhina, 1961); frontal lobotomy carried out in the caudal area will, in some instances, increase food intake, and the increase is proportional to the increased activity these animals usually show (Ruch and Shenkin, 1943). In the aggregate, the frontal lobes have an inhibitory influence on food intake. The amygdala is also heavily concerned and is also considered to have an inhibitory effect on food intake: aphagia (and adipsia as well) lasting 5 months was encountered, however, in a dog after complete removal of the amygdala bilaterally (Brutkowski and others, 1962). Not only the amygdala but also other limbic structures appear to exert an influence on food intake. Moreover, the view has been put forward that modification of food intake through a discriminative mechanism ("appetite") is a function of limbic structures of the frontal and temporal lobes, and that the primitive urge to eat ("hunger") originates at the hypothalamic level.

Studies in rats and mice have revealed two hypothalamic centers, one concerned in feeding and the other in satiety. The "feeding center" is situated in the lateral hypothalamic area at the level of the ventromedial nucleus, just in front of the "drinking center," while the "satiety (stop-feeding) center" lies in the ventromedial nucleus. (Oomura and others, 1967.) The term "satiety center" is used with some reservation, inasmuch as it has been shown that lesions in this region (ventromedial nucleus) can also reduce "hunger" if the latter be measured in terms of the work the animal will do or the noxious experiences it will accept in order to obtain and ingest food (Teitelbaum, 1957).

Destruction of the ventromedial nucleus bilaterally in the rat leads to hyperphagia and obesity. The gain in weight is not the outcome of a metabolic defect, but, instead, is the result of overeating. The rats do not overeat indefinitely, but only during a "dynamic" phase (until they become obese); after that a "static" phase ensues in which food intake levels off. The overeating is not accompanied by an increase in hunger drive. The animals are, in fact, in a relatively low drive state; they will not work as hard as other hungry rats, nor are they as willing to accept unpalatable food. (Hetherington and Ranson, 1942; Mayer and others, 1955.) Disruption of the "satiety center" (the ventromedial nucleus)—following which eating occurs at a different point in the scale of satiety than normally—seems basically at fault, but the coexistence of voracious behavior with a relatively low drive state remains to be explained. That the ventromedial nucleus in cats is a "satiety center" was shown graphically by Oomura and his associates (1967): the cats stopped chewing and food fell from their mouths during feeding when the ventromedial nucleus was electrically stimulated.

By contrast, destruction of a very small amount of tissue in the extreme part of the lateral hypothalamic area bilaterally leads to a cessation of eating (Anand and Brobeck, 1951; Morrison, Barrnett, and Mayer, 1958). Rats previously rendered hyperphagic by means of lesions in the ventromedial nucleus will cease eating when lesions are made in the lateral hypothalamus. Cats will eat to excess when this area is stimulated electrically through indwelling electrodes. Repetitive stimulation of the ventromedial nucleus results in disappearance of spontaneous unit discharges from the lateral hypothalamic center, and the reverse occurs when the latter center is stimulated, indicating a reciprocal relationship between the two (Oomura and others, 1967). A fiber system running from the ventromedial nucleus directly to the lateral hypothalamic area has been demonstrated (Arees and Mayer, 1967).

Two hypotheses have been advanced as to the means by which these centers are activated. One is the *thermostat hypothesis*. Ingestion of food, by increasing heat production, leads to satiety. Specific dynamic action of ingested food appears to be the main signal of satiety received by the hypothalamic feeding mechanism. By contrast, cooling of the body as heat is dissipated from the skin brings about activation of the feeding mechanism. (Brobeck, 1957.) This hypothesis could account for short-term food-intake regulation. Long-term regulation of food intake would require integration with additional mechanisms. The other hypothesis is the *glucostat hypothesis* (Mayer, 1953). This is described in the following section.

In man, hyperphagia (megaphagia, polyphagia, morbid hunger, bulimia, each having a different connotation) occurs in hypothalamic lesions (Dott, 1938; Poeck, Risso, and Pilleri, 1963), in frontal lobe glioma or trauma and in pontile glioma (Frazier, 1936; Terzian and Ore, 1955), and, further, as a component of the Kleine-Levin syndrome (p. 386). Thus numerous mechanisms must be involved. Hyperphagia can occur regardless of blood sugar level, whether it be low, in the usual range, or at a high level, as in obesity.

CARBOHYDRATE METABOLISM

Evidence exists that neural mechanisms of the hypothalamus are specifically sensitive to the glucose reaching them. On food ingestion, or on administering glucose intravenously, the electrical activity of the ventromedial region ("satiety center") has been found to increase, and glucose utilization (A-V difference) as well. Conversely, on food deprivation, or on creating hypoglycemia, electrical activity and glucose utilization in this region were shown to decrease. Electrical activity in the far-lateral hypothalamus ("feeding center") tended to vary in the opposite directions. (Anand, Chhina, and Singh, 1962; Anand, Dua, and Singh, 1961; Anand and others, 1961.) Associated with the increase in electrical activity of the ventromedial nucleus when blood-glucose level and glucose utilization were increased was an inhibition of gastric hunger contractions; following destruction of the ventromedial nucleus, the inhibition was no longer evident (Sharma and others, 1961). In animals in a state of hypoglycemia, the rate of blood-sugar fall rather than the absolute glucose level appears to be the major determinant in the hypothalamic response (Reichlin, 1967). In diabetes mellitus, food intake increases despite high blood sugar. In explanation of this paradox it has been postulated that "glucoreceptor" cells of the hypothalamus, unlike other neurons of the CNS, require insulin for the uptake and metabolism of glucose (Stevenson, 1969). For long-term regulation of food-intake, a "lipostatic mechanism" has been proposed (Mayer, 1960).

Electrical stimulation at various levels of the neuraxis results in alterations in blood-glucose level. In the cat, some increase in blood-glucose level occurred on stimulating the posterior hypothalamic and mamillary regions medially and the anterior and tuberal regions laterally, and a fall on stimulating the anterior and tuberal regions medially (Anand and Dua, 1955). Much different results have been obtained by others in such stimulations; in general, the predominant response obtained was blood-sugar increase. Acute lesions of the hypothalamus likewise frequently give rise to hyperglycemia and commonly to glycosuria as well. Transection of the midbrain (in dogs) decreases carbohydrate metabolism, as evidenced by a diabetic type of glucose tolerance curve (Anderson, Rioch, and Haymaker, 1952). As is well known, puncture of the floor of the fourth ventricle in the region of the dorsal nucleus of the vagus results in hyperglycemia and glycosuria. Under all the conditions cited, the response is usually transitory.

The glucose increase observed in these various studies is generally considered due to activation of the sympathico-adrenomedullary system, glycogenolysis in the liver being accelerated through the medium of sympathetic fibers passing to that organ, and glucose in the liver being mobilized by epinephrine. In what way the hypothalamo-pituitary system contributes is not clear. It has been postulated that under acute hypoglycemic conditions, hypothalamic glucoreceptor neurons (particularly those in the ventromedial nucleus) trigger not only autonomic discharges but also the release of ACTH (Matsui and Plager, 1966) and growth hormone (Glick and others, 1965), the latter of which appears to antagonize insulin. Despite the presence of hypothalamopituitary connections in bringing this about, it is generally agreed that section of the hypophysial stalk in normal animals does not produce any derangement in carbohydrate metabolism (Harris and George, 1969); however, stalk section in diabetic patients can reduce the insulin requirement by as much as 50 percent, an effect presumed to be due to depression in the rate of secretion of a pituitary diabetogenic factor, possibly growth hormone (Lundbaek, Malmros, and Mogensen, 1960).

In human subjects, acute lesions of the hypothalamus may increase blood-sugar level. Where small lesions of a degenerative nature are found in the paraventricular or neighboring nuclei of the hypothalamus and/or infundibulum in association with diabetes mellitus, it is probable that the diabetes caused the pathological changes, rather than the reverse. Insulin-resistant diabetes mellitus in man is known to occur in association with cyst in the third ventricle or cyst in the caudal midbrain (Anderson, Rioch, and Haymaker, 1952).

HYPOTHALAMUS AND GASTROINTESTINAL TRACT

Quite distinct from hypothalamic mechanisms concerned in feeding are others having the function of secreting gastric hydrochloric acid in preparation for the reception of food. Hypoglycemia is one of the factors responsible for initiating this hypothalamic response; the effector mechanisms are, on the one hand, humoral and, on the other, neural via the brainstem. Both sympathetic and parasympathetic systems are involved in the secretion of the hydrochloric acid.

Electrical stimulation of the "sympathetic" area of the hypothalamus (mainly its caudolateral part) (in monkeys) induces gastric acid secretion after some delay; secretion is maximal in about 3 hours after the stimulation. This secretory response is not influenced by vagotomy. Prior bilateral adrenalectomy prevents the response. The assumption is that the sympathetic-induced effect is humoral and is mediated by the anterior pituitary and adrenal cortex. (Porter, Movius, and French, 1953.)

In contrast, electrical stimulation of the rostral hypothalamus (in monkeys) induces a prompt increase in the secretion of gastric acid, reaching a maximum in about 1 hour. The efferent pathway is by way of the vagus nerve, since vagotomy prevents the response. (French and others, 1953.) Mucosal ulceration (in dogs) appears to result from vagal hyperactivity, through which the gastrointestinal musculature undergoes contraction, leading to ischemia, hemorrhagic infarction, and, finally, ulcer formation. Ulceration has been produced by electrically stimulating the tuberal region (with the vagi intact) or by stimulating the vagi themselves. The sympathetic system is also concerned. Prior sympathectomy does not prevent the ulceration that usually occurs after damage of the tuber cinereum, but it does prevent the occurrence of mucosal hemorrhages. (Beattie and Sheehan, 1934.) Further, it has been found (in monkeys) that prolonged stimulation of the hypothalamus (daily for 4 to 10 weeks) through indwelling electrodes often leads to gastric hemorrhage and ulceration (French and others, 1954).

From the standpoint of the effect of hypothalamic *lesions,* it has been noted (in dogs) that lesions made in the anterolateral region bilaterally (but not lesions made in the region of the paraventricular nuclei) result in a statistically significant increase in basal acid secretion, whereas insulin-induced gastric secretion is inhibited for as long as 3 months. Presumably, according to the authors (Davis, Brooks, and Steckel, 1968), (1) interruption of the fornix and medial forebrain bundle (bilaterally) by the lesions destroyed fibers coming to the hypothalamus from the limbic system and the frontal cortex, which normally exert a tonic, inhibitory effect on basal gastric secretion, and (2) alterations in conduction in diffuse descending connections from the lateral hypothalamus extending caudalward in the lateral tegmentum to the lower brainstem autonomic (vagal) centers can be held accountable for the inhibitory effect.

In man, areas of hemorrhage together with erosion and ulceration are not uncommonly found in the mucosa of the stomach, and less so in the duodenum and esophagus, in association with lesions (mainly acute) situated almost anywhere in the central nervous system. The causative lesion is thus often not localizable. It appears that acute lesions involving the hypothalamus and brainstem are especially apt to give rise to the hemorrhage and/or ulceration, but in most cases the disease process is more generalized. Perforation of the ulcerated region is fairly common. (Cushing, 1932; Davey, Kaada, and Fulton, 1950.) The spinal cord is not immune, inasmuch as gastrointestinal bleeding has been noted in acute cervical cord injury in as high a proportion of cases as 20 percent (Perret, 1964). Men older than 40 years are most prone to esophageal ulceration; aneurysm of strategically located arteries has now and then been demonstrated in some cases (Edmondson, Gindin, and Peebles, 1968). Gastric acid hypersecretion occurs as a result of trauma, but, apparently, not an increase in circulating adrenocorticoids. Lack of food to buffer gastric hypersecretion is an important factor in ulcer development.

OBESITY AND GONADAL ATROPHY

When the ventromedial nucleus of the hypothalamus is severely damaged, obesity usually occurs. The obesity has been attributed by some workers to increased food intake relative to the degree of energy expenditure, and by others to a disturbance of a neural-visceral mechanism whereby fat mobilization is reduced. The fiber system mostly concerned extends caudally from the ventromedial nucleus and passes down the brainstem.

Normal functioning of the gonads is dependent upon the integrity of a cell aggregate, the infundibular nucleus (tubero-infundibular nucleus, or arcuate nucleus), situated at the base of the third ventricle in contact with the upper part of the neurohypophysis (Fig. 26-2), and also upon the integrity of its fibers, the *tubero-hypophysial tract.* Damage of this system may lead to gonadal atrophy and loss of gonadal function of varied degree. (Guillemin, 1965; Laqueur and others, 1955; McCann, Antunes-Rodrigues, and Dhariwal, 1965.)

Lesions of the tuberal region of the hypothalamus frequently give rise both to gonadal atrophy and to obesity; the reason for this is that the neural mechanism influencing gonadal activity and that concerned in the deposition of fat lie very close together and thus are likely to be damaged by a single lesion. The disorder characterized by gonadal atrophy and obesity is known as *adiposogenital dystrophy.* If the disorder occurs in preadolescence, as a consequence of failure of gonadal maturation, *Fröhlich's syndrome* is the term then applicable.

CHROMOPHOBE ADENOMA OF THE PITUITARY AND CRANIOPHARYNGIOMA

Both these tumors usually extend into the hypothalamus and adjacent parts of the brain, and in their growth upward produce visual field and other disturbances.

Spatial relations of the pituitary to the optic nerves and chiasm constitute an important factor in the nature of the initial visual field defect. The optic nerves and chiasm usually lie just above the hypophysis and sella turcica (Fig. 19-1).

As shown in Fig. 26-3, the optic chiasm is situated partly or wholly above the hypophysis in 96 percent of human brains, while in the remaining 4 percent it lies behind the sella, resting on the dorsum sellae (markedly postfixed chiasm). Of the 96 percent, there are 79 percent in which the anterior and often the greater part of the chiasm lies over the hypophysis, 12 percent in which the entire chiasm lies over the hypophysis (slightly prefixed chiasm), and 5 percent in which the anterior part of the chiasm is located on the chiasmatic sulcus and the posterior part over the hypophysis (moderately prefixed chiasm). (de Schweinitz, 1923.)

Chromophobe adenoma. Chromophobe adenoma of the anterior pituitary is slightly more frequent in males than in females. The maximum incidence of symptoms in patients seeking treatment is between 40 and 50 years. The tumor may, however, be clinically evident in persons from 10 to 70 years of age. (Elkington, 1968.) Headache may occur in earlier stages of tumor development. It may be bitemporal in distribution but is much more frequent in the region of the orbit and nose, unilaterally. Sometimes the onset of headache is sudden and severe and is accompanied by abrupt deterioration of vision and impairment of consciousness—as a result of tumor infarction. The headache is attributable to tension exerted on the lining of the sella turcica and on the diaphragma sellae. Except for headache and endocrine disturbances (such as underdeveloped genitals and beard and lack of libido, in males; amenorrhea and poor development of breasts and axillary and pubic hair, in females), visual failure is usually the first complaint.

On growing upward, the tumor initially compresses either the optic nerve(s) or the

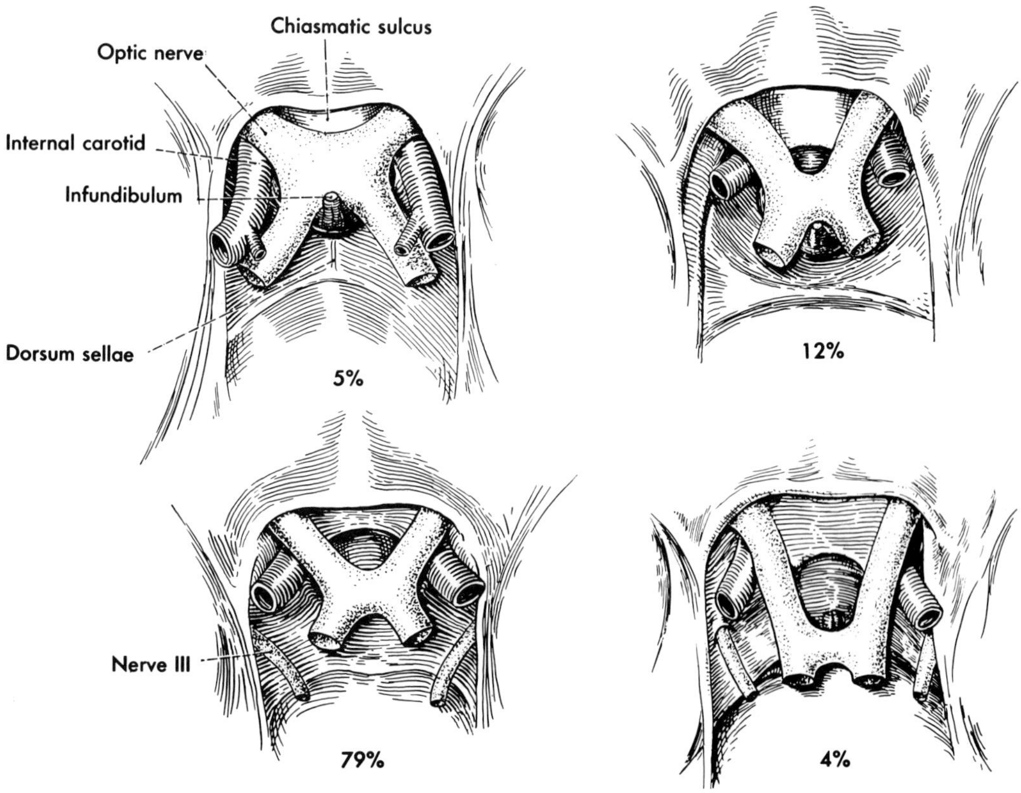

Fig. 26-3. Variations in the relationship of the optic chiasm to the pituitary gland.

chiasm. Reduction in the size of the fields is more marked than reduction in visual acuity, the loss often appearing initially in one or both of the upper temporal quadrants. The defects then enlarge. Complete more or less symmetrical, bitemporal hemianopia can occur, but is infrequent. "Atypical" field defects are common—for example, defects that are asymmetrical on the two sides (Espinosa and Randall, 1968; Rose, 1968). As the optic nerves and chiasm are displaced upward, the anterior cerebral and anterior communicating arteries are impinged upon, and since these arteries are incapable of yielding, the upper and temporal parts of the optic tracts and chiasm are compressed, then deeply indented (Rucker and Kernohan, 1954). Defects in the lower visual fields thus result. Ultimately all vision may be lost, especially if the lateral portion of the chiasm is trapped between the tumor (below) and the anterior cerebral arteries (above).

Since chromophobe adenomas tend to be nodular, they may implicate one optic nerve or one side of the chiasm more than the other, and thus produce a *predominantly unilateral field defect.* Under these conditions there may be pallor of the optic disk, a central scotoma, or blindness involving the field of the affected nerve. In seventy-eight cases of pituitary tumor or suprasellar cyst reported by Sachs (1938), blindness occurred in one eye in twenty-eight of the cases of pituitary tumor and in eighteen of the suprasellar cyst group. If, on the other hand, the tumor grows upward and backward and compresses the optic tract, as occasionally it does, *contralateral, incongruous homonymous hemianopia* will result. Occasionally noted are arcuate defects similar to those encountered in optic nerve or retinal lesions. Choking of the optic disks is rare. (Espinosa and Randall, 1968.)

In cases in which *central vision* has shown relatively early involvement, as documented by rapid loss of visual acuity, the optic chiasm has been found prefixed, with the tumor exerting its chief pressure on the caudal part of the chiasm.

Pallor of the optic disks followed by frank atrophy becomes evident when the optic nerves are encroached upon. The disks may, however, remain normal in appearance for some weeks despite advanced visual loss. Under such circumstances the tumor probably has extended posteriorly and implicated the optic tracts.

Depending on its growth proclivities, chromophobe adenoma may involve a number of structures in addition to the visual system. Among the vulnerable structures are the third nerve and related nerves. However, only in occasional instances are they affected. More commonly the diplopia complained of (by about 40 percent of patients) is the result of the bitemporal field defects and the consequent difficulty in accurately registering the image in each eye (Elkington, 1968).

Since the pituitary capsule is least resistant to expansion in its lateral part, the tumor, in its earlier stage of growth, may pierce the capsule and bulge into the cavernous sinus (unilaterally or bilaterally). If the tumor extends upward and backward into the cavernous sinus, above the carotid artery, it is likely to affect the third nerve. The palsy may involve, for example, the medial and superior recti and the levator palpebrae superioris, and spare or involve the intraocular muscles. In early stages the palsy may be intermittent, a characteristic attributed to varying congestion of the tumor, through which the sellar diaphragm is lifted to a greater or lesser extent, stretching the dural sheath that contains the third nerve. (François and Neetens, 1968.) In rare instances, third nerve palsy may be the only manifestation of an intrasellar tumor. The fourth and sixth nerves lie more inferolateral than the third (Fig. 16-1) and thus are less frequently affected. The fifth nerve may also be involved, giving rise to pain and sensory deficit in its region of distribution.

Uncinate seizures have been known to occur when the tumor extends still farther laterally, but are rare. Grand mal and psychomotor seizures may also occur, but they, too, are rare. The hypothalamus is usually encroached upon. Diabetes insipidus is, however, rare. When the tumor is sufficiently large to block the third ventricle, there will be internal hydrocephalus and associated signs of increased intracranial pres-

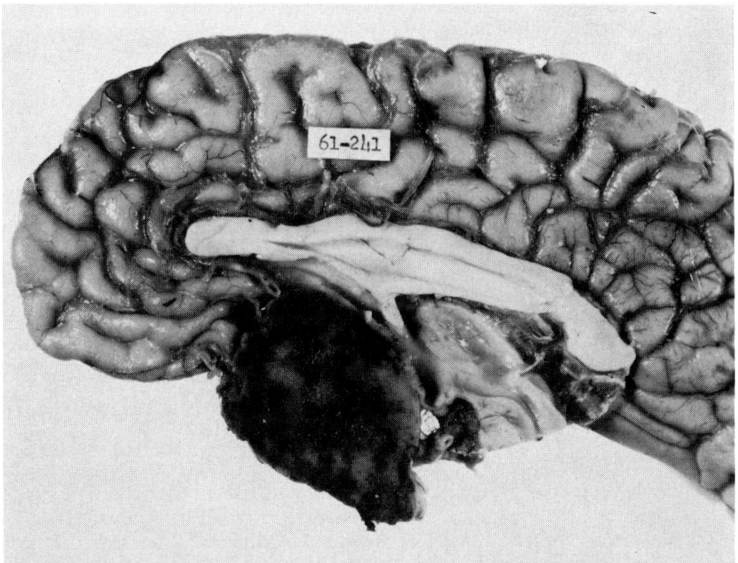

Fig. 26-4. Huge chromophobe adenoma of the pituitary, with fresh hemorrhages into the tumor tissue ("pituitary apoplexy"), causing sudden death. The tumor had grown upward into the region rostral to the lamina terminalis. The patient was 77 years old and bedridden. (Courtesy Dr. Richard Lindenberg, Baltimore.)

sure. If the tumor projects rostrally, involving the orbitofrontal and adjoining cortex, as frequently it does (Fig. 26-4), changes in temperament and personality may develop. Hyposmia or anosmia may also occur. (Bailey, 1948; Trumble, 1951.)

Increased intracranial pressure may in itself give rise to signs suggesting pituitary tumor. These include bitemporal hemianopia, distended sella turcica, reduction in pituitary function, and hypothalamic disturbances (Dott, 1936). However, the degree of increased pressure outweighs these disturbances.

Craniopharyngioma. Craniopharyngioma usually becomes clinically manifest in persons in their teens and twenties, but the disturbances may not set in until later on (Norstrand, 1955). The tumor is an encapsulated and cystic neoplasm which in 75 percent of cases undergoes conspicuous calcification. A characteristic example is shown in Fig. 26-5.

Symptoms and signs vary with the site of the tumor. When originating below the diaphragma sellae, the tumor, by damaging the anterior pituitary, may induce hypopituitarism as an early manifestation. On the other hand, a craniopharyngioma that is initially suprasellar may subsequently extend downward into the sella turcica and cause hypopituitarism relatively late.

During the course of its growth, craniopharyngioma almost always encroaches on the optic pathway. As a rule, the initial change consists of a paracentral scotoma in the upper temporal field on one side, then on the other. Later, bilaterally dissimilar defects develop in the inferior temporal quadrants of the visual field; still later they may enlarge and include all the visual field except the upper nasal quadrant bilaterally. Central vision of one or both eyes is ultimately lost. Probably playing an important role in the production of the visual field defects is upward displacement of the optic nerves by the tumor, so that they come to lie next to the unyielding anterior cerebral and anterior communicating arteries, producing a pincer effect. Sometimes at a later stage one eye is blind, while the other shows a temporal field defect. Homonymous hemianopia occurs with some frequency, and in some series of cases it is the visual field

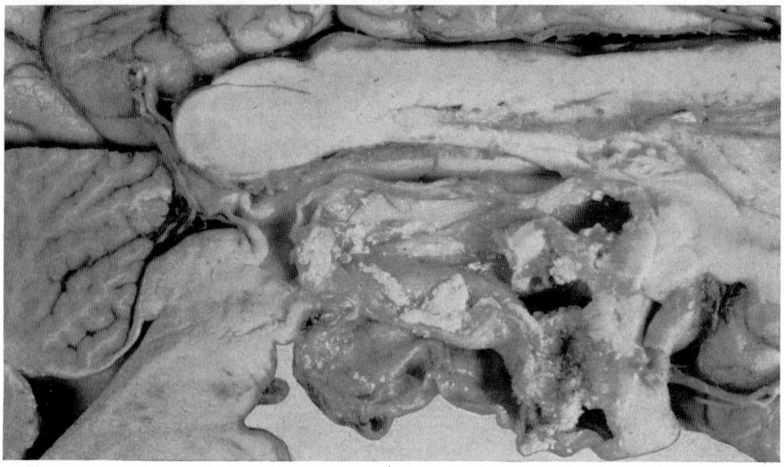

Fig. 26-5. Craniopharyngioma. Midsagittal view showing the cystic nature of the tumor. The cyst fills most of the third ventricle. The white flecks are calcific deposits, recognizable radiographically. The patient was a 19-year-old male. He had had headaches since childhood. Examination in the last week of life disclosed stiff neck, bilateral papilledema, right hemiparesis, and bilateral Babinski sign. (AFIP Acc. 138593.)

defect most often encountered. Concentric contraction of the visual field also occurs, but it is rare. Also rare is unilateral central scotoma without any other visual field defect, which may be difficult to distinguish from the scotoma occurring in retrobulbar optic neuritis (Schlezinger and Thompson, 1967). Incidence of optic atrophy varies (occurring in about 50 percent of adults with craniopharyngioma) and as the atrophy sets in, blindness for green, then for red, develops. In craniopharyngeal cyst, there may be binasal hemianopia, owing to outpouching of the cyst bilaterally. The reverse may also occur; there may be bitemporal hemianopic defects, with involvement of central vision unilaterally (Berry and Schlezinger, 1959).

In about one-third of cases, the tumor encroaches on or actually invades the hypothalamus. It may also invade the third ventricle. Not infrequently in such cases, the tumor extends sufficiently high in the ventricle to obstruct the interventricular foramen or sufficiently caudalward to obstruct the cerebral aqueduct. In such a case Korsakoff's syndrome was one of the most prominent disorders over several months prior to death; injury of the pars tecta of the fornix bilaterally due to compression by the tumor was considered the main factor in the production of the syndrome (Orthner and Rettinger, 1965).

In the presence of craniopharyngioma, if a state of pituitary insufficiency does not already exist, obesity may develop. Gonadal atrophy, which usually is evident, may result from damage inflicted either on the anterior pituitary or on the infundibular nucleus of the hypothalamus or both. Uncinate seizures may develop when the tumor extends into the temporal lobe. When growing into the interpeduncular fossa and through the incisura tentorii cerebelli, it may induce ataxia of the cerebellar type, pyramidal tract signs, or attacks of decerebrate rigidity. The first, third, and sixth nerves are occasionally affected.

The clinical course differs depending on the age of the patient. In children, the most common initial symptoms are headache and vomiting. Papilledema is also a characteristic feature. In adults, either visual disturbances or headaches mark the onset. Manifestations of increased intracranial pressure appear relatively late, and in elderly persons are rare. Diabetes insipidus is infrequent in children. In adults, particularly when beyond forty, diabetes insipidus, episodes of hyperthermia, somnolence, and dissociated pulse rate and temperature are fairly common. The thalamic syndrome and the Parkinson syndrome have occasionally been observed. (Critchley and Ironside, 1926; Frazier and Alpers, 1934; Wagener and Love, 1943.)

DIENCEPHALIC SYNDROME IN INFANCY AND CHILDHOOD

A series of paradoxes, the diencephalic syndrome (inanition syndrome, failure to thrive, athrepsia) results from extensive damage of the anterior hypothalamus by astrocytoma (or other glioma of low-grade malignancy). Sometimes the tumor originates in the optic chiasm. The tumor is "silent" in that it does not give rise to the disturbances ordinarily observed in later life from tumors in this region. Ocular nystagmus (to-and-fro oscillations of the eyes) occurs in about half the cases and may be a presenting sign. Profound emaciation is the chief manifestation, occurring despite food intake that is either adequate or in excess. Appetite is often ravenous. The infant usually has boundless energy, is constantly overactive, and is happy or euphoric. Most are "lovable clowns." The skin has a peculiar pallor, though no anemia exists. Lipid metabolism is disturbed. Occasionally a tendency toward hypoglycemia is observed, as is an elevation in the serum level of growth hormone. Bone growth is normal. Age of most of the subjects at the onset of the disorder is between 2 and 6 months. (Bain and others, 1966; Ciccarelli and Huttenlocher, 1967; Russell, 1951; Smith, Weinberg, and McAlister, 1965.)

ACROMEGALY

The tumor responsible for acromegaly —eosinophilic adenoma—is usually confined to the sella turcica; under such conditions this tumor gives rise to headache, usually bitemporal in distribution, which is aggravating and persistent. Following rupture of the diaphragm from upward growth of the tumor, the headache usually disappears. Involvement of the optic nerves and chiasm is no different than in chromophobe adenoma, but is less frequent. Since eosinophilic adenoma is a self-limited, circumscribed tumor, only now and then does it grow sufficiently large to involve the hypothalamus; it may also, on occasion, reach the gasserian ganglion, the frontal or temporal lobe, and even the superior part of the pars basilaris pontis (Kernohan and Sayre, 1955).

HYPOPITUITARY STATES

Hypopituitary states resulting from tumor have already been dealt with. Those observed in other conditions will now be considered.

Pituitary insufficiency in the adult

Profound pituitary insufficiency *(Simmonds' disease)* results when the anterior lobe of the pituitary is destroyed. The disorder is not infrequently due to craniopharyngioma or chromophobe adenoma (see foregoing). Meningioma situated just in front of the anterior clinoid processes and along the medial aspect of the sphenoid ridge may have the same effect, as may also chordoma or metastatic or invasive carcinoma. Also responsible are trauma (Daniel and Treip, 1966), chronic basal meningitis (most often tuberculous), granulomas of unknown etiology, epidemic hemorrhagic fever, and enlargement of the third ventricle in generalized hydrocephalus. The disorder may also occur postpartum (Sheehan's syndrome), in which case much of the anterior lobe of the pituitary becomes necrotic. The necrosis usually develops in association with obstetric hemorrhage; occasionally it is a sequela of eclampsia. The sella turcica may be small in some of these cases, and the smallness may be of etiological importance inasmuch as the pituitary gland enlarges during pregnancy. (Adams, Daniel, and Prichard, 1966; Harlin and Givens, 1968; Sheehan and Davis, 1968.) Fibrin thrombi reaching pituitary capillaries may be the causative factor in Sheehan's syndrome

(Beernick and McKay, 1962). The reversal of pituitary insufficiency observed in some cases may possibly be due to the vicarious activity of the pharyngeal hypophysis (Tönnis and others, 1954).

Pituitary insufficiency is manifested by loss of appetite and consequent reduction in body weight until cachexia ensues. When the responsible lesion is a chromophobe adenoma of the pituitary, there may be preliminary obesity brought about by initial pressure of the tumor on the base of the hypothalamus.

In women the disorder is also characterized by amenorrhea and atrophy of the genitalia, and in men by loss of libido and by atrophy of the testes and external genitalia. Other manifestations include loss of hair, dryness of the skin, muscular weakness, lowered blood pressure, slowing of heart rate, and a considerable reduction in the basal metabolic rate.

Pituitary insufficiency in childhood (pituitary dwarfism)

When occurring in children, pituitary insufficiency is most frequently due to craniopharyngioma. The bodily proportions remain infantile because of retardation of growth and maturation. There is a lack of sexual development and a reduction in 17-ketosteroids and follicle-stimulating hormone (FSH) in the urine. (Bailey, 1963; Launay and others, 1946.)

PUBERTAS PRAECOX

Lesions involving the hypothalamus or the diencephalic-mesencephalic transitional area of the brain account for about 15 percent of cases of pubertas praecox. Two groups may be distinguished; in one the disorder is associated with hamartoma of the hypothalamus (tumor-like malformation composed of redundant brain tissue), and in the other, with neoplasm or other pathological process. The hamartoma is almost invariably situated at the base of the brain in the region of the tuber cinereum or mamillary bodies; usually it is small and pedunculated, but it may be as large as a golf ball.

When occurring in association with hamartoma, pubertas praecox sets in during early childhood, from about the age of a few months up to 6 years. Males are almost exclusively affected. The penis and testes may be larger than normal at birth. The disorder is characterized by rapid growth of the genitalia, accelerated development of the secondary sex characteristics, precocious libido, and extraordinary muscular development and phenomenal strength. Bone age is accelerated. In cases in which mental disturbances have developed, disseminated cerebral malformations have been found.

In pubertas praecox in which some pathological process other than hypothalamic hamartoma is at fault, the onset of clinical disturbances is later in childhood. Responsible neoplasms include pineal tumor, hypothalamic glioma, and, rarely, suprasellar teratoma, craniopharyngioma, and chiasmal glioma; among infectious processes are poliomyelitis, epidemic encephalitis, measles encephalitis, and tuberculous meningitis. Hydrocephalus due to adhesive arachnoiditis may also be responsible. Occasionally the disorder is associated with cyst in the third ventricle, as in the case of a young girl described by Flicker (1943).

Varied clinical pictures have been observed. Hypergonadism is frequently the most conspicuous feature of pubertas praecox. In pineal tumor, the midbrain and brachium conjunctivum are often affected, giving rise to pupillary disturbances, paralysis of conjugate vertical gaze, ataxia, and so on (Northfield and Russell, 1967; Papez and Ecker, 1947; Schmidt, Hallervorden, and Spatz, 1958). Epileptic seizures are fairly common. Seizures of laughter, giggling, or chuckling occasionally occur in association with sexual precocity. A sense of amusement is experienced by some patients, but not by most. Now and then the hypothalamus is suggested as the responsible site when the patient complains that he experienced a feeling of alternate hot and cold during an attack of laughter. When such disorders as hyperphagia, hyperdipsia, hyperthermia, disturbances in conjugate ocular deviation, or facial flushing or pallor are components of a laughing seizure, the hypothalamus is probably the site at fault. (Daly and Mulder, 1957; Dott, 1938; Druckman and Chao, 1957; List and others, 1958; Poeck, Risso, and Pilleri, 1963.)

Normal onset of puberty is controlled by hypothalamic mechanisms, as experimentation has affirmed. Pubertas praecox is an expression of altered control.

Regarding the neural mechanisms involved, for tumors impinging on the hypothalamus such as pineal tumors, Weinberger and Grant (1941) have suggested that the tumor interrupts a posterior hypothalamic inhibitory system and thus releases, in the anterior hypothalamic area, a substance stimulatory to pituitary function. For hamartomas at the base of the hypothalamus, it has been suggested that the additional tissue might augment hypothalamopituitary function through an excess of nervous activity (Bauer, 1959) or that it might be deficient in mechanisms for neural inhibitory control (Richter, 1951).

REGULATION OF BODY TEMPERATURE

Dissipation of body heat, on the one hand, and the conservation and production of body heat, on the other, occurs in accordance with the thermal state of the body. The neural mechanisms concerned are widespread in the neuraxis, but the hypothalamus plays a leading role. Rostrally situated mechanisms in the hypothalamus can conveniently be viewed as concerned primarily with heat dissipation, and caudal mechanisms with heat conservation and heat production, but this oversimplifies the matter.

Experimental studies

The chief stimulus that determines the response of the hypothalamus is the temperature of the blood. Thermosensitive neurons, called *thermodetectors* (Ström, 1950), are present in the anterior and preoptic regions of the hypothalamus. Many are heat-sensitive units (Nakayama, Eisenman, and Hardy, 1961; von Euler, 1950). Cold-sensitive units are also located in this region. Since more thermal units exist than are present in the hypothalamus (Hardy, Hellon, and Sutherland, 1964), it is probable that the remainder are located in the brainstem and the spinal cord—a view in accord with clinical and experimental observations (Foerster, 1936; Kahn, 1963; Ström, 1960; Thauer, 1964) (pp. 482-484).

Thermodetector neurons in the anterior hypothalamic region serve in thermoregulation through biochemical means. It appears that one biogenic amine (serotonin) is selectively released for the activation of neural pathways for heat production when thermogenesis is required; at the same site in the anterior hypothalamus another biogenic amine (a catecholamine), in physiological opposition to the first, is released to deactivate the heat production systems and induce heat loss when cooling is needed. Individual serotonin-containing and norepinephrin-containing cells in this region have now been demonstrated. Cooler blood impinging on a "serotonin cell" releases serotonin, which triggers the efferent pathway for heat production. (Cooper, Cranston, and Honour, 1965; Cranston, 1966; Feldberg and Myers, 1963; Myers, 1968.) Serotonin when injected into the ventricular system (in cats) produces a marked and sustained rise in body temperature; catecholamines produce the reverse effect. In the brains of dying animals, Feldberg (1967) observed a great build-up in serotonin content, and he considered it possible that such increase may be responsible for the bouts of hyperthermia and shivering observed during neurosurgical intervention in hypothalamic and related regions.

The caudolateral part of the hypothalamus, on the other hand, is *temperature-blind* (Benzinger, 1964)—it possesses no capacity for thermostatic sensing of temperature changes in the blood (Freeman and Davis, 1959). Its importance in thermoregulation lies, instead, in its role in initiating vasomotor, sudomotor, and respiratory activity (Hardy, 1961); this region is also concerned in somatomotor function, for on electrical stimulation in various areas either augmentation or reduction in lumbosacral motoneuron activity can be elicited, both alpha motoneurons and gamma motoneurons being involved (Ishikawa and others, 1967). Cells in the caudolateral regulatory center appear to have a predetermined set-point of 98.6° F. and, by virtue of this quality, to control the magnitude of heat production and heat loss. Maintenance of the set-point and mobilization of reactions to defend this set-point appear to be achieved through effector signals coming from the anterior and preoptic regions of the hypothalamus (Benzinger, 1964; Cooper, 1966; Myers, 1969b). Impulses coming from the periphery are encoded by cutaneous and deeper-lying temperature receptors and then sent through ascending pathways to the caudolateral hypothalamic center (Benzinger, 1964; Thauer, 1964). Some may come from cutaneous "heat" receptors excitable only by radiant heat (Iggo, 1959, 1963). Others come from cold receptor systems in the skin; fibers—myelinated as well as nonmyelinated—issuing from these systems are excitable at skin temperatures between 68° and 95° F. but not at temperatures between 95° and 104° F. (Iggo, 1964). While temperature regulation in the "hot zone" of the caudolateral hypothalamus appears to be mostly under the control of local thermoreceptors (in the anterior hypothalamus), regulation in the "cold and neutral zones" appears to be largely effected by the action of afferent impulses from peripheral receptors (Hardy, 1961). Sharing in regulation through initiation or facilitation of shivering are the septal region, the caudolateral hypothalamus, and the subthalamus (Hammel, 1968; Hemingway, 1963; Ishikawa and others, 1967; Stuart, Kawamura, and Hemingway, 1961).

The main pathway through which impulses concerned both in heat dissipation and in heat conservation (and production) are conveyed takes its course through the caudolateral hypothalamus, tegmentum of the midbrain and pons, reticular formation of the medulla oblongata, and lateral columns of the spinal cord, then by way of sympathetic fibers to cutaneous vessels and sweat glands, and through somatic motor fibers to muscles. Another pathway, that concerned in hormonal aspects of thermal regulation, runs from various hypothalamic nuclei to the pituitary.

Clinical observations

Fever. In the febrile subject, qualitatively normal thermoregulatory responses to low and high ambient temperatures are preserved, but they vary about a new, elevated set-point. Pyrogens appear to act in a region identical with or close to the classic thermoreceptor area, that is, in the anterior hypothalamus. Endogenous pyrogen injected into this part of the hypothalamus induces fever at doses that are ineffective by systemic injection (Cooper, 1966). Mechanisms proposed in an effort to find an explanation are: (1) that the pyrogens depress the excitability of the thermoreceptor neurons to local heat stimuli, and in this way affect the set-point mechanism situated in the caudolateral part of the hypothalamus; and (2) that when a pyrogen impinges on a "serotonin cell" in the anterior hypothalamus, the cell releases serotonin, triggering the efferent pathway for heat production. (Myers, 1969a.) Considering the increase in basal metabolism in the presence of fever, one might expect an increase in appetite. Anorexia, however, occurs. This anorexia of fever may be the outcome of thermoreceptor reflex action on the food intake mechanism analogous to the change occurring in the temperature set-point. (Reichlin, 1967.)

Fulminant hyperthermia during anesthesia and surgery. It is not altogether rare for rapid increases in body temperature to occur, and be fatal, in apparently healthy persons during the administration of anesthesia for noncritical surgical procedures. Normally, anesthetics are an effective means for reducing body temperature. This lowering of temperature may be brought about by the action of the anesthetic on catecholamine-containing cells, causing a release of norepinephrine or perhaps dopamine from these cells, the catecholamine activating heat-loss systems by way of the efferent pathways delegated for this purpose (Myers, 1969b). It is possible that failure of a mechanism such as this, whereby the "thermostat" of the temperature regulator in the caudal hypothalamus is reset in an unopposed manner, is responsible for the hyperthermia that sometimes occurs. Uncoupling of oxidative phosphorylation in cells in this region by anesthetics has been suggested as a possible basis (Wilson and others, 1966). Sustained increase in muscle activity is noted in some of the subjects, and it could well be a secondary phenomenon. Further, there appears to be a deficit in the ability to hyperventilate in the face of increased tissue oxygen requirements. Atropine in excess, leading to temperature elevation as high as 109° F. when given to children, may be held accountable in some cases; suppression of sweating is one of the earlier manifestations. Introduction of pyrogens in intravenously introduced fluid should of course also be taken into consideration. Under all these circumstances the situation is serious because clinical abnormalities do not appear until the hyperthermic process is well established. (Ruscio and Marcus, 1968; Stephen, 1967.) Clarification of the disturbance awaits further information on hypothalamic chemostatic regulatory mechanisms.

Heat stroke. Excess heat load in the body is determined by climate, activity, body build, and by many other variables (Lee, 1964; Lee and Henschel, 1966). Considering the case of the resting body with zero heat exchange with the environment, and taking 0.83 as the specific heat of the body, storage of the metabolic heat would raise body temperature above 4° F. per hour, and if the subject were walking, the temperature increase would be two to three times this value (Schickele, 1947). Heat exchange between the body and the environment under ordinary conditions takes place through physical channels, mainly through radiation, convection, and conduction (65 percent), and evaporation of water from the skin and lungs (30 percent). Heat accumulates in the body and the temperature rises when the surrounding atmosphere is unable to absorb from the body surface the heat produced internally by metabolism. A "heat death line" for normal persons—in this case army personnel—taking into consideration the variables of environmental temperature, relative humidity, and degree of exercise is shown in Fig. 26-6. This chart indicates the wide range of relative humidity and temperature conditions under which normal persons, who may or may not be exercising strenuously, can become hyperthermic. Of particular interest are the fatalities occurring as a result of exercise at relatively low temperature.

The mechanisms responsible for the practically complete cessation of heat flow from the body to the environment under heat stroke conditions must be many and varied, and include failure of the secretory mechanism of sweat glands (Gottschalk and Thomas, 1966). It is likely that elevated blood temperature (above 105° F.) disrupts hypothalamic sensing and effector mechanisms, and so is instrumental in the deficit in heat dissipation that occurs. That the hypothalamus can be (and frequently is) damaged under conditions of heat stroke is evident from the decided reduction in thermoregulatory power in persons who have recovered. (The cerebellum also suffers permanent damage, p. 288.) Hemorrhages in many locations, including the hypothalamus, occur in fatal heat stroke, also prolongation of bleeding and clotting times and progressive thrombocytopenia (Malamud, Haymaker, and Custer, 1946). Endothelial cell damage and

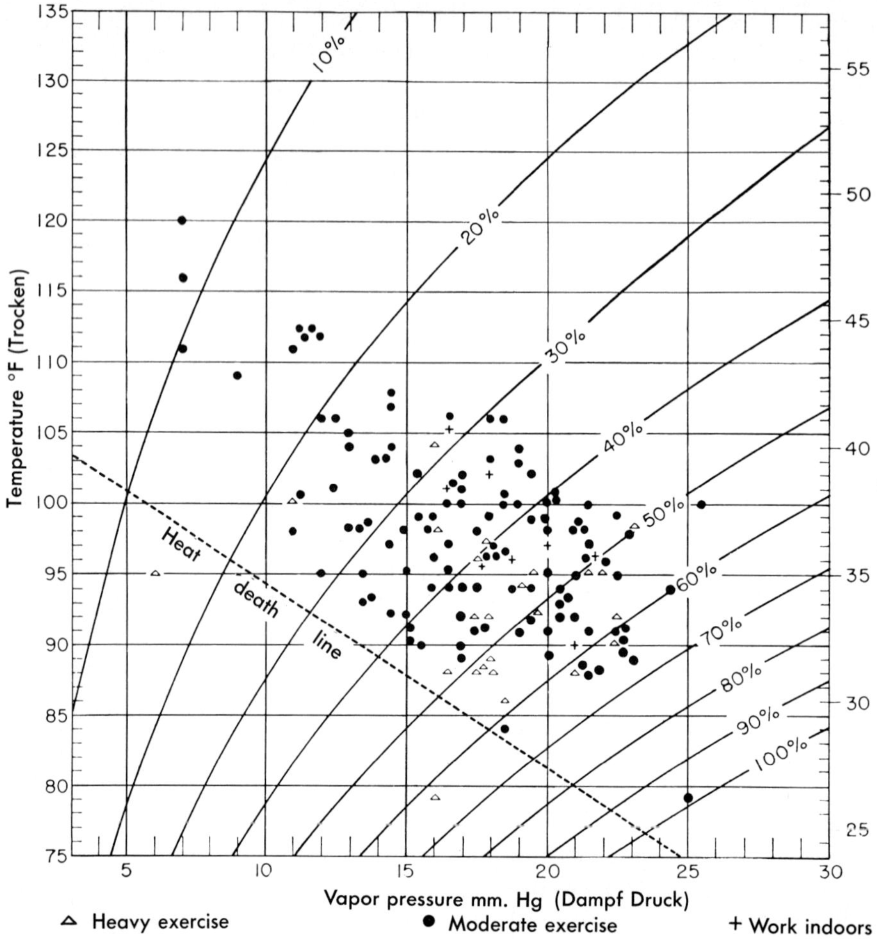

Fig. 26-6. Temperature and relative humidity conditions under which death from excess heat load occurred in 154 soldiers in World War II. A "heat death line" is plotted to indicate the atmospheric condition conducive to heat stroke in young men undergoing varied degrees of exercise. Many of the men were not acclimatized. Two of the fatalities occurred under atmospheric conditions beneath the heat death line. (From Schickele, 1947.)

the presence of thrombi in various organs have been noted electron microscopically in such a case, and the view put forward that fatal heat stroke may be considered an expression of acute coagulopathy (Sohal and others, 1968). Cause-and-effect relations of these phenomena, however, need yet to be ascertained, particularly when one considers that heat exhaustion may be fatal in the absence of a rise in body temperature (Malamud, Haymaker, and Custer, 1946). Disordered potassium metabolism has been suggested as a highly significant factor in creating conditions conducive to the development of the hyperthermic state (Vertel and Knochel, 1967).

Disruption of mechanisms concerned in heat dissipation or in heat production, coupled with adverse environmental conditions in some instances, account for the initiation of the hyperthermic and hypothermic states next to be described.

Thermal disturbances from trauma. Operations in the region of the third ventricle or the brainstem, by interfering with the central mechanism of thermoregulation, are hazardous because of the frequency with which acute hyperthermia occurs.

According to Erickson (1938), the body temperature begins to rise within 12 hours after operation. Tachycardia is among the earliest disturbances and often precedes the elevation in temperature. Usually the heart rate is about 140 per minute, but in severe cases it may rise to 180 or more. Death from heart failure may occur in about 36 hours. Respiratory rate also increases. The limbs are icy cold and the trunk relatively warm. Sweating is always absent. Hyperthermia occurs if not combated. However, according to Foerster (1935), under like conditions there may be no increase in heart rate or respiratory rate despite temperature elevation.

Softening in the preoptic and adjoining region from trauma from external sources can also result in hyperthermia (Beaton and Herrmann, 1945; Erickson, 1939).

Traumatic section of the cervical cord leads invariably to disturbances in body temperature, with the temperature either rising or falling.

In a study of 78 cases of traumatic section of the cervical cord, Gardiner and Pembrey (1912) observed that the body temperature in some instances rose, in others fell, and in still others remained at the normal level, although in the latter the capacity for temperature regulation was impaired. The fact that a certain degree of poikilothermia existed was evidenced by the facility with which high temperatures could be reduced by sponging the patients, and low temperatures elevated by applying blankets, hot water bottles, and other heating measures. In one instance the temperature fell terminally to 77.6° F. (Fig. 26-7).

Holmes (1915) has laid emphasis on the development of *hypothermia* following wounds of the cervical cord. Temperatures fell to low levels, sometimes to 80° F. There was a "coldness of death," dryness and cyanosis of the skin, slate color of the face, and stupor or lethargy. Except for the low rectal temperature and reduced pulse rate, the condition was not unlike that of shock.

Hyperthermia following cervical cord injuries was emphasized by Foerster (1935). Characteristically there was an intense reddening of the skin over the entire body, which he attributed to paralysis of vasoconstrictor nerves. Although the vasodilatation was conducive to the loss of body heat, the temperature remained high or continued to mount; hence the hyperthermia was ascribed to anhidrosis, which was a constant feature in all his cases.

Tumors. Tumors of the hypothalamus and upper brainstem are notable for the frequency with which they lead to disturbances in body temperature, and therefore should be suspected when fluctuations in temperature over prolonged periods of time cannot be accounted for by infective or other processes.

Hyperthermia commonly results from damage inflicted on the more rostral part of the hypothalamus, as in a case described by Martin and Cushing (1923) (their Case V).

On admission to the hospital, a man, aged 56, was disoriented and complained of headache and loss of vision. Projectile vomiting occurred. The man's temperature ranged up to 102° F., and postoperatively reached a high level. Death occurred shortly after operation. Postmortem examination revealed a chiasmal glioma that had invaded a considerable portion of the more rostral part of the hypothalamus.

Hypothermia in the presence of tumors involving the hypothalamus is less frequent (Davison and Selby, 1935; Sunderman and Haymaker, 1947).

Hypothermia of 93.2° to 95° F. lasting for weeks was noted by Foerster (1935) in a patient who harbored a pituitary tumor that involved the tuberal region of the hypothalamus. The body temperature fell still lower when the patient was exposed to cold, and gradually rose somewhat when warmth was applied. On occasion, and without apparent reason, the temperature ascended to hyperthermic levels for a day or two, then fell to its accustomed level.

Relative poikilothermia occasionally occurs under conditions in which the hypothalamus is widely occupied by tumor. Such a case was described by Davison and Friedman (1937).

Shortly after delivery, an infant was found to have a body temperature of 95° F., and during the 29 days of life his temperature fluctuated considerably, at times attaining a level above normal. Temperature could be raised by placing hot water bottles in the infant's crib or by placing

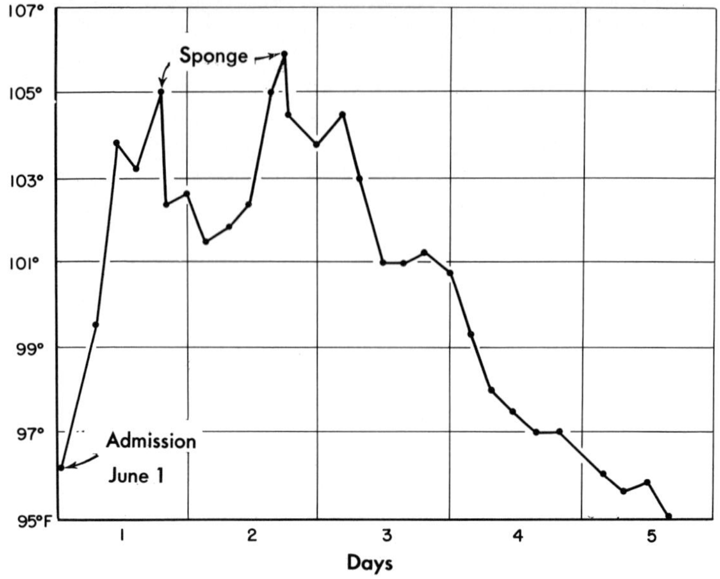

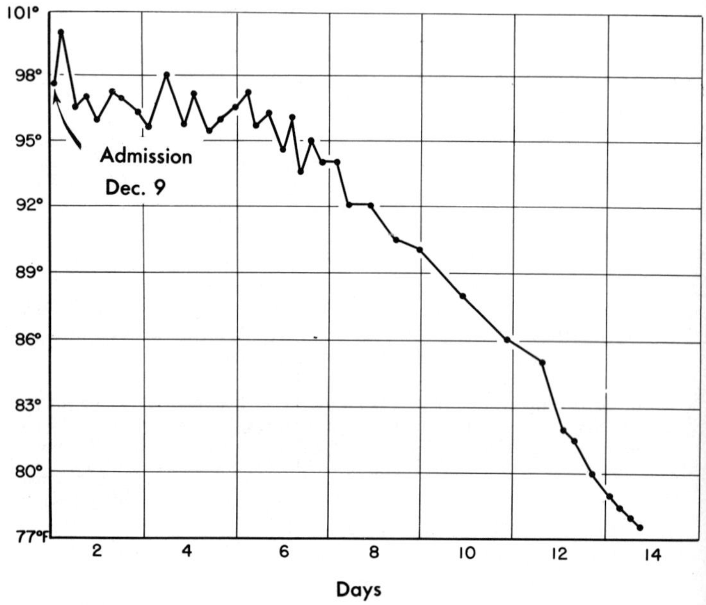

Fig. 26-7. Temperature recordings in two cases of traumatic injury of the cervical cord. Reduction of body temperature by means of sponging is illustrated in the first case (above), and a steady decline of temperature in the other. Injury in the first case occurred in June, and in the second, in December. (Redrawn from Gardiner and Pembrey, 1912.)

the crib near a steam radiator. When the infant was put into a cool room, his temperature promptly fell to below 94° F. Postmortem study revealed an infiltrating neuroblastoma that had destroyed virtually all of the hypothalamus, especially the medial and caudal group of nuclei, leaving intact only the supraoptic nuclei.

SLEEP-WAKEFULNESS AND RELATED STATES

Experimental studies

Wakefulness, light sleep, and paradoxical sleep are the three states of the nervous system recognized as existing in many vertebrates, with each state reflected in certain kinds of waves in EEG recordings (pp. 573-574). When a cat falls asleep it assumes a particular attitude. Often it adopts the attitude of a sphinx, its lowered head resting on its paws, signifying retention of muscular tonicity, at least tonicity of neck muscles. During this stage, cortical and subcortical electrical activity is reduced, and slow waves at high voltage at 3 to 5 c.p.s. appear (the stage of "slow wave" sleep; "light" sleep; "synchronized" sleep). After a lapse of 10 to 20 minutes another state of sleep sets in ("deep" sleep; "paradoxical" sleep; "activated" sleep; "desynchronized" sleep; "REM" [rapid eye movement] sleep; "D" [dreaming] state). The sleeping posture changes; if the head is on the paws, the head leans over until it touches the floor, and the animal may roll over on its side; all muscles are now atonic, including the neck muscles. Peripheral signs of central nervous *activity* then appear (constituting the "paradox"). Over a period of 6 to 7 minutes rapid eye movements, with coinciding pupillary widening, are noted. Twitches occur in distal muscles, the ears, whiskers, tongue, and tail move, and respiration becomes rapid and irregular. EEG waves follow suit in the form of rapid cortical activity. The activity phase over, quietude prevails for about 25 minutes, after which another activity phase of the cycle commences. Paradoxical sleep is deep; the threshold of wakening upon auditory stimulation, for example, is increased. The two states also characterize sleep in man, though electrical activity is much more varied in man than in the cat.

Falling asleep and waking up have been taken into account in varied studies utilizing three main approaches—neurophysiological, histochemical, and neuropharmacological.

Concepts formulated on the basis of results obtained from utilization of one or more of these approaches have varied widely. On the one hand it is held that the two stages of sleep arise from anatomically different structures, the synchronized stage from the neocortex and the desynchronized stage from the pontile region. Cortical action would be the trigger of synchronized sleep, the action being inhibitory on the reticular activating system. (Jouvet, 1962, 1965a, b.) "Sleep," according to this view, "is analagous to the withdrawal of the foot from the accelerator pedal of a car [deactivation of the waking system]; but waking is a more active process, analogous to the application of a brake" (Jouvet, 1967). An alternative hypothesis—the unitary hypothesis—is that the vigilance and the sleep systems are reciprocally connected through inhibitory tonic influences; presumably the two phases of sleep with different arousal thresholds result from different degrees of inhibition produced by the same functional hypnogenic neuronal system upon the vigilance neurons (Hernández Peón, 1965). Or, as postulated by Akert (1965), the determinant of the sleeping and the waking state is the excitatory level of cerebral nerve cells, especially the nerve cells of the cortex, further that this level is under the influence of both an inhibiting and an activating system in the brainstem, and that each, by reciprocal inhibition of its antagonist, can produce particular nuances of sleep-waking behavior. Integral parts of all hypotheses are (1) that the reticular activating system is under the influence of humoral factors and of impulses transmitted from peripheral receptors, (2) that the activating system, through ascending fibers, has an effect on behavior through the medium of the cerebral cortex (via corticobulbar and corticospinal tracts), and (3) that, through descending fibers, the activating system influences the reactivity of peripheral receptors (via the reticulospinal tracts).

The *hypothalamus* has been taken into account in neurophysiological studies. Here, the stream of impulses has been considered as moving in a downward direction. In monkeys a state that "resembled normal sleep" and that lasted 4 to 8 days was induced by lesions situated in the caudolateral part of the hypothalamus bilaterally; the animals had to be handled or shaken to be aroused (Ranson, 1939). The conclusion reached was that wakefulness is largely dependent on hypothalamic "drives," and also that if downward sympathetic discharge is abolished, then "waking" drives, which normally excite the cerebral cortex, are eliminated and somnolence ensues. Another concept came from Nauta (1946), whose work was carried out in rats. Sleep was produced by transection of the mamillary level, and irritability and hyperreactivity (to minor stimuli) by transection at the suprachiasmatic level. Leaving aside the evidence and the reasoning behind it, the conclusion reached was that the caudolateral hypothalamus contains a waking center, and the anterior hypothalamus an active sleep center that exerts an inhibitory influence on the waking center and not directly on the cerebral cortex or on any other major structure. Sleep or a sleep-like state has been induced in cats by electrical stimulation of anterior hypothalamus (Hess, 1925) and basal forebrain (preoptic and diagonal band areas) (Clemente and Sterman, 1963). The agitation and sleeplessness occurring when lesions are made in the anterior hypothalamus may be explainable on the basis that the anterior centers no longer inhibit the activity of the caudolateral hypothalamus (Akert, 1965).

Many investigations of a neurophysiological nature have been oriented to the *reticular activating system*, situated in the upper midbrain (p. 380) and known to induce a waking effect when electrically stimulated; the effect is recognizable both in behavior and in the electroencephalographic record (Magoun, 1958). Moreover, it is known that *sleep* can be induced by electrically stimulating the reticular formation at the midbrain level. Thus, in a monkey it was found that upon stimulating the reticular formation in the region just lateral to the red nucleus, the animal yawned, then fell asleep (Proctor, Knighton, and Churchill, 1957). Moreover, bilateral, circumscribed lesions in this region result in more or less severe impairment in attention and vigilance, both reversible with the passage of time (Sprague and others, 1963). In cats, Bremer and Terzuolo (1954) were able to induce irreversible (EEG) sleep in the forebrain by transecting the brainstem at a level just behind the oculomotor nuclei. To them, functional depression of the reticular formation plays a preponderant role in inducing sleep through the cumulative "defacilitation" of distant structures or, in other words, by the elimination of activating tonus.

The *pons and the medulla oblongata* are also concerned in sleep-wakefulness.

The rostral half of the pons appears to have an activating function, judging from the permanent sleep that occurs following hemisection at a pretrigeminal level (Rossi, Minobe, and Candia, 1963). However, in some completely transected pretrigeminal preparations, a waking, agitated state (with desynchronized rapid cortical activity) predominates, and from studies of such preparations it has been concluded that normally the dorsal part of the medulla oblongata inhibits the midbrain–pontile activating areas (Akert, 1965). In regard to other mechanisms, it is held that a synchronizing or deactivating, hypnogenic influence is tonically exerted by cell aggregates in the caudal brainstem, either through active inhibition of the reticular activating system or by triggering thalamic synchronizing mechanisms, and that sleep ensues when the deactivating influences become strong enough to overcome and supersede the antagonistic activating system of the brainstem (Moruzzi, 1960, 1962-63). Vago-aortic stimuli apparently lead to deactivation of the reticular activating system (Padel and Dell, 1965). There is strong evidence that neurons responsible for the induction of sleep (in the cat) are located within the limits of the nucleus reticularis pontis oralis: "All cats in which the lateral portion [of this nucleus] was injured, with sparing of the most medial areas, showed regular signs of deep sleep" (Zanchetti, 1967). Destruction of the middle third of this nucleus had a similar effect (Rossi, Minobe, and Candia, 1963). Jouvet (1965a, b), on the other hand, favored the nucleus reticularis pontis *caudalis* in this respect, and Hernández Peón (1965), felt that this part of the nucleus played an important role in the muscular hypotonia of the desynchronized phase of sleep.

The *thalamus* also comes into consideration. Sleep, many aspects of which were highly similar to those of natural sleep, has been produced (in cats and rabbits) by electrical stimulation of the intralaminar thalamic nuclei (Hösli and Monnier, 1962; Koella, 1967; Koella, Hess, Jr., and Akert, 1951). Similar results have been obtained from stimulation of other thalamic nuclei (Akimoto and others, 1956; Hess, 1949). Presumably, the sleep thus induced is the result of inhibitory action exerted by intralaminar nuclei on the cerebral cortex. Jouvet (1965a) has shown that frontal areas of the cortex are of particular importance for maintaining the synchronizing activity of thalamocortical systems.

The *caudate nucleus* (which has fiber connections with the intralaminar nuclei) is thought to have an inhibitory action on the cerebral cortex similar to that possessed by the intralaminar thalamic nuclei (Akert, 1965).

Other subsidiary systems are the *limbic cortex* and certain *deeper limbic structures,* such as the hippocampus. Electrical stimulation in these regions has produced sleep or sleep-like states (Parmeggiani, 1960).

Neuropharmacological and histochemical studies also indicate that sleep-wakefulness mechanisms are widespread in the central nervous system. Further, they have shown that cytological chemical factors play a role in sleep organization, sleep control, and the process of wakefulness.

By inserting microcrystals of various substances into numerous parts of the CNS of cats (such as *acetylcholine* and *eserine),* Hernández Peón (1965) was able to induce sleep lasting as long as 3 hours. Effective areas included cerebral cortex in various regions, parts of the limbic system including the cingulate cortex, medial forebrain bundle, medial preoptic region, medial thalamic nuclei, and certain brainstem nuclei. Flow of excitation in the hypnogenic system, according to Hernández Peón, was probably in the rostrocaudal direction.

That the sleep-waking apparatus is widespread is also suggested in studies on *serotonin* level in the CNS. Normally, serotonin level in the brain increases during sleep and is reduced considerably during periods of intense activity, as noted in the hamster (Matussek and Patschke, 1964). Lesions in various locations influence serotonin content in the brain. For instance, serotonin in the forebrain is depleted following lesions of the medial forebrain bundle (Heller, Harvey, and Moore, 1962). It is also depleted following electrical stimulation of the raphe nuclei, located in the lower brainstem (Aghajanian, Rosecrans, and Sheard, 1967). In cats, Jouvet and others (1967) paid particular attention to the *raphe nuclei.* Destruction of 80 percent of these nuclei led to almost complete insomnia over a period of 2 to 3 weeks (the cats sleeping only 6 to 10 percent of the time instead of the usual 60 percent). They noted a correlation between the extent of destruction of the raphe system and the duration of sleep loss, and also a correlation between magnitude of the lesion in this region and degree of reduction in serotonin level in the forebrain. With lesions in raphe nuclei, no significant modification of cerebral norepinephrine was observed. By carrying out stepwise transections of the brainstem and observing the animals for months afterward, it was found that the structures necessary for the periodic appearance of paradoxical sleep lay in the pons, in a region coinciding with the *locus coeruleus.* This locus is rich in monoamino oxidase, an enzyme playing a role in the catabolism of the monoamines. Its neurons contain a heavy concentration of norepinephrine. From their observations, Jouvet and his collaborators suggested that structures which simultaneously control the phasic and tonic phenomena of paradoxical sleep exist at the level of the pons, that the pontile reticular formation appears to be the keystone of paradoxical sleep, and that the role played by norepinephrine in paradoxical sleep probably supplements the part played by serotonin in slow sleep. By contrast, Zanchetti (1967) was able to rule out the raphe nuclei and the locus coeruleus as concerned in the induction of sleep.

In summary, it appears that a large hypnogenic core exists in the central nervous system and that different structures are specialized for the carrying out of different functions in the realm of sleep control. Major hypnogenic areas include thalamus, caudolateral hypothalamus, rostral midbrain, and pontile tegmentum. All other structures play a subordinate role. The trigger mechanism for the maintenance of wakefulness appears to be situated in the tegmentum of the rostral midbrain and the adjoining caudolateral hypothalamus and in the region extending from the mamillary bodies to the inferior surface of the more caudal thalamus.

Clinical observations

The relative importance of various components of the central nervous system to sleep-waking just outlined for animals applies, in the main, to man. However, for accurate localization of the responsible lesion, a greater number of factors need to be taken into consideration, such as type of lesion, rapidity of evolution of the lesion, whether intracranial pressure is increased, and whether, in the event of an expanding lesion, distant effects have been brought about through tissue compression.

Lesions of cerebral cortex and white matter. In cerebral hemispheric expanding tumors, a sleep-like state may be encountered (Davison and Demuth, 1945a), but because of the size of the tumor in most of these cases, it is likely that the somnolence represents a (distant) compressive effect on the upper brainstem. Extensive infarction of the cortex bilaterally has other consequences, for example, development of an akinetic syndrome.

Damage of the thalamus and environs. Sleep disturbances are frequent in parkinsonian patients. Many of them complain of nocturnal reduction in sleep, induction insomnia, and, occasionally, drowsiness during the daytime. Thalamotomy frequently modifies these disturbances. In the acute postoperative phase there may be changes ranging from a state of extremely prolonged vigilance to hypersomnia. During this phase, inversion of the sleep-wakefulness rhythm is also common. Total and irreducible insomnia may occasionally occur following thalamotomy. Bricolo (1967), who reported such a case, concluded that the thalamus is involved in the regulation of the sleep-wakefulness rhythm and that nonspecific nuclei (intralaminar nuclei) of the thalamus may be instrumental in the implementation of sleep-inducing mechanisms. After initial profound torpor following infarction of the intralaminar nuclei bilaterally, extending downward to the retromamillary level of both sides (in the bed of the thalamoperforating arteries), hypersomnia may be noted for a week or so, then apathy, indifference, and so on (Castaigne and Escourolle, 1967). As to hemorrhage limited to the thalamus and involving intralaminar nuclei, profound coma is the rule at the start, and transitory hypersomnia later on. Tumor of the thalamus and neighboring structures may, in occasional instances, lead to hypersomnia if situated bilaterally and medially and not far from the hypothalamus. However, other clinical disturbances overshadow the somnolence. (Castaigne and Escourolle, 1967; Davison and Demuth, 1945b.)

Infectious states. Von Economo (1929), in his account of the pandemics of encephalitis occurring in 1917 and 1920, described two chief clinical types of disturbance. One was characterized by prolonged somnolence and ophthalmoplegia; the responsible lesion was considered to be in the tegmentum of the midbrain. In the other type, insomnia, agitation, and hyperkinesias were described as the chief features; here, the responsible lesion was found to be located in the more anterior part of the hypothalamus. In analyzing all of von Economo's cases, Akert (1965) could find

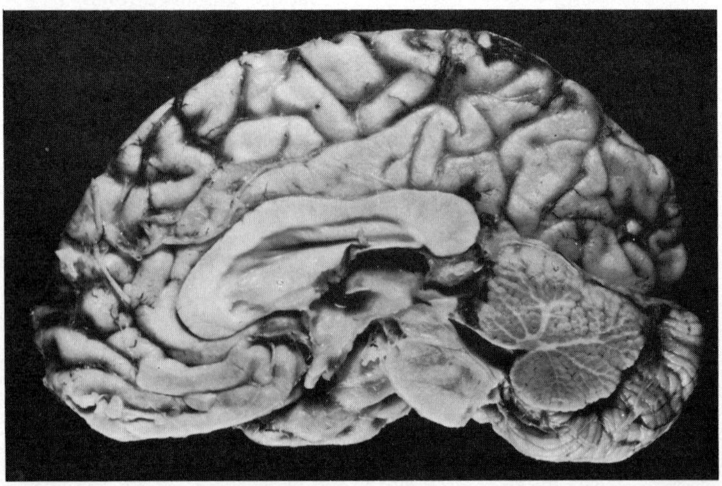

Fig. 26-8. The brain in a case of prolonged somnolence. The posterior part of the hypothalamus and the upper midbrain are extremely atrophic. The mamillary body has virtually disappeared. (Courtesy Dr. R. B. Richter and Dr. E. F. Traut, Chicago.)

no clear instance of insomnia. However, he was in agreement with von Economo with respect to the site of the damage responsible for the agitation and the hyperkinesias.

Probably the most extensive destruction of the hypothalamus in lethargic encephalitis was that reported by Richter and Traut (1940).

After several days of progressive drowsiness, the patient, a woman aged 26, sank into almost unbroken sleep that lasted 5 years. There were periods, varying from one-half to one hour, when she was awake and alert. When she was raised to the sitting position her head would fall forward on her chest, choking her, and her shoulders would slump toward her knees. She resisted any attempt to change her position. Temperature regulation was not altered but the pulse rate was persistently elevated. At autopsy, advanced atrophy was noted in the region of the caudal hypothalamus and rostral midbrain (Fig. 26-8). The anterior part of the hypothalamus was relatively free from damage (Fig. 26-9, *A*). In the lateral part of the hypothalamus the tuberomamillary nucleus was virtually intact, but some nerve cell loss together with gliosis was noted in the lateral tuberal nuclei. The ventromedial nucleus was suggestively atrophic. Caudally the changes were extreme, the posterior hypothalamic nucleus and the mamillary nuclei having completely disappeared (Fig. 26-9, *B*). Fornix and the fields of Forel (of the subthalamus) were the seat of gliosis. In the midbrain there was advanced demyelination of the tegmentum and considerable destruction of the substantia nigra. The globus pallidus was also severely injured. Thalamus and striatum were relatively spared.

Metastatic abscess in the hypothalamic-mesencephalic junctional area (in bacterial endocarditis) may also be a cause of hypersomnia (Lucksch, 1924).

Infarction. Infarction in the region of the tegmentothalamic axis may give rise to equally impressive disturbances in sleep-waking. In such a case, hypersomnia with inversion of the sleep-waking rhythm lasted 2 years, and complete hypersomnia for the following year. (Façon, Steriade, and Wertheim, 1958.) Cases of a similar nature are on record (Castaigne and Escourolle, 1967; van Bogaert, 1926).

Multiple sclerosis. Hypersomnia is rare in multiple sclerosis, but can occur as a

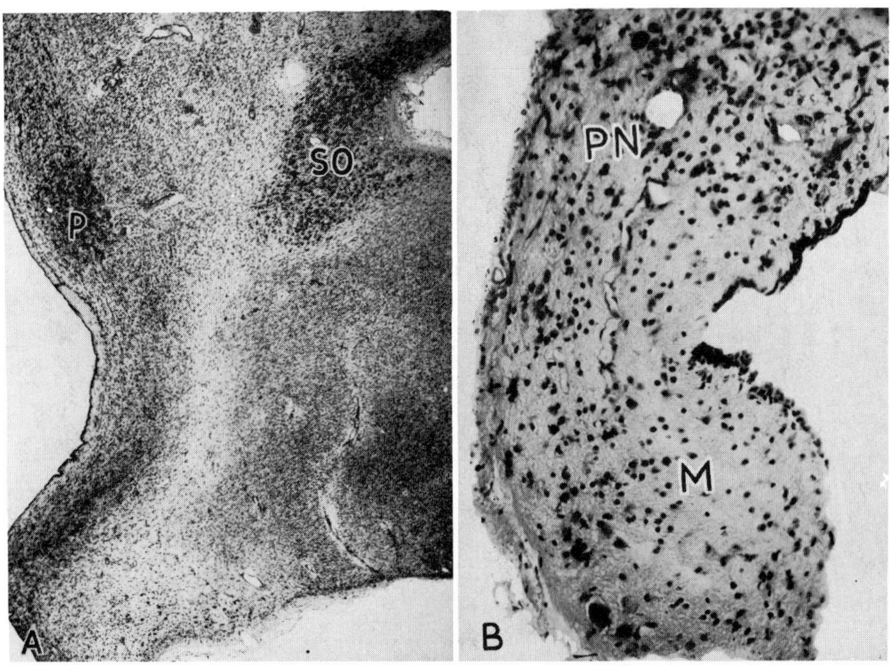

Fig. 26-9. From brain illustrated in Fig. 26-8. In **A,** which is a somewhat oblique section through the anterior part of the hypothalamus, the supraoptic *(SO)* and the paraventricular nuclei *(P)* are relatively intact. In **B,** the mamillary body *(M)* and the portion of the hypothalamus above it, including the posterior hypothalamic nucleus *(PN),* are converted into a glial scar. (Courtesy Dr. R. B. Richter and Dr. E. F. Traut, Chicago.)

leading symptom when lesions develop in the upper midbrain and adjoining diencephalon, as illustrated in Fig. 26-10. A case of a similar nature was described by Castaigne and Escourolle (1967).

Tumors. Hypersomnia as an initial or early symptom may occur in tumors involving hypothalamus, midbrain, or thalamus. Some examples follow.

In their monograph on pathological sleep associated with tumors in the region of the third ventricle, Fulton and Bailey (1929) record the case of a woman, aged 28, who for over a period of five years had had attacks of somnolence from which she could easily be aroused. (She also had polyuria and amenorrhea and was considerably obese.) While carrying on an animated conversation she would often drop off to sleep. During the month prior to admission to hospital, the somnolence had been almost continuous. The responsible lesion was found to be a meningeal sarcoma, situated in the floor of the third ventricle just above the pituitary stalk. Much of the tuberal region was destroyed. The mamillary bodies were infiltrated by tumor cells. The ventricles were of normal size.

Suprasellar craniopharyngioma destroying most of the hypothalamus and leading to dilatation of the rostral end of the aqueduct can have the same clinical effect (Gagel, 1936), as may also craniopharyngioma of smaller size, in the absence of an increase in intracranial pressure (Castaigne and Escourolle, 1967). Insomnia may also result from tumor in this region, for example, adamantinoma (Davison and Demuth, 1964a).

Cox (1937) records the case of a woman, aged 44, who for several months had been sleeping excessively (together with other disorders, such as hemiplegia and extraocular muscle palsy). When awakened she was alert. Her responses were intelligent, and memory was fully retained. Gradually the drowsiness became progressively worse and death ensued. A tumor (glioma), 3 cm. in diameter and cystic, was found in the midbrain. It extended to within 2 mm. of the uninvolved and patent aqueduct. The ventricular system was not dilated. The tegmental region, red nucleus, and substantia nigra of the right side were heavily damaged, and the tumor extended into the right side of the hypothalamus, encroaching on but not invading the mamillary body. Caudally it extended to the pons.

Tumor of the tectum of the midbrain may also be manifested by hypersomnia and other disturbances closely resembling those observed in encephalitis lethargica (Bornstein, 1933). Somnolence is said to occur in about 30 percent of cases of pineal tumor (in thirty-one of 105 cases) (Gabriel, 1935), but there is the question whether the disturbance was, instead, a reduction in consciousness brought about by a sudden increase in intracranial pressure from rapid blockage of the cerebral aqueduct.

Rowe (1935) described a case of hypersomnia in which a tumor occupied the thalamus and the rostral part of the midbrain but spared the hypothalamus. The periventricular system adjacent to the thalamus was bilaterally destroyed. The medial dorsal, centrum medianum, and anterior nuclei, as well as the pulvinar, were damaged, in that order of decreasing severity.

Damage of the pons and medulla oblongata. Infarction of the pons, especially

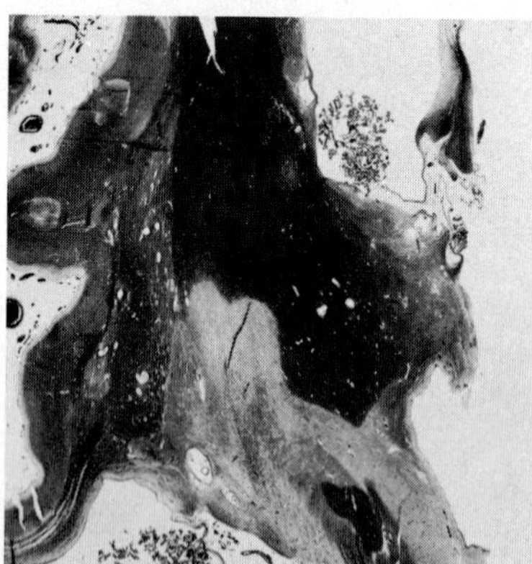

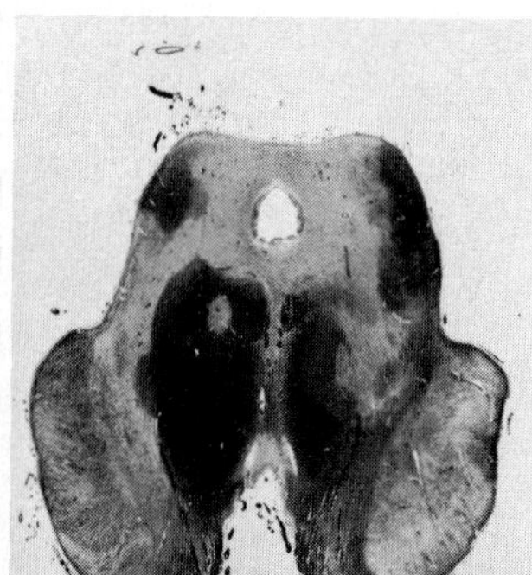

Fig. 26-10. Multiple sclerosis involving (to the left) the wall of the third ventricle, lower internal capsule and midbrain, and (to the right) the periaqueductal area, tegmentum of the midbrain, and basis pedunculi, bilaterally. (The plaques correspond to the pale areas, unstained by the myelin method used.) The oldest lesion is the one around the aqueduct. The patient, a woman aged 22 years at the time of death, became very sleepy at the age of 18, and a few months later she had diplopia (due to involvement of the third nerve and partly the fourth) and difficulty in walking. (Courtesy Dr. Richard Lindenberg, Baltimore.)

when widespread, usually leads to coma or to akinetic mutism, and to other disturbances as well; however, in rare instances, intermittent hypersomnia is a leading symptom (Castaigne and Escourolle, 1967). Tumors involving pons alone or both pons and medulla oblongata, and giving rise to an increase in intracranial pressure, occasionally are manifested by hypersomnia. In cerebellar hemangioblastoma involving the dorsal pons and/or medulla oblongata—sometimes predominantly the periventricular gray—spells of sleepiness, periodic deep dreamless sleep, and inversion of sleep-waking rhythm may be among the initial disturbances (Davison and Demuth, 1946b).

In summary, disturbances in sleep-waking result from lesions involving various levels of the neuraxis. This being so, localization of the responsible lesion requires that consideration be given to the clinical signs and symptoms that accompany the sleep-waking disturbances. In most cases the responsible lesion is situated in the upper midbrain.

REFERENCES

Adams, J. H., Daniel, P. M., and Prichard, M. M. L. 1966. Transection of the pituitary stalk in man: anatomical changes in the pituitary glands of 21 patients. J. Neurol. Neurosurg. Psychiat. **29**:545-555.

Aghajanian, G. K., Rosecrans, J. A., and Sheard, M. H. 1967. Serotonin: release in the forebrain by stimulation of midbrain raphé. Science **156**: 402-403.

Akert, K. 1965. The anatomical substrate of sleep. Progr. Brain Res. **18**:9-19.

Akimoto, H., Yamaguchi, N., Okabe, K., Nakagawa, T., Nakamura, I., Abe, K., Torii, H., and Masahashi, K. 1956. On the sleep induced through electrical stimulation on dog thalamus. Folia Psychiat. Neurol. Jap. **10**:117-146.

Allen, I. M. 1953. Variations of function in the hypothalamus and its neighbourhood following head injury. New Zeal. Med. J. **52**:478-487.

Anand, B. K., and Brobeck, J. R. 1951. Hypothalamic control of food intake in rats and cats. Yale J. Biol. Med. **24**:123-140.

Anand, B. K., Chhina, G. S., and Singh, B. 1962. Effect of glucose on the activity of hypothalamic "feeding centers." Science **138**:597-598.

Anand, B. K., and Dua, S. 1955. Blood sugar changes induced by electrical stimulation of the hypothalamus in the cat. Indian J. Med. Res. **43**:123-127.

Anand, B. K., and Dua, S. 1958. Hypothalamic control over water consumption in the rat. Indian J. Med. Res. **46**:426-430.

Anand, B. K., Dua, S., and Chhina, G. S. 1961. Effect of neocortical lesions over food intake. Indian J. Med. Res. **49**:491-497.

Anand, B. K., Dua, S., and Singh, B. 1961. Electrical activity of the hypothalamic "feeding centres" under the effect of changes in blood chemistry. EEG Clin. Neurophysiol. **13**:54-59.

Anand, B. K., Subberwal, W., Manchanda, S. K., and Singh, B. 1961. Glucoreceptor mechanism in the hypothalamic feeding centres. Indian J. Med. Res. **49**:717-724.

Anderson, E. 1966. Adrenocorticotrophin-releasing hormone in peripheral blood: increase during stress. Science **152**:379-380.

Anderson, E., Rioch, D. McK., and Haymaker, W. 1952. Disturbances in blood sugar regulation in animals subjected to transection of the brain stem. Acta Neuroveg. **5**:132-164.

Andersson, B., and McCann, S. M. 1956. The effect of hypothalamic lesions on the water intake of the dog. Acta Physiol. Scand. **35**:312-320.

Arees, E. A., and Mayer, J. 1967. Anatomical connections between medial and lateral regions of the hypothalamus concerned with food intake. Science **157**:1574-1575.

Bailey, P. 1948. Intracranial tumors, ed. 2. Springfield, Illinois, Charles C Thomas, Publisher, pp. 88-112, 185-192.

Bailey, P. 1963. Tumors of the nervous system. In Kelley, V., editor: Brennemann's practice of pediatrics, vol. 4, chap. 21. Baltimore, W. F. Prior Co., Inc.

Bain, H. W., Darte, J. M. M., Keith, W. S., and Kruyff, E. 1966. The diencephalic syndrome of early infancy due to silent brain tumor: with special reference to treatment. Pediatrics **38**: 473-482.

Barlow, E. D., and De Wardener, H. E. 1959. Compulsive water drinking. Quart. J. Med., n.s. **28**:235-258.

Bauer, H. G. 1959. Endocrine and metabolic conditions related to pathology in the hypothalamus; a review. J. Nerv. Ment. Dis. **128**:323-338.

Beaton, L. E., and Herrmann, J. D. 1945. Hyperthermia following injury of the preoptic region: report of a case. Arch. Neurol. Psychiat. **53**: 150-151.

Beattie, J., and Sheehan, D. 1934. The effects of hypothalamic stimulation on gastric motility. J. Physiol. **81**:218-227.

Beernink, F. J., and McKay, D. G. 1962. Pituitary insufficiency associated with pregnancy, panhypopituitarism, and diabetes insipidus. Amer. J. Obstet. Gynec. **84**:318-338.

Bellows, R. T., and Van Wagenen, W. P. 1939. The effect of resection of the olfactory, gustatory and trigeminal nerves on water drinking in dogs without and with diabetes insipidus. Amer. J. Physiol. **126**:13-19.

Benzinger, T. H. 1964. The thermal homeostasis of man. In Hughes, G. M., editor: Homeostasis and feedback mechanisms. Symposia of the Society for Experimental Biology, No. 18. New York, Academic Press, Inc., Publishers, pp. 49-80.

Berry, R. G., and Schlezinger, N. S. 1959. Rathke-cleft cysts. A.M.A. Arch. Neurol. **1**:48-58.

Biemond, A. 1949. Un nouveau syndrôme hypothalamique: oligurie intermittente avec oedeme du visage et troubles sexuels. Folia Psychiat. Neurol. Neurochim. Neerl. **52**:343-347.

Bornstein, B. 1933. Tumor des Tectum mesencephali unter dem Bilde der Encephalitis lethargica. Jahrb. Psychiat. Neurol. **49**:46-56.

Bremer, F., and Terzuolo, C. 1954. Contribution à l'étude des mécanismes physiologiques du maintien de l'activité vigile du cerveau. Arch. Internat. Physiol. **62**:157-178.

Bricolo, A. 1967. Insomnia after bilateral stereotactic thalamotomy in man. J. Neurol. Neurosurg. Psychiat. **30**:154-158.

Brobeck, J. R. 1957. Neural control of hunger, appetite, and satiety. Yale J. Biol. Med. **29**: 565-574.

Brutkowski, S., Fonberg, E., Kreiner, J., Mempel, E., and Sychowa, B. 1962. Aphagia and adipsia in a dog with bilateral complete lesion of the amygdaloid complex. Acta Biol. Exp. **22**:43-50.

Castaigne, P., and Escourolle, R. 1967. Etude topographique des lésions anatomiques dans les hypersomnies. Rev. Neurol. **1**:547-584.

Christ, J. F. 1966. Nerve supply, blood supply and cytology of the neurohypophysis. In Harris, G. W., and Donovan, B. T., editors: The pituitary gland, vol. 3. Berkeley, University of California Press, pp. 62-130.

Ciccarelli, E. C., and Huttenlocher, P. R. 1967. Diencephalic tumor: a cause of infantile nystagmus and cachexia. Arch. Ophthal. **78**:350-353.

Clemente, C. D., and Sterman, M. B. 1963. Cortical synchronization and sleep patterns in acute restrained and chronic behaving cats induced by basal forebrain stimulation. EEG Clin. Neurophysiol., suppl. **24**:172-187.

Cooper, K. E. 1966. Temperature regulation and the hypothalamus. Brit. Med. Bull. **22**:238-242.

Cooper, K. E., Cranston, W. I., and Honour, A. J. 1965. Effects of intraventricular and intrahypothalamic injection of noradrenaline and 5-HT on body temperature in conscious rabbits. J. Physiol. **181**:852-864.

Cox, L. B. 1937. Tumours of the base of the brain: their relation to pathological sleep and other changes in the conscious state. Med. J. Aust. **2**:742-774.

Cranston, W. I. 1966. Temperature regulation. Brit. Med. J. **2**:69-75.

Critchley, M., and Ironside, R. N. 1926. The pituitary adamantinomata. Brain **49**:437-481.

Crosby, E. C., and Woodburne, R. T. 1940. The comparative anatomy of the preoptic area and the hypothalamus. Res. Publ. Ass. Res. Nerv. Ment. Dis., Proc. **20**:52-169.

Cushing, H. 1932. Peptic ulcers and the interbrain. Surg. Gynec. Obstet. **55**:1-34.

Daly, D. D., and Mulder, D. W. 1957. Gelastic epilepsy. Neurology **7**:189-192.

Daniel, P. M., and Treip, C. S. 1966. Lesions of the pituitary gland associated with head injuries. In Harris, G. W., and Donovan, B. T., editors: The pituitary gland, vol. 2. Berkeley, University of California Press, pp. 519-534.

Darmady, E. M., Offer, J., Prince, J., and Stranack, F. 1964. The proximal convoluted tubule in the renal handling of water. Lancet **2**:1254-1257.

Davey, L. M., Kaada, B. R., and Fulton, J. F. 1950. Effects on gastric secretion of frontal lobe stimulation. Res. Publ. Ass. Res. Nerv. Ment. Dis., Proc. **29**:617-627.

Davis, R. A., Brooks, F. P., and Steckel, D. C. 1968. Gastric secretory changes after anterior hypothalamic lesions. Amer. J. Physiol. **215**:600-604.

Davison, C., and Demuth, E. L. 1945a. Disturbances in sleep mechanism: a clinicopathologic study. I. Lesions at the cortical level. Arch. Neurol. Psychiat. **53**:399-406.

Davison, C., and Demuth, E. L. 1945b. Disturbances in sleep mechanism: a clinicopathologic study. II. Lesions at the corticodiencephalic level. Arch. Neurol. Psychiat. **54**:241-255.

Davison, C., and Demuth, E. L. 1946a. Disturbances in sleep mechanism: a clinicopathologic study. III. Lesions at the diencephalic level (hypothalamus). Arch. Neurol. Psychiat. **55**: 111-125.

Davison, C., and Demuth, E. L. 1946b. Disturbances in sleep mechanism: a clinicopathologic study. IV. Lesions at the mesencephalometencephalic level. Arch. Neurol. Psychiat. **55**:126-138.

Davison, C., and Friedman, E. D. 1937. Poikilothermia with hypothalamic lesions: a clinicopathologic study. Arch. Neurol. Psychiat. **38**: 1271-1281.

Davison, C., and Selby, N. E. 1935. Hypothermia in cases of hypothalamic lesions. Arch. Neurol. Psychiat. **33**:570-591.

de Schweinitz, G. E. 1923. Concerning certain ocular aspects of pituitary body disorders, mainly exclusive of the usual central and peripheral hemianopic field defects. Trans. Ophthal. Soc. U.K. **43**:12-109.

Dott, N. 1936. Bitemporal hemianopia in relation to hydrocephalic distention of the third ventricle. Brit. Med. J. **2**:296.

Dott, N. 1938. Surgical aspects of the hypothalamus. In Clark, W. E. Le G., and others: The hypothalamus: morphological, functional, clinical, and surgical aspects. London, Oliver & Boyd, Ltd., pp. 131-185.

Druckman, R., and Chao, D. 1957. Laughter in epilepsy. Neurology **7**:26-36.

Dugan, S., and Holliday, M. A. 1967. Water intoxication in two infants following the voluntary ingestion of excessive fluids. Pediatrics **39**:418-420.

Edmondson, H. T., Gindin, R. A., and Peebles, G. C. 1968. Cerebral lesions as a cause of esophageal ulceration. Surgery **64**:720-727.

Elkington, S. G. 1968. Pituitary adenoma: preoperative symptomatology in a series of 260 patients. Brit. J. Ophthal. **52**:322-328.

Erickson, T. C. 1939. Neurogenic hyperthermia. (A clinical syndrome and its treatment.) Brain **62**:172-190.

Espinosa, R. E., and Randall, R. V. 1968. Early symptoms and signs of chromophobe adenoma. Med. Clin. N. Amer. **52**:827-834.

Façon, E., Steriade, M., and Wertheim, N. 1958.

Hypersomnie prolongée engendrée par les lésions bilatérales du système activateur médial: le syndrome thrombotique de la bifurcation du tronc basilare. Rev. Neurol. **2**:117-133.

Feldberg, W. 1967. Neue experimentelle Ergebnisse im Hypothalamus. Acta Neuroveg. **30**:169-189.

Feldberg, W., and Myers, R. D. 1963. A new concept of temperature regulation by amines in the hypothalamus. Nature **200**:1325.

Feldman, S. 1965. Excitability and projections of sensory pathways to the hypothalamus. Acta Physiol. Acad. Sci. Hung. **26**:161.

Fitzsimons, J. T. 1966. The hypothalamus and drinking. Brit. Med. Bull. **22**:232-237.

Flicker, D. J. 1943. Pubertas praecox in a female infant caused by ventricular cyst: report of a case. J. Nerv. Ment. Dis. **98**:42-47.

Foerster, O. 1935. Ueber Störungen der Thermoregulation bei Erkrankungen des Gehirns und Rückenmarks und bei Eingriffen am Zentralnervensystem. J. Psychiat. Neurol. **52**:1-14.

Foerster, O. 1936. Symptomatologie der Erkrankungen des Rückenmarks und seiner Wurzeln. In Bumke, O., and Foerster, O., editors: Handbuch der Neurologie, vol. 5. Berlin, Springer-Verlag, pp. 1-400.

François, J., and Neetens, A. 1968. Oculomotor paralyses and tumors of the pituitary gland. Confin. Neurol. **30**:239-252.

Frazier, C. H. 1936. Tumor involving the frontal lobe alone: a symptomatic survey of one hundred and five verified cases. Arch. Neurol. Psychiat. **35**:525-571.

Frazier, C. H., and Alpers, B. J. 1934. Tumors of Rathke's cleft. Arch. Neurol. Psychiat. **32**:973-984.

Freeman, W. J., and Davis, D. D. 1959. Effects on cats of conductive hypothalamic cooling. Amer. J. Physiol. **197**:145-148.

French, J. D., Longmire, R. L., Porter, R. W., and Movius, H. J. 1953. Extravagal influences on gastric hydrochloric acid secretion induced by stress stimuli. Surgery **34**:621-632.

French, J. D., Porter, R. W., Cavanaugh, E. B., and Longmire, R. L. 1954. Experimental observations on "psychosomatic" mechanisms: gastrointestinal disturbances. Arch. Neurol. Psychiat. **72**:267-281.

Fulton, J. F., and Bailey, P. 1929. Tumors in the region of the third ventricle: their diagnosis and relation to pathological sleep. J. Nerv. Ment. Dis. **69**:1-25, 261-277.

Futcher, T. B. 1904. A clinical report of nine cases of diabetes insipidus. Trans. Ass. Amer. Physicians **19**:247-286.

Gabriel, P. 1935. Les pinéalomes (étude anatomoclinique). Paris, Maloine et Cie.

Gagel, O. 1936. Symptomatologie der Erkrankungen des Hypothalamus. In Bumke, O., and Foerster, O., editors: Handbuch der Neurologie, vol. 5. Berlin, Springer-Verlag, pp. 482-522.

Gardiner, H., and Pembrey, M. S. 1912. Observations on the temperature of man after traumatic section of the spinal cord. Guy's Hosp. Rep., London **66**:87-108.

Glick, S. M., Roth, J., Yalow, R. S., and Berson, S. A. 1965. The regulation of growth hormone secretion. Recent Progr. Hormone Res. **21**:241-283.

Gonzalez, C. F., Finberg, L., and Bluestein, D. D. 1964. Electrolyte concentration during acute infections: observations in infants and children. Amer. J. Dis. Child. **107**:476-482.

Gottschalk, P. C., and Thomas, J. E. 1966. Heat stroke. Mayo Clin. Proc. **41**:470-482.

Green, J. R., Buchan, G. C., Alvord, E. C., Jr., and Swanson, A. G. 1967. Hereditary and idiopathic types of diabetes insipidus. Brain **90**: 707-714.

Guillemin, R. 1965. Hypothalamic polypeptides stimulating the secretion of pituitary hormones. Proc. 23d Internat. Congr. Physiol. Sci., Tokyo, abstr. 59.

Hammel, H. T. 1968. Regulation of internal body temperature. Ann. Rev. Physiol. **30**:641-710.

Hankiss, J., Keszthelyi, M., and Siro, B. 1961. A new type of diabetes insipidus due to increased hormone inactivation: its incidence in clinical material. Amer. J. Med. Sci. **242**:605-611.

Hardy, J. D. 1961. Physiology of temperature regulation. Physiol. Rev. **41**:521-606.

Hardy, J. D., Hellon, R. F., and Sutherland, K. 1964. Temperature-sensitive neurones in the dog's hypothalamus. J. Physiol. **175**:242-253.

Harlin, R. S., and Givens, J. R. 1968. Sheehan's syndrome associated with eclampsia and a small sella turcica. Southern Med. J. **61**:909-911.

Harris, G. W., and George, R. 1969. Neurohumoral control of the adenohypophysis and the regulation of the secretion of TSH, ACTH and growth hormone, In Haymaker, W., Anderson, E., and Nauta, W. J. H., editors: The hypothalamus. Springfield, Illinois, Charles C Thomas, Publisher, pp. 326-388.

Harris, G. W., Reed, M., and Fawcett, C. P. 1966. Hypothalamic releasing factors and the control of anterior pituitary function. Brit. Med. Bull. **22**:266-272.

Heller, A., Harvey, J. A., and Moore, R. Y. 1962. A demonstration of a fall in brain serotonin following central nervous system lesions in the rat. Biochem. Pharmacol. **11**:859-866.

Hemingway, A. 1963. Shivering. Physiol. Rev. **43**: 397-422.

Hernández Peón, R. 1965. Central neuro-humoral transmission in sleep and wakefulness. Progr. Brain Res. **18**:96-117.

Hess, W. R. 1925. Über die Wechselbeziehungen zwischen psychischen und vegetativen Funktionen: III, Zentrale Wirkung vegetativer Reizstoffe. Schweiz. Arch. Neurol. Psychiat. **16**:285-306.

Hess, W. R. 1949. Das Zwischenhirn: Syndrome, Lokalisationen, Funktionen. Basel, Schwabe & Co.

Hetherington, A. W., and Ranson, S. W. 1942. The relation of various hypothalamic lesions to adiposity in the rat. J. Comp. Neurol. **76**:475-499.

Holmes, G. 1915. The Goulstonian Lectures on spinal injuries of warfare. Brit. Med. J. **2**:769-774.

Hösli, L., and Monnier, M. 1962. Schlaf- und Wachwirkungen des intralaminaren Thalamus: Reizparameter und Koagulationsbefunde beim

Kaninchen. Pflügers Arch. Ges. Physiol. **275:** 439-451.

Iggo, A. 1959. Cutaneous heat and cold receptors with slowly conducting (C) afferent fibres. Quart. J. Exp. Physiol. **44:**362-370.

Iggo, A. 1963. An electrophysiological analysis of afferent fibres in primate skin. Acta Neuroveg. **24:**225-240.

Iggo, A. 1964. Temperature discrimination in the skin. Nature **204:**481-483.

Ishikawa, K., Ott, K., Eldred, E., and Stuart, D. 1967. Response of motoneurons to hypothalamic stimulation and its relation to thermoregulatory behavior. Amer. J. Phys. Med. **46:**1290-1301.

Jewell, P. A., and Verney, E. B. 1957. An experimental attempt to determine the site of the neurohypophysial osmoreceptors in the dog. Philos. Trans. Roy. Soc., B **240:**197-324.

Jouvet, M. 1962. Recherches sur les structures nerveuses et les mécanismes responsables de différents phases du sommeil physiologiques. Arch. Ital. Biol. **100:**125-206.

Jouvet, M. 1965a. Paradoxical sleep—a study of its nature and mechanisms. Progr. Brain Res. **18:**20-62.

Jouvet, M., editor. 1965b. Aspects anatomo-fonctionnels de la physiologie du sommeil. Paris, Publications du Centre National de la Recherche Scièntifique, pp. 613-650.

Jouvet, M. 1967. The sleeping brain. Science J. **3:** 105-110.

Jouvet, M., Bobillier, P., Pujol, J. F., and Renault, J. 1967. Suppression du sommeil et diminution de la serotonine cérébrale par lésion du système du raphé chez le chat. C. R. Acad. Sci. **264:** 360-362.

Kahn, E. A. 1963. Heat stroke and temperature control. J. Mich. Med. Soc. **62:**292-296.

Kastin, A. J., Lipsett, M. B., Ommaya, A. K., and Moser, J. M., Jr. 1965. Asymptomatic hypernatremia: physiological and clinical study. Amer. J. Med. **38:**306-315.

Kennaway, E. L., and Mottram, J. C. 1919. Observations upon two cases of diabetes insipidus: with an account of the literature relating to an association between the pituitary gland and this disease. Quart. J. Med. **12:**225-258.

Kernohan, J. W., and Sayre, G. P. 1955. Atlas of tumor pathology, sect. 10, fasc. 38; tumors of the pituitary gland and infundibulum. Washington, D. C., Armed Forces Institute of Pathology.

Kleeman, C. R., and Fichman, M. P. 1967. The clinical physiology of water metabolism. New Eng. J. Med. **277:**1300-1308.

Koella, W. P. 1967. Sleep, its nature and physiology. Springfield, Illinois, Charles C Thomas, Publisher.

Koella, W. P., Hess, R., Jr., and Akert, K. 1951. Zur Technik der Registrierung hirnelektrischer Erscheinungen im Rahmen des subcorticalen Reizversuches bei der Katze. Helv. Physiol. Acta **9:**316-325.

Laqueur, G. L., McCann, S. M., Schreiner, L. H., Rosenberg, E., Rioch, D. McK., and Anderson, E. 1955. Alterations in adrenal cortical and ovarian activity following hypothalamic lesions. Endocrinology **57:**44-54.

Launay, C., Ribadeau-Dumas, C., Maillard, L., and Chadoutand, L. 1946. La form cachectisante du craniopharyngiome. Arch. Franç. Pédiat. **3:**581-584.

Lee, D. H. K. 1964. Heat and cold effects and their control. Public Health Monogr. No. 72. Washington, D. C., U. S. Government Printing Office.

Lee, D. H. K., and Henschel, A. 1966. Effects of physiological and clinical factors in response to heat. Ann. N. Y. Acad. Sci. **134:**743-749.

Lee, J. 1966. Neurohypophyseal hormones: their role in oedema of man, with reference to their action on the alimentary canal and on metabolism. In Harris, G. W., and Donovan, B. T., editors: The pituitary gland, vol. 3. Berkeley, University of California Press, pp. 517-534.

List, C. F., Dowman, C. E., Bagchi, B. K., and Bebin, J. 1958. Posterior hypothalamic hamartomas and gangliogliomas causing precocious puberty. Neurology **8:**164-174.

Lucksch, F. 1924. Ueber das "Schlafzentrum." Z. Ges. Neurol. Psychiat. **93:**83-94.

Lundbaek, K., Malmros, R., and Mogensen, E. F. 1960. The effect of pituitary stalk section in man. Acta Med. Scand. **166:**9-15.

Magoun, H. W. 1958. The waking brain. Springfield, Illinois, Charles C Thomas, Publisher.

Malamud, N., Haymaker, W., and Custer, R. P. 1946. Heat stroke: a clinicopathologic study of 125 fatal cases. Mil. Surgeon **99:**397-449.

Martin, F. I. 1959. Familial diabetes insipidus. Quart. J. Med. n.s. **28:**573-582.

Martin, P., and Cushing, H. 1923. Primary gliomas of the chiasm and optic nerves in their intracranial portion. Arch. Ophthal. **52:**209-241.

Matsui, N., and Plager, J. E. 1966. Rate of blood glucose fall as determinant factor in insulin-induced adrenocortical stimulation. Endocrinology **79:**737-744.

Matussek, N., and Patschke, U. 1964. Beziehungen des Schlaf- und Wachrhythmus zum Noradrenalin- und Serotoningehalt im Zentralnervensystem von Hamstern. Med. Exper. **11:**81-87.

Mayer, J. 1953. Genetic, traumatic and environmental factors in the genesis of obesity. Physiol. Rev. **33:**472-508.

Mayer, J. 1960. The hypothalamic control of gastric hunger contractions as a component of the mechanism of regulation of food intake. Amer. J. Clin. Nutr. **8:**547-561.

Mayer, J., Hagman, N. C., Marshall, N. B., and Stoops, A. J. 1955. Fat metabolism in three forms of obesity: hepatic lipogenesis in vitro. Amer. J. Physiol. **181:**501-503.

McCann, S. M., Antunes-Rodrigues, J., and Dhariwal, A. P. S. 1965. Physiology and chemistry of hypothalamic factors which influence gonadotrophin secretion. Proc. 23d Internat. Congr. Physiol. Sci., Tokyo, abstr. 60, p. 42.

Montemurro, D. G., and Stevenson, J. A. F. 1956. The localization of hypothalamic structures in rat influencing water consumption. Yale J. Biol. Med. **28:**396-403.

Morrison, S. D., Barrnett, R. J., and Mayer, J. 1958. Localization of lesions in the lateral hypothalamus of rats with induced adipsia and aphagia. Amer. J. Physiol. **193**:230-234.

Moruzzi, G. 1960. Synchronizing influences of the brain stem and the inhibitory mechanisms underlying the production of sleep by sensory stimulation. EEG Clin. Neurophysiol., suppl. **13**: 231-256.

Moruzzi, G. 1962-63. Active processes in the brain stem during sleep. Harvey Lect. **58**:233-297.

Myers, R. D. 1968. Discussion of serotonin, catecholamines and fever. In Costa, E., editor: Symposium on the biological role of indol derivatives. Advances Pharmacol. **6**:318-332.

Myers, R. D. 1969a. In press. Chemical mechanisms in the hypothalamus mediating eating and drinking in the monkey. In Neural regulation of food and water intake. Ann. N.Y. Acad. Sci.

Myers, R. D. 1969b. Temperature regulation: neurochemical systems in the hypothalamus. In Haymaker, W., Anderson, E., and Nauta, W. J. H., editors: The hypothalamus. Springfield, Illinois, Charles C Thomas, Publisher, pp. 506-523.

Nakayama, T., Eisenman, J., and Hardy, J. D. 1961. Single unit activity of anterior hypothalamus during local heating. Science **134**:560-561.

Nauta, W. J. H. 1946. Hypothalamic regulation of sleep in rats: an experimental study. J. Neurophysiol. **9**:285-316.

Nauta, W. J. H., and Haymaker, W. 1969. Hypothalamic nuclei and fiber connections. In Haymaker, W., Anderson, E., and Nauta, W. J. H., editors: The hypothalamus. Springfield, Illinois, Charles C Thomas, Publisher, pp. 136-218.

Norstrand, I. F. 1955. Clinical study of craniopharyngiomas occurring in persons over 40. Neurology **5**:558-566.

Northfield, D. W. C., and Russell, D. S. 1967. Pubertas praecox due to hypothalamic hamartoma: report of two cases surviving surgical removal of the tumour. J. Neurol. Neurosurg. Psychiat. **30**:166-173.

Nothnagel, H. 1881. Durst und Polydipsie. Virchows Arch. Path. Anat. **86**:435-447.

Nyhan, W. L., and Cooke, R. E. 1956. Symptomatic hyponatremia in acute infections of the central nervous system. Pediatrics **18**:604-613.

Oomura, Y., Ooyama, H., Yamamoto, T., and Naka, F. 1967. Reciprocal relationship of the lateral and ventromedial hypothalamus in the regulation of food intake. Physiol. Behav. **2**:97-115.

Orthner, H., and Meyer, E. 1967. Der posttraumatischen Diabetes insipidus: Befunde am neurosekretorischen System beim stumpfen Schädeltrauma, nebst Bemerkungen zum posttraumatischen Hirnödem. Acta Neuroveg. **30**:216-250.

Orthner, H., and Rettinger, E. 1965. Ein intraventrikuläres Kraniopharyngeom, zugleich ein Beitrag zum hypothalamisch ausgelösten Korsakow-Syndrom: vergleichende Übersicht über die hypothalamisch auslösbaren Störungen der Merkfähigkeit und des Trieblebens beim Mensch und Tier. Fortschr. Neurol. Psychiat. **33**:299-331.

Padel, Y., and Dell, P. 1965. Effets bulbaires et réticulaires des stimulations endormantes du tronc vago-aortique. J. Physiol. (Paris) **57**:269-270.

Papez, J. W., and Ecker, A. 1947. Precocious puberty with hypothalamic tumor (infundibuloma): case report. J. Neuropath. Exp. Neurol. **6**:15-23.

Parmeggiani, P. L. 1960. Reizeffekte aus Hippocampus und Corpus mammillare der Katze. Helv. Physiol. Pharmacol. Acta **18**:523-536.

Perret, G. E. 1964. Stress ulcers and the neurosurgeon. J. Iowa Med. Soc. **54**:583-585.

Poeck, K., Risso, M., and Pilleri, G. 1963. Beitrag zur Pathophysiologie und klinischen Systematik des pathologischen Lachens und Weinens. Arch. Psychiat. Z. Ges. Neurol. **204**:181-198.

Porter, R. W., Movius, H. J., and French, J. D. 1953. Hypothalamic influences on hydrochloric acid secretion of the stomach. Surgery **33**:875-880.

Proctor, L. D., Knighton, R. S., and Churchill, J. A. 1957. Variations in consciousness produced by stimulating reticular formation of the monkey. Neurology **7**:193-203.

Ranson, S. W. 1939. Somnolence caused by hypothalamic lesions in the monkey. Arch. Neurol. Psychiat. **41**:1-23.

Reichlin, S. 1966. Functions of the median-eminence gland. New Eng. J. Med. **275**:600-607.

Reichlin, S. 1967. Editorial. Amer. J. Med. **43**: 477-485.

Richter, R. B. 1951. True hamartoma of the hypothalamus associated with pubertas praecox. J. Neuropath. Exp. Neurol. **10**:368-383.

Richter, R. B., and Traut, E. F. 1940. Chronic encephalitis, pathologic report of a case with protracted somnolence. Arch. Neurol. Psychiat. **44**:848-866.

Rose, F. C. 1968. Recent advances in neuro-ophthalmology. [Summary.] Proc. Roy. Soc. Med. **61**:2-3.

Rossi, G. F., Minobe, K., and Candia, O. 1963. An experimental study of the hypnogenic mechanisms of the brain stem. Arch. Ital. Biol. **101**: 470-492.

Rowe, S. N. 1935. Localization of the sleep mechanism. Brain **58**:21-43.

Ruch, T. C., and Shenkin, H. A. 1943. The relation of area 13 on orbital surface of frontal lobes to hyperactivity and hyperphagia in monkeys. J. Neurophysiol. **6**:349-360.

Rucker, C. W., and Kernohan, J. W. 1954. Notching of the optic chiasm by overlying arteries in pituitary tumors. Arch. Ophthal. **51**:161-170.

Ruscio, J. F., and Marcus, P. S. 1968. Sudden hyperthermia during anesthesia. Surg. Clin. N. Amer. **48**:415-421.

Russell, A. 1951. A diencephalic syndrome of emaciation in infancy and childhood. Arch. Dis. Child. **26**:274-275.

Sachs, E. 1938. The importance of ocular signs in the diagnosis of brain tumor. Ann. Intern. Med. **11**:1395-1400.

Schickele, E. 1947. Environment and fatal heat stroke: an analysis of 157 cases occurring in the army in the U. S. during World War II. Mil. Surgeon **100**:235-256.

Schlezinger, N. S., and Thompson, R. A. 1967. Pituitary tumors with central scotomas simulating retrobulbar optic neuritis. Neurology **17:** 782-788.

Schmidt, E., Hallervorden, J., and Spatz, H. 1958. Die Entstehung der Hamartome am Hypothalamus, mit und ohne Pubertas praecox. Deutsch. Z. Nervenheilk. **177:**235-262.

Sharkey, P. C., Perry, J. H., and Ehni, G. 1961. Diabetes insipidus following section of the hypophyseal stalk. J. Neurosurg. **18:**445-460.

Sharma, K. N., Anand, B. K., Dua, S., and Singh, B. 1961. Role of the stomach in regulation of activities of hypothalamic feeding centers. Amer. J. Physiol. **201:**593-598.

Sheehan, H. L., and Davis, J. C. 1968. Pituitary necrosis. Brit. Med. Bull. **24:**59-70.

Smith, K. R., Jr., Weinberg, W. A., and McAlister, W. H. 1965. Failure to thrive: the diencephalic syndrome of infancy and childhood; a case report. J. Neurosurg. **23:**348-351.

Smith, R. W., and McCann, S. 1961. Aphagia, adipsia and polydipsia following hypothalamic lesions in the rat. Fed. Proc. **20:**333.

Sohal, R. S., Sun, S. C., Colcolough, H. L., and Burch, G. E. 1968. Heat stroke: an electron microscopic study of endothelial cell damage and disseminated intravascular coagulation. Arch. Intern. Med. **122:**43-47.

Sprague, J. M., Levitt, M., Robson, K., Lin, C. N., Stellar, E., and Chambers, W. W. 1963. A neuroanatomical and behavioral analysis of syndromes resulting from midbrain lemniscal and reticular lesions in the cat. Arch. Ital. Biol. **101:** 225-289.

Stephen, C. R. 1967. Fulminant hyperthermia during anesthesia and surgery. J.A.M.A. **202:**178-182.

Stevenson, J. A. F. 1969. Neural control of food and water intake. In Haymaker, W., Anderson, E., and Nauta, W. J. H., editors: The hypothalamus. Springfield, Illinois, Charles C Thomas, Publisher, pp. 524-621.

Stevko, R. M., Balsley, M., and Segar, W. E. 1968. Primary polydipsia—compulsive water drinking: report of two cases. J. Pediat. **73:**845-851.

Stricker, E. M., and Wolf, G. 1967. Hypovolemic thirst in comparison with thirst induced by hyperosmolarity. Physiol. Behav. **2:**33-37.

Ström, G. 1950. Influence of local thermal stimulation of the hypothalamus of the cat on cutaneous blood flow and respiratory rate. Acta Physiol. Scand. **20:** suppl. 70: 47-76.

Ström, G. 1960. Central nervous regulation of body temperature. In Field, J., Magoun, H. W., and Hall, V. E., editors: Handbook of physiology, sect. 1, vol. 2. Washington, D. C., Amer. Physiol. Soc., pp. 1173-1196.

Stuart, D. G., Kawamura, Y., and Hemingway, A. 1961. Activation and suppression of shivering during septal and hypothalamic stimulation. Exp. Neurol. **4:**485-506.

Sunderman, F. W., and Haymaker, W. 1947. Hypothermia and elevated serum magnesium in a patient with facial hemangioma extending into the hypothalamus. Amer. J. Med. Sci. **213:**562-571.

Swanson, A. G., and Iseri, O. A. 1958. Acute encephalopathy due to water intoxication. New Eng. J. Med. **258:**831-834.

Szentágothai, J., Flerkó, B., Mess, B., and Halász, B. 1968. Hypothalamic control of the pituitary: an experimental-morphological study, ed. 3. Budapest, Akadémiai Kiadó.

Teitelbaum, P. 1957. Random and food-directed activity of hyperphagic and normal rats. J. Comp. Physiol. Psychol. **50:**486-490.

Teitelbaum, P., and Epstein, A. N. 1962. The lateral hypothalamic syndrome: recovery of feeding and drinking after lateral hypothalamic lesions. Psychol. Rev. **69:**74-90.

Terzian, H., and Ore, G. D. 1955. Syndrome of Klüver and Bucy reproduced in man by bilateral removal of the temporal lobes. Neurology **5:**373-380.

Thauer, R. 1964. Der nervöse Mechanismus der chemischen Temperaturregulation des Warmblutes. Naturwissensch. **51:**73-80.

Tönnis, W., Müller, W., Oswald, F., and Brilmayer, H. 1954. Kann die Rachendachhypophyse ein vikariierende Funktion ausüben? Klin. Wschr. **32:**912-914.

Trumble, H. E. 1951. Pituitary tumors: observations on large tumors which have spread widely beyond the confines of the sella turcica. Brit. J. Surg. **39:**7-24.

van Bogaert, L. 1926. Syndrome de la calotte protubérantielle avec myoclonies localisée et troubles du sommeil. Rev. Neurol. **1:**977-988.

Vertel, R. M., and Knochel, J. P. 1967. Acute renal failure due to heat injury: an analysis of ten cases associated with a high incidence of myoglobinuria. Amer. J. Med. **43:**435-451.

von Economo, C. 1929. Die Encephalitis lethargica, ihre Nachkrankheiten und ihre Behandlung. Wien, Urban & Schwarzenberg.

von Euler, C. 1950. Slow "temperature potentials" in the hypothalamus. J. Cell. Comp. Physiol. **36:**333-350.

Wagener, H. P., and Love, J. G. 1943. Fields of vision in cases of tumor of Rathke's pouch. Arch. Ophthal. **29:**873-887.

Weinberger, L. M., and Grant, F. C. 1941. Precocious puberty and tumors of the hypothalamus; report of case and review of literature, with pathophysiologic explanation of precocious sexual syndrome. Arch. Intern. Med. **67:**762-792.

Weir, J. F., Larson, E., and Rowntree, L. G. 1922. Studies in diabetes insipidus, water balance, and water intoxication. Arch. Intern. Med. **29:**306-330.

Williams, R. H., and Henry, C. 1947. Nephrogenic diabetes insipidus transmitted by females appearing during infancy in males. Ann. Intern. Med. **27:**84-95.

Wilson, R. D., Nichols, R. J., Dent, T. E., and Allen, C. R. 1966. Disturbances of oxidative phosphorylation mechanism as a possible etiology factor in sudden unexplained hyperthermia occurring during anesthesia. Anesthesiology **27:** 231-232.

Zanchetti, A. 1967. Brain stem mechanisms of sleep. Anesthesiology **28:**81-99.

Chapter 27

Cerebral artery occlusion, aneurysms, and arteriovenous malformations

GENERAL ORIENTATION

The major blood supply of the brain comes from two sources: the internal carotid arteries and the vertebral arteries. Actually these are two separate systems, which are connected in varying degrees of completeness by the arterial circle of Willis. The "circle" is formed by the anterior communicating artery rostrally, the anterior cerebral arteries rostrolaterally, the internal carotid and posterior communicating arteries laterally, and the basilar and posterior cerebral arteries caudally (Figs. 18-1 and 27-1). Incompleteness of the circle and hypoplasia of one or more of its components are common. On the other side of the ledger are persistent embryonic anastomoses between the internal carotid and the vertebral-basilar system; these are, however, rare. (Eadie, Jamieson, and Lennon, 1964; Lee and Hodes, 1967; Perryman and others, 1963.)

Incompleteness of the circle of Willis has been noted in 3 to 7 percent of brains, the posterior communicating artery being the one most often lacking (Fawcett and Blackford, 1905; Riggs and Rupp, 1963; Stopford, 1915). The anterior communicating artery, by contrast, is rarely absent; it is often doubled, tripled, or plexiform. Far more frequent than incompleteness of the circle of Willis is hypoplasia of some of its arteries (in 79 percent in one series in which the posterior communicating was the artery most often hypoplastic; Riggs and Rupp, 1963). As to defects in major vessels of the circle of Willis, one or both internal carotid arteries are occasionally absent (Fisher, 1913).

Embryologically, the posterior communicating artery arises from the internal carotid and is directly continuous with the posterior cerebral artery. As the cerebral hemispheres grow backward over the cerebellum, the posterior cerebral artery becomes elongated and its field of irrigation becomes farther and farther removed from the parent trunk. In meeting the increased functional demands on it, the posterior cerebral artery comes more and more to depend on a nearer source of blood, the basilar artery, to which it is connected from earlier embryonic stages by anastomotic channels. Ultimately the posterior cerebral becomes a branch of the basilar, and the posterior communicating becomes narrowed. The posterior communicating artery may, however, remain relatively large and be the only channel through which blood reaches the posterior cerebral artery (in 8 percent of brains). It may undergo regression and disappear. (Fawcett and Blackford, 1905; Stopford, 1916, 1917; Williams, 1936.)

The circle of Willis serves as a hemodynamic equalizer for the two sides of the cerebrum. Hemodynamic equalization is also carried out intracerebrally through precapillary arteriovenous anastomoses ("thoroughfare channels") and by way of anastomoses, in the pia, between terminal leptomeningeal branches of the major cerebral arteries (the latter are found in "junctional territories," or "border zones," uniting the anterior cerebral with the middle cerebral artery, and the middle cerebral with the posterior cerebral artery).

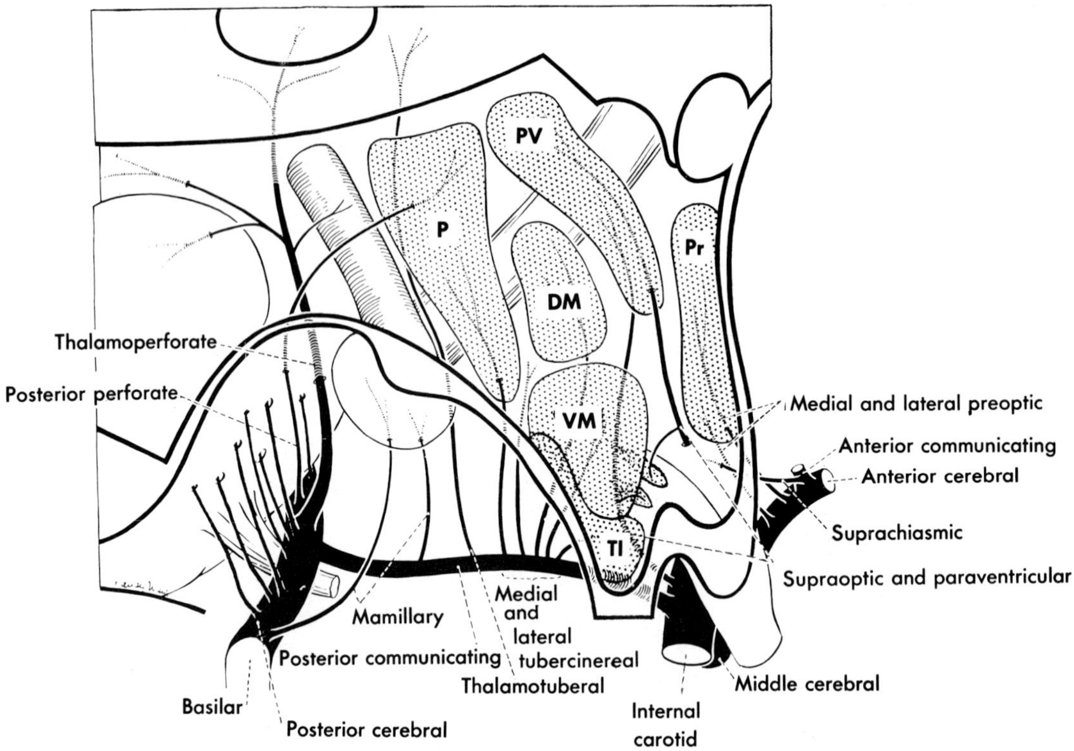

Fig. 27-1. Branches of the circle of Willis and their distribution to the hypothalamus and adjoining thalamus and midbrain. There are three groups of vessels for the supply of the hypothalamus: *anterior,* from the carotid, anterior cerebral and anterior communicating to the preoptic *(Pr),* paraventricular *(PV),* and supraoptic (not labeled) nuclei; *middle,* from the posterior communicating artery to the tuberoinfundibular *(TI),* ventromedial *(VM),* dorsomedial *(DM),* posterior *(P),* and lateral (not labeled) nuclei; and *posterior,* from the posterior communicating and posterior cerebral to the mamillary and caudolateral hypothalamic regions (not labeled). The vessels are named in accordance with their nuclei of supply. (Data based on observations of India ink-injected brains studied in collaboration with Dr. J. B. deC. M. Saunders, San Francisco.)

Despite all these rich interconnections, the two internal carotid arteries and the vertebral-basilar system function independently under conditions in which the subject is immobilized with his face front, as shown in angiograms. However, change in pressure relations between the two carotid arteries, or between the vertebral-basilar and the carotid system (such as may occur on turning the head), causes blood to shift immediately into the system with the lower pressure. (Toole, 1966.) The shunting occurs mostly through the circle of Willis and the leptomeningeal vessels. Manual compression of one internal carotid or one vertebral artery immediately increases blood flow through the other by more than 50 percent owing to these shunting mechanisms. (Ishikawa and others, 1965; Symonds, 1955; Toole, 1966; Vander Eecken, 1959; Vander Eecken and Adams, 1953.)

Where a major cerebral artery is occluded, remarkable shunts can develop intracranially and be sufficient to protect the brain tissue against ischemia (Alpers, 1959; Brain, 1957; Lee and Hodes, 1967; Lowe, 1962). However, when the potential for shunting is relatively low, cerebral infarction is prone to develop. Examples are given in the following.

Zones of anastomosis between branches of major vessels at the *pial level* may be the least adaptable to shunting, in which case adjacent "junctional territories" of brain tissue will be the most susceptible to ischemia (Fisher, 1957; Lindenberg, 1955; Zülch, 1955). Vascular hypotension occurring in association with occlusive disease proximally in arteries tends to give rise to infarcts in these territories. With occlusion of the internal carotid in the cervical region, blood continues to reach the cerebrum via the ophthalmic artery (through the external carotid) and via the posterior and anterior communicating arteries (through the vertebral-basilar arterial system). If blood flow is sufficiently reduced, infarction will occur at the border zone between anterior and middle cerebral artery, including the zone between the territories of supply of the artery of Huebner and the lenticulostriate artery. If the configuration of the circle of Willis is such that the posterior cerebral artery is continuous with the occluded carotid, then the blood flow in the posterior cerebral artery may also be so reduced that infarction occurs in the border zone between the middle cerebral and posterior cerebral artery. When the vertebral-basilar arterial system is occluded, a less than normal blood flow through the internal carotid may lead to infarction in the border zone between the middle cerebral and posterior cerebral arteries. Clinical disturbances vary accordingly. (Romanul and Abramowicz, 1964.)

If blood flow in the circle of Willis or in a major artery is impeded, as may occur in arteriosclerosis, the area of necrosis that develops following arterial occlusion will be correspondingly larger. For example, in the event of occlusion of the anterior cerebral artery, if the middle cerebral artery is narrowed by sclerosis, the infarct that develops will be of greater size than under conditions in which the middle cerebral artery is of normal caliber. This may be the basis of the relatively large infarct in the territory of anterior cerebral artery supply illustrated in Fig. 27-9.

Importance of collateral supporting blood flow between middle cerebral artery and leptomeningeal vessels is illustrated in the following two cases. During an operation a clip was placed on the middle cerebral artery distal to the origin of the striate arteries. Transient weakness occurred and was followed by complete recovery of function. Collateral circulation in this case was adequate. In a second case, occlusion occurred spontaneously in the middle cerebral artery proximal to the site of origin of the striate arteries. Hemiplegia developed immediately and persisted. Here the mouths of the striate arteries had inadequate collateral supply. (Rosegay and Welch, 1954.)

Notwithstanding the role of the circle of Willis and the leptomeningeal vessels as hemodynamic equalizers, these systems fall far short in equalizing acute ischemia occurring in one hemisphere (Dickinson, 1961).

A factor concerned in protecting the brain against vascular occlusion, particularly when the circle of Willis is incompetent, is the shunting of blood through *extracranial-intracranial anastomotic channels.* Toole (1966) cites three principal groups of anastomoses:

1. External to internal carotid arteries
   a. Through the orbit
   b. Through a network of external carotid arterial branches that perforate the dura and anastomose with surface branches of the internal carotid through the remains of the retia mirabilia
2. External carotid to vertebral-basilar artery through the occipital branch of the external carotid
3. Subclavian-vertebral to vertebral arteries
   a. Of the same side, by-passing segmental obstruction
   b. To the opposite side

Lee and Hodes (1967) propose the following classification of anastomoses through which shunts can occur:

1. Intracerebral anastomoses
   In middle cerebral artery occlusion, for example, enlarged lenticulostriate, thalamogeniculate, and anterior and posterior choroidal arteries often form intracerebral anastomoses enlarged enough to be demonstrated angiographically. (The main escape route is through the transcerebral venous system, a system connecting cortical veins with internal cerebral veins; Hasegawa, Ravens, and Toole, 1967, Kaplan, 1959.)
2. Extra-axial anastomoses
   a. Circle of Willis
   b. Cortical leptomeningeal anastomoses. There are end-to-end candelabra type anastomoses between the major arteries. Functionally they are second to the circle of Willis in importance.
   c. Retia mirabilia. These normally consist of rather small channels linking dural and cortical leptomeningeal arteries. (Enlargement has been particularly well demonstrated by Leeds and Abbott, 1965.)

To these local shunting mechanisms—circle of Willis and leptomeningeal, intracerebral, and extracranial-intracranial channels—another of a more general character is to be added. Reference is made to the borrowing-lending process reflected in the shifting of blood from one part of the body to another, a process that works to the detriment of blood flow to the brain. Most important and frequent in this regard is the *subclavian steal* phenomenon. This phenomenon is met with most commonly in thrombosis of the proximal part of the subclavian artery (on the *left* side). As a result of occlusion of the vessel, blood flow in the vertebral artery is reversed. The affected arm is thereby supplied with blood at the expense of the brain. In such thrombosis, resultant blood flow is as follows: aorta → innominate artery (on the right) → *right* vertebral artery → anterior communicating artery of the circle of Willis → *left* vertebral artery → *left* subclavian artery distal to the site of thrombosis. Certain arterial configurations or anomalies can also have this effect. Whether symptoms of intracranial vascular occlusion will occur depends upon the shunting capacity of the vascular system. Capacity of the circle of Willis is highly important, much more so than the functioning of the extracranial-intracranial anastomotic system. Varied subclavian steal syndromes occur. Examples are: (1) claudication of the left upper limb and vertigo, (2) nocturnal confusion followed later by prolonged loss of consciousness, and (3) acrocyanosis of the upper limb with no neurological disturbances. (Coder and others, 1965; Labauge, Thévenet, and Crouzet, 1967; Mishkin, 1967; Nicola and others, 1967; Patel and Toole, 1965; Reivich and others, 1961.)

Syndromes of arterial *occlusion,* which might be taken to mean either thrombotic or embolic occlusion, are described in the following text. This word *occlusion* is, however, used only as a matter of convenience in exposition. *Circulatory insufficiency* from arterial stenosis is equally at fault in the production of infarction (Fisher, 1954a, b; Samuel, 1956). Other causes of circulatory insufficiency also exist: in half or more cases of cerebral infarction neither thrombosis, embolization, nor significant arterial stenosis has been encountered (Torvik and Jörgensen, 1966; Yates and Hutchinson, 1961). Sometimes stricture of an extracranial artery is the cause of circulatory insufficiency, in which case the insufficiency is usually intermittent (Robicsek and others, 1967). Preexisting arterial stenosis may be aggravated by the formation of a hematoma in the arterial wall and probably by arterial spasm (Cohen, 1944); it may also be an immediate cause of brain infarction. Stenosis and thrombotic occlusion of a vessel are not mutually exclusive, since a thrombus may form at the site of arterial stenosis.

Pathologically speaking, in syndromes of vascular "occlusion" multiple infarcts within a given brain are the rule, making precise localization difficult clinically. Infarcts may occur in more than one territory of supply of a single vessel; both right and left side of a given brain may be infarcted. Infarcts in a given brain are not uncommonly found in the territory of supply of all three major arteries and of the vertebral-basilar arterial system as well. (Yates and Hutchinson, 1961.)

Considered in simplest terms, the cerebrum is supplied through its main trunks (anterior, middle, and posterior cerebral arteries) by three sets of arteries: the *paramedian,* which go to the wall of the third ventricle, the *short circumferential,* which pass to the other deep structures of the brain, and the *long circumferential,* which supply the surface of the brain. The same general plan holds also for the brainstem. (Foix and Hillemand, 1925b.)

INTERNAL CAROTID ARTERY

On reaching the base of the skull, the internal carotid artery enters the carotid canal. It ascends within this canal, then turns rostromedially to the apex of the petrous temporal bone, where it enters the foramen lacerum. After passing through this foramen, it ascends along the body of the sphenoid bone to enter the middle cranial fossa (Fig. 12-1). It then runs forward, in the lateral wall of the cavernous sinus (Fig. 16-1) to the small wing of the sphenoid. It turns backward along the medial border of the anterior clinoid process, which it grooves (Fig. 12-1); as it turns upward on the medial side of the anterior clinoid process, the internal carotid gives off the *ophthalmic artery,* which passes superior to this process. At the caudal extremity of the anterior clinoid process, the carotid turns upward, lateral to its termination, in the region in which it divides into the anterior and middle cerebral arteries. Near its termination the internal carotid gives off, in turn, the posterior communicating and anterior choroidal arteries (Fig. 27-3).

Upon emerging from the lateral wall of cavernous sinus, the carotid artery soon reaches the subarachnoid space. In this region it lies just lateral to the optic chiasm and nerve (Fig. 12-1).

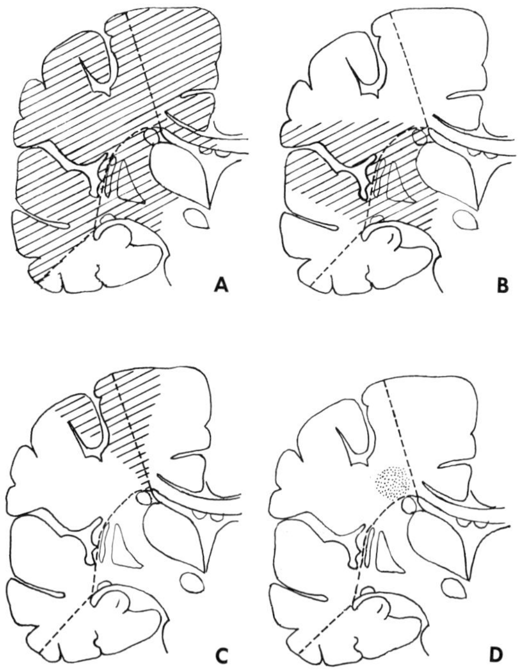

Fig. 27-2. Various types of infarct in carotid occlusion. **A,** Total infarct (in 55 percent of cases); **B,** proximal infarct (in 21 percent); **C,** watershed type of infarct (19 percent); **D,** terminal infarct (5 percent). (From Torvik and Jörgensen, 1966.)

While within the sinus or shortly after emerging, it provides branches for cranial nerves III through VI, the gasserian ganglion, the pituitary gland, and the dura of the anterior and middle cranial fossae.

Syndromes of occlusion vary, depending upon the level at which the lumen of the vessel is compromised, the number of arterial branches implicated, and the acuteness of occlusion. Clinical disturbances may be transient, slowly progressive, or catastrophic. Representative locations of infarcts are illustrated in Fig. 27-2.

Manifestations of *carotid insufficiency* include repeated attacks of unilateral impairment of motor and sensory functions and, in some instances, speech disorders and ipsilateral visual disturbances. Dysarthria may also occur. Altered consciousness and convulsive seizures are not features of this syndrome. (Millikan and Siekert, 1955.)

The *intermittency* may be of varied cause. Intermittent occlusion of the internal carotid artery from a detached intimal layer of the artery occurs and can be responsible for ischemic attacks; however, this is rare (Robicsek and others, 1967). *Thrombotic cerebral infarction,* which is common, often evolves in an intermittent, fluctuant fashion, frequently in association with transient attacks of an ischemic nature. Headache may be a prodrome; it is usually unilateral and situated in the lower forehead (Fisher, 1968). Most thrombi develop primarily in the extracranial part of the vessel; the others develop within intracranial segments of the vessel (Torvik and Jörgensen, 1964, 1966). Smaller cerebral infarcts are produced by thrombi in the region of origin of the internal carotid (rather than by thrombi in more distal portions), owing to more ample collateral circulation through the anterior communicating artery. Accordingly, focal cerebral manifestations may be few. Mental confusion is, however, common under such circumstances. If the occlusion is on the left side (in right-handed persons) aphasia is apt to develop.

Thrombotic occlusion of the *more distal part of the internal carotid* with advancement of a thrombus to the level of the cavernous sinus or farther forward, into the ophthalmic artery, may give rise to *carotid hemiplegia.* This is characterized by ipsilateral blindness and contralateral hemiplegia, in which the face and upper limb are usually more severely affected than the lower limb. (Blindness may not occur if the thrombus has not advanced far into the ophthalmic artery.) Homonymous hemianopia in the contralateral visual field may occur if the posterior communicating or the anterior choroidal artery is also occluded, but the hemianopia is usually transitory. Of regular occurrence in carotid hemiplegia are severe disturbances in spatial and discriminative sensibility of the contralateral side of the body and, when the left carotid is involved, motor and sensory aphasia. Though *karotides* means "vessels of unconsciousness," consciousness is usually preserved in unilateral occlusion. Palpation over the carotid in the neck and pharynx may or may not reveal diminished pulsations on the side of carotid thrombosis.

Embolic cerebral infarction usually occurs abruptly as a single monophasic event in which the symptoms reach a peak within a few seconds or minutes. The emboli commonly originate from the heart (from a mural thrombus or from an area of the endocardium affected in the course of subacute bacterial endocarditis). Symptoms vary in accordance with the site at which the embolus lodges. Unlike thrombotic infarction, embolic infarction conforms rather accurately to the entire territory of the occluded artery, and thus its location can often readily be determined. In numerous instances, however, embolic infarction closely resembles or is indistinguishable from thrombotic infarction clinically, though evolution of the former is usually the more rapid (in a day or so). Headache may precede embolic strokes by 24 to 36 hours. There may be transient attacks attributable to cerebral ischemia (such as dysarthria or numbness) a few hours prior to the stroke. Temporary arrest of embolic material in the carotid has been considered the basis of these premonitory disturbances. (Fisher, 1954a,b, 1958; Fisher and Pearlman, 1967.)

Hemorrhage occurring spontaneously into the brain of hypertensive persons takes place in the putamen or the rostral part of the base of the external capsule in some 60 percent of cases, in the thalamus in 10 percent, the pons in 10 percent, and the cerebellum in 10 percent. Fisher (1968) asserts that the putamen is the most common site of hemorrhage, Charcot (1883) and Abbie (1937) that the base of the external capsule is most subject to hemorrhage because there are relatively more vessels in this region to bleed from (Fig. 27-14). Whether the hemorrhage occurs in the putamen or in the environs, coma and hemiplegia ensue. If the hemorrhage is chiefly in the thalamus there will be a sensorimotor type of stroke with fixed pupils and impairment in vertical gaze (Fisher, 1968).

In *differential diagnosis between cerebral infarction and hemorrhage in the putamen or vicinity*, some guides may be offered (Schaafsma, 1968).

1. The occurrence of multiple previous "cardiovascular accidents" greatly favors cerebral infarction over cerebral hemorrhage.
2. Hyperacute onset is by far most frequent in hemorrhage.
3. A pulse rate less than 60/min. and a rectal temperature less than 97.5° F. (36° C.) indicate hemorrhage.
4. Decerebrate spasms are fairly common in hemorrhage but do not occur in infarction.
5. Bilateral absence of corneal reflexes may be noted in hemorrhage but not in infarction.
6. Nuchal rigidity and marked abnormality in pupillary reactions (presumably reflecting frequency of herniation of cerebral tissue) are much more common in hemorrhage than in infarction.
7. Conjugate deviation of the eyes is somewhat more frequent in hemorrhage than in infarction.
8. Blood in the cerebrospinal fluid is far more frequent in cerebral hemorrhage than in infarction.

About 10 percent of all cerebrovascular "accidents" are related to *atherosclerosis* of the internal carotid artery with or without carotid thrombosis. *Trauma* of the internal carotid artery in the region of the neck may also be responsible. Here the infarction is usually associated with carotid thrombosis. Or embolism may occur, or, occasionally, ischemia alone may be responsible.

Penetrating wounds in which a high velocity missile passes near the internal carotid without actually striking it may nonetheless induce thrombosis from indirect trauma of the vessel (Caldwell and Hadden, 1948; Ecker, 1945). The carotid may also be injured under conditions in which there is no penetrating wound in the neck. Forcible stretching of the carotid arteries of one side from trauma of the chin or angle of the jaw (with transverse fracture of the sternum) may be responsible. In such cases, hemiplegia sets in rapidly (within hours or in a day or two). Consciousness is relatively preserved. Postmortem studies have revealed a tear in the intima and tunica media of the carotid in association with thrombosis. (Hughes and Brownell, 1968.) Cerebral infarction sometimes follows a blow to the neck. It is thought that bruising of the artery may lead to sufficient vasospasm to bring this about. (Ecker, 1945; Houck and others, 1964; Yates and Hutchinson, 1961.) In support of this possibility is the observation (in monkeys) by Simeone, Ryan, and Cotter (1968) that vasospasm lasting 4 hours can occur in the entire field of distribution of the internal carotid following injury of this vessel (puncture of its intracranial portion with a 30-gauge needle). In children and adolescents trauma accounts for about 25 percent of proved cases of internal carotid thrombosis. Blunt trauma of the paratonsillar region, usually the result of falling on a foreign object carried in the mouth (for example, a toothbrush), can give rise to internal carotid thrombosis, resulting in hemiparesis or monoparesis either immediately or up to 24 hours after the accident. Intermittent blurring of vision may be an initial complaint, and there may be dysphasia. Embolization of thrombotic material formed at site of intimal or intimal-medial tear caused by the trauma has been suggested as the chief basis. Occasionally, such accidents are fatal. (Martin and Warren, 1969; Pitner, 1966.)

POSTERIOR COMMUNICATING ARTERY

The posterior communicating artery normally arises from the internal carotid at a level just behind the anterior clinoid process. Its branches arborize in the optic chiasm, optic tract, hypothalamus (in the tuberal region, between the preoptic area and mamillary body), thalamus (its anterior inferior quarter), infundibulum of the neurohypophysis (the internal carotid artery provides the main supply), subthalamus, the genu and a variable part of the anterior third of the posterior limb of the internal capsule, the basis pedunculi, and the interpeduncular region. Some of the territories of supply are illustrated in Figs. 25-6 and 27-1. (Abbie, 1937; Beevor, 1907, 1909; Dawson, 1958; Foley, Kinney, and Alexander, 1942; Lazorthes, 1961; Rubinstein, 1944.)

No cases of occlusion limited to the posterior communicating artery are known to us.

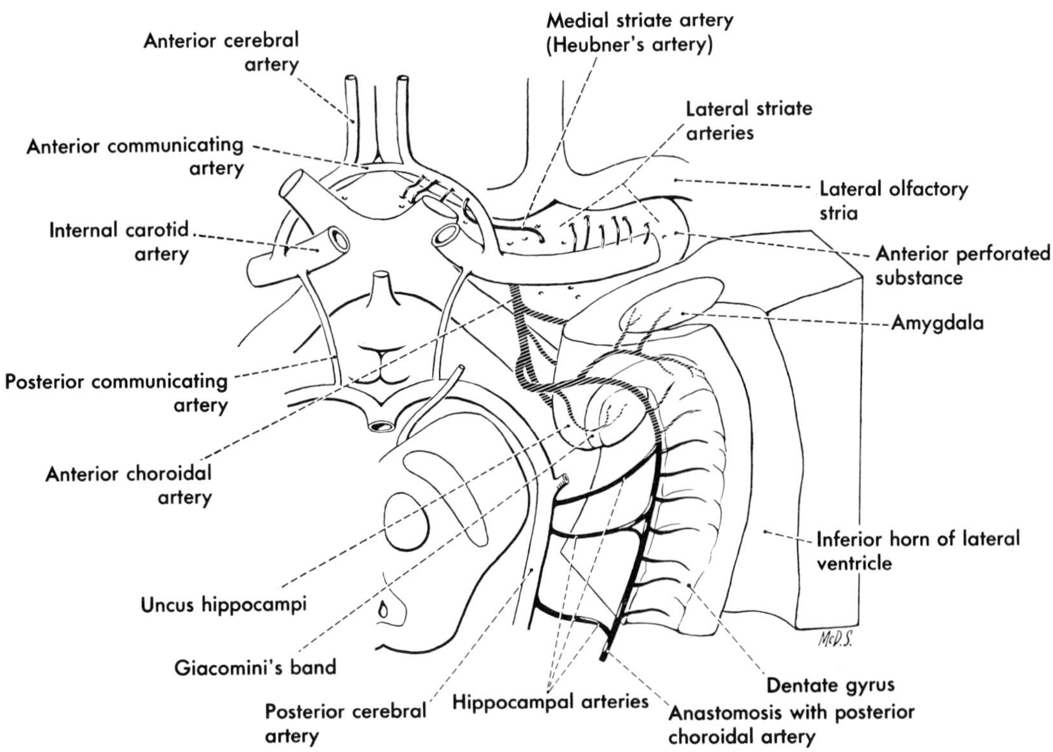

Fig. 27-3. The anterior choroidal and striate arteries. The anastomosis of the anterior choroidal with the posterior choroidal is inconstant. Vessels penetrating into the anterior perforated substances include the medial striate artery (from the anterior cerebral artery) and the lateral striate arteries (from the middle cerebral artery). In the medial group is Huebner's artery. (After Abbie, 1933a.)

ANTERIOR CHOROIDAL ARTERY

The anterior choroidal artery usually branches off the internal carotid a few millimeters from the latter's termination (Fig. 27-3), but not uncommonly arises from the middle cerebral (11.7 percent of brains), posterior communicating (6.7 percent), or the junctional area of the anterior and middle cerebral arteries (3.3 percent) (Carpenter, Noback, and Moss, 1954). It passes backward along the lateral aspect of optic tract, to which it sends a branch, and it reaches the lateral geniculate body, the lateral half of which it supplies (Fig. 18-6, *B*). In its earlier course, the anterior choroidal artery sends branches into the anterior perforated substance (together with lateral striate vessels from the middle cerebral artery) for the supply of part of the head of the caudate nucleus. Moreover, a branch of the anterior choroidal courses medial to the optic tract and ramifies in the middle third of the midbrain at rostral levels, including the basis pedunculi, substantia nigra, and red nucleus, and the subthalamic nucleus as well (Fig. 18-6, *B*). Another branch runs on to the medial surface of the temporal lobe and supplies the uncus hippocampi, amygdala, and the rostralmost part of the hippocampal formation. This branch usually anastomoses with hippocampal arteries (derived from the posterior cerebral artery) and in some instances with the posterior choroidal artery (Fig. 27-3); thus, the supply of these structures is shared by the posterior cerebral artery. Other branches of the anterior choroidal artery penetrate the brain to supply the globus pallidus, part of the putamen (in some instances), subthalamic region, parts of the thalamus (Fig. 25-6), and the posterior two-thirds of the posterior limb and retrolenticular part of the internal capsule (Figs. 27-6 to 27-8). In some 80 percent of brains another branch, which arises at the level of the lateral geniculate body, passes to the choroid plexus of the inferior horn of the lateral ventricle, and joins the posterior choroidal arteries in supplying parts of the thalamus (p. 460). Anastomosis of the anterior choroidal artery with other vessels must be rich, for following ligation of the artery little more than necrosis of the apical portion of the globus pallidus may be found. (Abbie, 1933a,b, 1937; Alexander, 1942; Balado and Franke, 1937; Carpenter, Noback, and Moss, 1954; Poppi, 1928.) Much of the area irrigated by the anterior choroidal artery and related vessels, including the posterior communicating artery, is indicated in Fig. 27-4.

Syndromes of occlusion vary depending on the site of the occlusion. There may be *contralateral* hemiplegia and hemianesthesia (to all sensory modalities, but in different degree) and, in some cases, partial or complete hemianopia (with sparing of the macula), *ipsilateral* pupillary dilatation, and sluggish reaction to light. "Coma vigil" may occur. The hemiplegia and hemianesthesia usually recede, while the hemianopic defects persist. Thalamic over-

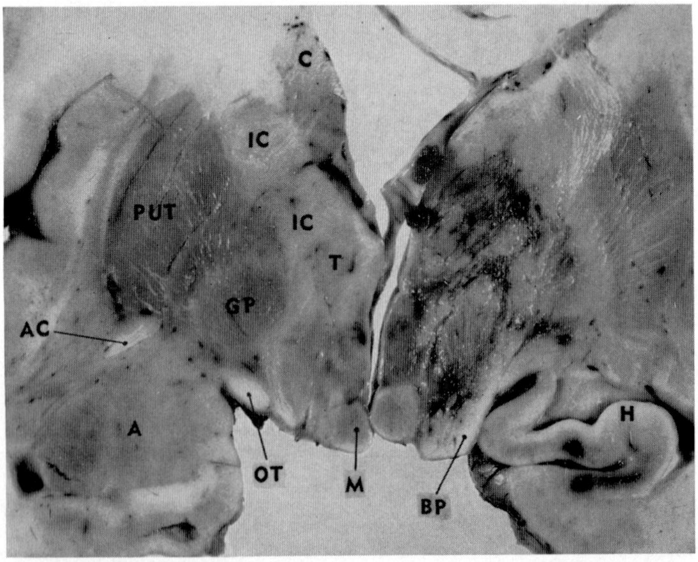

Fig. 27-4. Hemorrhagic softening in structures supplied by the anterior choroidal artery. The artery was compressed as the result of downward displacement of the brain following ipsilateral traumatic subdural hematoma that occurred one month previously. *A*, Amygdala; *AC*, anterior commissure; *B*, basis pedunculi; *C*, caudate nucleus; *G*, globus pallidus; *H*, hippocampal formation; *IC*, anterior limb and genu of internal capsule; *M*, mamillary body; *OT*, optic tract; *PUT*, putamen; *T*, anterior nucleus of thalamus. (From Lindenberg, 1955.)

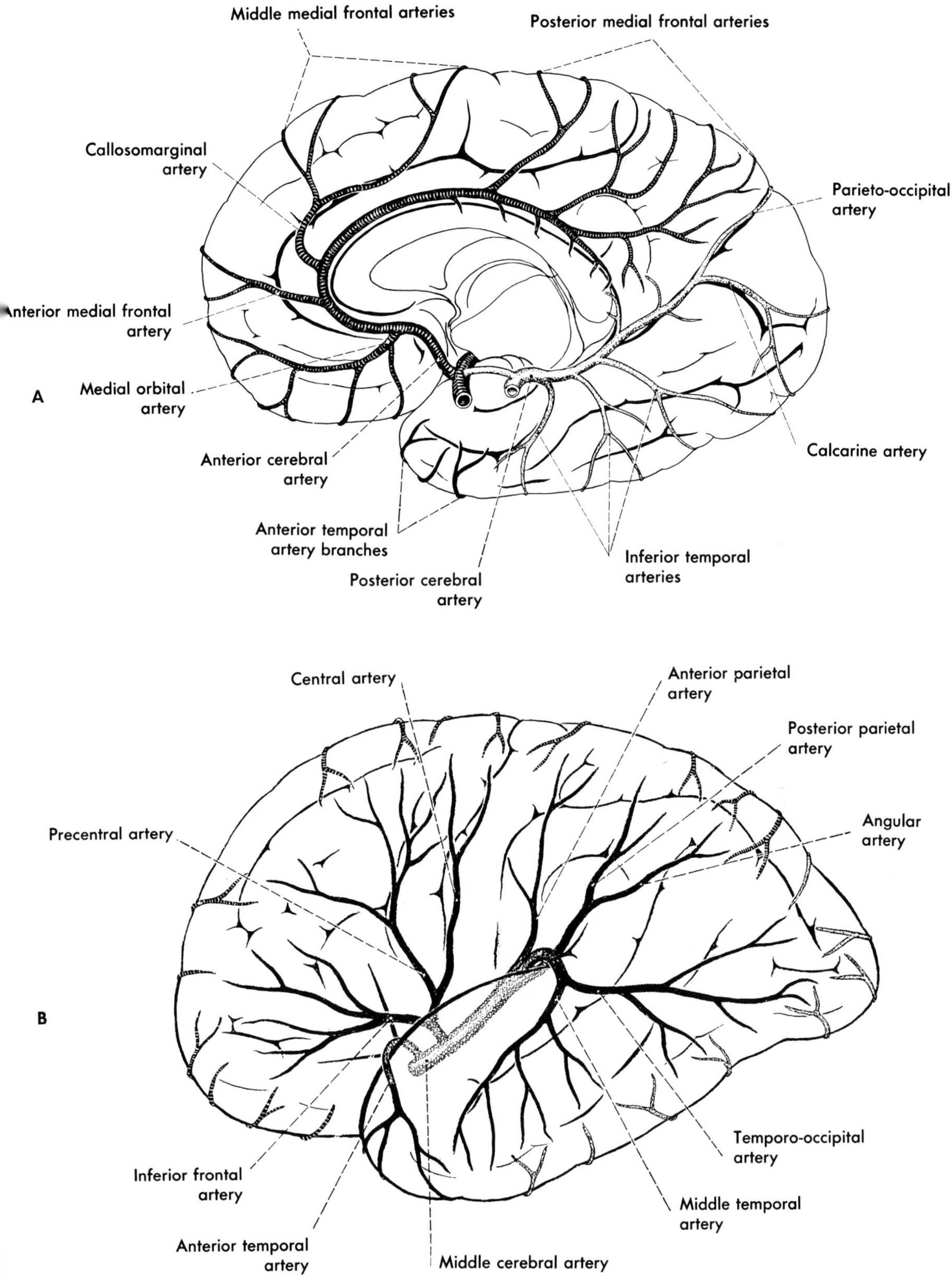

Fig. 27-5. The arterial supply of the brain as seen from the medial inferior and lateral aspects.

reaction may occasionally develop, as may also a "thalamic hand," characterized not only by an accoucheur attitude but also by vascular congestion and edema. (Abbie, 1933a; Poppi, 1928; Steegmann and Roberts, 1935.) Other aspects of occlusion of the anterior choroidal artery are described on pages 462 and 463.

ANTERIOR CEREBRAL ARTERY

The anterior cerebral artery extends forward and medially above the most proximal part of the optic nerve (Fig. 12-1), gains the genu of the corpus callosum around which it bends, then courses in the sulcus of the corpus callosum or on the medial surface of the hemisphere not far from the falx (or, occasionally, in the angular sulcus) and terminates in the region of the inferior end of the parieto-occipital fissure (Fig. 27-5, *A*). The artery sends branches to the corpus callosum, the medial aspect of the frontal and parietal lobes (including the paracentral lobule), and the adjoining narrow strip of cortex (about 2 cm.) of the convex surface of these lobes (Fig. 27-5, *B*). The subcortical white matter in these regions is also irrigated by this artery.

En route, the anterior cerebral artery gives off (1) the anterior communicating artery, (2) branches for the supply of the optic chiasm and olfactory tract and bulb, (3) branches to the parolfactory and septal regions, fornix, anterior commissure, and the rostral wall of the third ventricle, and (4) a recurrent branch, the medial striate or lateral perforating artery (Heubner's artery) (Fig. 27-3). The medial striate artery runs laterally and dorsally; its branches course into the cerebral substance in the region immediately rostral to the site of entrance of perforating branches of the middle cerebral artery. These branches extend upward to supply the anterior perforated substance, the rostromedial aspect of the head of the caudate nucleus and adjoining putamen, part of the septal region, the anterior limb of the internal capsule, and, in some brains, the rostral part of the globus pallidus (Figs. 27-6 to 27-8). (Abbie, 1937; Critchley, 1930; Kaplan, 1965.) The medial striate artery was absent in four of thirteen brains studied by Alexander (1942); entering the brain in its place were lateral striate arteries. Other

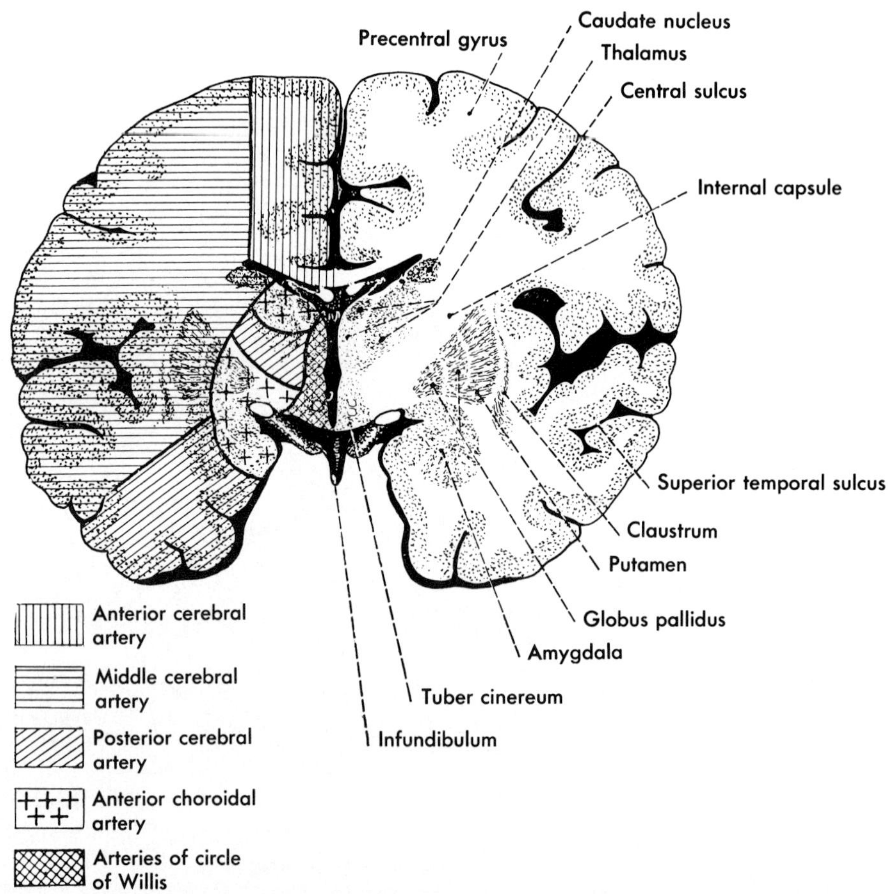

Fig. 27-6. Arterial supply of the brain at the level of the tuber cinereum (coronal section).

anomalies exist—for instance, union of the two anterior cerebral arteries to form an azygos (unpaired) artery, a third anterior cerebral artery, and an artery which, in its course, sends a branch to the opposite side (Baptista, 1963; LeMay and Gooding, 1966).

Occlusion of the anterior cerebral artery is relatively uncommon. Occasionally, akinetic mutism occurs (p. 391). Occlusion of the medial striate artery (Heubner's artery) is manifested by paresis of the contralateral lower part of the face, tongue, and upper limb. The occlusion may be attributable to any one of a number of factors, such as compression of the artery by a protruding edematous gyrus rectus. When occlusion occurs in the anterior cerebral artery at any point proximal to the paracentral lobule, the contralateral lower limb may

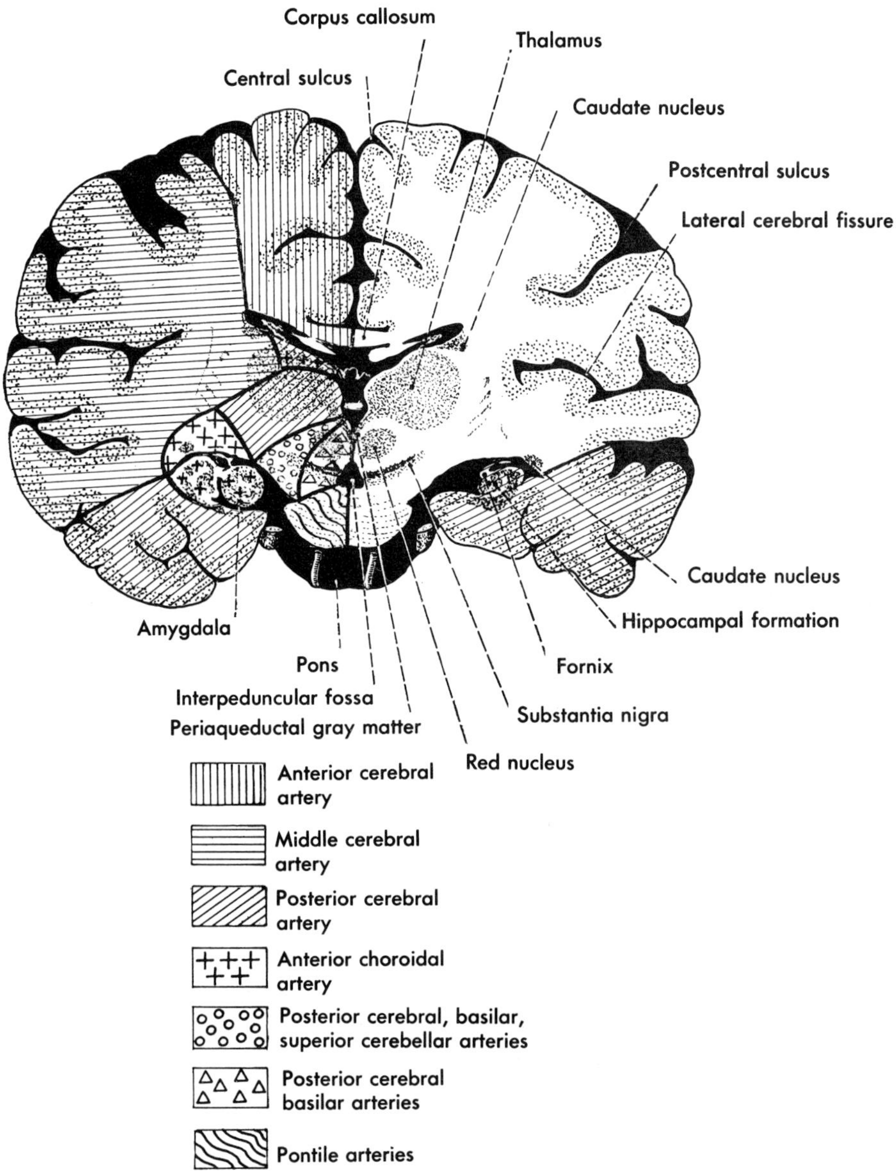

Fig. 27-7. Arterial supply of the brain at the level of the red nucleus (coronal section). The section is somewhat tangential, with the amygdala and hippocampal formation showing on the left and the hippocampal formation alone on the right.

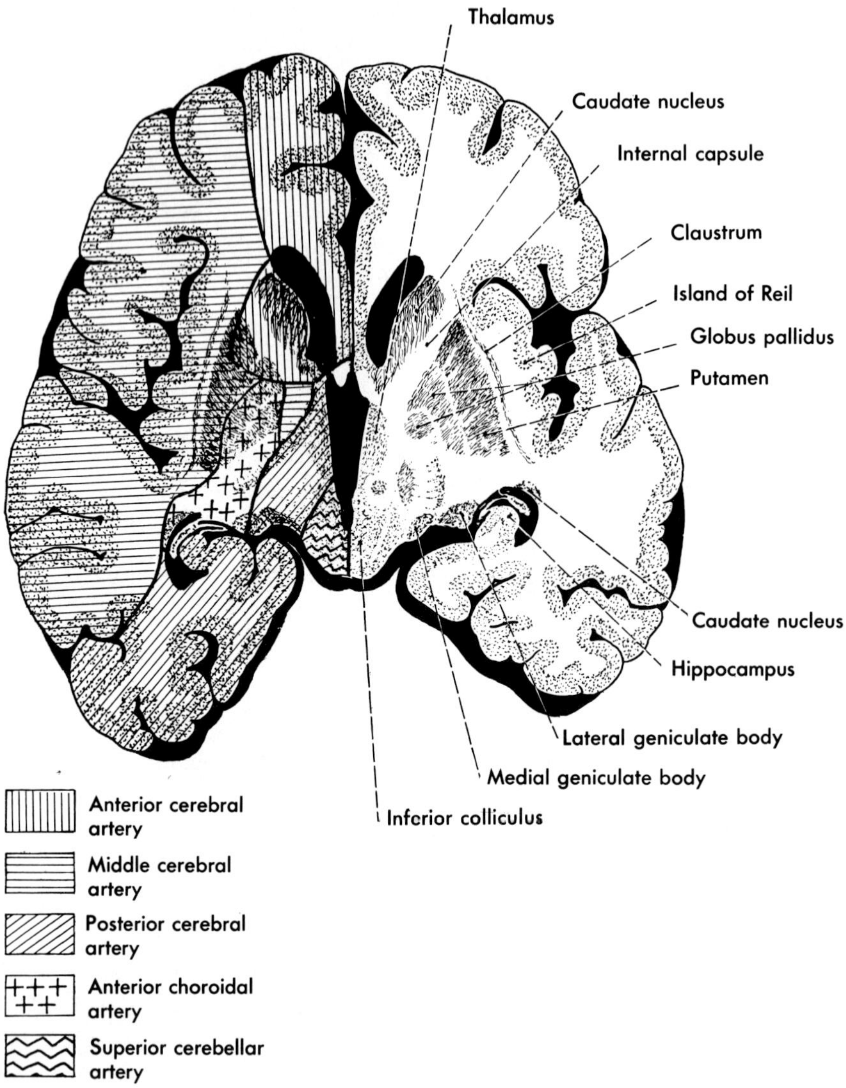

Fig. 27-8. Arterial supply of the brain at the level of the inferior colliculus (longitudinal section).

become paretic, and the Babinski sign can usually be elicited. There may be sensory disturbances of the cortical type. Sphincter control may also be lost. Rather numerous cases are characterized at the outset by hemiplegia, particularly when the infarction is widespread, as illustrated in Fig. 27-9. The hemiplegia is practically always of the spastic type; only rarely is it flaccid. A few days after the occlusion, the paresis of the upper limb usually recedes. Occlusion of the artery may sometimes result from compression from thrust of the artery against the free edge of the falx cerebri brought about by a unilateral expanding lesion in the vicinity.

Involvement of the corpus callosum may give rise to ideomotor apraxia of the left side owing to interruption of fibers extending from the left supramarginal gyrus to the right precentral gyrus; regardless of whether the right or the left anterior cerebral artery is occluded (in right-handed persons), the apraxia always involves the left side (Foix and Hillemand, 1925a). Motor aphasia (in the right-handed) is apt

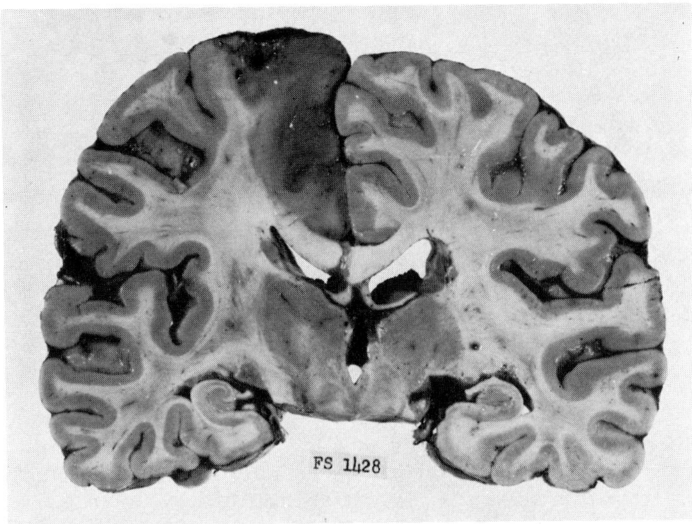

Fig. 27-9. Recent infarct in the territory of supply of the left anterior cerebral artery, involving both cortex and white matter, due to embolus from the region of a myocardial infarct. Paralysis and sensory loss developed in the right lower limb, and some weakness of the right upper limb. (Courtesy Dr. Richard Lindenberg, Baltimore.)

to occur when the occlusion is on the left side. Disorders also referable to the frontal lobe are indifference, euphoria, and grasping and groping movements. Mental clouding may occur and, occasionally, deep coma. Olfactory disturbances have sometimes been encountered. In bilateral anterior cerebral artery occlusion, there may be spastic paraplegia with some increase in tonus of the arms together with a tendency to catatonia. When clinical disturbances are bilateral, occlusion of an anomalous artery supplying the medial side of both hemispheres may be at fault. (Baptista, 1963; Chavany and others, 1955; Critchley, 1930; Davison, 1949.)

MIDDLE CEREBRAL ARTERY

The middle cerebral artery runs along the mouth of the lateral cerebral fissure (of Sylvius), adjacent to the lesser wing of the sphenoid bone, and extends to the island of Reil where it divides into several terminal branches (Fig. 27-5, *B*). In its early course, it begins to give off branches 1 to 4 cm. from its origin from the internal carotid. These vessels, the *lateral striate arteries,* come off the parent vessel at a right angle. They penetrate the lateral part of the anterior perforated substance (Fig. 27-3) and extend upward in the brain substance to supply various structures.

While traversing the brain substance, the *lateral striate arteries* pursue a dorsomedial course. They supply the dorsolateral part of the head of the caudate nucleus and adjacent superior half (or more) of the putamen, all the putamen at more caudal levels, and much of the body of the caudate nucleus. The lateral third of the globus pallidus is supplied by one of the lateral striate arteries (Fig. 27-12). Furthermore, the lateral posterior and lateral dorsal nuclei of the thalamus receive their blood supply from these branches. In extending to the caudate nucleus and thalamus, the lateral striate arteries course through the putamen and supply the part of the internal capsule adjacent to the lenticular nucleus (Figs. 27-6 to 27-8); they also supply the ansa lenticularis. Supply of the internal capsule is shared by branches from other vessels (Fig. 27-10) (Abbie, 1937; Rubinstein, 1944).

In its course the middle cerebral artery gives off branches to the orbitofrontal cortex, island of Reil, external capsule and claustrum, inferior and middle frontal gyri, the lower four-fifths of the precentral and postcentral gyri, supramarginal gyrus, angular gyrus, most of the convex surface of the temporal lobe, including its tip, and the anterior part of the convex surface of the occipital lobe (Figs. 27-5 to 27-8). It also irrigates the white matter of the centrum semiovale and the tapetum of the corpus callosum in the region corresponding to its cortical supply.

Thus, the middle cerebral artery supplies the motor and sensory speech centers, most of the sensorimotor cortex, and the cortical center for hearing. In a considerable proportion of brains the middle cerebral artery extends backward along the convexity of the hemisphere to the region of the occipital pole, supplying a small caudal segment of the calcarine cortex above the calcarine fissure.

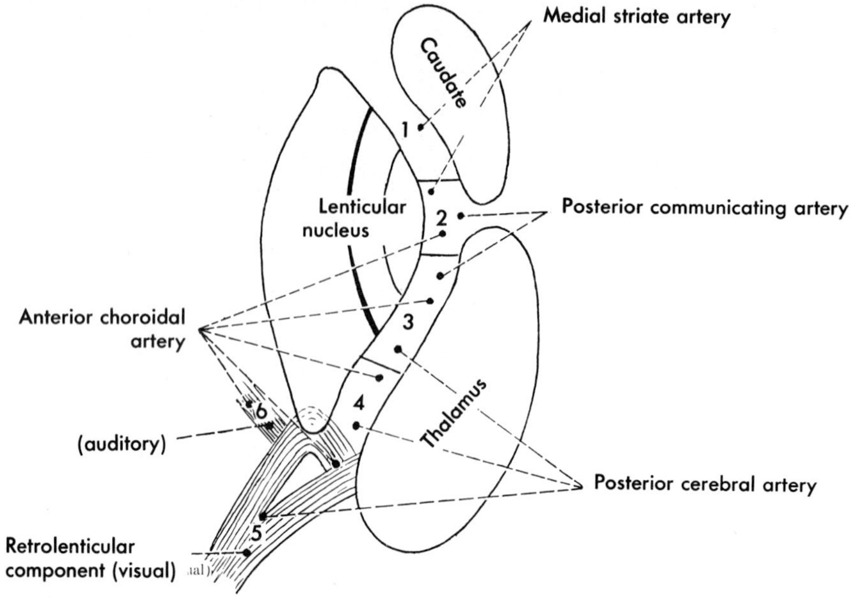

Fig. 27-10. The arterial supply of the internal capsule (longitudinal section). *1,* Anterior limb; *2,* genu; *3,* anterior two-thirds of the posterior limb; *4,* posterior third of the posterior limb; *5,* the retrolenticular fibers; and *6,* the sublenticular fibers. (Modified from Abbie, 1937, and Rubenstein, 1944.) According to Abbie (1937), the lateral striate arteries (derived from the middle cerebral artery) supply all parts of the internal capsule.

The field irrigated by the middle cerebral artery is more subject to infarction than that of any other major intracranial artery (Berry and Alpers, 1957; Lee and Hodes, 1967). Sclerosis of the stem of the middle cerebral artery, whether a thrombus has formed in it or not, accounts for only 15 percent of the infarctions; embolization of the artery from internal carotid, cardiac, and other extracranial sources accounts for the other infarctions (Lhermitte and others, 1968).

Headache may precede the infarction or occur as the attack is developing. In thrombosis of the stem of the middle cerebral artery the pain is typically behind, in, or above the corresponding eye, and the pain is usually steady. In embolism, headache is less frequent; when occurring, the pain is usually experienced in the region above the ipsilateral temple. The headache in middle cerebral arterial occlusion is usually lateralized, and it is more frequent in anterior locations than the headache in internal carotid arterial occlusion. (Fisher, 1968.)

Occlusion of the entire bed of the middle cerebral artery gives rise to profound disturbances: contralateral hemiparesis (involving chiefly the face, tongue, and upper limb), hemianesthesia of the cortical type, hemianopia or upper quadrantanopia, and, when on the left side (in right-handed persons), total aphasia as well. With complete occlusion of the middle cerebral artery, spastic hemiplegia eventually ensues, except in a minority of cases, in which flaccidity persists (Davison, 1949).

In most cases individual branches are occluded. Occlusion of *lateral striate arteries* results in hemiplegia of internal capsular origin. If the *precentral artery,* which supplies the operculum and posterior part of the inferior frontal gyrus (Broca's area), is occluded, there will be crossed paresis of the lower part of the face and the tongue of the opposite side, and motor aphasia as well if the occlusion is on the left. If occlusion involves the *central artery,* which supplies the major part of the precentral gyrus, there will be paresis of the contralateral arm or the arm and face. Occlusion distal to the point where the central artery arises cuts off

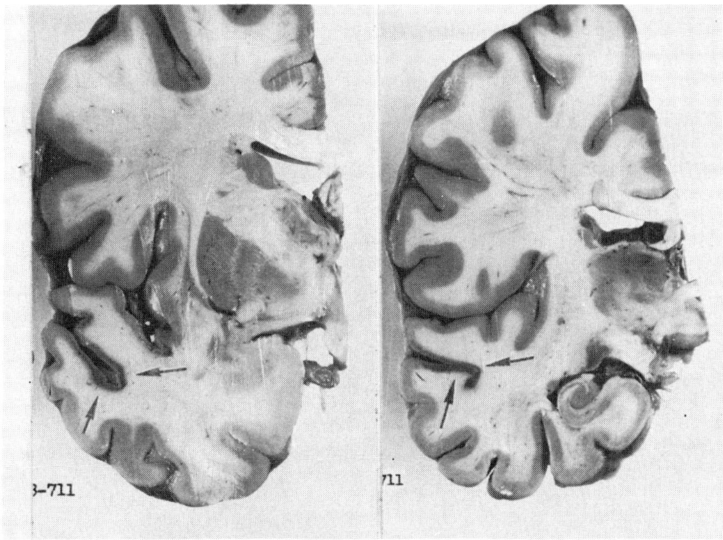

Fig. 27-11. Softening of cortex of the superior temporal gyrus *(arrows)*, of 8 weeks' duration, due to embolus originating from infarcted area in the heart in coronary disease. During a telephone conversation the patient was suddenly unable to understand what was said to him and he was unable to express himself. There were no other neurological disturbances. The sensory aphasia persisted. (Courtesy Dr. Richard Lindenberg, Baltimore.)

blood flow in the parietal, occipital, and temporal branches; this results in contralateral sensory disturbances of the cortical type, contralateral homonymous visual field defects (hemianopia or upper quadrantanopia), and, if the occlusion is on the left side, sensory aphasia and ideational apraxia as well. Occlusion of the *posterior temporal branch* extending to the superior temporal gyrus (Fig. 27-11) gives rise to sensory aphasia.

Infarction in the *border zone* between the anterior cerebral and middle cerebral arteries results in recurrent episodes of weakness and numbness of an arm (with grasp reflex), of an arm and leg, or, occasionally, of a leg alone. Conjugate deviation of the eyes to the opposite side may also occur. There may also be "parietal lobe signs." The face remains unaffected. With infarction in the territory of anastomosis between the middle cerebral and posterior cerebral arteries, the initial and often the only manifestations are those of parietal lobe dysfunction. (Romanul and Abramowicz, 1964.)

POSTERIOR CEREBRAL ARTERY

The origin of the posterior cerebral arteries and their branches to the midbrain is discussed elsewhere (pp. 304 and 460). The vessel rounds the basis pedunculi, gains the cisterna ambiens, passes adjacent to the upper surface of the tentorium, extends backward along the medial aspect of the temporal and occipital lobes, and terminates in the region of the occipital pole (Figs. 27-5 and 27-12).

Early in its course, the posterior cerebral artery gives off a vessel, the *medial posterior choroidal artery;* in the region of the cisterna ambiens it gives off other vessels, the *lateral posterior choroidal arteries.* All pass through the choroidal fissure with vessels from the anterior choroidal artery and reach the choroid plexus of the inferior horn of the lateral ventricle. Some of these vessels participate in the supply of the thalamus (Fig. 25-6).

As a rule, springing directly from the posterior cerebral artery in the latter's course through the cisterna ambiens are two or three fairly stout vessels, the *hippocampal arteries* (Figs. 27-3 and 27-13). Anastomosis between these branches prior to their passage into the hippocampal formation has been described as sparse (Lindenberg, 1955) or abundant. When abundant, the branches form an imposing anastomotic arcade from which a series of "rake-like" vessels penetrates the hippocampal formation (Heiman, 1938; Uchimura, 1928); or there may be hardly any arcade at all (Muller and Shaw, 1965). Either directly or by the mediation of arcades, a branch is given off to the subiculum,

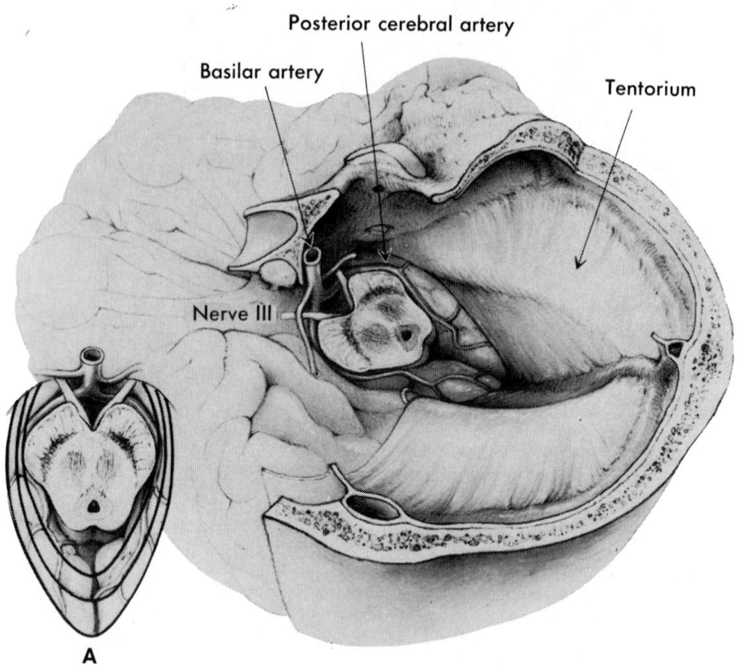

Fig. 27-12. Proximal course of the posterior cerebral artery, as viewed basally. The vessel partly encircles the midbrain, and its branches extend through the incisura tentorii. Inset **A** indicates variation in size of the incisura. (From Hoyt, 1960.)

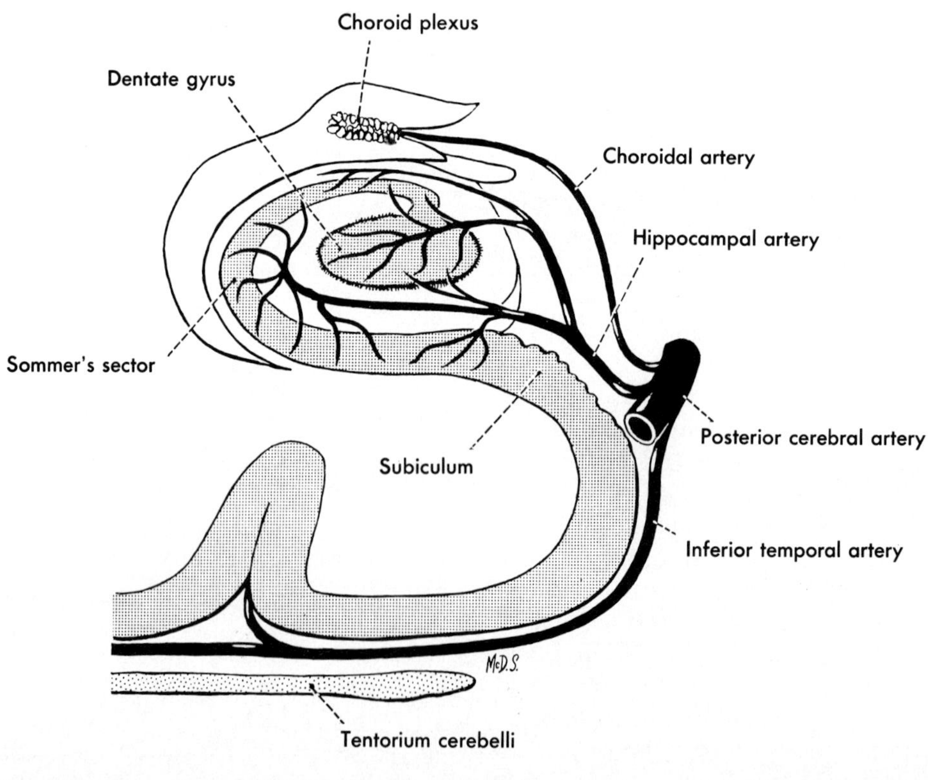

Fig. 27-13. Arterial supply of the hippocampal formation. (Redrawn from Lindenberg, 1955.)

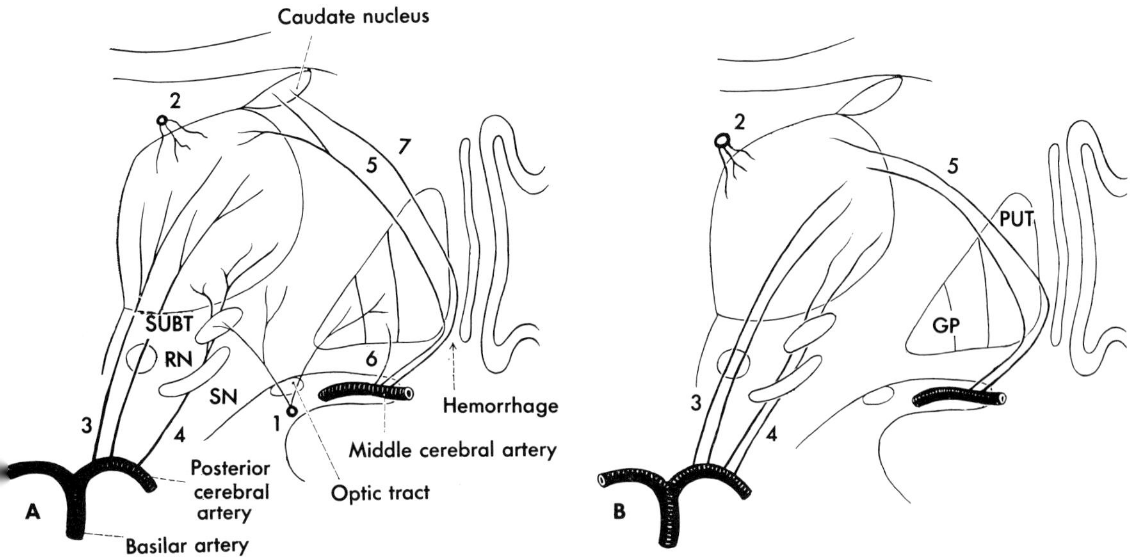

Fig. 27-14. Diagrams of arterial supply of the thalamus. **A,** Redrawn from Foix and Nicolesco (1925); **B,** redrawn from Foix and Hillemand (1925b). *1,* Anterior choroidal artery; *2,* anterior and posterior choroidal arteries; *3,* posterior thalamoperforate arteries; *4,* thalamogeniculate arteries; *5,* lateral striate arteries; *6,* supply of lateral part of globus pallidus according to Abbie (1937); *7,* course of lateral striate artery through base of external capsule according to Abbie (1937). The most common site of cerebral hemorrhage is indicated. *GP,* globus pallidus; *PUT,* putamen; *RN,* red nucleus; *SN,* substantia nigra; *SUBT,* subthalamus.

medial to which the artery divides into (1) the *dorsal* (or short) *branch,* which supplies the dentate gyrus and the dorsal part of the pyramidal layer, and (2) the *ventral* (or long) *branch,* which supplies the presubiculum and Sommer's sector of the pyramidal layer. An independent branch sometimes extends to the uncus hippocampi and the adjoining temporal cortex (Muller and Shaw, 1965; Vander Eecken, 1959).

The posterior cerebral artery also gives off a number of *penetrating branches* for the thalamus and environs (Figs. 25-6, 27-7, 27-8, and 27-14). Since the subject is handled elsewhere (pp. 460-461), only a few points will be made.

Thalamoperforate arteries. Blood supply provided by these vessels is not limited to the thalamus. They probably provide the chief blood supply for the subthalamic nucleus, with the anterior choroidal artery a subsidiary source. Another structure supplied by these arteries is the rubrothalamic tract, which also receives tributaries from a paramedian midbrain artery (Fig. 27-14). *Occlusion of the posterior cerebral artery* results in infarction, usually bilaterally, in the subthalamic region and in various thalamic nuclei supplied by the thalamoperforate and related arteries (medial dorsal [MD], especially its inferior and medial parts; centrum medianum [CM]; ventral posterolateral [VPL]; and others) and also, in occasional instances, infarction of the midbrain tegmentum. In such cases the hypothalamus has shared consistently in the damage, the dorsal periventricular region being most seriously affected. (Jakimowicz, Stefanko, and Pajak, 1968.)

Superficial branches of the posterior cerebral artery. These branches pass to and supply the medial and inferior aspects of the temporal lobe (except the tip of the temporal lobe, which is irrigated by the middle cerebral artery), the more caudal part of the uncus hippocampi, and most of the occipital lobe. The visual area is supplied by a separate branch, the calcarine artery (Fig. 27-5, A).

Signs of *occlusion of superficial branches of the posterior cerebral artery* are rather few because of the richness of their collateral circulation with adjoining vascular beds. The anterior choroidal artery, for instance, aids materially in the supply of the uncus and gyrus hippocampi, and thus these structures tend to be spared in anterior choroidal or middle cerebral artery occlusion. Furthermore, since the middle cerebral artery anastomoses with the posterior cerebral artery over the occipital pole, central vision, represented on the mesial side of the occipital pole, tends to be spared in occlusion of either vessel.

Occlusion of the posterior cerebral artery is characterized initially by bilateral blindness of the cortical type and within a few days by crossed homonymous hemianopia with sparing of central vision. Occlusion resulting from compression of the posterior cerebral artery at the free edge of the tentorium is usually unilateral but may be bilateral (Lindenberg, 1955). Such compression may result from birth injury. As a rule, involvement of the *calcarine artery* alone gives rise to a contralateral homonymous and congruous quadrantic defect. The occurrence of scintillations clinches the diagnosis, whether the calcarine artery alone, or a more proximal part of the posterior cerebral artery, is occluded. Headache occurring at the time of the stroke (sometimes before) is usually in the lower forehead and region of the eye, ipsilateral to the vessel occluded; pain in other regions (for example, the entire frontal region and the occipital region) is fairly common. (Fisher, 1968.)

For a description of the syndromes of *occlusion of the thalamoperforate arteries,* see page 461.

ANEURYSMS

Within the brain and brainstem the most common sites at which microaneurysms develop are the putamen, globus pallidus, and thalamus (Cole and Yates, 1967). As observed on the brain surface, micro- and larger aneurysms form predominantly in basal cerebral arteries, most commonly in vessels forming the anterior part of the circle of Willis. Incidence of aneurysm is rather high if aneurysms 5 mm. in diameter or less are included—in 7 percent of normotensive persons and in 46 percent of hypertensives (Cole and Yates, 1967). Figures generally cited are in the 0.5 to 0.8 percent range. Frequency of aneurysm is very low in persons less than 20 years of age; in persons beyond 20 their occurrence is age-dependent. They are somewhat more common in women than in men. Aneurysms may be multiple. In an analysis of 2,000 cases of intracranial aneurysm cited in the literature, Bigelow (1955) noted that the incidence of multiple aneurysm was about 10 percent; in his own experience they came to 25 percent.

Most aneurysms are saccular; the remainder are fusiform or arteriovenous. The most frequent saccular type is the "berry" aneurysm. Its development has commonly been laid to a combination of congenital and arteriosclerotic factors. In this connection, numerous aneurysms arise from circles of Willis that have retained their fetal form or are associated with anomalies of the circle of Willis, coarctation of the aorta, and congenital polycystic renal disease. Defects in the arterial media have been held accountable. Evidence thereof, however, is not strong, since such defects are commonly found at lateral angles of a point of branching, while aneurysms form at the distal angle of a point of branching (Sahs, 1966). The suggestion has been made that many berry aneurysms are not of congenital origin or attributable primarily to a medial defect, but instead to some alteration occurring secondarily in the arterial wall—some acute degenerative change that goes on to overt atheroma (du Boulay, 1967).

Larger *saccular* aneurysms are usually atherosclerotic in origin. About 12 percent of aneurysms of this kind are said to result from the lodgement of mycotic emboli in the arterial wall or its vasa vasorum. An incidence of about 6 percent for syphilitic aneurysms has been cited in the past, but an incidence this high does not hold currently; very few aneurysms can be proved to be syphilitic in origin. Trauma as an etiological factor is rather uncommon; it occurs most frequently, however, when there is skull fracture. In most cases the trauma may be viewed as a precipitating influence operating upon preexisting disease of the vessel wall. *Fusiform* aneurysms are comparatively uncommon and involve chiefly the internal carotid, basilar, and vertebral arteries. Such aneurysms are virtually always found in association with atherosclerosis of intracranial vessels and commonly in cardiovascular hypertension. (Araki and others, 1965; Bigelow, 1955; Crawford, 1959; Daly and others, 1964; Hamby, 1952; Krainer, 1947; Riggs and Rupp, 1943.)

Focal manifestations of aneurysm

Like any other mass, an aneurysm may stretch the leptomeninges or compress nerves or brain tissue sufficiently to become clinically manifest. However, only 10 to 15 percent act in this way. The great majority of aneurysms remain asymptomatic until leakage of blood or frank rupture occurs. The aneurysms most likely to produce clinical disturbances prior to hemorrhage are internal carotid aneurysms. In aneurysms involving this artery or a neighboring artery the most common complaint is severe headache; the next most common complaint is pain in the region of the orbit (Locksley, 1966). The region of the inner canthus is most apt to be painful (Jefferson, 1947). Migrainous headache may occur, mainly in internal carotid aneurysm, but is rare. In no aneurysm is palsy of the fourth or sixth nerve an isolated or a presenting disturbance (Daly and others, 1964). Visual field defects occurring in aneurysm in various locations are almost always bilateral (Jefferson, 1953, 1955).

Infraclinoid part of the internal carotid artery. Aneurysm, usually saccular, in the part of the artery lying in the lateral wall of the cavernous sinus (Fig. 16-1) commonly compresses adjacent nerves. Most frequently there is ipsilateral severe and persistent pain in the region of distribution of the ophthalmic division of the fifth nerve (or the maxillary division as well) and palsy of the third nerve; the sixth nerve and sometimes the fourth as well may also be involved. Now and then the fifth nerve is spared; occasionally, however, it alone is involved. Horner's syndrome may also occur. Edema of the eyelids and dilatation of the retinal veins are commonly noted; preretinal hemorrhage and occlusion of the central retinal vein may also occur. Total blindness in the affected eye is said ultimately to occur in some 20 percent of cases. By ballooning into the sella turcica, an aneurysm of this kind may, in rare cases, involve predominantly one side of the chiasm and cause homonymous hemianopia, with the blindness most pronounced in the eye ipsilateral to the site of major compression. Otherwise the optic pathway is usually not directly affected. Simmonds' disease is an occasional complication. (Brouwer, 1918; Daly and others, 1964; Jefferson, 1953; Schlezinger, 1950.)

Exophthalmos, usually pulsating, commonly occurs when a carotid aneurysm, by breaking into the cavernous sinus, becomes arteriovenous. A fistula between the two develops. Pounding headaches occur, and the patient may complain of a roaring noise in the head and decrease in visual acuity. The eyelids, cornea, and conjunctivae usually become edematous and

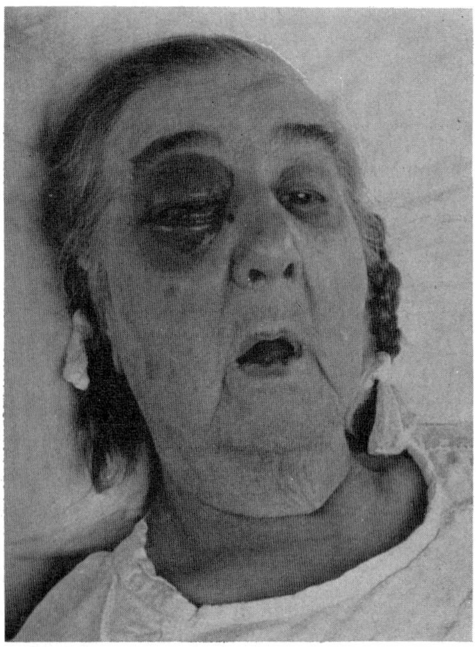

Fig. 27-15. Severe hemorrhagic edema of the eyelids together with proptosis in 80-year-old patient, resulting from spontaneously occurring carotid-cavernous fistula. (Courtesy Dr. A. Ornsteen, Philadelphia.)

A 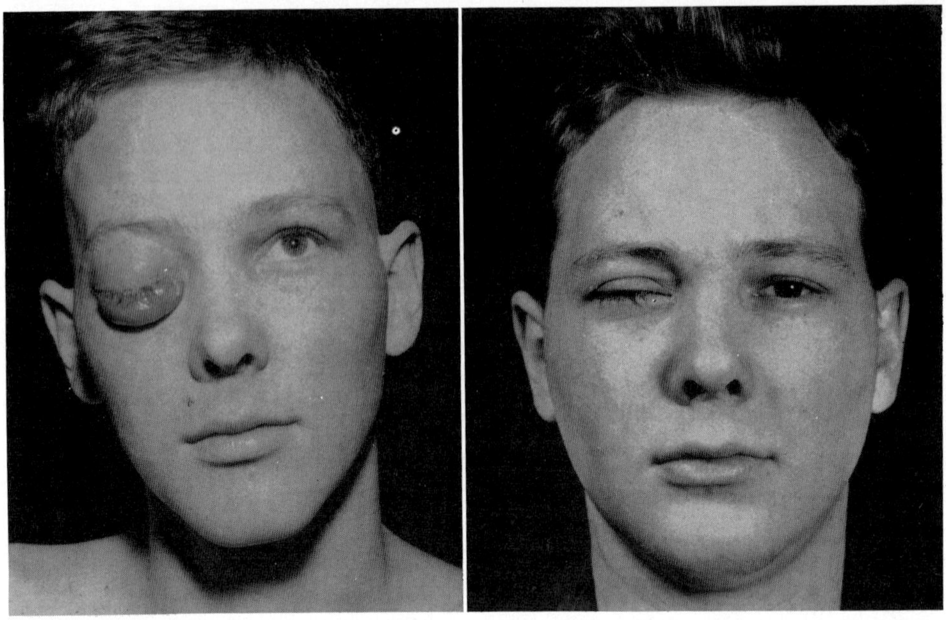 B

Fig. 27-16. A, Ectropion about 6 weeks after the development of a carotid-cavernous fistula following an automobile accident. **B,** Six months later, following operation. (From Walter Reed Army Hosp.; Negs. 9028C and 9028L.)

hemorrhagic. Papilledema may be noted. A bruit can be heard over the bulging eye in most cases. Rapidly progressive ophthalmoplegia occurs on the affected side and may develop also on the contralateral side, owing to a rush of blood by way of the intercavernous sinus system into the venous system of that eye. Epistaxis, which may be severe, occurs in some cases. Hemiplegia will develop immediately if there is insufficient collateral circulation by way of the anterior and posterior communicating arteries.

Carotid artery–cavernous sinus fistula may develop spontaneously not only from rupture of carotid aneurysm but also from rupture of an atheromatous carotid, such as occurred in the patient illustrated in Fig. 27-15. A patient in whom head trauma preceded fistula formation is shown in Fig. 27-16. Fistula development is preceded by head trauma in some 80 percent of cases, and basal skull fracture involving the sphenoid bone occurs in most of them (Daly and others, 1964). Sooner or later, arterialized veins become evident in the bulbar conjunctiva (Fig. 27-17). (Graf, 1965; Hamby, 1966; Martin and Maybon, 1943; Perret and Nishioka, 1966; Stern, Brown, and Alksne, 1967.)

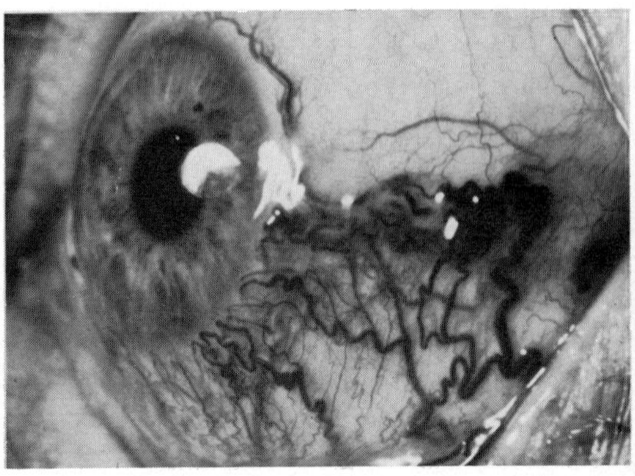

Fig. 27-17. Arterialized veins in the bulbar conjunctiva in a patient with carotid-cavernous fistula. The patient had pulsating exophthalmos. (Courtesy Dr. William F. Hoyt, San Francisco.)

Bilateral carotid aneurysms within the cavernous sinus are rare. Bilateral carotid artery–cavernous sinus fistulas are somewhat more common. Either may become clinically manifest at different times and lead to bilateral ophthalmoplegia of varying degree. Some 20 percent of cases associated with pulsating exophthalmos are of traumatic origin and about 10 percent are "idiopathic." Pulsating exophthalmos in the second eye almost never results from rupture of the second carotid vessel but is caused in the manner already indicated, namely, overflow of the arterial blood into the second intercavernous sinus, and through the second cavernous sinus into the venous system of the second orbit. Involvement of the second eye may develop in a few days, weeks, or months after the original rupture. (Alpers, Schlezinger, and Tassman, 1951.)

Supraclinoid part of the internal carotid artery. Both fusiform and saccular aneurysms arise from this part of the artery. Optic nerve chiasm or tract, singly or in combination, may be compressed by the aneurysm. Visual field defects vary accordingly, and optic atrophy occurs. Characteristic in optic nerve compression is a central scotoma that, in time, enlarges toward the periphery. The Paton-Kennedy syndrome is occasionally encountered. In aneurysm exerting pressure on the anterolateral angle of the optic chiasm from below (right), the visual loss is initially in the peripheral upper temporal field of the opposite eye (left). Partial or complete third nerve paralysis commonly occurs, and there may also be disturbances referable to the ophthalmic division of the fifth nerve. Commonly preceding visual disturbances is the occurrence of headaches, which are either generalized or limited to one side of the head. Sooner or later, excruciating pain in the region of one eye and the forehead above it sets in. Either pain or disturbances in vision in one eye may mark the onset. (Hughes, 1954; Jefferson, 1947; Schlezinger, 1950.)

Anterior cerebral and anterior communicating arteries. Aneurysms at or near the junction of the anterior cerebral and anterior communicating arteries may first compress the optic chiasm and thus lead to visual disturbances. By indenting the

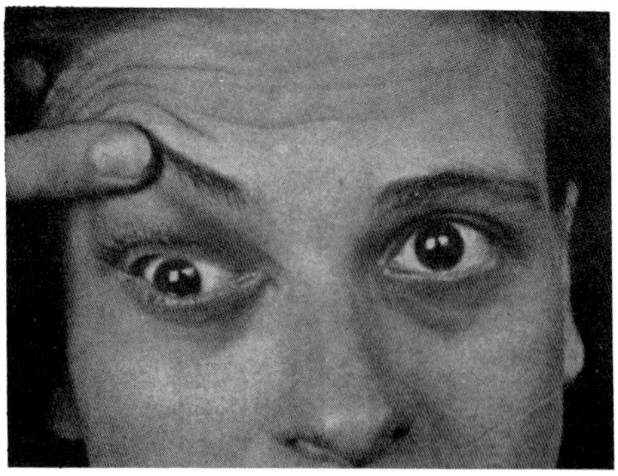

Fig. 27-18. Palsy of third nerve due to aneurysm of anterior part of circle of Willis. (Courtesy Dr. A. Ornsteen, Philadelphia.)

superior surface of the chiasm they are likely to produce bilateral inferior field defects with involvement of central vision (Jefferson, 1953). They may produce bitemporal hemianopic defects, with the defect most marked unilaterally. Headache mounting in severity, dizziness, and hyposmia occur, but their incidence is rather low. Mental and behavioral disturbances are prominent in some cases. (Courville and Olsen, 1938; Walker, 1956.)

Middle cerebral artery. Aneurysms of the middle cerebral artery at the base of the cerebrum, often as much as 1.0 cm. in diameter, tend to burrow into the brain substance. They are usually asymptomatic. Aneurysm of branches of this artery in their course in the region of the convex surface of the hemisphere is rare and becomes clinically evident only when large; then, like any other tumor, it may give rise to jacksonian attacks, hemiparesis, aphasia, and so on.

Region of junction of the internal carotid and posterior communicating arteries; posterior communicating artery. Aneurysms arising in the region of junction of these two arteries are small and flasklike, and through local pressure frequently produce isolated third nerve palsy, with ptosis, pupillary dilatation, and lateral strabismus resulting (Fig. 27-18). It is the sudden appearance and completeness of the third nerve palsy that point to involvement by aneurysm. There may, however, be no disturbance other than headache. Optic chiasm or optic nerve involvement by an aneurysm in this location is rare, but in aneurysm of more caudal parts of the posterior communicating artery homonymous visual field defects referable to compression of the optic tract are fairly common. (Bramwell, 1934; Jefferson, 1947; Sachs, 1938.) In aneurysm limited to the posterior communicating artery, recurrent third nerve palsy and pain (or headache) in the region of distribution of the ophthalmic division of the fifth nerve are the most common manifestations (Alpers and Schlezinger, 1949).

Posterior cerebral artery. Aneurysm in this location can be manifested by Weber's or some other crossed syndrome, a result

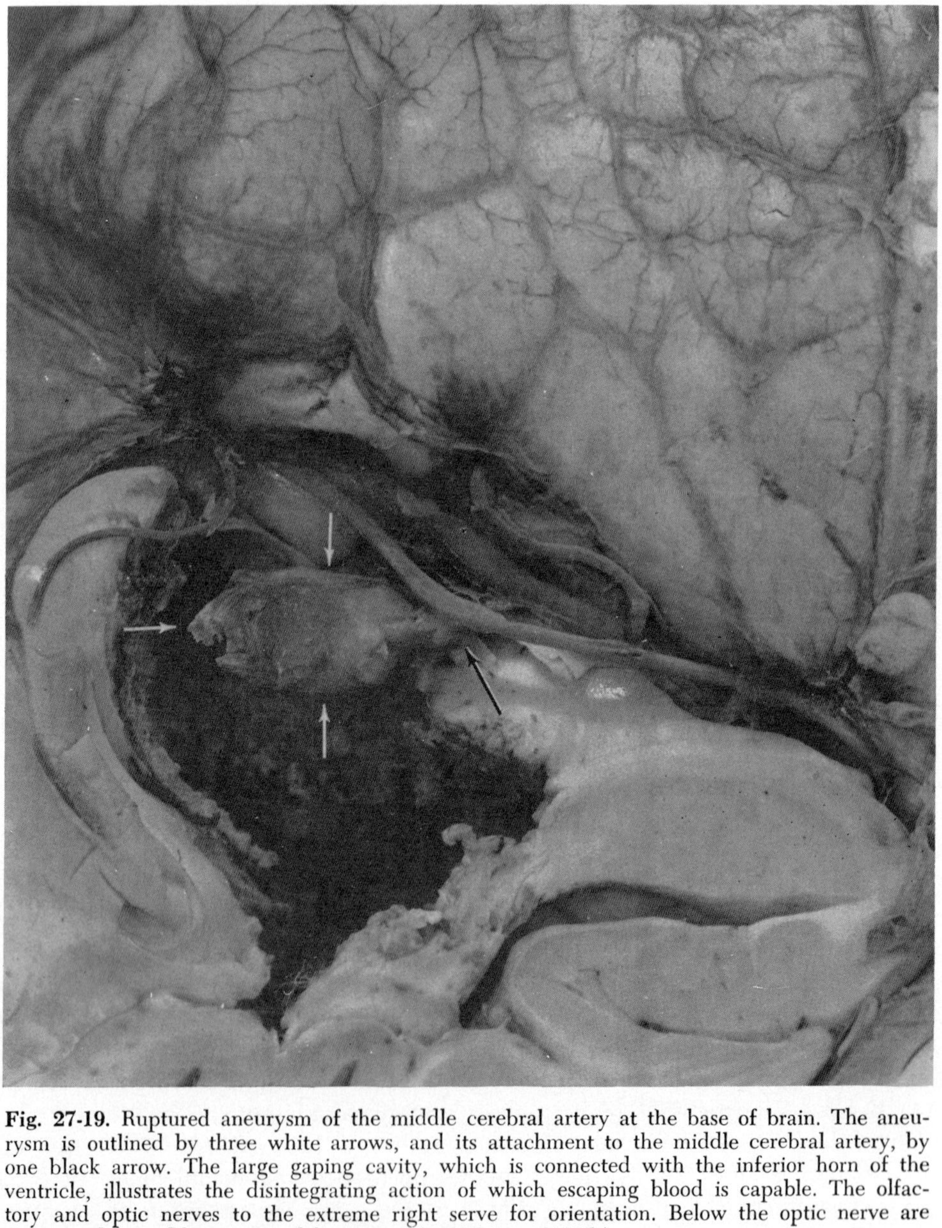

Fig. 27-19. Ruptured aneurysm of the middle cerebral artery at the base of brain. The aneurysm is outlined by three white arrows, and its attachment to the middle cerebral artery, by one black arrow. The large gaping cavity, which is connected with the inferior horn of the ventricle, illustrates the disintegrating action of which escaping blood is capable. The olfactory and optic nerves to the extreme right serve for orientation. Below the optic nerve are the amygdala and hippocampal formation. (AFIP Acc. 94867.)

of pressure exerted on the basis pedunculi and third nerve. Associated contralateral homonymous hemianopia appears to result from compression of the optic tract. Palsy of the third, fourth, and sixth nerves may occur and, in occasional instances, palsy of both third nerves. The fifth nerve is unaffected. Aneurysms of the posterior cerebral artery are usually quite large and may be indistinguishable from neoplasms in the region until arteriography is carried out (Dandy, 1944).

Manifestations of rupture of an aneurysm

Asymptomatic berry aneurysm will rupture only in about 1 case in 20 (du Boulay, 1967). When a person has his first subarachnoid hemorrhage, there is a 54 percent chance that it is due to ruptured aneurysm (Locksley, 1966). He may be active or not at the time of rupture; cranial trauma commonly precipitates rupture (Freytag, 1966). Hemorrhage, once it occurs, may remain limited to the subarachnoid space, or it may extend directly into the brain substance, disintegrating the tissue (Fig. 27-19) (Sahs and others, 1966). In the series of 88 cases of ruptured aneurysm, Williams, Bahn, and Sayre (1955) noted that the hemorrhage extended into the brain substance in 57 cases and broke into one of the ventricles in 43 cases. Hemorrhage may occur from a "symptomatic" aneurysm. For instance, in berry aneurysm situated at the junction of the carotid and posterior communicating artery, manifested by third nerve palsy, the sudden development of sixth nerve palsy and supraorbital pain can be taken as suggestive evidence of leakage from the aneurysm. Usually, however (in 85 to 90 percent of cases), hemorrhage from aneurysmal rupture occurs without prior warning signs.

The manifestations of rupture of an aneurysm may be subdivided into those caused (1) by rapidly increasing intracranial pressure with signs of meningeal irritation and (2) by focal compression. Both vary in intensity depending on the degree of hemorrhage and its site. Sometimes the initial hemorrhage is fatal within a few hours or days, but as a rule the patient recovers, only to have subsequent leakage or frank hemorrhage, most commonly in the week after the first hemorrhage (Locksley, 1966), though the incidence remains high for 2 to 3 weeks (Trumpy, 1967).

If hemorrhage is massive, consciousness is rapidly lost and vomiting may occur. Respiration becomes irregular and the pulse is slowed. When the patient remains conscious he usually complains of excruciating headache. A few complain of "a sudden snap in the head" or "a feeling of cold water rushing down the neck" as the initial symptom. In a very small proportion of cases, convulsive seizures mark the onset. The patient may assume an attitude of generalized flexion, but if hemorrhage is sufficient, there will be cervical rigidity. Semiconsciousness and irritability prevail. Depending on the degree of hemorrhage, there may be papilledema (but it is uncommon). When the hemorrhage involves the optic nerves, retinal and/or subhyaloid hemorrhages occur.

In hemorrhage emanating from an aneurysm of the circle of Willis, pain suddenly develops in and above one eye. Visual defects may occur, their nature being dependent on whether the optic nerves, chiasm, or tracts have been affected. These defects develop rapidly and tend to recede within a few days. Ocular palsies referable to involvement of the third, fourth, or sixth nerve may also occur and usually persist in some degree. (Collier, 1931; French and Blake, 1950; Symonds, 1923.)

In leaking aneurysm, blood is almost always present in the *cerebrospinal fluid*, but its appearance may be delayed for as long as 5 days. In intracerebral hemorrhage, the fluid is blood-stained in about 70 percent of cases. In cerebral thrombosis and intracranial tumor this is comparatively rare.

Subarachnoid bleeding can readily be distinguished from normal fluid contaminated by blood during lumbar puncture, for in accidental puncture of a vein there will be decreasing amounts of blood in the three tubes in which the fluid is collected. A streak of blood rather than uniform staining can be seen in the dripping cerebrospinal fluid. Clotting of blood in a tube is strong evidence for accidental bleeding.

Blood within the subarachnoid space begins to hemolyze in 12 to 24 hours, though shorter (4 hours) and longer (3 or 4 days) periods have been claimed. Hemolysis, as manifested by xanthochromic fluid, is maximal about the fifth day and is generally complete about the ninth day, but longer periods (up to 19 days) may be required if the hemorrhage is large. The xanthochromia vanishes in 16 to 39 days, depending upon the size of the hemorrhage.

If the white and red cells are in normal blood proportions (1:500), it may be assumed that hemorrhage is active or at least very recent. The neutrophil count falls on the third to fifth day, and during the same time the "lymphocytes" (probably mobilized arachnoidal histiocytes, not lymphocytes) increase in number both relatively and absolutely. The "lymphocytosis" is apparent within 2 hours of the bleeding and persists up to 4 weeks.

During the first 3 or 4 days, before hemolysis has occurred, about 1000 erythrocytes in the cerebrospinal fluid account for approximately 1.0 to 1.5 mg. percent of protein. If the erythrocyte count is 10,000 and the protein content 15 mg. percent, it may be concluded that the cerebrospinal fluid was normal when the bleeding commenced and that there is no appreciable hematoma. But if the number of erythrocytes comes to 7500 and the protein 70 mg. percent, the assumption is that the protein was elevated before the bleeding occurred or that a sizable hematoma is present. (McMenemey, 1954.)

ARTERIOVENOUS MALFORMATIONS

Arteriovenous malformations (hemangiomas) are frequent, comprising about 1.5 to 4.0 percent of all intracranial tumors. As compared with "symptomatic" aneurysms, "symptomatic" arteriovenous malformations are considerably fewer. These malformations appear to originate as a congenital malformation of blood vessels early in embryogenesis. Primitive arteriovenous sinusoids—shunts—persist in areas that normally would be replaced by an intervening capillary bed. Each component of the malformation responds to the altered local hemodynamics incident to these shunts. Arteries open directly into the sinusoids or alter their state so that the arteries may become veins without an intervening capillary bed. In the cerebrum and cerebellum the sinusoids lie within or below the cortex. The malformations are wedge-shaped, with the base parallel with the cortex and the apex frequently extending as far medially as the edge of the ventricle. Their configuration thus mimics that of transcerebral veins. Blood flow to and from the malformation is through large, normally situated channels, which can be seen in the leptomeninges (Fig. 22-1). Branches of the external carotid artery may contribute to the blood supply of the malformations. Various parts of the cerebrum may be involved, such as midline structures (found in about 10 percent of cases), but the most frequent site of involvement is the parietal lobe, in the territory of the middle cerebral artery. The cerebellum is also commonly affected.

These malformations usually become clinically manifest in patients in their teens and twenties, but there may be a delay in the appearance of the disturbances until the forties or the fifties. In about 10 percent of cases the initial clinical disturbances develop in persons up to 10 years old. The clinical course is usually prolonged over many years. Arteriovenous malformations situated near the central sulcus frequently manifest themselves first by jacksonian seizures. Subsequently there may be transitory, then permanent, monoparesis or hemiparesis. Some cases are characterized by sensory seizures followed by sensory deficit. Generalized seizures and psychomotor seizures may also occur. Aphasia may also develop. Throbbing and severe headache occurs in about 20 percent of cases, and audible bruit in about 50 percent. Arteriovenous malformations involving the occipital lobe may be associated with scintillating scotoma. Other manifestations (prior to hemorrhage) are sudden visual disturbances, sudden dysphagia, transient fainting episodes, attacks of dizziness or vertigo, and, occasionally, truncal ataxia and progressive proptosis. Generalized increased intracranial pressure can occur in cerebral arteriovenous malformation, but this is rare. By contrast, malformations in the cerebellum give rise relatively early to signs and symptoms of increased intracranial pressure, especially papilledema.

Hemorrhage into the subarachnoid space is the initial manifestation in 30 to 40 percent of cases. Recurrent hemorrhage is uncommon, and the intervals between hemorrhage often a matter of years. Seizures (generalized, psychomotor) occurring in association with hemorrhage are frequent. Just prior to hemorrhage (24 hours or more) headaches are fairly common, and they are also encountered over longer intervening periods, as already indicated. (Cushing and Bailey, 1928; Kaplan, Aronson, and Browder, 1961; MacKenzie, 1953; McCormick, 1966; Perret and Nishioka, 1966; Sahs and others, 1966.)

REFERENCES

Abbie, A. A. 1933a. The clinical significance of the anterior choroidal artery. Brain **56**:233-246.

Abbie, A. A. 1933b. Blood supply of the lateral geniculate body, with a note on morphology of choroidal arteries. J. Anat. **67**:491-521.

Abbie, A. A. 1937. The anatomy of capsular vascular disease. Med. J. Aust. **2**:546-568.

Alexander, L. 1942. The vascular supply of the strio-pallidum. Res. Publ. Ass. Res. Nerv. Ment. Dis., Proc. **21**:77-132.

Alpers, B. J. 1959. Compensatory mechanisms in occlusive vascular disease of the brain. Arch. Neurol. **1**:531-534.

Alpers, B. J., and Schlezinger, N. S. 1949. Aneurysm of the posterior communicating artery. Arch. Ophthal. **42**:353-364.

Alpers, B. J., Schlezinger, N. S., and Tassman, I. M. 1951. Bilateral internal carotid aneurysm involving cavernous sinus: right carotid artery—cavernous sinus fistula and left saccular aneurysm. Arch. Ophthal. **46**:403-407.

Araki, C., Handa, H., Handa, J., and Yoshida, K. 1965. Traumatic aneurysm of the intracranial extradural portion of the internal carotid artery. J. Neurosurg. **23**:64-67.

Balado, M., and Franke, E. 1937. Das Corpus geniculatum externum: eine anatomisch-klinische Studie. Berlin, Springer-Verlag.

Baptista, A. G. 1963. Studies on the arteries of the brain: anterior cerebral artery: some anatomic features and their clinical implications. Neurology **13**:825-835.

Beevor, C. E. 1907. The cerebral arterial supply. Brain **30**:403-425.

Beevor, C. E. 1909. On the distribution of the different arteries supplying the human brain. Philos. Trans. Roy. Soc. London **200**:1-55.

Berry, R. G., and Alpers, B. J. 1957. Occlusion of the cerebral circulation: pathologic considerations. Neurology **7**:223-237.

Bigelow, N. H. 1955. Multiple intracranial arterial aneurysms: an analysis of their significance. Arch. Neurol. Psychiat. **73**:76-99.

Brain, R. 1957. Order and disorder in the cerebral circulation. Lancet **2**:857-862.

Bramwell, E. 1934. Upon leaking aneurysm of cerebral arteries as cause of third nerve paralysis, etc. Trans. Ophthal. Soc. U.K. **54**:205-221.

Brouwer, B. 1918. Klinisch-anatomische Untersuchung über den Oculomotoriuskern. Z. Ges. Neurol. Psychiat. **40**:152-193.

Caldwell, H. W., and Hadden, F. C. 1948. Carotid artery thrombosis: report of eight cases due to trauma. Ann. Intern. Med. **28**:1132-1142.

Carpenter, M. B., Noback, C. R., and Moss, M. L. 1954. The anterior choroidal artery; its origins, course, distribution, and variations. Arch. Neurol. Psychiat. **71**:714-722.

Charcot, J.-M. 1883. Lectures on the localisation of cerebral and spinal diseases, translated and edited by W. B. Hadden. London, New Sydenham Society, pp. 49-64.

Chavany, J. A., Messimy, R., Pertuiset, B., and Hagenmuler, D. 1955. Les fonctions du territoire cortical de l'artère cérébrale antérieure; parentés séméiologiques des syndromes vasculaires, traumatiques et tumoraux. Presse Méd. **63**:512-514.

Coder, D. M., Frye, R. L., Bernatz, P. E., and Sheps, S. G. 1965. Symptomatic bilateral "subclavian steal." Proc. Mayo Clin. **40**:473-476.

Cohen, S. M. 1944. Traumatic arterial spasm. Brit. Med. Bull. **2**:144-145.

Cole, F. M., and Yates, P. O. 1967. The occurrence and significance of intracerebral microaneurysms. J. Path. Bact. **93**:393-411.

Collier, J. 1931. Cerebral haemorrhage due to causes other than arteriosclerosis. Brit. Med. J. **2**:519-521.

Courville, C. B., and Olsen, C. W. 1938. Miliary aneurysm of the anterior communicating artery: a clinical and pathologic report of nineteen cases, eighteen with fatal hemorrhage. Bull. Los Angeles Neurol. Soc. **3**:1-21.

Crawford, T. 1959. Some observations on the pathogenesis and natural history of intracranial aneurysms. J. Neurol. Neurosurg. Psychiat. **22**:259-266.

Critchley, M. 1930. The anterior cerebral artery and its syndromes. Brain **53**:120-165.

Cushing, H., and Bailey, P. 1928. Tumors arising from the blood vessels of the brain: angiomatous malformations and hemangioblastomas. Springfield, Illinois, Charles C Thomas, Publisher.

Daly, E. J., Holloway, J. A., Murto, R. E., and Schlezinger, N. S. 1964. Evaluation of ocular signs and symptoms in cerebral aneurysms. Arch. Ophthal. **71**:463-474.

Dandy, W. E. 1944. Intracranial arterial aneurysms. Ithaca, Comstock Publishing Associates.

Davison, C. 1949. Pathology. In Bucy, P. C., editor: The precentral motor cortex, ed. 2. Urbana, University of Illinois Press, pp. 425-457.

Dawson, B. H. 1958. The blood vessels of the human optic chiasma and their relation to those of the hypophysis and hypothalamus. Brain **81:** 207-217.

Dickinson, C. J. 1961. Functional efficiency of the circle of Willis; implications for reconstructive surgery of the main cerebral arteries. Brit. Med. J. **1:**858-859.

du Boulay, G. H. 1967. The natural history of intracranial aneurysms. Amer. Heart J. **73:**723-729.

Eadie, M. J., Jamieson, K. G., and Lennon, E. A. 1964. Persisting carotid-basilar anastomosis. J. Neurol. Sci. **1:**501-511.

Ecker, A. D. 1945. Spasm of the internal carotid artery. J. Neurosurg. **2:**479-484.

Fawcett, E., and Blackford, J. W. 1905. The circle of Willis: an examination of 700 specimens. J. Anat. **40:**63-70.

Fisher, A. G. T. 1913. A case of complete absence of both internal carotid arteries, with a preliminary note on the developmental history of the stapedial artery. J. Anat. Physiol. **48:** 37-46.

Fisher, C. M. 1957. Cerebral thromboangiitis obliterans. Medicine **36:**169-209.

Fisher, C. M. 1958. Cerebrovascular diseases: pathophysiology, diagnosis and treatment. J. Chron. Dis. **8:**419-447.

Fisher, C. M. 1968. Headache in cerebrovascular disease. In Vinken, P. J., and Bruyn, G. W., editors: Handbook of clinical neurology, vol. 5. Amsterdam, North-Holland Publishing Company, pp. 124-156.

Fisher, C. M., and Pearlman, A. 1967. The nonsudden onset of cerebral embolism. Neurology **17:**1025-1032.

Fisher, M. 1954a. Concerning cerebral arteriosclerosis. J. Amer. Geriat. Soc. **2:**1-18.

Fisher, M. 1954b. Occlusion of carotid arteries: further experiences. Arch. Neurol. Psychiat. **72:** 187-204.

Foix, C., and Hillemand, P. 1925a. Les syndromes de l'artère cérébrale antérieure. Encéphale **20:** 209-232.

Foix, C., and Hillemand, P. 1925b. Les artères de l'axe encéphalique jusqu'au diencéphale inclusivement. Rev. Neurol. **2:**705-739.

Foix, C., and Nicolesco, J. 1925. Les noyaux gris centraux et la région mésencephalo-sous-optique. Paris, Masson et Cie., pp. 323, 495-546.

Foley, J. M., Kinney, T. D., and Alexander, L. 1942. The vascular supply of the hypothalamus in man. J. Neuropath. Exp. Neurol. **1:**265-296.

French, L. A., and Blake, P. S. 1950. Subarachnoid hemorrhages and intracranial aneurysms. J. Lancet **70:**459-466.

Freytag, E. 1966. Fatal rupture of intracranial aneurysms. Arch. Path. **81:**418-424.

Graf, J. C. 1965. Spontaneous carotid-cavernous fistula. Arch. Neurol. **13:**662-672.

Hamby, W. B. 1952. Intracranial aneurysms. Springfield, Illinois, Charles C Thomas, Publisher.

Hamby, W. B. 1966. Carotid-cavernous fistula. Springfield, Illinois, Charles C Thomas, Publisher.

Hasegawa, T., Ravens, J. R., and Toole, J. F. 1967. Precapillary arteriovenous anastomoses: "thoroughfare channels" in the brain. Arch. Neurol. **16:**217-224.

Heiman, M. 1938. Über Gefässstudien am aufgehellten Gehirn: die Gefässe des Ammonshornes. Schweiz. Arch. Neurol. Psychiat. **40:**277-301.

Houck, W. S., Jackson, J. R., Odom, G. L., and Young, W. G. 1964. Occlusion of the internal carotid artery in neck secondary to closed trauma to head and neck: report of two cases. Ann. Surg. **159:**219-221.

Hoyt, W. F. 1960. Vascular lesions of the visual cortex with brain herniation through the tentorial incisuria: neuro-ophthalmologic considerations. Arch. Ophthal. **64:**44-57.

Hughes, B. 1954. The visual fields. Springfield, Illinois, Charles C Thomas, Publisher.

Hughes, J. T., and Brownell, B. 1968. Traumatic thrombosis of the internal carotid artery in the neck. J. Neurol. Neurosurg. Psychiat. **31:**307-314.

Ishikawa, S., Handa, J., Meyer, J. S., and Huber, P. 1965. Haemodynamics of the circle of Willis and the leptomeningeal anastomoses: an electromagnetic flowmeter study of intracranial arterial occlusion in the monkey. J. Neurol. Neurosurg. Psychiat. **28:**124-136.

Jakimowicz, W., Stefanko, S., and Pojak, B. 1968. Ramollissements du thalamus dans le territoire des pédicules artérielles venant de la cérébrale postérieure. Acta Med. Polona **9:**447-454.

Jefferson, G. 1947. Isolated oculomotor palsy caused by intracranial aneurysm. Proc. Roy. Soc. Med. **40:**419-432.

Jefferson, G., 1953. Concerning injuries, aneurysms and tumours involving the cavernous sinus. (The Bowman Lecture.) Trans. Ophthal. Soc. U. K. **73:**117-152.

Jefferson, G. 1955. Further concerning compression of the optic pathways by intracranial aneurysms. Clin. Neurosurg. **1:**55-103.

Kaplan, H. A. 1959. The transcerebral venous system: an anatomical study. Arch. Neurol. **1:** 148-152.

Kaplan, H. A. 1965. The lateral perforating branches of the anterior and middle cerebral arteries. J. Neurosurg. **23:**305-310.

Kaplan, H. A., Aronson, S. M., and Browder, E. J. 1961. Vascular malformation of the brain; an anatomical study. J. Neurosurg. **18:**630-635.

Krainer, L. 1947. Cerebral thrombosis in young adults. Lancet **1:**738-741.

Labauge, R., Thévenet, A., and Crouzet, G. 1967. Les hémodétournements dans les artères du cou à destinée encéphalique: à propos de six cas opérés de "subclavian steal syndrome." Rev. Neurol. **1:**5-30.

Lazorthes, G. 1961. Vascularisation et circulation cérébrales. Paris, Masson et Cie.

Lee, K. F., and Hodes, P. J. 1967. Intracranial ischemic lesions. Radiologic Clin. N. Amer. **5:** 363-393.

Leeds, N. E., and Abbott, K. N. 1965. Collateral circulation in cerebrovascular disease in childhood via rete mirabile and perforating branches of anterior choroidal and posterior cerebral arteries. Radiology **85:**628-634.

LeMay, M., and Gooding, C. A. 1966. The clinical

significance of the azygos anterior cerebral artery (A.C.A.). Amer. J. Roentgen. **98**:602-610.

Lhermitte, F., Gautier, J. C., Derouesné, C., and Guiraud, B. 1968. Ischemic accidents in the middle cerebral artery territory: a study of the causes in 122 cases. Arch. Neurol. **19**:248-263.

Lindenberg, R. 1955. Compression of brain arteries as pathogenetic factor for tissue necroses and their areas of predilection. J. Neuropath. Exp. Neurol. **14**:223-243.

Locksley, H. B. 1966. Natural history of subarachnoid hemorrhage, intracranial aneurysms and arteriovenous malformations: based on 6368 cases in the cooperative study. J. Neurosurg. **25**:219-239, 321-368.

Lowe, R. D. 1962. Adaptation of the circle of Willis to occlusion of the carotid or vertebral artery: its implication in caroticovertebral stenosis. Lancet **1**:395-398.

MacKenzie, I. 1953. The clinical presentation of the cerebral angioma: a review of 50 cases. Brain **76**:194-214.

Martin, J. D., Jr., and Mabon, R. F. 1943. Pulsating exophthalmos; review of all reported cases. J.A.M.A. **121**:330-335.

Martin, N., and Warren, G. C. 1969. Thrombosis of the internal carotid artery due to intra-oral trauma. Southern Med. J. **62**:103-107.

McCormick, W. F. 1966. The pathology of vascular ("arteriovenous") malformations. J. Neurosurg. **24**:807-812.

McMenemey, W. H. 1954. The significance of subarachnoid bleeding. Proc. Roy. Soc. Med. **47**:701-704.

Millikan, C. H., and Siekert, R. G. 1955. Studies in cerebrovascular disease: the syndrome of intermittent insufficiency of the basilar arterial system. Proc. Staff Meet., Mayo Clin. **30**:61-68.

Mishkin, M. M. 1967. Extracranial ischemic lesions which secondarily involve the brain. Radiologic Clin. N. Amer. **5**:395-408.

Muller, J., and Shaw, L. 1965. Arterial vascularization of the human hippocampus. Arch. Neurol. **13**:45-47.

Nicola, G. C., Ferrazzi, D., Faggioli, L., and Nizzoli, V. 1967. Occlusion bilatérale de l'artère carotide interne (à propos de trois observations). Psychiat. Neurol. (Basel) **154**:106-117.

Patel, A., and Toole, J. F. 1965. Subclavian steal syndrome—reversal of cephalic blood flow. Medicine **44**:289-303.

Perret, G., and Nishioka, H. 1966. Arteriovenous malforations: an analysis of 545 cases of craniocerebral arteriovenous malformations and fistulae reported to the cooperative study. J. Neurosurg. **25**:467-490.

Perryman, C. R., Gray, G. H., Brust, R. W., Jr., and Conlon, P. C. 1963. Interesting aspects of cerebral angiography with emphasis on some unusual congenital variations. Amer. J. Roentgen. **89**:372-384.

Pitner, S. E. 1966. Carotid thrombosis due to intraoral trauma: an unusual complication of a common childhood accident. New Eng. J. Med. **274**:764-767.

Poppi, U. 1928. Sindrome talamo-capsulare per rammollimento nel territorio dell'arteria coroidea anteriore. Riv. Pat. Nerv. **33**:505-542.

Reivich, M., Holling, H. E., Roberts, B., and Toole, J. F. 1961. Reversal of blood flow through the vertebral artery and its effect on cerebral circulation. New Eng. J. Med. **265**:878-885.

Riggs, H. E., and Rupp, C. 1943. Miliary aneurysms: relation of anomalies of circle of Willis to the formation of aneurysms. Arch. Neurol. Psychiat. **49**:615-616.

Riggs, H. E., and Rupp, C. 1963. Variation in form of circle of Willis: the relation of variations to collateral circulation: anatomic analysis. Arch. Neurol. **8**:8-14.

Robicsek, F., Daugherty, H. K., Sanger, P. W., and Galluci, V. 1967. Intermittent cerebrovascular insufficiency: a frequent and curable cause of stroke. Geriatrics **22**:96-108.

Romanul, F. C. A., and Abramowicz, A. 1964. Changes in brain and pial vessels in arterial border zones: a study of 13 cases. Arch. Neurol. **11**:40-65.

Rosegay, H., and Welch, W. K. 1954. Peripheral collateral circulation between cerebral arteries; demonstration by angiography of meningeal arterial anastomoses. J. Neurosurg. **11**:363-377.

Rubinstein, H. S. 1944. Relation of circulus arteriosus to hypothalamus and internal capsule. Arch. Neurol. Psychiat. **52**:526-530.

Sachs, E. 1938. The importance of ocular signs in the diagnosis of brain tumor. Ann. Intern. Med. **11**:1395-1400.

Sahs, A. L. 1966. Observations on the pathology of saccular aneurysms. J. Neurosurg. **24**:792-806.

Sahs, A. L., Perret, G., Locksley, H. B., Nishioka, H., and Skultety, F. M. 1966. Preliminary remarks on subarachnoid hemorrhage. J. Neurosurg. **24**:782-788.

Samuel, K. C. 1956. Atherosclerosis and occlusion of the internal carotid artery. J. Path. Bact. **71**:391-401.

Schaafsma, S. 1968. On the differential diagnosis between cerebral haemorrhage and infarction. J. Neurol. Sci. **7**:83-95.

Schlezinger, N. S. 1950. Cerebral aneurysm. In Piersol, G. M., editor: The cyclopedia of medicine, surgery, specialties, vol. 2. Philadelphia, F. A. Davis Co., pp. 425-443.

Simeone, F. A., Ryan, K. G., and Cotter, J. R. 1968. Prolonged experimental cerebral vasospasm. J. Neurosurg. **29**:357-366.

Steegman, A. T., and Roberts, D. J. 1935. Syndrome of the anterior choroidal artery; report of case. J.A.M.A. **104**:1695-1697.

Stern, W. E., Brown, W. J., and Alksne, J. F. 1967. The surgical challenge of carotid-cavernous fistula: the critical role of intracranial circulatory dynamics. J. Neurosurg. **27**:298-308.

Stopford, J. S. B. 1915. The arteries of the pons and medulla. M.D. Thesis, University of Manchester.

Stopford, J. S. B. 1916. The arteries of the pons and medulla oblongata. J. Anat. **50**:131-164.

Stopford, J. S. B. 1917. The arteries of the pons and medulla oblongata. J. Anat. **51**:250-277.
Symonds, C. P. 1923. Contributions to the clinical study of intracranial aneurysms. Guy's Hosp. Rep. **73**:139-158.
Symonds, C. 1955. The circle of Willis (Harveian oration). Brit. Med. J. **1**:119-124.
Toole, J. F. 1966. Interarterial shunts in the cerebral circulation. Circulation **33**:474-483.
Torvik, A., and Jörgensen, L. 1964. Thrombotic and embolic occlusions of the carotid arteries in an autopsy material: prevalence, location and associated diseases. J. Neurol. Sci. **1**:24-39.
Torvik, A., and Jörgensen, L. 1966. Thrombotic and embolic occlusions of the carotid arteries in an autopsy series: cerebral lesions and clinical course. J. Neurol. Sci. **3**:410-432.
Trumpy, J. H. 1967. Subarachnoid hemorrhage; time sequence of recurrences and their prognosis. Acta Neurol. Scand. **43**:48-60.
Uchimura, J. 1928. Über die Gefässversorgung des Ammonshornes. Z. Ges. Neurol. Psychiat. **112**:1-19.
Vander Eecken, H. 1959. Anastomoses between the leptomeningeal arteries of the brain. Springfield, Illinois, Charles C Thomas, Publisher.
Vander Eecken, H. M., and Adams, R. D. 1953. The anatomy and functional significance of the meningeal arterial anastomoses of the human brain. J. Neuropath. Exp. Neurol. **12**:132-157.
Walker, A. E. 1956. Clinical localization of intracranial aneurysms and vascular anomalies. Neurology **6**:79-90.
Williams, D. J. W. 1936. The origin of the posterior cerebral artery. Brain **59**:175-180.
Williams, R. R., Bahn, R. C., and Sayre, G. P. 1955. Congenital cerebral aneurysms. Proc. Staff Meet., Mayo Clin. **30**:161-168.
Yates, P. O., and Hutchinson, E. C. 1961. Cerebral infarction: the role of stenosis of the extracranial cerebral arteries. Med. Res. Council Rep. No. 300. London, Her Majesty's Stationery Office.
Zülch, K. J. 1955. Kreislaufstörungen an der Grenzlinie von Hirn- und Rückenmarksgefässen. Proc. 2d Internat. Congr. Neuropath., London. Amsterdam, Excerpta Medica Foundation, pp. 613-615.

Chapter 28

Trauma, brain shifts, intracranial neoplasms, and hematomas

TRAUMA

Brain injuries from trauma may be subdivided into three groups: (1) closed head injuries due to impact of the stationary skull, (2) open head injuries resulting from penetrating objects, such as a missile, and (3) closed head injuries due to impact of the moving skull (Lindenberg, 1966; Lindenberg and Freytag, 1960; Spatz, 1950).

Considering first the stationary skull to which a blunt force is applied, an area of tissue damage develops in the region of the impact ("coup"). This area of damage ("contusion focus") is wedge-shaped, with its base at the surface of the brain and its apex in the subcortical white matter. In time the involved tissue disintegrates, leaving a crater-like defect (Fig. 28-1). The lesion is attributable to tissue cavitation resulting from local negative pressure occurring at the instant of rebound of the skull following preliminary inbending (Unterharnscheidt and Sellier, 1966). Should the inbending at the moment of impact exceed the elastic properties of the skull, depressed fracture results. In this kind of injury little brain shift occurs. In the line of force there may be a few foci of tissue damage in intermediate parts of the brain ("intermediate coup"), but none in remote areas (no "contre coup"). Clinical manifestations vary in accordance with sites injured; usually they are milder than in closed head injury due to impact of the moving skull. Signs of concussion may develop; they are usually evanescent.

In open head injuries resulting from the penetration of an object, such as a missile, the nature of the brain wound is the same whether or not the head is in motion at the time of the injury. "Contre coup contusion" of the brain does not occur unless the head receives an impact when the person falls. Damage of the brain usually remains local, in the path of the missile or other penetrating object. In the case of high velocity missiles, which produce shock waves in tissue, there may, however, be indirect effects, such as fracture of the orbital roof or ethmoid cells (with damage of adjacent brain tissue) caused by abrupt increase in intracerebral pressure. Common in missile wounds are intracranial hematomas, situated most frequently within the path of the missile or of indriven fragments. Brain edema is usually more severe in this type of injury than in closed head injuries. (Meirowsky, 1954, 1966; Spatz, 1950.) Seizures resulting from high velocity missile wounds are three times more common than the seizures following blunt head injuries (Caviness, 1966).

In closed head injuries due to impact of the moving skull on a firm, stationary object, the mechanisms of brain damage differ from those just described. With sudden deceleration of the head, the impact

A 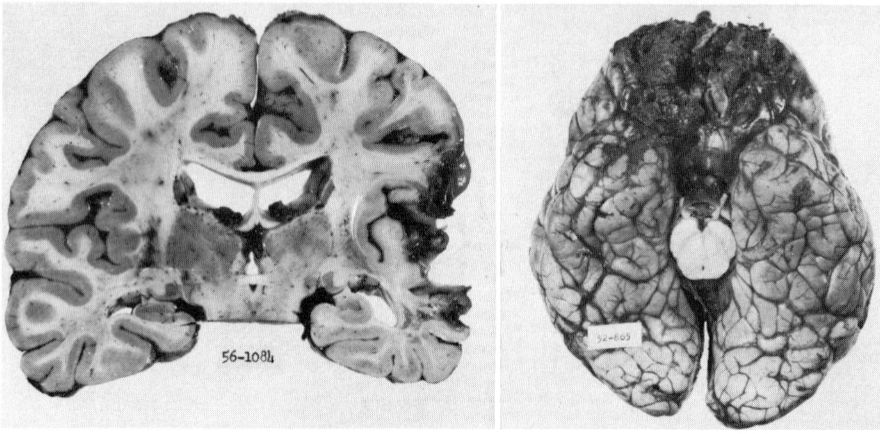 B

Fig. 28-1. To the *left,* crater-shaped defect in the lateral aspect of the cerebrum (lower parietal lobe and superior and middle temporal gyri). Three years earlier the temple had been struck a blow by a piece of lumber. Depressed fracture occurred in this region. Damaged tissue has been completely resorbed. The body of the ventricles and the inferior horn on the injured side are dilated. To the *right,* extensive damage of the orbitofrontal surface of the brain from recent contre coup contusion received in a fall on the back of the head. Olfactory bulbs and stalks (tracts) are also destroyed. The temporal poles are less affected. (Courtesy Dr. Richard Lindenberg, Baltimore.)

area is relatively wide, the velocity of the impact relatively moderate, and the energy load per unit area rather small. On collision of the head with a large, solid mass, the skull will be abruptly decelerated. Through inbending, however, the whole skull will itself reaccelerate, and the brain as a whole decelerate, with rebound of both then occurring. Cavitation from the negative pressure developing at the "contre coup" site produces an area of injury called a "contusion focus"; positive pressure created in the brain in the region of impact—the "coup" site—is much less pathogenic than negative pressure, and thus the "contusion" in this region of head impact tends to be minor. (Unterharnscheidt and Sellier, 1966.) The large proportion of energy transmitted deep into the brain results in shear strain and tensile forces, creating torsion movements of the brain and circulatory disturbances (Denny-Brown and Russell, 1941; Hallervorden and Quadbeck, 1957; Scheiddeger, 1948).

"Contre coup" sites vary with the region of the head receiving the impact. Such sites are related spatially to bone surfaces and other unyielding structures such as the falx cerebri and the tentorium cerebelli. With a fall on the *occiput,* "contre coup" contusions predominate in the orbitofrontal cortex, olfactory bulb, and temporal poles (Fig. 28-1, *B*). With impact on the *forehead or the vertex of the skull,* contusions occur in intermediate positions in the line of force, while contre coup contusions occur in structures in the region of the free edge of tentorium cerebelli, that is, in the region of the incisura tentorii (Fig. 28-2, *A* and *B*). Impact at the *base of the skull* near the foramen magnum also results in contusions of structures in the region of the incisure. The contusions occurring at the latter site are caused by shearing forces originating from sudden shifts in position both of deeper cerebral structures and midbrain relative to the incisure. To produce contusions of structures in the region of the incisure, the impact force must be directed toward the tentorium and it must be of a magnitude sufficient to deform the skull. On the other hand, lesions at these sites seldom occur in falls on the occiput or in the region of the temple. (Lindenberg and Freytag, 1960.)

Signs of *cerebral concussion* following

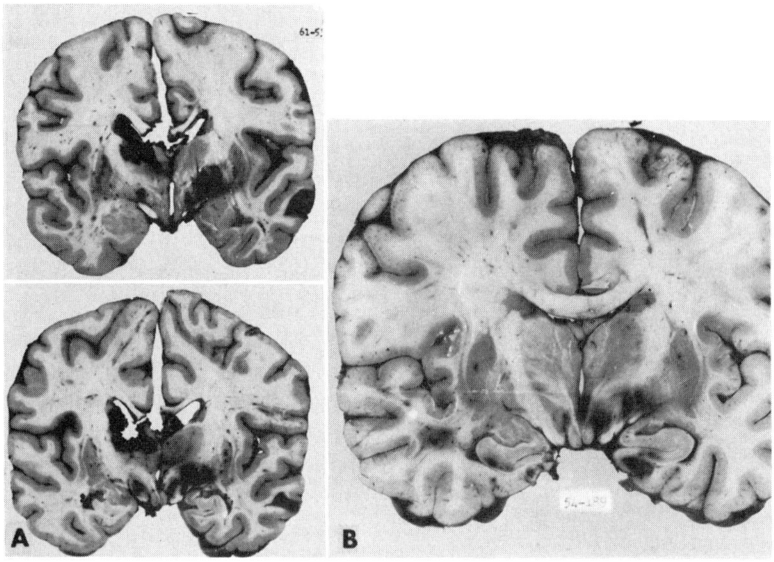

Fig. 28-2. Impact on forehead and adjoining vertex from sudden halt of head in motion. **A**, Fresh contusion hemorrhages involve central structures of the brain predominantly. The corpus callosum is ruptured and hemorrhages are present in the septum pellucidum and fornices and elsewhere. Deeper structures affected by contre coup contusion include the lower part of the internal capsule and the subthalamic and lateral hypothalamic regions. **B**, Cluster of fresh contusion hemorrhages in region of medial tip of right pallidum, adjacent inferior part of the internal capsule, and the region of the right mamillary body associated with contusions of both hippocampal gyri, and, on the left, hemorrhage in the hippocampal formation. (Courtesy Dr. Richard Lindenberg, Baltimore.)

skull impact consequent to sudden deceleration of the head, and some of the neural structures involved, are as follows: unconsciousness (reticular activating system); bilateral contraction of limb muscles followed by paralysis (corticospinal tracts); respiratory arrest and generalized vasoconstriction (medullary centers); loss of the corneal reflex (circuits of nerves V and VII); paralysis of deglutition (circuits of nerves IX and X) (Taylor, 1966). On "stabilization" of the injury in the acute phase of *craniocerebral trauma in general,* still other disturbances may be encountered, their proportional representation being dependent on mode, site, and extent of the injury: retrograde amnesia, anterograde amnesia, aphasia, and mental aberrations; also visual and auditory disturbances and alterations in somatomotor, somatosensory, and cerebellar function (Caveness, 1966). The unconsciousness occurring as a result of craniocerebral trauma may be evanescent or it may be of long duration, as in the apallic syndrome (p. 391); the unconsciousness, whether brief or prolonged, is attributable to concussion, that is, to tissue damage occurring at the time of impact, not (in any significant measure) to epiphenomena or to secondary cerebral complications (Ommaya, 1966; Spatz, 1950; Symonds, 1962). Loss of consciousness is closely linked with the length of amnesia: the harder the blow, the greater the duration of both (Taylor, 1966).

Probably of greatest pathogenic importance in the development of *concussion* are torsional movements of the brain associated with shear strain and tensile forces initiated at the time of the impact. In postmortem studies of chronic cases in which concussion occurred initially, Strich (1956, 1961) noted fragmented axis cylinders in much of the white matter, and considered shearing of nerve fibers the main basis. But as revealed by the symptomatology of concussion, the brainstem appears particularly concerned. Spatz (1950) states that the mamillary bodies are at the center of the crossing of "compression waves" regardless of the site of impact, and concluded that the diencephalon and mesencephalon are consequently most injured in concussion. Unterharnscheidt and Sellier (1966) considered that immediate unconsciousness results from "irritation" of the damaged part of cerebral cortex and that positive and negative pressure effects in the brain substance produced by skull deceleration and acceleration cause mechanical damage of the brainstem secondarily. Sudden extreme flexion or extension of the neck on impact, by interfering with function of the medulla oblongata, may also give rise to signs of concussion. Unconsciousness, for example, can result from sudden flexion-extension movements of the neck ("whiplash") without head impact (p. 97). From studies in cats, Friede (1961) concluded that the primary lesion in concussion is in the cranial-cervical junctional area. The lesion (snapped vertically running nerve fibers), he contended, resulted from a combination of cervicomedullary stretch and impact against the odontoid process. The snapping of fibers in this region was attributed to sagittal rotational forces in the course of head movement through an arc of 100 degrees from the neutral to the position of full neck flexion. To what extent such data can be extrapolated to concussion in man remains to be ascertained.

Epidural hemorrhage, usually arterial in origin, may occur in association with closed head injuries. When taking place in the *posterior cranial fossa,* the hemorrhage originates most commonly from a tear in the lateral dural sinus or torcular Herophili. The scalp in the region of the occiput is contused or lacerated, and in most cases (but not in all), suture separation is noted or a fracture line can be found crossing the foramen magnum or a venous sinus. Most patients become rapidly comatose, and when in this state they exhibit few if any localizing or lateralizing signs. Other patients recover consciousness for a time; they complain of headache of increasing severity and nausea; vomiting sets in, and after a period of drowsiness and restlessness they again lose consciousness. During the lucid period, nuchal rigidity occurs, deep reflexes disappear, and nystagmus may or may not develop. In addition to nystagmus (which occurs on extreme lateral gaze), there may be ataxia, hypotonia, hyporeflexia, and "cerebellar fits." Not infrequently the hematoma is situated over the occipital poles as well as over the cerebellum. In such cases, anisocoria, hemiparesis, and pyramidal tract signs may be noted. (Schneider, Kahn, and Crosby, 1951.) The *subfrontal region* is another site at which epidural hemorrhage may occur. Trauma from blunt impact on the forehead is the usual basis. Or the hemorrhage may result from a fall on the back of the head. Manifestations of the hemorrhage appear after the lapse of a few days, at a time when the patient is conscious. Persistent headache and bilateral retro-orbital pain are the chief complaints. Also of common occurrence are symptoms attributable to damage of the orbitofrontal cortex: unpredictable behavior, character change,

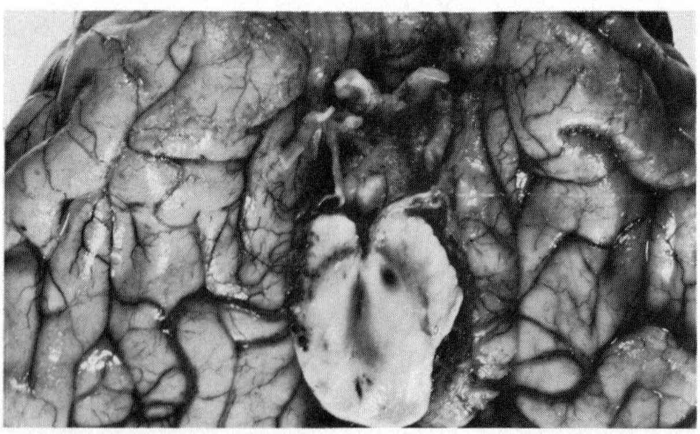

Fig. 28-3. Case of *left* subdural hematoma. Destruction of lateral part of basis pedunculi on the *right* side resulted from pressure exerted against the tentorial edge. Shift on the midbrain to the right was associated with impaction of the *left* hippocampal gyrus in the incisura cerebelli. (The tentorial pressure groove can be seen.) Edema of the tegmentum has occurred and hemorrhages have appeared in the median plane and are extending toward the nuclei of the third and fourth nerves; these complications are attributable, in part at least, to midbrain distortion and to compression of the contents of the interpeduncular fossa. (Courtesy Dr. Richard Lindenberg, Baltimore.)

defective memory and recall, and intermittent disorientation. (Jackson, 1966.)

EFFECTS OF BRAIN SHIFTS

Brain shift is predominantly downward following head impact and either downward or medialward in the presence of a supratentorial expanding mass, depending on its location. Complicating cerebral edema from an expanding mass, by increasing cerebral volume, is often as important a factor in brain shift as the size of the primary cerebral mass (Evans and Scheinker, 1943). In the case of brain infarction following vascular occlusion, such massive swelling may occur in the affected hemisphere as to suggest neoplasm radiologically (Riishede, 1957).

Mechanisms involved and effects of local pressure

Shift of the brain may lead to local brain compression at any site at which contact is made with a nonyielding structure. This occurs, for instance, in the region of the gyrus cinguli where the latter is thrust against the free edge of the falx cerebri, or along the upper surface of the cerebellum where it abuts against the free edge of the tentorium as a result of increased pressure in the posterior cranial fossa. Shift of the brain and brainstem downward leads to impaction mainly in two regions, the incisura tentorii and the foramen magnum. (Lindenberg, 1966.)

Fig. 27-12 illustrates the tentorium cerebelli and the structures that lie adjacent to its free border. Four points with respect to this region are worth emphasis.

(1) The incisura varies in size (see inset in Fig. 27-12), so that with downward shift there may or may not be significant herniation of tissue through the incisura (Corsellis, 1958).

(2) The basis pedunculi lies very close

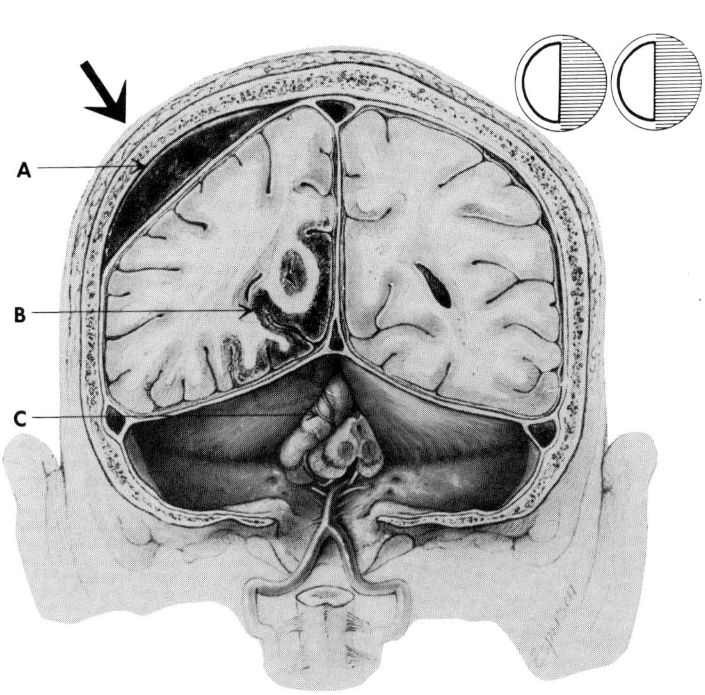

Fig. 28-4. Herniation of the left hippocampal gyrus, with compression of branches of the left posterior cerebral artery *(C)*, resulting from epidural hematoma *(A)*. The brainstem is displaced to the right. The calcarine cortex *(B)* is infarcted. Resulting right homonymous hemianopia is indicated at the upper right. (From Hoyt, 1960.)

to the free edge of the tentorium, as do also the tegmental and tectal regions of the midbrain if the incisura is narrow.

(3) Branches of the posterior cerebral artery, as they course along the surface of the temporal and occipital lobes, come into close spatial relation to the free edge of the tentorium.

(4) The fourth nerve courses near the free edge of the tentorium.

With shift either downward or medialward, damage may be incurred by the hippocampal gyrus and its uncus and the upper brainstem. Impaction of the hippocampal gyrus deeply indents the surface of the gyrus, producing a *tentorial pressure groove* (Fig. 28-3), and leads to herniation of the gyrus through the incisura *(tentorial pressure cone)* (Fig. 28-4). Damage incurred by the hippocampal gyrus under these conditions is direct, and, because of compression and angulation of hippocampal arteries (branches of the posterior cerebral artery) against the free edge of the tentorium, secondary changes of an ischemic nature may occur in the hippocampal formation, mainly in Sommer's sector (Fig. 28-5).

Under normal conditions, with the brain perfused *in situ* there is always a shallow groove in the uncus hippocampi in the region where it abuts against the free edge of the tentorium (Symington, 1906).

Another, and important, effect of downward or medialward shift is infarction—usually hemorrhagic—of the lower and mesial parts of occipital lobe (Fig. 28-6) from compression of branches of the posterior cerebral artery against the free edge of the tentorium (see Fig. 27-12 for topography in this region). The calcarine cortex is commonly affected, in which case contralateral homonymous hemianopia occurs (Fig. 28-4) (Moore and Stern, 1938; Sunderland, 1958). As emphasized by Hoyt (1960), impaction at a posterior incisural level may involve only a single calcarine branch, producing a crossed homonymous

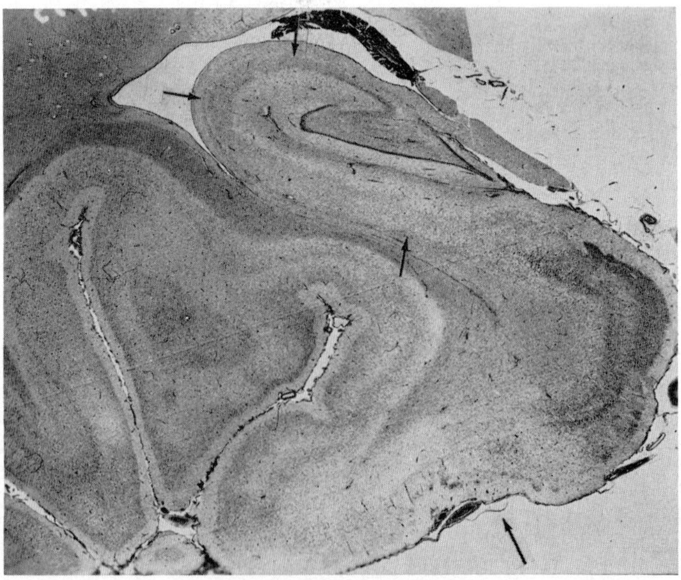

Fig. 28-5. Complete neuronal necrosis of the pyramidal layer of the hippocampus *(three arrows)* and of the cortex of the inferior surface of the temporal lobe *(one arrow)* resulting from compression of branches of the posterior cerebral artery (including the hippocampal arteries) at the free edge of the tentorium secondary to brain swelling following brain trauma 2 days previously. (From Lindenberg, 1955.)

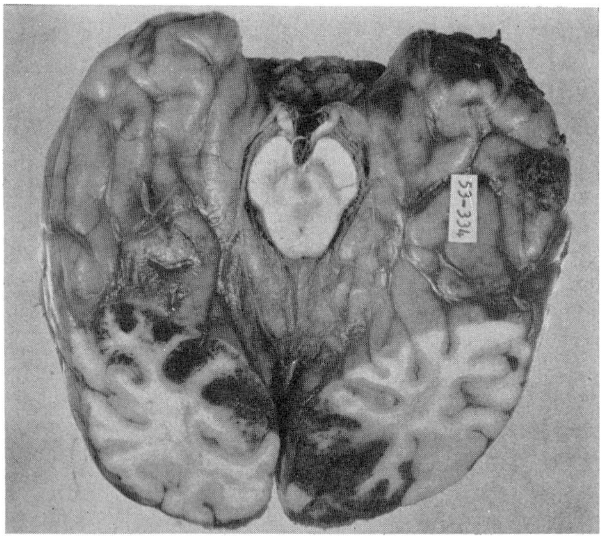

Fig. 28-6. Bilateral hemorrhagic softening of both occipital lobes due to compression of branches of both posterior cerebral arteries at the edge of the tentorium following traumatic subdural hemorrhage. (From Lindenberg, 1955.)

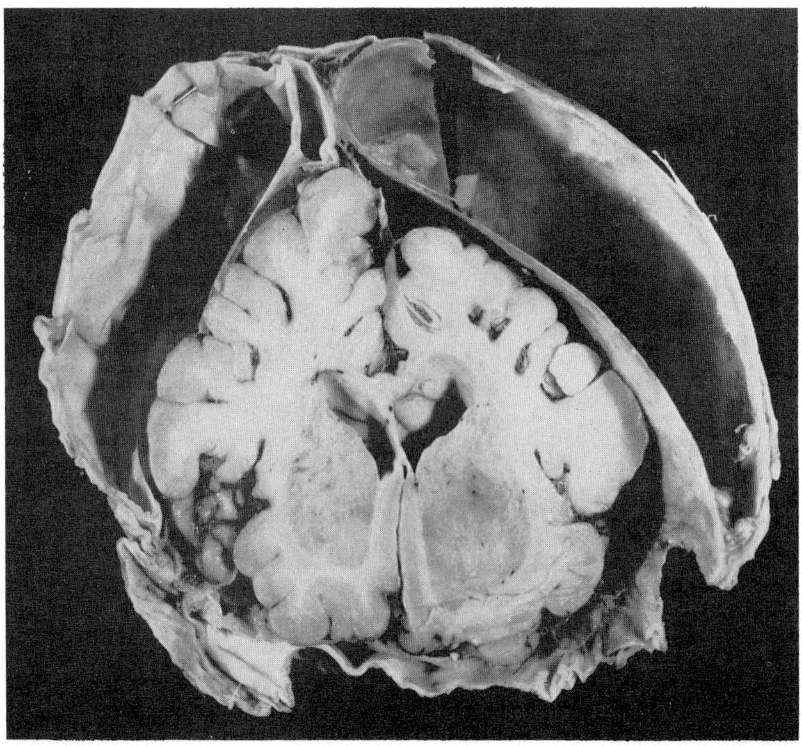

Fig. 28-7. Long-standing bilateral subdural hematoma with severe atrophy of the hemispheres, particularly the right. (AFIP Acc. 530476.)

quadrantic or similar field defect. Another result of downward shift of the cerebrum is compression of the anterior choroidal artery, resulting in widespread damage in its field of irrigation (Fig. 27-4). The optic tract may also be directly compressed, giving rise to contralateral homonymous field defects (Lindenberg and Walsh, 1964; Sunderland, 1958).

The multifocal ischemic necrosis sometimes found in basal ganglia in the presence of a rostrally situated mass may be caused by kinking of penetrating vessels or by circulatory disturbances brought about locally through brain tissue distortion. Unilateral tremor, choreoathetosis, or parkinsonism occurring in occasional cases after the passage of time may be laid to some such circulatory disturbance. Another late effect may be dementia from hemispheric atrophy, particularly in bilateral subdural hematoma such as is illustrated in Fig. 28-7.

With shift associated with a mass in one cerebral hemisphere—for example, temporal lobe abscess complicated by edema—or with rapidly developing subdural hematoma, the contralateral basis pedunculi may be compressed, notched, or lacerated (Fig. 28-3), giving rise to pyramidal tract signs ipsilateral to the mass (a false localizing sign). (The damaged area is called the *Kernohan notch;* its significance was documented by Kernohan and Woltman in 1929 and by Groeneveld and Schaltenbrand in 1927.) Moreover, crowding of the uncus and hippocampal gyrus into the incisura on one side may flatten the cerebral peduncle and compress the adjacent part of the optic tract, giving rise to crossed hemiparesis and crossed homonymous hemianopic field defects. Rapid downward shift of the brainstem with resultant brainstem contusion frequently gives rise to hemorrhage into the tegmentum of the midbrain or pons, or both, with ensuing signs of decerebration, loss of consciousness, and early death (Lindenberg, 1955; Meyer, 1920). This occurs, for example, in severe traumatic impact on the forehead (Fig. 28-8), in intracerebral hemorrhage, in hemorrhage into a glioma of a hemisphere, or in rapidly growing glioblastoma multiforme, all of which are associated with a severe edematous process in the hemisphere. Stretching of paramedian pontile arteries, or compression of them against the clivus owing to forward buckling of the pons, has been suggested as the basis of hemorrhage into the pontile tegmentum (Lindenberg, 1955). Mesencephalic perforating arteries have also been implicated in midbrain and pontile tegmental hemorrhage. The risk of secondary brainstem

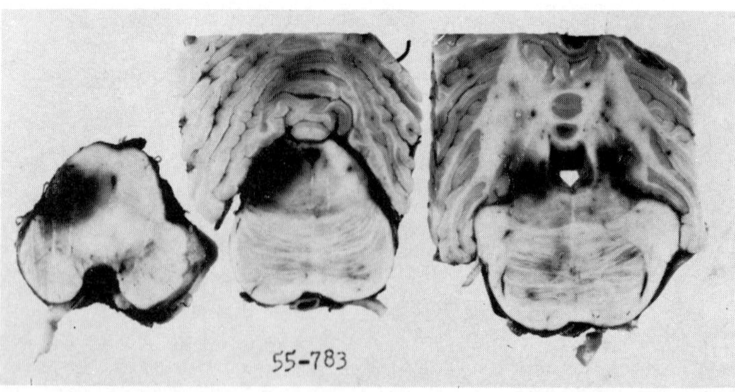

Fig. 28-8. Fall on the forehead, resulting in contusion of the lateral midbrain tegmentum on the right side, also of the pons and the superior cerebellar peduncle bilaterally. This was due to shift of central brain structures into the incisura tentorii, with propagation of the force into the midbrain and upper pons. Sudden rubbing of the lower midbrain along the edge of the tentorium accounts for the lesion in the midbrain. (Courtesy Dr. Richard Lindenberg, Baltimore.)

hemorrhage appears to be a function of the growth velocity of the primary space-occupying lesion and the volume this lesion ultimately attains. Age of the patient is also a factor: incidence of the hemorrhage is low in the young (younger than 16 years) owing to the availability of adequate compensatory mechanisms—for example, suture separation—and low also in the aged (persons more than 75 years old) owing presumably to brain atrophy. (Cohen and Aronson, 1968.)

Impaction and herniation of the hippocampal gyrus in the region of the incisura tentorii may result not only in arterial occlusion but also in obstruction in venous return. Reference is made to compression of pontile veins and of veins entering the superficial petrosal sinus. The suggestion has been made that stagnation of venous flow in this region can account for sudden death occurring, for example, in a patient with epidural hemorrhage in the parieto-temporal region who was conversing normally a few minutes earlier. (Jackson, 1966.)

Cranial nerve disturbances are commonly observed in brain shift. Most frequently the third or sixth nerve ipsilateral to the mass is damaged, and occasionally the third nerve on the contralateral side (pp. 262 and 534). Downward displacement of the brainstem with stretching of the sixth nerve may account for the palsy of the lateral rectus now and then observed under these conditions (Fischer-Brügge, 1951; Sunderland, 1958). Paralytic fourth nerve palsy develops in occasional cases; the palsy has been known to occur after the subject returns to work following slight head injury. Moreover, the root of the contralateral fifth nerve may be distorted because of thrust against an adjacent artery, and be manifested by trigeminal neuralgia or hypesthesia (Ehnig, 1950).

Downward displacement of the brainstem leads to impaction of the cerebellar tonsils in the foramen magnum *(cerebello-medullary pressure cone),* so that the tonsils compress the medulla oblongata. As a result of the displacement, kinking of the brainstem at its junction with the spinal cord may occur, particularly in children with severe brain edema. This kinking results from lack of "give" by the spinal cord, for it is held rigid by the dentate ligaments (Emery, 1967). Another effect of impaction of the cerebellar tonsils in the foramen magnum when the impaction is severe is ischemic necrosis of the undersurface of the cerebellum owing to compression of the posterior inferior cerebellar artery against the edge of the foramen magnum. Signs of cerebellar deficiency result.

With total obstruction of the foramen magnum, the passage of cerebrospinal fluid downward from the intracranial into the spinal subarachnoid space comes to a halt, giving rise to acute hypertensive hydrocephalus. Particularly in expanding lesions in the posterior cranial fossa, acute hydrocephalus thus induced starts a vicious cycle. Acute dilatation of the lateral ventricles occurs, resulting in downward impaction of the hippocampal gyrus in the region of the incisura tentorii; this in turn obstructs the flow of cerebrospinal fluid upward beyond the midbrain. Another cause of acute hydrocephalus is blockage of the third ventricle or the cerebral aqueduct by the hippocampal gyrus as a result of shift of a hemisphere far to the opposite side.

Posterior fossa tumors are particularly apt to displace the cerebellar tonsils downward into the foramen magnum. Withdrawal of spinal fluid by lumbar puncture under these conditions leads to further impaction. Death often ensues, usually within a few hours, with respiration ceasing a considerable time before the heart stops beating. Removal of cerebrospinal fluid by lumbar puncture when a tumor lies above the tentorium also carries an element of risk because the reduction in C.S.F. pressure may induce or aggravate hippocampal impaction in the region of the incisura and lead also to tonsillar herniation into the foramen magnum. This complication is manifested by signs of rapidly increasing intracranial pressure and by disturbances referable to the midbrain and the third and sixth nerves, such as fixed and anisocoric pupils and ptosis, irregular respiration, somnolence, and hyperthermia. Decerebrate rigidity may also occur. (Collier, 1904; Jefferson, 1938; Lindenberg, 1955; Moore and Stern, 1938; Wolman, 1953.)

Syndromes

In brain shift caused by mass lesions located supratentorially, two syndromes are commonly encountered, a *central syndrome* (due to involvement of the diencephalon bilaterally) and an *uncal syndrome* (due to involvement of midbrain and third nerve unilaterally) (McNealy and Plum, 1962). The former is the more frequent. As the syndromes develop, signs of respiratory, ocular, and motor disturbances appear and gradually progress as the associated edematous process becomes worse locally or spreads downward. The pathological process leads first to dysfunction of the diencephalon, then the pons, and finally the medulla oblongata. Lacking decompressive procedures, involvement of the latter may be lethal.

In the *central syndrome* the pupils are small and reactive in the diencephalic stage (from injury of hypothalamic mydriasis centers), slightly dilated and fixed in the midbrain stage, and widely dilated in the medullary stage. The "doll-head phenomenon" is usually elicitable in the diencephalic stage (the eyes turn conjugately when vestibular stimulation is induced by rapidly turning the head to the side). At this stage there may also be roving conjugate eye movements. In the midbrain (decerebrate) stage the doll-head ocular movements may be sluggish or dissociated, and in the pontile stage they no longer occur. In the diencephalic stage, irrigation of the ear with cold water brings out sluggish nystagmus; in the midbrain stage the same reaction occurs and the head undergoes tonic deviation toward the irrigated side; in the pontile stage these responses fail to occur. Both in the midbrain and the pontile stage the ciliospinal reflex (p. 42) may be lost.

In the *uncal syndrome*, the diencephalic stage is brief. Ocular signs are characterized initially by unilateral (ipsilateral) pupillary dilatation and extraocular muscle disturbances. The doll-head response in the uninvolved eye is elicitable until the pons becomes affected, when it can no longer be obtained.

Mechanisms proposed as the cause of third and sixth nerve involvement in the various conditions under discussion are: (1) pressure exerted on the nerve (third) through thrust against the sphenoid bone, (2) compression of the nerve (third) through downward thrust of the posterior cerebral artery, (3) strangulation of the nerve (third) in the region where it passes between the superior cerebellar and posterior cerebral arteries, (4) stretching of the nerve (sixth) in its passage over the clivus of the sphenoid bone, (5) pressure exerted on the nerve (sixth) by transverse branches of the basilar artery (Clark and Gooddy, 1953; Cushing, 1910; Spatz and Stroescu, 1934).

TYPES OF INTRACRANIAL TUMOR IN TERMS OF THEIR LOCATION

Clues as to the type of tumor one may be dealing with in a given patient are obtained from location of the tumor, its growth characteristics—whether it is rapidly and widely destructive or merely locally compressive—and whether or not it obstructs the ventricular system (and if so, at what level). Nature of the symptoms, the results of the physical examination, findings on roentgenographic examination and by scanning, and changes that may be found in the cerebrospinal fluid all help in ascertaining the type of the tumor in question. Age and sex are also determinants in the location of a tumor and its type.

In children and adolescents, tumors of the cerebellum and region of the fourth ventricle head the list, with cerebral hemisphere tumors second and subchiasmal tumors third. In the middle- and old-age groups, frontal tumors come first, then temporal, parietal, subchiasmal, cerebellopontile angle, and cerebellar and fourth ventricle tumors, in that order of decreasing frequency. As to sex, for most tumor types the incidence is highest in males—5:2 in medulloblastoma, 5:4 in oligodendroglioma, 3:2 in astrocytoma, 2:1 in glioblastoma multiforme, 4:3 in ependymoma, 3:1 in pinealoma, 2:1 in craniopharyngioma, 5:2 in epidermoids, 7:4 in teratomas, 2:1 in vascular tumors, and 6:5 in metastatic tumors. Women predominate over men in the incidence of meningioma (7:6) and neurinoma (2:1). (Zülch, 1951.)

Meningiomas

Meningiomas constitute from 12 to 20 percent of all intracranial growths. They are most commonly observed in adults up to middle age. Since meningiomas arise in close relation to arachnoidal villi, they are usually found along the course of the dural venous sinuses. Sites of greatest incidence are the convex surface of the brain (convexity meningiomas) and the region of the superior sagittal sinus (parasagittal meningiomas). They arise less commonly in the region of the ridge of the lesser wing of the sphenoid bone (sphenoid ridge meningiomas), the venous sinuses around the sella turcica (suprasellar meningiomas, tuberculum sellae meningiomas), and the olfactory groove (olfactory groove meningiomas). Most meningiomas are found over the anterior half of the cerebrum.

Meningiomas usually indent and compress the brain without invading it. Comparatively little damage is done to the indented region unless the tumor arises within or in close relation to the pia mater, in which case there may be cortical softening from interference with blood supply (Noetzel, 1951). Infiltration of tumor cells into the brain does, however, occasionally occur.

Convexity meningiomas, which as a rule develop in the region of the frontal lobe, are characterized by "frontal ataxia," hemiparesis or monoparesis (upper limb or face), and defects in the visual fields. The field defects, which are difficult to explain,

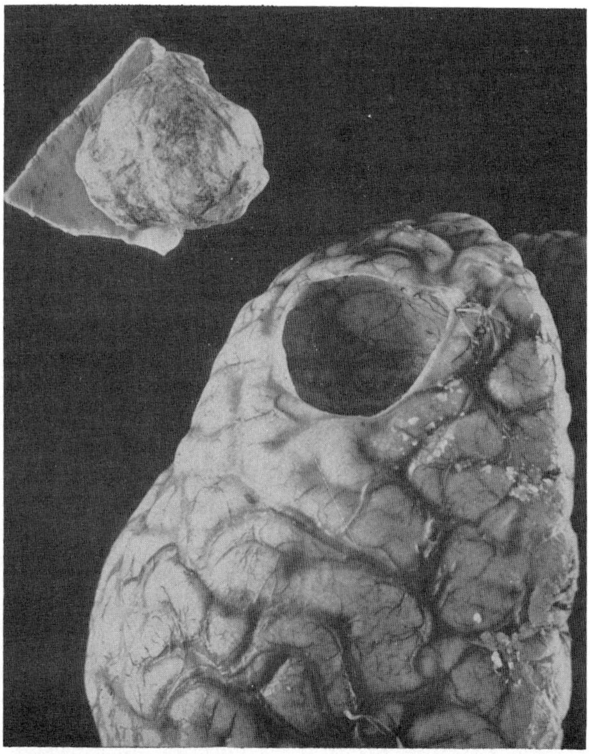

Fig. 28-9. Meningioma in the prefrontal region. The tumor, which is adherent to the dura, has pushed the brain substance ahead of it but has not invaded the cortex. (From the Deutsche Forschungsanstalt für Psychiatrie, Max-Planck-Institut, München.)

are usually of the homonymous type. Generalized or jacksonian seizures may occur, and there may be personality changes. Convexity meningioma is illustrated in Fig. 28-9. Compression of both paracentral lobules by parasagittal meningioma usually results in bladder disturbances and paresis of both lower limbs (more pronounced in one limb than in the other). In the expansion of growths in this region, alterations in deep and superficial reflexes occur relatively late, and paresis still later.

Sphenoid ridge meningiomas are apt to produce exophthalmos and bulging of the temporal region of the face as a result of proliferative changes in the sphenoid bone (incidence is about 20 percent). Those meningiomas of the lesser wing of the sphenoid ridge (this wing is situated medially) are characterized in earlier stages by reduction in vision unilaterally. Severe primary optic atrophy may occur; development of the Paton-Kennedy syndrome is not uncommon. Homonymous hemianopia has also been noted. Moreover, third nerve palsy gradually develops in occasional patients. Meningiomas of the greater wing (situated laterally) may give rise to papilledema as an early manifestation. Tumors in both locations are characterized by unilateral headache, which may be of migrainous type. Now and then, neuralgia involving the ophthalmic division of the fifth nerve occurs. Other disturbances include hemiplegia, parkinsonian syndrome, anosmia (rarely bilateral), and grasping movements. The symptomatology is usually of slow evolution but may be apoplectiform, suggesting the occurrence of a "vascular accident." Ataxia and mental disturbances occur in some patients. Meningiomas in this location are found predominantly in young women. (Guyot, Vouyouklakis, and Pertuiset, 1967.)

Suprasellar meningiomas usually lead to progressively failing vision. Bitemporal hemianopia or other field defect is noted; there may also be primary optic atrophy which is more pronounced on one side than on the other. The pituitary gland is not appreciably involved. Headache usually appears but is seldom severe. Psychomotor or generalized epilepsy has occasionally been noted. When developing in the region of the tuberculum sellae, meningioma may cause unilateral optic atrophy and blindness. Pains occur periodically in the region of the affected eye and may be such as to simulate trigeminal neuralgia. This and other types of meningioma are commonly found in persons 60 years of age or older. (Forster and Bonzarth, 1967; Jane and McKissock, 1962.)

Olfactory groove meningiomas, an example of which is shown in Fig. 28-10, are often manifested by anosmia on one side and later on the other. Hyperostosis also occurs. Visual field defects and papilledema are common; however, primary optic atrophy is infrequent. Psychomotor disorders may also occur.

Intraventricular meningiomas are occasionally encountered, and although most frequent in one lateral ventricle, they may, in a given case, be found in both lateral ventricles or in the third or the fourth ventricle. They originate either in the tela choroidea or in the stroma of the choroid plexus (Russell and Rubinstein, 1963), apparently from arachnoidal meningothelial cells that have migrated in the course of invagination of the mesenchyme that will form the choroid plexus (Arseni, Ionescu, and Maretsis, 1968). Frequently the tumor becomes sufficiently large to expand and occlude the ventricle. In occasional cases calcific material in the tumor is visible in plain x-ray radiographs.

In meningioma occupying one lateral ventricle, the clinical manifestations vary greatly from case to case and include disturbances involving pyramidal, extrapyramidal, special sense, sensory, and association pathways. Headache (in no special region, but commonly on the side of the tumor) may open the clinical tableau, and may be associated with episodes of muscular hypertonia. According to Abbott and Courville (1942), there may be hemiparesis, pain in the legs, dysphagia, dysarthria, convulsive seizures, and psychic disturbances. Homonymous hemianopia has been encountered (Cushing and Eisenhardt, 1938). Signs of a space-occupying process involving the optic chiasm has led to surgical exploration in this re-

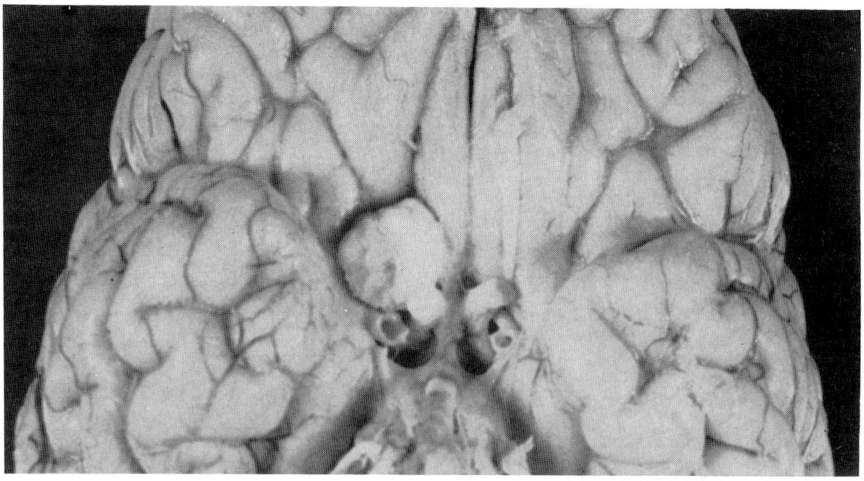

Fig. 28-10. Olfactory groove meningioma. (AFIP Acc. AMH-13488A. A-5825.)

gion. The signs and symptoms of meningioma in the lateral ventricle may be such as to suggest a mass in the posterior cranial fossa; for example, there may be ataxia and other "cerebellar" disturbances, hearing loss, and fifth nerve involvement. Intraventricular meningioma (or other intraventricular tumor) may be suspected in syndromes having both cerebral hemispheric and posterior fossa components, particularly when paroxysmal. The attacks are characterized by (1) headache and vomiting, obliging the patient to lie motionless without speaking as long as an attack lasts (usually for 10 to 15 minutes); (2) generalized or partial muscular hypertonia, with the head thrust backward; (3) a feeling of constriction (angor) together with suffocation, congestion of the face, and restlessness; (4) unilateral or bilateral paresthesia; and (5) in prolonged attacks, loss of consciousness and convulsions. (Arseni, Ionescu, and Maretsis, 1968.)

Posterior fossa meningiomas are uncommon. They are usually situated in the cerebellopontile angle. Characteristic symptoms are headache, unsteadiness, tinnitus and hearing defects, and, most frequent, trigeminal hypalgesia and hypesthesia, reduction or loss of the corneal reflex, and weakness of facial muscles. In one series (Markham and others, 1955) the incidence of supratentorial extension of the tumor was about 25 percent.

In meningiomas, cerebrospinal fluid changes tend to occur early, and increased intracranial pressure relatively late. Eventually the pressure increase is greater than is to be expected from the nature of focal signs and symptoms. A considerable proportion of the meningiomas undergo calcification and thus can be detected roentgenographically. The same is true of the 20 percent of meningiomas that actively invade the skull, causing bony rarefaction and, in about 5 percent of cases, new bone formation. Since vascularization of meningiomas is frequently rich, arteriography may also be of decided value in localization. (Cushing and Eisenhardt, 1938; Frazier, 1936; Globus, 1937; Horrax, 1939; Russell and Rubinstein, 1963; Stender, 1933.)

Pineal tumors

Pineal tumors are relatively uncommon. The majority occurs in males, most often in early adulthood. They may be classified as teratoid pinealomas, true pinealomas, and teratomas. Teratomas usually grow as an autonomous mass in or adjacent to the pineal body. Some originate from the edge of a primary teratoid pinealoma (Tompkins, Haymaker, and Campbell, 1950). Teratoid pinealoma cells commonly extend into the third ventricle and seed in the region of the infundibular recess (Fig. 28-11), sometimes resulting in diabetes insipidus, which, for a time, may be the only manifestation of the tumor. All three forms usually compress or invade the tectum of the midbrain and, to a less degree,

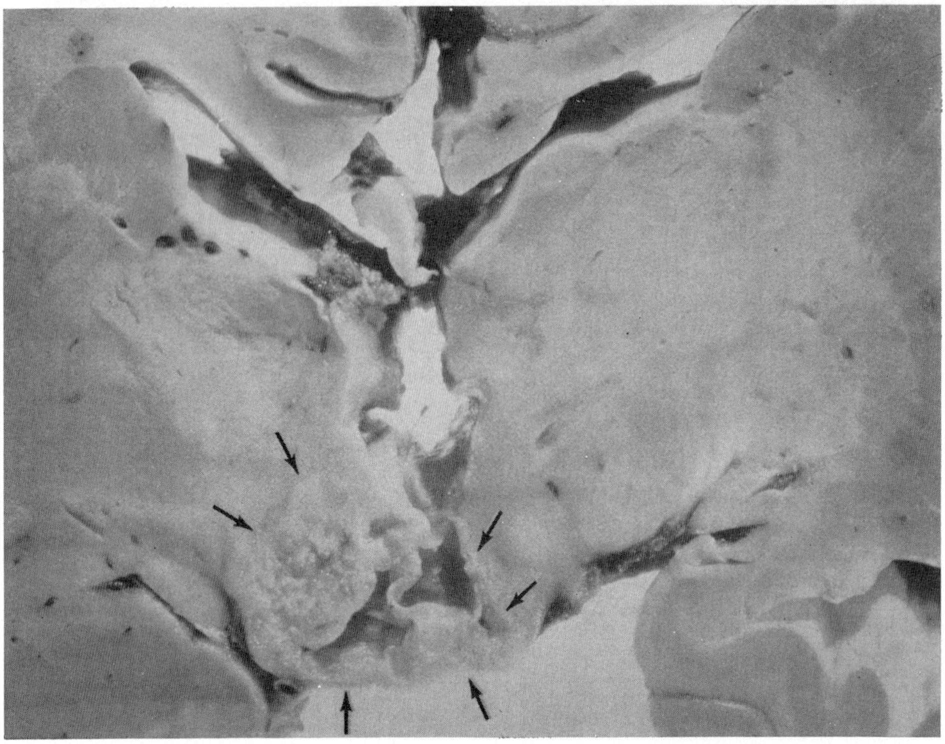

Fig. 28-11. Teratoid pinealoma invading the tuber cinereum of the hypothalamus. The pineal body was highly neoplastic but not appreciably enlarged. (Courtesy Dr. William Bernhard; AFIP Acc. 283653.)

the tegmentum, with resulting diplopia and loss of pupillary constriction to light. Paralysis of vertical gaze, usually in the upward direction, occurs in about 50 percent of cases. The aqueduct is commonly compressed early in the course of the growth, causing headache from internal hydrocephalus. Occasionally there is bilateral hypacusis. Pineal tumor often extends downward and compresses or invades the brachium conjunctivum or vermis of the cerebellum, giving rise to signs of cerebellar deficiency. Signs referable to the pyramidal and long sensory tracts are sometimes elicitable. Pubertas praecox occasionally develops in boys and rarely in girls. Roentgenographic films often reveal a pineal shift. It is rare for pineal tumors to undergo calcification. (Baggenstoss and Love, 1939; Ford and Muncie, 1938; Russell and Sachs, 1943; Stringer, 1934.)

Gliomas of the cerebrum and brainstem

Astrocytoma. Astrocytoma (grade 1 astrocytoma of Kernohan and others, 1949) is among the most common gliomas. The cerebrum is the site of predilection in adults, and the cerebellum in children. In adults, in whom the peak of incidence is in the middle thirties, the tumor develops most frequently in the frontal or the temporal lobe and less frequently in the parietal lobe. No part of the brain is immune. The tumor grows slowly. The majority are microcystic. A few contain a large cyst with or without an astrocytomatous mural nodule (Fig. 28-12, *B*). Now and then the tumor may be difficult to detect with the naked eye, but the enlargement of the hemisphere and the induration of the white matter it involves (Fig. 28-12, *A*) are reliable clues to its nature. A fair number contain calcific deposits visible roentgenographically.

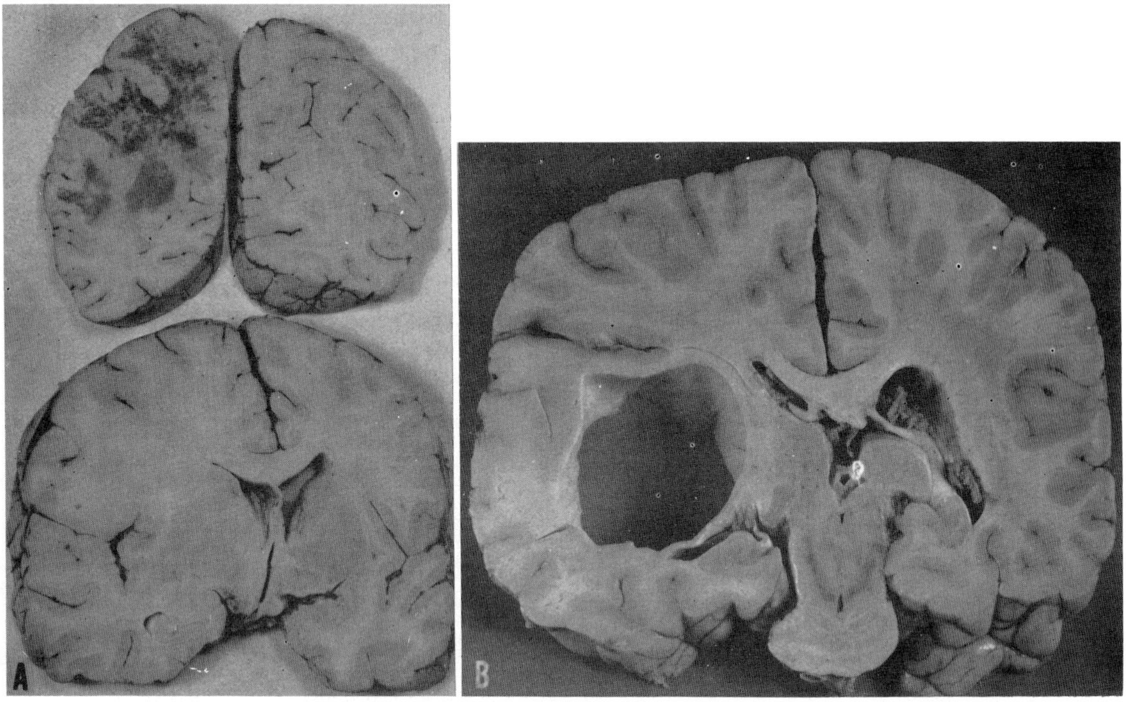

Fig. 28-12. Two cases of astrocytoma. In **A,** the characteristic enlargement of a hemisphere and induration are to be seen. Note the distortion of the ventricular system. (AFIP Acc. 102212.) **B,** Cystic astrocytoma. (AFIP Acc. 331317.)

Consistent with the slowness of growth, the clinical manifestations of astrocytoma are usually (in some 60 percent of cases) furtive for months or years, no clinical signs of an intracranial expanding lesion being discernible. Epileptic seizures may be the only manifestation during this time; such has been noted in 48 percent of cases (Gonzales and Elvidge, 1962). Hemiplegia, if it develops, is usually incomplete. Once the tumor reaches a significant size, "frontal ataxia," motor and reflex changes, and mental disturbances are as common as in other gliomas of the frontal lobe. When hemorrhage occurs into a cyst cavity, as it not infrequently does, the symptoms and signs are manifold and the course stormy. Hemiplegia is occasionally the presenting sign of astrocytoma in the absence of associated hemorrhage. (Cushing, 1932; Elvidge, Penfield, and Cone, 1935; Frazier, 1936; Knox and Adams, 1969; Teltscharow and Zülch, 1947.)

Anaplastic astrocytoma. Astrocytomas commonly undergo anaplasia; in one small series the incidence was 53 percent (Russell and Rubinstein, 1963). Those with advanced anaplasia are classified as grade 3 or grade 4 astrocytoma (Kernohan and others, 1949), or *glioblastoma multiforme.* They develop mostly in the cerebrum, either subcortically or in the region of the basal nuclei. Sites of predilection are frontal, temporal, parietal, brainstem, and occipital, in that order of decreasing frequency. The tumor sometimes originates in the corpus callosum and extends into both hemispheres, giving a butterfly pattern. It may also arise in the centrum semiovale of one side and extend across the corpus callosum to the other side. In 10 to 35 percent of cases the tumor remains limited to one side, confined, as a rule, to cortex and white matter. The tumor often contains brown-tinted necrotic areas and, occasionally, flocculent calcifications,

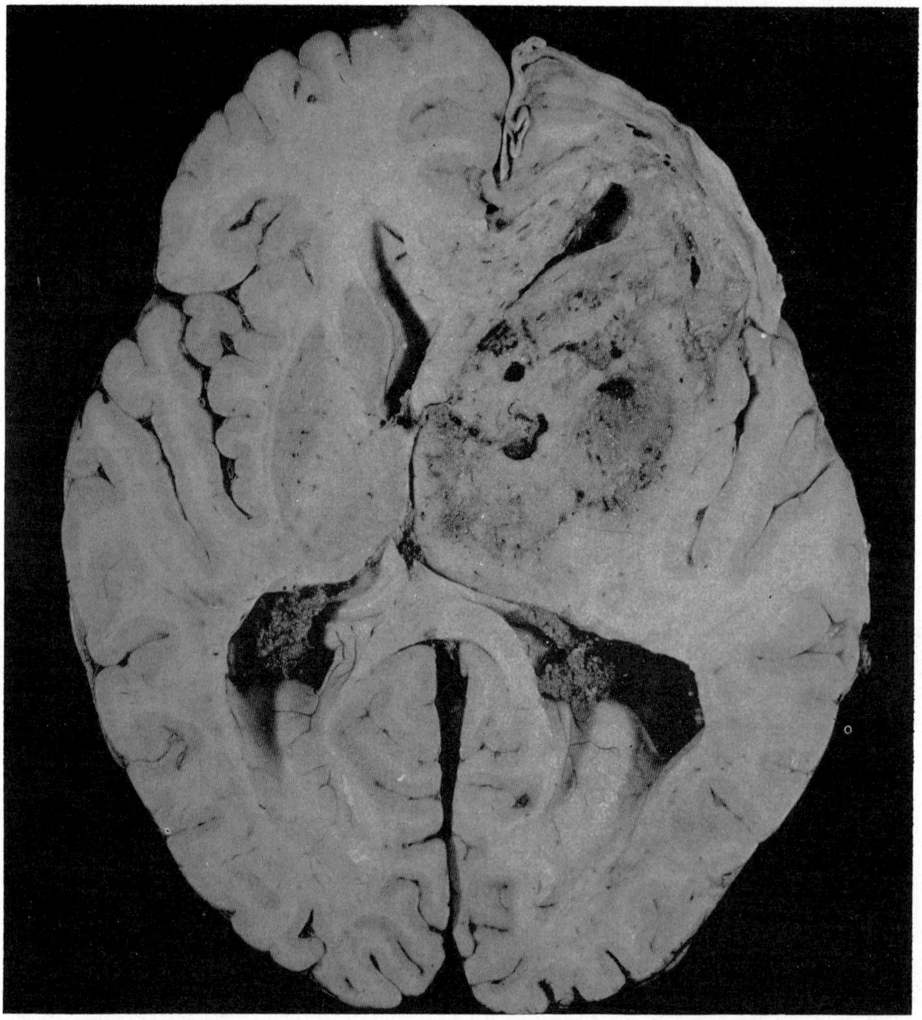

Fig. 28-13. Glioblastoma multiforme of the frontal lobe, striatum, and thalamus. The tumor is advancing to the opposite side by way of the corpus callosum. (AMH 11994C. A-54-59.)

and it usually has an ill-defined border (Fig. 28-13). Tumor growth is by contiguity, that is, neoplastic transformation of normal glia occurs over an ever widening area; the neoplastic cells seldom if ever "infiltrate." The neoplasm compresses and destroys structures in its vicinity and markedly enlarges the hemisphere, partly through the development of an edematous process. Tumor cells commonly enter the cerebrospinal fluid (Wieczorek and Greger, 1965) but do not take hold and grow in regions in which they might lodge.

Anaplastic astrocytoma develops mostly in young and middle-aged adults. The clinical course is stormy. Rapidly developing, pronounced hemiplegia goes hand-in-hand with severe general symptoms and signs (such as papilledema) and syncopal attacks. The incidence of epileptic seizures is somewhat less than in grade 1 astrocytoma, but once seizures appear, their frequency is greater. Death usually occurs within 1 year. (Bailey, 1948; Henschen, 1955; Zülch, 1951.) However, some patients survive 6 or 8 years or longer. In such cases the tumor has commonly been found circumscribed. Younger age seems to be significantly related to longer survival. (Busch and Christensen, 1947; Jelsma and Bucy, 1969; Roth and Elvidge, 1960.)

Oligodendroglioma. This tumor, which constitutes 5 to 8 percent of gliomas, arises in various locations: one hemisphere (most often the frontal lobe); both hemispheres; basal ganglia; wall of the lateral ventricle; occasionally the wall of the third ventricle. The site of predilection is the frontal lobe; the temporal lobe is a poor second, and the parietal, a trailing third; corpus callosum, occipital lobe, region of the optic chiasm, midbrain, and cerebellum are unusual as primary sites. Some 10 percent are infratentorial, the tumor being situated in the vermis, cerebellar hemisphere, wall of the fourth ventricle, or cerebellopontile angle (Earnest, Kernohan, and Craig, 1950). Rarely the tumor originates in the spinal cord. In the cerebrum the subcortical white matter is predominantly affected. The tumor has a distinct propensity to spread by way of the ventricular system or to extend into the cortex and be propagated in the cerebrospinal fluid via the subarachnoid space. As viewed in the fresh brain, the tumor is red-gray or "fleshy," with opaque calcific flecks. These flecks are visible in roentgenograms in 50 to 60 percent of cases. Cysts in the tumor are fairly common. Spontaneous hemorrhage seems a special liability in this kind of glioma. Well over 50 percent of oligodendroglial tumors are *oligodendroblastomas*, or grade 2 to grade 4 oligodendiogliomas. Sometimes they are more sharply circumscribed than oligodendroglioma. Cytologically speaking, they are obviously more active than the oligodendroglioma.

Oligodendroglioma and oligodendroblastoma usually become manifest in persons in their thirties or forties, but no age group is spared. The clinical course is prolonged, sometimes lasting several years. Epileptic seizures occur in 75 to 80 percent of cases. (Bailey and Bucy, 1929; Bormann and Schiefer, 1951; Cushing, 1932; Earnest, Kernohan, and Craig, 1950; Russell and Rubinstein, 1963; Weir and Elvidge, 1968.)

Ependymoma. Among the gliomas, ependymoma carries an incidence of about 3 to 7 percent. It occurs most commonly in childhood and during adolescence. In this age range, its favorite site is the region of the roof of the fourth ventricle in the vicinity of the inferior vermis. The tumor is nodular and cystic; it frequently extends into the fourth ventricle and may grow down into the foramen magnum and adjoining vertebral canal. The clinical manifestations are referable to both the medulla oblongata and the cerebellum (vermis syndrome; p. 286). Early symptoms include vomiting and suboccipital pain.

As in any other tumor growing in or into the fourth ventricle, pain in the neck may be induced by moving the head. The head may occasionally be bent forward and flexed, or it may be retracted and overextended. Any sudden change in posture induces vertigo *(Bruns' sign)*. So-called *cerebellar fits* (p. 289) may occur. Now and then the cerebellopontile angle syndrome is simulated. A conspicuous feature is the periodicity with which the symptoms appear and disappear. (Craig and Kernohan, 1938.)

In adults, the ependymomas have as their site of predilection the wall of the lateral ventricle. They frequently bulge into the ventricular lumen and may, on occasion, fill the ventricle; however, the main mass almost always extends into and occupies the cerebral white matter. Large cysts may form within the tumor.

Most ependymomas grow slowly, and they are usually well circumscribed. Their location is, however, such that the clinical course is usually relatively short. Calcification is visible roentgenographically in 40 to 50 percent of ependymomas in the cerebellar region and in about 20 percent in the cerebrum. Some 5 to 10 percent of ependymomas are (or become) anaplastic; they are called *ependymoblastomas* or grade 2 to 4 ependymomas. Spreading to distant parts by way of the cerebrospinal fluid is fairly common (Fig. 28-14), as it is also for ependymoma. (Cox, 1932; Craig and Kernohan, 1938; Jefferson and Jackson, 1937.)

Brainstem gliomas. Relatively rare

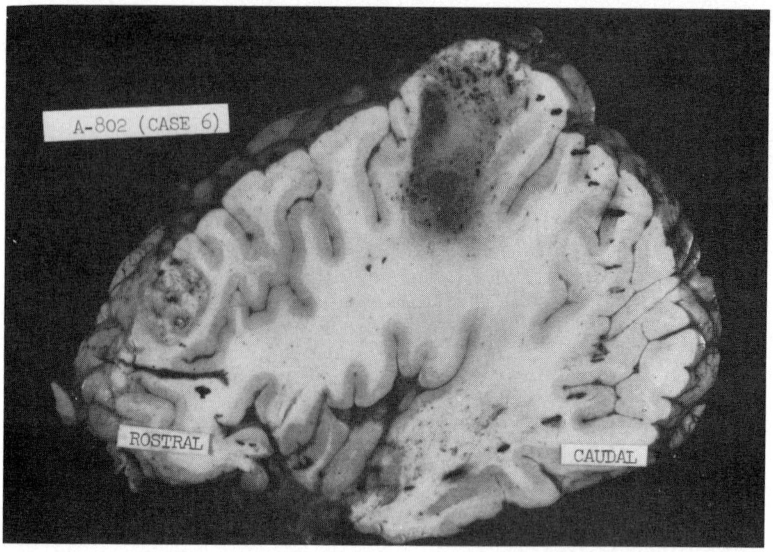

Fig. 28-14. Multiple ependymoblastomas originating from seedlings brought to the cerebrum by the cerebrospinal fluid from the primary growth, situated in the region of the roof of the fourth ventricle. The patient was 61 years old. Much of the mass in the temporal lobe is necrotic tissue. Proton radiation was given therapeutically in the area indicated by ink dots. (Courtesy Dr. Sten Graffman, Uppsala.)

(making up less than 1 percent of gliomas), brainstem gliomas constitute a heterogeneous group that consists chiefly of anaplastic astrocytoma and spongioblastoma polare. These tumors originate mostly in the pons, which they diffusely involve. The pons becomes asymmetrically enlarged, sometimes strikingly so, and presents an uneven nodular or verrucose surface. Occasionally the tumor is limited to one side of the pons. Children are chiefly affected, with the highest incidence at about 7 years. Adults in considerable number may also harbor the tumor (White, 1963).

The clinical course is characteristically progressive. Diplopia is a common sign in early stages and is of diagnostic importance if progressive. Strabismus and ptosis are also common. Manifestations of increased intracranial pressure are usually lacking until later stages. Although the tumor is characteristically diffuse, unilateral involvement of cranial nerves is not uncommon, with the sixth, seventh, and fifth nerves affected in that order of decreasing frequency. Often these nerves are affected bilaterally. Upward extension of the tumor may implicate the third nerve, and downward extension the eighth, tenth, and twelfth nerves. Ipsilateral tonic spasm of the masseter muscle and the facial muscles or ipsilateral facial twitching has occasionally been observed, as has also spastic paretic facial contracture. Disturbances referable to involvement of ascending pathways are rare in some series of cases and fairly common in others. Hemiplegia, when it occurs, is usually slight. Hemiplegia alternans has been noted in about 60 percent of cases. Quadriplegia occasionally develops. Since these tumors advance widely in the tissue, sometimes extending into the cerebellum, signs thereof, such as ataxia, intermittent tilting of the head ("torticollis"), and fixation nystagmus, are evident in a sizable proportion of cases. (Alpers and Yaskin, 1939; Horrax and Buckley, 1930; Pool, 1968; Rasdolsky, 1935.)

The tumors in point—for example, glioblastoma multiforme—may now and then

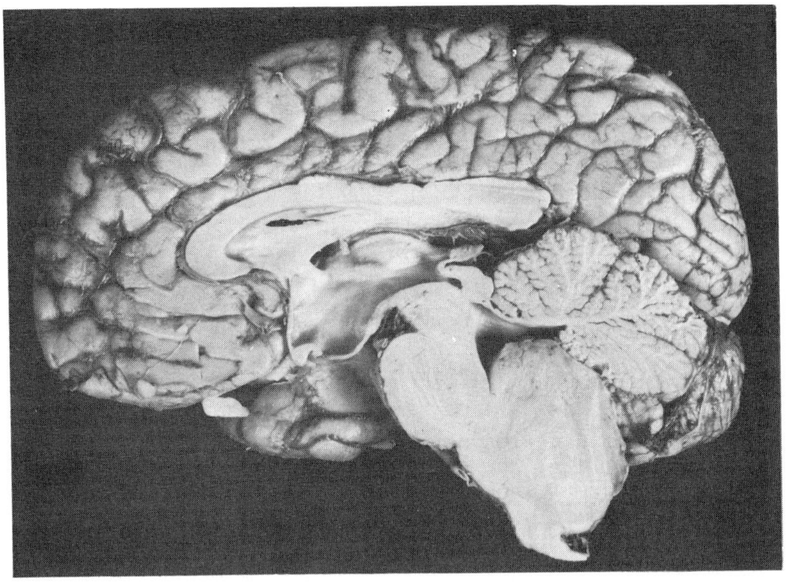

Fig. 28-15. Glioblastoma multiforme originating from the medulla oblongata. There is moderate dilation of the third and fourth ventricles. During the last 2 weeks of life the temperature frequently fell to 97° F. (AFIP Neg. 89294.)

originate in the medulla oblongata (Fig. 28-15) rather than from the pons. Signs and symptoms vary accordingly.

Cerebellar tumors

Astrocytoma. Astrocytoma, also called "spongioblastoma," is the most common cerebellar tumor. Its frequency is greatest in childhood, although a considerable proportion become clinically evident in adolescence. After the age of twenty its incidence recedes sharply. The tumor grows slowly. Clinical manifestations are episodic. About 60 percent of these tumors occupy the superior vermis, and the others occupy a hemisphere. In vermis astrocytoma, signs of cerebellar deficiency are rather few and limited to the lower limbs, while in hemisphere astrocytoma the signs of cerebellar involvement are full blown and unmistakable. Signs and symptoms of increased intracranial pressure tend to develop early. The head is often tilted toward the side occupied by the tumor. However, when the ipsilateral fourth nerve is implicated the head is usually tilted to the opposite side so that better vision may be obtained.

Frequently the tumor is macrocystic, especially when it is situated in a hemisphere of the cerebellum. Large cysts may contain a mural tumor nodule. Calcification visible in roentgenograms is rare, but it may be detected microscopically in about one-third of cases. Tumor cells often extend into the cerebellar meninges but are rarely, if ever, carried further by the cerebrospinal fluid. Now and then the tumor compresses the cerebral aqueduct, causing internal hydrocephalus; in rare instances it may invade the fourth or the third ventricle. (Bergstrand, 1939; Bucy and Gustafson, 1939; Ringertz and Nordenstam, 1951.) The tumor is benign, for when it is completely removed, the patient may remain in good health for over a quarter of a century (Bucy and Thieman, 1968).

Medulloblastoma. This is a tumor mainly of early childhood, with the highest incidence at about 5 years of age. Boys are affected about twice as frequently as girls. The tumor usually arises in the vermis, often from the region of the inferior medullary velum. The earliest clinical manifestations are referable to generalized increased intracranial pressure, with projectile vomiting particularly frequent. As in midline astrocytoma, signs of cerebellar deficiency in medulloblastoma are rather few and are referable chiefly to the lower limbs, but the signs are manifold if the tumor invades or initially occupies a cerebellar hemisphere.

Medulloblastoma frequently extends into the meninges, from which seedlings may be carried by the cerebrospinal fluid to distant regions—in the spinal direction as far as the cauda equina. The resulting compression often causes motor and sensory deficit in the lower limbs and urinary and fecal incontinence. The tumor may also spread directly upward and compress or invade the lamina quadrigemina, causing pupillary dilatation and paresis of upward conjugate deviation of the eyes. It may spread along the base of the brainstem, producing clinical disturbances referable to cranial nerves. It often encroaches on the fourth ventricle, and if it invades this cavity and compresses its floor there may be coarse tremor of the fingers and arms, resulting, presumably, from interruption of reticulospinal fibers. Compression of the medulla oblongata may cause opisthotonos, extensor rigidity of the limbs, and quadriplegia. (Abbott and Kernohan, 1943; Bailey and Cushing, 1925; Elvidge, Penfield, and Cone, 1935; Jenkin, 1969.)

Medulloblastoma may also occur in adolescents and young adults, and rarely in older adults. At this age level, no sex preference has been demonstrated. The tumor usually originates in a cerebellar hemisphere, and occasionally centrally in the cerebellum. The clinical course is slow in evolution and the patient may live for years after operative removal of the tumor. As in medulloblastoma occurring in childhood, many of these tumors seed to distant parts and now and then metastasize to vertebrae, cervical lymph nodes, and even the lungs. (Bailey, 1929; Berger and Elvidge, 1963; Penfield and Feindel, 1947; Spitz, Shenkin, and Grant, 1947.) Tumors having much the same clinical and pathological characteristics have been called *primary cerebellar sarcoma* and *circumscribed arachnoidal sarcoma of the cerebellum* (Kernohan and Uihlein, 1962; Zimmerman, Netsky, and Berkmann, 1951). However, a prevalent view is that these tumors are variants of medulloblastoma, reticulum fibers being acquired through some influence connected with meningeal invasion (Rubinstein and Northfield, 1964)—a response not essentially different from that aroused in cerebral glioma which has extended into the meninges. Cerebellar sarcomas occur, but the reticulum-containing tumor under discussion appears not to be among them.

Capillary hemangioblastoma. This tumor is uncommon, has a familial incidence—in about 20 percent of cases—and usually becomes clinically manifest in persons aged 30 to 45 years. It is most frequently situated in the angle between the inferior part of the roof of the fourth ventricle and the cerebellar vermis or tonsil. These tumors originate either from vascular adventitia or from pia, probably the latter. They remain loosely adherent to the cerebellum. The tumor varies in diameter from 1 cm. to as large as 6 cm. It is solid, though microcystic in places, and its surface is irregularly nodular and covered with blood vessels. The next most common site is the cerebellum, where it occupies the cortex of one of the hemispheres (Lindau, 1931). Here the tumor may be solid but is usually associated with a cyst, often many times larger than the tumor itself. The tumor, in the form of a brown or red-stained nodule, projects into the lumen of the cyst. The tumor thus constitutes a "mural" nodule. Such hemangioblastomas, which represent about 15 percent of cerebellar tumors, are frequently associated with *angioma of the retina* (von Hippel, 1911). In some cases there are cysts in the kidneys and pancreas and, rarely, polycystic kidneys and "benign hypernephroma"; capillary cutaneous naevi are also present but are rare. The clinical manifestations of cystic hemangioblastoma of the cerebellum are no different from those of other hemispheric tumors. Finally, some capillary hemangioblastomas arise in the area postrema, and they tend to invade the medulla oblongata. (Bailey, 1948; Cushing and Bailey, 1928; Henschen, 1955; Russell and Rubinstein, 1963.)

ALTERATIONS IN THE CEREBROSPINAL FLUID

Lack of protein increase in the cerebrospinal fluid (withdrawn by lumbar puncture) in the presence of intracranial tumor signifies that the tumor probably lies deep in the brain. Conversely, protein content is invariably elevated in tumors that occupy or project into one of the ventricles or into the subarachnoid space; under these conditions the degree of increase in protein may be taken as a reflection of tumor vascularization. Glioblastoma multiforme, ependymoma, and medulloblastoma are characterized by an increase in protein, and in choroid-plexus papilloma the increase is usually pronounced. Elevation in protein level is also encountered in acoustic neuroma, other cerebellopontile angle tumors, and most meningiomas. Tumors within the cerebellum are associated with an elevation in protein in about 50 percent of cases. Pleocytosis is common in most kinds of intracranial tumor; neutrophilic leukocytes are noted most frequently in glioblastoma multiforme, astrocytoma, meningioma, and neurinoma.

Blood in the spinal fluid traceable to intracranial tumors is comparatively rare, being noted in about 1 percent of tumors. In 25 to 50 percent of cases of tumor in which seepage of blood occurs into the subarachnoid space, the tumor is a glioma, most commonly glioblastoma multiforme. Next in incidence of blood seepage come pituitary tumors, then vascular tumors. Xanthochromia, abnormal colloid gold curve, and number of cells run more or less parallel with the protein increase. (Glass and Abbott, 1955; Jefferson and Jackson, 1939; Van Wagenen, 1930.)

Tumor cells are not uncommonly found in the cerebrospinal fluid, and may provide the diagnosis where other investigative means fail. Metastatic growths are thus revealed more frequently (in 25 to 70 percent of cases) than primary intracranial growths (in 10 percent). Of the latter, cells from medulloblastoma and glioblastoma multiforme are among the most commonly found. (Wieczorek and Greger, 1965.)

REFERENCES

Abbott, K. H., and Courville, C. B. 1942. Intraventricular meningiomas: review of the literature and report of two cases. Bull. Los Angeles Neurol. Soc. **7**:12-28.

Abbott, K. H., and Kernohan, J. W. 1943. Medulloblastomas: concerning the problems of spinal metastasis and malignancy: a report of six cases and discussion of the problems involved. Bull. Los Angeles Neurol. Soc. **8**:1-10.

Alpers, B. J., and Yaskin, J. C. 1939. Gliomas of the pons: clinical and pathologic characteristics. Arch. Neurol. Psychiat. **41**:435-459.

Arseni, C., Ionescu, S., and Maretsis, M. 1968. Meningiomas of the lateral ventricle. Psychiat. Neurol. Neurochir. **71**:319-336.

Baggenstoss, A. H., and Love, J. G. 1939. Pinealomas. Arch. Neurol. Psychiat. **41**:1187-1206.

Bailey, P. 1929. Intracranial sarcomatous tumors of leptomeningeal origin. Arch. Surg. **18**:1359-1402.

Bailey, P. 1948. Intracranial tumors, ed. 2. Springfield, Illinois, Charles C Thomas, Publisher.

Bailey, P., and Bucy, P. C. 1929. Oligodendrogliomas of the brain. J. Path. Bact. **32**:735-751.

Bailey, P., and Cushing, H. 1925. Medulloblastoma cerebelli: a common type of midcerebellar glioma of childhood. Arch. Neurol. Psychiat. **14**:192-224.

Berger, E. C., and Elvidge, A. R. 1963. Medulloblastomas and cerebellar sarcomas: a clinical survey. J. Neurosurg. **20**:139-144.

Bergstrand, H. 1939. Weiteres über sogenannte Kleinhirnastrocytome. Virchows Arch. Path. Anat. **299**:725-739.

Bormann, H., and Schiefer, W. 1951. Krampfanfälle bei Tumoren des Grosshirns. Deutsch. Z. Nervenheilk. **166**:1-16.

Bucy, P. C., and Gustafson, W. A. 1939. Structure, nature and classification of the cerebellar astrocytomas. Amer. J. Cancer **35**:327-353.

Bucy, P. C., and Thieman, P. W. 1968. Astrocytomas of the cerebellum: a study of a series of patients operated upon over 28 years ago. Arch. Neurol. **18**:14-19.

Busch, E., and Christensen, E. 1947. The three types of glioblastoma. J. Neurosurg. **4**:200-220.

Caveness, W. F. 1966. Posttraumatic sequelae. In Caveness, W. F., and Walker, A. E., editors: Head injury. Philadelphia, J. B. Lippincott Company, pp. 209-219.

Caviness, V. S. 1966. Epilepsy and craniocerebral injury of warfare. In Caveness, W. F., and Walker, A. E., editors: Head injury. Philadelphia, J. B. Lippincott Company, pp. 220-234.

Clark, E. S., and Gooddy, W. 1953. Ipsilateral third cranial nerve palsy as a presenting sign in acute subdural haematoma. Brain **26**:266-278.

Cohen, S. I., and Aronson, S. M. 1968. Secondary brain stem hemorrhages: predisposing and modifying factors. Arch. Neurol. **19**:257-263.

Collier, J. 1904. The false localizing signs of intracranial tumour. Brain **27**:490-508.

Corsellis, J. A. N. 1958. Individual variation in the size of the tentorial opening. J. Neurol. Neurosurg. Psychiat. **21**:279-283.

Cox, L. B. 1932. Ganglioneuroma of cerebrum, with additional case. Med. J. Aust. **1**:347-351.

Craig, W. McK., and Kernohan, J. W. 1938. Tumors of the fourth ventricle. J.A.M.A. **111**:2370-2377.

Cushing, H. 1910. Strangulation of the nervi abducentes by lateral branches of the basilar artery in cases of brain tumor: with an explanation of some obscure palsies on the basis of arterial constriction. Brain **33**:204-235.

Cushing, H. 1932. Intracranial tumors: notes upon

a series of two thousand verified cases. Springfield, Illinois, Charles C Thomas, Publisher.

Cushing, H., and Bailey, P. 1928. Tumours arising from the blood vessels of the brain: angiomatous malformations and hemangioblastomas. Springfield, Illinois, Charles C Thomas, Publisher, pp. 105-203.

Cushing, H., and Eisenhardt, L. 1938. Meningiomas: their classification, regional behaviour, life history, and surgical end results. Springfield, Illinois, Charles C Thomas, Publisher.

Denny-Brown, D., and Russell, W. R. 1941. Experimental cerebral concussion. Brain **64**:93-164.

Earnest, F., III, Kernohan, J. W., and Craig, W. McK. 1950. Oligodendrogliomas: a review of two hundred cases. Arch. Neurol. Psychiat. **63**:964-976.

Ehnig, G. 1950. "False" localizing signs in intracranial tumors: report of a patient with left trigeminal palsy due to right temporal meningioma. Arch. Neurol. Psychiat. **64**:692-698.

Elvidge, A., Penfield, W., and Cone, W. 1935. The gliomas of the central nervous system: a study of the two hundred and ten verified cases. Res. Publ. Ass. Res. Nerv. Ment. Dis., Proc. **16**:107-181.

Emery, J. L. 1967. Kinking of the medulla in children with acute cerebral oedema and hydrocephalus and its relationship to the dentate ligaments. J. Neurol. Neurosurg. Psychiat. **30**:267-275.

Evans, J. P., and Scheinker, I. M. 1943. Histologic studies of the brain following head trauma: post-traumatic infarction of cerebral arteries, with consideration of the associated clinical picture. Arch. Neurol. Psychiat. **50**:258-278.

Fischer-Brügge, E. 1951. Das "Klivuskantensyndrom." Acta Neurochir. **2**:36-68.

Ford, F. R., and Muncie, W. 1938. Malignant tumor within the third ventricle: three cases of unusual type of invasion of the ventricular walls. Arch. Neurol. Psychiat. **39**:82-95.

Forster, H. W., and Bonzarth, W. F. 1967. Meningioma and the tuberculum sellae as a cause of optic atrophy. Amer. J. Ophthal. **64**:908-910.

Frazier, C. H. 1936. Tumor involving the frontal lobe alone: a symptomatic survey of one hundred and five verified cases. Arch. Neurol. Psychiat. **35**:525-571.

Friede, R. L. 1961. Experimental concussion acceleration: pathology and mechanics. Arch. Neurol. **4**:449-462.

Glass, B., and Abbott, K. H. 1955. Subarachnoid hemorrhage consequent to intracranial tumors: review of literature and report of seven cases. A.M.A. Arch. Neurol. Psychiat. **73**:369-376.

Globus, J. H. 1937. The meningiomas: their origin, divergence in structure, and relationship to contiguous tissues in the light of phylogenesis and ontogenesis of the meninges; with a suggestion of a simplified classification of meningeal neoplasms. Res. Publ. Ass. Res. Nerv. Ment. Dis., Proc. **16**:210-265.

Gonzales, D., and Elvidge, A. R. 1962. On the occurrence of epilepsy caused by astrocytoma of the cerebral hemispheres. J. Neurosurg. **19**:470-482.

Groeneveld, A., and Schaltenbrand, G. 1927. Ein Fall von Duraendotheliom über der Grosshirnhemisphäre mit einer bemerkenswerten Komplikation: Läsion des gekreuzten Pes pedunculi durch Druck auf den Rand des Tentoriums. Deutsch. Z. Nervenheilk. **97**:32-50.

Guyot, J. F., Vouyouklakis, D., and Pertuiset, B. 1967. Meningiomes de l'arête sphenoidale: à propos de 50 cas. Neuro-Chir. (Paris) **13**:571-584.

Hallervorden, J., and Quadbeck, G. 1957. Die Hirnerschütterung und ihre Wirkung auf das Gehirn. Deutsch. Med. Wschr. **82**:129-142.

Henschen, F. 1955. Tumoren des Zentralnervensystems und seiner Hüllen. In Lubarsch, O., Henke, F., and Rössle, R., editors: Handbuch der speziellen pathologischen Anatomie und Histologie, vol. 13 (edited by Scholz, W.). Berlin, Springer-Verlag, pp. 413-1040.

Horrax, G. 1939. Meningiomas of the brain. Arch. Neurol. Psychiat. **41**:140-157.

Horrax, G., and Buckley, R. 1930. A clinical study of the differentiation of certain pontile tumors from acoustic gliomas. Arch. Neurol. Psychiat. **24**:1217-1230.

Hoyt, W. F. 1960. Vascular lesions of the visual cortex with brain herniation through the tentorial incisura: neuro-ophthalmologic considerations. Arch. Ophthal. **64**:44-57.

Jackson, F. E. 1966. The pathophysiology of head injuries. CIBA Clin. Sympos. **18**:67-93.

Jane, J. A., and McKissock, W. 1962. Importance of failing vision in early diagnosis of suprasellar meningioma. Brit. Med. J. **2**:5-7.

Jefferson, G. 1938. The tentorial pressure cone. Arch. Neurol. Psychiat. **40**:857-876.

Jefferson, G., and Jackson, H. 1939. Tumours of the lateral and 3rd ventricles. Proc. Roy. Soc. Med. **32**:1105-1137.

Jelsma, R., and Bucy, P. C. 1969. Glioblastoma multiforme: its treatment and some factors effecting survival. Arch. Neurol. **20**:161-171.

Jenkin, R. D. T. 1969. Medulloblastoma in childhood: radiation therapy. Canad. Med. Ass. J. **100**:51-53.

Kernohan, J. W., Mabon, R. F., Svien, H. J., and Adson, A. W. 1949. A simplified classification of the gliomas. Proc. Mayo Clin. **24**:71-75.

Kernohan, J. W., and Uihlein, A. 1962. Sarcomas of the brain. Springfield, Illinois, Charles C Thomas, Publisher.

Kernohan, J. W., and Woltman, H. 1929. Incisura of the crus due to contralateral brain tumor. Arch. Neurol. Psychiat. **21**:274-287.

Knox, E. W., and Adams, G. F. 1969. The hemiplegic onset of brain tumors. Gerontol. Clin. **11**:1-12.

Lindau, A. 1931. Vascular tumours of the brain and spinal cord. Proc. Roy. Soc. Med. **24**:1-8.

Lindenberg, R. 1955. Compression of brain arteries as pathogenetic factor for tissue necroses and their areas of predilection. J. Neuropath. Exp. Neurol. **14**:223-243.

Lindenberg, R. 1966. Significance of the tentorium in head injuries from blunt forces. Clin. Neurosurg., Congr. Neurol. Surgeons **12**:129-142.

Lindenberg, R., and Freytag, E. 1960. The mech-

anism of cerebral contusions: a pathologic-anatomic study. Arch. Path. **69**:440-469.
Lindenberg, R., and Walsh, F. B. 1964. Vascular compressions involving intracranial visual pathways. Trans. Amer. Acad. Ophthal. Otolaryng. **68**:677-694.
Markham, J. W., Fager, C. A., Horrax, G., and Poppen, J. L. 1955. Meningiomas of the posterior fossa: their diagnosis, clinical features, and surgical treatment. Arch. Neurol. Psychiat. **74**: 163-170.
McNealy, D. E., and Plum, F. 1962. Brainstem dysfunction with supratentorial mass lesions. Arch. Neurol. **7**:10-32.
Meirowsky, A. M. 1954. Penetrating craniocerebral trauma: observations in Korean War. J.A.M.A. **154**:666-669.
Meirowsky, A. M. 1966. Penetrating craniocerebral trauma. In Caveness, W. F., and Walker, A. E., editors: Head injury. Philadelphia, J. B. Lippincott Company, pp. 195-202.
Meyer, A. 1920. Herniation of the brain. Arch. Neurol. Psychiat. **4**:387-400.
Moore, M. T., and Stern, K. 1938. Vascular lesions in the brain-stem and occipital lobe occurring in association with brain tumours. Brain **61**:70-98.
Noetzel, H. 1951. Über Meningeome und ihre unterschiedlichen Auswirkungen am Gehirn. Beitr. Path. Anat. **111**:391-406.
Ommaya, A. K. 1966. Experimental head injury in the monkey. In Caveness, W. F., and Walker, A. E., editors: Head injury. Philadelphia, J. B. Lippincott Company, pp. 260-275.
Penfield, W., and Feindel, W. 1947. Medulloblastoma of the cerebellum, with survival for seventeen years. Arch. Neurol. Psychiat. **57**:481-484.
Pool, J. L. 1968. Gliomas in the region of the brain stem. J. Neurosurg. **29**:164-167.
Rasdolsky, I. 1935. Dorsal-pontines Tumorsyndrom. Z. Ges. Neurol. Psychiat. **152**:530-537.
Riishede, J. 1957. Cerebral apoplexy: an arteriographical and clinical study of 100 cases. Acta Psychiat. Neurol. Scand. **32** (suppl. 118):1-210.
Ringertz, N., and Nordenstam, H. 1951. Cerebellar astrocytoma. J. Neuropath. Exp. Neurol. **10**:343-367.
Roth, J. G., and Elvidge, A. R. 1960. Glioblastoma multiforme: a clinical survey. J. Neurosurg. **17**:736-750.
Rubinstein, L. G., and Northfield, D. W. C. 1964. The medulloblastoma and the so-called "arachnoidal cerebellar sarcoma": a critical re-examination of a nosological problem. Brain **87**: 379-412.
Russell, D. S., and Rubinstein, L. J. 1963. Pathology of tumours of the nervous system, ed. 2. London, Edward Arnold (Publishers) Ltd.
Russell, W. O., and Sachs, E. 1943. Pinealoma: a clinicopathologic study of seven cases with a review of the literature. Arch. Path. **35**:869-888.
Scheidegger, S. 1948. Pathologisch-anatomische Untersuchungen bei posttraumatischen Gehirnveränderungen und Encephalosen. Schweiz. Z. Path. Bakt. **11**:225-255.
Schneider, R. C., Kahn, E. A., and Crosby, E. C. 1951. Extradural hematoma of the posterior fossa. Neurology **1**:386-393.
Spatz, H. 1950. Brain injuries in aviation. In German aviation medicine, World War II, vol. 1. Washington, D. C., U. S. Government Printing Office, pp. 616-640.
Spatz, H., and Stroescu, G. J. 1934. Zur Anatomie und Pathologie der äusseren Liquorräume des Gehirns. (Die Zisternenverquellung beim Hirntumor.) Nervenarzt **7**:481-498.
Spitz, E. B., Shenkin, H. A., and Grant, F. C. 1947. Cerebellar medulloblastoma in adults. Arch. Neurol. Psychiat. **57**:417-422.
Stender, A. 1933. Über das Meningiom des Keilbeinrückens. Z. Ges. Neurol. Psychiat. **147**:244-262.
Strich, S. J. 1956. Diffuse degeneration of cerebral white matter in severe dementia following head injury. J. Neurol. Psychiat. **19**:163-185.
Strich, S. J. 1961. Shearing of nerve fibers as a cause of brain damage due to head injury: a pathologic study of 20 cases. Lancet **2**:443-448.
Stringer, S. W. 1934. Diabetes insipidus associated with pinealoma transplant in the tuber cinereum. Yale J. Biol. Med. **6**:375-383.
Sunderland, S. 1958. The tentorial notch and complications produced by herniations of the brain through that aperture. Brit. J. Surg. **45**:422-438.
Symington, J. 1906. A note on the topographical anatomy of the caput gyri hippocampi. J. Anat. **40**:244-246.
Symonds, C. 1962. Concussion and its sequelae. Lancet **1**:1-5.
Taylor, A. R. 1966. Slowing of cerebral circulation following concussional head injury: its relationship to symptoms and the etiology of concussion. In Caveness, W. F., and Walker, A. E., editors: Head injury. Philadelphia, J. B. Lippincott Company, pp. 235-241.
Teltscharow, L., and Zülch, K. J. 1947. Das Astrocytoma des Grosshirns vom pathologischanatomischen Standpunkt aus. Arch. Psychiat. Z. Ges. Neurol. Psychiat. **179**:691-720.
Tompkins, V. N., Haymaker, W., and Campbell, E. H. 1950. Metastatic pineal tumors: a clinicopathologic report of two cases. J. Neurosurg. **7**:159-169.
Unterharnscheidt, F., and Sellier, K. 1966. Mechanics and pathomorphology of closed brain injuries. In Caveness, W. F., and Walker, A. E., editors: Head injury. Philadelphia, J. B. Lippincott Company, pp. 321-341.
Van Wagenen, W. P. 1930. Papillomas of the choroid plexus: report of two cases, one with removal of tumor at operation and one with "seeding" of the tumor in the ventricular system. Arch. Surg. **20**:199-231.
von Hippel, E. 1911. Die anatomische Grundlage der von mir beschriebenen "sehr seltenen Erkrankung der Netzhaut." Arch. Ophthal. **79**: 350-377.
Weir, B. W., and Elvidge, A. R. 1968. Oligodendrogliomas: an analysis of 63 cases. J. Neurosurg. **29**:500-505.
White, H. H. 1963. Brain stem tumors occurring in adults. Neurology **13**:292-300.

Wieczorek, V., and Greger, J. 1965. Erfahrungen mit der Liquorzelldiagnostik: eine Analyse von etwa 5000 liquorzytologischen Untersuchungen. Psychiat. Neurol. (Basel) **150**:42-55.

Wolman, L. 1953. Ischaemic lesions in the brainstem associated with raised intracranial pressure. Brain **76**:364-377.

Zimmerman, H. M., Netsky, M. G., and Berkmann, J. 1951. Primary cerebellar sarcoma. Trans. Amer. Neurol. Ass. **76**:84-86.

Zülch, K. J. 1951. Vorzugssitz, Erkrankungsalter und Geschlechtsbevorzugung bei Hirngeschwulsten als bisher ungeklärte Formen der Pathoklise. Deutsch. Z. Nervenheilk. **166**:91-102.

Chapter 29

Roentgenographic localization of intracranial lesions

Bernard S. Epstein

DIAGNOSIS WITH PLAIN FILMS

Radiographic examination of the skull is essential in the investigation of neurological disorders. Suitable plain film examinations provide information about the integrity of the vault and base of the skull and the facial bones. Changes in size, configuration, and density of the sella turcica offer evidence of increased intracranial pressure or of the existence of a tumor of the pituitary gland. The condition of the mastoids, the orbits, the optic foramina, and the facial bones can readily be examined, as can the status of the paranasal sinuses. Calcifications within the cranial cavity can be identified and often localized. The position of the calcified pineal body is most important in demonstrating the influence of a space-filling lesion, because in the presence of such a lesion the pineal is shifted to the contralateral side. In the lateral projection, displacement of the pineal forward, backward, upward, or downward can be demonstrated by appropriate measurements (Vastine-Kinney method) or through some other method of pineal localization.

It is difficult to describe a "routine" skull examination. Suffice it to say that the procedure should be performed in order to answer pertinent questions based on the history and physical examination. All too often, however, the plain skull roentgenograms, no matter how carefully planned and taken, offer no definite information when there is little doubt that a pathological condition exists. At this time further methods available to the neuroradiologist come into play, including pneumoencephalography, cerebral angiography, angiography of the vessels of the neck, echoencephalography, and brain scans. While at times any one of these offers reliable evidence, it is not uncommon to have to call on two or more of these procedures to arrive at a diagnosis. The procedures should be considered as complementary. The neuroradiologist must be familiar with the performance, advantages, and disadvantages of all of them. (Bucy and Ciric, 1965; Di Chiro, 1961; Epstein, 1966; Quinn, 1965; Taveras and Wood, 1964.)

The position of the pineal body is one of the more important bits of information available from plain skull roentgenograms. The need for accurately positioned roentgenograms is obvious. Occasionally one may also find it advantageous to use body-section roentgenograms for the delineation of the pineal body. The most common anticipated change is contralateral displacement by a supratentorial mass. Occasionally the pineal body is shifted ipsilaterally when one side of the cerebrum is atrophic.

Posterior and downward displacement suggests the possibility of dilatation of the ventricular system, whereas upward and contralateral displacement may indicate the possibility of a temporal or occipital lesion. Choroid plexus calcification also occurs quite frequently, and occasionally the upward and lateral or medial shift of one glomus points to the existence of a tumor. Calcification of the falx cerebri is also frequent, but offers little diagnostic help. Indeed, the falx usually remains in the mid-

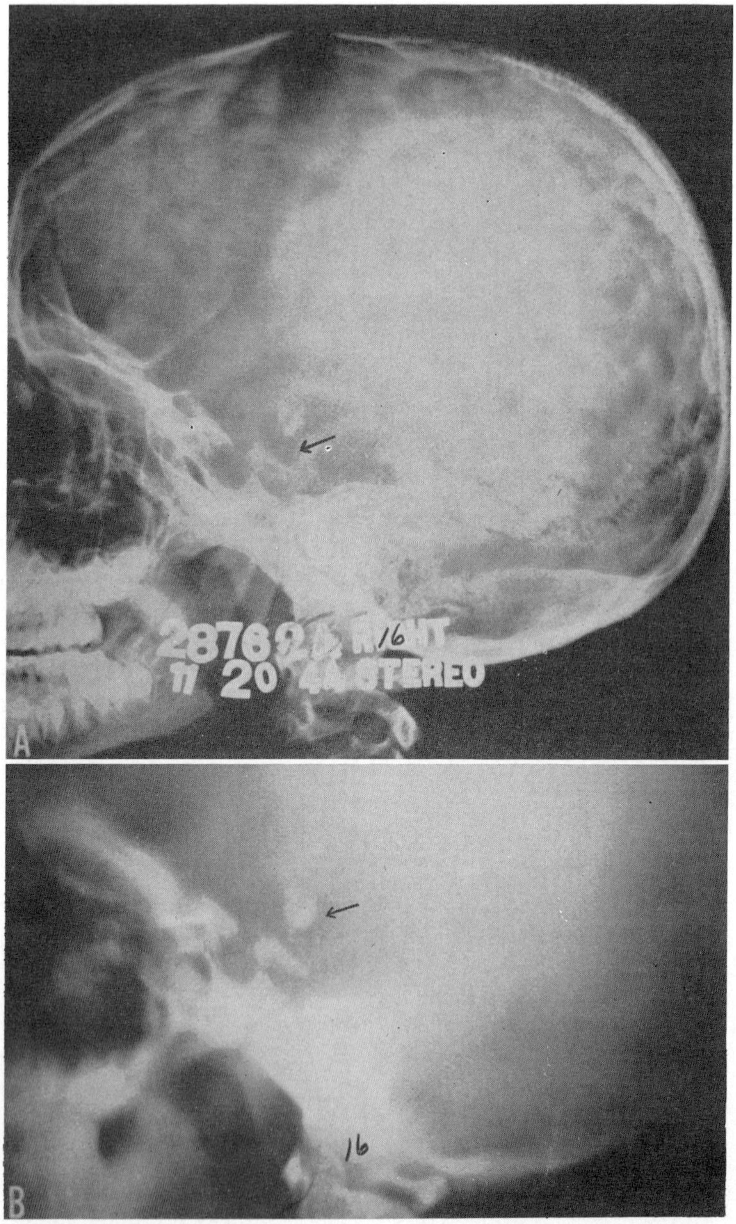

Fig. 29-1. A, Markedly increased intracranial pressure due to craniopharyngioma. The coronal suture is widely separated. The convolutional markings on the skull are increased, giving the skull a "hammered-silver" appearance. Calcification is present just above the dorsum sellae. Also the dorsum sellae is shortened. **B,** Midline laminagram, same patient. The calcifications above the sella turcica are evident.

line despite the presence of even a large tumor mass.

Increased intracranial pressure in children manifests itself by separation of the sutures and an increase in the convolutional pattern of the inner table of the skull, producing a "hammered silver" appearance. Often these changes are obvious, especially with slowly growing tumors in the midline (Fig. 29-1) or in the posterior cranial fossa, and with closure of the aqueduct of Sylvius or the foramina of Magendie and Luschka. In infants and children the sella turcica usually retains its normal bony density even when increased intracranial pressure is advanced. This appears to be due to the fact that the increased pressure is relieved by widening of sutures. Often there is difficulty in evaluating the appearance of the cranial sutures in children up to about 4 years of age, because the sutures may be rather wide even under normal circumstances. Increased convolutional markings also vary considerably, and unless the change is marked, caution should be exercised in interpretation.

In older persons, widening of the sutures is less likely to occur, and significantly deepened convolutional skull markings are infrequent. This is particularly true when increased intracranial pressure is rapid in its onset, such as may occur in the presence of certain gliomas. Under such conditions plain skull roentgenograms usually appear normal and are therefore unreliable. With slowly progressive increased intracranial pressure the dorsum sellae becomes demineralized and later the floor of the hypophysial fossa loses its osseous density. Prolonged increased intracranial pressure, such as may occur with a falx meningioma or aqueductal block, eventually leads to considerable bony loss and even to an increase in the size of the hypophysial fossa. Once in a while this reaches such proportions that an intrasellar tumor is suspected. With lesions close to the vault of the skull one occasionally encounters localized bulging and thinning of the overlying bone. Should there be visible calcifications near such a site, the lesion can be accurately localized, and an educated guess can be made as to tumor type. Lesions obstructing the flow of cerebrospinal fluid in or behind the sylvian aqueduct result in marked dilatation of the third ventricle. This produces enlargement of the sella

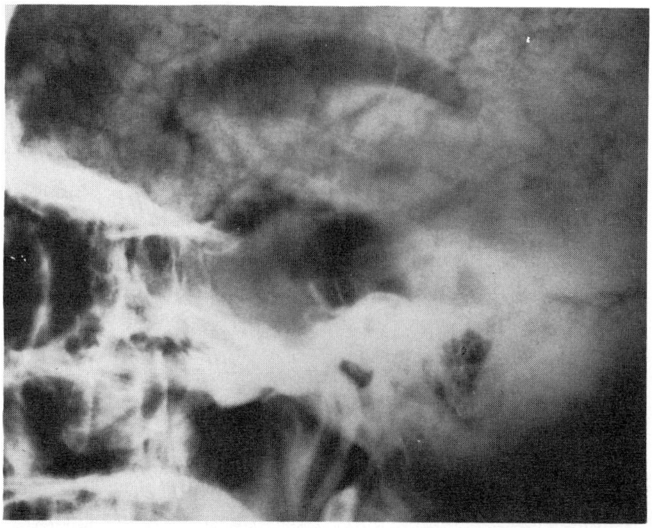

Fig. 29-2. Lumbar pneumoencephalogram in patient with a chromophobe pituitary adenoma. Extrasellar extension of the tumor into the cisterna interpeduncularis has occurred.

turcica, often with truncation and shortening of the dorsum sellae.

Intrasellar tumors, of which the chromophobe pituitary adenoma is the most frequent, produce ballooning of the hypophysial fossa (Fig. 29-2). The extent of this change is proportional to the size of the tumor. In some, the sella turcica may be symmetrically but only moderately enlarged; at the other end of the scale is advanced enlargement and actual destruction of the sellar confines. The anterior clinoid processes are involved, as a rule, only in the presence of large tumors that extend laterally for some distance. Occasionally, dilatation of the third ventricle may be so pronounced that the floor of the fluid-filled chamber comes to lie close to the dorsum sellae. This may result in an increase in the size of the hypophysial fossa, simulating the enlargement brought about by an intrasellar mass. Erosion of the sella turcica incident to aneurysm of the internal carotid is occasionally observed. This tends to be unilateral, but in the presence of large aneurysms the change may be difficult to distinguish from that resulting from an intrasellar tumor. Angiography is essential in solving this problem. Cavernous sinus aneurysms may also erode the sphenoid bone and enlarge the superior orbital fissure. Calcification of the wall of an aneurysm can be a clue in diagnosis.

Craniopharyngiomas are situated in or near the sella turcica (Fig. 29-1). In young people intrasellar and parasellar calcifications usually indicate the nature of the lesion. In older persons the sella may be normal, tumor calcification may be absent, and the tumor may be identified in an extrasellar position only on pneumoencephalographic study.

Body section roentgenograms are helpful in demonstrating hyperostotic changes in the bone or calcifications in the vicinity of the sella turcica. Extrasellar extension of pituitary adenomas and craniopharyngiomas is best revealed in pneumoencephalograms. Displacement of the interpeduncular and chiasmatic cisterns is diagnostic, as is upward or posterior displacement of the anteroinferior aspect of the third ventricle. These tumors sometimes grow large enough to extend into the foramen of Monro and produce marked hydrocephalus. They have also been observed to grow into the inferior portions of the lateral ventricles. So far as pituitary adenomas are concerned, intratumoral calcific deposits are rare, but occasionally small calcific plaques appear on the capsular surface. The size of a craniopharyngioma cannot be estimated from the disposition of the calcific material. The presence of such calcific deposits at some distance from the sella turcica is indicative of a large tumor (Fig. 29-1).

Alterations in the vault of the skull sometimes point to the presence of an intracranial tumor. For example, meningiomas may cause rarefactive or hyperostotic changes in the adjacent bone or changes in the vascular pattern of the inner table of the skull overlying the tumor. The tumor may invade bone, producing stippled areas of destruction that occasionally extend through the outer table and resulting in a visible bulge. Radiographic demonstration of a radial arrangement of bone spicules helps indicate the nature of the lesion (Fig. 29-3). Meningiomas en plaque produce severe bony reaction, for instance, in sphenoid wing meningiomas. Tuberculum sellae and clivus meningiomas may also be recognizable because of the bony changes produced by the tumor or by the presence of intratumoral calcific deposits.

Destruction of bone also constitutes an indication of adjacent tumor. Acoustic nerve tumors manifest themselves by destruction of the petrous tip and erosion of the internal auditory canal (Schmitz and Haveson, 1960). Advanced destruction in the region is illustrated in Fig. 13-11. Chordomas and occasionally nasopharyngeal tumors destroy the basisphenoid; bony erosion is at times extreme. Olfactory groove meningiomas may indent the cribriform plate. In these situations body section radiography is helpful.

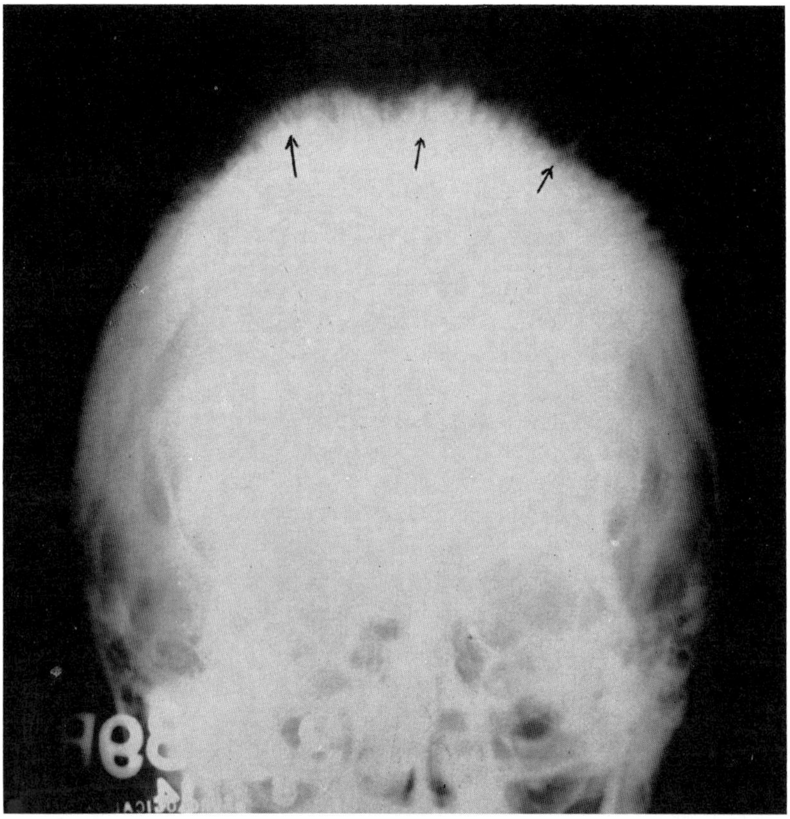

Fig. 29-3. Meningioma causing pronounced calcification of the vertex of the skull. The tables of the skull are thickened, and the outer table shows vertical striations (arrows).

Tumors of the optic nerve and chiasm are associated with enlargement of the involved optic foramen and identation of the optic groove (Taveras and Wood, 1964). No gross bone destruction is visible. It is believed that these tumors are of congenital origin, so that the optic foramen and the groove accommodate to the tumefied optic nerve.

Metastatic disease of the skull is frequently recognized from plain skull roentgenograms. A wide variety of tumors involve the cranium, mostly tumors metastasizing from lung, breast, thyroid, or kidney. Bone involvement by myeloma often presents a characteristic pattern of rarefied localized areas of destruction that vary considerably in size and distribution. It is interesting that patients with extensive bone destruction quite often have little or no involvement of the brain, while others with no visible osseous invasion have extensive brain metastases.

Many nonmalignant changes manifest themselves on plain skull roentgenograms. Paget's disease often affects the skull. The increased density produced by fibrous dysplasia is also characteristic in some instances. Benign tumors such as cholesteatoma, eosinophilic granuloma, and hemangioma can be demonstrated. Various metabolic diseases are revealed in skull roentgenograms—for example, granular porosity in hyperparathyroidism and in Cushing's disease.

Abnormal calcifications occur in the basal ganglia in some patients with hypoparathyroidism, although calcifications may occasionally appear without any reliable indication of this condition. In infants, small scattered calcifications are observed with toxoplasmosis, torulosis, cytomegalic inclusion disease, and coccidioidal infection. Characteristic of cysticercosis are widely scattered, tiny calcifications. Tuberous sclerosis produces fairly characteristic spotty calcification, most often in the ependyma of the lateral ventricles. Occasionally, calcifications are seen in tuberculoma, old subdural or intracerebral hematoma, or within neoplasms such as oligodendroglioma. Psammomatous calcifications in meningiomas are occasionally visible on plain skull roentgenograms. A diagnosis of lipoma of the corpus callosum is suggested by parenthesis-like streaks of calcification at the periphery of an otherwise radiolucent tumor. The streaky calcifications of Sturge-Weber's disease situated in subcortical areas present a serpiginous appearance that is often diagnostic.

PNEUMOENCEPHALOGRAPHY

Pneumoencephalography is performed either by the lumbar route or by means of ventricular puncture, and only infrequently by injection of gas into the cisterna magnum by the suboccipital route. As a rule, ventriculograms are obtained when intracranial pressure is increased, for example in cases of posterior fossa tumor. However, there is a tendency today to use the lumbar route even under such conditions, providing that little or no cerebrospinal fluid is withdrawn and providing that every precaution, such as seeing to it that a neurosurgeon is immediately available, is conscientiously observed. Even then, there are those who prefer to perform ventriculography when obviously increased intracranial pressure exists, especially in the presumed presence of a posterior fossa or midbrain tumor. Much depends on judgment in choosing the method best applicable to the patient under examination.

Knowledge of the pattern of the C.S.F. circulation is necessary for the interpretation of pneumoencephalograms (Liliequist, 1956). Perhaps even more important is an awareness of what happens when alterations occur in the C.S.F. passageways, including the subarachnoid cisterns. Tumors of the convex part of the brain produce fairly characteristic changes in the configuration of the lateral and third ventricles. Much depends on the size of the tumor and the degree of associated cerebral edema. Patients with relatively small tumors may have sufficient brain swelling to lead to narrowing of the (ipsilateral) lateral ventricle such as to prevent insertion of air into it. Other patients with far larger tumors may, however, have a dilated ipsilateral lateral ventricle, particularly if there is partial obstruction to the flow of C.S.F. through the foramen of Monro. Under these conditions the callosal sulcus may be dilated (Jacobson and others, 1965).

Frontal lobe tumors deform the anterior horns in a variety of ways. They may cause truncation of the chamber, displacement, or a "silver fork" or mushroom-like deformity of the horns. Extension to the contralateral side is sometimes suggested by bilateral deformities. Large tumors, however, also produce bilateral deformities without actually invading the opposite hemisphere. Parasagittal tumors depress the ipsilateral ventricle and shift the entire system contralaterally if sufficiently large (Fig. 29-4). Displacement of the third ventricle contralaterally is often noted even with moderate-sized masses. Usually the superior aspect is shifted more than the inferior aspect. Parietal and occipital tumors similarly deform the ventricular system in accordance with their size and location. Temporal lobe tumors displace the temporal horn as well as the bodies of the lateral ventricles. Displacement of the tip of the ipsilateral temporal horn indicates involvement medial or lateral to the involved chamber. If sufficiently large, tumors of the convex part of the hemisphere cause herniation of the brain under the falx cerebri, so that it is not uncommon to find that the roof of the ipsilateral ventricle is lower than that of the contralateral

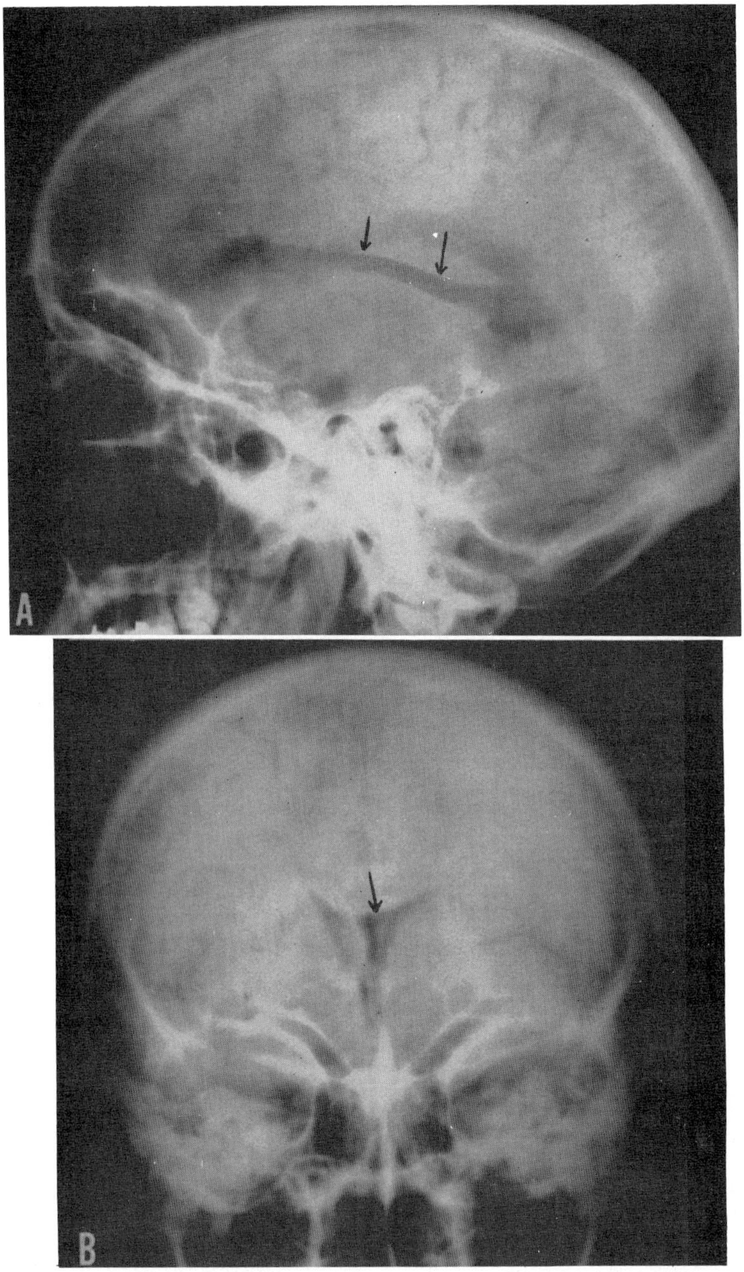

Fig. 29-4. **A,** Right prone lateral pneumoencephalogram. The left lateral ventricle is depressed and flattened (arrows). Operation revealed a left parasagittal meningioma. **B,** Anteroposterior view, same patient. The lateral ventricles are normal in size. There is a shift from left to right, and the roof of the left lateral ventricle is slightly flattened and elongated (arrow).

chamber. This should not be misinterpreted as indicative of a parasagittal tumor. Tumors of the corpus callosum, the septum pellucidum, and the walls of the lateral ventricles protrude into and deform the ventricular cavities in accordance with their size, their location, and their influence on C.S.F. circulation.

Midline tumors, especially those in the third ventricle, such as colloid cyst (Fig. 29-5), are found most easily in ventriculograms, and the same is true for thalamic

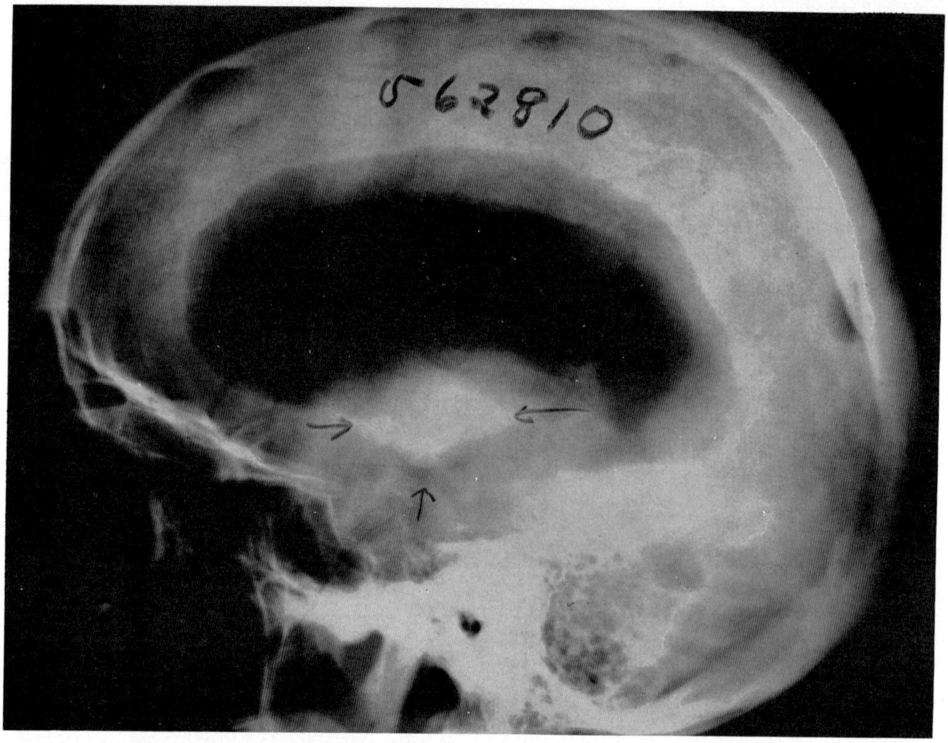

Fig. 29-5. Right lateral ventriculogram. A spherical mass (colloid cyst) is to be seen in the third ventricle (arrows). The lateral ventricles are greatly dilated. (AFIP Acc. 562810.)

tumors (Tovi, Schisano, and Liliequist, 1961). Impingement either on the foramen of Monroe or on the sylvian aqueduct may interfere with filling of the third or lateral ventricle, so that a tumor in that area may be difficult to identify on lumbar pneumoencephalograms. The demonstration of a filling defect in the third ventricle and displacement of the chamber are quite diagnostic. Obstruction in the region of the sylvian aqueduct produces pronounced dilatation of the third ventricle and the lateral ventricles. This is brought about, for example, by pineal tumor (Fig. 29-6), rostrally situated superior cerebellar tumor (Fig. 29-7), and aqueductal stenosis (Fig. 29-8). A characteristic funnel-like defect is occasionally found in the caudal part of the third ventricle. This deformity points to closure of the aqueduct of Sylvius, and quite often can be easily seen on body section roentgenograms made in the midline by encephalography. Sometimes, however, it becomes necessary to obtain positive contrast ventriculograms by instilling iophendylate (Pantopaque) into the lateral ventricles and passing this medium into the third and fourth ventricles in order to identify aqueductal obstruction. This can be accomplished sometimes by using a positive contrast agent introduced by the lumbar route.

Posterior fossa tumors such as hemangioblastoma (Fig. 29-9), medulloblastoma, and astrocytoma (Fig. 29-10) cause internal hydrocephalus when they interfere with C.S.F. passage from the foramina of Magendie and Luschka, or when they deform the sylvian aqueduct (McRae and Elliot, 1958). Such tumors can sometimes be localized by displacement of the fourth ventricle to one side or the other. Occasionally, upward indentation of the posterior aspect of the third ventricle produces some lateral displacement, which is helpful in diagnosis. Other significant changes in-

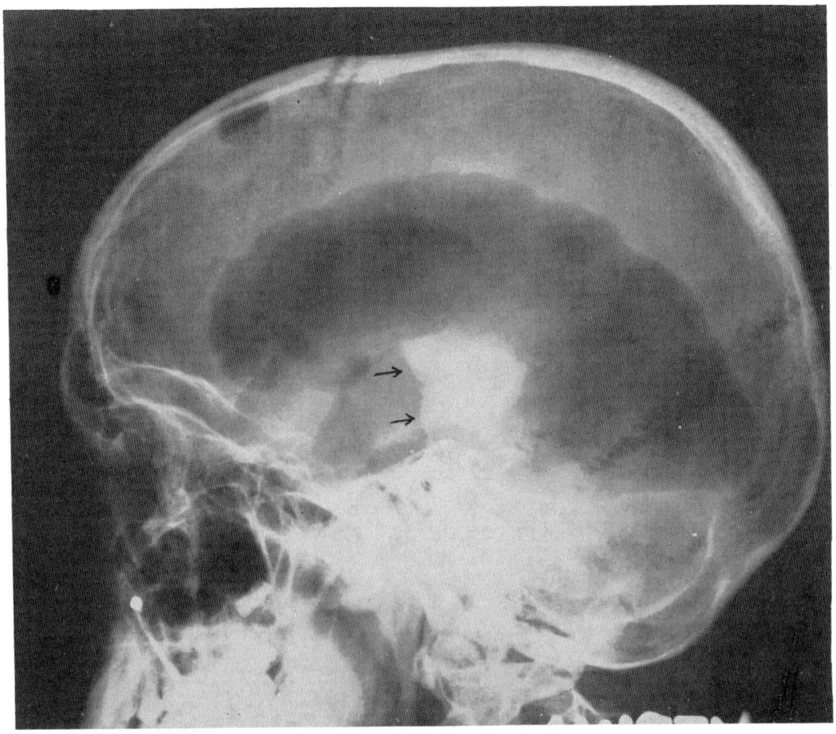

Fig. 29-6. Right lateral ventriculogram. A large mass (pinealoma) occupies the posterior half of the third ventricle (arrows). The lateral ventricles are markedly dilated. The coronal suture is widened.

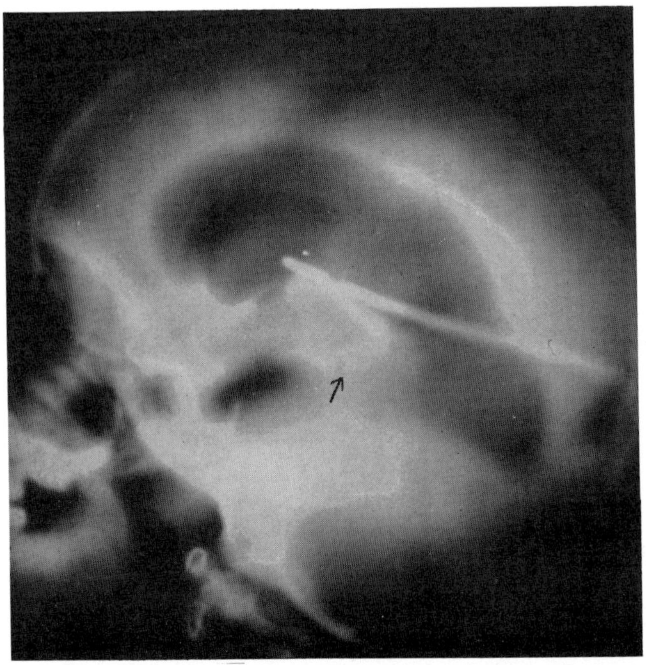

Fig. 29-7. Midline laminagram-ventriculogram. The third ventricle is dilated, and the aqueduct is blocked at the junction of its anterior and middle thirds (arrow). Inspection at operation disclosed a tumor in the superior part of the cerebellum.

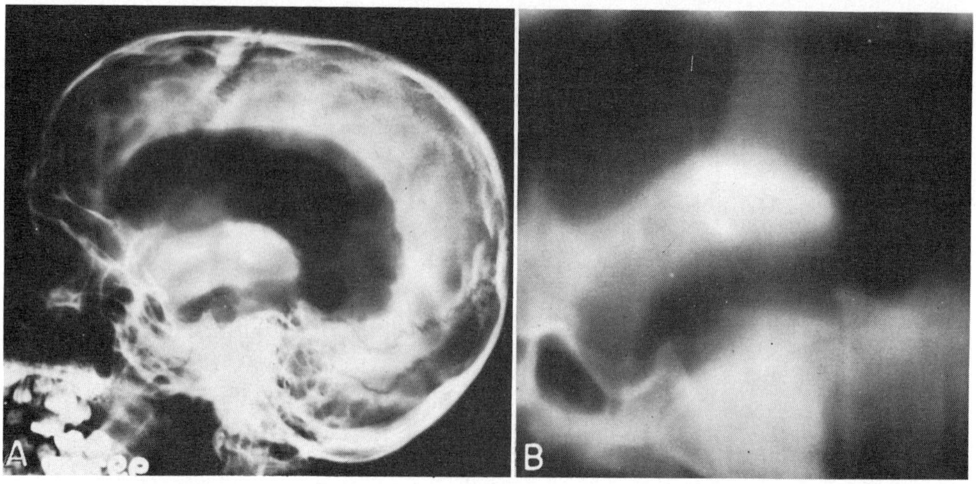

Fig. 29-8. A, This ventriculogram reveals hydrocephalus, with dilatation of the ventricles. The sutures are separated. The third ventricle is difficult to identify, but can be made out as a dilated structure. **B,** A midline laminagram demonstrates the third ventricle to better advantage. The ventricle is dilated and its floor is displaced downward into the sella turcica, causing deformity of the sella. The ventricular floor is displaced downward into the pontile cistern. The aqueduct of Sylvius terminates in a funnel-like configuration, consistent with the diagnosis of aqueductal stenosis.

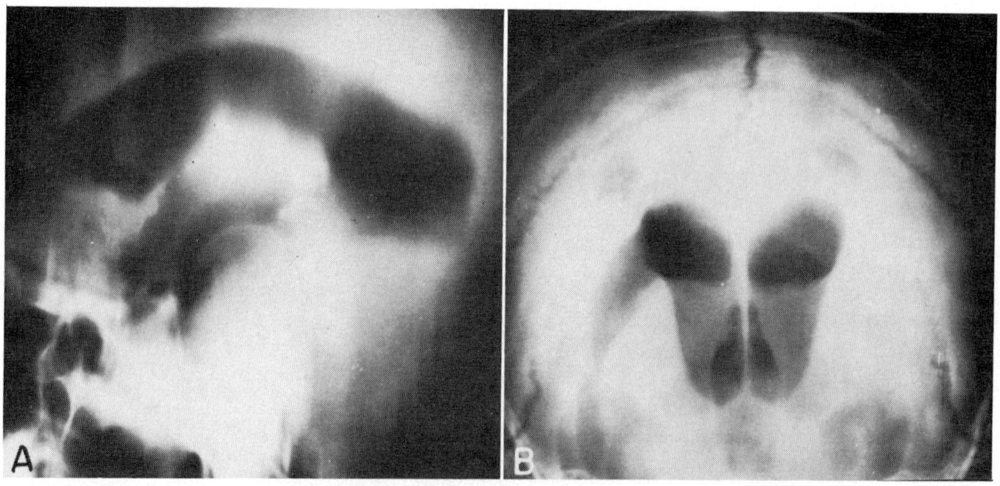

Fig. 29-9. A, Lateral body-section roentgenogram in a patient with hemangioblastoma of the vermis. The lateral and third ventricles are dilated. The aqueduct of Sylvius is dilated, bent forward, and is cut off in its proximal portion. **B,** Anteroposterior roentgenogram reveals diffuse dilatation of the lateral and third ventricles.

clude displacement of the fourth ventricle in the ventral direction, narrowing of the space between the fastigium and floor of the fourth ventricle, narrowing of the cisterna pontis (Fig. 29-10), and downward displacement of the cerebellar tonsils (Ralston, Gross, and Newman, 1959). Not uncommonly an axial pressure cone results (Liliequist, 1960). Tumors within the fourth ventricle itself distort or enlarge the chamber, and sometimes these changes are demonstrable particularly well in body section studies. Pontile tumors displace the fourth ventricle and the sylvian aqueduct

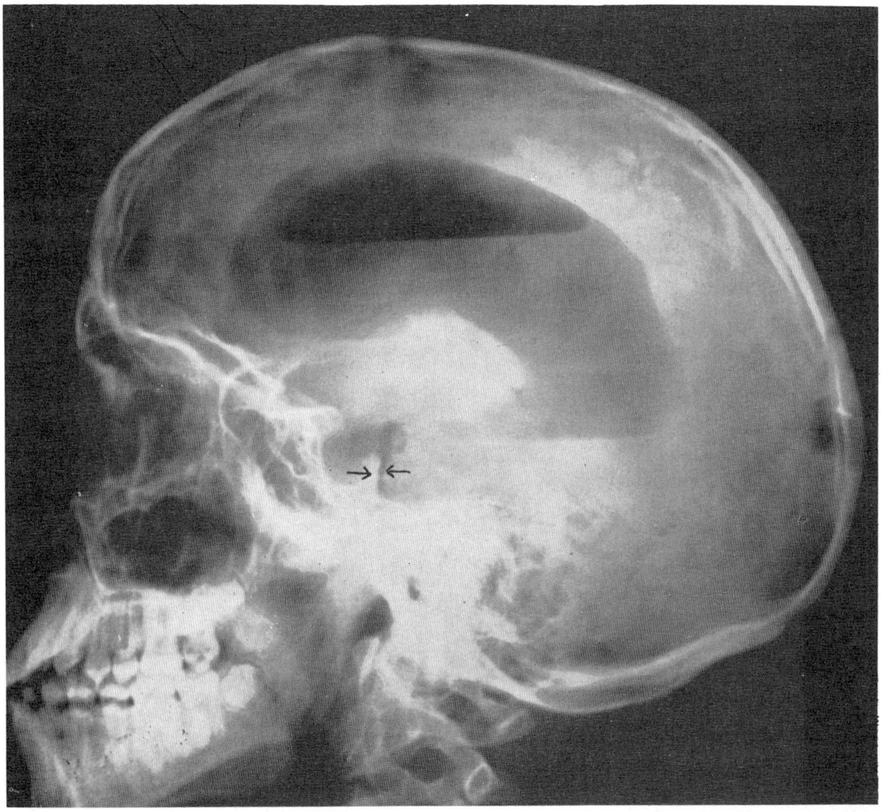

Fig. 29-10. Right erect ventriculogram. The lateral ventricles are dilated. The cisterna pontis (arrows) is narrowed to a thin slit by a cerebellar astrocytoma.

dorsally and result in a characteristic curvilinear configuration of the floor of the chamber. The floor-to-fastigium distance is narrowed. Acoustic nerve tumors and tumors involving the petrous pyramid—for example, tentorial meningioma—displace the fourth ventricle and the sylvian aqueduct contralaterally. Being situated in the ventral aspect of the posterior fossa, they push the fourth ventricle and the sylvian aqueduct dorsad (Taveras, 1960).

Cerebral atrophy and congenital malformations of the ventricular system are best diagnosed by means of pneumoencephalography. Agenesis of the corpus callosum and absence of the septum pellucidum are interesting but infrequent congenital conditions that can be readily identified.

CEREBRAL ANGIOGRAPHY

Cerebral angiography is a standard radiologic procedure for the diagnosis particularly of brain tumors, vascular malformations, and intracranial aneurysms. The contrast materials in use today, for example, meglumine iothalamate 60 percent (Conray) and orthodiatrizoate sodium 50 percent (Hypaque), are far less toxic than those in use several years ago.

In the presence of a suspected supratentorial mass that can be lateralized clinically as well as by a shift in the pineal and by a positive brain scan or echoencephalogram, the contrast material is injected into the common carotid on the affected side, and serial roentgenograms are then made in the lateral and frontal positions. These are best done with the use of the biplane technique, and at least two films per second are made during 6 seconds. This permits visualization of the arterial, arteriovenous, and venous phases. Whenever possible it is advisable to include the bifurcation of the common carotid artery

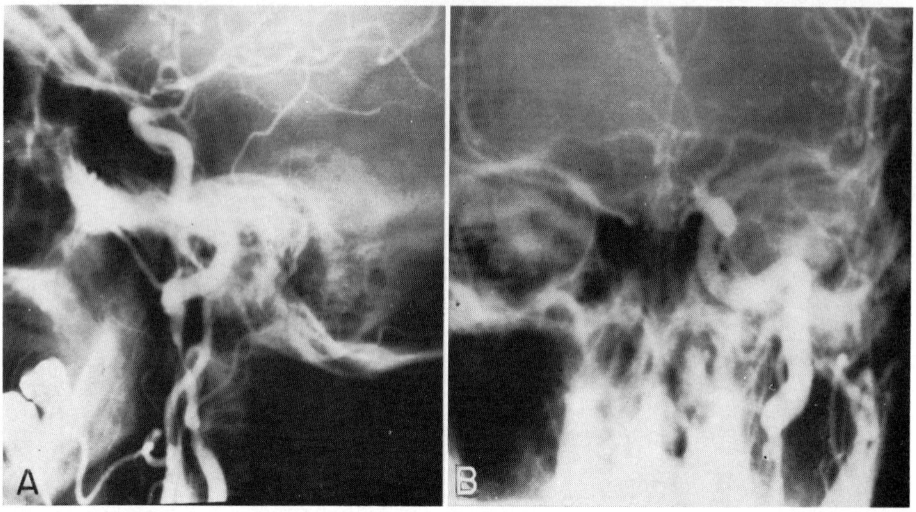

Fig. 29-11. A, The patient had symptoms diagnosed clinically as stroke. A carotid angiogram reveals extensive alteration of the internal carotid artery in its cervical portion. **B,** The anteroposterior angiogram shows some degree of poststenotic dilatation of the internal carotid as it enters the petrous bone and passes toward the cavernous sinus.

in the films, as illustrated in Fig. 29-11, because of the tendency for vascular disease in the neck to give rise to C.N.S. disorders. The vertebral and basilar arteries are examined by means of brachial angiography. Excellent visualization of the left vertebral artery can usually be obtained from left brachial angiograms, while right brachial angiograms portray the right vertebral as well as the carotid arterial system. The basilar artery derives its blood both from the right and the left vertebral artery, and adequate visualization sometimes requires both right and left brachial arteriograms. Catheter techniques and direct vertebral artery puncture have their many advocates, but inasmuch as satisfactory opacification can be obtained by a simpler method, I seldom use a catheter for visualization of the intracranial or vertebral artery circulation. Should there be a question as to the state of the major vessels at their origins from the aortic arch, a catheter is introduced into the arch by way of the femoral artery. As a rule, such a study provides excellent opacification of the great vessels up to the bifurcations of the common carotids and relatively unsatisfactory visualization of the upper cervical or intracranial circulation.

Cerebral angiograms are ideal for the diagnosis of aneurysms of the intracranial vessels. Most aneurysms originate at the dendritic points of the circle of Willis, but some arise from the internal carotid within or proximal to the cavernous sinus, or distally on smaller branches of the various intracerebral vessels. They also occur in the basilar artery, usually its distal tip, and also in the vertebral arteries and occasionally in their secondary branches. Angiographic study with the possibility of aneurysm in mind should include opacification of the circulatory tree of both carotids and the basilar artery. This can be done quite adequately by means of a right brachial and a left carotid angiogram, which leaves out only the left vertebral artery. For completeness a left brachial angiogram may be done. A protruding sac is diagnostic. Occasionally, intra-aneurysmal clotting is suggested by filling defects within the sac. More rarely, the entire sac is filled with clot, and if this reaches sufficient size it may mimic a tumor.

Congenital arteriovenous malformations

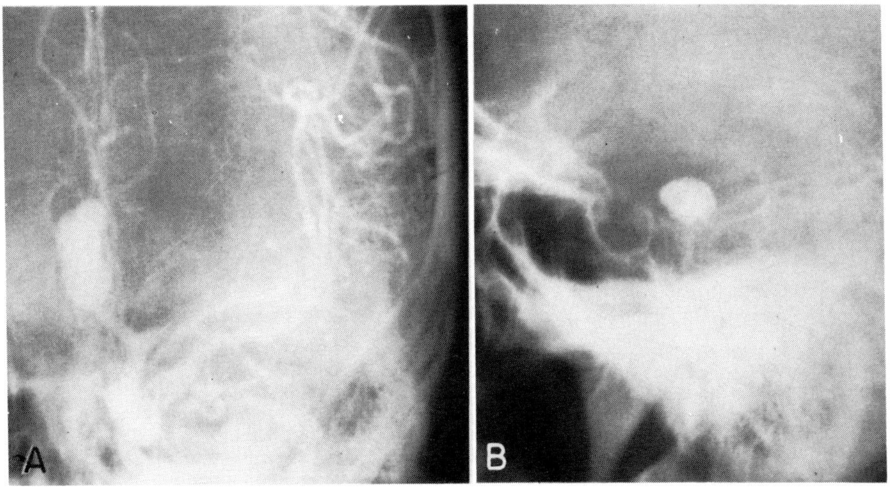

Fig. 29-12. A, Subarachnoid hemorrhage due to large aneurysm of the anterior communicating artery in a 35-year-old patient. **B,** Subarachnoid hemorrhage due to an aneurysm of the distal tip of the basilar artery in another patient.

are most satisfactorily opacified by means of carotid angiography in the supratentorial area and by means of vertebral angiograms in the infratentorial spaces. Such malformations are not identifiable on pneumoencephalograms unless a hematoma forms as a consequence of bleeding in the area. Such a hematoma displaces the ventricles or impinges on the subarachnoid space, simulating a mass lesion. Blood seeping from a small arteriovenous or other vascular malformation may obliterate the malformation so that it cannot be identified on angiograms, or indeed at necropsy without thorough investigations, including postmortem angiography.

Angiography is relied upon greatly for the detection of hemorrhage. Displacement of the cerebral cortex from the inner table of the skull as a result of subdural hemorrhage is readily demonstrated if the quantity of blood is fairly large. In the event of a recent hemorrhage the displacement will be fairly uniform. With subacute and chronic subdural hematomas the underlying part of the brain tends to be flattened; a straight-line or curved-line deformity is found along the edge of the depressed part of the brain. Epidural hematomas can occasionally be recognized by the characteristic downward indentation in the brain in the direction of the ventricle. Identification of the displaced middle meningeal artery is in itself sufficient to make the diagnosis. In addition, if the examination is performed during active bleeding, one can occasionally demonstrate contrast agent passing from the torn vessel. The vessel may be rendered visible by the presence of contrast agent on either side of it (the "track" sign), or traumatic arteriovenous communications may be established. Subarachnoid hematoma is also recognizable by angiography (Fig. 29-12).

Carotid angiography for the identification of hemispheric tumors is in everyday use. By this method the circulation within the tumor and the position of the adjacent vessels are visible (Torkildsen, 1949). Patterns observed in meningiomas are illustrated in Figs. 29-13 and 29-14, and for glioblastoma multiforme in Fig. 29-15. At times it is possible to make a fairly accurate statement as to the nature of the tumor. Meningiomas, for instance, may present a rich vascular bed with evidence of extracerebral vessels feeding into the tumor. Glioblastoma multiforme is suggested by the presence of increased circulation and small and rapidly filling

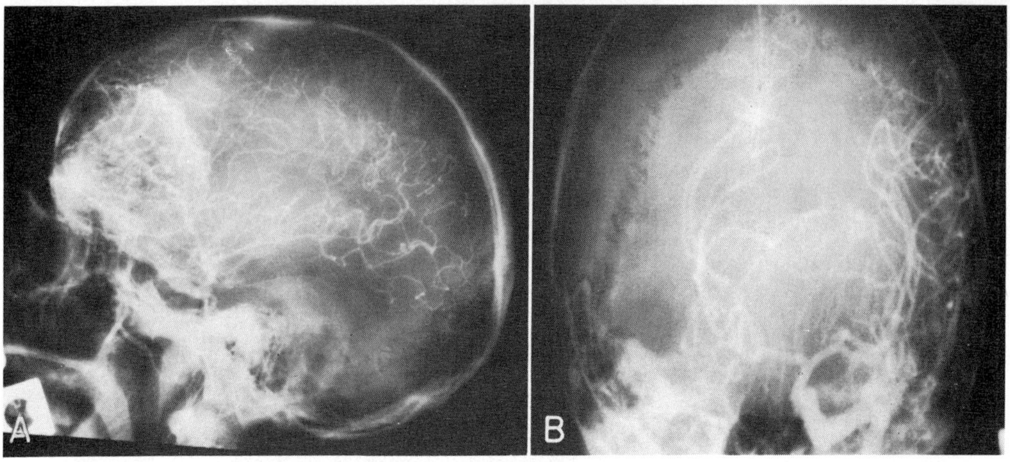

Fig. 29-13. **A,** Large olfactory groove meningioma. Note the abnormal vascular pattern in the frontal area, with a rim of condensed vessels resulting from pressure exerted by the mass. **B,** This anteroposterior angiogram reveals marked displacement of the anterior cerebral artery. The frontopolar artery is displaced medially. Vessels within the tumor can be seen between the displaced anterior cerebral artery and the middle cerebral artery.

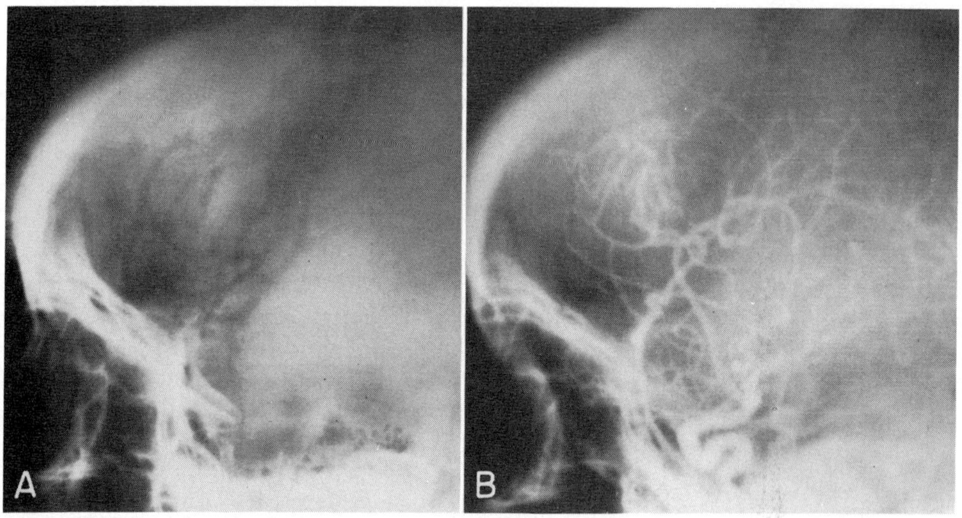

Fig. 29-14. **A,** Right lateral roentgenogram of skull. The vascular markings in the right frontal area are markedly increased. There is pronounced sella atrophy. **B,** Right lateral carotid angiogram. A large, highly vascularized tumor is visible in the frontal area. At operation the tumor proved to be a frontal convexity meningioma.

arteriovenous connections within the mass. However, one should exercise some restraint in venturing an opinion as to tumor type. Not at all infrequently metastatic deposits have been mistaken for meningiomas, or meningiomas have been considered to be glioblastomas. If a decision to operate is based entirely on vascular pattern there will almost surely come the occasion when one has cause for regret.

Useful information as to tentorial or tonsillar herniation is afforded by inspection of the posterior communicating and anterior choroidal arteries and of the posterior inferior cerebellar artery (Epstein, 1966; Liliequist, 1960). Demonstration of

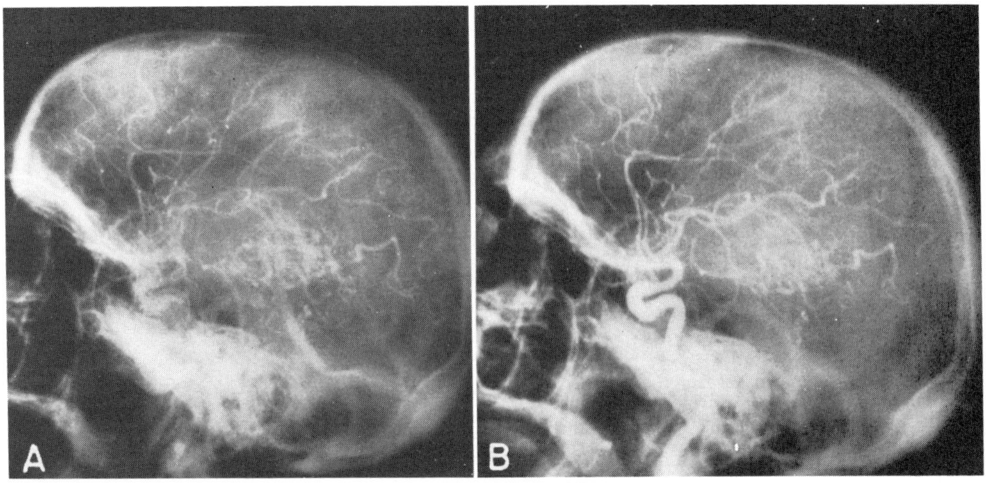

Fig. 29-15. Deep temporal lobe glioblastoma multiforme in a 50-year-old man. Lateral angiograms show large, prominent arteriovenous connections that become filled shortly after introduction of the contrast material (**A**). The vessels are derived mainly from the anterior cerebral artery. In the arteriovenous phase (**B**) the arteriovenous communications are more clearly demonstrated.

the septal vein is helpful, as its status is a good indicator of masses in the anterior cranial fossa (Zimmer and Annes, 1966). The thalamoperforate region of the thalamus artery is displaced by masses in the region of the thalamus and also by growths in the midbrain or in the posterior cranial fossa (Hara and Fujino, 1966).

Tumors in the midline are fairly difficult to define on angiograms. Nevertheless, the demonstration of changes characteristic of hydrocephalus, together with alterations in the position of the deep midline veins, is sometimes diagnostic and calls for further study by means of pneumoencephalograms. Similarly, tumors in the posterior fossa often can be accurately defined by means of vertebral angiograms. Nevertheless, a "negative angiogram" in a patient who presents a clinical picture of a posterior fossa lesion should not be considered conclusive, and pneumoencephalographic evidence should be obtained. I have often found it appropriate to perform angiographic examinations initially, and to continue with a pneumoencephalogram immediately afterward if any question as to diagnosis is raised. Here, too, one may seek help from brain scans. With today's technique for this procedure highly important evidence can be obtained. The neuroradiologist is well advised to seek information from all methods at his disposal—angiography, pneumoencephalography, brain scanning, and echoencephalography. While one method alone may suffice, there are times when all of them together leave one still in doubt. The various techniques should be considered complementary and should be selected carefully, quickly, and accurately, with due regard to the clinical diagnosis and the patient's welfare.

REFERENCES

Bucy, P. C., and Ciric, I. S. 1965. Brain scans in diagnosis of brain tumors: scanning with chlormerodrin Hg^{203} and chlormerodrin Hg^{197}. J.A.M.A. **191**:437-443.

Di Chiro, G. 1961. An atlas of detailed normal pneumoencephalographic anatomy. Springfield, Illinois, Charles C Thomas, Publisher.

Epstein, B. S. 1966. Pneumoencephalography and cerebral angiography. Chicago, Year Book Publishers, Inc.

Hara, K., and Fujino, Y. 1966. The thalamoperforate artery. Acta Radiolog. (Diagn.) **5**:192-200.

Jacobson, H. G., Zimmer, A. E., Schechter, M. M., and Shapiro, J. H. 1965. The dilated callosal sulcus sign. Amer. J. Roentgen. **94**:547-565.

Liliequist, B. 1956. The anatomy of the subarachnoid cisterns. Acta Radiol. **46**:61-71.

Liliequist, B. 1960. Encephalographic changes in

the axial pressure cone syndrome. Acta Radiol. **54**:369-378.

McRae, D. L., and Elliot, A. W. 1958. Radiological aspects of cerebellar astrocytomas and medulloblastomas. Acta Radiol. **50**:52-65.

Quinn, J. L. 1965. Tc-99m pertechnetate for brain scanning. Radiology **84**:354-355.

Ralston, B. L., Gross, S. W., and Newman, C. W. 1959. Pantopaque ventriculography in the localization of surgical lesions of the posterior fossa. Amer. J. Roentgen. **81**:972-983.

Schmitz, A. L., and Haveson, S. B. 1960. The roentgen diagnosis of eighth nerve tumors. Radiology **75**:531-543.

Taveras, J. M. 1960. The roentgen diagnosis of intracranial incisural space occupying lesions. Amer. J. Roentgenol. **84**:52-69.

Taveras, J. M., and Wood, E. H. 1964. Diagnostic neurology. Baltimore, The Williams & Wilkins Co.

Torkildsen, A. 1949. Carotid angiography with special reference to the diagnosis of cerebral gliomas, Acta Psychiat. Neurol., suppl. 55.

Tovi, D., Schisano, G., and Liliequist, B. 1961. Primary tumors of the region of the thalamus. J. Neurosurg. **18**:730-740.

Zimmer, A. E., and Annes, G. P. 1966. The septal vein. An indicator of space-occupying lesions in the anterior cranial fossa. Radiology **87**:813-823.

Chapter 30

Echoencephalography

Hans R. Müller
Jorge Huertas

Since its introduction by Leksell (1956), echoencephalography has become of such clinical importance that it is difficult to think of modern neurology or neurosurgery without its employment as an auxiliary diagnostic method. Its use permits recognition of side displacements of supratentorial midline structures as well as enlargement of ventricles, and is therefore of considerable value for topical diagnosis of intracranial space-occupying lesions. Furthermore, tumors, hematomas, and abscesses can occasionally be localized and outlined by applying two-dimensional sonographic techniques.

Echoencephalography is based on the principle of ultrasonic flaw detection, well known through wide industrial application. A beam of pulsed ultrasound is produced by a piezo-electrical crystal and transmitted through the object to be examined. At interfaces of media with different acoustical impedance, there is reflection. The relation of the reflected amount (Lr) of ultrasonic energy to the acoustic impedances (R_1 and R_2) of the two media in the case of perpendicular incidence of the sound beam to the interface is given by the equation

$$L_r = L \cdot \left(\frac{R_2 - R_1}{R_1 + R_2}\right)^2,$$

the acoustic impedance R of a substance being the product of its density ρ and its specific sound velocity c (Table 30-1).

When a beam of ultrasound strikes an interface at a right angle, the reflected energy travels back to the transducer, which acts as transmitter and receiver alternately (Fig. 30-1). The distance between the probe and the reflecting interface can be calculated from the time used by the acoustical signal to travel the distance to this interface and back to the transducer, and from the specific sound velocity in the particular medium. The echo is displayed on an oscilloscope either as vertical deflection of the cathode ray, proportional to the intensity of the signal (A-scope), or as a bright dot the intensity of which depends on the signal strength (B-scope).

When two or more interfaces are situated one after the other the echoes are seen on the cathode ray oscilloscope in a sequence; the distance between two neighboring echoes corresponds to the time necessary for the sound signal to travel from one interface to the next and back again. Since the specific sound velocities of the different soft tissues and body fluids (such as white and gray matter of the brain and cerebrospinal fluid) are very similar to one another, the same scale can be used to measure the distance between structures causing the various echoes.

The beam of ultrasonic waves depends on the proportion of wave length to the diameter of the transducer. At a given

Table 30-1. Specific sound velocities and acoustical impedances of normal brain tissue, cerebrospinal fluid, and brain tumors (from Schiefer, Kazner, and Kunze, 1965)

	Sound velocity m/sec.	*Acoustic impedance g/cm.² sec.*
Brain tissue	1532	1.59×10^5
Cerebrospinal fluid (ventricular)	1499-1502	1.51×10^5
Gliomas	1525-1547	$1.57\text{-}1.61 \times 10^5$
Meningiomas	1540-1550	$1.61\text{-}1.64 \times 10^5$

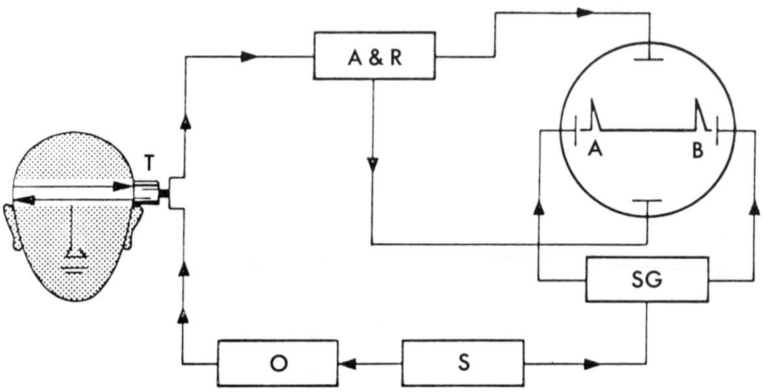

Fig. 30-1. Block diagram of ultrasonic equipment. *T*, transducer; *A*, initial blip; *A & R*, amplifier and rectifier; *O*, high frequency oscillator; *S*, synchronizer; *SG*, sweep generator. (From Grossman, 1966.)

crystal diameter, less divergency arises when higher frequencies are used. On the other hand, absorption of the ultrasonic waves by soft tissues is approximately proportional to the frequency. Since the energy loss by absorption can be compensated for only within certain limits with regard to the possibility of tissue damage, the improvement of directionality of the beam, by using higher frequencies, results in a better resolution only at small distances. For examinations through greater tissue depths, lower frequencies must be used. The optimal frequency and probe diameter should be carefully chosen for each sonographic technique. For brain examinations, probes of 10 to 15 mm. in diameter, and frequencies from 1 to 2.5 mcs., have been shown to give the best results.

The echoencephalographic method in general use at present is based on the *A-scope* technique. The standard procedure used in determining the position of midline structures consists in sounding of the third ventricle from the temporal region, as follows: The transducer is held against the patient's head just above the attachment of the ear or near by; polyethylene-glycol or some other contact jelly is used as a coupling medium. The walls of the third ventricle, which are almost parallel with the temporal bone, are struck by the ultrasonic beam nearly perpendicularly. A further advantage of the temporal region for sonography is that the bone is fairly thin; therefore it offers a minimum of absorption and refraction. In most cases, clear-cut echoes can be obtained from the third ventricle, forming a complex of two to four spikes. In normal subjects, this midline complex is located a bit farther away from the zero point than the middle between the initial complex and the far-side echo, caused by the inner surface of the opposite bone of skull (Figs. 30-2 and 30-3). The midline echoes are of a higher and less pulsating

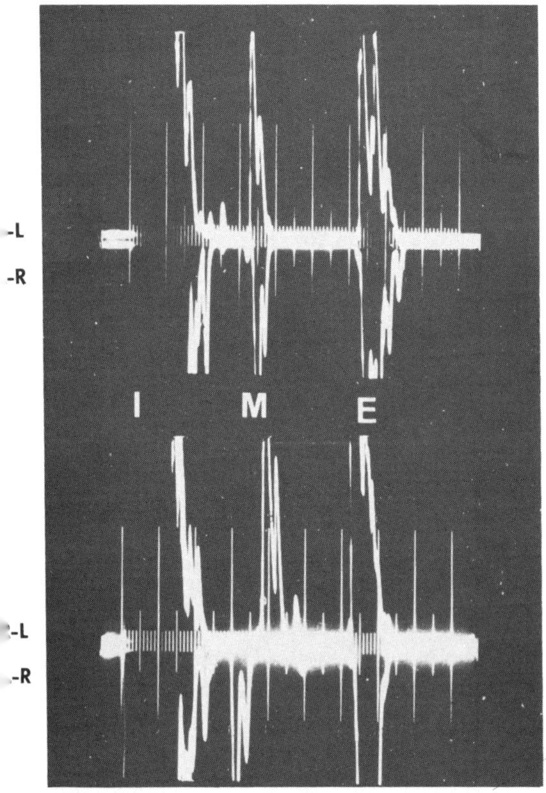

Fig. 30-2. A-scope echoencephalogram of a normal subject (upper tracing) and a patient with a neoplasm of the right hemisphere (lower tracing). The sonograms taken from the right side are represented by upward deflections, those taken from the the left side by downward deflections of the signals. *I*, initial complex; *M*, midline complex (third ventricle); *E*, end complex, starting with reflexion from the internal table of the skull. Owing to the presence of the tumor the two midline echoes are separated, the midline structures being displaced from right to left. (SEG No. 2754a, 2754.)

amplitude than the echoes from blood vessels, so that they can be differentiated without difficulty by a trained observer.

An echo scan is performed from both the right and the left side. The two echoencephalograms are generally registered on the same photograph. The deflection of the right side trace is upward, that of the left side trace downward. In normal subjects, the base point of the midline echo deflection on both right and left sonograms is at the same point on the time scale (indicating distance). When a displacement exists, as in the case of a space-occupying lesion, the two midline echoes are separated, and the *side displacement of the third ventricle* corresponds to half the distance between the two signals on the scale (Figs. 30-2 and 30-3).

Using this technique, Raskind (1965) studied six hundred patients. Abnormal echoencephalograms were found in twenty-eight, of which six were false positives. In the other twenty-two patients subdural hematomas and, less commonly, brain tumors, cerebral infarctions, and abscesses were localized.

Enlargement of the third ventricle in hydrocephalus can be recognized from a broadening of the midline complex; the echoes from the two walls of the ventricle show an abnormally wide separation from each other (de Vlieger and Ridder, 1959). By placing the probe 3 cm. above and 3

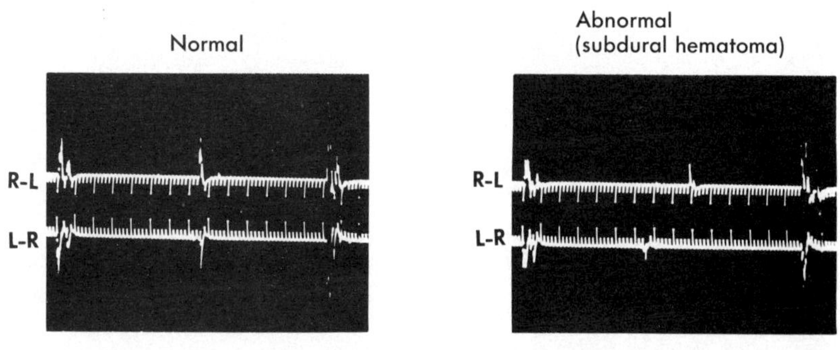

Fig. 30-3. The echoencephalogram on the right shows considerable shifting of the midline spikes. This shifting is due to a subdural hematoma on the right side, which has caused a displacement of the brain across the midline to the left. With the transducer on the right side the distance to the walls of the third ventricle is found to be increased. Transmission of the signal is thus delayed. With the transducer located on the left side, the converse occurs. The results are much the same as indicated in Fig. 30-2, but the technique of recording differs. (Courtesy Dr. D. R. Raskind, Oakland, California.)

cm. anterior to the superior attachment of the ear, the *size of the lateral ventricles* can be estimated (Ford and McRae, 1966).

Extracerebral hematomas can sometimes be identified by a "hematoma echo," which in the case of epidural hematoma originates from the detached dura (ter Braak, Grandia, and de Vlieger, 1959). The hematoma echo is much less frequent in subdural than in epidural hemorrhage and is only rarely found in either type when located in the frontal or the occipital region. Echoencephalography is particularly helpful in the diagnosis of hematomas that displace the cerebrum across the midline.

Direct sounding of *brain tumors* is also possible, when they can be reached by the ultrasonic beam (Tanaka, Kikuchi, and Uchida, 1959). Especially good conditions for tumor localization are presented by neoplasms of the upper brainstem; in these tumors additional echoes occur near the expected midline complex (Kazner and Kunze, 1968). Other techniques of direct tumor sounding—for example, transoral sonographic exploration of the posterior fossa (Wagai and others, 1965)—remain reserved for examiners with special experience. One of the authors has obtained considerable information on supratentorial tumors by transorbital sonoencephalography (Müller, 1969, 1970a, b). The use of this approach appears most rewarding for ultrasonic exploration of the parieto-occipital region, especially for chronic subdural hematomas.

Time changes of vessel echoes with respect to amplitude can be registered as *pulse-curves*. This method (Freund, 1965) may prove to be of clinical value in the diagnosis of intracranial or extracranial vessel obstructions. Time changes in the depth of an individual echo can also be registered (Müller and Blauenstein, 1968). This might be a valuable method of supervision of skull injuries.

B-scan techniques (Howry and Bliss, 1952; Wild and Reid, 1952), first applied in neurology by Kikuchi and co-workers (1957), are being used more and more in the investigation of intracranial lesions. They are of special value in outlining the cerebral ventricles (de Vlieger and others, 1963) and may show tumor complexes as

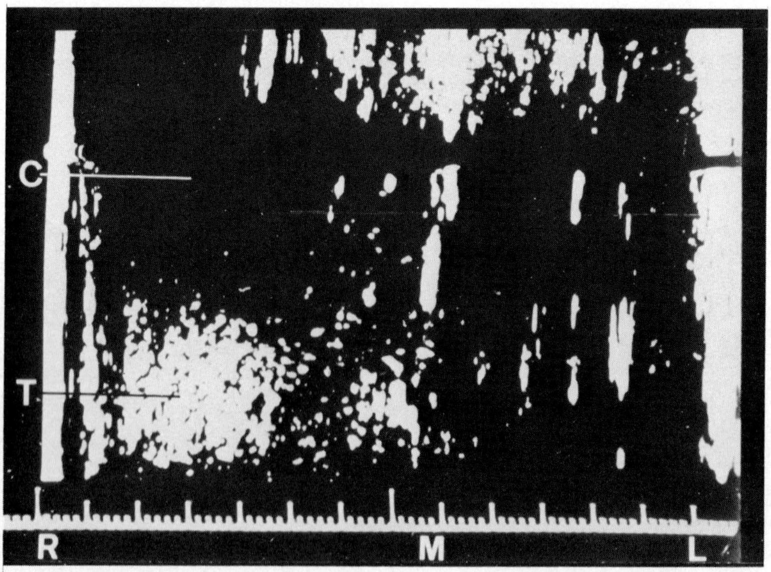

Fig. 30-4. B-scan-sonogram of an astrocytoma that has undergone necrosis. The tomogram represents a horizontal section, located 5 cm. above the external acoustic meatus. *M*, Displaced midline echoes. *T*, Solid portion of the tumor. *C*, Site of "cystic" tumor necrosis (SEG No. 3074.)

well (Grossman, 1964) (Fig. 30-4). In the B-scan techniques the probe is moved during the examination either along a straight line (linear B-scanning), or on a circular path around the object to be scanned (linear circular B-scanning). The beam axis may also be altered within one plane at a fixed point of placement (sector B-scanning). The combination of linear and sector scanning techniques is referred to as compound scanning. In all these techniques the echoes are displayed as spots of light corresponding in position to the distances of the reflecting interfaces. Each change of position or direction of the probe is displayed on the screen as an analogous change in the position of the zero-point and the direction of the time base. The shutter of the camera remains open during the entire examination; it registers all the spots and thereby produces a tomogram. The same effect can be created by use of a storage oscilloscope.

For intraoperative localization of brain tumors, intracerebral hematomas, and abscesses a tomographic method utilizing the A-scan presentation has proved to be more useful than B-scan techniques (Müller and Lévy, 1968; Müller, 1970a, b). Tumor outlines can be well defined by sounding through the intact dura at the site of a craniotomy, thus permitting more optimal surgical intervention.

REFERENCES

de Vlieger, M., de Sterke, A., Molin, C. E., and van der Ven, C. 1963. Ultrasound for two-dimensional echoencephalography. Ultrasonics **1**: 148-151.

de Vlieger, M., and Ridder, H. J. 1959. Use of echoencephalography. Neurology **9**:216-223.

Ford, R. M., and McRae, D. L. 1966. Echoencephalography—a standardized technique for the measurement of the width of the third and fourth ventricles. In Grossman, C. C., and others, editors: Diagnostic ultrasound. New York, Plenum Press, pp. 117-129.

Freund, H. J. 1965. Ultraschallregistrierung einzelner intrakranieller Arterien zur Diagnostik von Gefässverschlüssen. Arch. Psychiat. Nervenkr. **207**:247-253.

Grossman, C. C. 1964. Clinical diagnostic application of ultrasound in brain disorders (sonoencephalography). Dis. Nerv. Syst. **25**:403-411.

Grossman, C. C. 1966. The use of diagnostic ultrasound in brain disorders. Springfield, Illinois, Charles C Thomas, Publisher, p. 23.

Howry, D. H., and Bliss, W. R. 1952. Ultrasonic visualization of soft tissue structures of the body. J. Lab. Clin. Med. **40**:579-592.

Kazner, E., and Kunze, S. 1968. Echo-encephalographic findings with midline tumors and tumors of the base of the skull. In Krazner, E., Schiefer, W., and Zülch, K. J., editors: Proc., Echo-encephalography. Berlin, Springer-Verlag, pp. 71-75.

Kikuchi, Y., Uchida, R., Tanaka, K., and Wagai, T. 1957. Early cancer diagnosis through ultrasonics. J. Acoust. Soc. Amer. **29**:824-833.

Leksell, L. 1956. Echo-encephalography: detection of intracranial complications following head injury. Acta Chir. Scand. **110**:301-315.

Müller, H. R., 1969. Transorbitale B-Sonencephalographie. Schweiz. Med. Wschr. **99**:1022-1025.

Müller, H. R. 1970a. Transorbital sonoencephalography: a new approach to ultrasonic examination of the parieto-occipital region. Europ Neurol. **3**: (in press).

Müller, H. R. 1970b. Transdurale echoenzephalographie. Bern/Stuttgart/Wien, Huber.

Müller, H. R., and Blauenstein, U. 1968. Monitoring of midline-echo by use of a new probeholder. Europ. Neurol. **1**:28-30.

Müller, H. R., and Lévy, A. 1968. A simple method of two-dimensional intraoperative sonoencephalography employing the A-scan technique. Europ. Neurol. **1**:31-40.

Raskind, R. 1965. Clinical studies in echoencephalography. J. Internat. Coll. Surgeons **44**: 153-158.

Schiefer, W., Kazner, E., and Kunze, S. 1965. Ergebnisse der Echoenzephalographie bei supratentoriellen Geschwülsten. Zbl. Neurochir. **26**: 281-295.

Tanaka, K., Kikuchi, A., and Uchida, R. 1959. Ultrasonic diagnosis of brain tumor. Amsterdam, Elsevier Publishing Co., pp. 1291-1294.

ter Braak, J. W. G., Grandia, W. A. M., and de Vlieger, M. 1959. "Echo-encephalography" as an aid in the diagnosis of subdural and extradural haematomas. In Biemond, A., editor: Recent neurological research. Amsterdam, Elsevier Publishing Co., pp. 37-45.

Wagai, T., Miyazawa, R., Ito, K., and Kikuchi, Y. 1965. Ultrasonic diagnosis of intracranial disease, breast tumors and abdominal diseases. In Kelly, E., editor: Utrasonic energy. Urbana, University of Illinois Press, pp. 346-364.

Wild, J. J., and Reid, J. M. 1952. Applications of echo-ranging techniques to determination of structure of biological tissues. Science **115**:226-230.

Chapter 31

Electroencephalography

Jorge Huertas

Much is known of the electrical currents produced in organs of the human body, in the brain, in peripheral nerves, and in muscular tissues. An understanding of the organic process involved and of the electronic principles of recording and amplification of those currents is essential to the evaluation of bioelectrical potentials. Recordings of currents produced in organs are presently carried out for clinical purposes. Signals received from nervous tissue in general and from the muscular tissue have become essential tools for the neurologist.

The term *electroencephalography* is used particularly to describe the electrical phenomena occurring in the brain and recorded by means of scalp electrodes. Since the principles applied in electroencephalography, in electrocorticography, and in the recording from the deeper structures of the brain follow the same technical logic, a general description for such procedures will follow.

Recording of the electroencephalogram (EEG) is based upon the property of the brain to vary constantly its intrinsic electrical potentials in different areas simultaneously. If two electrodes are positioned on the scalp at two different places they will "pick up" the *relative* difference in electrical potential from those two areas.

Potential differences arise at the single neuron level, where the electrical currents flow in opposite directions inside and outside the cell, and it is here that the cell membrane plays a paramount role. A simplified model for this phenomenon is the electric dipole (Fig. 31-1). If the conductive milieu around the two poles is assumed to have a uniform resistance, then it is understandable that the voltage of the current will be lower as the distance between the source and recording electrode is increased. This equipotential distance represented in the drawing of circles of increasing radii assumes definite values at each circle at a specific time. These values serve to plot a curve representing the gradual changes of the electrical potentials in the dipole field. They are largest at the source and smallest at the periphery. The positive values will deflect in one direction, and the negative values in the opposite direction. The result will be a sinusoidal curve, providing that the dipole is studied parallel to its longest axis. If the dipole is studied perpendicular to its axis, only a positive or a negative deflection can be observed (Fig. 31-1).

As the electricity in the brain is generated at the membrane level of neurons, undoubtedly all the neurons of the brain (there are 2.6 billion in the cerebral cortex alone—Pakkenberg, 1966) contribute to the formation of brain waves when they are physiologically active. The genesis of the EEG must be a complicated matter. Obvi-

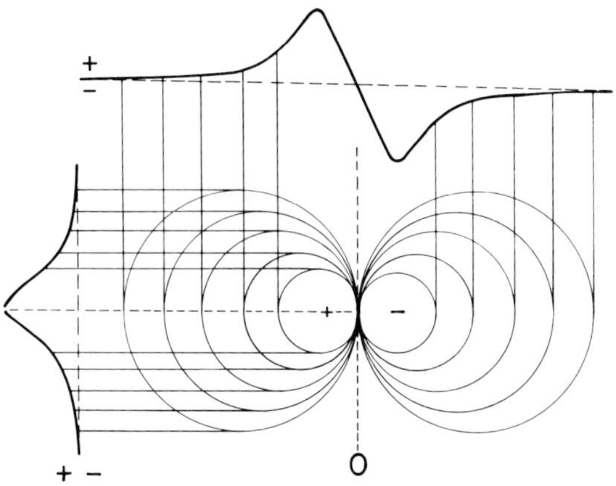

Fig. 31-1. Electric dipole, illustrating how the intensity of the electrical current is inversely proportional to the distance from the source. According to the relative position of the recording electrodes to the axis of these sources, the changes in potentials will be either monophasic or biphasic.

ously, the brain waves originate from the pulsed discharges of neurons (*action potentials*) and from the interconnections and distribution of their electrical energies. Current research on the origin of the EEG is very active but the basic mechanisms are still unknown. The integrated value of the primordial membrane potentials, the potentials from the neuronal cell bodies, potentials from the axons, dendrites, and perhaps the neuroglia, together account for a major part of the EEG tracing. Nevertheless, neurophysiologists are puzzled as to why the EEG is made up of relatively slow frequencies.

The EEG is characterized by a constant, continuous change in regional potentials. Such potentials are manifested by a slowly changing direct current (D.C.) in the background and by waves of frequencies that range from 0.5 per second* to more than 30 per second. In routine electroencephalography the slow D.C. potential is ignored. The amplitude of the waves of the scalp EEG is about a tenth the amplitude of the waves of the electrocorticogram. The main reason for this variation is not the resistance in series presented by the dura mater, bone, and scalp, but instead the parallel resistance presented by the tissues, particularly by the galea, which short-circuits the electrodes. The result is a distortion of the electromagnetic field.

RECORDING METHODS

The EEG needs an amplification of about one million times. The specifications for such amplifiers have been described in international conventions. The EEG should be obtained with adequate recording equipment. Input impedance, type of preamplifier, and band width are some of the factors that must be carefully weighed. Positioning of the electrodes over the scalp is also highly important. In order to render comparable tracings from different laboratories, the so-called "10-20 system" has been adopted internationally; it serves to obtain coinciding consecutive EEGs in one subject. It is based upon percentages of the actual measurements of the head. The electrodes must be relatively small. Their electrical characteristics must comprise good conductivity of electricity and yet have little tendency toward polarization. Strict care must be taken to keep the electrodes and conductive jellies in good condition. (Jasper, 1958.)

There are two main methods for recording the EEG. In one, both electrodes are placed over an electrically active surface of the scalp (bipolar). In the other, one electrode is placed over an active surface of the scalp and the other is placed at a distant location where presumably the electric value is relatively zero (monopolar) (Fig. 31-2). Such distant places may be the ears, the sternum, or the mandible. Both types of tracing have advantages and *each clinical record should have samples of both.* A computer can change a monopolar into a bipolar record provided that two or more leads can be compared.

THE NORMAL EEG

The EEG varies constantly in frequencies and amplitudes in different areas of the scalp. However, the different areas are characterized by a predominant EEG pattern. The general distribution of frequencies and patterns changes also with normal changes in consciousness (Bates, 1953).

Awake state. If a person is sitting in a chair or lying down relaxed with his eyes closed, a monopolar or a bipolar tracing will show the tendency of the waves to form groups characterized by frequencies lasting from 8 to 13 per second. This is the *alpha rhythm* (Fig. 31-3). Alpha

---

*The low frequency cutoff depends on the time constant of the preamplifier input.

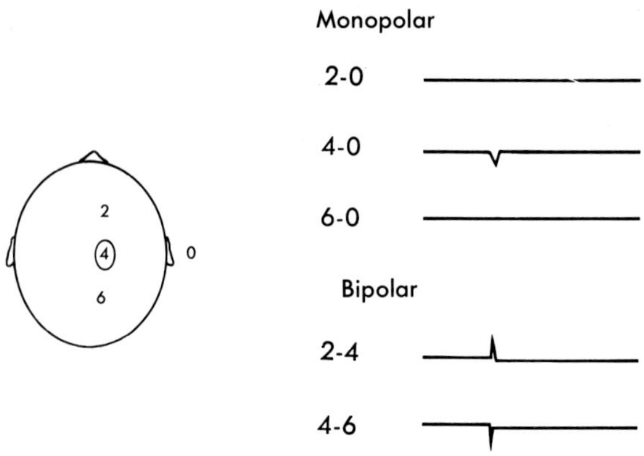

Fig. 31-2. The monopolar recording shows that one electrode is placed over the active area of the scalp and another electrode at a distance, in this case the ear *(0)*. At *4* on the scalp the brain has an abnormality that will be shown only in the tracing *4-0*. In the bipolar mode all electrodes are over an active area but only *4* has a special type of wave. Since the current in one instance will flow from *2-4* and in the other instance from *4-6*, the deviation of the tracing will occur in the direction of the flow of current, and since *2* and *6* are negative in reference to *4*, the deflection will point in opposite directions.

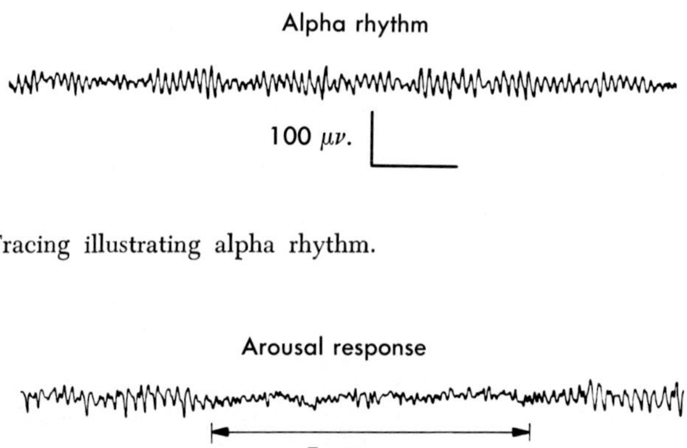

Fig. 31-3. Tracing illustrating alpha rhythm.

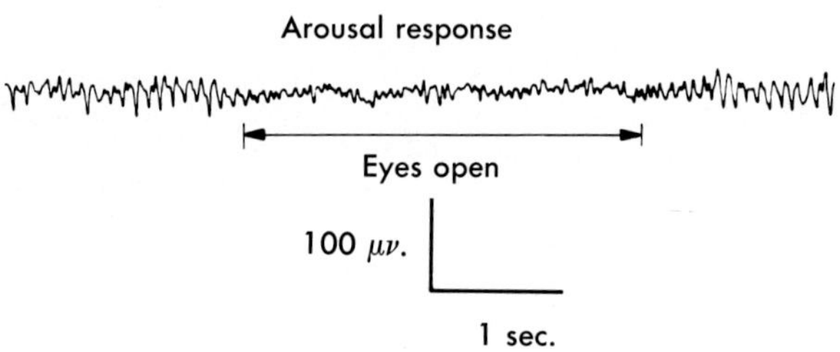

Fig. 31-4. EEG arousal response.

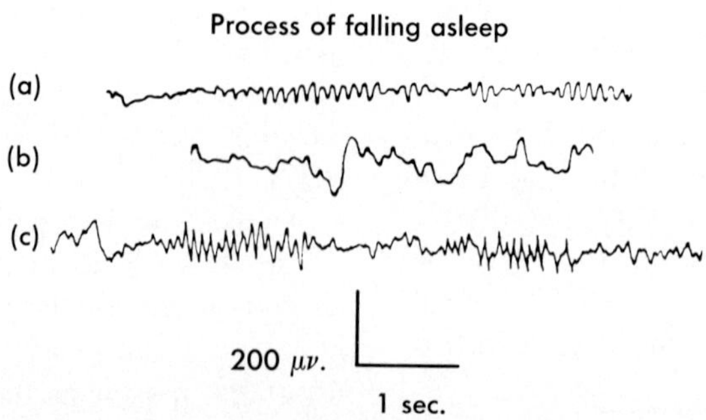

Fig. 31-5. Tracings from a person falling asleep.

rhythm is preponderant in the occipital areas, where it waxes and wanes constantly. If the individual is asked to open his eyes, to perform an active intellectual task, or if his attention is attracted by an external stimulus, there is a sudden change from alpha rhythm to a faster rhythm and the amplitude of the waves is decreased by about half or less. This new rhythm is called *beta rhythm.* The change from alpha to beta rhythm elicited in this manner is called the *arousal response* (Fig. 31-4). Beta rhythm is also observed in anterior regions of the head. The usual resting EEG has alpha rhythms toward the occipital poles and beta rhythms toward the frontal poles. Beta rhythm is composed of low voltage waves (10 to 40 μvolts) ranging in frequency from 14 to more than 30 per second.

Sleep. As in the awake state, sleep is characterized by specific patterns in the EEG. When sleep is setting in, the alpha rhythm becomes more common as other rhythms diminish (*a* in Fig. 31-5). As the process of falling asleep progresses, irregular, very short bursts of slow waves of low voltage can be noted in the parietal, temporal, and occipital areas (*b* in Fig. 31-5) (biparietal humps, K-complex, occipital slow waves). As the process continues, theta activity (4-8/sec. slow waves) begins to be more common in all leads. Appearance of theta activity in the EEG signifies not only a sleep process but also fatigue, and is used as an index of fatigue in aviation and space medicine. As sleep stabilizes, suddenly the frequency of the waves is increased, to be replaced by faster activity of 12 to 14 per second (*c* in Fig. 31-5). These waves of relative high amplitudes are called *sleep spindles.* The sleep spindle stage is prolonged, while the other described changes occur only during the period in which the person is falling asleep. Very deep sleep is manifested by generalized slow activity. After the person has been asleep for some time (beyond the 12-14/sec. spindle stage), fast activity reappears. This fast activity is similar to that of beta rhythms even though the person is asleep. If tracings from

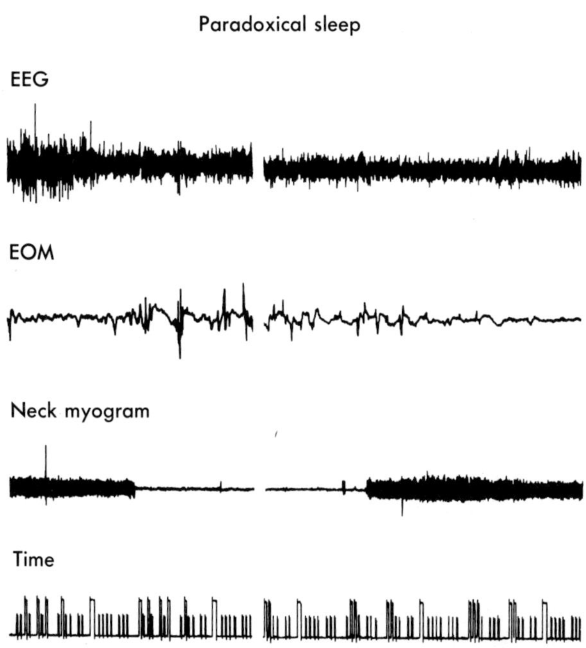

Fig. 31-6. Tracing illustrating paradoxical sleep. (*EOM,* **extraocular movements.**)

striated muscles of the body are taken during this time, they show typical concomitant activity. Moreover, muscles in the limbs twitch, the limbs move slightly, and the eyes perform searching movements, but no myogram is obtainable from the neck muscles (Fig. 31-6). This state is called *paradoxical sleep*. Despite the fact that the electroencephalographic record gives the appearance of an awake state, the subject is actually asleep (Dement and Kleitman, 1957). It is at this stage of sleep that dreaming occurs. (Note that the time scale in Fig. 31-6 is much altered in order to show minutes instead of seconds as the unit.)

Types of EEG waves. As already described, the frequency of the EEG varies normally. The different frequencies are as follows:

Delta rhythm	0.5 to 4 c.p.s.
Theta rhythm	4 to 8 c.p.s.
Alpha rhythm	8 to 13 c.p.s.
Beta rhythm	more than 13 c.p.s.

Other frequencies are also expressed in Greek (μ rhythms, γ waves), but these designations serve more to confuse than to clarify.

Generally speaking, when evaluated from the written record of the oscillograph, the rhythms appear symmetrical on the two sides of the midsagittal plane. Thus, the right frontal lobe and the left frontal lobe will have almost identical records at the same time. This symmetry is not as marked during sleep.

Recent advances in instrumentation, particularly in electronic computation, permit a more adequate and meaningful evaluation of the normal (and abnormal) wave frequencies and forms. A brief description of such methods will be found at the end of this chapter.

CYCLIC VARIATIONS OF THE EEG

From the preceding description, it follows that the EEG will vary during the 24 hours of a day according to the normal cyclic variation in metabolism and consciousness. These circadian variations are important in many ways. Experiments in mammals in higher stages of phylogenetic development have revealed a constant pattern and constant rates of electroencephalographic frequencies during the 24 hours. The circadian variations in the EEG should be kept in mind in interpretation of a record. The time of day in which a record was taken should always be noted. The advent of fast transportation by jet airplane has brought about the possibility of "desynchronizing" a person when travelling eastward or westward, but thus far no significant information on the EEG following intercontinental flights appears to be available. However, the behavior of such a desynchronized person might appear grossly abnormal during adaptation because while he is in one time zone his biological rhythms are set to his geographical departing point (Halberg, 1962, 1965).

THE EEG IN CHILDREN

The patterns described so far have been the normal patterns found in an adult. After birth, the EEG is characterized by slow frequencies of very low voltages. They are grossly symmetrical but markedly arrhythmic. Sleep is characterized by slightly higher voltages. At the age of 2 years indications of future organization appear. The occipital pole begins to show faster rhythms, which at the age of 5 years might approach the characteristics of alpha rhythm. This rhythm is confined to a small area in the occipital pole. From here it spreads slowly forward, displacing the delta rhythms from the temporal and parietal regions. By the end of puberty beta rhythms are well established and shortly afterward the EEG is that of a mature person.

ACTIVATION OF THE EEG

Provocation techniques. Since some electroencephalographic anomalies show up mainly during a particular phase of consciousness, it is sometimes desirable to enhance artificially the proportion of a certain rhythm over another. This en-

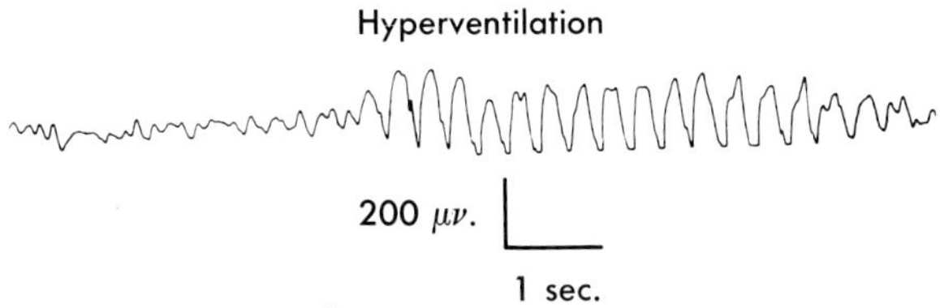

Fig. 31-7. Effect of hyperventilation.

hancement can remain within normal limits or point toward an abnormality. The techniques used clinically for the purpose of enhancement of the EEG are hyperventilation, induced sleep, the use of certain excitatory drugs (such as analeptics), and photostimulation.

Hyperventilation. If a person overbreathes for some time he will become hypocapnic, and hypocapnia produces changes in the EEG. These changes, which are symmetrical in the two hemispheres, consist in a progressive fluctuating increase in the total percentage of theta activity that will predominate over the normal background activity until it reaches three cycles per second or less. These changes appear about a minute after initiating voluntary hyperventilation (100 breaths) and may persist for 2 to 4 minutes in adults after hyperventilation has stopped. In children they sometimes last for 20 minutes (Fig. 31-7).

Sleep. Sleep is considered a provocation phenomenon because during sleep certain new rhythms appear. These rhythms often originate in the temporal lobes. In some types of epilepsy, EEG activation occurs while the individual is falling asleep. During the electroencephalographic examination, sleep is produced either after deprivation of sleep for many hours or by the administration of a short-acting barbiturate (for example, secobarbital).

Analeptics. Analeptics are used only in those cases in which need exists to diagnose certain types of seizures or to observe the pattern of an epileptic attack. This procedure is resorted to only in cases in which epilepsy is in question and where either diagnosis or treatment depends on the results obtained. The drug used most frequently is pentylenetetrazol (Metrazol), given intravenously. Septazol and probenecid (Benemid) have also been used.

THE ABNORMAL EEG

Sometimes the smooth flow of the EEG can be interrupted by single or by multiple waves of such characteristics that they indicate an abnormality.

Spikes. Perhaps the best known abnormality is the spike, which may appear randomly during a tracing or in bursts or in trains. An electroencephalographic spike is a fast wave with steep slopes on each side, which lasts for milliseconds (20 to 60 msec.). It stands out when a tracing is inspected. However, due to the inertia and dampening effect of the writing pens its configuration is somewhat altered depending on the machine used. These spikes should not be mistaken for the much faster spike recorded with microelectrodes from single nerve fibers, also known as *action potentials.*

According to the characteristics and polarity of such spikes they may indicate a local cortical disturbance, a local intracerebral disturbance, or a generalized disturbance.

Because spikes are so typical and relatively easy to detect they will be taken as an illustration of the techniques used for localization of abnormal foci in the brain. Fig. 31-2 illustrates the simplest situation. A spike originates at lead 4; in monopolar recording the downward deflection occurs when the indifferent and active electrodes are connected. In the bipolar configuration the relative exchange between the two recording areas plays a

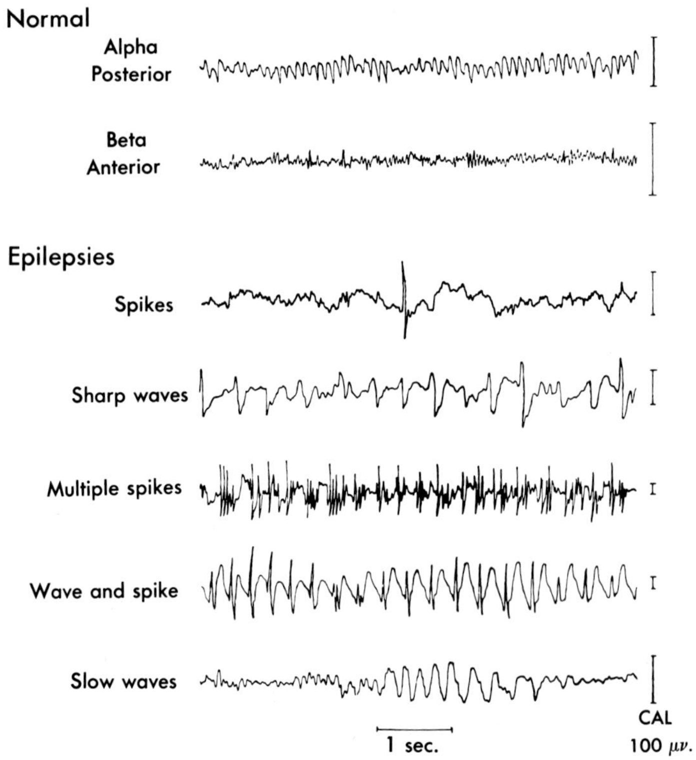

Fig. 31-8. Types of abnormal waves. (From Penfield and Jasper, 1954.)

role. Conventionally a downward deflection occurs when the active electrode is positive and an upward deflection when the active electrode is negative.

In some persons, spikes appear "randomly" (single spikes). In others they appear in bursts (multiple spikes), which may consist of a few spikes grouped together for a short time or many spikes lasting for hours, as might be seen in status epilepticus (Fig. 31-8).

Sharp waves. Sharp waves are also spiky wave forms, with duration from 60 to 500 msec. (Fig. 31-8). They can be solitary or paroxysmal. They indicate abnormal foci of electrogenesis in the brain tissue, possibly in the deep structures away from the electrodes. Collections of abnormal tissue in the cranial cavity that displace the brain do not have electrical waves of their own but they do alter the EEG, and the adjacent brain can become irritated. The EEG in such cases may show sharp waves. If a brain tumor is displacing brain tissue the short waves can be solitary or paroxysmal. They might emerge from a small area (focal), or they may be dispersed over a large portion of a hemisphere or over the whole brain (generalized). A sharp wave may be essentially a spike that originates in deeper structures of the brain but has expanded in time before reaching the surface. If sharp waves appear constantly over only one area the EEG abnormality is called a *slow focus*, whose meaning will be described later. Localization of a slow focus is carried out according to the same principles as for a spike.

Slow waves. Slow waves are characterized by low frequencies. They are indicative of disturbed function at the cortical level. A decrease in the number of cells participating in electrogenesis, as in cortical atrophy, can result in the occurrence of slow waves. Intracranial tumors, such as meningioma, that displace the cortex from its position next to the dura, can also

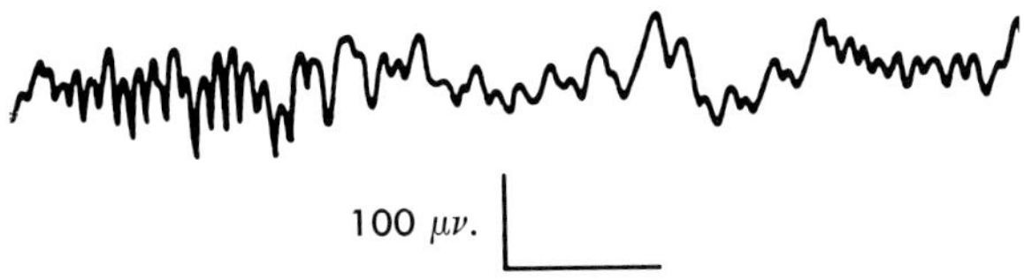

Fig. 31-9. Ctenoids.

give rise to slow waves, as may also subdural hematoma. Slow waves in most cases are not random, and they appear in long-lasting chains that are amplitude modulated (Fig. 31-8).

Spike-wave complexes, sharp-slow wave complexes. Spikes, sharp waves, and slow waves are sometimes found in combination with one another. These combinations are characteristic of certain abnormalities of the brain. Special associations, of constant encephalographic appearance, occurring under certain pathological conditions, will be dealt with in the subsequent text.

14- and 6-c.p.s. positive spikes (ctenoids). This type of electroencephalographic disturbance is characterized by a comb tooth configuration (Fig. 31-9). Correlation with the clinical state has not been achieved. Suffice it to say that these waves may occasionally occur in association with thalamic or hypothalamic dysfunction.

EPILEPSY

Diagnosis, treatment, and the understanding of epilepsy are closely tied to electroencephalography and it is in these areas that the EEG has gained a major place as a clinical tool. Classification of the epilepsies is most satisfactory when correlated with clinical signs and the electroencephalographic record. Ignoring the etiological factors contributory to the development of epileptic activity in the brain, the epilepsies can be classified from the electroencephalographic point of view into two large groups: focal and generalized. A focal attack can lead to a generalized attack. Many generalized attacks have a very brief focal phase. In fact, some epileptologists maintain that all epilepsies are focal in origin.

Focal epilepsy. Focal epilepsies usually originate in the cerebral cortex. They are expressed as random spikes arising in the cortical area in question. At this point it is very important to call attention to the fact that a conventional EEG is a record obtained mostly from the easily accessible convex surface of the cerebrum, and that abnormal waves originating in the hidden cortex in contact with the basal areas of the cranial cavity express themselves weakly or not at all during an ordinary scalp recording. Special electrodes have been designed for recording from the basal areas of the brain (nasal, tympanic, sphenoidal). Sometimes it is necessary to implant electrodes directly into the deeper structures of the brain to detect such foci. The focal epilepsies are usually characterized by spikes localized only in one area of the brain, as in the case of classical jacksonian epilepsy, or by spikes and sharp waves, as might be the case in epilepsy originating in the temporal lobe.

Many apparently primary generalized seizures clearly originate in either hemisphere and are therefore focal in nature (secondarily generalized seizures). Provoking an attack and using a specialized electroencephalographic technique is sometimes indicated. For this purpose, Metrazole is most widely used. EEG evidence for focal cortical epileptogenic lesions may be obtained in about half of all epileptic patients, if sufficiently complete studies are carried out. (Penfield and Jasper, 1954.)

Generalized epilepsy. This type of seizure has also been called—and appropriately so—*subcortical epilepsy,* because it originates in the deeper conglomerations of neurons (upper brainstem, diencephalon, basal nuclei). The electroencephalographic expression of (primarily) generalized epilepsy is bilateral both in the ictal and the interictal tracing. The discharges are essentially synchronous and usually symmetrical. With the use of certain highly specialized recording techniques, the EEG in some cases might reveal a deep focal origin of such seizures.

The EEG in a *grand mal* attack is seldom obtained in a routine EEG examination because of muscular activity during the seizure. A grand mal record shows the following gross electroencephalographic changes (Fig. 31-10): the activity in the whole record begins to drift toward the faster frequencies and the amplitude of the faster rhythms is abnormally higher until it reaches a stage in which high voltage generalized spikes dominate the picture (*a* in Fig. 31-10). The amplitude of such spikes can be so large that they exceed the limits of the oscillographic excursion and take on the appearance of a succession of square waves occurring at frequencies of 8 to 12 per second. A few seconds later the amplitude of the spikes becomes even larger *(b)* and the frequency diminishes; then the spikes appear in groups separated by slow waves (*c* and *d*) until a period of electroencephalographic slow activity sets in *(f)*. The duration of such an attack can vary from a few minutes to hours (status epilepticus).

Petit mal, a type of generalized epilepsy clearly related to genetic factors, is observed mainly in children but is not alien to adults. It is characterized by a very typical stereotype of waves called the spike-and-wave complex (Fig. 31-11). Electroencephalographically, this form of epilepsy is easily recognized by the typical pattern of the tracing. The spike-and-wave activity usually appears in paroxysms lasting a few seconds, generalized over all areas of the brain, but sometimes the activity is more

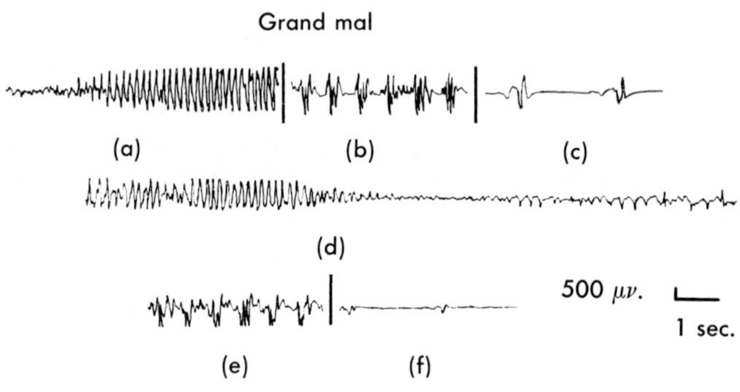

Fig. 31-10. Electroencephalographic tracing of a grand mal seizure. Samples of the different phases.

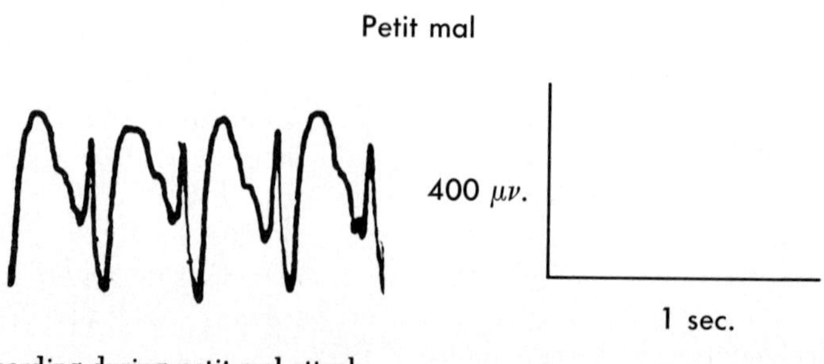

Fig. 31-11. Recording during petit mal attack.

prominent in the frontal areas. The repetition rate of the spike-and-wave complex is characteristic at 3 per second; sometimes the rate is slightly faster. Other repetition rates of spike-and-wave complexes, especially those of about 2 c.p.s. ("petit mal variant"), have nothing in common with true petit mal, being, instead, the expression of secondarily generalized epilepsy in the presence of acquired brain damage. They occur frequently only during the waking state; sometimes more than two hundred attacks occur in a day. Some authors consider *myoclonic epilepsy* as a subtype of petit mal even though the characteristics of the EEG are somewhat different. The myoclonic attack is characterized by a simultaneous burst of widespread slow waves lasting for about a second. These bursts are highly similar morphologically and care should therefore be taken not to mistake them for the so-called K-complex, which can appear normally during the initial stages of sleep (*b* in Fig. 31-5).

Interseizure patterns. Perhaps the most sought after electroencephalographic clue to clarify the presence of epilepsy is the interseizure pattern. A pattern of this kind consists of short-duration bursts of abnormal waves. Sometimes the waves reveal a focus or a subcortical anomaly. The bursts are usually not accompanied by abnormal clinical signs, although the patient's history points toward a clinically established convulsive disorder. The abnormal waves can be spikes, slow waves, spike and waves, and so on. However, when spikes and sharp waves are observed without a clinical history of convulsions, care must be taken to determine their meaning befor labeling a person an epileptic. Other studies, particularly provocation studies, should be undertaken before transferring the electroencephalographic phenomenon to a clinical fact. On the other hand, a normal interseizure EEG does not rule out epilepsy, but repeated recordings and sufficient activation procedures will demonstrate definite EEG abnormalities in about 90 percent of cases (Penfield and Jasper, 1954).

OTHER CONDITIONS IN WHICH THE EEG SERVES AS A DIAGNOSTIC TOOL

Head injury. The EEG in head injuries has not only clinical value but it might also become a legal record. In this connection, it is wise not to depend on the EEG alone in evaluating the extent of a head injury. Some records having an appearance highly suggestive of cerebral damage might merely reflect the preinjury state of the patient. Other apparently normal records might misguide the clinician and dismiss a serious case on electroencephalographic grounds. Those head injuries in which the brain has been directly affected obviously will show electroencephalographic changes, while for those in which the trauma is slight, evaluation may be difficult. A slowly bleeding vessel or a gradual build-up of hydrostatic intracranial pressure might induce encephalographic changes long after the injury. In severe head injuries the most useful application of electroencephalography is in the diagnosis of compressive phenomena, such as occur in subdural hematoma, subdural hygroma, and intracerebral hemorrhage. The most common finding is a focus of slow waves over the affected area (*d* in Fig. 31-8).

Post-traumatic epilepsy appears from weeks to months after head injury, usually in the form of focal cortical epilepsy. The opposite might also occur—the appearance, in time, of a generalized highly abnormal (slow wave) EEG, in which the waves then gradually revert to normal.

Lesions of vascular origin. Cerebral infarction occurring in association with vascular thrombosis is very common. Under such conditions the EEG is indicative either of generalized disease or of local damage. The EEG serves also to ascertain the course of the pathological process through consecutive tracings (Birchfield, Wilson, and Heyman, 1959).

In case of thrombosis of a main vessel,

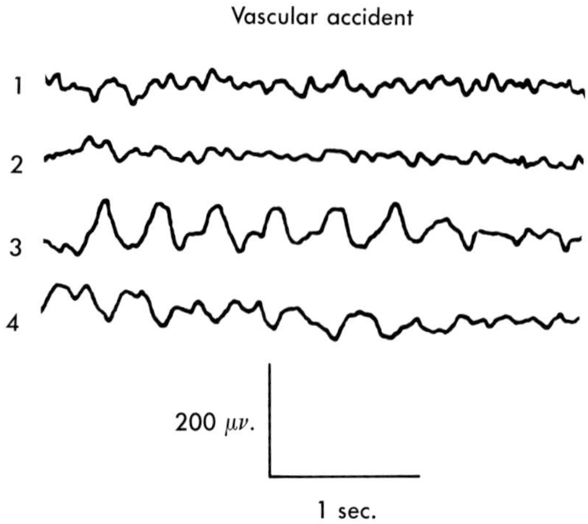

Fig. 31-12. Tracings following "vascular accident."

such as the middle cerebral artery, the tracing will show slow waves over the affected area (the region irrigated by the vessel). Generalized decreased activity over the rest of the brain is sometimes indicative of secondary injury, for example, from generalized atherosclerosis or cerebral edema (Fig. 31-12). Here again, the EEG has both diagnostic and prognostic value if consecutive examinations are performed.

Space-occupying lesions. Brain tumors, subdural hematomas, intracerebral hematomas, and other localized space-occupying masses alter the EEG. The changes are not always the same. There may, for example, be slow- and sharp-wave foci, rythmes à distance (Dreyfus-Brisac and others, 1950), and depression of the physiological alpha rhythm. The wave form depends very much on the fashion in which the normal tissue is displaced or damaged by the extraneous mass. If the brain is displaced away from the recording electrodes, or if neurons in the subjacent cerebral cortex undergo degeneration, slow waves will usually appear. On the other hand, if the cortex is irritated, spikes and epileptic-like discharges will be preponderant. Masses of abnormal tissue that displace the brain do not have electrical waves of their own. Yet the EEG may show marked changes. Intracranial tumors can be located anywhere (dura, hemispheres, ventricles). They can be intrinsic or extrinsic with respect to the brain tissue, and they can destroy, invade, or displace the tissue. The electroencephalographic characteristics will depend on the location of the space-occupying lesion, the amount of displacement, extent of destruction, degree of secondary edema, and obstruction of the intracranial fluids. The electroencephalographer's judicious study of the patient's history is the basis for interpretation of the tracings (Arfel and Fishgold, 1961; Daly and Thomas, 1958). Echoencephalography is in many cases an indispensable complementary diagnostic tool.

The EEG is not a direct means for the study of the electrical activity of the structures located in the posterior fossa. However, when the aqueduct of Sylvius and other outlets are obstructed, a uniform increase of the intracranial pressure in the anterior fossa (obstructive hydrocephalus) is produced. The EEG may show characteristically almost perfect sine waves in all leads. The frequencies vary; in children they range between 2 to 3 c.p.s. and in the adult they are somewhat faster, 4 to 7 c.p.s. A general increase of fast rhythms in posterior fossa tumors has also been found (van der Drift, 1957).

Other entities. The EEG has also been used for the diagnosis of certain diseases, such as those of an infectious or metabolic nature. It may be of special value in the examination of the comatose patient. Ordinarily in coma there is generalized irregular slow activity. However, the EEG may show laterality differences or focal abnormalities due to intra- or extracerebral hematoma, brain abscess, and so on, and give the indication for carotid angiography. In such cases echoencephalography may be an additional aid in establishing the sites of localized pathological changes.

Electroencephalography in the determination of death. An active electroencephalogram leaves no doubt that the complicated biological phenomena concerned with electrogenesis are functioning at least to some extent and that the brain cells are therefore alive. A flat EEG taken with A.C. coupled amplifiers does not signify that electrical activity cannot return. It has been demonstrated that activity can return after hypothermia, barbiturate intoxication, or shock (Brid and Blum, 1968; Callahan and others, 1954; Huertas, Portera, and Massulo, 1956). The electroencephalogram alone, without consideration given to other physiological parameters and to clinical factors is not a useful tool for the determination of brain death, even in the case of a real isoelectric line (Schwab, Potts, and Bonazzi, 1962; Silverman, 1969).

NEWER APPROACHES TO THE ANALYSIS OF THE EEG*

The basic concept required for the understanding of mathematical approaches to the analysis of the EEG is that of the periodic function of time. A function of time in this context is a set of measurements of some physical variable obtained at successive points in time. The EEG record is an example of such a time function, where successive measurements of voltage are made at successive points in time. In the dipole illustrated in Fig. 31-1 each circle constitutes a point in time.

At each point in time *t,* this voltage has the value v(t)—read, voltage at time *t,* or *v* of *t.* A function of time is periodic with a period T, if v(t) is identical with v(t+T), whatever the value of t. In other words, if the function repeats itself in such a way that any two values T sec. apart are the same, the function is periodic. Periodic functions are often described in terms of their frequency rather than in terms of their period. A function with a period of 1 second obviously repeats itself once per second and is said to have a frequency of one cycle per second (c.p.s.). A function with a period of 0.5 second would thus represent a frequency of 2 c.p.s., and if the period is T seconds, the frequency is 1/T c.p.s. A convenient property of complicated periodic functions is that they can be resolved into a sum of simpler periodic functions. The most useful set of simple functions used for the decomposition of periodic functions is the sinusoidal functions. Fourier has shown that any periodic function can be represented as a weighted sum of simple sinusoidal functions. The determination of the weights to be assigned in this sum to the sinusoidal functions of different frequencies is known as frequency or Fourier analysis.

Frequency analysis. Since its inception, clinical electroencephalography has made use of informal frequency analysis. The description of the various EEG rhythms and their diagnostic implications has already been discussed. Many have sought to automate and quantify the analysis of the EEG. This would entail the ability, for example, to tell with some degree of certainty whether or not there is "a lot of alpha" or "considerable amount of theta activity," and would also entail precise definition of these terms. The mathematical techniques developed for the analysis of periodic time functions into their sinusoidal components appear to be a natural solution to this problem. These techniques can be implemented in one or two ways.

A set of electronic filters can be constructed, each of which permits passage of activity in a very small number of frequencies (say, from 8 to 10 c.p.s.). If the EEG is passed through all these filters, and if their output is integrated, over some period the outputs will represent the relative weight of each constituent frequency in original function. One of the more popular devices that performs this analysis was developed by Grey Walter. The Grey Walter analyzer is an analog computing device because it operates on actual physical entities rather than on their numerical representations. Obviously the value of a physical entity at any instant can be represented as a number (Shipton, 1961). This *digitizing* process can be accomplished in many ways. One might apply a ruler to the graphic record of the function and read off the scale, or one might use any one of a large number of mechnical or electronic devices that can digitize the data. If the EEG is digitized and available as a list of numbers that can be fed into a digital computer, frequency analysis can be performed by the computer. The process is equivalent to analog filtering. Each of these techniques has advantages and disadvantages (Shipton, 1961).

A term often encountered in discussions of EEG analysis is *correlation functions.* When two functions of time are multiplied and the cross-products are summed, and the sum normalized, the value obtained is defined as the correlation between the two functions. The correlation can be used as

*Dr. E. Donchin, of the University of Illinois, Urbana, contributed to the preparation of this section.

a measure of the similarity of two function. When they are precisely identical the correlation is equal to 1.00; when they are precisely out of phase (whenever one increases, the other decreases by the same ratio) the correlation is equal to –1.00. Intermediate values represent intermediate situations. To ascertain the period at which a function repeats itself we can determine the correlation between this function and the same function shifted in time by various amounts. The correlation can then be plotted as a function of the shifts (this is the *autocorrelation function*) and the shift at which the correlation is equal to 1.00 is the period of the function. Only rarely is the situation that simple, particularly when the analyzed function is a sum of periodic functions. But it is possible to use the autocorrelation function to resolve the function into its frequency components.

Correlation functions can also be obtained for two different functions. They are then known as *cross correlation functions* and are useful in studying the relations between the two functions.

Averaging techniques. It is well known that the presentation of specific stimuli to an organism, which can excite a specific sensory end-organ for that stimulus, produces in various cerebral structures a series of voltage changes that are maintained for about 500 to 1,000 msec. These changes, called *evoked potentials*, can readily be observed when recording directly from cortical structures. However, in scalp recordings of the EEG, the evoked potentials are very difficult to detect because their amplitude relative to the ongoing EEG activity is small (about a fifth). Fortunately, the evoked potential tends to have a stable pattern in time (time series) when the same stimulus is presented to the same subject under the same conditions. If the stimulus is repeatedly presented at irregular intervals, the EEG segment following the stimulus will contain both the small evoked response and the ongoing activity. It is possible to extract the evoked response by the simple maneuver of superimposing these segments, as evoked response components tend to follow the same pattern in time after application of the stimulus, the many small superimposed evoked responses will accumulate to a considerable amplitude (Jasper and Li, 1953). On the other hand, in the ongoing activity having no particular relation to the stimulus, positive and negative amplitudes (that are presumably random) will cancel each other over the presentations and thus in the superimposed records the evoked response will be enhanced by additions. Superimposition can best be effected by adding corresponding points in the different post-stimulus periods. If a flash of light is presented one hundred times, we can digitize the EEG record immediately following each flash—for example, once every millisecond. The half-second following a stimulus is thus represented by a sequence of five hundred numbers. The first number would represent the first millisecond, the second number the second millisecond, and so forth. In other words, we have a usual plot of a curve in which the abscissa represents time in milliseconds. If we now take the first point from all one hundred records and average them, and do the same for all other points, we obtain a sequence of five hundred averages that represent the superimposed one hundred records. This sequence of averages is known as the *average evoked potential* and is a good estimate of the minute evoked potential that could not be seen in any of one hundred separate records.

To perform the foregoing we have had to digitize one hundred records and perform five hundred summations—a time-consuming and tedious procedure. This task can however, be performed by a computer. A number of computers that can perform this task have been developed. They accept the EEG as input and perform the digitization and the required summations. They provide as output the average evoked response in some conveniently accessible manner. The same task can, of course, be performed by a large-scale general purpose computer though most computer facilities at the present time lack the capability to digitize the EEG.

REFERENCES

Arfel, G., and Fishgold, F. 1961. EEG signs in tumors of the brain: electroencephalography and cerebral tumors. EEG Clin. Neurophysiol., suppl. **19**:36-51.

Bates, J. A. V. 1953. A technique for identifying changes in consciousness. EEG Clin. Neurophysiol. **5**:445-446.

Birchfield, R. I., Wilson, W. P., and Heyman, A. 1959. An evaluation of electroencephalography in cerebral infarction and ischemia due to arteriosclerosis. Neurology **9**:859-870.

Brid, T. D., and Blum, F. 1968. Recovery from barbiturate overdose coma with a prolonged isoelectric electroencephalogram. Neurology **18**: 456-460.

Callahan, J. C., McQueen, D. A., Scott, J. W., and Bigellow, W. G. 1954. Cerebral effect of experimental hypothermia. A.M.A. Arch. Surg. **68**:208-218.

Daly, D. D., and Thomas, J. E. 1958. Sequential alterations of the electroencephalogram of patients with brain tumors. EEG Clin. Neurophysiol. **10**:395-404.

Dement, W., and Kleitman, N. 1957. Cyclic variations in EEG during sleep and their relation to eye movements, body mobility and dreaming. EEG Clin. Neurophysiol. **9**:673-690.

Dreyfus-Brisac, C., Lairy-Bounes, G. C., Fischgold, H., and Scarpalegos, S. 1950. Rhythmes pathologiques détectés à distance des tumeurs des hémisphères cérébraux. Sem. Hôp. (Paris) **54**: 2623-2628.

Halberg, F. 1962. Physiologic 24-hour rhythms: a determinant of response to environmental agents. In Schaefer, K. E., editor: Man's dependence on the earthly atmosphere. New York, The Macmillan Company, pp. 48-49.

Halberg, F. 1965. Some aspects of biologic data analysis; longitudinal and transverse profiles of rhythms. In Aschoff, J., editor: Circadian clocks. Proc. Feldafing Summer School, Sept., 1964, Amsterdam, North-Holland Publishing Co., pp. 13-22.

Huertas, J., Portera, A., and Massulo, E. A. 1956. Effects of hypothermia on the electrical activity of the central nervous system. Bull. Georgetown Med. Center **9**:135-141.

Jasper, H. H. 1958. Report of the Committee on Methods of Clinical Examination in Electroencephalography. EEG Clin. Neurophysiol. **10**: 370-375.

Jasper, H., and Li, C. L. 1953. Microelectrode studies of "spontaneous" and evoked potentials of cerebral cortex. Fed. Proc. **12**:73.

Pakkenberg, H. 1966. The number of nerve cells in the cerebral cortex of man. J. Comp. Neurol. **128**:17-20.

Penfield, W., and Jasper, H. H. 1954. Epilepsy and the functional anatomy of the human brain. Boston, Little, Brown and Co.

Schwab, R. S., Potts, F., and Bonazzi, A. 1962. EEG as an aid in determining death in the presence of cardiac activity. EEG Clin. Neurophysiol. **15**:147-148.

Shipton, H. W. 1961. Engineering considerations in the design of waveform analyzers of the Walter type: computer techniques in EEG analysis. EEG Clin. Neurophysiol., suppl. **20**: 25-27.

Silverman, D. 1969. In press. Cerebral death and and the electroencephalogram. EEG Clin. Neurophysiol.

van der Drift, J. H. A. 1957. The significance of electroencephalography for the diagnosis and localisation of brain tumours. Leiden, H. E. Stenfert Kroese N.V.

Chapter 32

Radioactive-nuclide scanning

Jorge Huertas

In normal brain tissue the blood-brain barrier prevents many substances from being metabolized or deposited even temporarily in the brain tissue. However, the abnormal cytological, vascular, and interstitial fluid conditions that prevail, for example, in a brain tumor, allow many substances to remain temporarily or permanently in altered areas.

Among substances that penetrate the blood-brain barrier under these conditions (but not normally) and remain in the affected tissue for a time are certain radioactive nuclides (isotopes), of which radioactive mercury (Hg-203) and radioiodinated serum albumin (RISA) are in most common use. All these nuclides have the property of emitting gamma rays.

Modern scanning and counting techniques have been applied to detect and localize radioactive nuclides in cases of suspected intracranial space-occupying lesions. The technique is complicated and requires experience in all phases, including the handling of the nuclides and the methods of measurement used. After administration of the radioactive material, scanning is performed. Several types of automatic scintillation machines are available that can produce photoscans or printout records or both. (Afifi and others, 1965; McAfee and Fueger, 1964; Mealey, Dehner, and Reese, 1964.)

Scanning is used for the localization of brain tumors, intra- or extracerebral (Blahd, 1965; Moore, 1948). The scanning is an adjuvant, not a substitute, for arteriography or pneumoencephalography in ascertaining the presence of tumors and their location. Its main advantage is that it outlines tumor size and shape. Tumors in certain locations, however, may not be revealed in brain scans, particularly those in the region of the foramen magnum, the base of the skull, or in structures close to the midline. Malignant gliomas, metastatic tumors, and meningiomas are most easily identified. A "negative" scan does not necessarily mean that no tumor exists. In 104 cases of proved intracranial tumor, scanning failed to disclose the presence of tumor in 28; on the other hand, there were no false positive scans in this series (Myre, Andersen, and Kristiansen, 1965). Fig. 32-1 illustrates a scan in a case of meningioma. Gradual uptake of the radioactive material has occurred. Serial scans provide a more adequate delineation of the tumor than one view alone. An area with complete absence of radioactivity can also be meaningful. Such is noted in some subdural hematomas, subdural effusions, and in porencephaly. The contention that subtentorial tumors do not become evident in a scan does not always hold. Fig. 32-2 illustrates a well-outlined medulloblastoma.

Cerebral angiodynamics and regional cerebral blood flow can be assessed with the use of scintiangiophotography (Kennedy, Chin, and Potter, 1968). This method reveals only the qualitative distribution of

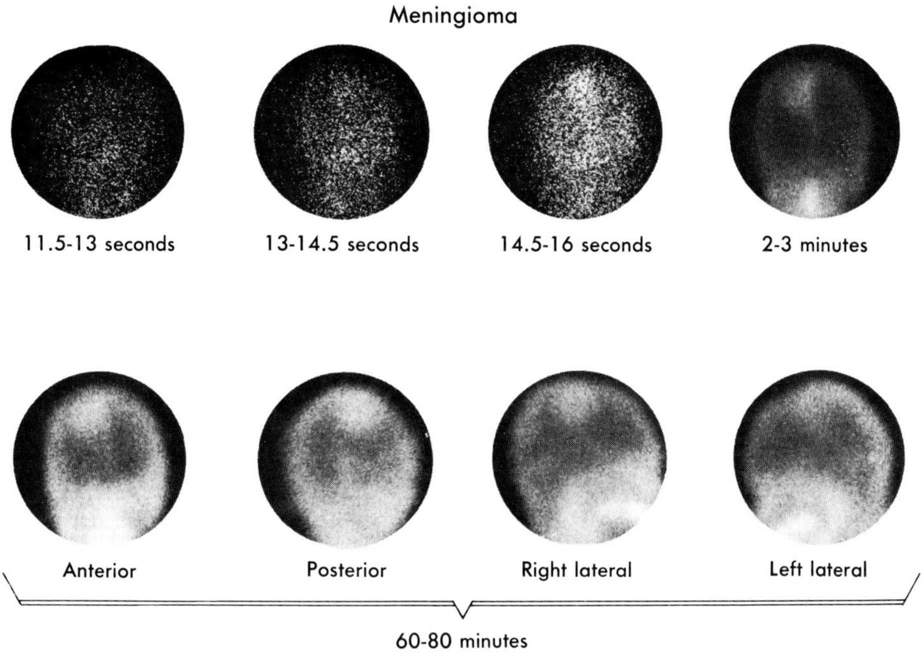

Fig. 32-1. Scintiphoto of a meningioma following injection of ^{99m}Tc-pertechnetate into the right anterior cubital vein. The upper row shows the sites of the nuclide, as follows: 11.5 to 13 seconds—arterial distribution in major anterior vessels; 13 to 14.5 seconds—capillary distribution; 14.5 to 16 seconds—venous distribution; 2 to 3 minutes—concentration of radioactive material in region of tumor, with some of the material in the torcular Herophili. The lower photos were made 60 to 80 minutes after the injection. Each photo was taken during a 2-minute exposure period. Each reveals altered permeability in the right parietal area due to the meningioma. (Courtesy Dr. Paul M. Weber, Oakland, California.)

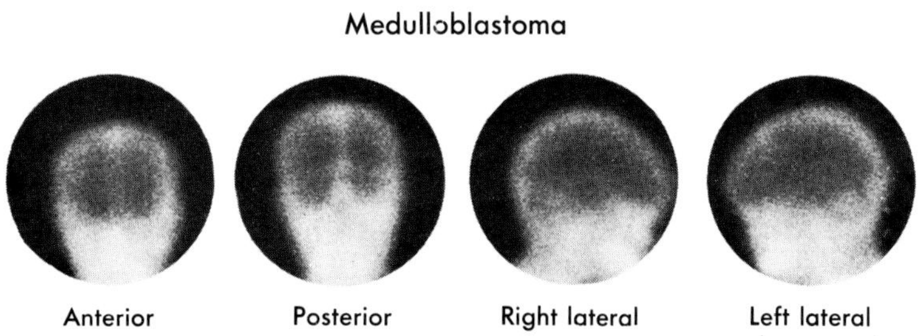

Fig. 32-2. Scintiphotos of medulloblastoma following intravenous injection of 2 mCi ^{99m}Tc-pertechnetate. The photos are equivalent in time periods to those in the lower row of Fig. 32-1. They show a focal lesion in the posterior fossa just below the torcular Herophili—a reflection of altered permeability of the blood-brain barrier. The tumor is best visualized in the lateral views. (Courtesy Dr. Paul M. Wetber, Oakland, California.)

radioisotopes in different regions of the brain. Zierler (1965) has, however, described a method for quantitative external measurement of cerebral blood flow with the use of radioactive nuclides. The mathematical analysis is time-consuming. The isotopes usually employed for this purpose are xenon-133 in saline, and, more recently, technetium-99 in labeled albumin (^{99m}TcAA) and ^{99m}Tc-pertechnetate.

Cerebral circulation studies by means of radioactive nuclides provide information in four general areas. *First,* the method provides a photographic record of the cerebral hemispheres and the hemodynamic features of regional circulation.

Scintiangiophotography for cerebral blood flow is carried out with use of time-lapse photographic techniques. Serial photographs taken at a frequency of 0.03 per second give adequate data on filling and depletion of cerebral tissue by tagged blood. *Second,* the method provides information of the circulatory bed in intracranial tumors. For instance, in meningioma a clear idea of the routes by which a tumor receives its blood supply can be obtained by injecting a radioactive nuclide into the external and internal carotid arteries of the suspected side. Some cerebral metastases not demonstrable by regular angiography may be brought out by this method. *Third,* in head trauma, the method allows the localization of hematomas and blood extravasations. Cerebral edema can also be disclosed. *Fourth,* in cerebrovascular disease, changes in radiodensity in serial time reveal infarcted or otherwise affected areas of the brain. If the injection is done cardially to the lesion, the secondary changes in regional cerebral blood flow will serve as a monitor of the site of the damage and point to the therapeutic measures that need to be taken, for example in "ischemic attacks."

REFERENCES

Afifi, A. K., Morrison, R. R., Sahs, A. L., and Evans, T. C. 1965. A comparison of chlormerodrin Hg-203 scintiencephaloscanning with neuroradiology and electroencephalography for the localization of intracranial lesions. Neurology **15**:56-63.

Blahd, W. H. 1965. Brain tumors. In Blahd, W. H., editor: Brain tumors in nuclear medicine. New York, McGraw-Hill Book Company, pp. 484-495.

Kennedy, J. C., Chin, F., and Potter, R. 1968. Visualization of cerebral blood flow with the scintillation camera in man. Scand. J. Clin. Lab. Invest. (Copenh.), suppl. 102.

McAfee, J. G., and Fueger, G. F. 1964. The value and limitations of scintillation scanning in the diagnosis of intracranial tumors. In Queen, J. L., III, editor: Scintillation scanning in clinical medicine. Philadelphia, W. B. Saunders Co., pp. 183-217.

Mealey, J., Jr., Dehner, J. R., and Reese, I. C. 1965. Clinical comparison of two agents used in brain scanning. J.A.M.A. **189**:260-264.

Moore, G. E. 1948. Use of radioactive diiodofluorescein in the diagnosis and localization of brain tumors. Science **107**:569.

Myre, K., Andersen, M. G., and Kristiansen, K. 1965. Isotope encephalometry. In Gilland, O., editor: Technical progress in neurological diagnostics. Amsterdam, Elsevier Publishing Company, pp. 22-26.

Zierler, K. L. 1965. Equations for measuring blood flow by external monitoring of radioisotopes. Circulation Res. **16**:309-315.

Index

A

Abadie's sign, 82
Abdominal reflex, 68
Abducens nerve, 255
  palsy, 159, 255, 264
Achromatopia, 372
Acoustic neuroma, 209
Acromegaly, 477
Acroparesthesia, 26
Adiposogenital dystrophy, 472
Adipsia, 467
Aerodontalgia, 240
Affect, disorders of, 384
Ageusia, 179
Agnosia, 402
Agraphia, 400
Air myelography, 129
Alexia, 373, 398, 400
  lesions, 374
Allochiria, tactile, 339
Allocortex, 312
Amaurosis, 358
Amaurosis fugax, 359
Amyotrophic lateral sclerosis, 76, 166, 429
  bulbar form, 164
Amyotrophy
  diabetic, 87
  syphilitic, 86
Anacusis, 206
Analgesia, 25
Anesthesia
  cutaneous, 50
  radicular, 50
  tactile, 24, 80
Anesthesia dolorosa, 26, 81, 245
Aneurysms
  affecting extraocular nerves, 104, 263
  of anterior cerebral and anterior communicating arteries, 517
  of basilar artery, 308
  fistula formation, 516
  focal manifestations, 515
    exophthalmos, 515
  fusiform, 514
  incidence, 514
  of internal carotid artery, 177, 515, 517
  manifestations of rupture, 519
  of middle and posterior cerebral arteries, 517, 518
  saccular, 514
  sites in brain and brainstem, 514
Anhidrosis, 38
Anisocoria, 101
Ankle clonus, 72
Anterior ethmoid nerve syndrome, 240
Anterior horn lesions, manifestations, 75
  abolition of reflexes, 75
  flaccid paralysis, 75
  vasomotor disturbances, 75
Antibiotics toxic to internal ear, 211
Antidiuretic hormone (ADH)
  conservation of body water, 468
  diabetes insipidus, 467
Aphagia, 469
Aphasia, 397
  anterior or Broca's area, 399
  and dementia, 401
  distinguishing features, 401
  motor, 398
  posterior or Wernicke's area, 400
  sensory, 399, 400
  subcortical lesions of dominant hemisphere, 400
  types and localization, 398
  verbal, 398
Apneustic ventilation, 41
Apraxia, 402
  constructional, 402
  for dressing, 402
  ideational, 402
  kinetic, 402
Archicortex, 312
Area striata, 350
Argyll Robertson pupil, 259, 260
Arm paralysis, 51
Arterial occlusion, brainstem, 294, 307, 308
  basilar artery, 298
    anterior inferior cerebellar artery, 299
    basis pedunculi syndrome, 304
    combined paramedian and laterosuperior midbrain syndrome, 306
    dorsolateral midbrain syndrome, 304
    internal auditory artery, 300
    lateral pons syndrome, 301
    laterosuperior midbrain syndrome, 306
    midbrain tegmentum syndrome, 304
    paramedian midbrain syndromes, 305
    paramedian pons syndrome, 300
    pontile arteries, 300
    pontile syndromes in general, 302
    pontile tegmental syndrome, 305
    superior cerebellar artery, 304

Arterial occlusion—cont'd
red nucleus syndromes, 305
vertebral arteries
anatomy, 294
bulbar syndromes, 295
effects of aneurysm, 298
occlusion, 297, 307, 308
Arteriosclerotic disease, involving spinal cord, 87
cerebral, 165
Arteriovenous malformations (hemangiomas), 520
Arteritis, giant cell, 360
Asterixis, 411
Astrocytoma, 538
anaplastic, 549
cerebellar, 543
Ataxia
cerebellar *(q.v.)*, 281
Friedreich's, 79
from cord lesions, 82
frontal, 289
and hypotonia, associated disorders
arm and leg deviation, 285
assessment of weight of objects, 284
laterality of disturbances, 284
pointing test, 285
parietal, 291
sensory, 29, 79, 81
Ataxic respiration, 41
Athetosis
disorders characterized by, 413, 415
double, 413
Atypical neuralgia, 243, 244
Auriculotemporal syndrome, 224
Automatic bladder, 107
Automatisms from frontal lobe lesions, 332
Autonomic nervous system
overall view, 33
parasympathetic division, 34
sympathetic division, 33
Avellis' syndrome, 183

B

Babinski reflex (sign), 73
Babinski-Nageotte syndrome, 154
Bacterial infections, source of vertigo and hearing loss, 211
Ballism, 416
Basilar artery, 298
aneurysm, 308
occlusion; *see* Arterial occlusion
Basis pedunculi
divisions, 142
lesions involving, 159
Bathesthesia, 23
Behavior, disorders, 382
Bell's palsy, 223; *see also* Facial palsy
complications, 224, 225
Bending reflex, 330
Benedikt's syndrome, 153
Biernacki's sign, 82
Blink reflex, 224
Body image, disturbances, 339
Botulism, 264
Brachial plexus, 51
Brain shifts following head impact, 529
central and uncal syndromes, 534
cranial nerve disturbances, 533
Brain shifts following head impact—cont'd
impaction and displacement of cerebellar tonsils, 533
mechanisms and effects of local pressure, 529, 534
Brain trauma
cerebral concussion, 526, 527
closed head injuries, 525
contre coup sites, 526
epidural hemorrhage, 528
open head injuries, 525
Brainstem
basic architectural plan, 146
caudal nerve group, 170
defined, 130
disturbances
basal lesions, 158, 159
bulbar paralytic, 164
destruction of nuclei and interruption of ascending pathways, 149
hemiplegia alterna, 153
interruption
of cranial nerves, from basal lesions, 158
at level of corticobulbar and corticospinal fibers, 150
of midbrain, 156
of nuclei and tracts of fifth nerve, 158
of pontile tegmentum, 158
structural features, 130, 145
course
of corticopontile and corticobulbar fibers, 149
of medial longitudinal fasciculus, spinal tract of fifth nerve, and spinocerebellar tracts, 149
of pyramidal (corticospinal) fibers, 149
intramedullary course of cranial nerve fibers, 148
midbrain, 141, 143, 144
medulla oblongata, 130, 132, 137
nuclear pattern, 145
pons, 138, 140
relation of cranial nerve nuclei to medial lemniscus and spinothalamic tracts, 148
Brissaud-Sicard syndrome, 153
Bronchogenic carcinoma and recurrent laryngeal nerve, 176
Brown-Séquard syndrome, 89, 90
Bruns' sign, 203
Buccal neuralgia, 242
Bulbar poliomyelitis, 164
Bulbothalamic tract, 236

C

Calcarine cortex, 349, 350
Caloric test for nystagmus, 197
Carpal tunnel syndrome, 26
Catalepsy, 385
Catatonia, 385
Cauda equina, lesions, 108
Causalgia, 25
Central vision, 351
Cerebellar ataxia, 281
associated disorders, 284
disturbed function of upper limbs, 282
disturbed gait and static adaptation, 281
as sign of cerebellar disturbance, 281

Cerebellar atrophy, subacute diffuse, 286
in alcoholic malnutrition, 288
associated conditions, 288
Cerebellar fits, 158, 541
Cerebellar hypotonia, 283
associated disorders, 284
Cerebellar tumors, 543
Cerebellopontile angle syndrome, causes, 209
Cerebellum, 277
anatomy and functional scope
afferent and efferent connections, 278
pathways, 279-280
cerebellofugal fibers, 280
synaptic stations, 280
synergy, 281
lesions, clinical manifestations, 281, 286
ataxia, 281, 284
frontal, 289
parietal, 291
hypotonia, 283, 284
involving extracerebellar structures *(q.v.)*, 288
Cerebral artery occlusion
anterior choroidal artery, 504
cerebral artery
anterior, 506
middle, 509
posterior, 511
general orientation
circle of Willis, 497
circulatory insufficiency, 500
development of shunts, 498
internal carotid artery, 500
posterior communicating artery, 503
subclavian steal syndrome, 499
Cerebral concussion following skull impact, 526
Cerebral cortex
components of corona radiata and internal capsule, 324
corticofugal fiber systems
corticonuclear tracts, 324
corticosubcortical fibers, 324
corticopetal fiber systems, 324
cytoarchitectural areas, 311
fiber pathways between hemispheres, 326
functional subdivisions, 314
for adversive movements, 317
association or parasensory areas, 322
cortically originating extrapyramidal system (COEPS), 317-318
input from visceral structures, 324
limbic lobe, 323
prefrontal and orbitofrontal areas and psychic function, 324
sensibility, 319
special senses, 320
vestibular function, 322
voluntary motor functions, 315
lesions, motor deficit; *see* Motor deficit from lesions
noncallosal, 326
Cerebral peduncle, 141
Cervical cord, traumatic transection, 38
Cervical spondylitis, 80
Cervical spondylosis, 88, 97
Cervical and upper thoracic spinal segments, lesions and autonomic disturbances, 97
Cervical and upper thoracic spinal segments, lesions and autonomic disturbances—cont'd
Horner's syndrome and associated disturbances, 101
prolapsed intervertebral disk, 63, 98, 99
respiratory disturbances, 100
slowing of pulse, 100
tumor in foramen magnum, 99
vasomotor and sudomotor paralysis, 100
whiplash injury, 97
Cestan-Chenais syndrome, 183
Cheyne-Stokes respiration, 41
Chorda tympani, 217
syndrome, 224
Chorea, 410, 411
Chorea gravidarum, 411
Choreoathetosis, 411
Chromophobe adenoma of pituitary, 472, 473
Chronotaraxis, 340
Chvostek's phenomenon, 229
Ciliary neuralgia, 242
Ciliospinal reflex, 42, 103
Circulatory deficiency of vertebral-basilar arterial system, 307
clinical syndromes, 307
dizziness and vertigo, 308
ophthalmoplegia, 308
Clarke's nucleus of spinal cord, 1
Clonic facial spasms, 228
Cluster headache, 242
Cochlear end-organ and nerve
anatomy and functions, 203
clinical disturbances, 206; *see also* Deafness; Hearing loss
damage, 206
physical properties of basilar membrane, 206
reduction of auditory threshold, 205
sites of damage and symptomatology, 211
COEPS; *see* Cortically originating extrapyramidal system
Cogwheel phenomenon, 424
Collet-Sicard syndrome, 183
Coma vigil, 390, 462
Compulsive water drinking, 468
Concussion
in brain trauma, 526, 527
cause of hearing loss, 211
following skull impact, 526
Conduction time in electrical stimulation, 120
Conduction velocity in electrical stimulation, 120
Congenital syphilis, hearing disturbances, 211
Conjugate ocular disturbances
compulsive eye opening, 271
convergence or divergence paralysis, 271
in eye centering, 268
in fixation away from center position, 268-269
in horizontal gaze, 269
internuclear ophthalmoplegia, 272
nystagmus, 271
spasmodic deviation, 271
sylvian aqueduct syndrome, 272
vertical paralysis, 270
Consciousness, disturbances, 389
Conus syndrome, 110
Cordotomy, 8, 12, 100
Corneal reflex, 238

Cortically originating extrapyramidal system (COEPS), 317-318, 404-405
Corticopontocerebellar pathway, 279
Corticospinal (pyramidal) tract, 3, 315
  anterior, 14
  lateral, 13
Cranial neuralgias, 179, 241
Craniocerebral topography, 311
Craniocerebral trauma, 527
Craniopharyngioma, 472, 475
  clinical course, 476
Cremaster reflex, 68
Creutzfeldt-Jakob's disease, 421
Cristae, 186
Crocodile tear phenomenon, 224
Crossed reflexes, 72, 332
Cupulometry for nystagmus, 197
Cutaneous reflexes, 73
Cystic arachnoiditis, 286

D

Deafness; *see also* Hearing loss
  from antibiotics, 211
  from brainstem lesions, 210
  cortical, 380
  middle-ear, 206
  sensorineural, 206, 207
  speech discrimination, 207
  tests, 206
  and/or tinnitus of peripheral origin, 208
Decerebrate rigidity, 156
Decompression sickness, 89
Deep muscle reflexes, 72
Defecation, reflex intermittent, 109
Déjà vu phenomenon, 372, 383
Dejerine-Klumpke's paralysis, 102
Dejerine-Roussy syndrome, 461
Deltoid paralysis, 51
Dementia, 391
  and aphasia, 401
Dermatomeres, 47, 50
Dermatomes, 47, 50
Dermographia dolorosa, 37
Dermographia peripherica, 37
Diabetes insipidus and adipsia, 467
Diabetes mellitus
  amyotrophy, 87
  bladder disturbances, 108
  facial palsy, 225
  involving ocular nerves, 262
Diagonal reflex, 332
Diencephalic syndrome in infancy and childhood, 477
Digastric muscle paralysis, 239
Diphtheria, source of palsy, 264
Diplegia, spastic, in infancy, 341
Disk, intervertebral, prolapsed, 63, 98, 99
Diskography, 129
Dizziness; *see* Vertigo and dizziness
"Dry eye," 228
Duchenne-Erb upper plexus paralysis, 51
Dumbbell tumors, 125
Dural neuralgia, 244
Dysarthria, 397
Dysautonomia, familial, 385
Dysesthesia, 26
Dysglobulinemia, source of cranial nerve palsies, 263
Dyshomeostasis syndrome of neuraxis, 390
Dysphonia, spastic, 176
Dyslexia, developmental, 398; *see also* Alexia
Dyssynergia cerebellaris myoclonica, 163
Dyssynergia cerebellaris progressiva, 163
Dystonia musculorum deformans, 416
  formes frustes, 417

E

Echoencephalography
  basic principle, 565
  brain tumors, direct sounding, 568
  compound scanning, 569
  hematoma echo, 568
  procedure, 565
  pulse-curves, 568
  techniques
    A-scope, 566
    B-scan, 568
Edinger-Westphal-Perlia complex, 42, 253, 254, 260
Ejaculation, 109
Electroencephalography
  change in regional potentials, 571
  cyclic variations, 574
  defined, 570
  in determination of death, 580
  electroencephalograms
    abnormal, 575, 576, 577
    activation
      analeptics, 575
      hyperventilation, 575
      provocation techniques, 574
    in children, 574
  in epilepsy, 577, 578, 579
  in head injury, 579
  newer approaches
    averaging techniques, 582
    frequency analysis, 581
  normal, 571
    awake state, 571
    sleep, 573
    wave types, 574
  recording, 570
  in space-occupying lesions, 580
  in vascular lesions, 579
Electromyography
  observations, 114
    during electrode insertion, 116
    during muscle rest, 117
      fasciculations and fibrillations, 117
      muscle cramps, 117
  physiology and function of muscle, 116
  recording, 116
Electronystagmography, 197
Eminentia teres, 110
Emotional expression, loss of, 231
Emotional over-activity, 167
Enophthalmos, 102
Ependymoma, 541
Epiconus, 110
  lesions, 110
  syndrome, 111
Epicritic sensory system, 24

Epilepsy
electroencephalography (*q.v.*), 577
facial, 334
focal, 334
focal sensory, 336
jacksonian, 334, 335
local, 334
myoclonus, 163
partialis continua, 335
temporal lobe, 383
uncinate, 382
Epiphora, 223
Erotomania, 383
Erythropia, 372
Erythroprosopalgia, 242
Etat lacunaire, 164
Extensor responses, 73
Exteroreceptors, 23
Extraocular nerves, lesions involving, 251
clinical disturbances, 268; *see also* Conjugate ocular disturbances
conjugate ocular movements, 266
defective pupillary response, 261
infranuclear and nuclear palsies, 255
in disease states, 258
innervation of ocular muscles, 251
Marcus Gunn and related synkineses, 265
miscellaneous disorders, 262
muscle functions, 255
neoplasms, 262
progressive external ophthalmoplegia, 264
trauma, 261
Extrapyramidal motor system, 404, 405
clinical syndromes, pathology, mechanisms, 409
athetosis, 413
ballism, 416
chorea, 410
Creutzfeldt-Jakob's disease, 421
dystonia, 416
Hallervorden-Spatz's disease, 420
hepatolenticular degeneration, 418
parkinsonian states, 423; *see also* Parkinsonism and parkinsonian states
subacute spongiform encephalopathy, 421
COEPS, 404-405
connections
cerebellum, 409
pallidum, 405
red nucleus, 407
reticular formation, 409
striatum, 405
substantia nigra, 407
subthalamic nucleus, 407
thalamus, 409
disorders
classification, 410
distinguishing features, 404
mechanisms involved, 409-410
superimposed neuron systems, 404
Eyelid vibration sign, 223

F

Face, "onion peel" sensory distribution, 247
Facial colliculus, 139
Facial epilepsy, 334
Facial myokymia, 227
Facial nerve
anatomy and functions, 217
autonomic pathways, 100, 219-222
blood supply, 217
chorda tympani, 217
clonic spasms, 228
disorders, 221
disturbances in supranuclear innervation, 229
infranuclear and nuclear palsies, 227; *see also* Bell's palsy; Facial palsy
interruption, 222, 225
involvement in cerebellopontile region, 228
irritation, 215
pontile lesions, 226
salivary secretion, 220
taste sensation, 219
tear secretion, 219
trauma, 226
Facial palsy; *see also* Bell's palsy
causation, 225
intermittent, 228
in pathological processes, 159, 226, 227
persistent tonic, 228
progressive, 226
in systemic disorders, 225
unilateral, 228
Facial spasms, clonic, 228
Fanning phenomenon, toes, 73
Fasciculation
facial, 227
muscular, 33, 117
Fasciculus retroflexus of Meynert, 143
Fibrillation, muscular, 32, 117, 118
Figure writing for tactile testing, 29
Finger flexor reflex, 74
Finger paralysis, 51
Flexor withdrawal reflex, 69, 74
Foramen magnum, neoplasms and aneurysms, 99
Forearm paralysis, 51
Foville's syndrome, 153
Friedreich's ataxia, 79
Frontal ataxia, 289
Frontal leukotomy syndrome, 462
Frontal lobe lesions, release and allied phenomena
automatisms, 332
bending reflexes, 330
crossed flexion reflex, 332
diagonal reflex, 332
diagonal rigidity, 332
forced grasping and groping, 329
localizing importance, 330
gait disorders, 332
persistence of induced movements, 332
tonic plantar reflex, 330
test, 331
tonic spasms of fingers and toes, 332
traction response and grasp reflex, 329, 330

G

Gag reflex, 175
Gait disorders, 332
Galvanic nystagmus test, 197
Gasperini's syndrome, 154
Gasserian ganglion, involvement, 245
Gastrectomy and cord lesions, 82
Gastric crises, 82

Geniculocalcarine tract, 349
Genital organs, innervation and function, 109
Gerstmann's syndrome, 339
Gestalt dissolution, visual, 374
Glioblastoma multiforme, 539, 542
Gliomas
  of brainstem, 541
  of cerebrum, 538
Glossopharyngeal nerve, 177
  baroreceptive function, 178
  chemoreceptive junction, 177
  disturbances, 179
  neuralgia, 179
  parasympathetic fibers, 179
Glossopharyngeal neuralgia, 179
Glossoplegia, 170
Golgi tendon organs, 31
Gowers' syndrome, 359
Gradenigo's syndrome, 244, 259
Grasp reflex, 329, 330
  in frontal lobe lesions, 402
Gustatory hyperhidrosis, 224

H

H fields of Forel, 42, 102
Habenulo-interpeduncular fasciculus, 143
Hallervorden-Spatz's disease, 420
Hallucinations, lilliputian, 372; *see also* Metamorphopias
Head-retraction reflex, 166
Head's hyperesthesia, 23, 26
Hearing loss, 206, 380; *see also* Deafness
  in aging process, 212
  from antibiotics, 211
  in hemiplegics, 211
  sources of end-organ damage, 211-213
  tests, 206
  transitory and permanent, 380
  in trauma, 208
Hemangioblastoma, capillary, 544
Hemangiomas, 520
Hemianopia
  from optic chiasm involvement, 363
    caudal aspect, 366
    lateral aspect, 365
  from visual tract involvement, 369
Hemiathetosis, 415
Hemiballism, 416
Hemichorea, 416
Hemiplegia, 289
  hearing loss, 211
  spastic, in infancy, 341
  spinal, 90
  striatal, 341
Hemiplegia alterna, 153
Hemiplegia alternans infima, 295
Hemiplegia cruciata, 295
Hemispheric dominance, 397
Hepatolenticular degeneration, 418
Heredofamilial spinocerebellar degeneration, 286
Herpes zoster, 88
  geniculate, 225
  trigeminal, 245
Heterochromia iridis, 102
Heterogenetic cortex, 312
Histaminic neuralgia, 242
Hoffmann's sign, 74
Holmes-Adie syndrome, 260
Homogenetic cortex, 312
Hook bundle of Russell, 280
Horner's syndrome and associated disturbances, 101, 246
H-reflex, 120
Huntington's disease, 412
Hunt's neuralgia, 243
Hydrocephalus, 392
Hypacusis, 206
  neural versus non-neural, 207
Hypalgesia, 25
Hyperacusis, 223
Hyperalgesia, 25
Hyperesthesia
  of Head, 23, 26
  tactile, 24
Hyperhidrosis, 38
  gustatory, 224
Hyperphagia, 469
Hyperventilation, 41
Hypesthesia, tactile, 24
Hypoglossal nerve, 170
Hypohidrosis, 38
Hypothalamus
  ADH release, 468
  blood temperature as determinant of response, 479
  carbohydrate metabolism, 470
  centers
    feeding, 469
    glucostat hypothesis, 470
    satiety (stop-feeding), 469
    thermostat hypothesis, 470
    thirst, 468, 469
  effects of lesions
    diencephalic syndrome, 477
    food consumption, 469
    glycosuria, 471
    hyperglycemia, 471
    obesity and gonadal atrophy, 472
    pubertas praecox, 478
    water balance, 467
      adipsia, 467, 469
      diabetes insipidus, 467
  fiber systems, 464
  gastrointestinal tract, 471
  hormone release, 467
  influence on behavior, 465
  longitudinal zones, 465
  nuclei, 465
  regulation of body temperature, 479
  in sleep-wakefulness, 485
  supraopticohypophysial tract, 467
  tuberohypophysial tract, 467
Hypoventilation, 41

I

Inattention
  tactile, 339
  visual, 372
Innervation of muscles
  peripheral and radicular, 47-50
  radicular anesthesia, 50

Innervation of muscles—cont'd
segmental, 47
extremity muscles (table), 57
trunk muscles (table), 58-59
sensory fibers, 49
Interoceptors, 23
Intracranial tumors, localization by types, 534
cerebral angiography, 559
pneumoencephalography, 559
roentgenography, plain films, 549
Intramedullary (spinal) tumors, 69
distinguished from extramedullary, 92
Intraneural plexuses, 48
Island of Reil, 379
Isocortex, 312

J

Jacksonian epilepsy, 334
Jackson's syndrome, 153, 183
Jaw-winking phenomenon, 265

K

Kakopia, 372
Kalopia, 372
Kennedy's syndrome, 359
Kernohan notch, 532
Kinesthesia, 23
Klüver-Bucy syndrome, 385
Koniocortex, 312
Korsakoff syndrome, 387

L

Labyrinth, 186
Lacunar stroke, 345
Lagophthalmos, 223
Laminectomy for spinal cord tumor, 69
Landry-Guillain-Barré syndrome, 225, 264
Latent reflexes, 74
Laughter and crying, 167
Lead poisoning, chronic, 176
Limbic lobe, 323
Little's disease, 340
Liver flap, 411
Long spinal tracts, cross-sectional topography, 13
"Lower-half" headache, 242
Lumbosacral plexus, 51

M

Macropia, 372, 383
Macula, ocular, 351
fibers, 351-352
Macular fan, 355
Marcus Gunn phenomenon, 265
inverted, 266
Marin-Amat syndrome, 266
Masseter reflex, 239
Mastication reflex, 166
Masticatory muscle paralysis, 239
Masticatory spasms, 244
Measles, hearing loss, 211
Medial longitudinal fasciculus (MLF) syndrome, 272, 273
Medulla oblongata, structural features; *see* Brainstem
Medulloblastoma, 543
Memory disturbances, 387
Mendel-Bechterew's sign, 74
Ménière's disease, 199, 212, 226
Meningiomas, 535
convexity, 535
intraventricular, 536
olfactory groove, 536
posterior fossa, 537
sphenoid ridge, 536
suprasellar, 536
Mesencephalic nucleus, 237
Metameres, 47
Metamorphopias, 340, 372
classification, 372
hemangiopic, 372-373
Micropia, 372, 383
Microtelopia, 383
Midbrain, structural features; *see* Brainstem
Middle-ear deafness, 206
Migraine, 360
ophthalmoplegia in, 263
Migrainous neuralgia, 242
Millard-Gubler syndrome, 153
Miosis, 101
Mirror movements, 344
Mitral valve disease, 176
Mixed spinal nerves, 48
Monoplegia, 332
Monospasms, 334
Motility, 29
Motor deficit from lesions, 322
jacksonian epilepsy, 334
monoplegia, 232
monospasms, 334
muscle atrophy and related disorders, 334
seizures, 334
voluntary movement, muscle tonus, reflexes, 333
Motor innervation; *see* Innervation of muscles
Motor and sensory disturbances combined
lesions involving posterior and lateral spinal columns, 82
partial versus complete transection, 86
transverse lesions, 83
Mouth-opening reflex, 166
Movements, associated, 74, 344
Multiple sclerosis, 39, 211, 227, 247, 489
source of ocular nerve palsies, 263
Mumps infection
facial palsy, 225
hearing loss, 211
ophthalmoplegia, 264
Muscles
atrophy, 33
of denervation, 33
of disuse, 33
clonus, 72
electrical stimulation, 121
fasciculation, 33, 117, 118
fibrillation, 32, 117, 118
innervation; *see* Innervation of muscles
paralysis; *see* Paralysis
tonus and reflexes, 29
central nervous system responses, 31
localizing value, 31
Mutism
akinetic, 390, 401, 462
distinguished from total aphasia, 401

Myasthenia gravis, 177, 263
Myelinolysis, central pontile, 388
Myelitis, subacute necrotic, 88
Myelography
  air, 129
  with water soluble substances, 129
Myelomeningocele, spinal, 108
Myelopathy from carcinoma, 88
Myelopathy, progressive, 87
Mylohyoid muscle paralysis, 239
Myoclonus, 161
Myokymia, 33
  facial, 227
Myomeres, 47
Myotomes, 47

N

Neocortex, 312
Nervus intermedius, 217, 218
  neuralgia, 243
Neuralgias; *see* specific types
Neurogenic bladder
  autonomous, 107
  uninhibited, 107
Neuromeres, 47
Neuronitis, vestibular, 212
Neuroparalytic (neurotrophic) keratopathy, 246
Neurosyphilis, 86; *see also* Syphilis
  meningomyelitic, 86
Neurotomes, 47
Noise, hearing loss from, 212
Nothnagel's syndrome, 154
Nutritional deficiency
  and extraocular muscle palsy, 263
  and facial palsy, 225
Nymphomania, 383
Nystagmus
  defined, 196
  fixation, 196
  gaze, 197
    dissociated, 197
  induced, 196
  jerky, 196
  from lesions involving the labyrinth and neuraxis, 199
  optokinetic, 371
    abnormalities in, 371-372
  pendular, 196
  positional, 196
  provoked, 196
  related disorders, 199
  retraction, 196
  rotary, 196
  spontaneous, 196
  tests
    cupulometry, 197
    electronystagmography, 197
    of otolithic function, 198
    parallel swing, 198
    for positional nystagmus, 198
    of semicircular canal function, 197
  vertical, 196
  vestibular, 196

O

Ocular bobbing, 162
Ocular fixation, disturbances, 268
Ocular posture, mechanisms concerned, 194
Oculomotor nerve, 251
  palsies, 159, 255
  parasympathetic innervation, pupillary response, accommodation, convergence, 253
  subdivisions of nucleus, 251
    Edinger-Westphal nucleus, 253
    lateral group, 252
    nuclei of Perlia, 253
Oculosensory reflex, 42
Olfactory acuity
  functional disturbances, 381
  stimulation and response, 381
  threshold of sensitivity, 381
Oligodendroblastoma, 541
Oligodendroglioma, 541
Olivocerebellar tract, 279
Olivospinal tract, 5
Ophthalmic zoster, 245
Ophthalmoplegia
  from circulatory deficiency, 308
  diabetic, 262
  internal, 256
  internuclear, 272
  in migraine, 263
  progressive external, 264
  total, 257
Opsoclonus, 285
Optic atrophy, 358
Optic chiasm, 363, 473
Optic nerve
  anatomy, 349
  lesions, 355, 359
  syphilis, 360
  trauma, 360
Optic neuritis
  intraocular, 356-358
  retrobulbar, 357, 358
Optic system; *see* Visual system
Optic tract involvement, 366
Orbicularis oculi reflexes, 223, 238
Orbicularis oris reflex, 166
Orbitofrontal cortex
  lesions, 386
  respiratory, function, 41
Organ of Corti, 203; *see also* Cochlear end-organ and nerve
Oscillopia, 196
Osteitis deformans and deafness, 208
Otalgia, 213
Otalgic neuralgia, 243
Otitis media, 208
Otolithic function tests, 198
Otoliths, 186
Otosclerosis, 208, 210

P

Pachymeningitis, 81, 86
  rheumatoid, 98
  syphilitic, 86
Pachymeningitis cervicalis hypertrophica, 86
Pain
  deep, 27
  facial, pathways, 237
  fibers of spinal cord, 7, 15
  girdle, 81, 82

Pain—cont'd
  insensitivity to, 79
  from malocclusion of teeth, 240
  odontogenic, 240
  paranasal sinus, 240
  pressure, 27
  referred, 7, 63, 213; *see also* Referred pain
  temporomandibular joint or muscle, 213, 240
Palatal reflex, 238
Pallanesthesia, 25, 338
Pallesthesia, 25
Palsies, infranuclear and nuclear, 222, 255; *see also* Bell's palsy; Facial palsy
  abducens nerve, 159, 255, 264
  in disease states, 258
  oculomotor nerve, 159, 254
  third, fourth, and sixth nerves, 160, 257
  trochlear nerve, 254
Papilledema, 355
  causes, 361-363
  in hematological disorders, 362
Papillitis, 356
Papillomacular bundle, 351
Paracusis, 207
  Willisiana, 207
Parallel swing test for nystagmus, 198
Paralysis; *see also* specific forms
  contracture in opposing muscle groups, 56
  extent by level of lesion, 56
    tables, 57-59
  of facial nerve, 222; *see also* Facial palsy
  limb involvement, 51
  radicular versus peripheral nerve, 51, 57
  sensory disturbances, 57
  site of spinal cord lesion, 51
  from spinal canal tumor, 56
  spinal segments involved, 47, 51
  sudomotor, 100
  vasomotor, 100
  from vertebral fracture or dislocation, 56
Paralysis agitans, 423, 425
  hereditary, 426
Paramyoclonus multiplex, 162
Paraplegia
  Pott's, 88
  spastic, 86
  traumatic, 85
Parasympathetic system, 34, 219
Paresthesia, 26
Parietal ataxia, 291
Parietal lobe lesions, sensory and related disturbances, 336
Parinaud's syndrome, 156
Parkinsonism and parkinsonian states
  amyotrophic lateral sclerosis, 429
  arteriosclerotic, 427
  atrophies with Parkinson variants
    progressive pallidal atrophy, 430, 431
    striatonigral degeneration, 429
  in carbon monoxide poisoning, 428
  contrasted with cerebellar disorders, 425
  damage of substantia nigra, 430
  distinguishing features, 423
  in manganese poisoning, 428
  neural mechanisms, 430
  paradoxical kinesis, 424
  phenothiazine medication, 429
Parkinsonism and parkinsonian states—cont'd
  postencephalitic, 423
  posttraumatic, 427
  punch-drunk state, 428
  resting tremor, 423, 432
  rigidity, akinesis, and postural disturbances, 430
  sequence of signs, 424
  tests, 424
Paradoxical vertigo, 201
Patellar clonus, 72
Pathological laughter and crying, 167
Paton's syndrome, 359
Periostitis, source of ocular nerve palsy, 258
Peripheral nerve injury, 37, 38
  trophic disturbances, 39
Pernicious anemia, 82
Perseveration
  in aphasia, 401
  tactile, 339
Petrosal neuralgia, 243
Pharyngeal reflex, 175
Photomas, 372
Photopia, 372
Pick's visions, 158
Pilomotor function, 39, 100
Pilomotor reflex, 69
Pineal tumors, 537
Piriform cortex, 312
Pituitary dwarfism, 478
Pituitary insufficiency
  in adults, 477, 478
  in childhood, 478
Plantar reflex, 68
  tonic, 330, 331
Pneumoencephalography, 554
Poliomyelitis, 39
  bulbar, 164
Polydipsia, 468
Pons
  structural features; *see* Brainstem
  syndromes, 300
Pontile lesions involving seventh nucleus, 226
  fasciculation, 227
Posttraumatic neuralgia, 24, 26
Postural disorders, 384
Pott's paraplegia, 88
Presbycusis, 212
Pressure pain, 27
Proprioception, 23
Proprioceptors, 23
Prosopagnosia, 374
Prosopalgic neuralgia, 243
Protopathic sensory system, 24
Pseudobulbar palsy, 164, 167
  reflexes, 166
Pseudopapilledema, 356
Pseudosclerosis, 418
Psychomotor seizures, 382
  extirpation of temporal cortex, 384
Ptosis, 102, 255
Pubertas praecox, 478
Pupillary dilatation, 42
  pain-induced, 43
Pupillary reactions, 353
Pyramidal (corticospinal) tract, 3, 13, 14, 315
  lesions, 72; *see also* Spastic syndrome

Q

Quadriceps femoris reflex, 66
Queckenstedt test, 93
Quintothalamic tract, 236

R

Radial nerve paralysis, 51
Radicular artery of Adamkiewicz, 17
Radicular finger paralysis, 51
Radioactive-nuclide scanning, 584
  areas of information, 585
  scintiangiophotography, 584
  uses, 584
Raeder's paratrigeminal syndrome, 103
Ramsay Hunt syndrome, 225
Raymond-Cestan syndrome, 154
Receptor unit, 24
Rectum
  innervation and function, 108
  spinal lesions, 109
Recurrent laryngeal nerve, 175
  paralysis, 175
  thyroidectomy, 176
Referred pain, 7, 63, 213, 240
  mechanisms, 7, 64
  sites, 66, 67
  somatic and visceral afferents, 65-68
Reflex bladder, 107
Reflex changes, localization, 66, 72
Reflex erythema, 37
Reflex intermittent defecation, 109
Reflexes; *see* specific reflexes
Respiratory distrubances, 41, 100
Reticular formation, 5, 11, 380
  activating and integrating systems, 380
  functional connotation, 390
Reticulocerebellar atrophy, 390
Reticulospinal tracts, 5, 14
Retina
  blood supply, 354
  emboli, 359
  fibers for central vision, 351
  occlusion
    of central artery, 359
    of central vein, 360
  thrombosis, 359
Retrocollis, 417
Rheumatoid disease complex, 98
Riley-Day syndrome, 385
Rinne's test of hearing, 206
Romberg's test for ataxia, 29
Rossolimo's sign, 74
Rotation test for nystagmus, 197
Rubella, hearing loss, 211
Rubrospinal tract, 5, 14

S

Saccadic tracking system, 266
Sagittal stratum, external, 351
Salivary secretion, 220, 228, 246
Schmidt's syndrome, 183
Schwabach's test of hearing, 206
Scintiangiophotography, 584
Scotomas
  arcuate, 359
Scotomas—cont'd
  awareness of, 370
  negative and positive, 350
Semicircular canal tests, 197
Sensibility
  combined (cortical sensory function), 27
    discrimination of weights, 29
    figure writing, 29
    location of tactile stimuli, 28
    somatic sense of space, 29
    stereognosis, 27
  disturbances; *see* Sensory disturbances
  epicritic, 23, 24
  exteroceptive (superficial)
    pain, 25
    tactile, 24
    temperature, 26
    vibration, 25
  fibers conveying, 218
  proprioceptive (deep), 27
  protopathic, 23, 24
  somatic, 23
Sensorineural deafness, 206, 207
Sensory disturbances
  in parietal lobe lesions
    body image, 339
    chronotaraxis, 340
    Gerstmann's syndrome, 339
    irritative phenomena, 336
    metamorphopias, 340
    sensory deficit, 336
    tactile inattention, perseveration, and allochiria, 339
  of spinal origin
    ataxia, 29, 79, 81
    combined ataxia, sensory loss, and irritative phenomena, 81
    irritative phenomena, 63, 80, 81
    overlap of radicular fields, 57
    posterior root lesions, 78
    referred pain, 63
    reflex changes, 66
    spinal lesions involving pain and thermal sensibility, 78
    tactile sensibility, 79
Sensory function, 23; *see also* Sensibility
  classification, 23
  cortical, 27; *see also* Sensibility, combined
Serratus magnus palsy, 173
Sexual function, lesions and disturbances, 111
Sheehan's syndrome, 477
Sigmoid, innervation and function, 108
Simmonds' disease, 477
Simultanagnosia, 374
Sleep-wakefulness and related states, 484
  clinical observations
    damage
      of pons and medulla oblongata, 490
      of thalamus and environs, 488
    infarction, 489
    infectious states, 488
    multiple sclerosis, 489
    tumors, 490
  experimental studies, 484
  hypnogenic core of central nervous system in sleep control, 487

Smooth-pursuit tracking system, 268
Sneeze reflex, 238
Snout reflex, 166
Social attitudes, disorders, 384
Somesthesia, 23
Somites, 47
Space perception, disturbances, 158, 383
Spastic contracture of face, 228
Spastic diplegia and hemiplegia, 340
Spastic dysphonia, 176
Spastic paraplegia, 86
Spastic syndrome, 72, 75
Special senses, functional disturbances, 380
Speech; *see also* Aphasia; Apraxia
  as acquired social skill, 397
  clinical signs of breakdown, 397
  correlation with cerebral structures, 397
  discrimination, 207
  dysarthria, 397
  reception threshold, 207
Sphenoid sinusitis, source of ocular nerve palsy, 259
Sphenopalatine neuralgia, 242
Spinal accessory nerve, 170
  intermedullary lesions, 172
  interruption, 172
Spinal artery occlusion
  anterior, 88
  posterior, 88
Spinal cord
  blood supply
    arterial, 15
    venous return, 19
  conus lesions, 110
  "distant" effects following trauma, 83
  fibers; *see also* Tracts of spinal cord
    anterior root, 15
    pain, 7
    posterior root, 11
  neoplasms, 91; *see also* Spinal tumors
  nerve cell groups, 1, 2
  pathways, 15, 77
  radiation necrosis, 89
  segments; *see* Spinal segments
  sudomotor centers, 38
  thrombophlebitis, 88
  tracts; *see* Tracts of spinal cord; specific tracts
  trauma, 38, 56, 85, 89, 97
  unilateral lesions, 89
Spinal hemiplegia, 90
Spinal reflexes, 68
Spinal segments
  alignment with vertebral spinous processes, 69
  innervation in terms of, 47; *see also* Innervation of muscles, segmental
  involved in spinal cord lesions
    localization
      of motor disturbances, 51
      of reflex changes, 66
      of sensory disturbances, 57
    motor functions of peripheral nerves (table), 60
Spinal shock, 85
Spinal thrombophlebitis, 88
Spinal transection, 86
Spinal tumors, roentgenography, 123
  atrophy of cord, 124
Spinal tumors, roentgenography—cont'd
  bony changes on scout films, 123
  cervical cord tumors, 98
  diskography, 129
  image intensification control, 128
  intraspinal tumors, 69, 123
  localized tumors of nerve roots, 124
  metastatic tumors of vertebral column, 127
  methodology, 123
  myelography, 129
  neurofibromas and meningiomas, 125
  special procedures, appraisal, 123
  vertebral tumors, 127
Spinocerebellar tracts, 279
  dorsal (of Flechsig), 9, 14
  ventral (of Gowers), 10, 15
Spino-olivary tract, 10
Spinoreticular systems, 11, 15
Spinotectal tract, 15
Spinothalamic tracts
  anterior, 9, 14
  lateral, 6, 14
  lesions, 79
Spondylosis, cervical, 97, 298
Spongiform encephalopathy, subacute, 421
Statoacoustic nerve, 186
  membranous labyrinth, 186
  nystagmus; *see* Nystagmus
  vestibular end-organs and nerve (*q.v.*), 189
Stereoanesthesia, 28
Stereognosis, 27
Stilling's nucleus of spinal cord, 1
Streptomyces toxic to internal ear, 211
Styloid process, elongated, 244
Subacute combined degeneration of cord, 82
Subclavian steal syndrome, 499
Subdural hematoma, 391
Sudomotor function, 37
  centers in spinal cord, 38
  lesions, 37
  paralysis, 100
  testing, 38
Superficial muscle reflexes, 73
Suprarubal syndrome, 461
Sydenham's chorea, 410
Sylvian aqueduct syndrome, 272
Sympathalgies faciales, 242
Sympathetic system, 33, 219
Syndromes; *see* specific syndromes
Synesthesialgia, 339
Synkinesias, 344
Syphilis
  and deafness, 208, 211
  involving spinal cord, 86
  of optic nerve, 360
  source of ocular nerve palsy, 258, 259
Syphilitic pachymeningitis, 86
Syringobulbia, 164, 227
Syringomyelia, 12, 39, 78, 88
Systematic vertigo, 201

T

Tabes dorsalis, 39, 81, 82, 177
Tapia's syndrome, 183
Tarsal tunnel syndrome, 26

Taste sensation
  fibers conveying, 179, 219
  functional disturbances, 224, 246, 380
Tear secretion
  "dry eye," 228
  epiphora, 223
  fibers concerned, 219
  loss from injury of nerve V, 246
Tectospinal tract, 4, 14
Tectotegmentospinal tract, 4, 14
Teichopsias, 372
Teleopia, 372
Temperature regulation, 479
  clinical observations
    fever, 480
    fulminant hyperthermia, 480
    heat stroke, 481
    thermal disturbances from trauma, 482
    tumors, 483
  experimental studies, 479
  hypothalamic control, 479
Temporal lobe
  anatomy, 379
  epilepsy, 383
    paroxysmal, 384
Temporomandibular joint disease, 213
Tensor tympani muscle paralysis, 239
Teres minor paralysis, 51
Tetanus, 244
Thalamic syndromes, 461
Thalamotomy, 9, 42
Thalamus
  anatomical definitions, 441
  functional considerations, 455
    dorsolateral and posterior zones, 458
    paramedian zone, 457
  functional considerations—cont'd
    reticulate component and median zone, 456
  nuclei of dorsolateral and posterior zones (homotypical)
    cortical projection, 454
    development, 453
  nuclei of paramedian zone (heterotypical), 447
    rostral or limbic group, 450
      projections, 452
  reticulate and nucleate components, 446
  in sleep-wakefulness, 486
  syndromes
    coma vigil, 390, 462
    Dejerine-Roussy, 461
    frontal leukotomy, 462
  vascularization, 459
Thermoanesthesia, 26
Thermohyperesthesia, 26
Thermohypesthesia, 26
Thyroidectomy and inferior laryngeal nerve, 176
Thrombophlebitis, spinal, 88
Tinnitus, 208, 209
Todd's paralysis, 333
Toe flexor reflex, 74
Tonic neck reflex, 74
Tonic plantar reflex, 330
  test, 331
Tonic postural reflex, 424
Tonic pupil, 260
Topagnosis, 28
Torticollis, 417
  stationary, nonspasmodic, 417
Tracts of spinal cord, 3
  ascending, 5
    spinocerebellar, 9, 10, 14, 15
    spino-olivary, 10
    spinoreticular systems, 11, 15
    spinotectal, 11, 15
    spinothalamic, 6, 9, 14
  descending
    corticospinal (paramedial), 3, 14
    olivospinal, 5
    reticulospinal, 5, 14
    rubrospinal, 5, 14
    from subcortical structures, 4
    tectospinal, 4, 14
    tectotegmentospinal, 4, 14
  intersegmental, 12
  Lissauer, 1
  long, cross-sectional topography, 13
  Morin, 11, 12, 15
Transection of spinal cord, partial versus complete, 86
Trapezius palsy, 172
Trauma
  involving lower cranial nerves, 183
  involving nerves III, IV, and VI, 261
  involving nerve V, 239
  involving nerve VII, 226
Traumatic paraplegia, 85
Triceps reflexes
  humerus, 66
  sural, 68
Trigeminal nerve
  anatomy, 234
  central distribution, 235
  disorders of autonomic components, 246
  distal level involvement, 239
  interruption, 238
  lesions of spinal nucleus, 247
  motor changes, 239
  proximal level lesions, 244
  sensory and reflex changes, 238
  supranuclear lesions, 247
  tumors, 245
Trigeminal neuralgia, 180, 241
Trismus, 244
Trochlear nerve, 254
  palsies, 256, 257
Trophic disturbances, 39, 40
  etiology, 40
Tuberculous meningitis, source of ocular nerve palsy, 258
Tumors
  brainstem, 227, 541
  foramen magnum, 99
  intracranial, 534, 538, 543, 544, 549, 559
  involving extraocular nerves, 262
  spinal, 56, 61, 91, 92, 98, 100, 123
Two-point threshold for tactile testing, 8

U

Ulnar paralysis, 51
Uncal syndrome in brain shift, 534
Uncinate epiplepsy, 382, 383
Uncinate fasciculus, 280
Unverricht-Lafora disease, 163

Urinary bladder
innervation and function, 105
lesions and disturbances
above sacral level (reflex bladder, automatic bladder), 107
cauda equina, 108
interruption of higher suprasegmental systems (uninhibited neurogenic bladder), 107
lower spinal levels in myelomeningocele, 108
posterior lumbar roots, 108
sacral segments (autonomous neurogenic bladder), 107

V

Vagal neuralgia, 179
Vagotomy, 176
Vagus nerve, 173
interruption, 175
motor components, 174
progressive damage, 175
reflexes, 175
sensory fibers, 174
Vascular headaches, 241
migraine type, 242
Vasoconstrictor fibers, 219
Vasodilation with anhidrosis, of face, 102
Vasodilator fibers, 219
Vasomotor functions
control systems, 15
disturbances and lesions, 36
involving face, 100
reflexes, 37, 69
Vasomotor reflex, 69
Vergence tracking system, 268
Vernet's syndrome, 154, 183
Vertigo and dizziness
causation, 201, 210
from circulatory insufficiency, 308
differential diagnosis, 202
influencing factors, 203
paroxysmal, 201
positional, 199
subjective, 201
sustained, 201
vestibular, 201, 382
Vestibular apparatus, functional disturbances, 380
Vestibular end-organs and nerve
anatomy and functions, 189
factors in conjugate ocular movements and nystagmus, 194
fixation mechanisms, 196
gaze mechanisms, 196
labyrinthine activation, 194
neuronitis, 212
pathological ocular nystagmus, 196; *see also* Nystagmus
Vestibular end-organs and nerve—cont'd
pathways in central nervous system, 192
Vestibular function, 381
disturbed equilibrium, 382
symptoms of temporal lobe lesions, 381
vertigo, 382
Vestibulocerebellar pathway, 279
Vestibulospinal tract, 5, 14
Vidian neuralgia, 242
Villaret's syndrome, 183
Viral infections, source of end-organ damage, 211
Virchow-Robin space in visual system, 349
Visceral motor functions
autonomic nervous system, 33
pilomotor, 39
pupillary dilatation, 42
respiratory, 41
sudomotor, 37
trophic, 39
vasomotor, 35
Visual agnosia, 373
apperceptive, 374
associative, 374
classification, 374
Visual cortex involvement, 369
Visual extinction, 372
Visual fields, 351
Visual illusions, 158
Visual inattention, 372
Visual pathways, 349
Visual system
anatomy, 349
central and peripheral field representation, 351
fibers subserving reflex responses, 352
fields, 351
pathways, 349
blood supply, 353
lesions and clinical disturbances; *see also* specific conditions
optic chiasm, 363
optic nerve and retina, 355, 359
optic tract, 366
visual cortex, 369
visual radiation, 368
Vitamin B_{12} deficiency, 82

W

Wartenberg's sign, 74
Weber's syndrome, 153, 159
Weight discrimination for tactile testing, 28
Wernicke's encephalopathy, 388
Westphal's paradoxical reaction, 424
Westphal's pseudosclerosis, 418
Whiplash injury, 97
Wilson's disease, 418